NATIONAL ASSOCIATION OF ORTHO

Core Curriculum for Orthopaedic Nursing

7th Edition

Lorry Schoenly, PhD, RN
Editor
Visiting Professor
Chamberlain College of Nursing
Graduate Nursing Program
Downers Grove, IL

This text is funded in part
by an educational grant from
Lilly USA, LLC.

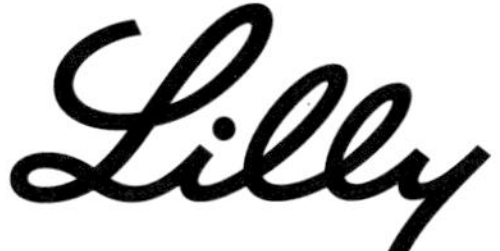

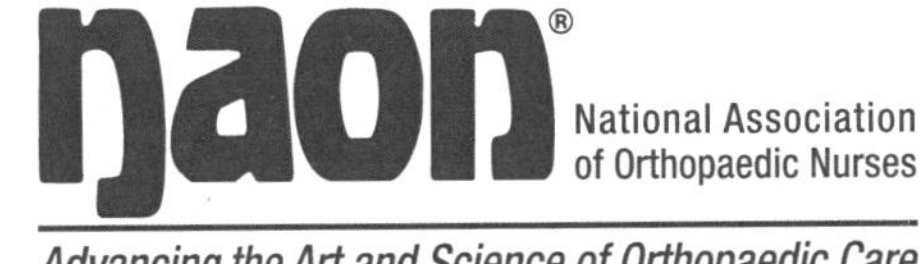

Production Credits
Project Director: Jan Foecke, MS, RN, ONC®
Copy Editor: Erin Larson
Creative Designer: Patrick Williams
Editorial Coordinator: Katie DenHollander

National Association of Orthopaedic Nurses
330 N Wabash Ave, Suite 2000
Chicago, IL 60611
1.800-289.6266
www.orthonurse.org

ISBN: 978-0-9790408-5-6

Table of Contents

Contributors

Lori E. Abel, MEd, RN, ONC
Joint Care Program Director, Orthopedic Service Line
WellSpan Health
York, PA

Linda Alitzer, RN, MSN, ONC, D-ABMDI
Health Professions Manager, Contining Education
Hagerstown Community College
Hagerstown, MD

Donna M. Barker, APRN, ANP-BC, ONC, RN-C
Pain Management Nurse Practitioner
St. Alexius Medical Center
Hoffman Estates, IL

Deborah A. Brown, MSN, APRN-BC, ONP-C
Orthopaedic Nurse Practitioner
Dartmouth Hitchcock Medical Center
Department of Orthopaedic Surgery
Lebanon, NH

Rebecca L. Buti, MS, ANP-C, ONP-C
Nurse Practitioner
UCSF Medical Center
San Francisco, CA

Laura M. Criddle, PhD, RN, ACNS-BC, ONC, FAEN
Clinical Nurse Specialist
The Laurelwood Group
Scappoose, OR

Jack Davis, MSN, RN, ONC
Manager, Patient Education Programs
Hospital for Special Surgery
New York, NY

Jan Foecke, MS, RN, ONC
Director of Programs
National Association of Orthopaedic Nurses
Chicago, IL

Linda R. Greene, RN, MPS, CIC
Director Infection Prevention
Rochester General Health System
Rochester, NY

Kate Hill, RN
Director of Clinical Services
The Compliance Team
Spring House, PA

Barbara Kahn-Kastell, RN, ONC
Nurse Clinician
Hospital for Special Surgery
New York, NY

Patricia A. Krieger, MSN, RN, ONC, CNOR
OR Service Group Manager, Ortho/Spine/ Podiatry/Dental
Hanover Hospital - Operating Room
Hanover, PA

Cathleen E. Kunkler, MSN, RN, ONC, CNE
Associate Professor, Nurse Education
Corning Community College
Corning, NY

Christina Kurkowski, MS, ONC, CNOR, ANP-C, ONP-C
Nurse Practitioner
Marshfield Clinic
Wausau, WI

Kelly A. McDevitt, RN, MS, ONC
Clinical Nurse Manager Orthopaedics/ Surgery
University of Colorado Hospital
Aurora, CO

Patti Murray, DNP, RN-BC
Nurse Practitioner - Pain Management
Loyola University Medical Center
Maywood, IL

Marianne K. Ostrow, RN, MSN, ONC
Clinical Nurse Specialist, Pennsylvania Orthopaedic Foot and Ankle Surgeons
University of Pennsylvania Health System
Philadelphia, PA

Debra M. Palmer, DNP, FNP-BC, ONP-C
Assistant Professor
Azusa Pacific University, School of Nursing, San Diego Regional Center
San Diego, CA

Rebecca Parker, MSN, RN, CNL, ONC
RN Clinician
Saint Mary's Health Care
Grand Rapids, MI

Angela N. Pearce, RN, MS, FNP-C, ONP-C
Trauma/Orthopaedic Nurse Practitioner
Parkland Memorial Hospital
Dallas, TX

Rebecca A. Perz, MSN, NP-C, ONP-C
Orthopaedic Nurse Practitioner
Tomah Memorial Hospital
Tomah, WI

Dottie Roberts, MSN, MACI, RN, CMSRN, OCNS-C, CNE
Nursing Instructor
University of South Carolina
Columbia, SC

Susan C. Ruda, MS, APN, RN, NP-C, ONC
Nurse Practitioner
Parkview Musculoskeletal Institute
Joliet, IL

Penny Saulog-Wendel, BSN, RN, ONC
Nurse Clinician
Hospital for Special Surgery
New York, NY

Mary Jane Smalley, MSN, CRNP, CPNP-PC
Nurse Practitioner
Shriners Hospitals for Children-Erie
Erie, PA

Elizabeth Turcotte, MSN, RN-BC, ONC
Nurse Manager
Orthopaedic Institute of Central Maine
Lewiston, ME

Colleen R. Walsh, DNP, RN, CS, ONP-C, ACNP-BC
Clinical Assistant Professor, Nursing
University of Southern Indiana
Evansville, IN

Reviewers

Linda D. Abella, MSN, RN, ONC

Elizabeth Abrahams, RN, MSN, ONC

Diane L. Agpaoa, RN, MNE, ONC

Ann Berndtson, MA, RN, ONC

Joyce Blau, MS, APN, ONC

Marie Boltz, PhD, RN, GNP-BC

Frederick M. Brown, Jr., DNP, RN, ONC

Lori Ann Clark, RN, MSN, ONC

Tara A. Cortes, PhD, RN, FAAN

Pamela A. Cupec, BSN, MS, RN, ONC, CRRN, ACM

Denise Curtis, RN, MSN, APN-C, FNP-C

Mary R. Evans, MS, RN, ONC, OCNS-C

Barbara Fauth, RN, ONC, CNOR

Cathy A. Femmer, RN, ONC, MSN

Susan Girdhari, APRN-BC, ONP-C

Carol V. Harvey, MSN, RN, ACNS-BC, ONC

Melissa Herlein, MSN,FNP-BC

Sherry M. Lawrence, DNP, RN, CNOR, ONC

Mary Lyons, MSN, RN-BC, APN, ONC

Miki M. Patterson, PhD, APRN, ONP

April Paulson, RN, MS, FNP-BC, ONP-C

Susan Wright Selman, RN, MS, ONC

Suzanne Frey Sherwood, MS, RN

Renee Silver, RN, MSN, CNRN

Carol M. Simon, MS, RN, ONC

Kimberly A. Stauffer, MS, CRNP

Diana Weinel, MS, RN

Lynn Whelan, DNP, RN, NEA-BC, ONC

Melissa Yager, MS, RN, CNS, ONC

Anita M. Zehala, MS, RN, ONC, CNS

Foreword

Serving as NAON's 33rd President has been a phenomenal opportunity and honor. When I was asked to write the forward for this 7th edition to the *Core Curriculum of Orthopaedic Nursing,* I was given a preview of this 7th edition. After that review, I firmly believe the new *Core Curriculum* will prove to be one of NAON's premiere products for many years.

This text connects back to NAON's mission and demonstrates our commitment to excellence. The dedication placed upon our mission to "advance the specialty of orthopaedic nursing through excellence in research, education, and nursing practice" is revealed throughout this textbook because each chapter is grounded in evidenced-based practice and research. Orthopaedic nursing implications are included in all areas of discussion, providing an exceptional forum to educate all nurses on the specialty of orthopaedics.

One of the greatest attributes about this book is that NAON listened to our members and readers while developing the 7th edition. Previous editions were written in an outline format. Feedback from our customers and nurses taking the certification exam informed NAON that those earlier editions were difficult to read, review, and utilize as a study guide. As a certified orthopaedic nurse, I echo the same comments. I used a very early *Core Curriculum* for my primary study guide and recall the struggle of grasping concepts while reading an outline textbook. Another reason why NAON embarked on this extensive journey to bring our colleagues a new *Core* was time. Our last edition was published in 2006, and it was basically time for a renewal so that the information remains relevant to orthopaedic nursing practice.

I am confident that readers will be pleased with the new 7th edition *Core.* There are several updates within this version. First, the new contents have additional topics that all orthopaedic nurses require in their knowledge base as we care for increasingly more complex patients. Clearly the most exciting update in this new edition is the narrative format. As I was reading the new book, I realized how easy and enjoyable the chapters were to read. The information flowed in a logical manner, was descriptive yet succinct, and left me with a positive impression.

There is an old idiom which states "A picture paints 1000 words"; that expression came full circle when I reviewed one of many illustrations and tables in this impressive text. I believe that the inclusion of pictures is one of the most significant improvements to this edition. The online resources are another example of the continued excellence in this adaptation.

Why should the 7th edition *Core Curriculum for Orthopaedic Nursing* be on your book shelf? There are many reasons. It is an extraordinary reference for all nurses. The text is a momentous work that will expand nursing knowledge. Professional nursing practice includes continuous self-improvement through education, along with an understanding of best practice that this text clearly provides. Nurses are consistently trusted by our patients as leaders in health care delivery. This book secures the foundation to enhance and maintain our position as those experts. Finally, our 7th edition places NAON as the leader in orthopaedic nursing. I can't think of any reason why a nurse would not want to be associated with such distinction. On behalf of the National Association of Orthopaedic Nurses, I want to extend my thanks and appreciation to all nurses who purchase this book. Your commitment and dedication to excellence is gratifying.

Christy E. Oakes, MSN, RN, ONC
2012-2013 President, National Association of Orthopaedic Nurses

Preface

Welcome to the 7th edition of the *Core Curriculum for Orthopaedic Nursing*. If you have read prior editions, you will notice a difference right away. After six prior editions using an outline format, reader feedback moved us to create the first full-text edition of the Core. Full-text writing allows for more complete information and referencing. Increased tables and figures enhance the text and improve understanding. Key terms are now defined in a glossary. In addition, an extensive appendix provides a listing of common orthopaedic NANDA nursing diagnosis along with a listing of nursing interventions and outcomes to make care planning and documentation easy and trouble-free.

Great thought was given to the new features of this text, and I am delighted to have edited this expanded edition of the primary clinical resource for orthopaedic nurses. Having chartered in 1980, the National Association of Orthopaedic Nurses (NAON) has supported the specialty practice for more than 4 decades. The first *Core Curriculum for Orthopaedic Nursing* (published by the Orthopaedic Nurses Association in 1980) established the boundaries of the specialty. This 7th edition represents the current state of the practice of orthopaedic nursing, building on this foundation.

Over the last 2 years, I have had the pleasure of being in contact with orthopaedic nursing experts as chapter authors and reviewers. What a wonderful group of dedicated professionals. A review of the author and reviewer list is all that is needed to see the extensive knowledge and experience represented in the pages of this text.

The information shared here is of huge importance to the nursing profession and the specialty practice of orthopaedic nursing.

Between these covers is information that will benefit patients experiencing a wide variety of medical conditions, disease processes, and surgical interventions related to bones, muscles, and connective tissues. The expanded emphasis on understanding these conditions and the appropriate nursing interventions allows the reader to confidently practice in any setting requiring orthopaedic nursing care. Of particular benefit is the increased information on NANDA, Nursing Interventions Classification (NIC) and Nursing Outcomes Classifications (NOC) terminology. Use of these naming structures helps to validate the impact of nursing care on patient outcomes and is advantageous in creating a valid electronic documentation system.

All nurses caring for orthopaedic patients, whether practicing in clinical, education, management, or researcher roles, will want to have access to this text. Nurses new to the specialty of orthopaedics have a one-stop source for all major conditions. Reading this publication can jump-start entry into the specialty. Nurse experts can find information to validate their current practice, expand knowledge in areas of orthopaedic nursing that are not a part of their background, and use in developing publication and speaking materials. Nurses seeking certification in orthopaedics can use this book as a primary text for certification preparation. Health care institutions and libraries can add the text to their shelves and use the book as a unit resource. Educational institutions and nursing instructors will find this publication invaluable for undergraduate and graduate courses involving orthopaedic nursing content. Staff educators can use this resource to develop introductory courses and provide in-services. The online chapter CE option is particularly helpful for staff development, as well as individual nurse recertification or re-licensure purposes.

Enjoy this edition of the *Core Curriculum for Orthopaedic Nursing*, and use it regularly in your nursing practice. Orthopaedic nurses make a difference in the lives of their patients. Make today count for good!

Lorry Schoenly, PhD, RN
Editor

Chapter 1

Practice Settings & Roles of Orthopaedic Nurses

Susan C. Ruda, MS, APN, RN, NP-C, ONC

Objectives

- Identify various practice settings for the nurse specializing in orthopaedic nursing.
- Define the role of the orthopaedic nurse in multiple practice settings.
- Discuss the responsibilities of the orthopaedic nurse in various settings and roles.
- Discuss the knowledge base required for the orthopaedic nurse in various settings and roles.

Nursing is a dynamic, ever-changing profession that remains a high-growth job field. The United States Bureau of Labor Statistics (BLS) *Occupations with Largest Job Growth* (n.d.) projects that more than 518,000 new registered nurse (RN) positions will be created through 2018. Domrose (2010) estimates that governmental regulations may open opportunities for nurses in all areas. Due to the aging nursing population, many nurses will be retiring in the upcoming years, which will create new openings in the profession.

The aging baby boomer population will continue to require health care needs in the upcoming years (Stringer, 2010). By the nature of orthopaedic care, these baby boomers will be seeking care for treatment of musculoskeletal disorders such as arthritis and osteoporosis. Opportunities will abound for the nurse who specializes in orthopaedics. The orthopaedic nurse may practice in a wide variety of settings, including but not exclusive to hospitals, clinics, office settings, academic settings, and skilled nursing facilities (National Association of Orthopaedic Nurses [NAON], 2002).

The term "orthopaedics" is derived from the Greek words *orthos* (to correct or straighten) and *paideion* (child). The symbol for orthopaedics depicts a tree with a crooked trunk, with a stake attached to it in order to stabilize or straighten it. Orthopaedics is the branch of nursing that specializes in the care and treatment of persons with musculoskeletal disorders. These may be congenital or acquired disorders. These include musculoskeletal trauma, sports-related injuries, infections and tumors. Orthopaedic disorders span the continuum of life. They range from disorders such as congenital hip dysplasia in the newborn to osteoarthritis in the older adult. While many disorders require surgical intervention, conservative management with interventions such as casting or drug therapy may also be appropriate.

Hospital, Long-Term Care, and Extended Care Facilities

Setting Characteristics

The acute care or extended care facility is the most common area of practice for orthopaedic nurses. (See Table 1.1.) Within these settings, there may be a unit dedicated to orthopaedic or rehabilitation patients. Patients with musculoskeletal disorders are also seen on medical-surgical, pediatric, intensive care, ambulatory surgery, post-anesthesia, and operating room and rehabilitation units. These patients may have undergone surgery, including total joint arthroplasty, spinal surgery, or fixation of fractures. Nonsurgical patients may be seen for musculoskeletal pain management or conservative treatment of fractures.

The orthopaedic nurse in the acute care or extended care facility practices on a specific unit. While the titles of the nursing and management personnel may vary depending upon the institution, the roles will be similar. The nursing unit is managed by a head nurse who reports to a division director who reports to the director of nursing. Other disciplines involved in the orthopaedic care of the patient include the physical therapist, occupational therapist, social worker, dietitian, clinical nurse specialist (CNS), and case manager.

Nursing Roles

Staff Nurse. The staff nurse is the entry-level position. The orthopaedic staff nurse provides direct bedside care for the patient with an orthopaedic disorder. In the acute care setting, a nursing unit may be dedicated specifically to the care and treatment of orthopaedic patients. The staff nurse serves as a liaison between the patient and

Table 1.1. Nursing Roles in the Hospital Setting

Staff Nurse	Completion of Registered Nurse program with state licensure	ONC certification recommended	Acute and extended care facilities
Clinical Nurse Specialist	Registered Nurse with advanced degree	ONC certification with ONCNS-C recommended	Acute and extended care facilities
Case Manager	Registered Nurse with advanced degree	ONC certification recommended. Certification as case manager recommended	Acute and extended care facilities. May also work in insurance setting.
Nurse Practitioner	Registered Nurse with advanced degree	ONC certification with ONCNP-C recommended. Certification as Nurse Practitioner required	Acute and extended care facilities. May also work in office or clinic setting
Nurse Executive	Registered Nurse with advanced degree	ONC certification recommended	Acute and extended care facilities

Table 1.2. Common Nursing Certifications			
Orthopaedic Nurse Certified (ONC)	Registered Nurse license 1,000 hours orthopaedic nursing care per year	Successful exam completion Recertification every 5 years	www.oncb.org
Orthopaedic Nurse Clinical Nurse Specialist Certified ONCNS-C	Registered Nurse license 3 years nursing experience Completion of master's degree in nursing with emphasis as clinical nurse specialist	Successful exam completion Recertification every 5 years	www.oncb.org
Orthopaedic Nurse Practitioner Certified ONP-C	Registered Nurse license 3 years nursing experience Completion of master's degree in nursing with emphasis as nurse practitioner	Successful exam completion Recertification every 5 years	www.oncb.org
Clinical Nurse Specialist (CNS) ***Several different CNS specialties***	Registered Nurse license Completion of master's degree in nursing with emphasis as clinical nurse specialist	Successful exam completion Recertification every 5 years	www.nursecredentialing.org
Nurse Practitioner (NP) ***Several different specialties***	Registered Nurse license Completion of master's degree in nursing with emphasis as nurse practitioner	Successful exam completion Recertification every 5 years	www.nursecredentialing.org or www.aanp.org
Nurse Case Manager (NCM)	Registered Nurse license 2,000 clinical hours in past 3 years	Successful exam completion Recertification every 5 years	www.nursecredentialing.org
Nurse Educator	Registered Nurse license Master's or doctoral degree with emphasis on nursing education 2 years of full-time employment in faculty position in past 5 years	Successful exam completion Recertification every 5 years	www.nln.org
Nurse Executive	Registered Nurse license Completion of master's degree in nursing Administrative position as nursing executive	Successful exam completion Recertification every 5 years	www.nursecredentialing.org
School Nurse	Registered Nurse license Bachelors degree in nursing 3 years nursing practice as school nurse	Successful exam completion Recertification every 5 years	www.nbcsn.com

the physician, mid-level practitioner, and other health care personnel. The orthopaedic staff nurse administers therapies, treatments, and medications as prescribed by the physician or mid-level practitioner. This nurse collaborates with other disciplines including physical and occupational therapy.

The staff nurse specializing in orthopaedic nursing must possess a basic knowledge of anatomy and physiology of the musculoskeletal system. Knowledge of preoperative, perioperative, and postoperative nursing care aids in the treatment of the orthopaedic surgical patient. The nurse must demonstrate good body mechanics to prevent personal injury while participating in patient care. The staff nurse must remain updated on current research, medications, and treatment plans to provide optimum care for the orthopaedic patient. This knowledge can be obtained from hospital in-services, scholarly journals, and workshops. Networking with other orthopaedic nurses provides an ongoing source of information. Attending local, state, or national meetings and seminars, such as those sponsored by the National Association of Orthopaedic Nurses (NAON), will offer current information and opportunities for networking.

Teaching about musculoskeletal conditions is an essential role of the staff nurse. Education includes disease prevention, medication side effects, safety, and home care.

The staff nurse utilizes the nursing process as a systematic way to organize the care of the patient. The orthopaedic nurse employs a holistic approach to obtain data via direct sources including interview, observation, and physical assessment (NAON, 2002). Indirect data is gathered from records, labs, and other diagnostic data, or it may be obtained from the family and other health care providers. Objective data is measurable or observed, and includes vital signs, laboratory results, and physical exam findings. Subjective data, such as statements by the patient, is not measurable.

Once the nurse gathers and analyzes the data, nursing diagnoses are developed and goals can be formulated. These goals will determine the plan of care for the patient. Goals must be measurable and focus on promoting, maintaining, and restoring musculoskeletal health in order to evaluate whether the outcomes have been achieved. A plan is developed with the mutual agreement of the patient and family. Interventions are implemented, and outcomes are evaluated.

To become an RN, one must successfully complete education from an accredited associate degree or baccalaureate program, then apply for the state licensure examination. A current state license in the state of employment is required to practice nursing. Refer to the state of licensure for renewal and maintenance requirements, as these requirements will vary from state to state.

Orthopaedic certification is offered by the Orthopaedic Nurses Certification Board (ONCB®). Certification requires the applicant to have practiced in nursing for a minimum of 2 years and a minimum of 1,000 hours in orthopaedic nursing within the past 3 years. Successful completion of a multiple choice written exam provided by the ONCB® allows the orthopaedic nurse to refer to her- or himself as "Orthopaedic Nurse Certified" and use the credentials ONC. Renewal is required every 5 years and can be obtained by completing either continuing education in orthopaedics or the exam (ONCB®, n.d.). (See Table 1.2 for a comparison of certifications offered.)

Licensed Practical Nurse. The Licensed Practical Nurse (LPN) is also known as the licensed vocational nurse in Texas and California. The LPN completes an 18- to 24-month program from an accredited program. The LPN will be required to complete a state licensure examination. Refer to the state of licensure for renewal and maintenance requirements, as these will vary depending up the state.

The LPN can practice in the hospital, skilled nursing facility, or office setting. The LPN practices under the direct supervision of the RN or physician. The LPN provides basic bedside care including assessing vital signs and assisting with activities of daily living (ADLs). In some states, the LPN can administer medications. Refer to the Nurse Practice Act of the individual state for specific types and routes of medication administration that are allowed.

Clinical Nurse Specialist. The Clinical Nurse Specialist (CNS) role is an Advanced Practice Nurse (APN) role designed to provide enhanced patient care. The CNS does this by incorporating the primary components of expert orthopaedic clinical practice consultation, education, and research into practice. The CNS typically is employed by the hospital (National Association of Clinical Nurse Specialists [NACNS], n.d.).

The CNS possesses experience in orthopaedic nursing. The CNS also has advanced knowledge in nursing diagnoses, clinical pathways, and evidence-based practice. Knowledge of research design and statistical analysis is required. Strong leadership skills and communication skills are necessary.

The CNS is required to have completed a minimum of a master's degree in nursing. Certification as a CNS is offered by the American Nurse Credentialing Center (ANCC). ONC and ONCS-C certification is strongly recommended for the ONCS-C that specializes in orthopaedics. ONCS-S certification is offered by the ONCB®. The ONCS-C must refer to the state board of nursing and the Nurse Practice Act of the state of licensure for further information regarding licensure requirements. Advanced practice licensure may be required.

The CNS offers direct care by the actual interactions that occur with clients, families, and patient groups. Indirect care is offered in the form of education and consultation services for both nurses and client families. The CNS also participates in community-wide education about musculoskeletal conditions with an emphasis on safety, health promotion, and illness/injury prevention.

The CNS utilizes research findings in orthopaedic nursing practice. Researchable problems are explored, and solutions are offered based upon findings. The CNS will interpret literature and research findings for the nursing personnel and clients. The CNS will also collaborate with other hospital disciplines to participate in research studies. The CNS will publish research-based and nonresearch-based journal articles related to orthopaedic nursing. Presentations will be made on various topics related to orthopaedic nursing and patient care at local, state, and national meetings.

In some institutions, administration is also incorporated into the role. The CNS assists administration with management of nursing personnel. The CNS will offer feedback for personnel evaluations, aid in staff development and education, and assist with the implementation and evaluation of institutional policies.

Nurse Case Manager. The Nurse Case Manager (NCM) serves as a patient advocate for the orthopaedic patient. The NCM may be employed by a hospital or insurance company. The NCM is responsible for ensuring that the hospitalized orthopaedic patient is receiving appropriate and timely care. The NCM also aids in the development of the discharge plan for hospitalized patients to ensure the patient receives the appropriate equipment and services once the patients are discharged.

Experience and knowledge in orthopaedic nursing care, orthopaedic equipment, and home health care is beneficial. The NCM will communicate with the insurance companies to ensure that patients are receiving timely care and are adhering to length-of-stay restrictions. The NCM will interface with the patient and family to ensure that their expectations are in line with hospital and insurance expectations. The hospital-based NCM also collaborates with the physicians, nurses, and health care personnel to certify that goals are achieved and discharge needs are met.

The NCM who is employed by the insurance company is responsible for guaranteeing that subscribers receive the benefits they are entitled to based upon their individual insurance policies. The NCM will interface with the insurance company and the individual policy-holder. Interpretation of insurance policy benefits and restrictions is a primary role of the insurance NCM. The NCM acts as an advocate for the policy-holder and family, while offering cost-effective solutions that fit within policy guidelines.

A current state nursing license in the state of practice is required. A bachelor's or master's degree may be required, depending upon institution policies. NCM certification may be required by the institution and is highly recommended. Nursing Case Management Certification is offered by the ANCC. Two years of full-time RN practice and 2,000 hours of clinical nursing practice within the last 3 years is required to apply for the certification examination. There is no specific orthopaedic NCM specialty certification (American Nurses Credentialing Center [ANCC], n.d.).

Nurse Manager. The nurse manager may be referred to as the Head Nurse, Unit Manager, or Nursing Supervisor, depending upon the institution. The nurse manager is responsible for supervising the care provided by nursing and other health care personnel. The nurse manager serves as a liaison between the orthopaedic staff and administration. The nurse manager implements hospital policies and governmental laws for nursing personnel, patients, and families. Budgeting, scheduling, and staffing decisions are incorporated into the role of the nurse manager.

The nurse manager is responsible for creating an environment of professional growth for the nursing staff by participating in evaluation of nursing personnel. The role of coach/mentor to newer and less-experienced staff helps create an environment that promotes the development of staff. A strong background in leadership and supervision of personnel is required. Strong communication skills and knowledge of budgeting is recommended.

The nurse manager on the orthopaedic unit must possess knowledge of orthopaedic disorders. Depending upon the institution, a bachelor's or master's degree may be required. ONC certification is strongly recommended. Current state licensure is also required. Membership in an organization of nurse executives will offer networking opportunities and the ability to enhance leadership skills.

Nurse Executive. As a member of the senior nursing leadership team, the nurse executive is a nurse leader in the hospital setting. The role of the nurse executive includes collaborating, mentoring, co-creating, communicating, and coordinating outcomes management. The nurse executive participates in the facilitation and design of patient care delivery, advances the discipline of nursing; builds relationships and connections with staff and colleagues, and fosters stewardship.

In addition to an orthopaedic background, the nurse executive must possess knowledge in business and health care management. A master's degree in business or healthcare administration may be required. Knowledge of federal, state, and local health care policy is beneficial. Membership in the American Organization of Nurse Executives (AONE), for example, is beneficial. Certification as a nurse executive may not be required but is highly recommended. Certification is offered by the ANCC (ANCC, n.d.).

Combined Inpatient and Office Settings

Setting Characteristics

Several orthopaedic roles incorporate employment in both the inpatient and outpatient settings. Orthopaedic nurses in these roles may be employed by either an institution or physician practice.

The orthopaedic nurse who practices in a combined setting typically has roles in the office, hospital, and clinic. This nurse may be employed by the hospital or medical center or a physician practice. The nurse has privileges to practice in all settings. Typically this nurse practices in the role of a Nurse Practitioner (NP) or Registered Nurse First Assistant (RNFA). These roles are viewed as advanced practice roles and possess a higher degree of autonomy.

Nursing Roles

Nurse Practitioner. The NP is an advanced practice nurse who provides nursing and medical care as a licensed independent practitioner. The NP administers primary care to the patient with an orthopaedic disorder within the acute care or extended care setting, clinic, office setting, or home environment (American Academy of Nurse Practitioners [AANP], n.d.). The NP enhances the delivery of affordable health care services for clients with orthopaedic disorders (NAON, 2002). The Nurse Practice Act of each state delineates the classifications of medications the NP can prescribe, as each state varies on the extent of physician involvement that is required to maintain the state standards.

The NP has completed a specialty program in family health, adult health, pediatrics, or acute care, and may serve as a hospitalist. In the hospitalist role, the NP performs comprehensive histories and physical exams (Hummer-Bellmyer, 2002). The NP formulates medical diagnoses and develops a treatment plan based upon national standards of practice (Klein, 2007). The NP is qualified to prescribe diagnostic tests, treatments such as physical therapy, and certain medications. The NP can perform procedures such as joint aspiration, injection, and closed reduction of simple fractures. The NP may see patients in an office or clinic setting where the role varies widely based upon job requirements. An NP employed by a physician practice may work in both the office and hospital setting. The NP may also serve as first surgical assistant during orthopaedic surgical procedures, although restrictions and degree of autonomy vary among states.

Because the NP can bill for services, knowledge of reimbursement requirements for services rendered is necessary, as some secondary insurance agencies do not cover NP services. Commercial insurance companies may reimburse for services rendered; however, each insurance company differs in the amount of reimbursement. Medicare pays for health services to patients registered, the majority of whom are age 65 and older. Medicaid is funded by federal and state governments to reimburse for health care services and is administered solely by the state of the residency. The Civilian Health and Medical Program for the Uniformed Services (CHAMPUS) may provide reimbursement for NP services rendered. Worker's Compensation reimbursement varies by states, and payment is based upon a fee-for-service system.

Becoming an NP requires earning a degree from an accredited NP program and successfully passing the certification examination. The NP program focuses upon the specialty of adult health, acute care, pediatric health, family health, or gerontological health. NP programs grant the graduate a master's or doctoral degree. Effective in 2015, the minimum entry-level to complete the certification exam will be the doctoral degree (AACN Position Statement, 2004).

The NP is required to have a current RN license. In addition to state licensure, current national certification in the area of NP practice is required. NP certification is offered by ANCC and American Association of Nurse Practitioners (AANP, 2010). Once certification as an NP is obtained, the NP can complete ONC-NP certification offered by the ONCB (Klein, 2007).

The NP practicing in the hospital setting will require hospital credentialing. The hospital credentialing committee will differentiate the specific roles and tasks the NP can perform within the hospital facility, according to the guidelines of the hospital's policies and procedures.

The NP requires a strong clinical background in orthopaedic nursing. Excellent communication skills, the ability to function in an autonomous role, strong physical assessment skills, and current knowledge of advanced pathophysiology and pharmacology are mandatory. The NP should publish manuscripts on various orthopaedic topics and may be involved in research; therefore, experience in grant writing and statistical experience would also be beneficial. Active participation in professional associations such as ANA, NAON, and AANP enables the NP to remain current with information. The NP should attend state, local, and national meetings to obtain continuing education hours that are required to maintain certification and licensure.

The NP may be employed as a salaried employee or per contractual agreements. Contracts, to include work hours, are negotiated at the time of employment and may include incentive clauses and bonuses.

Registered Nurse First Assistant. The RNFA is an expanded practice role. The RNFA is an RN who serves as the first surgical assistant at surgery. The RNFA collaborates with the orthopaedic surgeon and other health care team members to perform safe surgical procedures and achieve optimal outcomes for the orthopaedic patient. The RNFA works in an expanded peri-operative nursing role under the supervision of the surgeon.

Because the RNFA is responsible for performing preoperative, perioperative, and postoperative assessments of the surgical patient, the RNFA must possess expanded knowledge of all three of these nursing phases. Knowledge of common orthopaedic surgical procedures, surgical anatomy, physiology, and operative techniques are required. The RNFA aids in proper positioning, skin preparation, and draping of the surgical patient. During the surgical procedure, the RNFA performs activities including hemostasis, wound exposure, tissue suturing, and sterile surgical dressing application (AORN, n.d.).

Working as an orthopaedic RNFA can be physically demanding. The RNFA must practice good body mechanics and proper transfer techniques. Because the operating room can be a stressful setting, the RNFA must have the ability to work effectively in emergency situations. Emergency room experience is helpful. The RNFA must be able to work harmoniously with the operating room staff.

The RNFA requires a valid RN nursing license in the state of practice. Knowledge of state board requirements, Nurse Practice Act specifications, and hospital policies is mandatory. CPR certification is required, with advanced cardiac life support (ACLS) recommended.

Certification in perioperative nursing and separate certification as a RNFA is highly recommended (AORN, n.d.). Certification is offered from the Association of Operating Room Nurses (AORN). A minimum of 3 years of perioperative nursing experience, working as a scrub and circulating nurse, is required in order to apply for certification. Programs offer both a didactic and clinical component to prepare for the certification exam.

The RNFA may be employed by a hospital, may work in a physician practice, or may be self-employed. The RNFA employed by the hospital must be familiar with all hospital policies. The institution may incorporate the charge for the hospital-employed RNFA into the surgical room charge or may use a line-item charge for the fee. The RNFA employed by the physician practice may work in the hospital, same-day surgery, or office setting. The RNFA must be familiar with policies and procedures at each facility with staff privileges. The facility may require attendance at orientation and regular staff meetings. The self-employed RNFA requires knowledge of claims processing for reimbursement. Marketing of services offered to various facilities and physician practices is crucial to maintain a steady income flow.

Knowledge of reimbursement requirements for services rendered is necessary for the RNFA. Reimbursement of services provided by the RNFA vary by company and coverage plan. Medicare only recognizes the RNFA who is certified as an advanced practice nurse or certified midwife. Most state medical programs do not recognize RNFAs as surgical assistants; however, provider numbers may be issued by the state, and claims may be considered for preoperative and postoperative care. Florida provides direct Medicaid reimbursement of the RNFA at the same rate that is paid to the physician for the same service. The Civilian Health and Medical Program for the Uniformed Services (CHAMPUS) may provide reimbursement for the RNFA services for preoperative and postoperative services. Worker's Compensation reimbursement varies by states, and payment is based upon a fee-for-service system.

Office and Outpatient Setting

Setting Characteristics

The office or clinic nurse provides care in an outpatient setting. RNs and LPNs frequently work in these settings. The BLS *Occupational Outlook Handbook 2010-2011 Edition* (n.d.) projects a 48% growth rate in nursing jobs in the offices of physicians, as the decreasing length of hospital stays and increased use of outpatient services creates an increased demand for nurses to practice in these settings.

Nursing Roles

Office Nurse. Responsibilities for the office nurse include treatments or therapies education, triage, and some business operations. Treatments may include intramuscular medications, dressing changes, and cast application and removal. The nurse may assist with minor procedures such as closed reductions in the office setting. Patient education is a vital role for the orthopaedic office nurse. The nurse will educate patients and families about proper preparation for surgery, outcomes about their surgical procedures, and follow-up care.

A strong background in physical assessment, pharmacology, and rehabilitation of the orthopaedic patient is necessary to do telephone triage. The office nurse may also be involved in communication with insurance companies to obtain necessary approval for procedures and equipment that is needed by the patients; knowledge of office coding may be required by the employer.

Job requirements and hours will vary widely among employers, based upon the specific needs of the physician and office. The orthopaedic nurse may practice in the office of an orthopaedic physician, a podiatrist, a physiatrist, or a sports medicine practitioner. The nurse may also practice in an HMO office or clinic setting.

Other Settings and Roles

Setting Characteristics

While the majority of nurses work in the office or hospital setting, opportunities are available in other areas. These roles are unique and may not have traditional job descriptions. The orthopaedic nurse may be required to define the role and negotiate job tasks based upon the specific needs of the practice, individual, or corporation. Benefits, hours, and salary will be negotiated between the nurse and the employer.

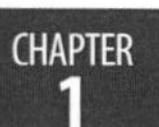

Nursing Roles

School Nurse. The school nurse participates in the care of children within the school setting. This role includes the care of children with non-orthopaedic disorders. Specific schools may be designed to provide services for a specific school population such as children with special needs.

The role of the school nurse includes maintaining records of vaccinations and immunizations, allergies, and medical histories on all children in attendance. The nurse will administer prescribed medications and treatments during school hours. The school nurse will educate the students and parents on health promotion and disease prevention, including participating in scoliosis, vision, and hearing screenings. The school nurse will encounter children with musculoskeletal disorders including but not limited to scoliosis, juvenile rheumatoid arthritis, chondromalacia, osteogenesis imperfecta, Osgood Schlatter disease, and a wide variety of sprains, strains, and fractures; therefore, an orthopaedic background will be beneficial.

The school nurse position requires a strong pediatric background. Knowledge of growth and development, pediatric pharmacology, pathophysiology and physical assessment skills is necessary. The school nurse must have knowledge of first aid. CPR certification and Pediatric Advanced Life Support (PALS) may be required. The school nurse must be able to interface with parents, students, and other medical offices.

The school nurse is required to have an RN license for the appropriate state. National, state, and local legislation, state nursing boards, and school district policies will guide the practice of the school nurse. A bachelor's degree may be required, based upon state or local school district requirements. The school nurse may participate in professional organizations including NAON, the Society of Pediatric Nurses, or the National Association of School Nurses (NASN). Certification is offered through NASN; refer to www.nasn.org for further information.

The position may only be part-time, and the salary will vary depending upon the school district. Depending upon specific school needs and budget constraints, the school nurse may be responsible for several schools and travel among them.

Camp Nurse. The camp nurse provides care for clients at a camp setting. According to the Association of Camp Nurses, it is estimated that over 5 million children attended camp last year (Minority Nurse, n.d.).

The focus and goals for the camp experience will define the campers who attend a specific camp. While most camp settings are geared for the child or adolescent with no pre-existing health conditions, a camp can also provide services for a specific age group with special health needs. The camp setting may be in a remote rural area or in an urban setting. Residential camps require campers to stay overnight for a specified length of time, ranging from several days to several weeks, while day camp participants return to their homes each evening. Camp nursing opportunities are available in all states and may also be available in Canada. The American Camp Association (ACA; www.acn.org) offers accreditation for camps to ensure a professional camping experience.

A passion for outdoor activities will be necessary for the camp nurse to ensure a positive experience. The camp nurse must have first aid training. School, pediatric, and emergency nursing experience is helpful because the majority of clients are children. A physician may not be present at the campsite; therefore, nursing autonomy is high. The specific camp policies and protocols will provide practice guidelines for specific situations. Licensure in the state or country of the camp location is required. This will further help define the camp nurse's scope of practice.

Camp nurses may be in high demand, especially during the summer months. These positions are often temporary employment. Salary and benefits will vary depending upon the camp setting.

Nurse Educator. The nurse educator is employed by an educational institution, such as a community college or university, to instruct nursing students in the classroom and clinical settings. The nurse educator is a position currently in high demand because recent increases in enrollment in nursing programs have created a shortage in nurse educators (Allen, 2008).

The nurse educator requires a minimum of a master's degree in nursing, with a doctoral degree strongly recommended. Certification as a nurse educator is offered by the ANCC; this is a general certification. There is no current certification as an orthopaedic nurse educator.

The nurse educator must have experience in nursing research and grant writing. The nurse educator may be required to regularly participate in nursing research based upon university requirements. Writing for journal publication is often required. These requirements are negotiated with the employer.

Nurse Researcher. The nurse researcher is typically employed by a medical center, university, or government agency. Changes in the health care climate have created a need for nurse researchers. It is estimated that there will be a high demand for nurse researchers in the upcoming years (Domrose, 2010). The nurse researcher is responsible for performing scientific research on subjects related to orthopaedic nursing practice, as well as publishing research findings. The nurse researcher aids in the implementation of orthopaedic research findings in the health care setting. The nurse researcher must have knowledge of grant and proposal writing to obtain funding from federal, public, and private sources for research.

Statistics, research design, theory development, informatics, health policy, and outcomes measurement are necessary for the nurse researcher (Ivey, 2007). A master's degree is the minimum requirement, and a doctoral degree is required for most positions.

Nurse Consultant. The nurse consultant provides expertise and direction to hospitals, insurance companies, physician practices, and corporations in the area of direct patient care or the revision of a patient care delivery system. The nurse consultant requires RN licensure in the state of practice. Certification in orthopaedic nursing will offer additional credentials. The nurse consultant may be an independent practitioner or employed by a consulting firm.

The nurse consultant relies on networking to obtain referrals for additional employment and prospective contracts. Attending local and national nursing meetings and working with local business organizations provides networking opportunities and potentially new referrals. The nurse consultant must have knowledge of legal aspects of self-employment, bookkeeping, and taxes. A business attorney and an accountant will be beneficial in providing direction regarding federal, state, and local regulations, financial records tax documents, and proper bookkeeping. Courses in business may be beneficial. Funding and low-interest loans may be available through small business organizations.

A legal nurse consultant (LNC) reviews records and provides expert advice regarding a patient or health care worker who is typically being sued by another party. While there is no certification for a LNC who specializes in orthopaedics, a general certification is offered by the American Legal Nurse Consultant Certification Board (ALNCCB), which is a branch of the American Association of Legal Nurse Consultants (AALNC). See www.aalnc.org/lncc/about/board.cfm for information. The LNC participates in an accredited program to quality for certification.

Salary for a nurse consultant varies based upon services provided and time spent on services. Employment may be full-time, part-time, or intermittent.

Nurse Entrepreneur. The nurse entrepreneur is an independent nurse who provides a unique service or product. The nurse may provide this service or product to nurses, physicians, patients, families, or the general public.

The nurse entrepreneur must first determine the need for the service or product by performing a needs assessment. Once the need has been established, the product or service must be marketed to the target audience. This may be done via advertising, website, phone, or personal contact with the target audience. Networking with professional organizations such as NAON, AAOS, and ANA is invaluable in maintaining a demand for the product or service. The nurse entrepreneur may advertise or sell the product at local and national exhibits held by such organizations.

The nurse entrepreneur must possess a strong knowledge of the product or service being provided. Networking and sales skills are necessary to successfully market the product or service. A strong sense of autonomy with excellent leadership skills will aid in successful business strategy.

Consultation with an attorney will provide proper direction, especially in seeking a patent. Consultation with an accountant will aid in maintaining financial records and tax documents. Courses in business and knowledge of federal, state, and local legal regulations will be necessary. Funding and low-interest loans may be available through small business organizations. Experience in grant writing will help the nurse entrepreneur in writing proposals for funding. Knowledge of Food and Drug Administration (FDA) product testing may be required if approval is needed for a new product.

The nurse entrepreneur may provide the service or product on either a part-time or full-time basis. The nurse entrepreneur may be self-employed and use the financial benefits to supplement income. Salary and work hours for the nurse entrepreneur will vary based upon services provided and time spent on services.

Summary

Ongoing continuing education is necessary for the orthopaedic nurse at all levels to maintain credibility. Advanced education at the baccalaureate, master's, or doctoral level provides opportunities for new roles and advancement. Maintaining orthopaedic certification provides credibility at all levels. Additional certification such as the RNFA, NP, or case manager may be required for ongoing employment is specific roles.

Opportunities in orthopaedic nursing abound. The orthopaedic nurse has the power to choose the role that meets personal preferences. Different personal needs will suit different nursing preferences. As the orthopaedic nurse's priorities change, other orthopaedic nursing roles may better meet personal and professional needs. Orthopaedic nursing is an exciting nursing specialty with a wide variety of roles. A passion for orthopaedic nursing empowers the nurse to actively pursue its subspecialties and career opportunities for career fulfillment.

References

Allen, L. (2008). The nursing shortage continues as faculty shortage grows. *Nursing Economics, 26*(1), 35-40.

American Association of Colleges of Nursing (AACN) *Nursing Shortage Fact Sheet.* (n.d.). Retrieved from www.aacn.org.

American Association of Colleges of Nursing (AACN) *Position Statement on the Practice Doctorate in Nursing 2004*. Retrieved from www.aacn.nche.edu.

American Academy of Nurse Practitioners (AANP). (2010.) *The Standards of Practice for Nurse Practitioners*. Retrieved from http://www.aanp.org.

American Nurses Credentialing Center. *ANCC Nurse Certification.* (n.d.). Retrieved from http://www. ancc.org.

Association of Perioperative Registered Nurses (AORN). *AORN Position Statement on RN First Assistants.* (n.d.). Retrieved from http://www.aorn.org/PracticeResources/AORNPositionstatements/Position_RNFA/.

Bureau of Labor Statistics (BLS). *Occupational Outlook Handbook 2010-2011 Edition.* (n.d.). Retrieved from http://bls.gov/oco/pdf/ocos083.pdf.

Bureau of Labor Statistics (BLS). *Occupations with Largest Job Growth.* (n.d.). Retrieved from http://bls.gov/emp/ep_table_104.htm.

Domrose, C. (2010). What's in store. *Advance Practice 2010 Specialty Guide*, 16-17.

Hummer-Bellmyer, J. (2002). The collaborative role of the perioperative nurse practitioner in assessing perioperative patients. *Orthopaedic Nursing, 21*(1), 39-44.

Ivey, J.B. (2007). The preparation of nurse faculty: Who should teach the students? *Topics in Advanced Practice Nursing eJournal, 7*(2).

Klein, T.A. (2007). Scope of practice and the nurse practitioner: regulation, competency, expansion, and evolution. *Topics in Advanced Practice Nursing eJournal, 7*(2).

Minority Nurse. *Camp Nurse Jobs.* Retrieved from http://www.minoritynurse.com/camp-nurse-jobs.

National Association of Clinical Nurse Specialists (NACNS). (n.d.) *What is a Clinical Nurse Specialist?* Retrieved from www.nacns.org.

National Association of Orthopaedic Nurses (NAON). (2002). Position Statement: Role and value of the orthopaedic nurse. *Orthopaedic Nursing, 21*(6), 6.

Orthopaedic Nurses Certification Board (ONCB). (n.d.) *Orthopaedic Nurses Certification Board Exam Eligibility.* Retrieved from www.oncb.org.

Stringer, H. (2010). Unlocking opportunities. *Advance Practice 2010 Specialty Guide*, 22-23.

Chapter 2
Anatomy & Physiology

Linda Altizer, RN, MSN, ONC, D-ABMDI

Objectives

- Describe the various types of bones in the human body.
- Explain the basic functions of the musculoskeletal system.
- Identify the characteristics of muscle tissue.
- List the various joint movements.
- Describe how bone is remodeled.
- Explain the physiology of muscle tissue.

CHAPTER 2

A thorough understanding of orthopaedic anatomy and physiology is the basis of accurate nursing assessment, diagnosis, treatment, and evaluation. Normal anatomy and physiology principles provide an improved understanding of injury and disease processes. In turn, this leads to improved evaluation of healing and disease prevention.

Anatomic Terminology

Body position and anatomic planes are used to identify orthopedic injury and deformity. Standard anatomic body position is standing upright, facing forward with feet positioned straight ahead and separated slightly. Arms are positioned on each side of the torso with palms facing anterior. From this position, the areas of the body, the body's mobility, and the patient's range of activity can be identified. Anatomic planes of the body intersect from three primary angles (see Figure 2.1):

1. The sagittal or lateral plane separates the left and right sides of the body;
2. The coronal or frontal plane separates the body from ear to ear; and
3. The transverse or axial plane separates the top and bottom of the body.

Figure 2.1. Anatomic Planes of the Body

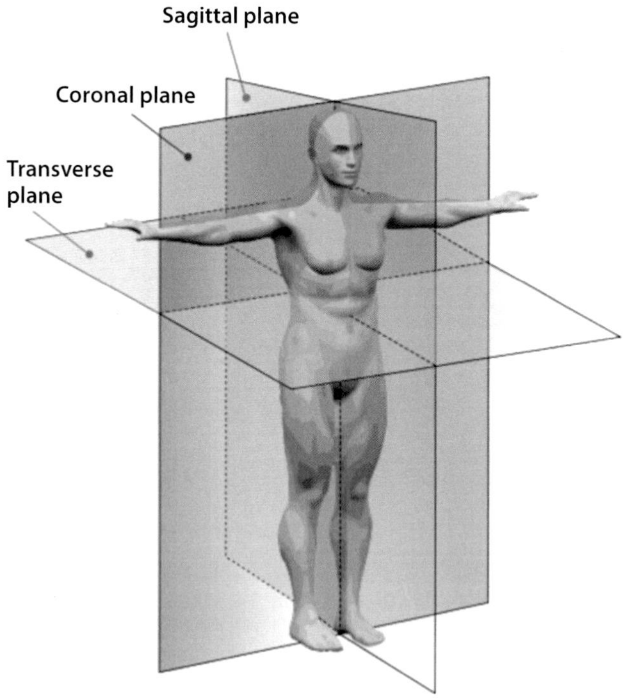

From Human Anatomy Planes *by YassineMrabet, 2008, http://en.wikipedia.org/wiki/File:Human_anatomy_planes.svg. Reproduced with permission.*

Table 2.1. Common Anatomic Terms

Term	Definition
Prone	Lying horizontally with anterior body and face downward
Supine	Lying on the back with anterior body and face upward
Anterior	Ventral or front
Posterior	Dorsal or back
Ventral	Anterior or front side of the body
Dorsal	Back or posterior side of the body
Superior	Above another structure; above midline
Inferior	Below another structure; below midline
Medial	Toward the midline of the body; toward the center
Lateral	Away from the midline
Proximal	Closer to the structural midline of the body
Distal	Farther from the structural midline of the body
Articular area	Surfaces within the joint
Intra-articular	Space within the joint
Extra-articular	Outside the joint space
Ligament	A strong fibrous tissue connecting bone to bone at the joint
Tendon	A strong fibrous tissue connecting muscle to bone
Meniscus	Intra-articular fibrous cartilage of crescent shape within the knee
Condyle	Protuberance that is rounded at the end of a bone, which forms an articulation
Medulla	In the middle of something; inner-most part
Intermedullary canal	Canal in the center of long bones
Synovial membrane	Lining the capsule of a joint
Synovial fluid	Fluid secreted by the synovial membrane that lubricates the joint
Articular cartilage	Cartilage formed at the articulating ends of bones
Epiphysis	Secondary ossification center in developing infants and children that is separated from a parent bone by cartilage
Diaphysis	Shaft or mid-section of a long bone
Periosteum	Fibrous membrane that covers the outside of the bone, except at the articular surfaces

Data from Core Curriculum for Orthopaedic Nursing *(6th ed., p. 17), by the National Association of Orthopaedic Nurses (NAON), 2007, Boston: Pearson.*

Anatomic terms (Table 2.1) specifically define the location of a body part in relation to the position of the body. In addition, anatomic action terms (Table 2.2) define the movement activity or position of various body parts. Some movements are without clear opposites. For example, rotation refers to turning on an axis such as the head turning from right to left on the spine. Opposition takes place when the thumb and fingers grasp an objection. Reposition is the release of an object by spreading the fingers and thumb, while reciprocal motion of a joint involves alternating motion in opposing directions such as an elbow alternating between flexion and extension (Gosling, Harris, Humpherson, Whitmore, & Willan, 2008).

Table 2.2. Common Anatomic Action Terms

Term	Definition
Dorsiflexion	Upward motion of foot and ankle
Plantar flexion	Downward motion of the foot and ankle
Lateral flexion	Bent to either side
Extension	Backward or posterior, the opposite of flexion; usually straightens out a bent part
Hyperextension	Extension beyond 0 degrees
Abduction	Away from the midline
Adduction	Toward the midline
Circumduction	Combination of adduction, abduction, extension, and flexion: to make a circular motion
Pivot	Rotation, to turn
Medial rotation	Rotation toward the midline
Lateral rotation	Rotation away from the midline
Eversion	Sole of foot turned outward, laterally
Inversion	Sole of foot turned inward, medially
Pronation	Forearm turned so palm faces posteriorly, or down
Supination	Forearm turned so palm faces anteriorly, or up

Bone

Bones serve protective and supportive functions for the entire body. They are continually remodeling and renewing to fit a body's daily needs. Bones store vital nutrients, minerals, and lipids, and produce blood cells that provide nourishment to the body and help protect the body from infections. The musculoskeletal system mainly contains bone, cartilage, connective tissue, nervous tissue, muscles, tendons, and ligament.

Bones are inherently multifunctional, providing the following functions highlighted by Davenport (2006):

- Protection: Encase and shield important organs (such as the ribs protecting the lungs and heart or the skull protecting the brain).
- Support: Provide a framework for muscles, ligaments, and other tissue to attach and provide support and action.
- Motion: Enable leverage for attachment of muscles and ligaments to provide movement.
- Storage: Accumulate calcium, phosphorus, and other minerals for cellular activities, and store lipids in the adipose cells of the yellow marrow for energy.
- Production: Produce blood cells consistently within certain bone cavities.

Bone Anatomy

There are 206 bones in the human skeleton, not including teeth and sesamoid bones (small bones found within cartilage). The 80 axial bones are found in the head, hyoid, auditory, torso, ribs, and sternum. The remaining 126 appendicular bones include those in the arms, shoulder girdle, wrists, hands, legs, hips, ankles, and feet. Bones are classified by their shape: long, short, flat, or irregular. Primarily, they are referred to as either long bones (such as the femur) or short bones (such as the phalanx) (Clarke, 2008). Figure 2.2 illustrates various elements of long bones.

Figure 2.2. Long Bone

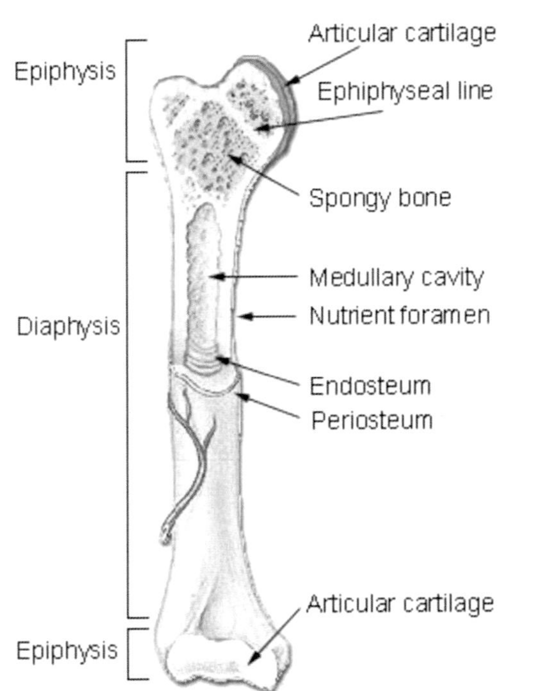

From Long Bone *(public domain), 2005, http://en.wikipedia.org/wiki/File:Illu_long_bone.jpg.*

There are ***three types of bone tissue***, defined as follows:

1. Compact tissue: Harder, outer tissue of bones.
2. Cancellous tissue: Sponge-like tissue inside bones.
3. Subchondral tissue: Smooth tissue at the end of bone, covered with another type of tissue called cartilage. Cartilage is the specialized, gristly connective tissue that is present in adults, and the tissue from which most bones develop in children.

Compact and cancellous tissues join together to form the periosteum. Beneath the hard outer shell of the periosteum are tunnels and canals through which blood and lymphatic vessels flow to carry bone nourishment (Davidson, 2010). Muscles, ligaments, and tendons may attach to the periosteum.

Bone Physiology

Bone is living and growing tissue with porous mineralized structure, comprised of cells, vessels, and crystals of calcium compounds. Bone cells are separated into two classifications: osteoblasts make bone, and osteoclasts resorb/dissolve bone. A subcategory of bone cells, bone lining cells, are the inactive osteoblast that actually cover bone surfaces.

There are ***four major bone surfaces,*** defined as follows:

1. Periosteal: outer surface of all bones.
2. Endosteal: inner surface of cortical bone.
3. Haversian: inner surface of Haversian canals within osteons.
4. Trabecular: outer surface of all individual trabeculae.

The human skeletal system has ***two types of bones***, categorized as follows:

1. Cortical bone (also called compact bone) forms the outer shell of the bone for protection. It has a high resistance to torsion and bending. It is especially strong at the midpoints of the long bones and the skull. Osteons within the bone are composed of central vascular channel surrounded by the Haversian canal (Clarke, 2008).
2. Cancellous bone (also called trabecular bone) is less dense and more elastic than cortical bone, and helps to maintain the shape of the bone. It is 80% of the bone surface (Clarke, 2008). Its center (in the medulary canal) contains red and yellow marrow, bone cells, and other tissue (Davenport, 2006). Cancellous bone is located in the epipheseal and metaphyseal areas of long bones and interior area of short bones. It is also in the skull, ribs, hip, femur, and spinal areas.

Clarke (2008) defines the three major processes during which bone can be changed:

1. Osteogenesis: Bone can be formed on soft tissue and usually occurs during embryonic development and during the early stages of growth. It may also occur during a healing process. Two subclassifications are intramembranous (bone formed on soft tissue) and endochodral (bone formed on cartilage).
2. Modeling: Bone forms on existing bone tissue and usually occurs during the growth phase and the healing phase. Osteoclasts and osteoblasts act independently in different areas.
3. Remodeling: Bone can be resorbed and developed at the same site, which can occur during the entire lifetime.

Hormonal Impact on Bone

Several hormones have an effect on bone growth and density. Post-menopausal osteoporosis attributed to estrogen loss highlights the importance of this hormone in maintaining bone density. Research continues as to the exact mechanism of estrogen's effect on bone strength, but studies suggest that this hormone may prevent apoptosis (programmed cell death) in osteoblasts, thereby sustaining demineralization (Bradford, Gerance, Roland, & Chrzan, 2010). In addition, estrogen stimulates growth factors and influences antiresorptive action (Meczekalski, Podfigurna-Stopa, & Genazzani, 2010).

Parathyroid hormone (PTH) has been found to have a strong anabolic effect on the central skeletal system in patients on hormone replacement therapy. PTH has also been found to increase total-body bone mineral, with no effects that are detrimental at any bone site (Lindsay et al., 1997). An increase in the vertebral mass is associated with a reduced rate of vertebral fractures. Thyroid hormone increases osteoclast resorption activity and has a critical role in bone maturation (Abe et al., 2007). In addition, a thyroid-stimulating hormone produced by the pituitary gland promotes bone growth in ways other than the stimulation of the thyroid (Mount Sinai School of Medicine, 2011).

Muscle

Muscle is classified into the following three categories:

1. Cardiac muscle is only found in the heart. It works automatically, and does not get tired or take a break.
2. Smooth muscle is located in the hollow organs such as the intestines and the stomach. The smooth muscles in the intestines and stomach contract to circulate food through the gastrointestinal system.

Smooth muscles also tense the bladder to excrete urine and contract the uterus to deliver a baby (Hall, 2012).

3. Skeletal muscle is tailored for force generation and movement at both the macroscopic and microscopic levels. This chapter will focus on skeletal muscles, as the focus is on orthopaedics.

Muscle Anatomy

Skeletal muscle differs from cardiac and smooth muscles in its biological structure-function relationship. Skeletal muscle is comprised of many cylindrical muscle fibers that often run from point of origin to point of insertion. Connective tissue binds the fibers and provides a path for blood vessels and nerves. The muscle fibers contain myofibrils, mitochondria, smooth endoplasmic reticulum (SER), and nuclei. The fiber numbers are usually fixed early in life and regulated by myostatin and acytokine, which is synthesized in muscle cells and later in life circulates as a hormone. Myostatin may suppress skeletal muscle development (Hall, 2012).

Because muscle fiber is not a single cell, it is divided into the following specific titles based on contents:

- Sarcolemma: plasma membrane;
- Sarcoplasmic reticulum: endoplasmic reticulum;
- Sarcosomes: mitochondria; and
- Sarcoplasm: cytoplasm.

The motor neurons that lead into the skeletal muscles have axons that branch out and terminate in the neuromuscular junction with a single muscle fiber (Hall, 2012). Nerve impulses that go down through a single motor neuron will initiate contraction to all the muscle fibers at which the branches of that neuron terminate. This unit of contraction is termed the motor unit.

Muscle Physiology

There are at least two phases in the process of development of the neuromuscular system. Myogenesis describes the fusion of the precursor myoblasts into the true muscle fibers during the first phase. Synaptogenesis is the second phase when nerves attach to fibers, which results in increased muscle innervation. With multiple axons in contact with each fiber, there is competition for control during the synapse elimination until each fiber is synapsed with just one axon. Single innervation is very significant, as the axon is considered to have a strong influence on the fiber properties (Hall, 2012).

Each muscle cell is embedded in a basal lamina of collagen and large glycoproteins. The large number of satellite cells between the fiber and the basal lamina play a significant role in the growth and repair of the fiber. The fiber contains structures for excitation-contraction, joining together to provide balanced communication to the entire fiber. While contractile and performance characteristics vary, both are closely linked to the myosin-heavy chain isoform expressed by the fiber. Myofibrils produce forceful actions, which are chains of sarcomeres running from one end of the fiber to the other. Metabolism of fats and sugars generate the energy for contraction (Hall, 2012).

Muscle properties depend on (a) the properties of the fibers and (b) the organization of the fibers. For example, fibers do not always run the entire length of the muscle and may run oblique to the muscle's line of action. The peak force production is related to the physiological cross sectional area (PCSA), which estimates the cross sectional area of all the fibers. Fiber length relates to the contraction velocity and excursion range. While each fiber has one axon, a motorneuron may have over a hundred axons; therefore; a motorneuron is termed a motor unit, controlling many fibers. During a maximal voluntary contraction, it would be unlikely that all motor units would be activated (Hall, 2012).

Joints

A joint, or articulation, is the place where two bones come together. Principle joints of the human body are summarized in Table 2.3. Davidson (2010) defines three types of joints classified by the amount of movement they allow: immovable, slightly movable, and freely movable.

Immovable joints are called synarthroses. In this type of joint, the bones are in very close contact and are separated only by a thin layer of fibrous connective tissue. The suture in the skull between skull bones is an example of a synarthrosis.

Slightly movable joints are called amphiarthroses. This type of joint is characterized by bones that are connected by hyaline cartilage (fibrocartilage). The ribs that connect to the sternum are an example of an amphiarthrosis joint.

Freely movable joints are called diarthroses. Most of the joints in the adult human body are freely movable. There are six types of diarthrosis joints, as follows:

1. Ball-and-socket: The ball-shaped end of one bone fits into a cup-shaped socket on another, allowing the widest range of motion (ROM), including rotation. Examples include the shoulder and hip.
2. Condyloid: An oval-shaped condyle of one bone fits into an elliptical cavity of another, allowing angular motion but not rotation. This occurs between the metacarpals (bones in the palm of the hand) and phalanges (fingers) and between the metatarsals (foot bones excluding heel) and phalanges (toes).

3. Saddle: The touching surfaces of two bones have both concave and convex regions, with the shapes of the two bones complementing one other and allowing a wide range of movement. The only saddle joint in the body is in the thumb.
4. Pivot: Rounded or conical surfaces of one bone fit into a ring of another bone or tendon, allowing rotation. An example is the joint between the axis and atlas in the neck.
5. Hinge: A convex projection on one bone fits into a concave depression in another, permitting only flexion and extension as in the elbow joints.
6. Gliding: Flat or slightly flat surfaces move against each other, allowing sliding or twisting without any circular movement. This happens in the carpals in the wrist and the tarsals in the ankle (Davidson, 2010).

Table 2.3. Principle Joints of the Human Body	
Acromioclavicular	Radioulnar, distal
Ankle (tibia-fibula and talus)	Radioulnar, middle
Atlas and axis	Radioulnar, proximal
Atlas and occipital	Radius-ulna and carpals (wrist)
Calcaneocuboid	Ribs, heads of
Carpometacarpal	Ribs, tubercles and necks of
Elbow (humerus, radius, and ulna)	Sacrococcygeal
Femur and tibia	Sacroiliac
Hip bone and femur	Shoulder (humerus and scapula)
Humerus and ulna	Symphysis
Intercarpal: Carpal, proximal Carpal, distal Carpal bones (two rows with each other)	Sacroiliac Scapula and humerus Skull Sternoclavicular
Intermetacarpals	Sternocostal
Intermetatarsals	Subtalar
Interphalangeal	Talus and calcaneus
Knee (femur, tibia, and patella)	Talus and navicular
Mandible (jaw) and temporal	Tarsometatarsal
Metacarpophalangeal	Tiobiofibular
Metatarsophalangeal	Vertebral arches
Pubic bones	Vertebral bodies
	Wrist (radius-ulna and carpals)

The Skull

The skull is the bony framework of the head and a protector of the brain (Figure 2.3). In humans, the adult skull is normally comprised of 22 bones: eight cranial bones form the neurocranium (braincase), a protective vault surround the brain, and 14 facial bones form the splanchnocranium, the bones supporting the face.

Figure 2.3.
The Skull

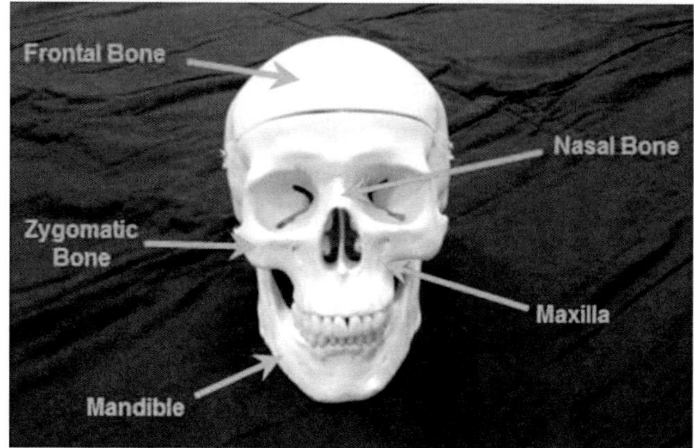

Author creation. Reproduced with permission.

Encased within the temporal bones are the six ear ossicles of the middle ears, though these are not part of the skull. The hyoid bone, supporting the tongue, is usually not considered as part of the skull either because it does not articulate with any other bones (Davidson, 2010).

The skull contains the sinus cavities, air-filled pockets lined with respiratory epithelium, which also lines the large airways. The exact functions of the sinuses are unclear; they may contribute to decreasing the weight of the skull with a minimal decrease in strength, or they may be important in improving the resonance of the voice (Davidson, 2010).

Cranial Bones. The eight cranial bones make up the protective frame of bone around the brain, as follows:

1. The frontal bone forms part of the cranial cavity as well as the forehead, the brow ridges and the nasal cavity.

2, 3. The left and right parietal bones form much of the superior and lateral portions of the cranium.

4, 5. The left and right temporal bones form the lateral walls of the cranium and house the external ear.

6. The occipital bone forms the posterior and inferior portions of the cranium. Many neck muscles attach here, as this is the point of articulation with the neck.

7. The sphenoid bone forms part of the eye orbit and helps form the floor of the cranium.

8. The ethmoid bone forms the medial portions of the orbits and the roof of the nasal cavity.

Except for the mandible, all of the bones of the skull are joined together by sutures, or rigid articulations between bones that permit very little movement. The parietal bones are joined by the sagittal suture. The parietal bones meet the frontal bone at the coronal suture. The parietals and occipital bone meet at the lambdoidal suture. The parietals and the temporal bone join at the squamous suture. These sites are the common location of fontanels, or the "soft spots" on a baby's head (Kiesler & Ricer, 2003).

Facial Bones. The 14 facial bones make up the upper and lower jaw and other facial structures:

- 1. The mandible is the lower jawbone. It articulates with the temporal bones at the temporomandibular joints and forms the only freely moveable joint in the head. It provides the chewing motion.
- 2, 3. The left and right maxilla are the upper jaw bones. They form part of the nose, orbits, and roof of the mouth.
- 4, 5. The left and right palatines form a portion of the nasal cavity and the posterior portion of the roof of the mouth.
- 6, 7. The left and right zygomatics are the cheek bones. They also form portions of the orbits.
- 8, 9. The left and right nasal bones form the superior portion of the bridge of the nose.
- 10, 11. The left and right lacrimals help to form the orbits.
- 12. The vomer forms part of the nasal septum (the divider between the nostrils).
- 13, 14. The left and right inferior turbinates form the lateral walls of the nose and increase the surface area of the nasal cavity.

In humans, the anatomic position for the skull is the Frankfurt plane, where the lower margins of the orbits and the upper borders of the ear canals are all in a horizontal plane (Cassiopia, 2003). In this position, the subject is facing forward.

The Shoulder

The shoulder joint is the most mobile joint in the human body. The shoulder can abduct, adduct, rotate, be raised in front of and behind the torso, and move through a full 360 degrees in the sagittal plane. This mobility also makes the shoulder extremely unstable, far more susceptible to dislocation than other joints (Kishner, Munshi, & Black, 2011). The muscles and joints of the shoulder provide the upper extremity with the capacity to move through complete ROM.

The rotator cuff is a term given to the group of muscles and tendons that stabilize the shoulder. It is composed of the tendons and muscles (supraspinatus, infraspinatus, teres minor, and subscapularis) that sustain the head of the humerus in the glenoid fossa. Two filmy sac-like structures called bursae allows smooth motion between bone, muscle, and tendon. They cushion and protect the rotator cuff from the bony arch of the acromion.

Individual Shoulder Joints

The shoulder is made up of three joints: glenohumeral, acromioclavicular, and sternoclavicular. These joints connect the upper extremity to the body (Kishner, Munshi, & Black, 2011).

Glenohumeral Joint. The glenohumeral is the main joint of the shoulder, and the generic term "shoulder joint" usually refers to it. It is a ball (humeral head) and socket (glenoid fossa) joint that allows the arm to rotate in a circular (circumduction) fashion or to hinge out and up away from the body. It is formed by the articulation between the head of the humerus and the lateral scapula (specifically the glenoid fossa of the scapula).

The shallowness of the fossa and soft tissue connections allows the arm to have tremendous mobility, at the expense of being much easier to dislocate than most other joints in the body (AAOS, 2007b). The capsule is a soft tissue envelope that encircles the glenohumeral joint and attaches to the scapula, humerus, and head of the biceps. It is lined by a thin, smooth synovial membrane. This capsule is strengthened by the coracohumeral ligament that attaches the coracoid process of the scapula to the greater tubercle of the humerus.

Three other ligaments, collectively called the glenohumeral ligaments, attach the lesser tubercle of the humerus to lateral scapula. The ligamentum semicirculare humeri is a transversal band between the posterior sides of the tuberculum minus and majus of the humerus. This band is one of the most important strengthening ligaments of the joint capsule (Davidson, 2010).

Acromioclavicular Joint. The acromioclavicular attaches the clavicle to the acromion of the scapula and assists in the ability to raise the arm above the head. This joint functions as a pivot point (although technically it is a gliding synovial joint), operating to assist with scapular movement for greater degree of arm rotation. This joint, like most joints in the body, has a cartilage disk (or meniscus) inside, and the ends of the bones are covered with cartilage. The joint is held together by a capsule, and the clavicle is held in the proper position by the two heavy coracoclavicular ligaments (Kishner, Munshi, & Black, 2011).

Sternoclavicular Joint. The sternoclavicular is stationed at the medial end of the clavicle with the manubrium (or the top portion of the sternum). The clavicle is triangular and rounded, and the manubrium is convex; the two bones articulate. The joint consists of a tight capsule and complete intra-articular disc that ensure the stability of the joint (Davidson, 2010). The costoclavicular ligament is the main limitation to movement and, therefore, the main stabilizer of the joint. A fibrocartilaginous disc present at the joint increases ROM.

The Upper Extremity

The upper extremity can be divided into three distinct sections. The upper arm, or brachium, is the region between the shoulder and elbow. The forearm is the area between the elbow and the wrist. The wrist, hand, and fingers round out the extremity.

Bones of the Upper Extremity

The upper extremity consists of three bone groups: the humerus in the upper arm; the radius and ulna in the forearm; and the carpals, metacarpals, and phalanges in the wrist, hand, and fingers.

Humerus. The upper arm consists of a single long bone called the humerus. This is the longest bone in the upper extremity (Davidson, 2010). The proximal humerus (or head) is large, smooth, and rounded, and it fits into the scapula at the shoulder. The distal portion of the humerus contains two areas where the humerus connects to the ulna and radius of the forearm. The radius is connected on the lateral side and the ulna is connected on the medial side when standing in the anatomic position. Together, the humerus and the ulna make up the elbow joint. The distal humerus protects the ulnar nerve and is called the "funny bone" because striking the elbow on a hard surface stimulates the ulnar nerve and produces a tingling sensation.

Radius and Ulna. The forearm is formed by the radius on the lateral side and the ulna on the medial side when the forearm is viewed in the anatomic position. The ulna is longer than the radius and connected more firmly to the humerus. The radius is, however, a stronger bone and contributes more to the movement of the wrist and hand. When the hand pronates (or is turned over so that the palm is facing downward), the radius crosses over the ulna. The top of each bone connects to the humerus of the arm and the bottom of each connects to the bones of the hand.

Carpals, Metacarpals, and Phylangs. There are 27 bones in the wrist and hand. The wrist itself contains eight small bones, called carpals. The carpals join with the two forearm bones, the radius and ulna, forming the wrist joint. Further into the palm, the carpals connect to the metacarpals. There are five metacarpals forming the palm of the hand. One metacarpal connects to each finger and thumb. Small bone shafts called phalanges line up to form each finger and thumb (Wilhelmi, 2011).

The main knuckle joints, called the metacarpophalangeal (MCP) joints, are formed by the connections of the phalanges to the metacarpals. The MCP joints work like a hinge when the fingers are flexed and extended. The three phalanges in each finger are separated by two joints, called interphalangeal (IP) joints, that also work like hinges (Davidson, 2010). The middle joint, closest to the knuckle, is called the proximal IP (PIP) joint. The joint near the end of the finger is called the distal IP (DIP) joint. The thumb only has one IP joint between the two thumb phalanges.

The joints of the hand and fingers are covered on the ends with articular cartilage. This white, shiny material has a rubbery consistency. The function of articular cartilage is to absorb shock and provide an extremely smooth surface to facilitate motion. There is articular cartilage essentially everywhere that two bony surfaces move against one another, or articulate (Wilhelmi, 2011).

Muscles of the Upper Extremity

Muscles of the Upper Arm and Forearm. The muscles in Figure 2.4 mobilize the upper extremity in every motion and enable activities of daily living (ADLs). The deltoid muscle provides abduction of the arm; the pectoralis major provides flexion, adduction, and internal rotation of the arm; and the latissimus dorsi provides adduction, extension, and internal rotation of the humerus. The teres major provides adduction, extension, and internal rotation of the arm. The coracobrachialis provides flexion and adduction.

Figure 2.4.
Muscles, Ligaments, and Nerves of the Upper Arm and Forearm

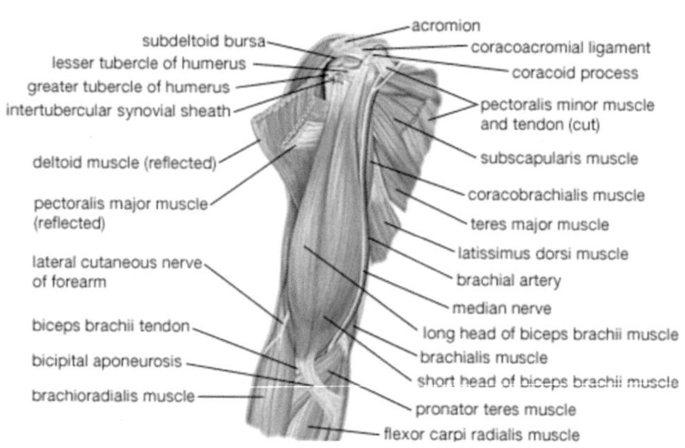

From Encyclopedia Britannica, Inc., 2008, http://media-1.web.britannica.com/eb-media/37/113037-004-D4CF5BB4.jpg. Reprinted with permission.

Additional muscles in the upper extremity include the biceps, which allows flexion and supination of the forearm, and the triceps, which provides extension of the forearm.

Muscles of the Hand and Wrist. Many of the muscles that control the hand start at the elbow or forearm. They run down the forearm and cross the wrist and hand. Some control only the flexing or extending the wrist. Other tendons affect the motion of the fingers or thumb. Many of these muscles help position and maintain the wrist and hand while the thumb and fingers flex or perform fine motor actions.

Many of the small muscles that provide action for the thumb and fifth finger start on the carpal bones. These muscles connect to allow the hand to grip and hold. Two muscles allow the thumb to flex across the palm of the hand (Wilhelmi, 2011). The smallest muscles that originate in the wrist and hand are called the intrinsic muscles. The intrinsic muscles guide the fine motions of the fingers by getting the fingers positioned and holding them steady during hand activities.

Ligaments & Tendons of the Upper Extremity

Ligaments and tendons are similar in that they are both fibrous tissues made of collagen and serve as connectors.

Ligaments join bone to bone, and tendons join muscle to bone. Ligaments limit the mobility of articulations or prevent certain movements altogether, while tendons are capable of withstanding tension.

Ligaments and Tendons in the Upper Arm and Forearm. The ligaments and tendons of the upper arm and forearm provide strength and support to the elbow and wrist joints. The radial collateral ligament, ulnar collateral ligament, and annular ligament provide strength and stability to the elbow joint. In addition, the common extensor tendon and common flexor tendon are attached at this joint assisting in rotational movements of the forearm, wrist, and hand.

Ligaments and Tendons in the Wrist, Hand, and Fingers. The collateral ligaments are two important structures, found on either side of each finger and thumb joint, that prevent those joints from abnormal sideways bending. In the PIP joint, the strongest ligament is the volar plate. This ligament connects the proximal phalanx to the middle phalanx on the palm side of the joint. The ligament tightens as the joint is straightened and keeps the PIP joint from bending back too far (hyperextending). Finger deformities can occur when the volar plate loosens from disease or injury.

The tendons that allow each finger joint to straighten are called the extensor tendons. The extensor tendons of the fingers begin as muscles that arise from the back of the forearm bones. These muscles travel towards the hand, where they eventually connect to the extensor tendons before crossing over the back of the wrist joint. As they travel into the fingers, the extensor tendons become the extensor hood. The extensor hood flattens out to cover the top of the finger and branches out on each side that connect to the bones in the middle and end of the finger. The site where the extensor tendon attaches to the middle phalanx is called the central slip. When the extensor muscles contract, they pull on the extensor tendon and straighten the finger. Problems occur when the central slip is damaged, as can happen with a tear.

Nerves of the Upper Extremity

The innervations are what actually activate the muscle to move. These nerves carry signals from the brain to the muscles that provide motion for the entire arm, hand, fingers, and thumb. The nerves also carry signals back to the brain about sensations such as touch, pain, and temperature. Sensation location based on innervation is graphically presented in Figure 2.5. The three dynamic nerves in the upper extremity begin at the shoulder and run all the way down into the fingers: the median nerve, the radial nerve, and the ulnar nerve.

Figure 2.5.
Upper Extremity Dermatome

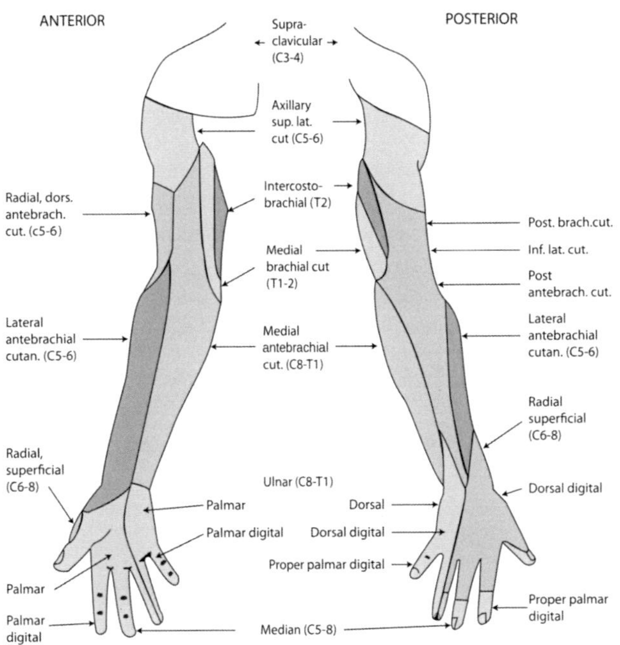

From Gray812and814 (public domain), 2010, http://en.wikipedia.org/wiki/File:Gray812and814.svg.

Median Nerve. The median nerve runs down the anteromedial aspect of the arm and at the elbow. It lies medial to the brachial artery on the brachialis muscle. It passes through the cubital fossa, deep to the bicipital aponeurosis and medial to the brachial artery. The median nerve enters the forearm between the humeral and ulnar heads of the pronator teres muscle, passes between the flexor digitorum superficialis and the flexor digitorum profundus muscles, and then becomes superficial by passing between the tendons of the flexor digitorum superficialis and flexor carpi radialis near the wrist.

The median nerve innervates all anterior muscles of the forearm except the flexor carpi ulnaris and the ulnar half of the flexor digitorum profundus. It also innervates the lateral two lumbricals, the skin of the lateral side of the palm, and the palmar side of the lateral three-and-a-half fingers and the dorsal side of the index finger, middle finger, and half of the ring finger (Tank, 2009).

The median nerve travels through a tunnel within the wrist called the carpal tunnel. This nerve gives sensation to the thumb, second finger, third finger, and half of the fourth finger. It also sends a nerve branch to control the thenar muscles of the thumb. The thenar muscles move the thumb and let the thumb touch the tips each of each finger on that hand, called opposition (Wilhelmi, 2011).

Radial Nerve. The radial nerve comes from the posterior cord and the largest branch of the brachial plexus. It descends posteriorly between the long and medial heads of the triceps, after which it passes inferolaterally with the profunda brachii artery in the spiral groove on the back of the humerus. It pierces the lateral intermuscular septum to enter the anterior compartment and descends anterior to the lateral epicondyle between the brachialis and brachioradialis muscles to enter the cubital fossa, where it divides into superficial and deep branches (Tank, 2009).

The radial nerve travels down along the lateral forearm. It wraps around the distal radius bone toward the back of the hand and gives sensation to the dorsum of the hand from the thumb to the third finger. It also supplies the back of the thumb and just beyond the metacarpal joint of the back surface of the fourth finger and the third finger (Wilhelmi, 2011).

Ulnar Nerve. The ulnar nerve begins at the medial cord of the brachial plexus, runs down the medial aspect of the arm, pierces the medial intermuscular septum at the middle of the arm, and descends together with the superior ulnar collateral branch of the brachial artery. It descends behind the medial epicondyle in a groove or tunnel where it is readily palpated and most commonly injured. The ulnar nerve enters the forearm by passing between the two heads of the flexor carpi ulnaris and descends between and innervates the flexor carpi ulnaris and flexor digitorum profundus muscles (Mazurek & Shin, 2001).

The ulnar nerve travels through a separate tunnel, called Guyon's canal. This tunnel is formed by two carpal bones (the pisiform and hamate) and the ligament that connects them. After passing through the canal, the ulnar nerve branches out to supply sensation to the fifth digit and the medial half the fourth digit. Branches of this nerve also supply the small muscles in the palm and the muscle that pulls the thumb toward the palm (Wilhelmi, 2011).

The Thoracic Cage

The thoracic cage is a bony and cartilaginous structure that surrounds the chest and supports the pectoral girdle, forming a core portion of the human skeleton. A typical human rib cage consists of 24 ribs, the sternum, costal cartilages, and the 12 thoracic vertebrae The thoracic wall provides attachments for the muscles of the neck, thorax, upper abdomen, and back (Halim, 2008b).

Rib Cage

The rib cage encloses and protects the thoracic cavity content, which contains the lungs, trachea, esophagus, and heart. When inhaling, the muscular diaphragm contracts and flattens, and contraction of the intercostal muscles lifts and expands the rib cage. These actions produce an increase in volume and a partial vacuum (or negative pressure) in the thoracic cavity, resulting in atmospheric pressure pushing air into the lungs to inflating them. When exhaling, the diaphragm and intercostal muscles relax, and elastic recoil of the rib cage and lungs expels the air.

Human Rib Parts. The head is the end of a rib closest to the vertebral column. The costovertebral joints, the articulations that connect the heads of the ribs to the thoracic vertebrae, form the costotransverse joint. The neck is the flattened portion that extends laterally from the head. The tubercle is the prominence on the posterior surface, and the angle is the flexed portion. The costal groove is a groove between the ridge of the internal surface of the rib and the inferior border (Davidson, 2010)

All ribs are attached to the posterior thoracic vertebrae. They are divided into three classifications:

1. The *true ribs* are the superior seven ribs (costae verae, vertebrosternal ribs, I-VII). These are attached to the anterior sternum by means of costal cartilage. Their elasticity allows movement when inhaling and exhaling.
2. The *false ribs* are the eight, ninth, and tenth ribs (costae spuriae, vertebrochondral ribs, VIII-X). These connect with the costal cartilages of the ribs above.
3. The *floating ribs* are the eleventh and twelfth ribs (costae fluitantes, vertebral ribs, XI-XII) because they do not have any anterior attachment to the sternum. The spaces between the ribs are known as intercostal spaces and contain the intercostal muscles, nerves, and arteries (Halim, 2008b).

The first, second, eleventh, and twelfth are called atypical ribs. The first rib shaft is wide, nearly horizontal, and has the sharpest curve. Its head has a single facet to articulate with the first thoracic vertebra (T1). It also has two grooves for the subclavian vessels, which are separated by the scalene tubercle. The first rib forms the superior thoracic aperture together with the manubrium and T1. The second rib is thinner, less curved, and longer than the first rib. It has two facets to articulate with T2 and T1, and a tubercle to attach to muscles. The eleventh and twelfth ribs have only one facet on their head; they are short with no necks or tubercles and terminate in the abdominal wall before fusing with the costal cartilages (Davidson, 2010).

Sternum

The sternum is composed of the following three sections:

1. The manubrim, also called the handle, is located at the superior sternum and moves slightly. It is connected to the first two ribs.
2. The body, also called the blade or the gladiolus, is located in the middle of the sternum and connects the third to seventh ribs directly and to the eighth through tenth ribs indirectly.
3. The xiphoid process, also called the tip, is located on the bottom of the sternum. It is often cartilaginous but becomes bony in later years.

These three segments of bone are usually fused in adults (Davidson, 2010).

Thoracic Muscles and Nerves

The thorax muscles include the intercostals between the ribs, which consists of three layers (the external, the internal, and the intermost layer), and the diaphragm, which closes the thoracic outlet and separates the thoracic cavity from the abdominal cavity (Halim, 2008b). Table 2.4 lists primary muscles of the thorax, along with innervation and blood supply.

The Spine

Vertebral Column

The vertebral column is composed of a series of 31 separate bones known as vertebrae (Figure 2.6). The vertebrae are referred to by their name and number, counting down from the top of the spinal column, as follows:

- The seven cervical vertebrae are C1 - C7
- The 12 thoracic vertebrae are T1 –T12
- The five lumbar vertebrae are L1 – L5

The sacrum and coccyx are not numbered, as they are each considered one bone. The sacrum is composed of

Table 2.4. Primary Muscles of the Thorax

Muscle	Origin	Insertion	Action	Innervation	Artery
External intercostal	Rib - lower border within an intercostal space	Rib elbow - upper border - coursing downward and medially	Monitor the intercostal space from blowing out or sucking in during respiration	T1-T11 - Intercostal nerves	Intercostal
Innermost intercostal	Rib - upper borders	Rib - fibers course up and medially to insert on the inferior margin	Monitor the intercostal space from blowing out or sucking in during respiration	T1-T11 - Intercostal nerves	Intercostal
Internal intercostal	Rib - upper borders	Rib - lower border above, coursing up and medially	Monitor the intercostal space from blowing out or sucking in during respiration	T1-T11 - Intercostal nerves	Intercostal
Serratus posterior inferior	Spines of vertebrae T11-T12 and L1-L2 - thoracolumbar fascia	Ribs 9-12, lateral to the angles	Pulls down lower ribs	Ventral primary rami of spinal nerves T9-T12 - branches	Lowest posterior intercostal subcostal first two lumbar
Serratus posterior superior	Spines of vertebrae C7 and T1-T3 - ligamentum nuchae	Ribs 1-4, lateral to the angles	Raises upper ribs	Ventral primary rami of spinal nerves T1-T4 - branches	Posterior intercostal 1-4
Subcostalis	Rib - angle	Rib 2-3 ribs above origin	Compresses the intercostal spaces	Intercostal nerves	Intercostal
Transversus thoracis	Sternum- posterior surface	Costal cartilages 2-6 - inner surfaces	Create forced expiration by compressing the thorax	Intercostal nerves 2-6	Internal thoracic

five fused vertebrae, and the two coccygeal vertebrae are sometimes fused (Davidson, 2010). Spinal nerves exit the sacrum and coccyx at levels within the main structure of each vertebra (Gilroy, Macpherson, & Ross, 2008).

Figure 2.6.
The Vertebral Column

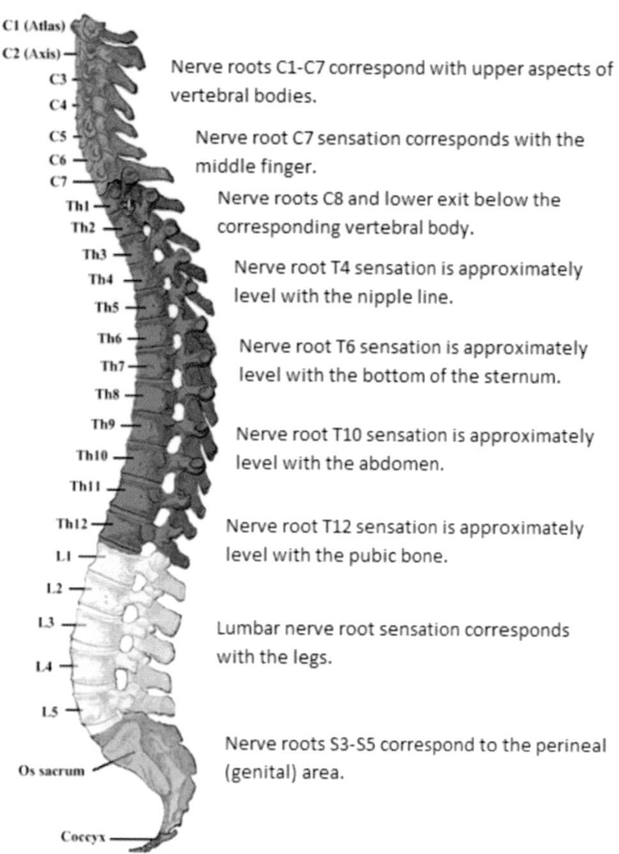

From Vertebral Column-Coloured *(public domain), 2007, http://en.wikipedia.org/wiki/File:Gray_111_-_Vertebral_column-coloured.png.*

Typical *cervical vertebrae* have large spinal canals, oval shaped vertebral bodies, and articular facets oriented obliquely. Their most characteristic features are their bifid spinous processes and a foramen in their transverse processes. These foramina transversaria contain the vertebral artery and vein. The first and second cervical vertebrae are atypical. The first cervical vertebra, the atlas, is remarkable for having no body. It contains an anterior tubercle instead. Its superior articular facets articulate with the occipital condyles of the skull and are oriented in a roughly parasagittal plane. The head thus moves forward and backwards on this vertebra. The second cervical vertebra contains a prominent odontoid process, or dens, which projects superiorly from its body. It articulates with the anterior tubercle of the atlas, forming a pivotal joint. Side-to-side movements of the head take place about this joint. The seventh cervical vertebra is sometimes considered atypical because it lacks a bifid spinous process (Windsor et al., 2011).

Thoracic vertebrae form a transition between cervical vertebrae above and lumbar vertebrae below. The upper four thoracic vertebrae are like cervical vertebrae in some respects. They have vertically oriented articular facets and posteriorly directed spinous processes. The lower four thoracic vertebrae contain more lumbar features, like large bodies, robust transverse and spinous processes, and lateral projecting articular facets. The middle four thoracic vertebrae have characteristics between these two regions. These include vertically oriented articular processes and long, slender, and inferiorly inclined spinous processes.

Lumbar vertebrae consist of moveable vertebrae L1 thorough L5. Flexion, extension, rotation and side bending are possible through the functioning of this structure. They provide considerable strength to the spinal column through the interworkings of the vertabae, flexible ligaments and tendons, and large muscles. In addition to providing strength, the lumbar vertebrae protect the lower section of spinal innervation.

Spinal Curvatures. The normal adult has four curvatures in the vertebral column in an anteroposterior plane. These serve to align the head with a vertical line through the pelvis. In the thoracic and sacral regions, these curves are oriented concave-anterior, and each is known as a kyphosis. The thoracic and sacral curvatures are the same in the adult as they are in fetal life, and they are known as primary curvatures.

In the lumbar and cervical regions, the curves are convex-anterior, and each is known as a lordosis. These normal curvatures develop during childhood in association with lifting the head (cervical) and assuming upright sitting (lumbar), and they are thus known as secondary curvatures.

Exaggerated kyphosis or lordosis can occur under some normal conditions (e.g. increased lumbar lordosis in pregnancy). A curvature of the vertebral column in a mediolateral plane can occur pathologically and is known as a scoliosis (Kishner, Moradian, & Morello, 2011).

The Pelvic Girdle

The pelvis is the part of the skeleton that connects the sacrum region of the spine to the femurs, subdivided into the pelvic girdle and the pelvic region of the spine (sacrum and coccyx). The pelvic girdle, also called the hip girdle, serves several important functions in the body. It supports the weight of the body from the vertebral column. It also protects and supports the lower organs, including the urinary bladder, the reproductive organs, and the developing fetus in a pregnant woman.

The pelvic girdle differs between men and women. The male pelvis is more massive, with iliac crests that are closer together. The female pelvis is more delicate, and the iliac crests are farther apart (Halim, 2009).

A network of ligaments connects the various components of the pelvic girdle to anchor it in place, provide support to the spine and legs, and create articulation for the hips so that they bend and flex. The space inside the pelvis creates a hollow that protects the reproductive organs and some of the lower abdominal organs. When viewed from above, the pelvic girdle strongly resembles a bowl in shape (Halim, 2008a).

The pelvic girdle is composed of two coxal (hip) bones. The coxal bones are also called the ossa coxae or innominate bones (Figure 2.7). During childhood, each coxal bone consists of three separate parts: the ilium, the ischium, and the pubis. In an adult, these three bones are firmly fused into a single bone. In the back, these two bones meet on either side of the sacrum. In the front, they are connected by a muscle called the pubic symphysis (Davidson, 2010).

Illium

The highest and largest of the three pelvic bones is designed with a crest, angles, and spines, which are distinctively obvious for the attachment of various muscles. The prominence associated with the hip is created by the iliac crest. As the crest reaches the anterior portion, it alters into the anterior superior iliac spine. Just below this rests the anterior and inferior iliac spine. As the posterior portion of the iliac crest terminates, it forms the posterior superior iliac spine. Just below this, the greater sciatic notch provides passage for the sciatic nerve. The rough auricular surface located on the medial portion of the illium joins with the sacrum. Adversely, the smooth concave portion of the anterior surface belongs to the iliac fossa that joins to the iliacus muscle. Posterior to the iliac fossa, the iliac tuberosity provides the point of attachment for the sacroliliac ligament. The gluteal surface is represented by three roughened ridges on the posterior portion of the iliac. Presented anterior, inferior, and posterior, these roughened ridges attach gluteus muscles (Gilroy et al., 2008).

Ischium

The posterior and inferior portion of the hip is known as the ischium. The distinguishing spine of the ischium is an obvious projection immediately posterior and inferior to the illium's great sciatic notch. The lesser sciatic notch belonging to the ischium is then just inferior to this spine. The body's weight is supported in the seated posture by the ischial tuberosity. Located on the inferior section of the acetebulum is the seething acetubular notch. The inferior ramux of this unique bone forms the large obturator foramen. This comes together at the conjoining of the pubis. This foramen is additionally saturated with obturator membrane to allow the attachment of several surrounding muscles (Gilroy et al., 2008).

Pubis

The anterior bone of the hip is the pubis. The supportive structure of the pubis is created by superior and inferior ramus. The joint structure located between the two ossa coxae, the symphisys pubis, is created by this entire structure. The inguinal ligament is then attached to the pubic tubercle, which is created at the latter end of the anterior border (Davidson, 2010).

Figure 2.7.
Pelvic Girdle

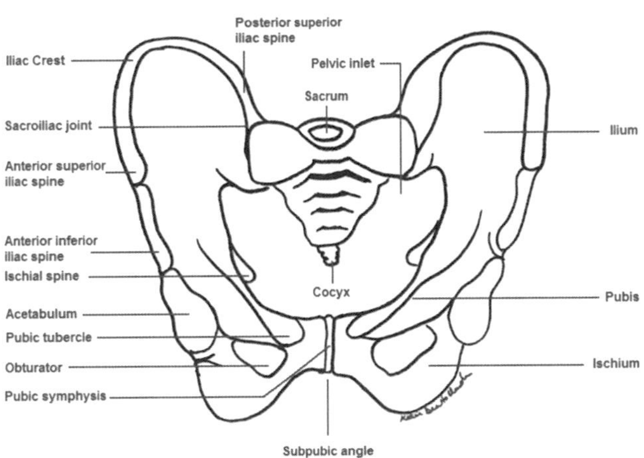

Author creation. Reproduced with permission.

Lower Extremity

In human anatomy, Medicine.Net, (n.d.) defines the term "lower extremity" as encompassing the thigh (from hip and knee), the leg (from knee to ankle), and the foot. The lower extremity comprises the hip, knee, and ankle joints, and includes the bones of the thigh, leg, and ankle and foot. (For clarity, the particulars of the ankle and foot will be discussed separately in this chapter.)

Bones of the Lower Extremity

The major (long) bones of the lower extremity are the femur (thighbone), tibia (shinbone), and fibula (rear calf bone). The patella (kneecap) is the bone anterior to the knee. (See Figure 2.8.)

Most of the lower extremity skeleton has bony prominences and margins that can be palpated, notable exceptions being the hip joint and the neck/shaft of femur. Many of these anatomic landmarks are used to define the extent of the lower extremity, most notably the anterior superior iliac spine, the greater trochanter, the superior margin of the medial condyle of tibia, and the medial malleolus.

Figure 2.8.
Bones of the Lower Extremity

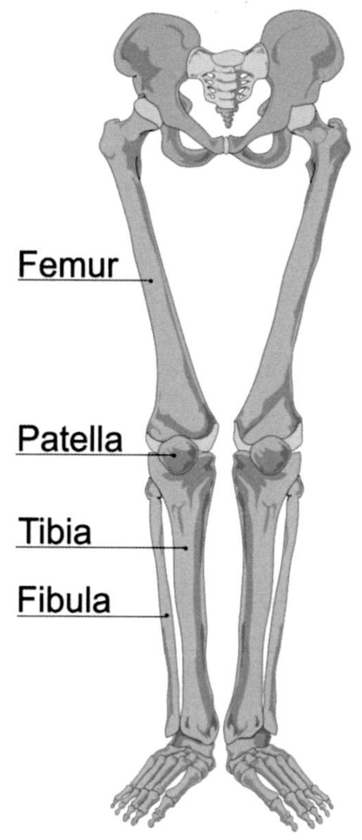

From Human Leg Bones Labeled *(public domain), 2010, http://en.wikipedia.org/w/index.php?title=File:Human_leg_bones_labeled.svg&page=1.*

Muscles of the Lower Extremity

Various muscles, highlighted in Figure 2.9, make up the lower extremity. These muscles allow an individual to stand, walk, run, jump, and kick. The lower extremities make up a significant amount of total body strength and power of mobility.

The Hip. (See Chapter 21—The Hip.) There are several ways to classify the muscles of the hip: by location or innervation, by development on the basis of their points of insertion, and by function. (See Table 2.5.) Because the area of origin and insertion of many of these muscles are very extensive, these muscles are often involved in several very different movements. Some hip muscles also function on either the knee joint or the vertebral joints. Lateral and medial rotation occurs along the axis of the limb; extension and flexion occur along a transverse axis; and abduction and adduction occur about a sagittal axis (Platzer, 2004).

Table 2.5. Major Hip Muscles

Muscle	Insertion	Action
Gluteus minimus	Greater trochanter	Hip abduction and extension
Gluteus medius	Greater trochanter	Hip abduction and rotation
Gluteus maximus	Gluteal tuberosity of the femur	Hip extension and rotation
Iliopsoas	Lesser trochanter	Hip flexion
Adducter magnus, longus and brevis	Linea aspera of femur	Hip adduction
Gracilis	Medial surface of tibia	Hip adduction
Pectineus	Line between lesser trochanter and linea aspera of femur	Hip adduction and flexion

From Core Curriculum for Orthopaedic Nursing *(4th ed., p. 488) by the National Association of Orthopaedic Nurses (NAON), 2001. Pitman, NJ: NAON. Reprinted with permission.*

The *anterior dorsal hip muscles* unite to form the iliopsoas muscle, which is inserted on the lesser trochanter of the femur (Kishner & Chowdhry, 2011).

- The psoas major originates from the last vertebra and along the lumbar spine to stretch down into the pelvis.
- The iliacus originates on the iliac fossa on the interior side of the pelvis.

The *posterior dorsal hip muscles* are inserted on or directly below the greater trochanter of the femur.

- The tensor fascia latae, stretching from the anterior posterior illiac spine down into the iliotibial tract, presses the head of the femur into the acetabulum but also flexes, rotates medially, and abducts the hip joint.
- The piriformis originates on the anterior pelvic surface of the sacrum, passes through the greater foramen, and inserts on the posterior aspect of the tip of the greater trochanter. In a standing posture, it is a lateral rotator but also assists in extending the thigh.
- The gluteus maximus begins between (and around) the iliac crest and the coccyx from where one part radiates into the iliotibial tract and the other stretches down to the gluteral tuberosity under the greater trochanter. The gluteus maximus is primarily an extensor and lateral rotator of the hip joint, and it comes into action when climbing stairs or rising from a sitting to standing posture. Furthermore, the part inserted into the fascia latae abducts and the part inserted into the gluteal tuberosity adducts the hip.

Figure 2.9.
Muscles of the Lower Extremity

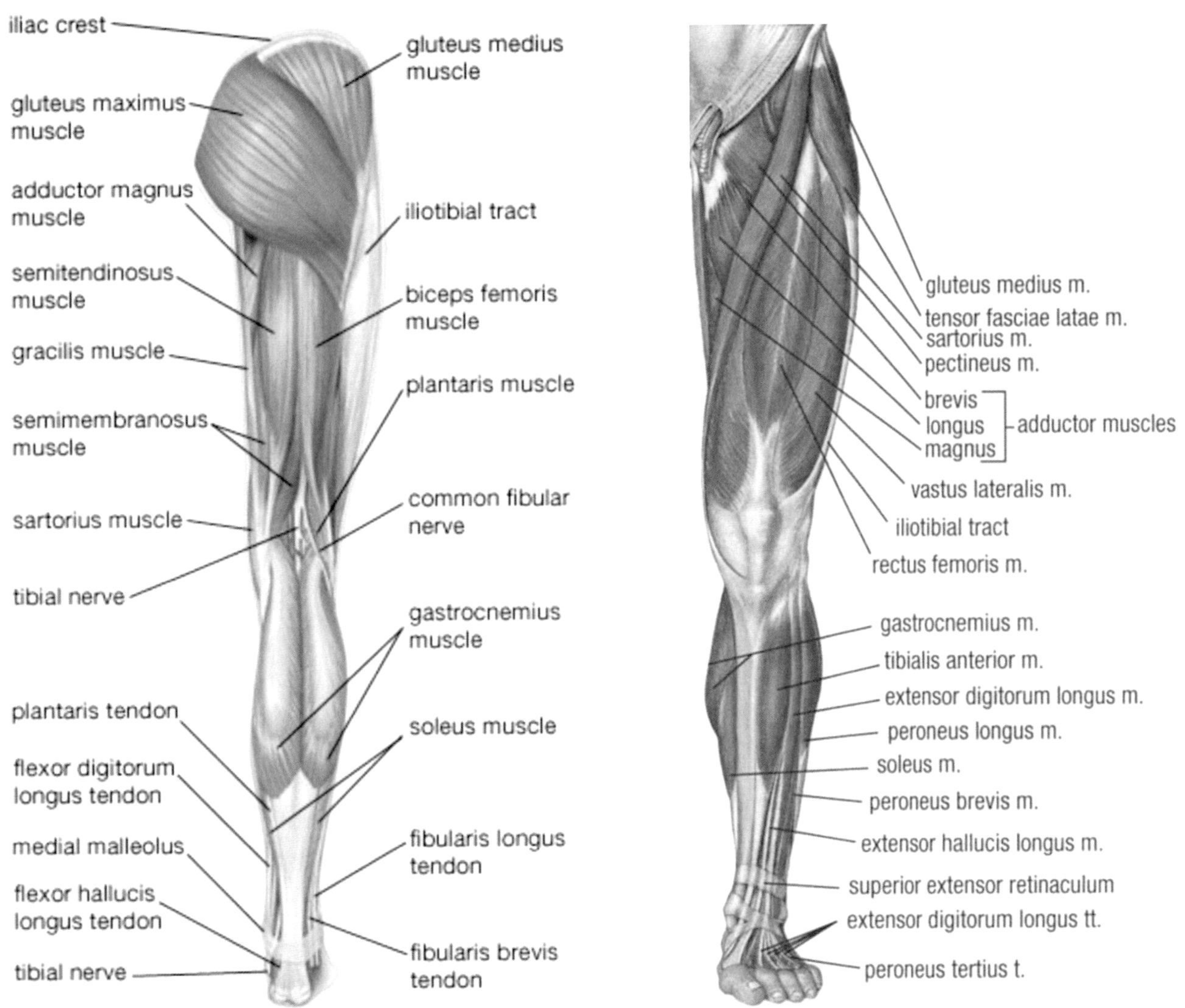

From Image Gallery: The Leg *by Encyclopedia Britannica, Inc., 2007, http://www.britannica.com/EBchecked/media/101369/Posterior-view-of-the-right-leg-showing-the-muscles-of. Reproduced with permission.*

- The two deep glutei muscles, the gluteus medius and the gluteus minimus, both originate on the lateral side of the pelvis. The medius muscle is shaped like a cap. Its anterior fibers act as a medial rotator and flexor; the posterior fibers as a lateral rotator and extensor; and the entire muscle abducts the hip. The minimus has similar functions and both muscles are inserted onto the greater trochanter (Halim, 2008a).

The *ventral hip muscles* function as lateral rotators and play an important role in the control of the body's balance. Because they are stronger than the medial rotators, in the normal position of the leg, the apex of the foot is pointing outward to achieve a better the support.

- The obturator internus originates on the pelvis on the obturator foramen and its membrane, passes through the lesser sciatic foramen, and is inserted on the trochanteric fossa of the femur. "Bent" over the lesser sciatic notch, which acts as a fulcrum, obturator internus forms the strongest lateral rotator of the hip (together with the gluteus maximus and quadratus femoris). When sitting with the knees flexed, it acts as an abductor.
- The obturator externus has a parallel course with its origin located on the posterior border of the obturator foramen. It is covered by several muscles and acts as a lateral rotator and a weak adductor.
- The inferior and superior gemelli represent marginal heads of the abturator internus and assist this muscle. The three muscles have been referred to as the triceps coxae.

- The quadratus femoris originates at the ischial tuberosity and is inserted onto the intertrochanteric crest between the trochanters. This flattened muscle acts as a strong lateral rotator and adductor of the thigh (Kishner & Chowdhry, 2011).

The *adductor muscles* of the thigh are innervated by the obturator nerve, with the exception of pectineus (that receive fibers from the femoral nerve) and the adductor magnus (that receive fibers from the tibial nerve).

- The gracilis arises from near the pubic symphysis and is unique among the adductors in that it reaches past the knee to attach on the medial side of the shaft of the tibia, thus acting on two joints. It shares its distal insertion with the sartorius and semitendinosus, all three muscles forming the pes anserinus. It is the most medial muscle of the adductors, and with the thigh abducted, its origin can be clearly seen arching under the skin. With the knee extended, it adducts the thigh and flexes the hip.
- The pectineus has its origin on the iliopubic eminence laterally to the gracilis. Rectangular in shape, it extends obliquely to attach immediately behind the lesser trochanter and down the pectineal line and the proximal part of the linea aspera on the femur. It is a flexor of the hip joint, and an adductor and a weak medial rotator of the thigh.
- The adductor brevis originates on the inferior ramus of the pubis below the gracilis and stretches obliquely below the pectineus down to the upper third of the linea aspera. Except for being an adductor, it is a lateral rotator and weak flexor of the hip joint.
- The adductor longus has its origin at superior ramus of the pubis and inserts medially on the middle third of the linea aspera. Primarily an adductor, it is also responsible for some flexion.
- The adductor magnus has its origin just behind the longus and lies deep to it. Its wide belly divides into two parts: one is inserted into the linea aspera, and the tendon of the other reaches down to adductor tubercle on the medial side of the femur's distal end to form an intermuscular septum that separates the flexors from the extensors. Magnus is a powerful adductor, especially active when crossing legs. Its superior part is a lateral rotator, but the inferior part acts as a medial rotator on the flexed leg when rotated outward and also extends the hip joint.
- The adductor minimus is an incompletely separated subdivision of the adductor magnus. Its origin forms an anterior part of the magnus and distally inserts on the linea aspera above the magnus. It acts to adduct and lateral rotate the femur (Halim, 2008a).

The Thigh. The muscles of the thigh can be classified into three groups, according to their location.

Anterior (front) muscles: Of the anterior thigh muscles, the largest are the four muscles of the quadriceps femoris. The central rectus femoris is surrounded by the three vasti: intermedius, medialis, and lateralis. Rectus femoris is attached to the pelvis with two tendons, while the vasti are inserted to the femur. All four muscles unite in a common tendon inserted into the patella, from where the patellar ligament extends it down to the tibial tuberosity. The quadriceps is the knee extensor, but the rectus femoris additionally flexes the hip joint. The articular muscle of the knee protects the articular surface of the knee joint that runs superficially and obliquely down on the anterior side of the thigh, from the anterior superior iliac spine to the pes anserinus on the medial side of the knee, from where it is further extended into the crural fascia. The sartorius acts as a flexor on both the hip and knee but, due to its oblique course, also contributes to medial rotation of the leg as one of the pes anserinus muscles (with the knee flexed) and to lateral rotation of the hip joint (Davidson, 2010).

Posterior (back) muscles: There are four posterior thigh muscles. The biceps femoris has two heads. The long head originates on the ischial tuberosity, together with the semitendinosus, and acts on two joints. The short head originates from the middle third of the linea aspera on the shaft of the femur and the lateral intermuscular septum of thigh and acts on only one joint. These two heads unite to form the biceps, which inserts on the head of the fibula.

Adductors (on the medial side): All adductors except gracilis insert on the femur and act exclusively on the hip joint, so functionally they qualify as hip muscles (Davidson, 2010). As such, they are detailed under the section "The Hip."

The majority of the thigh muscles, the "true" thigh muscles, insert on the leg (either the tibia or the fibula) and thus act primarily on the knee joint. Functionally, the extensors lie anteriorly on the thigh and are distinguished from flexors on the posterior side. Even though the sartorius flexes the knee, it is ontogenetically considered an extensor due to its secondary displacement.

The Knee. (See Chapter 22—The Knee.) The quadriceps femoris extends the knee, while the articular muscle protects the articular capsule of the knee joint during extension (Platzer, 2004). The biceps femoris flexes the knee joint and rotates the flexed leg laterally. It is the only lateral rotator of the knee and thus has to oppose all medial rotators. Additionally, the long head extends the hip joint.

The semitendiosus and the semimembranosus share their origin with the long head of the biceps femoris, and both attach on the medial side of the proximal head of the tibia together with the gracilis and sartorius to form the pes anserinus. The semitendinosus has three functions: extension of the hip, flexion of the knee, and medial rotation of the leg. Distally, the semimembranosus tendon is divided into three parts, referred to as the pes anserinus profondus. Functionally, the semimembranosus is similar to the semitendinosus and thus produces extension at the hip joint and flexion/ medial rotation at the knee.

Posteriorly below the knee joint, the popliteus stretches obliquely from the lateral femoral epicondyle down to the posterior surface of the tibia. The subpopliteal bursa is located deep to the muscle. The popliteus flexes the knee joint and medially rotates the leg (Davidson, 2010).

The Lower Leg. The lower leg is divided into the following four compartments that contain the various muscles:

1. The anterior compartment holds the tibilais anterior, the extensor digitorum longus, the extensor hallucus longus, and the peroneus tertius muscles. These muscles dorsiflex the foot and toes (pull the foot and ankle upward). The tibialis anterior also assists turning the foot inward. To feel these muscles contract, place a hand just to the outside the tibia and pull the foot up (Halim, 2008a).
2. The lateral compartment is along the outside of the lower leg. It contains the peroneus longus and peroneus brevis muscles. These muscles pull the foot outward. They also help with plantarflexion.
3. The posterior compartment holds the large muscles that are most commonly known as the calf muscles (the gastrocnemius and soleus). It also contains plantaris muscle. The gastrocnemius is shorter, thicker and has two attachments (inner and outer). It is the most visible of the calf muscles. The soleus lies underneath. These three muscles attach to the Achilles tendon. They all aid with plantarflexion (Halim, 2008a).
4. The deep posterior compartment is deep within the back of the lower leg. They are the tibialis posterior, flexor digitorum longus, and flexor hallucus longus. Tibialis posterior pulls the foot inward, flexor digitorum longus flexes the toes, and flexor hallucus longus flexes the first digit of the foot. All three aid in plantarflexion.

The Ankle & Foot

(See Chapter 23—The Foot & Ankle). The ankle enables the movements of the foot. The foot is the terminal end of the lower extremity. Together, these two complex structures combine mechanical complexity and structural strength to provide the body with the support, balance, and mobility that empower humans to stand upright and walk. Because of anatomic interdependence, an abnormality in the ankle or foot can cause orthopaedic difficulties in other parts of the body. Likewise, malfunction in other parts of the body can lead to problems in the feet (Health Communities, 1999).

Bones of the Ankle and Foot. The ankle and foot contain 26 bones. One fourth of all the bones in the human body are in found in the feet (Health Communities, 1999).

Ankle bones: The ankle comprises the true ankle and the subtalar joint (Figure 2.10). The true ankle, responsible for up and down motion of the foot, is a large joint made up of the following three bones:

1. The tibia, or shinbone, has two bony protrusions at its base. The medial malleolus is on the inside of the ankle, and the posterior malleolus is on the back of the ankle.
2. The fibula, or rear calf bone, is the thinner bone running alongside the tibia. The lateral malleolus, the bony protrusion on the outside of the ankle, is the low end of the fibula.
3. The talus, or ankle bone, is the bone that fits into the socket formed by the tibia and fibula, above the heel bone (WebMD, 2012).

The subtalar joint, which allows side-to-side motion of the foot, consists of the talus on top and calcaneus (heel bone) on the bottom (Southern California Orthopedic Institute, 2012).

Figure 2.10.
Ankle Anatomy

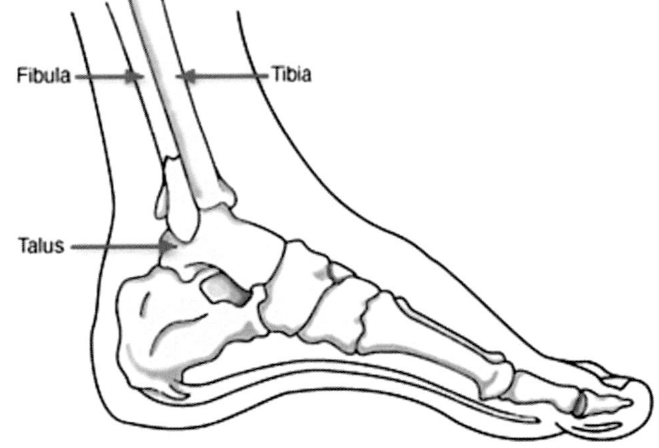

From "Ankle Fractures" by the American Academy of Orthopaedic Surgeons (AAOS), 2007, OrthoInfo, http://orthoinfo.aaos.org/topic.cfm?topic=a00391. Reproduced with permission.

Foot bones. The foot is made up of 26 bones (Figure 2.11 and Figure 2.12) in the following classifications:

- Calcaneus (or heel bone): The bone under the talus and behind the cuboid.
- Cuboid: The bone adjacent to the cuneiforms on the outside of the foot.
- Cuneiforms: The three bones in the middle of the foot, toward the center of the body.
- Metatarsals: The bones in the middle of the foot.
- Navicular: The bone behind the cuneiforms.
- Phalanges: The bones in the toes.
- Talus (or ankle bone): The bone directly behind the navicular bone (Merriam-Webster, n.d.)

Figure 2.11.
The Foot: Anterior and Posterior Views

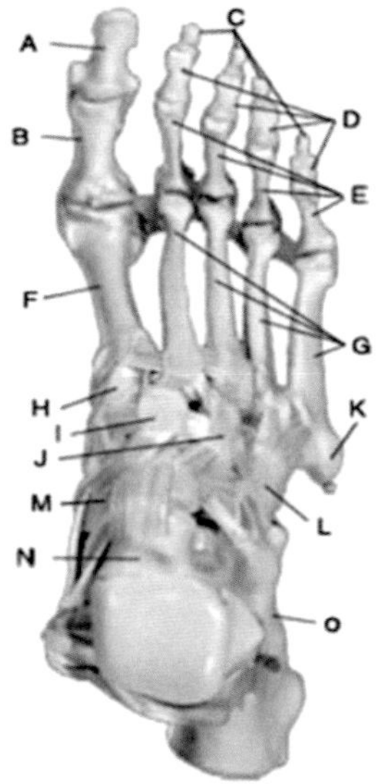

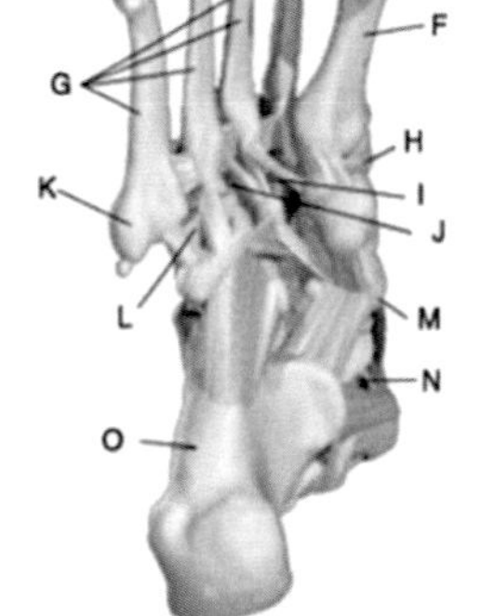

A. distal phalanx of the hallux
B. proximal phalanx of the hallux
C. distal phalanges
D. intermediate phalanges
E. proximal phalanges
F. 1st metatarsal
G. lesser metatarsals
H. medial cuneiform
I. intermediate cuneiform
J. lateral cuneiform
K. styloid process
L. cuboid
M. navicular
N. talus
O. calcaneus

From Foot and Ankle Anatomy *by Northcoast Footcare, 2011, https://www.northcoastfootcare.com/pages/Foot-and-Ankle-Anatomy.html. Reproduced with permission.*

Muscles of the Ankle and Foot. *Ankle muscles:* Movement of the ankle and foot is enabled through the stronger muscles in the lower leg, whose tendons pass by the ankle and connect in the foot. Contraction of the muscles in the lower extremity is the main way to attain movement in the ankle and foot.

The key ankle muscles (detailed in the section on "Muscles of the Lower Extremity—The Lower Leg") and their actions include the following:

- The peroneals (peroneus longus and peroneus brevis) bend the ankle down and out.
- The calf muscles (gastrocnemius and soleus) bend the ankle down when the calf muscles tighten.
- The tibialis posterior supports the arch and helps turn the foot inward.
- The tibialis anterior pulls the ankle upward (Orthopod, n.d.).

Figure 2.12.
Bones of the Foot

Phalanges distales (3)
Phalanges mediae (2)
Phalanges proximales (1)
Metatarsalia
Ossa tarsi

1. Talus
2. Calcaneus
3. Os naviculare
4. Os cuneiforme I
5. Os cuneiforme II
6. Os cuneiforme III
7. Os cuboideum

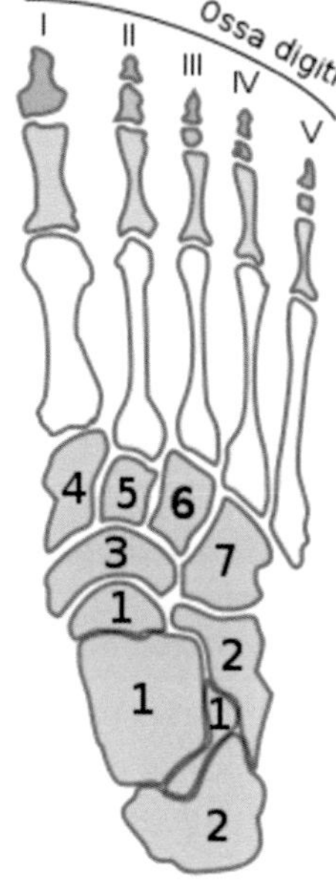

From Ospied *by U. Gille, 2010, http://en.wikipedia.org/wiki/File:Ospied-de.svg. Reproduced with permission.*

Foot muscles: There are 20 muscles in the foot that hold the bones in position enable movement by expanding and contracting. The lower extremity muscles that act on the foot are called the extrinsic foot muscles, while the muscles located in the foot itself are called the intrinsic foot muscles. Smaller muscles enable the toes to lift and curl. The main muscles of the foot are classified with the following motions:

- The anterior tibial muscle enables upward movement.
- The posterior tibial muscle supports the arch.
- The peroneal tibial muscle controls movement on the outside of the ankle.
- The extensors help the ankle raise the toes when stepping.
- The flexors stabilize the toes against the ground (Health Communities, 2000).

Ligaments and Tendons of the Ankle & Foot. Ligaments are the strong fibrous bands that connect the bones of ankle and foot. They are often susceptible to injury due to the excessive movement of the subtalar joint during activity (Inverarity, 2008). Tendons are the elastic tissues that connect the muscles in the ankle and foot to their bones and joints. Tendons in the ankle and foot function together to move the ankle and the toes.

Ligaments: Numerous ligaments surround the true ankle and subtalar joints, binding the bones of the leg to each other and to those of the foot (WebMd, 2012). The ankle ligaments can be divided into the medial ligaments and the lateral ligaments.

Figure 2.13.
Ligaments of the Ankle (Lateral Aspect)

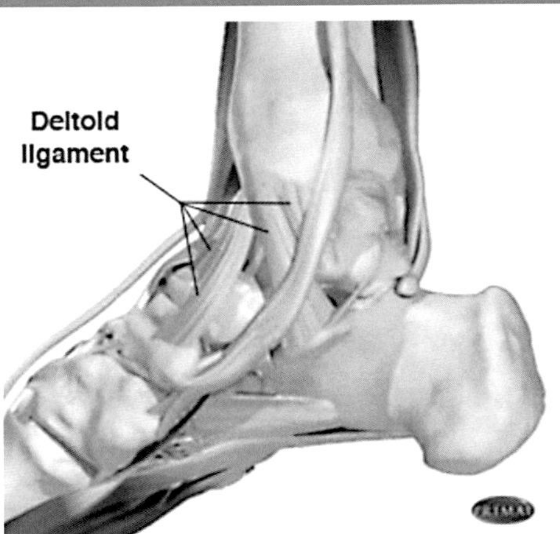

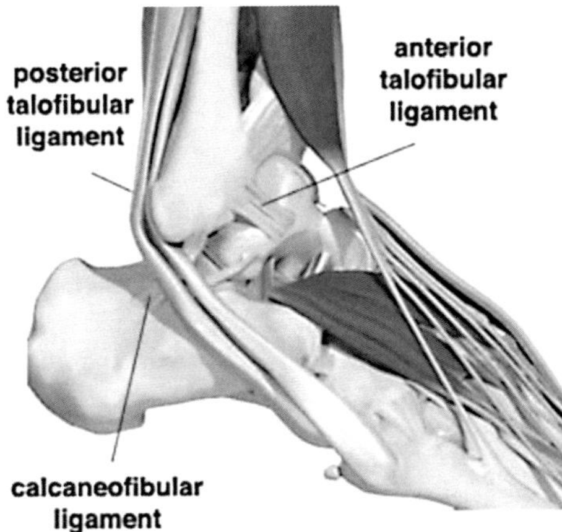

From Foot and Ankle Anatomy *by Northcoast Footcare, 2011, https://www.northcoastfootcare.com/pages/Foot-and-Ankle-Anatomy.html. Reproduced with permission.*

The deltoid ligament supports the *medial aspect of the ankle joint.* It is attached at the medial malleolus of the tibia and connects in four places to the sustentaculum tali of the calcaneus, the calcaneonavicular ligament, the navicular tuberosity, and the medial surface of the talus. The deltoid ligament is actually four separate ligaments: the osterior tibiotalar ligament, the tibiocalcaneal ligament, the tibionavicular ligament, and the anterior tibiotalar ligament.

Three ligaments (anterior talofibular ligament, posterior talofibular ligament, and calcaneofibular ligament) support the *lateral aspect of the ankle joint* (Figure 2.13). The anterior and posterior talofibular ligaments support the lateral side of the joint from the lateral malleolus of the fibula to the dorsal and ventral ends of the talus. The posterior talofibular ligament sits under the peroneal tendons. It attaches to the fibula on one end and the talus on the other, extending to the posterior ankle. The calcaneofibular ligament originates at the lateral malleolus and runs to the lateral surface of the calcaneus (Golanó et al., 2010). The lateral ankle ligaments are most commonly damaged in ankle sprains (Panchbhav, 2011).

The plantar fascia is a long ligament that works with the posterior tibial tendon to support the longitudinal arch when walking (Halim, 2008a). Figure 2.14 shows the three bands: medial, central, and lateral.

Figure 2.14.
Plantar Fascia

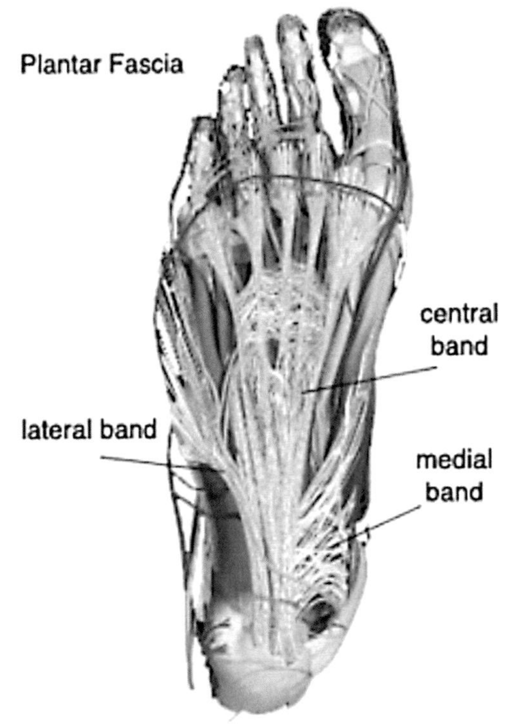

From Foot and Ankle Anatomy *by Northcoast Footcare, 2011, https://www.northcoastfootcare.com/pages/Foot-and-Ankle-Anatomy.html. Reproduced with permission.*

The ligaments in the foot include the Lisfranc, the intermetatarsals, and the joint capsule of the great toe. Lisfranc ligaments are very strong stabilizers for the small bones of the mid-foot and the transverse tarsal joint. The intermetatarsal ligaments, between the bones at the base of the toes, connect the neck of each metatarsal to the adjacent one and bind them together for fluid metatarsal motion. The joint capsule of the great toe, running from the inner portion of the first metatarsal head to the distal phalanx, stabilizes the great toe on the inside (Foot Education, 2009).

Tendons: Figure 2.15 illustrates the main ankle and foot tendons on the lateral side. The two peroneal tendons are responsible for flexing the foot down and rotating the foot outward. Both function to evert and plantar flex the foot and stabilize the arch when walking. The peroneal longus courses under the foot and attaches on the inside of the arch. The peroneal brevis attaches to the styloid process (see "K" in Figure 2.11) and is the more powerful everter of the two.

Figure 2.15.
Tendons of the Ankle (Lateral Aspect)

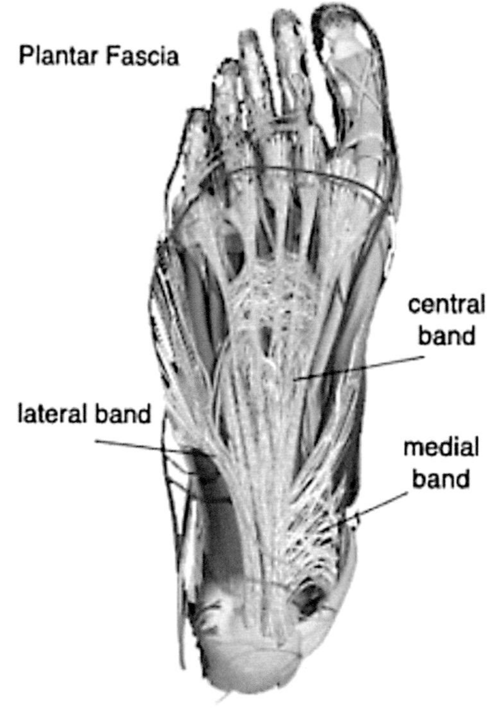

From Foot and Ankle Anatomy *by Northcoast Footcare, 2011, https://www.northcoastfootcare.com/pages/Foot-and-Ankle-Anatomy.html. Reproduced with permission.*

The extensor and flexor tendons (Figure 2.16) flex the ankle and move the toes. The extensors are the main tendons on the top of the foot that elevate the toes (dorsiflexion), while the flexors pulling the toes down (plantarflexion) (Halim, 2008a; Northcoast Footcare, 2011).

The Achilles tendon (Figure 2.17) plantarflexes the foot to bring it down and assist in "push-off" when walking. The Achilles tendon is the largest and strongest tendon in the body. It extends from the calf muscle all the way to the heel (Health Communities, 2000).

Figure 2.16.
Extensor and Flexor Tendons of the Foot

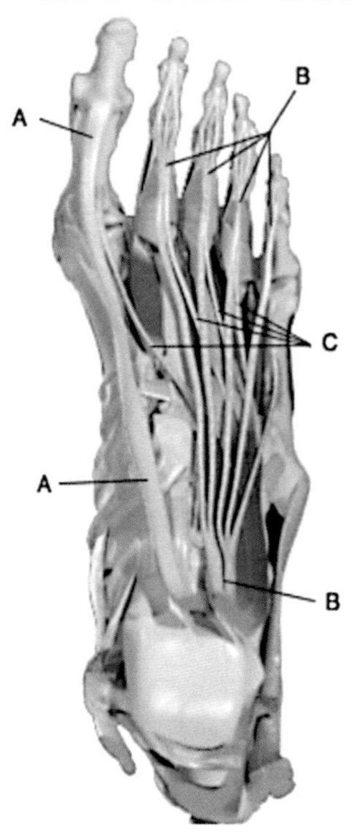

A. Extensor hallucis longus: dorsiflexes the great toe and foot
B. Extensor digitorum longus: dorsiflexes the small toes foot.
C. Extensor digitorum brevis: dorsiflexes the small toes.

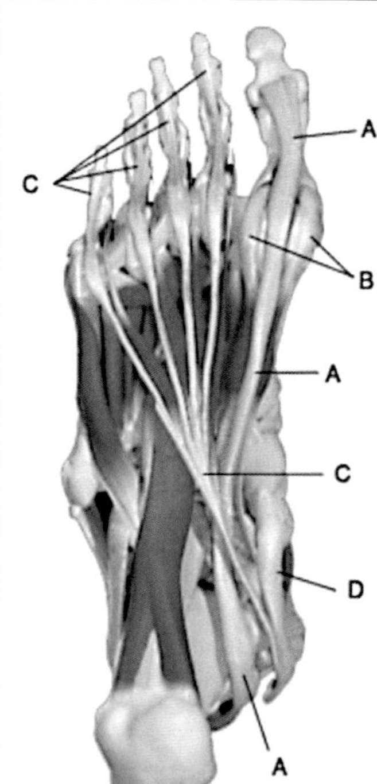

A. Flexor hallucis longus: plantarflexes the great toe and foot.
B. Flexor hallucis brevis: plantarflexes the great toe.
C. Flexor digitorum longus: plantarflexes the toes and the foot.
D. Posterior tibialis: inverts and plantarflexes the foot.

From Foot and Ankle Anatomy *by Northcoast Footcare, 2011, https://www.northcoastfootcare.com/pages/Foot-and-Ankle-Anatomy.html. Reproduced with permission.*

The posterior tibial tendon (Figure 2.18) originates in the back of the leg and courses around the inside of the ankle to attach on the inside and bottom of the arch. The main attachment is on the navicular, a tarsal bone in the midfoot, labeled in the image on the right, but the tendon extends across the base of the foot (Panchbhav, 2011).

Figure 2.17. Achilles Tendon

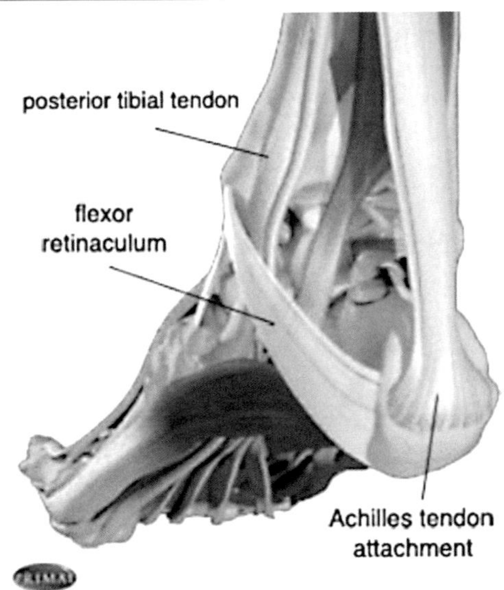

From Foot and Ankle Anatomy *by Northcoast Footcare, 2011, https://www.northcoastfootcare.com/pages/Foot-and-Ankle-Anatomy.html. Reproduced with permission.*

Figure 2.18. Posterior Tibial Tendon

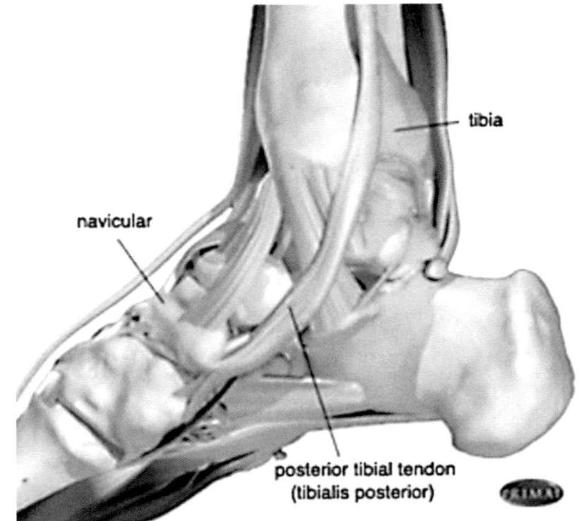

From Foot and Ankle Anatomy *by Northcoast Footcare, 2011, https://www.northcoastfootcare.com/pages/Foot-and-Ankle-Anatomy.html. Reproduced with permission.*

Summary

In order to successfully care for orthopaedic patients, the nurse must have a complete comprehension of the basics of orthopaedic anatomy and physiology. A thorough understanding of anatomy and physiology – along with the knowledge of the proper terminology – is critical for quality assessment, evaluation, and patient treatment manner. In addition, use of appropriate terminology is necessary for communication among care providers. Understanding orthopaedic anatomy and physiology will assist the nurse in developing expertise in caring for patients with a variety of orthopaedic conditions.

References

Abe, E., Sun, L., Mechanick, J., Iqbal, J.,Yamoah, Baliram, R.,… Zaidi, M. (2007). Bone loss in thyroid disease: Role of low TSH and high thyroid hormone. *Annals of the New York Academy of Science, 1116*, 383–391.

American Academy of Orthopaedic Surgeons (AAOS). (2007a). Ankle fractures. *OrthoInfo*. Retrieved December 2012 from http://orthoinfo.aaos.org/topic.cfm?topic=a00391

American Academy of Orthopaedic Surgeons (AAOS). (2007b). Shoulder trauma. *OrthoInfo*. Retrieved October 2012 from http://orthoinfo.aaos.org/topic.cfm?topic=A00394

Bradford, P.G., Gerace, K.V., Roland, R.L., & Chrzan, B.G. (2010). Estrogen regulation of apoptosis in osteoblasts. *Physiology Behavior, 99*(2), 181-5.

Cassiopia,V. (2003). *What Is the Frankfurt Plane?* Retrieved December 2012 from http://www.wisegeek.com/what-is-the-frankfurt-plane.htm

Clarke, B. (2008). Normal bone anatomy and physiology. *Clinical Journal of the American Society of Nephrology, 3*, S131-139. doi:10.2215/CJN.04151206

Davenport, S.G. (2006). *Anatomy and Physiology Text and Laboratory Workbook.* San Antonio: Link Publishing.

Davidson, G. (Ed). (2010). *Gray's Anatomy: With Original Illustrations by Henry Carter.* London: Arcturus.

Encyclopedia Britannica, Inc. (2007). *The Leg.* Retrieved from http://www.britannica.com/EBchecked/media/101369/Posterior-view-of-the-right-leg-showing-the-muscles-of

Encyclopedia Britannica, Inc. (2008.) *The Arm.* Retrieved from http://media-1.web.britannica.com/eb-media/37/113037-004-D4CF5BB4.jpg

Foot Education. (2009). *Ligaments of the Foot and Ankle Overview.* Retrieved October 2012 from http://www.footeducation.com/ligaments-of-foot-and-ankle-overview

Gille, U. (2010). *Ospied.* Retrieved from http://en.wikipedia.org/wiki/File:Ospied-de.svg

Gilroy, A.M., Macpherson, B.R., & Ross, L.M. (2008). *Atlas of Anatomy.* New York: Thieme Publishing.

Golanó, P.,Vega, J., de Leeuw, P., Malagelada, F., Manzanares, C., Götzens,V., & van Dijk, C. (2010, May). Anatomy of the ankle ligaments: A pictorial essay. *Knee Surgery, Sports Traumatology, Arthroscopy, 18*(5), 557–569. doi: 10.1007/s00167-010-1100-x

Gosling, J.A., Harris, P.F., Humpherson, J.R., Whitmore, I., & Willan, P.L. (2008). *Human Anatomy, Color Atlas and Textbook.* St. Louis, MO: Mosby.

Halim, A. (2008a). *Human Anatomy: Regional and Clinical Abdomen and Lower Limb.* New Delhi: I.K. International Publishing House.

Halim, A. (2008b). *Human Anatomy: Upper Limb and Thorax.* New Delhi: I.K. International Publishing House.

Halim, A. (2009). *Human Anatomy: Female Pelvis and Breast.* New Delhi: I.K. International Publishing House.

Hall, J.E. (2012). *Pocket Companion to Guyton and Hall Textbook of Medical Physiology.* Philadelphia: Elsevier Saunders.

Health Communities. (1999). *Anatomy of the Foot and Ankle.* Retrieved October 2012 from http://www.healthcommunities.com/foot-anatomy/foot-anatomy-overview.shtml

Health Communities. (2000). *Muscles, Tendons & Ligaments of the Foot & Ankle.* Retrieved October 2012 from http://www.healthcommunities.com/foot-anatomy/muscles-tendons-ligaments.shtml

Inverarity, L. (2008). *Ligaments of the Ankle Joint.* Retrieved October 2012 from http://physicaltherapy.about.com/od/humananatomy/p/ankleligaments.htm

Kiesler, J. & Ricer, K. (2003). The abnormal fontanel. *American Family Physician, 67*(12), 2547-52.

Kishner, S. & Chowdhry, M. (2011). *Hip Joint Anatomy.* Retrieved October 2012 from http://emedicine.medscape.com/article/1898964-overview

Kishner, S., Moradian, M., & Morello, J. (2011). *Lumbar Spine Anatomy.* Retrieved October 2012 from http://emedicine.medscape.com/article/1899031-overview

Kishner, S., Munshi, S., & Black, J. (2011). *Shoulder Joint Anatomy.* Retrieved October 2012 from http://emedicine.medscape.com/article/1899211-overview

Lindsay, R., Nieves, J., Formica, C., Henneman, E., Woelfert, L., Shen, V.,…Cosman, F. (1997.) Randomized controlled study of effects of parathyroid hormone on vertebral-bone mass and fracture incidence among postmenopausal women on oestrogen with osteoporosis. *The Lancet, 350,* 550-5.

Mazurek, M.T. & Shin, A.Y. (2001). Upper extremity peripheral nerve anatomy: Current concepts and applications. *Clinical Orthopaedics and Related Research, 383,* 7-20.

Meczekalski, B., Podfigurna-Stopa, A., & Genazzani, R. (2010). Hypoestrogenism in young women and its influence on bone mass density. *Gynecological Endocrinology, 26*(9), 652-657.

Medicine.Net. (n.d.). *Definition of Leg.* Retrieved from http://www.medterms.com/script/main/art.asp?articlekey=8739

Merriam-Webster Visual Dictionary Online. (n.d.). *The Foot.* Retrieved October 2012 from http://visual.merriam-webster.com/human-being/anatomy/skeleton/foot.php

Mount Sinai School of Medicine. (2011). *Pituitary Hormone TSH Found to Directly Influence Bone Growth.* Retrieved October 2012 from http://www.mssm.edu/about-us/news-and-events/pituitary-hormone-tsh-found-to-directly-influence-bone-growth

National Institute of Arthritis and Musculoskeletal and Skin Diseases (NIAMS). (2010). *Shoulder Problems.* Retrieved October 2012 from http://www.niams.nih.gov/Health_Info/Shoulder_Problems/shoulder_problems_ff.asp

Northcoast Footcare. (2011). *Anatomy: Foot and Ankle Tendons and Ligaments.* Retrieved October 2012 from http://www.northcoastfootcare.com/pages/Anatomy-Foot-and-Ankle-Tendons-and-Ligaments-.html

Orthopod. (n.d.). *A Patient's Guide to Ankle Anatomy.* Retrieved October 2012 from http://www.eorthopod.com/content/ankle-anatomy

Panchbhavi, V.K., (2011). Foot bone anatomy. *Medscape Reference.* Retrieved October 2012 from http://emedicine.medscape.com/article/1922965-overview

Phillips, B. & Schmidt, S. (2011). Wrist anatomy. *Medscape Reference.* Retrieved October 2012 http://emedicine.medscape.com/article/1899456-overview

Platzer, W. (2004). *Color Atlas of Human Anatomy, Vol. 1: Locomotor System* (5th ed.). New York: Thieme.

Southern California Orthopedic Institute. (2012). *Anatomy of the Ankle.* Retrieved October 2012 from http://www.scoi.com/ankle.php

Tank, P.W. (2009). *Nerves of the Upper Limb—Listed Alphabetically.* Retrieved October 2012 from http://anatomy.uams.edu/anatomyhtml/nerves_upperlimb.html

WebMD. (2012). *Fitness & Exercise: The Ankle.* Retrieved October 2012 from http://www.webmd.com/fitness-exercise/picture-of-the-ankle

Wilhelmi, B., Marrero, I., & Sahin, B. (2011). Hand anatomy. *Medscape Reference.* Retrieved October 2012 from http://emedicine.medscape.com/article/1285060-overview

Windsor, R.E., Malanga, G.A., Petre, B.M., Chawla, J. Goodrich, J.A, & Khan, A.N. (2011). Cervical spine anatomy. *Medscape Reference.* Retrieved October 2012 from http://emedicine.medscape.com/article/1948797-overview

YassineMrabet. (2008). *Human Anatomy Planes.* Retrieved from http://en.wikipedia.org/wiki/File:Human_anatomy_planes.svg

Chapter 3
Musculoskeletal Assessment

Debra M. Palmer, DNP, FNP-BC, ONP-C

Objectives

- Appropriately use terms used in describing musculoskeletal anatomy and assessment.
- Identify key questions to ask when taking a health history related to musculoskeletal injury or condition.
- Describe four key components of the musculoskeletal physical examination.
- Identify measurement tools used in performing a musculoskeletal physical examination.
- Document measurements of objective physical findings using a grading scale.
- Describe elements of the sensory exam that are included in the musculoskeletal physical assessment.
- Identify symptoms associated with abnormal gaits.
- Describe age-related variations in risks for bone, muscle, and tendon injury.
- Identify conditions recognized as contraindications for participation in contact sports.

The musculoskeletal assessment forms the basis for an individualized evaluation and intervention plan, which is readily documented in a consistent format for individuals with musculoskeletal complaints. A thorough understanding of anatomic structures, physiologic function, and changes through the life span forms the basis of an accurate physical assessment. (See Chapter 2—Anatomy & Physiology for background knowledge to support the musculoskeletal assessment.) Competence in the art of history-taking and physical assessment techniques contributes to the collection of pertinent data that are measured and described using specific descriptive terms, measurement tools, and tests unique to the orthopaedic examination. Table 3.1 includes definitions of key terms used in orthopaedics to assist in effective musculoskeletal assessment.

Table 3.1. Musculoskeletal Terminology
Abduction: motion in which a body part moves away from a defined line, for example, the midline of the body.
Adduction: motion in which a body part moves toward a defined line.
Ankylosis: abnormal fusion, immobility of a joint due to pathological changes; may occur if a joint is surgically fused.
Atrophy: deterioration, wasting, or degeneration of tissue.
Cardinal frontal: the plane that divides the body into front and back segments.
Cardinal horizontal: the plane that divides the body into top and bottom segments.
Cardinal sagittal: the plane that divides the body into left and right sides.
Causalgia: severe burning pain related to paresthesia or partial injury of peripheral nerves.
Circumduction: swinging motion or movement, abduction, adduction, flexion and extension totaling 360 degrees or a full circle of motion; this motion is seen in the shoulder, hip, and ankle.
Contracture: abnormal shortening or contraction of soft tissue and muscles surrounding a joint.
Coxa vara: deformity of hip associated with a decrease in the angle of the femoral neck.
Deformity: malformation or defect of any part of the body.
Dislocation: displacement of joint surfaces altering alignment, caused by traumatic injury, congenital defect, or pathology (disease, infection, or inflammation).
Dorsiflexion: movement of a body part up toward the dorsum as when the ankle moves to point the toes toward the head.
Dysplasia: abnormal development of tissue.
Eversion: turning outward of the foot and ankle.
Extension: motion involving an increase in the angle of a joint between two bones; pulling or extending.
External rotation: the rotating of a joint outward.
Flexion: motion involving a decrease in the angle of a joint between two bones; bending or contracting.
Gait: a definite pattern or style of achieving upright bipedal locomotion.
Goniometer: instrument used for measuring joint movement and angle.
Hallux valgus: lateral deviation of the great toe toward the second toe.
Hyperextension: excessive extension of a joint.
Internal rotation: rotating motion of a joint inward.
Inversion: turning inward of the foot and ankle.
Kyphosis (round back): excessive angulation, curvature, or convexity of the thoracic spine due to disease (osteoporosis, arthritis, rickets) or other pathological conditions.
Lateral: the area toward the outer aspect of the body away from the midline.
Leg-length discrepancy: inequality in the length of legs genetically or iatrogenetically induced.
Lordosis: concavity of the vertebral column; a normal curvature existing in cervical and lumbar areas, which may become pathologic if accentuated.
Medial: area nearest the midline of the body.
Midsagittal: divides the body in the cardinal sagittal plane.
Palmar flexion: motion of the wrist moving the hand down.
Palsy: inability to move a part as in paralysis.
Passive movement: any body movement that occurs without muscle contraction.
Plantar flexion (equinus): motion of the ankle moving the foot downward.
Pronation: motion of the forearm characterized by the palm down or movement toward the posterior of the body in the anatomic position.
Range of motion: the full motion a joint can move.
Recurvatum: hyperextension of the joint as in the knee or genu recurvatum.
Relaxation: stage during which the force of contraction is diminishing to inactivity.
Rotation: motion that involves turning on an axis in a circular movement.
Scoliosis: lateral curvature of the spine.
Subluxation: a sideways force causing splitting, shifting, or displacement, with partial or incomplete dislocation of the joint surfaces.

From Core Currriculum for Orthopaedic Nursing (6th ed., p. 40) by National Association of Orthopaedic Nurses (NAON), 2007, Boston, MA: Pearson. Reproduced with permission.

Health History

Obtaining the health history serves several purposes and usually precedes questions related to the review of systems, ordering of tests and performance of the physical examination. In addition to gathering information necessary to evaluate and treat the patient, the health history process establishes rapport with the patient; triages for conditions requiring immediate medical referral; and determines the patient's goals, preferences, and expectations. Information related to the patient health history can be obtained from multiple sources, including interviews with family members and significant others, review of past and current medical records, consultations with other care providers, and results of diagnostic studies (provided necessary permission has been obtained).

The value of a thorough patient history cannot be overstated, as approximately 80% of the information necessary to diagnose the presenting problem is obtained in history-taking (Dutton, 2008). This underscores the inherent value in identifying and eliminating potential barriers to a successful interview and a complete collection of objective and subjective data. Potential barriers include the patient's lack of language access, hearing or vision limitations, decreased mental capacity, or increased level of confusion, as well as misunderstandings and misperceptions secondary to cultural differences. In addition, it is necessary for the nurse to identify his or her own barriers to successful communication with the patient.

The patient history should be documented in a consistent and systematic fashion to avoid exclusion of necessary components of the history and to form a baseline for future evaluations of the presenting problem and response to treatment. Information generated from the patient history includes any or all of the information outlined in Table 3.2 as is pertinent to the individual patient and presenting complaint. Questioning should start open-ended and proceed with more specific closed-ended questions to guide the interview in a timely and relevant fashion. Nonverbal communication and the use of silence, confirmation, clarification, and reflection are all essential components to the interviewing process.

Table 3.2. Review of History Questions

OLD CART	
O	Onset of complaint
L	Location of symptoms
D	Duration of symptoms
C	Characteristics of the symptoms
A	Aggravating factors
R	Relieving factors
T	Treatment tried and timing of symptoms

Data from Orthopedic Physical Assessment *(5th ed., p. 29) by D. J. Magee, 2008, St. Louis, MO: Saunders Elsevier. Reproduced with permission.*

Components of the Health History

The general line of questioning in the patient interview begins with demographic data and the patient's primary reason for being seen, or "chief complaint" (CC). The patient's age and CC provides a high index of suspicion to the experienced clinician regarding likely diagnostic probabilities, which guides the line of questioning in the interview (Dutton, 2008). After the demographics and CC are established, the interviewer should collect a history of the present illness, past health history (medical, surgical, and psychosocial health), current lifestyle, family and social history, and a review of systems.

Chief Complaint (CC). Ascertain, in the patient's own words, their reason for seeking medical attention. Typical musculoskeletal complaints include pain, loss of function, joint instability or stiffness, loss of sensation, or a newly discovered deformity. The degree or severity of the problem, as perceived by the patient, should also be determined, especially as it affects the patient's activities of daily living (ADLs) and employment.

History of Present Illness (HPI). The pneumonic OLD CART (Table 3.2) can be used in directing questions related to the HPI, including the patient's usual state of physical, mental, and social health leading up to the CC. The CC should be evaluated as acute or chronic in nature. Knowing the onset of the injury, illness, or abnormal finding aids in defining the presentation as an acute or chronic condition. An acute condition alerts the provider to a different set of differential diagnoses than a chronic condition, which in turn influences the urgency and focus of the physical examination. Acute conditions involving trauma are suggestive of a fracture, dislocation, or rupture of tissue, which prompt a different line of questioning and testing than a chronic condition. Additionally, symptoms of chronic pain or dysfunction suggest an entirely different cause as compared to an acute injury or trauma. In addition to ascertaining the timing of a musculoskeletal injury, it is necessary to determine the mechanism of an injury for clues to the severity and type of injury.

When determining the mechanism of injury, inquire about forces that contributed to the injury (such as twisting or blunt force) and whether the injury was the result of a standing height fall or fall from a significant height. This information provides clues to the propensity for a fracture to be related to osteoporosis. For example, an ankle injury that occurs from a trip and fall versus a fall from 200 feet will have fewer concerns for adjacent spine trauma and or severe fractures. A shoulder injury sustained from blunt trauma in a high-speed motor vehicle accident would be more suspect for additional chest wall trauma than a shoulder injury occurring spontaneously while batting a ball. An injury that occurs as a result of violence or abuse must be documented as such and reported to the appropriate law enforcement authorities.

The time at which pain occurs may provide insight into possible diagnosis. Pain that worsens throughout the day with increased use of the affected joint is typical of osteoarthritis, whereas pain and stiffness that lessen throughout the day with increased use and/or exercise are commonly seen with Rheumatoid arthritis (RA) (see Chapter 13—Arthritis & Connective Tissue Disorders). Inquire about additional symptoms associated with the onset of the condition. Associated symptoms that may help guide a diagnosis may include the presence of swelling, hematoma, a wound, fever, or rash.

The location or distribution of pain provides clues that assist in formulating a diagnosis. Migratory joint pain that starts in one joint, improves, and moves to another joint, is typical for Rheumatoid pain, which tends to be symmetrical and starts in small peripheral joints. Pain associated with psoriatic arthritis, Rieter's syndrome, and gout becomes polyarticular in the late stages, presenting initially in one or two joints. Spondylitis presents first in the spine and moves to peripheral joints. The location of pain is best determined by directing the patient to point with one finger to the point of maximal tenderness. The intensity of pain should be graded on a scale from one to ten, with ten being the worst pain imaginable (Child, 2007). It is useful to ask the patient to document the location and severity of pain on a diagram. This initial pain documentation by the patient establishes a baseline for future response to treatment. The presence or absence of nocturnal pain should be included in the pain assessment.

The duration of symptoms is best described in specific measurements of time (minutes, day, months, or years). Symptom characteristics include descriptions of pain; encourage descriptive terms such as "stabbing," "burning," "throbbing," or "disabling." Pain resulting from nerve pathology includes numbness, tingling, radiating, electric shock sensation, or the feeling of "pins and needles." Pain originating in muscle tissue is often described as "pulled muscle," "charley horse," or "spasm." Descriptions of joint pain include "dull ache," "stiff," or "excruciating."

Aggravating or precipitating factors include but are not limited to movement, weight-bearing, or positioning; weather; time of day; stress; insomnia; and the intake of food, medications, or alcohol. Relieving factors are activities or conditions that relieve the symptoms, commonly including rest or sleep, assistive devices such as a cane or splint, and prescribed or over-the-counter (OTC) medications.

Treatment(s) that the patient has already tried—and their effect on symptom relief—should also be documented, along with length of time of treatment. Note the use of treatments such as medication, resting the affected limb with ambulatory aids or splints, elevation of the extremity, and adjunctive therapies (such as physical therapy, chiropractic care, electrical stimulation, massage, or surgical intervention).

Past Medical and Surgical History (PMH). The PMH is often related to the CC and is therefore included in the health history. The PMH can be obtained using a standard questionnaire followed by clarification/confirmation of responses. The PMH provides information with regards to allergies, immunizations, childhood illnesses, and congenital anomalies. In addition, prior episodes of illness, injury, or trauma and their respective treatments, surgeries, or hospitalizations are also included. Successive onset of symptoms in the past, which are similar to the current complaint, should be identified as a likely reoccurring injury or infection. If the current problem is related to a prior surgery, details related to surgical complications (such as malignant hyperthermia or hemorrhage) and postoperative protocol should be obtained through patient questioning and/or review of surgical records (Dutton, 2008).

Current Health Status (CHS). The key information related to CHS includes the patient's use of substances, occupational situation, exercise, sleep, and dietary habits. The CHS should also document the patient's hand dominance. The use of substances includes tobacco, alcohol, OTC and/or prescribed medications, and recreational drugs. Specifics related to the use of substances include type of product used, quantity, frequency of use, length of time used, and when the substance was last taken. Exercise habits include type, frequency, duration, and last time attempted. Sleep history includes the usual number of hours of sleep obtained nightly and use of sleep aids. Dietary habits include diet restrictions, intentional or unintended weight loss or gain, a 24-hour dietary recall, and use of dietary supplements such as vitamin D and calcium.

Family History (FH). FH provides clues about a patient's propensity of inheriting a familial disease. Many neurologic and orthopaedic problems can be traced to family members (Cipriano, 2003). Critical data include the age and health of parents, siblings, grandparents, and children. Major health problems or genetic disorders in the family unit should be included

Social/Occupational History (SH). SH includes factors that influence lifestyle. Social and occupational histories are important as they may lead to factors contributing to the patient's problem, such as overuse syndrome. Occupational history can be described as sedentary or physically demanding and includes the type of physical labor performed and number of years worked. If the patient is disabled, determine the reason for disability and number of years disabled. Information related to living arrangements, mode of transportation, presence of a significant other or family support system, religious affiliations, and ability to continue participation in desired activities is critical in planning the care and treatment of the patient with a musculoskeletal illness or injury (Dutton, 2008).

Review of Systems (ROS). The physiologic systems include the respiratory, cardiovascular, gastrointestinal, neurological, reproductive, musculoskeletal, endocrine, immune, and genitourinary systems. An orderly review of subjective symptoms in each physiologic system is necessary when assessing the patient's overall health in the context of the CC. The presence of a disease process can be gleaned through specific questioning of symptoms related to each system.

Physical Exam Techniques of the Musculoskeletal System

The technique of the physical examination (PE) includes the objective determination and documentation of physical findings in the context of the health history. The accuracy of the PE findings is dependent on the skill of the examiner, as well as reliability and validity of the examination tests included in the assessment (Chou, 2006). The PE, and the examiner's sense of urgency in completing it, is guided by the CC and pertinent information obtained in the history. According to Child (2007), the history should include the mechanism of the injury. The physical findings should be consistent with the stated mechanism of injury. When there is disparity between the history and physical findings, further questioning should assess for possible violence/abuse or other underlying pathology such as osteogenesis imperfecti, absence of pain receptors, or psychological disorders.

The PE should follow a universal and systematic approach, whether examining a single joint or multiple components of the musculoskeletal system. The PE should begin with inspection or observation, followed by palpation, measurement of range of motion, muscle strength testing, neurological assessment, reflex testing, diagnostic studies, and analysis of gait (Child, 2007).

Inspection

Inspection begins with the initial observation or general impression, as well as a focused examination of the affected body part. The initial impression influences the direction of the examination, noting such things as signs of general or specific distress, systemic disease, and level of patient engagement (Dutton, 2008). Any sign of potential loss of life or limb is an emergency requiring immediate medical intervention. Dividing the body into the four anatomic regions—anterior, posterior, medial, and lateral—facilitates a well-organized examination. Visualizing all four anatomic planes of the body is necessary, regardless of which body part is being evaluated, as this decreases the chance of overlooking an important finding. Care should be taken to achieve full visualization of both sides of the body in a setting that ensures privacy without undue exposure of the patient. The examination should proceed in an orderly fashion, either from head to toe or from proximal to distal, comparing one side of the body to the other and include the joint proximal and distal to the affected body part. A systematic inspection should be performed for each of the following features: attitude, alignment of a bone or joint, deformity, color, swelling, skin integrity, and muscle bulk or contour.

Attitude. Attitude refers to the position or posture in which the patient holds the involved body part or extremity when it is at rest. A side to side comparison is made to noting differences.

Alignment. Assessment of alignment includes both bones and joints, and should be distinguished from deformity. Mal-alignment suggests the presence of trauma from soft tissue injury, fracture or dislocation, or a congenital anomaly.

Deformity. Visual anomalies such as an absent body part, large tumor, or scars from previous surgeries or injuries should be noted.

Color. Discoloration provides clues to the cause of the symptoms or underlying systemic disease. Redness typically accompanies infection. Ecchymosis suggests disruption of soft tissue or bone, as in trauma. Pallor indicates local or systemic loss of blood flow from occlusion or vessel damage. Cyanosis points to a compromise in systemic oxygenation as in respiratory or cardiac disease.

Swelling. Swelling should be described as either diffuse or localized and intra- or extra-articular. Diffuse swelling should be differentiated from localized swelling and should be graded by severity. Swelling confined to a joint (intra-articular) suggests a distention of the joint with excess synovial fluid (effusion), blood (hemarthrosis), or pus (pyarthrosis). Diffuse swelling that extends beyond the joint (extra-articular) can occur with major infections, tumors, or problems with either venous or lymphatic drainage (McRae, 2004). It is important to determine when the patient first noticed the onset of swelling, as this may provide a clue to the source. For example, immediate swelling in the knee joint following a twisting injury of the knee is often due to an anterior cruciate ligament tear and suggests the presence of a hemarthrosis.

Skin Integrity. An inspection of skin integrity can provide evidence of systemic disease and localized trauma. Examples include diabetic patients with diabetic foot ulcers, rheumatoid patients with noted fragility of the epidermis, complex regional pain syndrome patients with cold shiny skin, and neurologically and/or vascular compromised patients with an absence of normal hair distribution in extremities. A break in the skin integrity near a potential surgical site must be noted and reported to the surgeon immediately. The trauma patient with a skin disruption overlying a bone should be suspect for an open fracture until proven otherwise and treated as a potential surgical emergency.

Muscle Bulk. Inspect the contour, size and, position of the muscles. In particular, note variations between the right and left sides. Use a tape measure to document side to side differences in size when indicated.

Palpation

Palpation is used to detect pain, tenderness, localized temperature changes, capillary refill, absence or presence of pulses, size of lymph nodes, muscle shape, tone, resistance to motion, bone and joint alignment, symmetry between sides, and the presence of bone or soft tissue masses and crepitus. Crepitus is also noted audibly. Pulses can be described as strong or weak, absent or present, or detected by Doppler. Care should be taken to ensure that infection control measures are followed, and the examiner's hands should be warm prior to palpating the patient.

It is helpful to examine the unaffected side first when palpating to detect pain, as this alerts the examiner to the patient's usual comfort level when pressure is applied. That pressure point is the patient's "zero" on a 1-10 scale. When palpating on the affected side, begin distal to the identified source of pain and gradually palpate toward the identified point. The maximal point of tenderness should be noted and described in relation to anatomy, as this often reveals the underlying anatomic structure involved in the symptom presentation (McRae, 2004). When pain or tenderness is noted, it is important to determine if it is diffuse or localized. The anatomic structures palpated include skin, subcutaneous soft tissue, and bony structures.

The *skin* should be evaluated first. Skin temperature differences noted between right and left sides are best determined using the back of the examiner's hand. Increased heat indicates an underlying inflammatory response, whereas decreased temperature suggests underlying vascular deficiency. Diffuse areas of increased heat suggest the involvement of a substantial amount of tissue mass. This is most commonly noted in joints with either infectious or noninfectious inflammatory responses. A localized asymmetric decrease in temperature, absence of a pulse, or delay in capillary refill suggests impaired circulation (McRae, 2004). Decreased skin mobility may indicate adhesions or collagen disease.

The assessment of *subcutaneous structures* requires significantly more applied pressure than skin assessment. Subcutaneous tissues include the fat, fascia, tendons, muscle, ligament, joint capsules, nerves, and blood vessels. Subcutaneous abnormalities include inflammation, soft tissue swelling, atrophy, or hypertrophy, which can be detected by comparing bilateral symmetry of the torso and extremity circumference measurements (Cipriano, 2003).

Palpation of *bony structures* is necessary when patients present with a functional abnormality or an alteration in range of motion (ROM). Palpating bone aids in detecting alignment problems such as fractures, subluxations, or dislocations. In addition to knowing which bone is being palpated, the attached tendons and ligaments should be identified (Cipriano, 2003).

Motion

An essential component of the orthopaedic examination includes the estimate and measurement of the ROM in a joint. Table 3.3 includes a listing of all joints and their respective types and range of normal motion in degrees. To determine deviation from "normal," the affected side is compared to the contralateral or unaffected side. The unaffected side is tested first when feasible. ROM is documented as degrees of motion from a neutral point or "zero."

Neutral points from which the angle is measured should be defined, and a goniometer (Figure 3.1) is used to measure angles of motion when practical. Another method for estimating ROM measures the distance reached in inches, centimeters, or finger-breadths between two locations. For example, the distance reached with forward flexion at the waist can be described as inches between fingertip and floor; the maximum distance reached by the thumb to the center of the back when internally rotating the shoulder can be described as number of inches reached above or below the bra line.

Figure 3.1
Goniometer

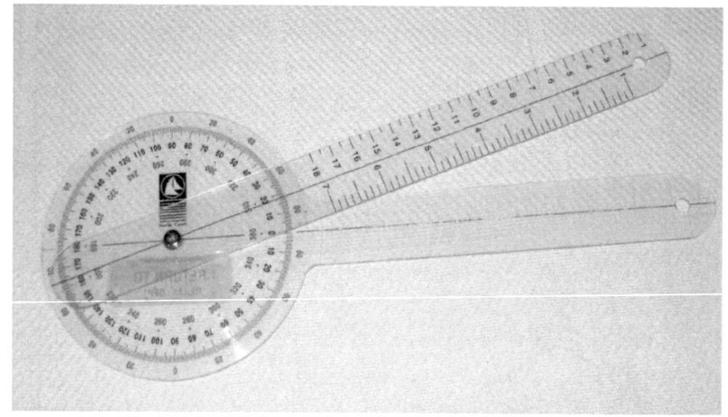

Photo by Mickey Haryanto. Reproduced with permission.

Table 3.3. Normal ROM for Joints

Joint	Range of Motion
CERVICAL SPINE	
Flexion	45 degrees
Extension	45 degrees
Lateral flexion	20-45 degrees
Rotation	70-90 degrees
LUMBAR SPINE	
Flexion	40-60 degrees
Extension	20-35 degrees
Lateral flexion	15-20 degrees
Rotation	3-18 degrees
SHOULDER	
Flexion	160-180 degrees
Extension	50-60 degrees
Abduction	170-180 degrees
Adduction	50-75 degrees
External rotation	80-90 degrees
Internal rotation	60-100 degrees
Circumduction	200 degrees
ELBOW	
Flexion	140-160 degrees
Extension	0-10 degrees
Supination	90 degrees
Pronation	80-90 degrees
WRIST	
Flexion	80-90 degrees
Extension	70-90 degrees
Ulnar deviation	35-45 degrees
Radial deviation	15 degrees
Pronation	85-90 degrees
Supination	85-90 degrees
HIP	
Flexion	110-120 degrees
Extension	10-15 degrees
Abduction	30-50 degrees
Adduction	30 degrees
External rotation	40-60 degrees
Internal rotation	30-40 degrees
KNEE	
Flexion	0-130 degrees
Extension	0-15 degrees
Medial rotation	20-30 degrees
Lateral rotation	30-40 degrees
ANKLE	
Plantar flexion	50 degrees
Dorsiflexion	20 degrees
Inversion	30 degrees
Eversion	20 degrees
Subtalar inversion	5 degrees
Subtalar eversion	5 degrees
Forefoot adduction	20 degrees
Forefoot abduction	10 degrees
Great toe flexion	45 degrees
Great toe extension	70 degrees

From Core Currriculum for Orthopaedic Nursing (6th ed., p. 44) by NAON, 2007, Boston, MA: Pearson. Reproduced with permission.

ROM is classified into active and passive joint ROM. The patient's own muscle power is used to produce motion when testing active ROM, whereas passive ROM testing is performed by the examiner at the extreme ranges. Resisted active ROM assesses both musculotendinous and neurological structures. Active ROM testing is deferred if small motions provoke intense pain, a sign of potential joint instability, or other serious condition (Dutton, 2008). When evaluating active ROM, note both the degree of motion and the amount of pain. Passive ROM testing occurs when the examiner moves the joint to the end of its range and applies pressure to the joint. The quality of the feel at the end point is assessed as normal ROM or abnormal ROM. Abnormal ROM indicates either hypo- or hypermobility. Pain on passive ROM often indicates a capsular or ligamentous lesion on the side of movement or a muscle lesion on the opposite side of movement.

Joints vary in both their range and plane of motion. Terminology used to describe joint motion and planes of motion is included in Table 3.1. Planes of motion vary between the freely movable joint types. Because muscle groups responsible for particular motions are often innervated by a single spinal nerve root, knowledge of motor nerve roots and associated muscle groups is necessary in accurately interpreting examination results. (See Chapter 2—Anatomy & Physiology for a description of freely movable joints, as well as the anatomy of spinal nerve roots and the muscles they innervate.) Muscle groups supplied by a single spinal nerve root are called myotomes. Myotomes are referred to according to their respective nerve root segments. Standard documentation includes use of relevant terminology and factors that limit active or passive ROM testing such as loss of strength, pain, or injury.

The absence or presence of pain can be described by patients using a rating scale from one to 10 with 10 being the worst pain ever experienced by the patient, or described using the following sensory rating scale described by Child (2007):

4 = Normal sensation. Detects light touch and able to discern two points 5mm apart.

3 = Two-point discrimination intact but diminished. Intact proprioception.

2 = Detects painful cutaneous stimulation only.

1 = Unable to detect any cutaneous stimulation. Comatose patient responds to sterna rub.

0 = No sensation in area affected by nerve.

Injuries to muscles (strains) or ligaments (sprains) may result in deformity, weakness, or loss of strength, which in turn effects ROM. Strains and sprains are classified by severity (Cipriano, 2003). See Table 3.4 for a description of the grading classification for these injuries. The degree of injury correlates with the degree of swelling, loss of function, and/or disability. Motion restriction may also be caused by a mechanical restriction in the joint (McRae, 2004).

Table 3.4. Categories of Sprains and Strains

Degree of Strain (Muscle)	
1st	Mild: Few muscle fibers torn.
2nd	Moderate: Almost half of muscle
3rd	Severe: All fibers torn (rupture)
Degree of Sprain (Ligament)	
1st	Mild: Few ligament fibers torn.
2nd	Moderate: Half of ligament torn
3rd	Severe: All ligament fibers torn (rupture)
Third degree injuries may include injuries to additional structures. Ligament attached to bone fragment pulled from bone is an avulsion fracture.	

Data from Orthopedic Physical Assessment *(5th ed.), by D.J. Magee, 2008, St. Louis, MO: Saunders Elsevier.*

Strength Testing

Muscle strength reflects peripheral neuromuscular function and is evaluated using manual muscle testing (MMT). Standardized classification systems for grading MMT have been developed based on the Medical Research Council 0-5 point scale (Nadler, Rigolosi, Kim, & Solomon, 2006), in which zero indicates no palpable muscle contraction and five indicates complete muscle contraction and ability to resist examiner throughout ROM testing in an individual muscle group. (See Table 3.5 for a description of the complete grading scale.) General strength testing is described in this section; testing specific to individual muscles and joints is described in "Head-to-Toe Physical Examination" later in this chapter.

Table 3.5. Strength Scale

Rank	Significance
5	Normal strength
4	Movement against gravity with some resistance
3	No resistance. Some movement against gravity is possible
2	Very weak motion Movement is dependent on position or gravity assisted
1	Muscles contract but are ineffective with no movement
0	No muscle contraction, no movement

From Basic Orthopedic Exams *(p. 4) by Z. Child, 2007, Baltimore, MD: Lippincott Williams and Wilkins. Reproduced with permission.*

The MMT scores are used for baseline assessments, as an indicator of disease progression, and to gauge response to interventions. Accurate MMT depends on the patient's ability to maximally exert muscle contraction. Objective measurements of strength are obtained using mechanical equipment such as a dynamometer, which is a hand-held device measuring grip strength (Dutton, 2008). Several factors influence the reliability of this strength test, including pain, fear, fatigue, quality of instructions, and motivation to cooperate with the examiner. The near-normal results of manual muscle testing is examiner-subjective, as it relies on the examiner's perception of force required to resist motion before the patient's contraction is "broken" (Nadler et al., 2006). Resistance to ROM evaluates both the strength and the state of muscles, ligaments, and tendons. Weakness may indicate neurological dysfunction. Pain may indicate a muscle strain, ligament sprain, or tendon tear or rupture. (See Chapter 2—Anatomy & Physiology for further description of nerves, muscles, ligaments, and tendons.)

Several principals must be observed to properly perform strength and motion assessments. The examiner should carefully hold the limb being tested to ensure stability without undue pressure that may inhibit muscle or tendon movement when assessing motion. The examiner should observe the entire ROM, from beginning to end, for even, steady speed throughout motion. Resistance to movements should be applied continuously against the direction of movement over one joint at a time. Resistance to isometric movement is performed with the joint in a neutral position. Muscles are noted for their ability to overcome resistance directed against movement and or gravity, their ability to work when gravity is eliminated, and their ability to cause movement when contracted.

Neurological Assessment

The neurological assessment assists the examiner in localizing a lesion within the peripheral or central nervous system (Nadler et al., 2006). This examination includes sensory, motor, reflex, and cerebella function testing. Spinal nerve roots are made of a dorsal root (sensory component) and ventral root (motor component). Knowledge of neurological anatomy allows the examiner to differentiate an injury involving a spinal nerve, the sensory or motor component of the nerve, or the associated peripheral nerve. (See Chapter 2—Anatomy & Physiology for further description of spinal nerve roots and their associated motor and sensory distributions.) The presence of pain and a decrease in or loss of extremity sensation, strength, or reflexes indicates nerve root pathology. Clinical presentation of nerve root pathology is dependent on the location and severity of the injury. The suspected location or level of the nerve root injury is narrowed down by grouping tests that assess sensation to the skin, muscle function, and deep tendon stretch reflexes. The degree or depth of necessary neurological testing depends on the patient's complaint and presenting symptoms.

Sensory Testing. A comprehensive sensory examination includes the patient's proprioception position sense and response to cutaneous stimulation. Proprioception is tested by moving a joint, such as repositioning a finger or toe, and asking the patient to describe the position of a joint without watching. Cutaneous stimulation is tested through one or more of the following: light touch, pin prick, two-point discrimination, temperature changes, and vibration with a tuning fork (Chou, 2006). Two-point discrimination testing is reliable for identifying peripheral nerve injuries that limit sensation, especially in the hand. The measurement between the two points is described in millimeters (Nadler et al., 2006); in general, discrimination greater than 6mm is suggestive of pathology. The affected side should be compared to the unaffected side, noting the presence or absence of normal sensation (or hyperparesthesia). The patient's response to stimulation is documented as one of four responses in Table 3.6. Diagnostic sensory testing (such as nerve conduction studies) has become more commonplace and is believed to be more sensitive than traditional subjective sensory examinations.

Table 3.6. Sensory Examination

Sensory Description	Significance of Finding
Sensitive to light touch	Appropriate screening exam, if intact likely a normal exam
Able to localize pain with protective sensation	Intact proprioception
Responds to deep pain only, no response to light touch or pin prick	Indicates a severe injury or comatose state
Absent response to all stimuli	Associated with loss of nerve function and complete nerve transection

From Basic Orthopedic Exams (p.4) by Z. Child, 2007, Baltimore, MD: Lippincott Williams and Willkens. Reproduced with permission.

Motor Testing. Motor examination is described under "Motion" and "Strength Testing." Balance testing with the eyes closed assesses for central nervous system discrepancies (Child, 2007).

Reflex Testing. A reflex is an involuntary motor response of the nervous system to a specific stimulus. Reflexes are categorized into deep tendon reflexes (DTRs) and superficial reflexes. The reflex consists of the following cycle: the stimulus travels along sensory nerve synapses in the spinal cord and then back along the motor nerve fiber. The neuromuscular junction stimulates muscle jerk, which is observed, graded, and documented by the examiner. DTR responses are often documented using a straw man diagram of the body, identifying the reflex responses on the diagram next to area tested using the Deep Tendon Reflex Rating Scale in Table 3.7.

Table 3.7. Reflex Grading Scale

Grade	Response
0+	Absent
1+	Hypoactive
2+	Normal
3+	Brisk
4+	Hyperactive with clonus

From Basic Orthopedic Exams (p. 5) by Z. Child, 2007, Baltimore, MD: Lippincott Williams and Wilkins. Reproduced with permission.

To test DTRs, the tendon must be partially stretched and lightly tapped, usually with a reflex hammer over a predetermined anatomic point. The resulting motor response should be compared with the opposite (unaffected) side and documented per a grading scale. It may be necessary to repeat the test and distract the patient when repeating the test to get a more accurate result. There is no universally accepted grading scale for documenting DTRs. A common five-point scale is from the National Institute of Neurologic Disorders and Strokes, which ranges from 0-4 where 0 implies an absence of response and 4 implies an enhanced response that is more than normal (Nadler et al., 2006). Observation of the reflex amplitude is the most important part of reflex testing. Asymmetric reflex amplitude suggests either lower motor neuron disease on the side with the diminished reflex or upper motor neuron disease on the side with an exaggerated reflex. The grading of DTR is variable: different observers for the same patient will often reach a different analysis due to examiner and patient factors. Consequently, DTR results should not be used in isolation as they may be misleading (Nadler et al., 2006).

Cerebella Function Testing. The cerebellum plays a role in muscle movements (such as tics and tremors) and general coordination and balance. Cerebella screening examinations include assessing the patient's balance when walking heel-to-toe, as well as when standing with arms stretched forward and eyes open compared to when eyes are closed (known as the Rhomberg test). The presence of poor balance or swaying to one side may indicate cerebella dysfunction. Additionally, extremity coordination can be evaluated by asking the patient to perform repetitive rapid motions. For example, the patient touches the examiners hand, held 2ft in front of patient's face, then his/her own nose repeatedly from slow to fast motion. The lack of a smooth, accurate response may indicate dysfunction (Springhouse, 2009).

Diagnostic Studies

Additional diagnostic tests compliment the PE findings. Blood and urine laboratory tests evaluate systemic effects on the musculoskeletal system. The following diagnostic studies identify more localized findings in bone and soft tissue: radiographs, joint fluid analysis, computerized tomography (CT), magnetic resonance imaging (MRI), MRI arthrograms with and without contrast, gadolinium scans, densometer or dexa scans, and nerve conduction studies.

Ordering, obtaining, and interpreting diagnostic studies in collaboration with the physician is included in the nurse practitioner's physical assessment, as approved by health care agency setting. An awareness of the indications for obtaining diagnostic test, and an understanding of the implications of abnormal test results, contributes to a more complete PE by the registered nurse and nurse practitioner. (See Chapter 1—Practice Settings and Chapter 4—Diagnostic Studies. Specific diagnostic studies indicated in the physical assessment of individual joints, extremities, and the spine are not included in this chapter, as they will appear in chapters specific to body parts and in Chapter 4—Diagnostic Studies.)

Analysis of Gait

Gait is a definite pattern or style of achieving upright bipedal locomotion. The two phases of gait are the stance phase (or weight-bearing phase) and the swing phase (or non-weight-bearing phase). The stance

Table 3.8. Abnormal Gait

Gait	Cause	Description
Antalgic	Multiple disorders	Pain or discomfort on weight bearing. Ambulates on affected extremity as little as possible. Shortened stride. Expresses pain verbally, by gesture, by expression on face, or by posture while walking.
Ataxic	Neurogenic (cerebellar)	Staggering, uncoordinated gait. Sway may be evident. Foot stomping, slapping, or double tap.
Festinating	Neurogenic (Parkinson disease)	Body held rigidly. Trunk leans forward. Short, quick, shuffling steps. Delayed start.
Quadriceps	Neurogenic (muscle or nerve injury)	Hand on thigh to support gait. Decreased quadriceps function. Knee flexion contracture.
Short leg	Structural (degenerative joint disease, congenital dislocated hip, fracture)	Leg-length discrepancy of 1 inch or more. Vertical telescoping with dip on affected side.
Senile	Aging	En bloc turning, hesitant, short steps. May need to support self to get started. Once started, able to ambulate with no apparent associated gait problems.
Spastic	Neurogenic (cerebral palsy, hemiplegia, dislocated hip)	Jerky, uncoordinated movement. Short steps with dragging or scraping of foot. Crossed knee (scissors) gait. Severe spasticity.
Steppage	Neurogenic (peroneal nerve injury, tertiary syphilis, paralyzed dorsiflexor muscles)	Increased hip and knee flexion in order to clear the floor.
Trendelenburg	Myogenic (coxa vara, congenital)	Foot slaps or drags along ground. Dropfoot evident. Known as the gluteus medial lurch. Typical gait associated with positive Trendelenburg test. Duck-like waddle or sailor's sway. Pelvis drops of unaffected side displaying the gluteus medius is not functioning.

From Core Currriculum for Orthopaedic Nursing (6th ed., p. 46) by NAON, 2007, Boston, MA: Pearson. Reproduced with permission.

phase includes heel strike, flat foot, mid-stance, and push off. Swing phase includes acceleration, mid-swing, and deceleration. Assessment of gait is an integral component of a comprehensive muscle skeletal examination and occurs throughout the patient visit. The use of assistive devices, splints, or special shoes should be documented in the gait assessment, as well as unusual shoe wear pattern. Visual signs of normal gait include the pelvis rotating forward 40 degrees while the arms swing in tandem with each step. The usual width of the gap between ankles while walking is 2-4 inches, and the average heel-to-heel length of a step is 15 inches (NAON, 2007). The body's center of gravity while walking is centered in the midline.

Evidence of abnormal gait is often detected audibly as in the foot-slapping gait, stomping gait, the toe box of the shoe scraping on the ground, or the unequal rhythm of steps. (See Table 3.8.) Abnormal gait patterns have various causes, which suggest underlying pathologies or injuries to a joint or compensation for injuries or pathologies. Knowledge of potential underlying pathology assists the examiner in directing the health history and PE. Abnormal gait is typically caused by pain; muscle weakness in the hip, knee, or ankle; structural deformities; and instability of ligaments and joints. The signs provide clues as to which areas the examiner should target during the PE.

Head-to-Toe Musculoskeletal Physical Assessment

The head-to-toe PE consists of the following primary components and their respective joints:

- The upper extremities: includes the shoulder, elbow, wrist, and hand joints.
- The lower extremities: includes the hip, femur, pelvis, knee, foot, and ankle joints.
- The spine: divided into neck (or cervical spine) and back. The back includes the thoracic, lumbar, and sacral segments.

The various steps in the overall exam format are integrated into a comprehensive exam that minimizes the need for the patient to repeatedly change positions. Including the joint or limb above and below the area being examined or the associated spine segment contributes to a more comfortable, complete, and efficient examination. For example, the shoulder exam includes the cervical and thoracic spine, as well as the shoulder and elbow. The components of the head-to-toe assessment that receive the majority of the examiner's attention are dependent on the patient's CC and health history (Magee, 2008).

Cervical Spine (Neck)

History. (See Chapter 2—Anatomy & Physiology, Chapter 15—Trauma, and Chapter 17—The Spine.) Of particular importance to note during the history-taking is a recent trauma or injury involving the head, as well as the quality and character of symptoms. Symptoms such as numbness, tingling, paralysis, and neck or arm positions that aggravate or induce the symptoms should be identified. The presence of radicular symptoms that spread down the arm should be evaluated for sensory or motor deficit.

Patients presenting with neck pain and no history of trauma should be further assessed for underlying degenerative osteoarthritis or RA and symptoms suggesting an infection or carcinogenic origin. Pain in the C spine region may originate in adjacent structures such as the teeth, jaw, cardiovascular system, or shoulders; therefore, the patient should be questioned about a history of symptoms involving these structures.

The more serious and less common conditions involving the head and neck include cervical fractures, dislocations, and cancer. Information noted on history suggestive of a possible fracture or dislocation includes a combination of head trauma and neck pain, with or without a loss of feeling or use of an extremity. The presence of nocturnal pain without a history of trauma and the presence of systemic symptoms suggestive of cancer should be noted.

Inspection. The general posture, spine curvature, and relationship of the neck to the trunk are noted with the patient in both seated and standing positions. To fully observe skin, symmetry, and motions of the head and neck, the patient must be viewed from all four sides. General movement of the head, neck, and eyes are assessed for ease of motion, guarding, or rigidity, which should be consistent throughout the interview and examination. Lack of consistency in movement may indicate malingering (Anderson, 2006).

Palpation. Palpate the musculature in the neck and shoulders with the patient in the supine position to ensure maximum relaxation of the muscles, noting tenderness, trigger points, or spasm. The remainder of the C spine exam occurs in the seated or standing position. With the head held in neutral position, the bony prominences, musculature, skin, pulses, and lymph tissue are palpated. From the anterior neck, palpate the hyoid bone that correlates with C3, thyroid cartilage (C4), sternocleidomastoid muscle, lymph node chains, and the supra clavicular fossa. The sternocleidomastoid should be palpated at both the clavicular and sternal heads (Landes, Malanga, Nadler, & Farmer, 2006). Carotid pulses are palpated one at a time, lateral to trachea and medial to sternocleidomastoid border (Child, 2007). The posterior bony prominences include the occiput, mastoid

CHAPTER 3

Table 3.9. Sensory Distribution of Nerves of the Cervical Spine			
Nerve	**Motor**	**Reflex**	**Sensory**
C5	Shoulder abduction/deltoid/biceps	Biceps, brachioradialis	Axillary nerve, lateral arm
C6	Wrist extension/biceps	Biceps, brachioradialis	Musculocutaneous nerve, lateral forearm, thumb, and index finger.
C7	Wrist flexion/finger extension/triceps	Triceps	Middle finger
C8	Finger flexion/hand	Triceps	Medial antebrachial cutaneous nerve, medial forearm, and ulnar nerve, fourth finger, little finger on ulnar side
T1	Finger abduction	None	Medial brachial cutaneous nerve, upper half medial forearm and elbow

From Core Currriculum for Orthopaedic Nursing *(6th ed., p. 50) by NAON, 2007, Boston, MA: Pearson. Reproduced with permission.*

processes, spinous processes of cervical vertebrae, and facet joints. Spinous processes are assessed for the presence of tenderness and alignment from C2-T1. The atlas vertebra (or C1) does not have a spinous process. Cervical vertebra C2-C7 have prominent, easily palpated spinous processes, best palpated with the neck slightly flexed passively (Magee, 2008). Slightly lateral to the spinous process lie the facet joints. Bone tenderness in the presence of trauma is suggestive of fracture, which requires further radiographs to confirm. The most often injured vertebrae are C5 and C6, which are also the most common sites for osteoarthritis (Parvizi, 2006). Posterior soft tissue structures include the supporting muscles of the neck (paraspinal and upper trapezial), lymph nodes, and superior nuchal ligament. The muscles are examined for tenderness, spasm, and their effect on flexion. Muscle spasm may indicate inflammation from torn muscle fibers and edema resulting from trauma, while palpable crepitus upon neck movement is suggestive of degenerative joint disease (Cipriano, 2003).

Motion. Cervical ROM should not be evaluated if neck trauma or instability is suspected, as in the case of head trauma from a motor vehicle accident. Begin passive ROM in a supine position, followed by active ROM and resisted isometric movements in a seated or standing position. (For normal ROM of the cervical spine in extension, flexion, lateral flexion, and rotation, see Table 3.3.) Passive ROM of the cervical spine may result in greater motion than active ROM due to more relaxed muscles. For passive flexion and extension ROM, gently push the back of the head forward, noting the distance from the chin to the chest and the forehead backwards. Active neck flexion tests cranial nerve XI and the C1-C2 myotomes.

Pain with active ROM signifies cervical muscle strain, whereas pain with passive ROM signifies a ligament sprain (Cipriano, 2003). The most painful motions are evaluated last. Cervical spine extension is commonly reported as a comparison to normal, while flexion is reported as the number of finger breadths between the chin and the sternum. Lateral flexion and rotation of the C-spine is reported as degrees from the midline. (See Table 3.3 for the normal ROM in the cervical spine.)

To ease the exam process and ensure completeness, neck and shoulder ROM are evaluated together. Rotation is assessed by having the patient turn the head from right to left. Normal rotation allows the ear to line up with the shoulder. Lateral flexion is achieved by reaching the ear toward the shoulder. Comparisons should be made contralaterally.

Strength Testing. The major muscle groups of the cervical spine are the intrinsics, primary and secondary flexors, primary and secondary extensors, primary and secondary rotators, and primary and secondary lateral benders (Rouscher, 2001). The muscles and their associated spinal and peripheral nerves contribute to motor function of the cervical spine (Landes et al., 2006) (see Table 3.9 and

Table 3.10. Major Peripheral Nerves		
Nerve	**Motor**	**Sensory**
Radial	Wrist, thumb extension	Dorsal web space between thumb and index
Ulnar	Abduction of all fingers. Ulnar deviation	Distal ulnar aspect of little finger (volar surface)
Medial	Thumb pinch, opposition, abduction, and wrist flexion	Distal fat pad or index finger (volar surface)
Axillary	Deltoid	Lateral arm and deltoid patch on upper arm
Musculocutaneous	Biceps	Lateral forearm

From Core Currriculum for Orthopaedic Nursing *(6th ed., p. 50) by NAON, 2007, Boston, MA: Pearson. Reproduced with permission.*

Table 3.10). Resistance to neck extension, flexion, and rotational ROM evaluates strength, the state of muscles, and motor nerve innervations. Weakness may indicate neurological dysfunction in C5-C8, which contributes to limited neck motion and strength. Pain may indicate a cervical strain or sprain.

Before initiating the strength test, the patient should be seated and comfortable with the head in neutral position. To assess resistance to neck extension, support the patient at the sternum while applying increasing resistance at patient's occipital area. When testing resistance, ensure that there is no patient movement and only muscle contraction. To evaluate the strength of the neck flexors, the patient flexes the head forward against resistance from the examiner's hand placed at the forehead. To assess rotational strength, the patient rotates the head to one side against resistance from the examiner's hand, which cups the patients' cheek. The patient's strength while flexing or bending the head from side to side against the examiner's resistance is also tested. All maneuvers are done bilaterally, and the grade of strength is documented using the 0-5 muscle reflex grading scale (see Table 3.7.).

Sensory. Neurologic assessment of the cervical spine includes the evaluation of motor function, sensation along dermatomes, peripheral nerve distributions, and deep tendon reflexes in the upper extremities. (See Table 3.9 for information related to sensation, motor function, and DTRs of cervical spine segments C5-T1 and Chapter 2—Anatomy & Physiology for details on muscles and their nerve innervations.) Additional sensation and motor function are provided by peripheral nerves. Cervical nerve root assessment of DTRs in the upper extremity (biceps, triceps, and brachioradialis) assesses sensory and motor function (Child, 2007).

Referred Pain. Pain from cervical spine abnormalities may radiate to other structures or be detected using tests such as distraction, compression, valsava maneuvers, and swallowing. The *distraction test* is performed to determine if traction will help relieve symptoms. This maneuver is done by placing one hand under the chin and one hand on the occiput while gently pulling up, increasing the space between vertebrae.

The *compression test* is used to locate the level of pathology by narrowing the foramen, increasing pressure on facet joints, and reproducing spasm. This test is performed by placing both hands on the patient's head and gently pushing down, reproducing symptoms. This may cause referred pain from neck to shoulder. The location and distribution of symptoms should be documented. Compression should not be performed if a fracture or dislocation from an injury is suspected.

The *valsalva maneuver* is performed to detect a lesion (such as tumor or herniated disc) that may cause increased intrathecal pressure and subsequent increased pain. The maneuver is performed by asking the patient to hold his/her breath while bearing down as if to evacuate the bowel. Have the patient describe pain. Patients may also note that their pain intensifies with coughing or sneezing.

The *swallowing test* assesses for dysphagia (or painful swallowing), which may occur when bony protrusions, osteophytes, or soft tissue involvement are present, secondary to tumor, infection, or hematoma in the anterior cervical spine region. Ask patient to swallow while fingers are gently pressed on either side of the throat, and document reports of pain or difficulty with swallowing.

Patients with upper extremity pain, a cold upper extremity, and upper extremity claudication or supraclavicular pain should be assessed with the *subclavian artery compromise test*. Blood flow in the subclavian artery may be hindered by a cervical rib, tumor, hematoma, or infection, causing tightness in the neck muscles. To test for subclavien artery patency, take the radial pulse while abducting, extending, and externally rotating the patient's arm. Have the patient take a deep breath while turning the head toward the arm being tested. If the subclavian artery is compromised, the radial pulse will be absent or decreased.

Diagnostics. Cervical spine x-rays are indicated for patients with radiculopathy, greater than 25% decrease in neck ROM, and/or a history of trauma. A cervical collar is left in place while obtaining a cross-table lateral x-ray for patients with a known head injury and neck pain. The lateral view provides useful clinical information to screen for loss of alignment, degree of osteoarthritis, disk space narrowing, and bony disorders (Anderson, 2006).

Lumbar Spine (Back)

History. (See Chapter 2—Anatomy & Physiology, Chapter 15—Trauma, and Chapter 17—The Spine.) The underlying cause of back pain is difficult to discern, even after careful history-taking followed by a detailed physical exam. Identifying the location of pain (primary back pain vs. back-and-leg pain) and noting a history of trauma contribute to defining a diagnosis. Back pain typically fits one of four categories: disk, facet, nerve root involvement, or neurogenic intermittent claudication (Magee, 2008). The index of suspicion for each of the four categories is based on the patient's age, occupation, description of symptoms, and pattern of symptom presentation. Serious spine pathology should be considered if the following red flags are present; symptoms occur younger than age 20 or older than age 55, a history of violent trauma, carcinoma, drug abuse, chronic systemic steroid use, human immunodeficiency virus (HIV), unintended significant weight loss, constant progressive nonmechanical symptoms, and neurologic compromise (Magee, 2008).

Inspection. Inspection begins wherever the examiner meets the patient, whether in the waiting room or exam room. Gait, stance, and posture while sitting, standing, or supine are observed from all sides, noting the normal curvatures of the spine. Observe for symmetry of the pelvic crests, scapula, and skin folds. Observe the skin for redness, hairy patches, café au lait spots, or birthmarks. Note any structural deformities, such as kyphosis, scoliosis, and spinous process step deformities.

Palpation. Beginning on the posterior surface, palpate each spinous process from the head to the coccyx, noting any tenderness or irregularities. Palpate each scapula and the soft tissue structures of the spine, beginning with supraspinous and interspinous ligaments. Note areas of firmness, tissue irregularities, or spasm in paraspinal muscles. Move down to the area of the iliac crests, noting the symmetry of the musculature. Palpate the sciatic nerve distribution for any irregularities and point tenderness. Palpate the ischial tuberosities, greater trochanters, and sciatic notches for irregularities or point tenderness. The ishial tuberosity may best be palpated with the patient lying on the side with the hip flexed. Moving to the anterior surface, palpate the structures of each rib to detect deformities or asymmetry. Palpate the musculature of the abdomen, and press gently in the inguinal areas.

Motion. (See Chapter 2—Anatomy & Physiology for muscles and nerve innervations responsible for hip motion.) The motion of the lumbar spine must be assessed in all planes, including flexion, extension, side-bending, and rotation. Active ROM is assessed with the patient standing. Side-bending should occur while patient stands against a wall. If there is no limit in active ROM, the examiner can apply pressure as the patient reaches full active ROM. There is more movement in the lumbar spine than in the thoracic spine.

To assess *active flexion*, the patient touches the toes while the knees are kept straight. If the patient is unable to touch the toes, the distance from the long fingertip to the floor is measured to establish a baseline. This is a combined movement of both lumbar spine and hip flexion. *Active extension* is assessed from behind the patient as the examiner supports the patient's lower back with open palms on the iliac crests. The patient bends back as far as possible, then moves laterally left and then right with the examiner's continued support.

Table 3.11. Sensory Testing of the Spine

Nerve	Motor	Reflex	Sensory	Deficit/Compression
T12, L1	Iliopsoas	None	Anterior thigh between the inguinal ligament and knee	Dysfunctional bladder. Anal reflex is hyperactive. Paraplegics with pelvic stability can ambulate with braces.
L1, L2, L3	Iliopsoas	None	Anterior thigh between the inguinal ligament and knee	No voluntary control of bowel or bladder. No sensation of two-thirds of thigh distally. Decreased patellar reflex, absent Achilles reflex.
L2, L3, L4	Quadriceps, hip abductor	Patellar	Medial side of leg L2: anterior thigh L3: knee L4: medial calf	
L4 (overlap)	Tibialis anterior	Patellar	From the knee down, medial side of leg	
L5	Extensor halluces, gluteus medius, extensor digitorum longus, and brevis	None	Lateral leg and medial aspect of dorsum of foot	
S1	Peroneus longus and brevis, gastrocnemius soleus, gluteus maximus	Achilles	Lateral malleolus, lateral aspect of foot, and plantar surface of foot	
S2, S3, S4	Bladder muscles, intrinsic mucles of the foot	None	Three concentric rings around the anus: S2: outermost ring S3: middle ring S4: innermost ring Also S2: posterior thigh and knee	

From Core Currriculum for Orthopaedic Nursing *(6th ed., p. 58) by NAON, 2007, Boston, MA: Pearson. Reproduced with permission.*

The presence of stiffness or pain is noted. *Active rotation* detects only major restrictions in motion. If patient has had a spinal fusion, there will be some limitation in motion. While standing behind the patient, the examiner places one hand on the patient's shoulder and the other hand on the opposite side iliac crest to stabilize the pelvis, while the patient twists the torso.

Sensory. The sensory exam includes assessment of bilateral lower extremities, evaluating areas of the skin innervated by single nerve roots (dermatomes) or specific peripheral nerves. Using a sharp object, lightly prick patient's skin along nerve distributions and dermatomes described in Table 3.11, documenting the patient's response to assess the spine.

Special Spine Tests. A number of tests help assess neurological and muscle dysfunction, pelvic joint dysfunction, and spine alignment, as well as identify the malingering patient. A positive response indicates dysfunction. The more common tests are described below.

The *Oppenheim test* is conducted using the handle of the reflex hammer to stroke the medial tibia distally. Normally there is no reaction; if the great toe extends dorsally, the test is positive (Magee, 2008).

The *Babinski reflex* is tested by running the handle of the reflex hammer or a key across the plantar surface of the foot from heel to toe, along the lateral border of the forefoot. The toes normally bunch together. If the great toe extends while the other toes plantar flex and splay, the test is positive (Magee, 2008).

The *Beevor's sign* indicates muscle paralysis and is usually positive in patients with polio and meningomyocele. The patient is asked to do a quarter sit-up with arms held behind the head, while the examiner observes the umbilicus for movement. Normally no movement is apparent. If movement is present, the umbilicus moves toward the weak abdominal segment (Cipriano, 2003).

FABERE (Patrick's) tests may indicate sacroiliac joint pathology. (This acronym stands for Flexion, Abduction, External Rotation, Extension.) With patient supine, the hip is abducted by placing the foot of the involved side on the opposite knee, with hip externally rotated, flexed, and abducted. The patient remains in this position while the examiner presses down on the flexed knee while stabilizing the opposite anterior iliac spine, noting the presence of groin pain. Pain may be caused by hip or sacroiliac joint involvement (Krabak, 2006).

Femoral nerve stretch aids in the diagnosis of a high lumbar nerve root herniation. It is tested with the patient in the prone position. The examiner places a palm at the popliteal space as the knee is dorsiflexed. If the test produces pain in the distribution of the patient's anterior thigh and back, it is positive (Solomon, 2006).

The *Hoover test* may be helpful in determining if voluntary effort is made by the patient during an examination. The patient is instructed to raise one leg as the examiner holds the heel of the opposite leg. If patient is genuinely making an attempt, increased pressure from the heel will be felt by the examiners hand (Magee, 2008).

The *Valsalva maneuver* is performed by asking the patient to hold his/her breath while bearing down as if to evacuate the bowel. If pain occurs down the legs or in the lower back or buttocks, the maneuver is positive (Magee, 2008). A positive valsava maneuver may indicate a bulging or ruptured intervertebral disc or spinal cord compromise.

The *Naffziger's test* is performed with patient supine. The examiner compresses the jugular veins for 10 seconds, causing the face to become flushed. The patient then coughs or performs the valsalva maneuver. The test is positive if the patient experiences pain in the low back (Magee, 2008, p. 567). A positive Naffziger's test may indicate the abnormal pressure on the spinal cord.

The *scoliosis test* detects abnormal curvature of the spine. The patient is inspected from behind for an abnormal lateral curvature, facing away from the seated examiner and then bending forward at the waist with the knees straight. The upper extremities are extended loosely in front of the body toward the floor with fingertips of each hand extended and touching. This position enables the examiner to note subtle rotational differences in the thorax; normally the sides of the thorax, scapula, and pelvis are symmetric. A shortening of one leg may be present in an upright and forward flexed position, indicating a structural deformity (Magee, 2008).

The *straight leg test* (SLT) evaluates the L5-S2 nerve roots. It is positive if pain occurs in the buttock, back, and leg when the supine leg is passively elevated to 30-70 degrees. Both legs are tested separately, with the unaffected side first. The patient is placed supine, with hips medially rotated and adducted, and the knee in extension. The examiner slowly lifts the extended leg off examination table and notes the position and degree of flexion in which pain occurs. Document the angle of elevation that causes severe pain (Solomon, 2006). Pain that occurs with less than 30 or more than 70 degrees of flexion is not due to sciatic nerve irritability; instead, it is most likely due to tight hamstrings or gluteal muscles.

The *Brudzinski's/Kernig test* is similar to the SLT except that the patient performs movements actively. The patient is supine with hands cupped behind the head and the head flexed onto the chest. The patient then raises one extended leg actively by flexing the hip until pain is felt. Pain is a positive sign that may indicate meningeal, nerve root, or dural irritability. If the pain disappears when the knee is flexed, the test is positive (Magee, 2008).

CHAPTER 3

Shoulder

History. (See Chapter 2—Anatomy & Physiology, Chapter 15—Trauma and Chapter 18—Shoulder.) Conditions intrinsic to the shoulder are presented as complaints of shoulder pain, loss of shoulder mobility, shoulder or arm weakness, deformity, or a combination of these symptoms. Inquiring about hand dominance and limitations in activities of daily living (ADLs) such as teeth-brushing, hair-combing or self-dressing is an important part of the shoulder evaluation (Magee, 2008). The shoulder evaluation with upper extremity pain or paresthesia includes an evaluation of the C-spine. Cervical spondylosis is the most common cause of pain in the shoulder and is referred pain caused by irritation to cervical nerve roots (McRae, 2004). Seventy percent of all shoulder diagnoses include tendinitis (Anderson, 2006). The most common outpatient shoulder conditions are rotator cuff tears; osteoarthritis of the acromioclavicular (AC) or glenohumeral (GH) joints; frozen shoulder; inflammation of subscapular bursa, biceps tendon, or rotator cuff tendons; and shoulder instability (Anderson, 2006). Other less common shoulder conditions include RA, fractures, dislocations, and infections. The presence of nocturnal pain may indicate rotator cuff tear or impingement syndrome. Pain relieved by raising the arm overhead may be caused by nerve root pain (Magee, 2008), whereas pain brought on by overhead reaching may be due to instability or inflammation. If an injury is reported, it is necessary to determine the exact mechanism. A fall on an outstretched hand (FOOSH) can result in a fracture or dislocation the hand, elbow, or shoulder. Blunt trauma or a fall on the tip of shoulder may result in a ligament injury to the AC joint or a fractured clavicle.

Inspection. Proper exposure of the entire shoulder, with draping at the bra line, is necessary for adequate inspection. Bra straps should be off the shoulder. The shoulder is inspected for scars, atrophy, erythema, ecchymosis, swelling, rashes, deformities, scapular positioning, and shoulder heights. Muscle bulk, scapular positioning, and ease of motion are best viewed posteriorly. The sternoclavicular joint, clavicle, and AC joint are noted in the anterior plane. Errythema, edema, and deformity are noted in the anterior and lateral views. Symmetry of the supraclavicular fossa is noted while standing over the patient looking downward. The patient's posture and upper extremity position held at rest are also noted.

Palpation. The four soft tissue zones palpated in the shoulder are the rotator cuff, subacromial and deltoid bursa, axilla, and muscles of the shoulder girdle (Parvizi, 2006). Palpation of the shoulder begins with the examiner standing behind the seated patient. Starting at the deltoid and moving proximal towards the C spine, the examiner palpates the bony processes—sternal notch, sternoclavicular joint, clavicles, and corocoid processes—one side at a time. The AC joint is palpated while the patient reaches across the body (adducts) and touches the opposite shoulder while lifting the elbow towards the ceiling. Next, the examiner ascertains irregularity or asymmetry between sides by palpating the acromion, lesser and greater tuberosities of the humerus, bicipital grooves, and outer borders of the scapula. (The spine of the scapula is at the level of the third thoracic vertebra, and the inferior border is at the seventh thoracic vertebra.) The subacromial and subdeltoid busae are palpated along with the musculature of the shoulder girdle (sternocleidomastoid, pectoralis major, biceps, deltoid, trapezium, rhomboids, latissimus dorsi, and serratus anterior), noting swelling, tenderness, deformity, or asymmetry. The axillary region is evaluated for presence and size of lymph nodes, masses and palpation of muscles. Ease of motion and patient expression is noted during all palpation maneuvers.

Motion. (See Table 3.3 for normal shoulder ROM.) The shoulder moves in the following planes of motion: forward flexion or elevation, extension, internal and external rotation, abduction and adduction, and a combination of movements called circumduction. Additionally, the scapula enables elevation, retraction, and protraction. (See Chapter 2—Anatomy & Physiology for further descriptions of the muscles of the shoulder, their actions and nerve innervations.) Shoulder ROM is usually noted in degrees from the neutral anatomic position of zero degrees. Passive ROM testing occurs as the examiner anchors the inferior angle of the shoulder and supports the patient's elbow while assisting the patient through abduction, adduction, flexion, extension, and rotation internally and externally.

Forward flexion/elevation of the shoulder is assessed via the Neer impingement test. The patient elevates the arm forward from the neutral anatomic position of zero. Pain upon passive forward flexion that causes the greater tuberosity of the humerus to jam against the underside of the acromion flexion is noted as a positive Neer sign.

Shoulder extension is measured with the goniometer (Figure 3.1) placed at the glenohumeral joint in the sagital plane. The patient's arm is dropped along the side of the body. The patient moves the arm backwards while elevating the arm posteriorly.

The neutral position for measuring *internal and external rotation* of the GH joint can be with arms at the side and elbows touching the body, or with the shoulder abducted 90 degrees away from midline and the elbow flexed at 90 degrees and palm facing the floor. Internal rotation with shoulders abducted is assessed by having the patient rotate the shoulder inward by moving the forearm so the palm of the hand faces posteriorly. External rotation is assessed by having the patient rotate the shoulder outward by moving the forearm so the palm faces forward or anterior.

Abduction and adduction measures begin in a neutral position with the arms held alongside the body. Abduction is measured as the patient raises the arm laterally away from the midline. Adduction is measured with the goniometer (Figure 3.1) placed anterior to glenohumerol joint. The patient is instructed to raise the arm toward the midline or medially following the movement with the goniometer.

Strength Testing. The usefulness of strength testing is enhanced when performed in conjunction with both a careful history and other special tests of the shoulder that evaluate rotator cuff and biceps tendon pathology, shoulder stability, and impingement of rotator cuff tendons in the subacromial space. Specific tests assist in evaluating the shoulder pathology that contributes to muscle weakness. Evaluating resistance to shoulder motion begins with the patient raising the arm forward in the sagital plane as the examiner provides resistance, holding the area anterior and proximal to the patient's flexed elbow and noting the grade of strength from 0-5. Next, while standing behind the patient, the examiner pushes against the patient's flexed elbow as the patient extends the shoulder in the posterior direction, again documenting strength from 0-5 and comparing it to the unaffected side. The patient then abducts the shoulder (moves it laterally away from the midline) with the elbow flexed at 90 degrees against the examiners hand, while the examiner stabilizes the lateral shoulder with other hand. Patient resistance to shoulder abduction assesses the integrity of the infraspinatous muscle. According to Kibler, Sciascia, Wolf, Warme, and Kuhn (2009), combining infraspinatus muscle strength testing with the Hawkins test, to produce pain upon shoulder forward flexion beyond 90 degrees, best predicts the presence of impingement syndrome (see "Special Shoulder Tests" for a description of the Hawkins tests). While the examiner continues to stabilize the lateral shoulder with one hand, the patient adducts (pulls their arm towards the midline of the body) with elbow flexed at 90 degrees and the examiner providing resistance on the medial arm. To evaluate resistance to internal and external rotation, stabilize the shoulder with one hand and hold the patient's wrist with the other hand while the patient flexes the elbow and pulls forearm inward and outward against examiner resistance.

Sensory Testing. See Table 3.12 for nerve roots responsible for the specific sensations in the arm and shoulder.

Special Shoulder Tests. Special tests are often done by the experienced examiner as a follow-up to confirm a tentative diagnosis (Magee, 2008) or findings such as ligament laxity, instability, impingement, or pathology in the ligaments, muscles, tendons, or labrum.

The *Apley scratch test* is accomplished by having the patient place the thumb as high up the midline of the back as possible, noting the location of the thumb. The degree of rotation can be quantified by the level of the spinous process that is reached in comparison to the opposite (unaffected) side performing the same maneuvers. The location of the thumb is described in relation to vertebra or as in centimeters above or below the bra line. The inferior border of the scapula is thoracic vertebra number seven. This maneuver is the most practical means of screening shoulder movement and objectively assessing shoulder rotation because it assesses the GH joint and the muscles and tendons of the rotator cuff (Anderson, 2006); however, there is no documented predictive value of this maneuver other than as a screening test to assess motion.

Table 3.12. Sensory Testing of the Shoulder

Nerve Root	Sensation
C5	Regimental patch area on lateral arm
T1	Medial arm
T2	Axilla
T3	Axilla to nipple
T4	Nipple

From Core Currriculum for Orthopaedic Nursing (6th ed., p. 52) by NAON, 2007, Boston, MA: Pearson. Reproduced with permission.

The *apprehension test* assesses anterior shoulder instability (laxity) and is best performed with the patient in a supine position with the examiner's hand under the GH joint to stabilize the shoulder. The examiner then abducts the arm 90 degrees and externally rotates the patient's shoulder (Magee, 2008). This test is positive if the patient looks or feels apprehensive.

The test for inferior shoulder instability is the *sulcus sign* (Magee, 2008). This maneuver is done with the patient standing or sitting with the arm by the side and the shoulder relaxed. The examiner grasps the forearm and pulls distally toward the floor, attempting to distract the GH joint. An observed sulcus or cleft at the anterolateral shoulder indicates inferior GH instability.

The two most common valid and reliable impingement tests include the *Neer test* and *Hawkins test*. The Neer test has a high sensitivity for identifying inflammation of the rotator cuff bursa and tendons, partial tears of tendons, and inflammation in the AC Joint (Magee, 2008). The patient elevates the arm forward from the neutral anatomic position. Pain upon passive forward flexion that causes the greater tuberosity of the humerus to jam against the underside of the acromion is noted as a positive Neer sign. For the Hawkins test, the examiner forward-flexes the patient's arm to 90 degrees and medially rotates the shoulder forcibly. Evidence of pain indicates a positive test for supraspinatus tendinosis/tendinitis or impingement (Magee, 2008).

CHAPTER 3

The *Lidocaine injection test* is performed to confirm rotator cuff tendinitis and to exclude rotator cuff tear or GH joint involvement. This is conducted on the patient with severe pain and guarding on examination. Anesthetizing the subacromial space assists in a more accurate examination of shoulder function (Anderson, 2006). This test is commonly performed by trained Registered Nurse Practitioners.

The following special testing maneuvers assess muscle-tendon pathology:

- The *Speeds test* detects potential bursitis, tendinitis, or tendon tears, especially of the biceps tendon (Magee, 2008) by stressing the biceps tendon in the bicipital groove. The patient is seated with the elbow in full extension, the forearm supinated, and the arm forward-flexed 45 degrees while the patient resists the examiner pushing downward at the wrist. Pain or tenderness at the bicipital groove indicates bicipital tendinitis.
- The *Yergason test* checks the transverse humeral ligament's ability to maintain position of the biceps tendon in the bicipital groove. The patient flexes the elbow to 90 degrees, holds the arm against the side with the forearm supinated while the examiner resists the patient's attempt to pronate the forearm.
- The *empty can test* measures rotator cuff pathology and is highly specific and sensitive to identifying partial and full tears of the supraspinatus tendon. The patient rotates the upper arm with the thumb pointing towards the floor. The arm is raised to 30 degrees of forward flexion and 90 degrees of abduction against resistance by the examiner. Unilateral weakness is a positive test finding (Magee, 2008).
- The *lift off maneuver* tests the muscle strength of the subscapularis and is highly predictive test of a subscapularis rupture. It is performed with the patient seated or standing, and the arm internally rotated behind the back. The patient is asked to lift the forearm off the back against the examiner's resistance. Inability to lift the dorsum of the hand off the back is a positive sign suggesting pathology (Bowen, 2006).
- The *drop arm test* is specific and sensitive for evaluating tears and inflammation of the rotator cuff (Magee, 2008). The examiner stands behind the patient and instructs the patient to abduct arms as high as possible. The patient then slowly lowers the arm while the examiner watches for a sudden drop of the arm, which indicates a probable tear of the rotator cuff. This test is incorporated into the shoulder abduction active ROM assessment.

Diagnostics. The three standard x-ray views of the shoulder are the anteroposterior view (AP) in internal and external rotation, lateral or scapular Y view, and axillary view. Posterior dislocations are best seen on the axillary and Y views. A forth view, the posterior oblique view, is useful to fully depict the GH joint (Child, 2007). Stress views to assess AC ligament disruption may be ordered, although they seldom influence treatment management. Undiagnosed mechanical problems or painful arc syndromes of the shoulder can be further examined by CT or MRI scans. A CT scan may be indicated to determine extent of fracture. Suspected rotator cuff tears can be confirmed with MRI, arthrogram, or MRI arthrogram.

Elbow

History. (See Chapter 2—Anatomy & Physiology, Chapter 14—Trauma, and Chapter 19—The Elbow.) Insidious onset of elbow symptoms with weakness and or pain necessitates an examination of the C-spine in addition to the elbow. Information specific to age, occupation, mechanism of injury, and changes in sensation of the upper extremity are essential in evaluating elbow complaints.

Inspection. As the patient enters the examining room, observe posture and carrying angle of the elbow. The patient's overall gait should be smooth, with arms moving in tandem. Expose both arms for comparison. Observe the patient in an anatomic position with the elbow fully extended and the forearm fully supinated to evaluate the carrying angle of the elbow. The normal carrying angle at the elbow is 5 degrees of valgus deformity in males and greater than 15 degrees in females (Magee, 2008). A carrying angle less than 5-10 degrees, cubitus varus, is also known as a gunstock deformity. A carrying angle greater than 15 degrees is called cubitus valgus. Observe the elbow for scars, deformity, contusion, and swelling. The absence of hollow areas on either side of the elbow may indicate a joint effusion, especially if the elbow is being held protectively in a semiflexed position (Magee, 2008). Swelling at the tip of the olecranon indicates infectious or inflammatory bursitis and/or gout.

Palpation. Pinpointing the exact area of tenderness is a key component to palpating the elbow as it aids in identification of pathology. (Easily palpated landmarks are described in Chapter 2—Anatomy & Physiology.) Palpation of bony landmarks includes the lateral epicondyle, radial head, medial epicondyle, olecronon process of the ulna, and olecronon fossa. Soft tissue is palpated with elbow flexed to 90 degrees and fully extended while supinating and pronating the forearm (Child, 2007). Anterior soft tissue structures of elbow include the biceps tendon, brachial artery, median nerves, and musculocutaneous nerves. Posterior soft tissue structures include the olecranon bursa and the triceps muscle. Laterally, the lateral collateral ligament, annular ligament, brachioradialis muscle, and wrist extensors are palpated. Medially palpated are the wrist flexor/pronator, the supracondylar lymph nodes, and the ulnar nerve (the soft tissue that lies in the sulcus between the olecranon and the medial epicondyle).

Motion. (See Table 3.3 for normal elbow motion.) Elbow motion includes active, passive, and resisted extension, flexion, supination, and pronation. (Resisted motion will be presented in the "Strength Testing" section.) Evaluating flexion includes assessment of muscle mass and tendon approximation in the arm and forearm. Normal ROM of the elbow rules out the likelihood of joint abnormality. ROM is rarely affected by bursitis or epicondylitis (Anderson, 2006).

Active flexion occurs as the patient flexes the elbow and touches the same shoulder with the hand. Active supination is assessed as the patient flexes the elbow to 90 degrees with arms held close to the body with a closed fist palm down. The patient is then asked to rotate wrist so palm points upward. Active pronation is evaluated with the patient in same position as for evaluating supination except the fist is closed with the palm up. The patient is then asked to rotate the wrist so the palm points downward.

Passive ROM occurs as the patient is assisted through the elbow's full range only if unable to independently complete the range. Passive flexion and extension is assessed with the elbow flexed and extended, while the examiner supports the wrist and cups the elbow. Passive supination and pronation occurs as the examiner supports the elbow with one hand and assumes the "shake hands" position; gently rotate the wrist so the palm faces up and then faces downward.

Strength Testing. Resistance to active ROM is tested with the patient seated or standing. Resistance to elbow flexion is evaluated with the forearm in a neutral position. Resisted supination and pronation occur with the elbow flexed 90 degrees. Pain with resisted elbow flexion is usually due to biceps involvement, while pain with resisted extension is often due to triceps pathology (Dutton, 2008). Supinator function is isolated by having the patient resist supination with the elbow fully extended. (The forearm muscles and their associated nerve innervations, which contribute to motor function in the elbow, are detailed in Chapter 2—Anatomy & Physiology.)

Sensory Testing. (See Table 3.13 for nerve roots supplying sensation to the arm and forearm.) The three main nerves found close to the elbow include the median, radial, and ulnar nerves. The ulnar nerve originating from C7-C8 is the most likely to be injured, compressed, or overstretched in the elbow. The radial nerve originates from C5-C8 and innervates all extensor muscles of the elbow, wrist, and fingers. The median nerve originates in cervical root levels C6-T1 and lies anterior to the elbow joint. Radial and medial nerve injuries near the elbow are associated with fractures of the distal humerus (Magee, 2008). Deep tendon reflexes in the elbow include the biceps aponeurosis and triceps tendon.

Table 3.13. Sensory Testing of the Elbow

Nerve Root	Sensation
C5	Lateral arm
C6	Lateral forearm
C7	Medial forearm
T1	Medial arm

From Core Currriculum for Orthopaedic Nursing *(6th ed., p. 54) by NAON, 2007, Boston, MA: Pearson. Reproduced with permission.*

Special Elbow Tests. Special tests are done to evaluate the elbow for ligament laxity and instability, nerve conduction, circulatory compromise, or inflammation at the condyles of the distal humerus. Entrapment or lesions of the median, radial, or ulnar nerves may be evaluated with nerve conduction studies. Ligament laxity is assessed using varus and valgus stress test maneuvers across the slightly flexed elbow to determine stability of medial and lateral collateral ligaments of the elbow. The examiner cups the elbow with one hand, using the thumb and index fingers as a fulcrum, and gently moves the forearm medially and laterally by holding the wrist. Ligament laxity is present if any gapping is palpated.

The presence of a nerve lesion or neuroma can be detected by tapping the area between olecranon and medial condyle to elicit tenderness over a possible neuroma within the ulnar nerve. If a neuroma is present, the patient will experience a tingling sensation along the ulnar nerve distribution to the hand (Cipriano, 2003).

Testing for inflammation at the medial and or lateral condyles of the distal humerus is performed with specific maneuvers relative to the location of pain. Lateral epicondyle pain is evaluated by first stabilizing the patient's elbow with the examiner's thumb resting on the lateral epicondyle. The patient makes a fist, pronates the forearm, and radially deviates and extends the wrist against the examiners resistance (Magee, 2008). To evaluate pain at the medial epicondyle, the examiner palpates the medial epicondyle with one hand, passively supinates the forearm, and extends the elbow while grasping the patient's wrist (Magee, 2008).

The olecranon bursa fluid is aspirated and tested to rule out infection, gout, inflammation, and hemarthrosis. Radiographs are ordered if fracture or dislocation of the elbow is suspected.

Hand and Wrist

History. (See Chapter 2—Anatomy & Physiology, Chapter 15—Trauma, and Chapter 20—The Hand & Wrist.) Evaluation of hand and wrist pain begins with questions that identify a history of either overuse or trauma using the OLD CART history-taking format (see Table 3.2). Determining the onset and length of time that symptoms have persisted, along with limitations in performing ADLs, aids in determining the functional limitations and sense of urgency required in evaluation and treatment of symptoms. Additionally, age makes certain conditions more or less likely. For example, persons older than age 40 with hand and wrist complaints are more likely to have degenerative conditions of joints and tendons. The dominant hand is more likely to be injured, and the functional loss in patients with dominant hand injuries initially is greater than for those who injure the nondominant hand. The more common conditions of the hand and wrist, as reported by Anderson (2006), include tendon pathology, ligament injuries, carpal tunnel syndrome, degenerative joint disease (DJD, or osteoarthritis), ganglions, and wrist sprains and fractures of the scaphoid (navicular) bone.

Inspection. While inspecting the anterior and posterior hand, forearm, and wrist, note the patient's willingness and ability to use the hand, and observe the "attitude" of the hand and fingers (their position at rest). In the normal resting position, the fingers are progressively more flexed moving from the radial side of the hand to the ulnar side (Magee, 2008). Both hands are compared throughout the examination. Observing active and passive joint motion is part of the inspection, noting the quality of movement. The dominant hand is usually larger than the nondominant. Begin the exam by having the patient place both hands in the lap with palms facing upward while looking for muscle wasting, webbing, ecchymosis, edema, and presence of sweat (absence of sweat could be indicative of nerve damage). Next, ask the patient to place the palms down to ascertain color, presence of hair on fingers, muscle wasting, joint deformity, alignment, presence of edema, or shiny skin. Color changes of significance include pallor and cyanosis (which may indicate decreased tissue oxygenation) and redness and erythema (which may indicate infection). The condition and color of fingernails and presence of onychomycosis (or fungal infection) is also noted.

Palpation. Palpation of the hand and wrist is directed to the area of perceived pathology in an attempt to localize injury. Palpation must follow a logical, consistent pattern to avoid overlooking important structures. The anterior or palmer surface assessment includes the fleshy thenar and hypthothenar areas near the base of the thumb, carpal tunnel, six wrist and digit flexor tendons, the hook of the hamate and pisiform carpal bones, and radial and ulnar pulses. (See "Special Hand/Wrist Tests" for evaluating Kanavel signs.) Soft tissue structures should be assessed for pain and deformity.

The dorsal wrist allows easier palpation than the palmer aspect. The ulnar styloid process is the most prominent dorsal feature in a normal wrist. The scaphoid bone can be palpated at the "anatomic snuff box," the depression noted on the dorsal surface of the hand at the base of the thumb. Tenderness at this site is classic for a scaphoid fracture. Near the tip of the radial styloid are the extensor pollicis brevis, extensor pollicis longus, and adductor pollicis tendons. Tenderness at their insertion and a positive Phalens test is suggestive of tenosynovitis (see "Special Hand/Wrist Tests"). Bony structures in the dorsal wrist include the lunate, capitates, and 3rd metacarpal base.

Motion. (See Table 3.3 for normal upper extremity joint ROM.) The presence of finger or wrist pain always warrants an evaluation of both active and passive motion. ROM can be measured with a goniometer (see Figure 3.1). Difficulty with active ROM is an indication for further passive ROM testing. Pain with passive stretch of a finger, in the presence of swelling and tenderness along a flexor tendon sheath, is suggestive of an infection of the flexor tendon.

Evaluation of active finger flexion and extension occurs with the wrist in a neutral position as the patient bends and straightens each metacarpal phalangeal (MCP) joint of each individual finger and thumb. The MCP joint is held in neutral as the interphalangeal and distal phalangeal joint is flexed one finger at a time while holding adjoining fingers in extension. Testing of active abduction and adduction occurs as the patient spreads the fingers as far apart as possible and then returns them to the neutral position. To evaluate active thumb movement, the patient moves the thumb across the palm to touch pad at the base of the little finger, spread the thumb as far from hand as possible, and touch thumb to each of the fingertips to test opposition.

To evaluate active wrist flexion and extension, the examiner stabilizes the forearm while the patient flexes and extends the wrist. Active ulnar and radial deviation is assessed with the patient rotating the hand side to side while the examiner stabilizes the forearm close to the wrist. Supination and pronation motions are the same as for the elbow.

Strength Testing. Strength is tested by applying resistance to active motions described above and comparing graded results to the opposite extremity. Hand grip strength is also tested using the dynometer, a hand-held mechanical device (Magee, 2008). To test strength associated with active finger extension, stabilize the wrist in neutral position while trying to force fingers into flexion with pressure on the dorsum of the PIP joint. Testing resistance to finger flexion occurs as the examiner tries to force fingers out of flexion. Resistance to active finger abduction occurs as the patient spreads the fingers, attempting to prevent the examiner from bringing them together. Resistance to active finger adduction is tested by placing a piece of paper between thumb and index finger and asking the patient to squeeze the paper tightly as the examiner attempts to pull the paper away. This maneuver is repeated for all fingers. To test resistance to thumb flexion, the patient touches the hypothenar eminence (the prominent fleshy part of the palm above the base of the little finger) with his/her thumb, while the examiner's thumb is hooked around patient's to pull it out of flexion.

Strength with active thumb extension is tested with resistance to thumb extension. Resisted active thumb abduction occurs with the metacarpal joints stabilized first and then pressure against the thumb pushing toward the palm. The thumb and wrist are stabilized before testing resistance to thumb adduction, which occurs as the thumb and index finger pinch to make an "o" while the examiner tries to break the circle. Thumb opposition is tested with the thumb and little finger pinched together while the examiner tries to pull apart the connection.

Sensory Testing. Table 3.14 identifies the individual nerve roots that supply sensation to the hand and wrist. Diminished sensation to light touch can be further evaluated by testing the patient's ability, without looking, to identify pressure along a sensory nerve via 2-point discrimination, a simple test where two objects (such as a caliper or two ends of a bent paper clip) are applied adjacent to one another simultaneously. The distance between the two points is measured. The ability to identify two points 6 millimeters apart or less is normal.

Table 3.14. Sensory Testing of the Hand and Wrist

Nerve Root	Sensation
C6	Thumb, index, and half of the middle finger
C7	Middle finger
C8 and T1	Ring and little finger

From Core Currriculum for Orthopaedic Nursing *(6th ed., p. 56) by NAON, 2007, Boston, MA: Pearson. Reproduced with permission.*

Special Hand/Wrist Tests. The common orthopaedic hand and wrist tests are described below. These tests identify problems using specific maneuvers designed to assess blood flow, tendon pathology, ligament laxity, and nerve compression in the hand and wrist.

The *Allen test* evaluates blood supply to the volar arch within the hand. The patient opens and closes the hand several times, pumping blood to the hand. With the hand closed in a fist, the examiner applies pressure to the radial and ulnar arteries, momentarily occluding the blood supply. As the patient opens the hand, pressure is released from the ulnar artery. The hand should flush immediately. If it does not, the ulnar artery may be impaired.

The *Finkelstein test* assesses for de Quervain's syndrome, tenosynovitis of the tendons that extend and adduct the thumb. The patient makes a fist with the thumb inside while the examiner stabilizes the forearm. The wrist actively deviates toward the ulnar side. The test is positive if this maneuver elicits pain.

Kanavel signs include the four cardinal signs of an acute infection of flexor tendons of the hand: 1.) Pain with passive extension of the digit; 2). Flexed position of the digit at rest; 3.) Symmetric swelling of the digit, which may extend to the palm; and 4.) Tenderness with palpation along the flexor tendon sheath (Bednar, 2006).

The *Phalens test* evaluates for carpal tunnel syndrome, which is the result of median nerve compression at the wrist. The patient pushes the dorsal surface of both wrists together for at least 1 minute. The generation of tingling in the first three fingers and radial side of ring finger indicates the probable presence of carpal tunnel syndrome.

Tinel's sign also tests for carpel tunnel syndrome. A positive Tinel's sign is elicited by gently tapping the volar surface of the wrist. A subsequent "tingling" sensation in the medial nerve distribution suggests carpal tunnel syndrome.

Trousseau's sign is assessed by inflating a blood pressure cuff on the patient's arm, creating enough pressure to stop venous circulation for 1-5 minutes. Contractions of the fingers and hands, collectively referred to as carpopedal spasms, indicate the presence of tetany.

Ligament, capsule, and joint instability tests are performed on both sides to compare differences. The application of valgus stress across the thumb, with MCP in extension and again in 30 degrees of flexion, is done to assess the ulnar collateral ligament for partial or complete tear. The examiner grasps the thumb proximal to the joint to eliminate MCP rotation and avoid a false interpretation (Agesen, 2006). A difference in laxity greater than 15 degrees between the two sides suggest partial tear and greater than 30 degrees suggests a complete tear or rupture of the ligament. Substantial differences between sides indicate the presence of "Gamekeeper's Thumb," commonly seen with a history of forced thumb abduction through trauma or repetitive overuse (Magee, 2008).

Diagnostics. Radiographs are indicated if the patient has a history of trauma or if the patient demonstrates painful joint swelling or point tenderness overlying a bone. A routine series of wrist radiographs includes the AP, true lateral, and scaphoid views. X-rays of individual fingers include AP and lateral views, plus scaphoid views for patients with a known trauma and point tenderness over the scaphoid bone. Other possible x-ray views include carpal tunnel, clenched fist, radial, and ulnar deviation views.

Bone scans should be considered for patients with unexplained diffuse hand or wrist pain, swelling, and discoloration, which suggest possible infection, fracture, or reflex sympathetic dystrophy, also known as complex regional pain syndrome.

Arthrograms assist in confirming ligamentous or fibrocartilage injury in the wrist; however, they are less specific and less sensitive than CT and MRI. CT enables highly specific three-dimensional views of bone and soft tissue. MRI is the best option for visualizing soft tissue in the hand. MRI and bone scans of the wrist are able to detect scaphoid fractures earlier than traditional radiographs.

Nerve conduction studies are indicated for patients with advanced carpal tunnel symptoms involving motor weakness and atrophy (Anderson, 2006). Translumenation along with palpation over a dorsal wrist soft tissue mass along a tendon confirms the presence of ganglion cyst (Anderson, 2006).

Hip

History. (See Chapter 2—Anatomy & Physiology, Chapter 14—Trauma, and Chapter 21—The Hip, Femur, & Pelvis.) Hip function and limitations in daily activities are included in the assessment. Assess for patient's ability to walk, ascend and descend stairs, tie shoes, perform foot hygiene, and rise from a seated position unassisted. The driving questions that guide the hip examination are related to patient age and the presentation of symptoms. The character, location, and description of pain are key elements in developing differential diagnosis for hip pain (Anderson, 2006). Groin pain suggests hip joint involvement, whereas lateral thigh pain is related to trochanteric bursitis and paresthetica meralgis. Diffuse posterior hip pain is the least common hip pain presentation and is often referred pain from the gluteus medius bursa, lumbar sacral joint, and lumbosacral spine. Pain related to trauma with abnormal physical findings is suggestive of a fracture and warrants diagnostic radiographs.

The most common outpatient hip problems are related to bursitis, arthritis, avascular necroses of the hip, fractures, metastatic disease, vascular occlusions, and or referred pain from the low back (Anderson, 2006). Trauma related hip pain in the elderly is highly suggestive of a hip fracture. Younger patients with trauma-induced hip pain in the absence of fracture are suspect for hip labral tears. Structures adjacent to the hip (such as the lumbar spine, knee, lower gastrointestinal, and reproductive tract) should be evaluated as sources for referred pain.

Inspection. The initial exam begins by observing the patient's gait and posture while standing. The use of ambulatory aids should be noted. The alignment of the lower extremity should be observed for excessive external or internal rotation (Krabak, 2006). According to Child (2007), the following observations could warrant emergency care: a shortened and internally rotated leg (a sign of a possible hip dislocation) and a shortened externally rotated leg (suspicious for hip fracture). This is especially true in elderly patients with a history of trauma. In the peripubescent child, a painful limp is a red flag for a slipped capitofemeral epiphysis (SCFE) (Child, 2007). The infant or young child should be examined for the presence of a congenitally dislocated hip. Abnormal gait (Table 3.8) may result from specific deficits related to muscle weakness. In the supine position, legs should be of near-equal length and in slight external rotation. In the standing position, hips and gluteal folds should appear symmetric. Examine the skin for possible bruising, or gross deformity.

Palpation. With the patient in supine position, palpate the anterior superior iliac spines, iliac crests, iliac tubercles, greater trochanters, and symphysis pubis. Abduct the hip and flex the knees so that the lower extremity crosses the opposite knee. This should allow full visualization of the area known as the "femoral triangle." There are three main structures in this area that should be palpated: the inguinal ligament, the sartorius muscle, and the adductor longus muscle. Next, palpate the femoral pulse. (The femoral nerve and vein are also in this area but are not palpable.) While the patient remains supine, palpate the iliopsoas, sartorius, and rectus femoris (hip flexors). Then palpate the medial hip adductors, the gracilis, the pectineus, the adductor brevis, and the adductor magnus.

With the patient prone, feel the superior iliac spines, the greater trochanters, the ischial tuberosities, and the sacroiliac joint, noting the presence of pain, swelling, or asymmetry. The sacral iliac (SI) joint is examined for pain or tenderness with the knee flexed 90 degrees and hip rotated externally.

With the patient side-lying, palpate the greater trochanter for increased skin temperature, the presence of pain, and a palpable trochanteric bursa. The ischeal tuberosity is palpated distal to the gluteal fold while side-lying with the hip flexed. Lateral muscles palpated include the gluteus medius, the gluteus maximus, and hamstrings (hip extensors).

Motion. The patient should be guided through the full range of active hip movements:

- *Active abduction.* Ask the patient to stand and spread the legs as far apart as possible. Be prepared to steady the patient.
- *Active adduction:* Ask the patient to cross one leg over the other while keeping the knee straight.
- *Active flexion.* Ask the patient to draw each knee up to the chest while lying supine.

- *Active extension.* Ask the patient to stand up from a seated position without using hands.
- *Active flexion and adduction.* Ask the patient to cross one leg over the other at the thigh in a seated position.
- *Active flexion, abduction, and external rotation:* Ask the patient, in a seated position, to place the lateral side of foot on top of the opposite knee.
- *Active internal and external rotation.* Ask the patient, while in supine position, to roll the legs so that the toes point in (internal) and then out (external).

Assist patient through the range of *passive* hip movements only if the active ROM was not full or if end-point resistance is not appreciated with resisted active motion. The passive movements are performed the same way as the active movements. All movements are performed with the patient supine except passive extension, which occurs with the patient prone. The pelvis should not move during testing of hip motion. The pelvis is stabilized by the examiner placing one hand on the opposite hip being examined. Passive extension may be limited by the presence of hip contractures. Passive abduction and adduction is also tested while stabilizing the pelvis. Passive internal and external rotation testing occurs with the legs extended while the examiner grasps above the ankle and rolls the leg inward (internal) and outward (external), noting the position of the patella as the movement is carried out. This should not be tested if the patient has had a total hip arthroplasty or hip prosthesis.

Strength Testing. Resisted isometric movements are performed to test strength in the flexors, extenders, adductors, abductors, and rotators of the hip, as well as in the extensors and flexors of the knee. This is done during ROM testing. The patient is instructed to resist the examiner's attempt to move the hip and knee, noting which motions cause pain or demonstrate weakness. See "Palpation" for descriptions of specific hip muscles and their motion.

Table 3.15. Sensory Testing of the Hip

Nerve Root	Sensation
T10	Transverse, slightly oblique band at the level of the umbilicus
T11	Transverse, slightly oblique band at the level between T10 and T12
T12	Transverse, slightly oblique band at the level above the inguinal ligament
L1	Lies below the inguinal ligament, parallel to the upper anterior portion of the thigh
L2	Lies below L1 area and most of the anterior thigh
L3	Knee including above and below the patella
Cluneal (L1, L2, L3)	Over the iliac crest between the posterior, suprailiac spine, the iliac tubercle, and the gluteus maximus

From Core Currriculum for Orthopaedic Nursing (6th ed., p. 61) by NAON, 2007, Boston, MA: Pearson. Reproduced with permission.

Sensory Testing. Using a sharp object, lightly prick the skin and document the patient's response over cutaneous nerve distribution in the hip and leg. Cutaneous sensory testing is done overlying anatomic structures, and correlates to the thoracic and lumbar nerve roots included in Table 3.15.

Special Hip Tests. In addition to grading strength during active resistance to motion, other tests have been designed to assess tightness or pathology in the muscles of the hip. Recent studies indicate that the commonly conducted Thompsons, FABERE, and Ober tests lack evidence to support their reliability, specificity, and sensitivity (Krabak, 2006).

The *Thompsons test* assesses flexion contractures in the hip. The patient is evaluated in supine position with the pelvis stabilized. The patient actively flexes the uninvolved hip to the chest, while the examiner observes the opposite leg. If opposite leg lifts off the examination table, a flexion contracture is present. The amount of flexion contracture is determined by measuring the angle between the posterior thigh and the table with a goniometer (see Figure 3.1) (Krabak, 2006).

FABERE (Patrick's) tests assess for evidence of pathology through Flexion, Abduction, External Rotation, and Extension of the hip. This positioning applies compressive forces to the cartilage of the hip. A positive text elicits pain and most likely indicates hip arthritis (Krabak, 2006).

A positive *Ober test* indicates a contracture of the illiotibial band or tensor fascia lata (Child, 2007). The patient is positioned side-lying with the involved leg up and the hip and knee flexed for stability. The leg is passively abducted, and the examiner slowly lowers the limb. Normally the leg should drop into an adducted position. If the leg remains abducted, the test is positive.

The *Trendelenberg test* evaluates the strength of the gluteus medius muscle. While standing behind patient, the examiner observes the dimples over the posterior iliac spines. The level of those dimples should be equal if the patient's weight is evenly distributed. When standing erect, the gluteus medius muscle should contract as the foot leaves the floor. When the pelvis is elevated on the unsupported side, the test is negative. If the pelvis on the unsupported side remains in position or descends, and the gluteal folds drop, the muscle is not functioning (a positive test result) (Krabak, 2006).

All newborns are screened with a *congenital dislocated hip test.* Congenital dislocated hip has two characteristics: abduction is limited on the involved side, and telescoping occurs when traction is applied to the knee. Abduction is tested in the supine position, with the infant's hips flexed to 90 degrees and abducted. Normal abduction is 90 degrees. Limited abduction of 20 degrees is an indication of abduction contracture (Magee, 2008).

The *Ortolani test* determines infant hip laxity in the first few weeks after birth. With the infant supine, the examiner flexes the hips while grasping the legs with the thumb against the inside of the knees and thighs, and the fingers placed on the outside of thigh and buttock. The thighs are gently abducted to reduce the hip. The examiner may feel or hear a click or clunk when abducting, as the femoral head relocates and slides over the acetabular rim. This crepitus indicates a positive test and that hip is reducible. The test is not accurate in a dislocated hip that is nonreducible (Magee, 2008).

Barlow's maneuver assesses the potential for the hip to dislocate in an infant up to 6 months of age (Child, 2007). Both the hip and knee is flexed to 90 degrees with the infant supine. Each hip is examined individually while examiner's other hand steadies the opposite femur. The examiner grasps the leg with the middle finger placed over the greater trochanter and the thumb along the inner knee and thigh. The hip is then abducted as the middle finger applies forward pressure against the greater trochanter. If the hip reduces (the femoral head slides into the acetabulum), a click or clunk may be heard or felt, indicating that the hip was dislocated (a positive test). This part of the exam is the same as the Ortolani test. Next, the examiner applies posterior pressure with the thumb against the thigh in an attempt to posteriorly dislocate the hip. If the hip relocates as pressure is removed, the hip is classified as unstable (Child, 2007). The sequence is gently repeated 1-2 times to establish the degree of laxity. This should not be repeated too often, however, as this may cause damage to or dislocate the femoral head.

Galeazzi's or Alli sign determines unilateral congenital dislocated hip in the 3-18 month old child. The child lies supine with the hips and knees flexed to 90 degrees and feet placed on the exam table. If one knee is higher than the other, the test is positive (Magee, 2008).

The child with a dislocated hip demonstrates a positive *telescoping sign*. The child is placed supine with the hip and knee flexed to 90 degrees. The examiner's hand is placed over the greater trochanter to detect movement as the femur is pushed backward toward the table and then forward away from the table. There is little movement with this action in a normal hip. Excessive motion indicates a positive telescoping sign (Magee, 2008).

The *leg length discrepancy test* determines if one leg is shorter than the other and whether the shortness occurs above or below the knee. A leg length difference of 1.5cm or less is considered normal. True leg length measurements are taken first with the patient lying supine, using a tape measure to measure from the anterior iliac spine to the medial malleolus. Apparent leg length measurements assess for functional shortening of the limb, which occurs as an adaptation to pathology or contracture in the spine, pelvis, or lower limb in the patient with equal bone lengths. After the test for true leg length measurement is complete, the patient is measured from the umbilicus to the medial malleolus. This method uses a nonfixed point (umbilicus) to a bony fixed land mark (medial malleolus). If the measurement of true leg length is equal and the apparent leg length is unequal, functional leg length discrepancy is present (Magee, 2008). Leg length asymmetry may also be determined visually at the same time as the true leg length test. With the patient supine, flex the knees so the malleoli are level, with the feet flat on the examination table. Note the level of the patellae. If one knee projects farther anteriorly than the other, the femur is the site of the discrepancy. If one knee is higher than the other, the tibia is the site of the discrepancy (Magee, 2008).

Diagnostics. Standard radiographic views of the hip include AP and axial (or "frog leg") views. Weight-bearing x-rays are indicated when full visualization of the joint space is necessary, as in ruling out DJD or when assessing leg length discrepancy. MRI may detect a hip fracture before it is evident on standard x-rays. The MRI arthrogram detects tears of the hip labrum and other soft tissue structures of the hip such as tendons and muscles.

Knee

History. (See Chapter 2—Anatomy & Physiology, Chapter 15—Trauma, and Chapter 22—The Knee.) The presence of knee pain associated with trauma requires an in-depth line of questioning related to the mechanism of the injury in determining a diagnosis. Magee (2008) suggests the following questions: Did the injury occur while suddenly accelerating or decelerating after moving at a constant speed? Was an audible pop heard? Did it occur while bearing weight and rotating the leg? Was it from a direct blow to the knee medially, laterally, or anteriorly? Knowing the timing of the injury and the onset of symptoms associated with the injury aids in developing a diagnosis. For example, swelling in the knee immediately following an injury signifies trauma within the joint rather than external to the joint. Inquire about functional limitations associated with the injury such as difficulty kneeling, cutting, pivoting, twisting, climbing, or straightening the leg due to catching or locking.

Questions of pain unrelated to trauma include those from the OLD CART line of questioning (see Table 3.2), as well as the following questions:

- Is pain worse after sitting for long periods of time? This indicates DJD and is described as a positive theater sign.
- Has this knee been previously injured? A prior injury may be the underlying cause of a new onset of pain.
- Do medications relieve symptoms? Pain relieved by anti-inflammatory medications may result from an inflammatory response, while pain unrelieved by narcotics may signify a more serious condition.
- Is there pain at rest or during the night? In the absence of a trauma, this pain may indicate an underlying arthritic condition or a malignancy.

Inspection. Observe the patient entering the exam room, noting gait and posture while standing, sitting, and lying down. If possible, observe ability to undress and whether the patient uses any strategies to make ADLs easier. Inspect the knees from all sides, noting alignment and symmetry, edema, atrophy, effusion, scars, and skin color changes. Note the presence of genu valgus (knock-knees), genu varus (bowlegs), or recurvatum (pushed-back) deformities. Assess alignment with the medial ankles positioned as close together as possible. Note the position of the patella in flexion and extension.

Palpation. It is best to place the knee in both extension and flexion during palpation. Palpate for abnormal swelling, tenderness, deformities, and temperature differences.

The following anterior structures should be palpated with the knee in extension: patella, associated patella, and infrapatellar tendons; patella, prepatella, and pes anserine bursa; peripatella areas; retinaculum, and quadriceps muscles; medial collateral ligament (MCL) and bony landmarks. Anterior bony landmarks include the anterior tibial tubercle, medial tibial condyle, adductor tubericle, and head of the fibula. The patella should be mobile without pain or guarding, and without ballotable fluid in the peripatella areas.

Meniscus tears are best palpated with the knee flexed 45 degrees, whereas the joint line is best palpated at 90 degrees of flexion. Flexing the knee slightly relaxes the knee and can be done with a folded towel behind the knee with the patient supine.

Anterior palpation continues with the knee in flexion, palpating the tibial femoral joint line, tibial plateau, femoral condlyes, and adductor muscles. Palpation of the lateral collateral ligament (LCL) is best accomplished with the knee flexed to 90 degrees, either sitting or lying supine, with the knee in varus position and the ankle resting on the opposite knee (Magee, 2008). Additional structures in the lateral knee include the joint line overlying the meniscus, anterior superior tibial fibular ligament, fibula head, and tendon attachments. The structures in the posterior knee, including hamstrings, gastocenemius muscle, popliteal artery, and lymph nodes, are examined in prone position. Tenderness and swelling posteriorly signify a Baker's cyst, commonly found in arthritic knee joints (Magee, 2008).

Motion. To assess active flexion, the patient performs a deep knee bend from standing, with the examiner prepared to steady the patient if needed. While sitting at the edge of the examination table, the patient fully extends the legs to assess active extension. Active internal and external rotation is observed with the patient seated on examination while internally and externally rotating the foot.

The patient is assisted through ROM only if unable to complete active ROM. Passive flexion and extension is tested with the patient seated at the edge of the examination table. Placing one hand on the ankle and the other supporting the knee, the examiner gently flexes the knee as far as possible. For passive extension testing, the examiner places one hand on the patient's thigh above the knee to stabilize the leg and pulls the leg out with the other hand at the ankle to fully extend the patient's leg. To assess passive internal and external rotation while the patient is seated, the examiner places a hand on the patient's thigh just above the knee to stabilize the femur, grasps patient's ankle, and gently rotates the tibia inward and outward.

Strength Testing. Muscles responsible for internal and external rotation cannot be separated for individual strength testing. (See Chapter 2—Anatomy & Physiology for muscles, lumbar nerve roots, and DTR in the knee associated with movement in the lower leg.) With the patient seated at edge of the exam table, the examiner applies resistance to the patient's calf while the patient attempts to actively flex and extend the knee. With the patient lying prone on the examination table, the examiner places a stabilizing hand on the patient's thigh and applies gentle resistance to the hamstrings and at the ankle joint, while the patient flexes the knee as if to try to lift leg off the table.

Sensory Testing. (See Chapter 2—Anatomy & Physiology for a discussion of the lumbar spine roots and DTR responsible for sensation and movement in the knee.) Using a sharp object, lightly prick the skin over the patient's knee and document the response to assess cutaneous nerve distribution in the knee. See Table 3.16 for sensory nerve testing in the knee.

Special Knee Tests. Special tests evaluate the knee joint for plane and rotational injuries of the ligaments, meniscus injury, and evidence of an effusion. The unaffected knee should be tested first to establish a

Table 3.16. Sensory Testing of the Knee

Nerve Root	Reflex	Sensation
L2		Lies below L1 area
L3		Lies above and below the patella
L4	Patellar or quadriceps	Anterior and posterior portion of medial knee, down the leg medially. The infrapatella branch of the saphenous nerve is the only sensory branch of the femoral nerve that continues in the leg. Often cut during surgical removal of the medial meniscus.
S2	None	A strip down the midline of the posterior thigh, covering the popliteal bursa and supplied by the posterior femoral cutaneous nerve.

From Core Currriculum for Orthopaedic Nursing *(6th ed., p. 64) by NAON, 2007, Boston, MA: Pearson. Reproduced with permission.*

baseline and to prepare the patient for what to expect when examining the affected knee. Muscles must be relaxed for tests to be valid. Resting the knee over a folded towel or pillow will assist in relaxing the knee in a slightly flexed position. Differences between knees of 3mm or more are considered abnormal.

Ligament testing: An intact ligament has an abrupt end point or stop. Ligament instability testing is less accurate in an acutely injured painful knee unless the knee is anesthetized (Magee, 2008). The best indicator of anterior cruciate ligament (ACL) injury is the Lachman test, which is done with the patient lying supine and the examiner holding the patient's knee between full extension and 30 degrees of flexion One hand stabilizes the femur while the other grasps the proximal tibia and pulls forward. A positive sign is appreciated with a soft end point or "mushy" feel when the tibia is moved forward on the femur. Modified versions of the Lachman test occur with the patient seated at the edge of the exam table, the femur stabilized with examiner's hand holding the thigh against the examination table, the patient's foot held between the examiner's knee, and the patient's knee flexed 25 degrees. Anterior translation force is applied with the examiner's other hand to the tibia.

The *anterior drawer sign* is a test for anterior or posterior ligament instabilities. The supine patient's knee is flexed to 90 degrees and the hip flexed to 45 degree. The patient's foot is placed on the exam table with the examiner holding it in place by leaning on the top of the foot to eliminate forward slide of the foot while the knees remain flexed between 60 and 90 degrees. The examiner cups the knee, placing the thumbs on the medial and lateral joint lines as the rest of the fingers grasp the posterior aspect of the knee. The tibia is gently pulled forward. If excessive forward movement of the tibia is observed or felt, the anterior drawer test is positive for probable ACL compromise (Magee, 2008).

The *posterior drawer test* indicates posterior cruciate ligament (PCL) compromise. Testing occurs in the same position as for ACL testing; however, the tibia is gently pushed backward onto the femur to assess for posterior motion. Other indications of a PCL tear include the presence of a step-off or sulcus observed at the anterior knee joint line when the knee is flexed 90-110 degrees: the tibia drops backward or sags posteriorly as compared to the unaffected knee held in the same position with feet flat on exam table. This same phenomenon occurs when the affected leg is lifted in extension and the knee sags into a "back knee" position (Magee, 2008).

The medial collateral ligament (MCL) is the most frequently injured ligament in the knee. The primary method used to diagnose a MCL injury is the *valgus stress test*. The knee is flexed 30 degrees and overhangs the side of the examination table with patient in a supine position. The examiner places one hand on the lateral aspect of the knee and the other one grasps the ankle. Valgus stress (away from the midline) is applied to the knee. The test is repeated in extension.

Injuries to the lateral collateral ligament (LCL) are less frequent than to the MCL. Patient positioning for testing the LCL is the same as for the MCL, but with the examiner's hand applying pressure to medial aspect of the knee and ankle with varus stress applied (toward the midline) (Andrus, 2006).) If collateral ligaments are compromised, the examiner is able to palpate and observe opening of the joint laterally and/or medially.

Patella testing: The *apprehension test* is performed to detect patella subluxation and dislocation; however, recent studies indicate that only 39% of patients with patella dislocation demonstrate a positive apprehension sign (Andrus, 2006). Patella stability is assessed with patient lying supine with the legs extended and the quadriceps muscle relaxed. The examiner presses the patella along the medial edge with the thumb. The patient's face is observed as the patella is pushed laterally. If the patient anticipates that the patella will dislocate upon applied pressure, they will become visibly apprehensive and try to stop further examination, indicating a positive test (Andrus, 2006).

Meniscus testing: Signs and symptoms of a meniscus injury include joint line pain, loss of extension and or flexion, joint swelling, crepitus, and one or more positive special tests or provocative maneuvers. Joint line tenderness provides more useful information than the provocative maneuvers designed for evaluating meniscus injuries (Andrus, 2006). The anterior half of each meniscus is best palpated with the knee flexed (Andrus, 2006).

The *McMurray test* is useful in evaluating the knee for meniscus injury if it is performed with other tests and in patients with a history suggestive of meniscus injury. It is less accurate as a single determinant of pathology, especially for lateral meniscus tears (Andrus, 2006). The patient lies on examination table with the knee completely flexed and the heel close to the buttock. The examiner cups the heel with one hand and places the other hand around the knee joint, with the fingers on the medial joint line and the thumb and thenar eminence on the lateral joint line. The examiner pushes the lateral knee to apply valgus stress to the medial side of the joint, while at the same time rotating the leg externally and slowly extending the leg as the medial joint line is palpated. If a click is heard or palpated within the joint, there is a probable tear in the medial meniscus (Child, 2007)

The *"bounce home" test* indicates probable cause of limited extension. With patient lying supine, the examiner cups the heel with one hand while supporting the knee with the other hand. The patient flexes the knee into full flexion, and then the knee is passively moved into extension. The knee movement will end with a bouncing motion into full extension. A loose body such as a torn meniscus or osteochondral fragment may impede the knee from fully extending.

The *compression test* (or "grinding" test) has been used to predict pathologic changes in the retropatellar cartilage associated with chondromalacia (Andrus, 2006); however, studies comparing arthroscopic findings of the compression test results indicate a poor correlation between a positive test and articular cartilage damage.

Effusion testing for knee joint swelling should be performed whenever examining the knee. The type and amount of swelling are indicators of the source of swelling and potential cause of pathology. Three types of fluid collect in the knee joint: blood, synovial fluid, and pus. Blood in the joint collects quickly, within 1-2 hours after injury. Synovial fluid collection occurs over 8-24 hours with joint irritation. Pus in a joint is often associated with other signs and symptoms of infection not trauma or irritation. Aspiration for joint fluid analysis may indicate blood-tinged fluid. Blood in synovial fluid usually indicates trauma as in a torn ligament, intra-articular fracture, or meniscus tear.

To test for swelling, the patient lies supine on the examination table. The examiner places one hand above the suprapatellar pouch and gently "milks" the pouch distally and medially. After the fluid collects in the medial side of the pouch, the examiner gently pushes the fluid to the lateral side. The presence of a wave of fluid within seconds of "milking" the joint suggests mild-to-moderate excess joint fluid (4-8mL). Large effusions (greater than 40mL) of fluid are detected with the patient lying supine and the knee extended as much as possible. It may be necessary to provide support under the back of the knee for comfort and to relax the quadriceps.

The patella is gently pushed into the trochlear groove and released causing the patella to float in the joint fluid. The fluid collected in the joint surrounds the patella and then resumes its previous shape. The action of floating the patella and causing it to rebound is known as ballottement.

Diagnostics. AP and lateral radiographs are ordered as weight-bearing when possible. Additional views include patellar femoral or sunrise views and tunnel views. Magee (2008) outlines the Ottowa Knee Rules, below, for ordering radiographs of the acutely injured knee:

- Patient age <55 or >18 years;
- Fibular head tenderness;
- Patellar tenderness;
- Inability to flex knee to 90 degrees; and
- Inability to bear weight and walk four steps when examined at time of injury.

Foot and Ankle

History. (See Chapter 2—Anatomy & Physiology, Chapter 15—Trauma, and Chapter 23—The Foot & Ankle.) The primary foot and ankle complaints are pain, instability, or deformity. Pain is either from a repetitive overuse injury, trauma, or inflammation. Identifying the cause of pain assists the examiner in determining a diagnosis. The history needs to include questions about the patient's need to stand or walk for long periods of time and the types of surfaces the patient walks on. If the patient was injured, it is important to note the mechanism of the injury, the position of the foot at the time of injury, and whether the patient was able to bear weight after the injury. If a deformity is noted, it is critical to determine whether it was acquired suddenly or gradually and what may have triggered the onset.

Inspection. Inspection begins with noting gait, posture, and stance. Evaluate the patient standing, seated, and supine. (See "Analysis of Gait" for normal stance and gait.) Note the use of ambulatory aids. Observe the condition of the patient's shoe soles, noting areas of excessive wear or special accommodation such as a wedge. The skin and nails of the foot should be evaluated with position dependent on gravity and elevated, noting edema, color changes and the presence of calluses and pressure areas. The arch of the foot should be evaluated for pes planus (or flat feet) both during weight-bearing and at rest. Assess for the presence of hair on dorsal surface of the foot. Absent or abnormal hair distribution may indicate underlying neurologic or vascular pathology.

Palpation. When inspecting the ankle following an injury, it is necessary to palpate the tibia and fibula proximal to the ankle joint for bone or syndesmosis tenderness. The following bony structures are palpated on the medial aspect of the foot and ankle: the first metatarsocuneiform joint, the navicular tubercle, the head of the talus, the medial malleolus, and the first metatarsophalangeal joint (MTPJ). The first MTPJ is assessed for hallux rigidus or hallux valgus. Palpate the sustentaculum tali and medial tubercle of the talus. The metatarsal shafts are palpated on the dorsum of the foot, noting the presence of tenderness indicative of a fracture. The space between the metatarsals is also palpated for tenderness indicative of a neuroma, most commonly found in the second intermetatarsal space.

On the lateral aspect, palpate the fifth metatarsal base and the fifth MTPJ, calcaneus, peroneal tubercle, and lateral malleolus. In the midfoot, palpate the inferior tibiofibular joint area and metatarsal tarsal joints. In the hindfoot, palpate the calcaneus and the medial tubercle. The heads of the metatarsal bones are palpated on the plantar aspect. Tenderness under the first MTPJ may be indicative of sesamoiditis or a fractured sesamoid.

The soft tissue is palpated medially in the area of the first MTPJ, noting a swollen bursa or joint. In the area of the medial malleolus, the deltoid ligament (often torn in ankle sprains) is palpated for evidence of tenderness and or swelling. Tendons are palpated for pain, disruption, or signs of inflammation, especially in the posterior Achilles and medial posterior tibialis tendons. Palpate the posterior tibial artery for a pulse.

The following tendons in the dorsum of the foot between the malleoli are palpated for tenderness, inflammation, or loss of function: tibialis anterior, extensor hallucis longus, and extensor digitorum longus tendon. Palpate the dorsalis pedis pulse on the dorsum of the foot.

In the area of the lateral malleolus, palpate the following ligaments for pathology: anterior talofibula, calcaneofibula, and posterior talofibular ligament. Lateral tendons include the peroneus longus and brevis tendons. Palpate the structures of the sinus tarsi, anterior to the lateral malleolus at the junction with the extensor digitorum brevis muscle (a common site for sprain). The head of the fifth metatarsal, the common site of a Tailor's bunion or inflamed bursa, is included in the lateral foot ankle exam.

In the posterior foot and ankle, palpate the length of the Achilles tendon, located at the distal third of the calf and attached to the calcaneus. This area is a common site for inflammation in the retrocalcaneal and the calcaneal bursa. This area is also a common site for blistering from footwear pressure over a bony prominence.

The plantar foot is evaluated for spurs at the MTPJ's and calcaneus, and for tenderness along the plantar fascia. Each toe is evaluated, beginning proximally and moving distally, for any deformity such as claw toes, hammertoes, corns, or calluses. The nails are inspected for fungal infections and ingrown toenails.

Motion. Normal ROM in the foot and ankle is found in Table 3.3. Dorsiflexion and plantar flexion of the ankle refers to motion in the tibiotalar joint. Inversion and eversion delineates subtalar or talocalcaneal motion. Supination and pronation involve the mid- and forefoot. Combined tibiotalar and talocalcaneal movements comprise internal and external rotations of the ankle. Limitations in any of these movements suggest pathology in one or more underlying anatomic structures. Differences between legs are not present in the normal ankle (Hyman, 2006). See Table 3.17 for muscles nerves and nerve roots responsible for foot and ankle motion.

Table 3.17. Sensory Testing of the Foot and Ankle

Nerve Root	Reflex	Sensation
L4		Medial aspect of calf and ankle
L5		Dorsum of the medial aspect of foot and lateral side of the leg
S1	Achilles	Lateral side of foot

From Core Currriculum for Orthopaedic Nursing *(6th ed., p. 68) by NAON, 2007, Boston, MA: Pearson. Reproduced with permission.*

Toe deformities can be flexible or mobile with passive stretch, or rigid and resistant to passive ROM (Magee, 2008). Toe deformities that affect ROM include claw toes, hammertoe, and mallet toe. A claw toe deformity combines hyperextension of the MTPJ with flexion of the proximal and distal interphalangeal joints. Underlying causes of claw toes include muscle imbalances and neurological causes. Hammertoe deformity results in extension contracture of the MTPJ and flexion contracture of the PIPJ. Underlying causes include muscle imbalance, mechanical complications, and hereditary factors. The primary mechanical factor is ill-fitting footwear. A mallet toe involves a flexion deformity at the distal inter phalangeal joint. Underlying causes include acute trauma or degeneration of the extensor tendon. (See Chapter 23—Foot & Ankle for further descriptions of these toe deformities.)

Active ROM: To assess active dorsiflexion and plantar flexion, the patient walks on heels and toes. Active inversion is assessed as the patient walks on the lateral sides of the feet, and eversion is assessed as the patient to walks on the medial sides of the feet. There are no isolated motions for assessing active forefoot adduction and abduction; they are presumed normal if all other active motion is normal. To assess flexion and extension, the patient flexes the tips of the toes downward and upward.

Passive ROM: Passive ankle dorsiflexion and plantar flexion are tested while stabilizing the subtalar joint by holding the calcaneus firmly and gripping the forefoot. The foot is pulled into dorsiflexion about 30 degrees and pushed down into plantar flexion about 50 degrees. Passive subtalar inversion and eversion of the heel is performed while stabilizing the patient's tibia distally and holding the patient's heel. This is followed by adducting and abducting the forefoot while continuing to hold the heel and gripping the forefootmoving it to the medial and lateral sides. Passive great toe flexion and extension is tested by flexing and extending the first MTPJ while holding the foot. Decreased passive dorsiflextion of the great toe due to arthritis is called hallux rigidus. A valgus deformity at the first MTPJ is hallux valgus, also known as a bunion.

Strength Testing. (See Table 3.17 and Chapter 2—Anatomy & Physiology for muscles and nerve innervations responsible for movement in the foot and ankle.) Grade and record muscle strength against resisted dorsiflexion, plantar flexion, inversion, and eversion. The presence of foot drop will occur if the deep peroneal nerve has been injured. Heel-walking is the primary means of assessing this group of muscles. Walking on toes and medial/lateral borders assesses general flexion strength.

Sensory Testing: (See Table 3.17 for nerve roots that supply sensation to the foot/ankle and Chapter Two—Anatomy & Physiology for muscles and peripheral nerves in the foot and ankle.) Sensation must be tested on both the affected and unaffected sides for symmetry. Test peripheral nerve sensation by applying light touch to the anterior, lateral, medial, and posterior surfaces of the patient's leg below the knee, on the foot, and on each toe to determine side-to-side differences. Differences should be noted and mapped in greater detail, according to L3-S3 nerve root distributions and dermatomes, using a sharp object, pinwheel, or wisp of cotton. Document the patient's response. Two reflexes are commonly checked in the ankle: the Achilles deep tendon reflex and the posterior tibial reflex. The Babinski reflex is tested by running the handle of the reflex hammer across the plantar surface of the foot along the lateral border of the forefoot. A positive Babinski response, in which the great toe extends while the other toes plantar flex and splay, is abnormal in adults. Although tested on the foot, it is actually used to screen for upper motor neuron disease or spinal conditions.

Special Foot/Ankle Tests. *Anterior drawer test:* This test is highly sensitive and specific for predicting a tear in the lateral ankle ligaments, particularly of the anterior talofibular ligament (Hyman, 2006). With the patient seated on the edge of the examination table and the ankle flexed 90 degrees to the leg, the examiner cups the heel with the palm on the plantar surface and gently grasps the distal tibia with the opposite hand. The heel is pulled forward while pushing posterior on the tibia in an attempt to draw the talus forward. Motion indicates disruption in the integrity of the ligament. Results are more accurate in the absence of pain.

Homan's sign: This exam indicates possible deep vein thrombosis (DVT) in the calf. With the patient lying in a supine position, the ankle is passively dorsiflexed with the knee in extension. If pain is elicited in the calf of the extended leg, further testing for DVT is indicated (Child, 2007).

Thompson test: This test assesses the Achilles tendon for possible rupture. It should be performed first on the unaffected side to prepare the patient for what to expect. The patient lies prone or kneels on a chair with the feet over the edge of the exam table or chair. The examiner squeezes both sides of the calf muscle. The absence of plantar flexion when the calf is squeezed indicates a positive test, which is indicative of a rupture to the Achilles tendon (Magee, 2008).

Diagnostics. X-rays are usually taken weight-bearing when possible. The usual series of radiographs includes AP, lateral, mortise, and oblique views. Mortise views are essential in assessing the ankle for joint displacement. CT assists in diagnosing fractures difficult to assess or evaluate with traditional x-ray. MRI assesses tissue with a high water content (such as ligaments, tendons, and bone marrow) and is able to detect avascular necrosis earlier than traditional x-rays.

Considerations Across the Life Span

The different stages of life carry with them their own set of considerations with regard to appropriate health care. Magee (2008) identifies populations that should have age-specific concerns addressed during the examination.

Infants

The newborn neurologic system is incomplete; therefore, sensory testing is limited to more primitive reflex testing. Infant examinations include screening for possible congenital anomalies of the hips and feet, as well as common delivery-related injuries such as clavicle fractures and brachial plexus injuries. Infant bones are primarily made of cartilage, which is softer than bone and not visible on x-rays. Reflexes are not fully developed. Gait pattern and foot, leg, and knee alignment do not normalize until ages 3-4. The examiner should keep in mind that physical abuse accounts for 10.6% of all blunt traumas in ages newborn to 4 years.

Young Children

A child with a limp should receive a complete musculoskeletal examination, especially of the hip, knee, and foot. Because the young child is unable to communicate symptoms, the examiner must rely on the parents' history and keen observation skills while distracting the child. The prepubescent child (ages 6-10) examination should include screening for congenital anomalies of the hip, foot, leg, and spine, which may not have been diagnosed earlier. Assessment of body mass index (BMI) for age in all children ages 2-18 should be included with the height and weight measurement as this identifies children who are obese and or at risk for obesity. A BMI index-for-age percentile greater than 80% and less than 90% implies a risk for obesity. A BMI index-for-age of 90% or more indicates obesity. Childhood obesity increases the risk for hip and knee problems, as well as chronic diseases (Barlow, 2007).

Adolescents

The 11-15-year-old's examination includes an evaluation of BMI index-for-age percentile, physical maturation, and preventive health practices. Older children may wish to be examined and interviewed alone, without the presence of a parent. Inquire about menstruation, and assess the chest, axillae, and pubic area for hair distribution to assist in determining skeletal maturation. The child with open growth plates heals fractures faster than those who have completed skeletal growth, and is more at risk for growth plate fractures and their potential growth complications. Older children with closed growth plates and young adults are more at risk for sprains than for fractures. The growth spurt of adolescents may trigger related skeletal symptoms associated with an imbalance in growth of bone at tendonous and ligamentous attachments. Examples include knee pain in Osgood Schlatter disease, hip pain in SCFE, and heel pain with calcaneal apophositis or Severs disease. Growth spurts occur approximately 2 years earlier in girls than boys. Bodily proportions change in regular sequence: first the legs lengthen, triggering growing pains, followed by a widening of the hips, chest, and shoulders. This is followed by a lengthening of the chest and trunk, with muscles increasing in size and strength, especially in boys.

Young Adults

Examinations of the young adult (ages 16-30) should identify a history of previous injuries and problems associated with specific physical activities or sports activities. This age group should be screened and counseled regarding the use of protective gear with sports, seat belts in automobiles, and the negative effects of tobacco and alcohol use on bone health. Dietary intake of calcium and vitamin D-enriched foods should be encouraged, and exercise level should also be assessed.

Adults

Examinations of those ages 30-60 should assess for possible overuse syndromes, general health concerns, and muscle conditioning. Degenerative and overuse syndromes occur more frequently in the over-40 age group (Dutton, 2006). Patients at risk for decreased bone health in this population include those with decreased thyroid, parathyroid, estrogen, and testosterone hormone levels.

The Elderly

The physical examination of the elderly population (ages 60 and older) should assess mental status, patient and environmental risk factors contributing to falls, and the presence or absence of a social support system or advocate. Fall risks include decreased muscle strength, balance, visual acuity, and the use of alcohol or medications that affect balance. Decreased muscle mass and bone density is a normal age-related phenomenon. A baseline Dexa Scan should be included in patients at risk for osteoporosis or older than age 65. The muscle skeletal exam in the elderly is more individualized as it includes assessment of underlying medical conditions that may limit the patient's ability to increase physical exercise. Environmental factors that contribute to fall risk include poor lighting, stairs, throw rugs, and other obstacles. Include a member of the patient's support group when obtaining the history, especially if there is a compromise in mental acuity.

Musculoskeletal changes continue through adult years. After maturity, height slowly decreases, especially in individuals with osteoporosis. A loss of height may be the first indication of osteoporosis. First the intervertebral bodies become less spongy and thin, followed by shortening or collapse of vertebrae, the result of osteoporosis. Additionally, increased flexion at knees and hips may contribute to shortened stature. Kyphosis, barreling of anterior chest with increased thoracic diameter (especially in women), signals osteoporosis. Skeletal muscles decrease in muscle mass, bulk, and power with age. Ligaments may lose tensile strength, and ROM may diminish. Pain, however, is not an expected "normal" result as one ages.

Assessing Sports Injuries

An emergency sports injury evaluation must first assess for life-threatening injuries prior to conducting the musculoskeletal examination. The musculoskeletal examination is conducted as previously outlined in this chapter, assessing for injury to bones, tendons, ligaments, muscles, and nerves. The history, as outlined earlier, includes the mechanism of the injury and provides approximately 80% of the information necessary for diagnosis. Additionally, the techniques of inspection and palpation over muscle skeletal structures contribute to narrowing down the possible diagnosis. Pain with direct palpation overlying a bone is suggestive of fracture. Fractures often missed in an emergency assessment include carpal, elbow, femoral neck, and pubic ramus fractures, as well as injuries to open growth plates (Magee, 2008). It is important to have a thorough grasp of adult and pediatric skeletal anatomy when assessing for fractures and growth plate injuries.

Sport injuries commonly result in sprains and strains. The PE should assess for the degree of injury and grade of the sprain or strain (see Table 3.4). Grade three ligament and muscle injuries, commonly seen in the ankle, knee, and AC joint, should be referred for medical evaluation. The Ottowa rules are helpful in determining when to order radiographs when assessing ankle and knee injuries (see "Knee—Diagnostics.")

Abnormal or asymmetric joints with a lack of motion may indicate a dislocation due to a tendon, joint capsule, or ligament injury. Posterior shoulder and lisfranc (tarsometatarsal) dislocations are commonly overlooked in an emergency (Magee, 2008). Radiographs confirm dislocation and possible associated fractures. Tendon ruptures, partial or complete, are suggested by an inability to move a joint with or without a palpable defect. Partial or complete ruptures of tendons or muscles may be palpated, as in the Achilles tendon or gastrocnemius muscle in the calf. Tendon injuries in the hand and at the patella tendon are also commonly missed (Magee, 2008).

Asymmetric deep tendon reflexes associated with a sport injury may indicate a spinal injury, which requires emergency medical referral. Neurological compromise to the sensory or motor nerves may indicate a spinal or peripheral nerve injury. Nerve injuries associated with hand fractures and lacerations are also frequently missed in an emergency (Magee, 2008). Hand injury evaluations include individual assessments of each finger to evaluate tendons for ruptures or lacerations and 2-point discrimination for partial or complete digital nerve injuries.

Compartment syndrome is a serious limb-threatening injury that may be missed in an emergency and requires emergency medical referral. The elbow and the leg are two of the more common locations for compartment syndrome caused by trauma (Magee, 2008). The warning signs for compartment syndrome are known as the five Ps (Pain, Paresthesia, Pallor, Poilkotherma (cold), and ultimately Pulselessness), which are the result of a vascular injury leading to increased pressure within a muscle compartment (Child, 2007).

Pre-Participation Athletics Evaluations

Pre-participation physicals for youth should identify 1.) the conditions that would predispose the participant to serious injury or worsening of current medical or psychological conditions; and 2.) the physical maturation level required to participate safely. Sports can be categorized as collision, contact, noncontact, and other. Participants should be channeled into the proper sport category based upon their unique physical circumstances and conditions. The nurse should be aware of conditions that exempt eligibility into certain levels of athletic participation when conducting pre-participation evaluations or when counseling parents and adolescents during sports physicals. A complete listing is included in Table 3.18. Predispositions to sports injuries include underdeveloped or unbalanced muscle strength, open growth plates, and inability to perceive pain.

The best way to evaluate muscle balance is to test the strength of opposing muscle groups through manual muscle testing and strength grading or via mechanical devices that measure strength. Athletics can also contribute to muscle imbalance. For example, runners may have weak, underdeveloped upper bodies and abdominal muscles, contributing to an imbalance with back muscle strength. Swimmers tend to have weak, underdeveloped hamstrings and more overpowering quadriceps. In the case of cyclists and sprinters, the quadriceps overdevelop in relation to the hamstrings, predisposing them to many sports-related injuries due to unbalanced muscle groups.

Summary

This chapter has provided the general overview of the musculoskeletal assessment and specific limb and joint examination principals, which can be applied in conjunction with the chapters addressing individual body parts. The assessment can be used in obtaining the musculoskeletal portion of the more extensive and comprehensive head-to-toe patient history and physical exam, or it can be applied to the specific muscle skeletal complaint as a component of the baseline or follow-up exam to monitor changes over time. This revised and lengthier format of overall assessment provides a more in-depth line of questioning in obtaining a muscle skeletal history and a more specific description of the physical exam and provocative tests used in examining extremities, joints, and the spine.

Table 3.18. Sports Participation Disqualifiers

Conditions		Types of Sport			
		Collision	Contact	Non Contact	Other
Eyes	Absence of one eye	??	??	—	—
	Congenital glaucoma	X	X	—	—
	Retinal detachment	X	X	—	—
	Severe myopia	?	?	—	—
Musculoskeletal	Acute inflammatory conditions	X	X	X	X
	Spinal instability	X	X	?	?
	Growth abnormalities incompatible				
	with demands of sport	X	X	X	—
	^Chronic or unhealed conditions	X	X	X	X
Neurological	Uncontrolled convulsive disorder	X	X	?	X
	Controlled Convulsive disorder	?	?	?	?
	Repeated concussions	X	X	—	—
	Serious head trauma	X	X	—	—
	Previous head surgery	X	X	—	—
	^Transient quadriplegia	X	X	—	—
Cardiovascular	Acute infection	X	X	X	X
	Cardiomegaly	X	X	X	X
	Enlarged spleen	X	X		
	Hemmorhage (bleeding) disorders	X	X	X	—
	^Heart abnormalities	X	X	X	X
	Organic Hypertension	X	X	X	X
	^Previous heart surgery	X	X	X	X
Pulmonary	Acute infection	X	X	X	X
	Pulmonary insufficiency	X	X	X	X
	^Uncontrolled asthma	X	X	X	X
Urogenital	Absence of one kidney	??	??	—	—
	Acute infection	X	X	X	X
	Enlarged liver	X	X	—	—
	^Hernia, inguinal or femoral	X	X	X	—
	Renal disease	X	X	X	X
	Absent or undescended testicle	?	?	—	—
Gastrointestinal	Jaundice	X	X	X	X
Dermatological	Acute infection, impetigo boils, herpes simplex	X	X	?	?
General or Systemic Disease	Acute systemic infection	?	?	?	?
	Uncontrolled diabetes	X	X	X	X
	Physical Immaturity (relative to level of competition)	X	X	—	—

X participation prohibited

? depends on MD clearance and individual case

?? inform athlete of risk, suggest protective gear

— participation permitted

^ unless cleared by MD or specialist

From Orthopedic Physical Assessment *(p.1059-60) by D. Magee, 2008, St. Louis, MO: Saunders. Reproduced with permission.*

References

Agesen, T.S.N. (2006). Physical examination of the elbow, wrist, and hand. In G.A. Malanga & S.F. Nadler, *Musculoskeletal Physical Examination: An Evidence-Based Approach* (pp. 119-187). Philadelphia, PA: Elsevier Mosby.

Anderson, C.B. (2006). *Office Orthopedics for Primary Care: Diagnosis*. Philadelphia, PA: Saunders Elsevier.

Andrus, S.G.M. (2006). Physical examination of the knee. In G.A. Malanga & S.F. Nadler, *Musculoskeletal Physical Examination: An Evidence-Based Approach* (pp. 279-314). Philadelphia, PA: Elsevier Mosby.

Barlow, S.E. (2007). Expert committee recommendations regarding the prevention, assessment, and treatment of child and adolescent overweight and obesity. Summary report. *Pediatrics*, 120, p.1692.

Bednar, M.T. (2006). Hand surgery. In H.B. Skinner (Ed.), *Current Diagnosis and Treatment in Orthopedics Fourth Edition* (pp. 535-96). New York, NY: McGraw-Hill/Lang Medical Books.

Bowen, J.E. (2006). Physical examination of the shoulder. In G.A. Malanga & S.F. Nadler, *Musculoskeletal Physical Examination: An Evidence-Based Approach* (pp. 59-118). Philadelphia, PA: Elsevier Mosby.

Child, Z. (2007). *Basic Orthopedic Exams*. Baltimore, MD: Lippincott Williams and Wilkins.

Chou, L.H. (2006). Reliability and validity of physical examinations. In G.A. Malanga & S.F. Nadler, *Musculoskeletal Physical Examination: An Evidence-Based Approach* (pp. 7-14). Philadelphia, PA: Elsevier Mosby.

Cipriano, J.J. (2003). *Photographic Manual of Regional Orthopaedic and Neurological Tests*. Baltimore, MD: Lippincott Williams and Wilkins.

Dutton, M. (2008). *Orthopaedic Examination, Evaluation, and Intervention* (2nd ed.). New York, NY: McGraw Hill Medical.

Hyman, G. (2006). Physical examination of the foot and ankle. In G.A. Malanga & S.F. Nadler, *Musculoskeletal Physical Examination: An Evidence-Based Approach* (pp. 315-343). Philadelphia, PA: Elsevier Mosby.

Kibler, W.B., Sciascia, A., Wolf, B. Warme, B., & Kuhn, J. (2009). Nonacute shoulder injuries. In AAOS, *Orthopaedic Knowledge Update: Sports Medicine* (p. 28). Rosemont, IL: American Academy of Orthopaedic Surgeons.

Krabak, B., Jarmain, S., & Prather, H. (2006). Physical examination of the hip. In G.A. Malanga & S.F. Nadler, *Musculoskeletal Physical Examination: An Evidence-Based Approach* (pp. 251-78). Philadelphia, PA: Elsevier Mosby.

Landes, P., Malanga, G., Nadler, S., & Farmer, J. (2006). Physical examination of the cervical spine. In G.A. Malanga & S.F. Nadler, *Musculoskeletal Physical Examination: An Evidence-Based Approach* (p 34). Philadelphia, PA: Elsever Mosby.

Magee, D.J. (2008). *Orthopaedic Physical Assessment* (5th ed.). St. Louis, MO: Saunders Elsevier.

McRae, R. (2004). *Clinical Orthopaedic Examination*. Edinburgh, Scotland, UK: Elsevier Churchill Livingstone.

Nadler, S., Rigolosi, L., Kim D., & Solomon, J. (2006). Sensory, motor and reflex examination. In G.A. Malanga & S.F. Nadler, *Musculoskeletal Physical Examination: An Evidence-Based Approach* (pp. 15-30). Philadelphia, PA: Elsever Mosby.

National Association of Orthopaedic Nurses (NAON). (2007). *Core Currriculum for Orthopaedic Nursing* (6th ed., pp. 37-66). Boston, MA: Pearson.

Parvizi, J. (2006) *Orthopaedic Examination Made Easy*. Edinburgh, Scotland, UK: Elsevier Churchill Livingston.

Rab, G.T. (2006). Pediatric orthopedic surgery. In H.B. Skinner (Ed.), *Current Diagnosis and Treatment: Orthopedics* (4 ed., p. 602). New York, NY: Lang Medical Books/McGraw.

Solomon, J.S.N. (2006). Physical examination of the lumbar spine. In G.A. Malanga & S.F. Nadler, *Musculoskeletal Physical Examination: An Evidence-Based Approach* (pp. 189-26). Philadelphia, PA: Elsevier Mosby.

Springhouse (2009). *Assessment: An Incredibly Easy Pocket Guide* (2nd ed.). Philadelphia, PA: Lippincott Williams & Wilkins.

Chapter 4

Diagnostic Studies in Orthopaedics

Deborah A. Brown, MSN, APRN-BC, ONP-C

CHAPTER 4

Objectives

- Explain the definition, purpose, parameters, and nursing considerations for common diagnostic studies.
- Specify the appropriate indication for each orthopaedic diagnostic study.
- Integrate the objective data for diagnostic and therapeutic purposes in the orthopaedic setting.
- Delineate applicable patient preparation for each orthopaedic diagnostic procedure.
- Recognize potential complications associated with each orthopaedic diagnostic procedure.
- Distinguish relevant nursing considerations for each diagnostic procedure.

The purpose of this chapter is to review common diagnostic studies utilized in the orthopaedic setting. This content will provide the orthopaedic nurse with a framework to review and evaluate the clinical significance, as well as a thorough understanding of current diagnostic studies available in the working environment. Secondly, this chapter will help integrate decision-making parameters of this content to better enable the nurse to provide expert and informed care. In addition, there is an emphasis on anticipating potential complications related to each diagnostic study, as well as a highlight of new diagnostic studies.

The orthopaedic nurse, an integral part of the health care team, can help demystify these diagnostic studies to alleviate the patient's anxiety. With the advent of managed care, aspects such as Point of Care Testing (POCT) allow the nurse to provide a collaborative, rapid approach to allow seamless, safe, and efficient care.

Blood Tests

Acid Phosphatase (ACP)

Defined as a lysosomal enzyme with an optimal acid pH~5 environment, these phosphatase enzymes free attached phosphatase groups from other molecules during digestion. These enzymes are found in bodily tissue and organs such as erythrocytes, platelets, bone marrow, prostate, liver, pancreas, spleen, and kidneys (Pagana & Pagana, 2011). ACP is found in large abundance in prostate tissue: Fischbach and Dunning (2009) report that it is 100 times higher than in the other aforementioned tissues and 1,000 times higher in seminal fluid. The term "prostatic acid phosphatase" (PAP) is most medically significant (Dunning and Fischbach, 2011).

There are numerous reasons for obtaining this lab value that include the following: to detect prostatic carcinoma that has metastasized, as a diagnostic "work-up" of Paget's disease (Sherwood, 2008), to check for hyperparathyroidism with skeletal involvement, and to monitor for metastatic involvement of neoplasms including breast cancer. Other medical indications for a ACP test could include infection, injury, hepatitis, and thrombophlebitis.

Normal adult values are 0.13-0.63 units/L or 2.2-10.5 units/L (SI units) (Pagana & Pagana, 2011). Value results are based on the individual lab, the particular method used, and the tissue or organs that have incurred cellular destruction (i.e., bone, prostate, and liver will contain higher levels of ACP). Elevated serum levels of acid phosphatase can be seen in patients with the following conditions:

- Acute renal impairment;
- Any carcinoma that has metastasized to the bone;
- Hepatitis;
- Hyperparathyroidism;
- Leukemia;
- Multiple myeloma;
- Obstructive jaundice;
- Paget's disease;
- Prostatic carcinoma;
- Sickle cell crisis; and
- Thrombocytosis.

According to Donofrio and Labus (2009), elevated levels of ACP and ALP (see below) in the setting of prostate cancer can signify that the cancer has metastasized outside the "prostate capsule" and into bone, producing increased osteoblastic activity. Also known as the test for "Lysosomal Storage Diseases" (such as Gauchers Disease and Niemman Pick Disease), the ACP test is important as ACP is stored in the lysosomes of blood cells (Van Leeuwen & Poelhuis-Leth, 2009). Lower levels of ACP could indicate an inborn error of metabolism, an autosomal recessive trait, caused by a deficiency of lysosomal ACP. This deficiency can be seen in the neonatal setting and is rapidly fatal. If indicated, prenatal analysis of amniotic fluid is a method of detecting this type of deficiency (Kruer & Steiner, 2008).

Nursing considerations include noting that a recent rectal exam such as prostatic massage (Blanchard, 2010), biopsy, or catheterization will increase ACP levels. Additionally, while obtaining labs, the blood sample should not sit at room temperature or hemolyze because these factors will lead to a falsely elevated ACP level. Furthermore, ACP levels will drop by 50% within 1 hour if the sample remains at room temperature or not frozen; therefore, if not analyzed in 30 minutes, this lab test should be frozen. The nurse should also consider that certain medications will alter test results. Specifically, patients should be advised (with physician consent) to hold fluorides, phosphates, and oxalates, which may all produce a falsely low test. Conversely, clofibrate may cause a falsely elevated test.

In regards to patient education and prostate cancer work up, this test has essentially been replaced with the Prostate-Specific Antigen (PSA) test. While the PAP is not the "gold standard" test for prostate cancer, it can be used to help monitor the disease process and response to therapy. According to Fischbach and Dunning (2009), persons with prostate cancer will invariably present with dramatically elevated ACP (PAP) when metastatic prostate cancer exists. This level will fall after the tumor is excised and reduced by treatment.

Aldolase (ALD)

The fructose glycolytic enzyme ALD catalyzes the division of fructose 1, 6-biphosphate, into the glyceraldehydes 3-phosphate and dihydroxyacetone phosphate (sugar metabolism) (Oneal, Schechter, Griffin, & Miller, 2010). The normal adult ALD values are <7.4 units/L (Van Leeuwen & Poelhuis-Leth, 2009). When muscle deteriorates and breaks open, ALD will flow into serum and allow levels to rise. Medical conditions in which there will be elevated ALD levels include the following:

- Carcinomatosis;
- Duchene's muscular dystrophy;
- Granulocytic leukemia;
- Hepatic necrosis;
- Myocardial infarction;
- Severe crush injuries;
- Skeletal muscle necrosis;
- Tetanus; and
- Trichinosis (related to myositis).

According to Van Leeuwen and Poelhuis-Leth (2009), in regards to carcinoma, this refers to breast, lung, genitourinary tract, and liver metastasis, and genitourinary tract involvement. A recent injury, infection, and gangrene can also increase the ADL level. According to Fishbach and Dunning (2009), ALD levels may be increased by diclofenac, cholesterol-lowering medications (simvastatin, niacin, and lovastatin), and corticotrophin, to name a few.

ADL levels may be decreased in patients with hereditary fructose intolerance (hereditary deficiency of the aldolase B enzyme is an autosomal recessive trait), as well as hemolytic (chronic) anemia that may require blood transfusions during acute blood loss (Oneal et al., 2010).

Nursing considerations regarding ALD include educating patients to avoid strenuous exercise prior to this test. Also, patients need to be NPO (no oral intake of food or fluids) for 8-10 hours before this test is obtained.

The purpose of obtaining this lab value is to monitor diseases affecting damaged cells in which ALD is stored such as muscle, heart, and liver. It should be noted that this test is no longer the gold standard for muscle disorders (Brancaccio, Maffulli, & Limongelli, 2007). It has essentially been replaced by the ALT, CK, and SGOT/AST tests (see separate sections below).

Alkaline Phosphatase (ALP)

This hydrolase enzyme is responsible for removing phosphate groups (dephosphorylation) from many types of molecules. This enzyme functions effectively in an alkaline environment, optimally at ~9 (Fischbach & Dunning, 2009). Serum levels of ALP are always present, primarily concentrated in the liver (kupffer cells [biliary tract epithelium] lining the bile tract), bone, placenta, kidney, and intestinal lining (Pagana & Pagana, 2011; Vahabzadeh & Early, 2010). According to Donofrio and Labus (2009) and Carey (2010), this enzyme is very sensitive to mild-to-moderate biliary obstruction, hepatic lesions (inflammation), viral hepatitis, mononucleosis, and inactive cirrhosis. According to Pagana & Pagana (2011), metastatic liver lesions will almost always have an increased ALP ("most sensitive"). Isoelectric focusing methods can identify 12 isoenzymes of ALP.

Three main isoenzymes are of clinical significance:

1. ALP-1—Liver origin;
2. ALP-2—Bone origin (bone-specific alkaline phosphatase [BSAP]); and
3. ALP-3 —Intestinal origin (Pagana & Pagana, 2011).

The purpose of obtaining an ALP is primarily as an indicator of both liver and bone diseases (i.e. Paget's disease and bone metastatic disease) when associated with other clinic findings (Whyte, 2006). ALP can be further fractionized to determine the tissue of origin (Van Leeuwen & Poelhuis-Leth, 2009).

Normal value ranges for both males and females are 30-120 IU/L. An immunoassay method is available for measuring bone-specific ALP, which is an indicator of increased bone turnover and estrogen deficiency in postmenopausal women (Sherwood, 2008; Van Leeuwen & Poelhuis-Leth, 2009). Normal bone-specific ALP levels are 6.5-20.1 IU/L for men, 4.5-16.9 IU/L for premenopausal women, and 7.0-22.4 IU/L for postmenopausal women. Potential health causes for abnormal levels, as summarized by Donofrio and Labus (2009), Fishbach (2009), and Pagana and Pagana (2011), are found in Table 4.1.

Table 4.1. ALP Abnormal Levels
Elevated Levels
Associated with increased osteoblastic activity: Paget's disease, osteitis deformans, rickets, osteomalacia, healing fractures, hyperparathyroidism, osteoblastic bone tumors, pregnancy, normal growth, biliary obstruction, sarcoidosis, heterotopic bone growth, amyloidosis
Associated with liver disease: Obstructive jaundice, abscesses of liver/biliary and hepatocellular cirrhosis, moderate increases in hepatitis
Associated with other etiologies: Pulmonary/myocardial infarction, Hodgkin's lymphoma, lung/pancreatic cancer, colitis, amyloidosis, chronic renal failure
Associated with medication: Anti-epileptic medications
Decreased Levels
Associated with health conditions: Scurvy, malnutrition, hypophatasia, hypothyroidism, magnesium deficiency, milk-alkali syndrome, severe anemia
Associated with medications: Oral contraceptives, Clofibrate®

Nursing considerations regarding ALP include educating patients that while NPO prior to testing is not required, recent consumption of a large meal could result in an incorrect ("false") elevation of ALP.

Anti-Nuclear Antibody (ANA)

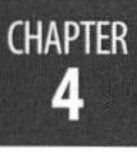

This analysis of gamma globulins (antibodies) react to specific nuclear antigens (Byrd & Brasington, 2010). These antibodies (anti-DNA, extractable antibody) are produced in response to the nuclear part of white blood cells (Van Leeuwen & Poelhuis-Leth, 2009). ANA forms antigen-antibody complexes (Donofrio & Labus, 2009) that cause tissue damage. The purpose of obtaining an ANA test is to detect the presence of antinucleoprotein factor associated with certain autoimmune diseases.

The indirect immunofluorescence microscopy (IFA) is still considered the gold standard test for ANA to detect systemic lupus erythematous (SLE) (Shur, 2009). If a positive ANA and the patient's history/physical are highly suggestive of SLE, more sophisticated studies (including the anti-"double stranded DNA" [anti-ds DNA], anti-Sm, anti-Ro/SSA, and anti-La/SSb tests) should be considered for further investigation (American College of Rheumatology [ACR] 2009; Schwartzman, Gross, & Putterman, 2010). Anti-ds DNA is highly specific for SLE in up to 70% of patients, whereas it is only positive in ~0.5% of the population without SLE. This level will decrease with appropriate lupus drug treatment. Renal involvement with SLE will have high levels of anti-ds DNA titers (Pagana & Pagana, 2011).

Normal ANA values are 1:320 or below (when mixed in the laboratory) for the negative titer and 1:320 or above for the positive titer. Positive titer tests in ANA are associated with connective tissue diseases such as SLE (Pagana & Pagana, 2011). This test is considered to have 95% sensitivity; however, low specificity as a positive ANA (high false positive result) will appear in many other types of diseases (rheumatoid arthritis, rheumatic fever, scleroderma, polyarteritits nodosa, dermatomyositis, Sjorgren's syndrome, and Raynaud's disease), thus resulting in lower specificity of this test (West, 2008).

Nursing considerations include the awareness that a positive ANA can occur in healthy individuals: Morehead (2008) notes that 5% of the population will have a false positive titer, more commonly among women and the elderly; therefore, more testing may be necessary to identify specific auto-antibodies (Fauci et al., 2009). Secondly, careful attention should be taken if recent radioactive scans have been obtained, as these may alter ANA test results. Finally, the phrase "drug-induced ANA" refers to certain medications that can produce an elevated ANA such as oral contraceptives, Procan SR® (procainamide), hydralazine, and dilatin (Donofrio & Labus, 2009).

Anti-Streptolysin O (ASO)

The ASO titer measures serum concentration of the antibody streptolysin O, an oxygen labile enzyme produced by the group A/B-hemolytic streptococcus extracellular (gram-positive) bacteria. The enzyme acts as an antigen that stimulates the immune system to develop streptolysin O antibodies. These antibodies usually occur as serial rising titers within 1 month of streptococcal infection (Fischbach & Dunning, 2009; Pagana & Pagana, 2011). The purpose of the ASO test is used primarily in the differential diagnosis of post-streptococcal diseases such as pneumonia, acute glomerulonephritis, acute rheumatic fever, bacterial endocarditis, and scarlet fever (Daniels, 2010).

Normal ASO values are as follows:

- Adults: <166 Todd units/mL
- Newborn: similar to mother's value
- Preschoolers: <60 Todd units/mL
- School-age children: 170 Todd units/mL

Highly elevated titers are seen in patients with post-streptococcal diseases, bacterial endocarditis, rheumatic fever, acute rheumatoid arthritis, acute glomerulonephritis, pyodermal streptococcal, and scarlet fever. Additionally, ASO titers may be elevated in uncomplicated streptococcal diseases (Pagana & Pagana, 2011).

Nursing considerations include educating patients to fast for 6 hours before serum is obtained. It is important to note that antibiotic therapy and corticosteroids may falsely lower results.

Calcium

The element calcium, a positively charged cation in musculoskeletal physiology, is one of the most abundant minerals in the body (Daniels, 2010; Dunning & Fischbach, 2011). The skeleton and the kidney are the two organs that help maintain calcium equilibrium. According to Straub (2007) and Sambrook (2008), the serum calcium levels are maintained through a complex synchronization of calcitonin, PTH, and 1-25 dihydroxycalciferol. Responsible for growth, maintenance, and radiopacity of bone, calcium is also a key piece in the development of lymphatic fluids.

The majority of bodily calcium (98%-99%) is stored in the skeleton in the form of hydroxyapatite, functioning to build and maintain the structure of the teeth and skeleton (Sambrook, 2008; Straub, 2007). Serum calcium is separated into the free ionized form and the portion that is bound to protein; however, both forms are measured in the serum calcium level diagnostic study (Pagana & Pagana, 2011). Free ionized calcium (the most physiologically active form ~50% of blood calcium) is involved in coagulation, neuromuscular conduction, intracellular regulation, and control of skeletal and cardiac muscle contractility (Fischbach & Dunning, 2009).

According to Dunning and Fischbach (2011), the main purpose of obtaining a calcium level is to measure parathyroid function, malignancy activity, and calcium metabolism. Calcium levels differ inversely with phosphorus. Normal adult values are 8.2-10.2 mg/dL for total calcium and 4.64-5.28 mg/dL for ionized calcium serum (Van Leeuwen & Poelhuis-Leth, 2009). Increased calcium values can most commonly with hyperparathyroidism and malignancy. Additional causes are primary hyperparathyroidism, parathyroid-producing tumors, Paget's disease, renal disease/transplant, multiple myeloma, metastatic cancers, multiple fractures, prolonged immobilization (because of bone resorption and risk of hypercalcemia), sarcoidosis, Addison's disease, and milk-alkali syndrome (Jones, 2009; Van Leeuwen & Poelhuis-Leth, 2009). The most common etiology for decreased calcium values is hypoalbuminemia. Other medical causes include hypoparathyroidism, hyperphosphatemia, Cushing's syndrome, osteomalacia, rickets, renal failure, acute pancreatitis, and peritonitis. Free ionized decreased levels of calcium can be associated with bicarbonate administration, sepsis, vitamin D and magnesium deficiency, and multiple organ failure (Fischbach & Dunning, 2009).

Nursing considerations include educating patients to avoid taking nutritional supplements/vitamins prior to phlebotomy. Medications that may alter calcium levels include androgens, calciferol-activacted calcium salts, progestins-estrogens, lithium, thiazide diuretics, dialysis resins, and long-term anticonvulsant use. Finally, bisphosphonates such as alendronate can increase the risk for "rebound hypercalcemia" (Jones, 2007).

Creatine Kinase (CK)

Also known as creatine phosphokinase (CPK), CK is an enzyme (or dimeric globular protein) that catalyzes the creatine-creatinine metabolic pathway in heart and skeletal muscles, and to a lesser amount in brain tissue (Fischbach & Dunning, 2009). According to Van Leeuwen and Poelhuis-Leth (2009), this enzyme is essential in intracellular storage and energy release. Clinically, this enzyme is assayed in blood tests as a marker for myocardial infarction, rhabdomyolysis, and muscular dystrophy. CK levels mirror normal tissue catabolism (Donofrio & Labus, 2009). Normal total CK values for adults are 38-174 U/L for men and 26-140 U/L for women. CK is divided into three isoenzymes (found in Table 4.2).

Table 4.2. CK Isoenzymes

Isoenzyme	Structure	Normal Values
CK-BB (CK1)	Brain tissue	Trace or absent
CK-MB (CK2)	Primarily in cardiac muscle (a small amount found in skeletal muscle)	0.00-0.06%
CK-MM (CK3)	Primarily in skeletal muscle	96-100

Data from Nurses' Quick Reference to Common Laboratory & Diagnostic Tests *by M. Dunning and F. Fischbach, 2011, New York, NY: Wolters Kluwer/Lippincott Williams & Wilkens;* A Manual of Laboratory and Diagnostic Tests *by F. Fischbach and M. Dunning, 2009, New York, NY: Wolters Kluwer/Lippincott Williams & Wilkins; and* Mosby's Diagnostic and Laboratory Test Reference *by K. Pagana & Pagana, 2011, St Louis, MO: Elsevier.*

The purpose for obtaining a CK level is to diagnose myocardial infarction (CK-MB). The test is a dependable measure of musculoskeletal conditions that do not have a neurological origin such dermatomyositis and Duchene's muscular dystrophy (CK-MM) (Van Leeuwen & Poelhuis-Leth, 2009). In Duchene's muscular dystrophy, mainly in the early stages, the amount of CK-MB may be increased, most likely due to skeletal muscle type II involvement, with CK-MM increased to a much greater degree. The CK-MB isoenzyme level begins to rise in 2-4 hours, and peaks in 12-24 hours, in myocardial infarction. According to Dunning and Fischbach (2011), however, cardiac troponins are considered the gold standard for recognizing injury to cardiac muscle and myocardial infarction, and have by and large been supplanted by the CK-MB marker for acute myocardial infarction (MI).

CK is increased in what Baer (2008) terms "muscle glycogenesis." Body builders will have higher values of CK. Elevations in CPK-MB and CPK-MM levels are associated with muscular dystrophy, polymyositis, rhabdomyolysis, and skeletal muscle injury; muscle damage from trauma such as surgery, crush injuries, and IM injections; myocardial damage; significant aerobic exercise; and blunt skeletal muscle trauma (Brancaccio et al., 2007; Daniels, 2010; Oddis, 2008). According to Daniels (2010), elevated CPK-MB also indicates Reye's syndrome, cardiac surgery, and myocarditis.

Decreased CK levels can be related to small physique and lower muscle mass (Brancaccio et al., 2007; Van Leeuwen & Poelhuis-Leth, 2009). Lower CK levels can also indicate an inactive lifestyle. Additionally, older individuals will have lower values due to decline of muscle mass normally associated with the aging process (Pagana & Pagana, 2011).

Nursing considerations regarding CK include educating patients to avoid strenuous activity or IM injections (Dunning & Fischbach, 2011) for at least 24 hours before the test. The patient's laboratory request form should document recent bruises or surgical procedures, as well as the exact time of specimen collection. The nurse should recognize that certain medications (including cholesterol-lowering medications and statins) can decrease CK levels, leading to statin-related myopathies (Joy & Hegele, 2009; Pagana & Pagana, 2011).

Creatinine

Creatinine is the end product of the catabolic reaction of creatine phosphate in primarily skeletal muscle during muscle contraction (Pagana & Pagana, 2011). The daily production of creatine (then creatinine) is generally constant and is proportionate to the mass of skeletal muscle (Fischbach & Dunning, 2009); however, if there is a severe crushing injury or massive muscle damage, the production is disrupted (Van Leeuwen & Poelhuis-Leth, 2009). Unlike creatine, creatinine is excreted entirely by the kidney and is proportional to kidney excretory function (Pagana & Pagana, 2011).

According to Fauci et al. (2009), the most common purpose for obtaining this lab value is to diagnose impaired renal function. Creatinine serum testing also assesses a known or suspected disorder of the muscles in the absence of renal disease, and it is an estimate of the glomerular filtration rate (GFR) (Donofrio & Labus, 2009).

Normal creatinine values range from 0.8-1.2 mg/dL or 71-106 umol/L. Increased levels occur in patients who suffer from trauma, muscular dystrophy, amyotrophic lateral sclerosis (ALS), poliomyelitis, glomerulonephritis, urinary obstruction, rhabdomyolysis, gigantism, and acromegaly (Daniels, 2010). Decreased levels occur in patients with late-stage muscular dystrophy, small stature, inadequate protein intake, and hyperthyroidism, as well as accompanying the natural aging process and weight loss (Chen, Rachakonda, & Caballon, 2010).

Nursing considerations include educating patients that a high-meat diet will elevate creatinine levels (Pagana & Pagana, 2011). According to Mobley (2009), creatinine serum results can vary with age, weight, gender, and race. A number of medications could increase levels of creatinine, including antibiotics such as gentamycin and cephalosporin, ace inhibitors, and angiotensin II blockers (ARBs) (Donofrio & Labus, 2009).

C-Reactive Protein (CRP)

This acute-phase protein is defined as a glycoprotein manufactured by the liver in response to inflammation (Dunning & Fischbach, 2011; Van Leeuwen & Poelhuis-Leth, 2009). This protein is known for its ability to bind to microbial polysaccharides and ligands exposed on damaged cells, which triggers the classical complement system that leads to the uptake of phagocytic cells allowing for precipitation of the somatic C substance polysaccharide of streptococcus pneumococcus (Capuzzi, 2007; Daniels, 2010). The presence of CRP in the blood serum can be detected 1-24 hours after the inception of tissue damage.

The CRP assay is a nonspecific marker that determines the presence—but not the cause—of inflammation (Pagana & Pagana, 2011; Peterson, 2006). This assay has approximately the same utility as the erythrocyte sedimentation rate (ESR) (see separate section); these tests are often ordered concurrently (Morehead, 2008).

The purpose for obtaining CRP levels is to diagnose and evaluate inflammatory diseases, specifically inflammatory arthritis and polyarthritis (Morehead, 2008), Rheumatoid arthritis, myocardial infarction, and active widespread malignant diseases. This test is often used to monitor the status of orthopaedic infections following joint replacements (Greidanus et al., 2007), as well as septic joints and septic arthritis (Margaretten, Kohlwes, Moore, & Bent, 2007). Recent studies suggest that the Interleukin-6 (IL-6) study may be a more significant marker for infection following joint replacement rather than the sed rate and CRP test. Cytokine-derived from activated T lymphocytes, IL-6 is also considered an acute phase inflammatory protein (Berbari et al., 2010). The high-sensitivity assay (hs-CRP) is used specifically for predicting ischemic episodes related to cardiovascular disease (Fischbach & Dunning, 2009; Pagana & Pagana, 2011; Van Leeuwen & Poelhuis-Leth, 2009).

Normal adult nephelometry values are 0-4.9 mg/L for CRP and 1.0-3.0 mg/dl for hs-CRP. Elevated CRP levels can occur in patients with rheumatoid arthritis, rheumatic fever, SLE, myocardial infarction, active widespread malignancy, inflammatory bowel disease, renal or bone marrow transplant rejection, and postoperative wound infections (Daniels, 2010; Van Leeuwen & Poelhuis-Leth, 2009). According to Greidanus et al. (2007) and Fischbach and Dunning (2009), CRP levels typically rise the fourth postoperative day and decrease at approximately 3 weeks after infection. Acute bacterial and viral infections are also considered causes, although Pagana and Pagana (2011) caution that elevation is not consistent in viral infections.

Conversely, lower levels of CRP can be associated with moderate alcohol use, certain cholesterol-lowering medications, and increased physical activity (Stolker, 2010). Additionally, some reports indicate that decreasing weight in postmenopausal women may lower CRP levels (Stewart, Earnest, Blair, & Church, 2010).

There are a number of nursing considerations when testing this lab value. Cigarette smoking and pregnancy can elevate CRP levels. Certain medications will affect CRP levels, including oral contraceptives, intrauterine devices, and estrogens (Daniels, 2010). Additionally, Donofrio and Labus (2009) note that CRP levels can rise more rapidly than ESRs and are less susceptible to error as the ESR. Unlike ESR, CRP is not affected by anemia.

D-Dimer Test

Fragment D-Dimer is produced from the action of plasmin on cross-linked fibrin (Dunning & Fischbach, 2011). This test indicates a high level of fibrin degradation products (Van Leeuwen & Poelhuis-Leth, 2009).

The D-Dimer assay detects conditions where hypercoagulability may exist. In the orthopaedic setting, this assay may be used in the assistance of diagnosing or screening for deep vein thrombosis (DVT) (Pagana & Pagana, 2011). This can occur following extremity surgery including arthroscopic surgery, fracture repair, lower extremity casting/immobilization, or joint arthroplasty (Van Leeuwen & Poelhuis-Leth, 2009). DVT risk involves primarily the lower extremities.

Quantitative normal D-Dimer values are <250 ug/L or 1.37 nmol/L, and for qualitative measurements, no D-Dimer fragments are present (Dunning & Fischbach, 2011). Increased D-Dimer levels can be associated with arterial or venous DVT and pulmonary embolism, sepsis, DIC, trauma, myocardial infarction, malignancy including metastatic carcinoma, and severe infection (Fischbach & Dunning, 2009; Gay, 2010).

Nursing considerations include the awareness that a rheumatoid factor lab result of >50 IU/ml could potentially result in an elevated D-Dimer level (Pagana & Pagana, 2011) and that liver disease may experience false positive results. Additionally, this test may be positive with patients who have experienced trauma or surgery (Donofrio & Labus, 2009). Although sensitive for DVT evaluation, D-Dimer does not necessarily indicate the location (Fauci et al., 2009); therefore, further diagnostic studies, including a duplex ultrasound, may be indicated to complete the DVT diagnostic evaluation (Yusen & Gage, 2010).

Enzyme-Linked Immunosorbent Assay Test (ELISA)

This assay tests for the exposure to surface antigens of killed human immunodeficiency virus (HIV): if antibodies are present, a positive reaction occurs. The test is simple to perform and is sensitive to the point of 99.8% accuracy. The purpose of this test is to screen donated blood and blood products for the HIV protein, or to detect the presence of Lyme disease or the spirochete borrelia burgdorferi (Donofrio & Labus, 2009; Dunning & Fischbach, 2011).

If the first ELISA test is positive, a second test "two-step process" is run (Fischbach & Dunning, 2009); if this test is positive, the more sensitive Western Blot test is used for confirmation (Pagana & Pagana, 2011; Savely, 2007). ELISA should be confirmed by immunofixation methods. A positive test does not diagnose acquired immunodeficiency syndrome (AIDS); it merely indicates exposure to the HIV virus at some time (Pozza, 2008). A false negative does exist, as the person's exposure may be recent and the disease could still be in the acute ("nonreactive") stage (Savely, 2010).

In regards to ELISA and Lyme disease indications, serological tests are the "mainstay" of diagnosis as they provide evidence of borrelia burdorferi exposure (Bockenstedt, 2008). According to Daniels (2010) and Van Leeuwen and Poelhuis-Leth (2009), however, this test may reveal a false negative (40%-60% of the time) when only erythema migrans is present (which can appear 3-30 days after a tick bite) but will convert to positive later in the disease. A false positive may result in the presence of other spirochete illnesses (such as syphilis) (Dunning & Fischbach, 2011); however, these patients will also have a positive *treponema* reagin test that Lyme disease patients will not (Donofrio & Labus, 2009).

Nursing considerations involve understanding that false positives can occur in patients with autoimmune diseases (such as rheumatoid arthritis), lymphoma, leukemia, syphilis, and alcoholism (Van Leeuwen & Poelhuis-Leth, 2009). Informed consent must be obtained before blood is drawn. Maintain a nonjudgmental attitude toward the patient, and allow time for questions or concerns.

Erythrocytes/Red Blood Cells (RBCs)

Erythrocytes, or red blood cells (RBCs) are nonnucleated, biconcave discs containing hemoglobin (the blood's oxygen-carrying capacity; see separate section) (Platt & Eckman, 2006). The primary purpose of the erythrocytes is the transport of hemoglobin, which in turn carries oxygen to bodily tissues and carbon dioxide away from the lungs (Fischbach & Dunning, 2009). RBC production occurs in healthy adults in the following anatomic locations: pelvis, ribs, sternum, skull, proximal ends of the femur and humerus, and bone marrow of the vertebrae. Conversely, the breakdown of RBCs occurs in the liver and spleen. Erythropoietin (see separate section), a glycoprotein hormone, is responsible for RBC regulation and production. The hemoglobin in the RBCs combines exclusively with oxygen and carbon dioxide (Daniels, 2010). The highly oxygenated blood from the hemoglobin/oxygen combination gives the blood a bright red appearance. This combination also contributes to acid-base balance. According to Donofrio and Labus (2009), the RBC count can be used to compute two erythrocyte indices: mean corpuscular volume (MCV) and mean corpuscular hemoglobin (MCH).

The test measures the level of mature RBCs as part of the complete blood count (CBC) (Pagana & Pagana, 2011), which is one of the most common diagnostic studies found in the laboratory setting. The purpose of obtaining a RBC is to evaluate for anemia or polycythemia, and measures the total number of erythrocytes (for example, in acute hemorrhage).

Normal RBC counts are 4.2-5.4 million/cubic mm for males and 3.6-5.0 million/cubic mm for females.

Increased erythrocytes are associated with the following conditions:

- Acute and chronic hemorrhage;
- Acute poisoning (acute carbon dioxide poisoning also referred to as polycythemia);
- Cardiac decompensation;
- Chronic obstructive pulmonary disease (COPD);
- Cirrhosis of liver;
- Congenital heart disease;
- Cor pulmonae;
- Hypernephroma;
- Hypothyroidism;
- Primary and secondary polycythemia vera as in erythropoietin-secreting tumors and renal disorders;
- Pulmonary fibrosis;
- Renal cell carcinoma;
- Scurvy;
- Severe diarrhea or dehydration;
- Splenomegaly; and
- Thalassemia trait (Fischbach & Dunning, 2009; Pagana & Pagana, 2011; Van Leeuwen & Poelhuis-Leth, 2009).

The life span of a normal red blood cell is ~120 days (Van Leeuwen & Poelhuis-Leth, 2009). In addition to this normal turnover, there are other influences that may play a role in decreased erythrocyte levels including but not limited to the following conditions:

- Adrenal dysfunction such as Addison's disease;
- Anemia (including sickle cell disease, aplastic or pernicious anemias, and hemolytic anemia);
- Cancer (including Hodgkin's disease, malignant lymphoma, and chronic lymphocytic leukemia);
- Chronic heavy metal exposure;
- Chronic renal disease;
- Hyperthyroidism;
- Infectious mononucleosis;
- Intoxication with chemical agents such as arsenic;
- Intravascular trauma from atherosclerosis;
- Most viral infections and chronic infections;
- Multiple myeloma;
- Nutritional deficits (particularly of vitamin B6 and B12, cobalt, amino acids, copper, folic acid, and iron)
- Overhydration;
- Pregnancy (due to anemia and "dilutional effect");
- Rheumatic fever; and
- SLE(Fischbach & Dunning, 2009; Pagana & Pagana, 2011; Van Leeuwen & Poelhuis-Leth, 2009).

Nursing considerations include ensuring proper documentation of the patient's age and gender (Dunning & Fischbach, 2011); female counts should be lower. Pregnancy can interfere with RBC production, while tobacco use and high altitude (low oxygen tension) can increase the RBC count. Many drugs/medications/chemical agents affect RBCs as well: gentamycin and methyldopa may increase RBC levels, whereas chemotherapy, quinidine, and arsenic can decrease RBC levels (Van Leeuwen & Poelhuis-Leth, 2009).

Erythrocyte Sedimentation Rate (ESR)

ESR is the most common measurement of acute-phase proteins in the rheumatic diseases (Pagana & Pagana, 2011). During the lab process, erythrocytes "settle out" of unclotted/anticoagulated blood within 1 hour (Fischbach & Dunning, 2009). An increased rate of settling/sticking together in vertical tubes (or stacks called *rouleaux*) due to circulating fibrinogen (asymmetric shape) levels indicates the presence of acute and chronic inflammation and/or necrotic processes (Cha, 2009; Donofrio & Labus, 2009). Inflammatory states can modify hepatic production of plasma proteins; hence, fibrinogen and immunoglobulin levels will be elevated during this acute phase response (Morehead, 2008; Van Leeuwen & Poelhuis-Leth, 2009). When RBCs interact with these proteins, they form clusters that sediment at a faster rate than individual RBCs. Morehead (2008) further states that in prolonged inflammatory states, reduced serum albumin and hematocrit levels can lead to amplified degrees of erythrocyte sedimentation.

This test has three main limitations:

1. ESR is sensitive but not specific for multiple or many inflammatory diseases;
2. ESR may present normal results during active disease; and
3. ESR results may be influenced by technical factors (Dunning & Fischbach, 2011; Morehead, 2008; Pagana & Pagana, 2011; Van Leeuwen & Poelhuis-Leth, 2009).

The purpose for obtaining an ESR lab value is to test for inflammatory diseases such as rheumatoid arthritis, polymyalgia rheumatica, temporal arteritis/giant cell arteritis, rheumatic fever, respiratory infections, and necrosis (Eamonn, Koening, & Hoffman, 2010; Pagana & Pagana, 2011). Additionally, this test can help to stage disease and/or monitor steroid treatment of inflammatory disease such as polymyalgia rheumatica (PMR) (Daniels, 2010). The most common method for testing ESR values, the Westergren (or modified Westergren) test, uses a 100-mm citrate diluted tube over a 1-hour period (Van Leeuwen & Poelhuis-Leth, 2009). Normal values for this method are found in Table 4.3. According to Morehead (2008), the higher normal limit for a man will be equivalent to the age divided by 2; for a woman, add 10 to the age and divide by 2.

Table 4.3. Normal ESR Values

Gender	Age	Range
Males	<50	0-15mm/hr
	> 50	0-20mm/hr
Females	<50	0-25 mm/hr
	>50	0-30mm/hr

Data from Davis's Comprehensive Handbook of Laboratory and Diagnostic Tests with Nursing Implications *(3rd Ed.) by A. Van Leeuwen & Poelhuis-Leth, 2009. Philadelphia, PA: F.A. Davis Company.*

RBCs fall in patients with the increased plasma volume (anemia) and increased plasma viscosity states such as multiple myeloma (very high ESR levels) (Dunning & Fischbach, 2011). In routine orthopaedic procedures, ESR increases 25-100mm/hr days after surgery and gradually decrease over the subsequent 1-2 weeks (Greidanus et al., 2007); however, joint arthroplasty/total hip replacement (THR) has been known to cause elevated ESR levels that may stay elevated for up to a year (Berbari et al., 2010). Increased ESR values are also seen in patients with acute sepsis and chronic infections (such as osteomyelitis). Elevated ESR is associated with increased levels of fibrinogen and other acute-phase reactant proteins that respond to inflammation such as PMR and giant cell arteritis (Fischbach & Dunning, 2009). Other indications of elevated ESR include tissue necrosis, collagen diseases such as SLE, inflammatory bowel diseases such as Crohn's disease, carcinoma and lymphoma, acute heavy metallic poisoning, Lyme disease, myocardial infarction, anemia, and renal disease such as nephritis (Byrd & Brasington, 2010; Daniels, 2010; Donofrio & Labus, 2009; Dunning & Fischbach, 2011; Van Leeuwen & Poelhuis-Leth, 2009).

Decreased ESR levels could occur in conditions with a high hemoglobin level and RBC count, evidence of cryoglobulins, and elevated blood glucose (Donofrio & Labus, 2009; Van Leeuwen & Poelhuis-Leth, 2009).

The ESR screener should be mindful of a number of nursing considerations. The ESR test should be run within 3 hours of sample collection. The screener should be aware that females naturally have slightly higher rates than males and that rates increase with age (Morehead, 2008). Women in the postpartum period (typically +12 weeks after pregnancy) often present with elevated ESR (Van Leeuwen & Poelhuis-Leth, 2009). Further considerations regarding ESR include knowing how certain medications affect the test: Heparin and oral contraceptives can produce elevated levels (Van Leeuwen & Poelhuis-Leth, 2009), while steroids and aspirin can cause lower ESR levels (Dunning & Fischbach, 2011).

Erythropoietin (EPO)

Defined as a glycoprotein, EPO is a renal hormone produced mainly in the kidney (Donofrio & Labus, 2009; Pagana & Pagana, 2011; Van Leeuwen & Poelhuis-Leth, 2009). This glycoprotein stimulates erythropoiesis that promotes differentiation and development of RBCs and helps initiate the production of hemoglobin (stem cells in the bone marrow) to produce RBCs in the bone marrow. EPO is very sensitive to changes in tissue oxygen levels. It is a cytokine for RBC erythrocyte precursors in the bone marrow. Tissue hypoxia stimulates production of erythropoietin, thereby increasing the production of RBCs (Pagana & Pagana, 2011).

The test measures renal hormone production in the peripheral circulation. The purpose of ordering this test is to help differentiate between primary and secondary polycythemia, renal tumors, and EPO-producing tumors. Additionally, this test is used to observe patients obtaining EPO therapy (Kurlander & Schechter, 2010; Van Leeuwen & Poelhuis-Leth, 2009). According to Donofrio and Labus (2009) and Green, Frankel, and Puffer (2010), it also assesses misuse of commercially (exogenously) prepared EPO by athletes who may have used "blood doping" to augment their sporting activity, which is a banned practice in professional sports.

Normal EPO values using the radioimmunoassay method are 5-36 U/L. Increased levels can be seen in patients with secondary polycythemia, moderate hemorrhage, hepatic carcinoma, COPD, chronic heart failure, and cyanotic congenital heart disease (den Elzen et al., 2010; Fauci et al., 2009). Additionally, low levels of oxygen will stimulate EPO production as in high altitude hypoxia (Levine & Stray-Gundersen, 2010), renal cysts (Daniels, 2010), and "anemias as a compensatory mechanism in the restoration of homeostasis" (Donofrio & Labus, 2009, p. 121). Inappropriate EPO elevations (when hematrocrit is normal to high) are seen in polycythemia and erythropoietin-secreting tumors such as hepatoma, nephroblastoma, pheochromocytoma, and polycystic kidney disease (Donofrio & Labus, 2009; Fischbach & Dunning, 2009; Pagana & Pagana, 2011). Pregnancy and kidney transplant rejection are elevation triggers (Van Leeuwen & Poelhuis-Leth, 2009). Anabolic steroids can also increase EPO levels (Pagana & Pagana, 2011).

Nursing considerations include the awareness that certain medications decrease EPO levels such as chemotherapies, estrogens, and theophylline (Van Leeuwen & Poelhuis-Leth, 2009). Also, blood transfusions can decrease EPO levels (Pagana & Pagana, 2011). Finally, "recent radioactive scans or radiation within one week before" the exam can hinder test outcomes when "radioimmunoassay is the testing" technique (Van Leeuwen & Poelhuis-Leth, 2009, p. 581).

Ferritin

This "ubiquitous" globular intracellular protein, a major iron storage protein, is referred to as an acute phase protein (Leitman & Bolan, 2010). This protein, produced in the spleen, liver, and bone marrow, is comprised of a protein casing, apoferritin, and an iron core. In terms of storage, this protein is found in all tissues but primarily in the reticuloendothelial system (Fischbach & Dunning, 2009). This system, commonly referred to as the macrophage system or mononuclear phagocyte system, systematically filters out bacteria, viruses, and foreign substances, and destroys worn-out or abnormal cells and tissues. There is a high level of ferritin found in the liver. The amount of ferritin stored in nontoxic form is proportional to the amount of stored iron (as ferritin and hemosiderin). Serum ferritin levels are typically very low (Donofrio & Labus, 2009), when absent iron stores at less than 10 ng/ml (Pagana & Pagana, 2011). Unlike iron levels, ferritin is not affected by "exogenous iron intake or subject to diurnal" differences (Van Leeuwen & Poelhuis-Leth, 2009, p.608).

This lab value measures the intracellular total body iron stores and is used as a work-up for restless leg syndrome and adult stills disease (Moses, 2007). This is a very specific test used to differentiate iron deficiency anemia from other types of anemia, particularly hypochromic and microcytic anemias (Fischbach & Dunning, 2009). Finally, this test can help support the diagnosis of hemochromatosis and other disorders of iron metabolism and storage (Van Leeuwen & Poelhuis-Leth, 2009). This test is often ordered along with an iron test and a total iron binding capacity (TIBC; see separate section) (Dunning & Fischbach, 2011).

Normal values of ferritin for males, measured with the immunoassay method, are 15-200 ng/mL. Normal levels for females are 11-22ng/ml <age 40 and 12-263 ng/mL >age 40. Decreased levels of ferritin can result from EPO, iron deficiency anemia, and hemodialysis (Fischbach & Dunning, 2009; Van Leeuwen & Poelhuis-Leth, 2009). Increased levels can occur with the following conditions summarized by Fischbach and Dunning (2009), Van Leeuwen and Poelhuis-Leth (2009), Kurlander and Schechter (2010), and Dunning and Fischbach (2011):

- Ethanol and iron exposure;
- Acute or chronic liver disease;
- Alcoholism;
- Breast cancer;
- Chronic inflammatory diseases;
- Chronic renal diseases;
- Hemolytic anemia;
- Hyperthyroidism;
- Infection;
- Iron overload from hemochromatosis or hemosiderosis;
- Malignancies;
- Megaloblastic anemia;
- Oral or parenteral administration of iron (overload);
- Thalassemia; and
- Type II diabete.

Nursing considerations include knowing that the test needs to be run within 3 hours of sample collection. Also, nurses should be aware of recent blood transfusions, which can affect test results (Pagana & Pagana, 2011). Use of oral contraceptives (Fischbach & Dunning, 2009), menstruation (Daniels, 2010), and pregnancy can also cause elevated ferritin levels. Finally, Dunning and Fischbach (2011) caution, "recent radiopharmaceuticals for nuclear scans can cause 'spurious' results" (p. 347).

Fluorescent Treponemal Antibody Absorption Test (FTA-ABS)

Also known as the early treponemal test (Sena, White, & Sparling, 2010), the fluorescent treponemal-specific antibody absorption test uses indirect immunofluorescence to detect the spirochete treponema pallidum in serum, which is the antibody that causes the venereal disease syphilis. As Donofrio and Labus (2009) caution, however, the antibody is not detected during the first 3-4 weeks of infection.

The purpose of ordering the FTA-ASB is to differentiate biologic false positives from true syphilis positives, as well as to diagnose syphilis when definite clinical signs of syphilis are present but other tests are negative. For this reason, it is described as a "confirmatory test" for syphilis (Van Leeuwen & Poelhuis-Leth, 2009). While this test is considered the most sensitive test for confirmation of antibodies in early infection, the treponemal serological tests generally have "lower sensitivities in primary syphilis compared with later-state syphilis" (Sena et al., 2010, p.702). Finally, when testing cerebrospinal fluid (CSF) fluid, the FTA-ABS test is sensitive but not specific (Fauci et al., 2009).

In normal test results, a particle agglutination assay comes back negative. In abnormal results, the serologic test for syphilis comes back positive. According to

Fishbach and Dunning (2009), the following is a list of sensitivity of FTA-ABS:

- Primary syphilis: 84%
- Secondary syphilis: 100%
- Latent syphilis: 100%
- Late syphilis: 96%

Affirmative results will permanently remain positive after "efficacious treatment," while a negative FTA-ABS eliminates neurosyphillis (Fauci et al., 2009). According to Van Leeuwen & Poelhuis-Leth (2009), biologic false positive for FTA-ABS can can occur with infections including mononucleosis, leprosy, Lyme disease, malaria, and relapsing fever. Noninfectious false positive scenarios include SLE and substance abuse.

Nursing considerations for this test includes knowledge that alcohol ingestion, excessive hemolysis, or excess blood chyle levels may alter results (Daniels, 2010; Dunning & Fischbach, 2011). It is important to verify the fasting protocol with the lab, as this varies between facilities.

Hematocrit

Hematocrit is defined as the "erythrocyte volume fraction" of the percentage of blood ("total blood volume") occupied by RBC mass (Daniels, 2010; Pagana & Pagana, 2011). Whole blood is made up of RBCs and plasma (Van Leeuwen & Poelhuis-Leth, 2009). Centrifugation is used with anticoagulated whole blood in a capillary tube with tightly packs RBCs (Fischbach & Dunning, 2009); the percentage and height of packed RBCs gives an indirect estimate of the number RBC per 100mL of whole blood. This test is also influenced by the size and shape of the RBC (Daniels, 2010). This test, a critical component of the complete blood count (CBC), is generally accompanied by a hemoglobin study (see separate section) (Fischbach & Dunning, 2009). If hemoglobin is normal and RBC shape/size is normal, a determination of hematocrit should be three times the hemoglobin (Pagana & Pagana, 2011).

The purpose of obtaining a hematocrit is to measure the percentage of RBC mass, as measured by its packed cell volume (PCV) to original blood volume (Fischbach & Dunning, 2009). The test is also indicated to diagnose polycythemia vera and anemia, to detect neoplasm, to monitor blood loss, and to track response to therapy such as blood transfusions in combination with a hemoglobin study. This test can help monitor chronic diseases including COPD, malabsorption syndromes, cancer, and renal disease.

Normal hematocrit levels are 40-54/100mL (42%-52%) for males and 37-47/100mL (37%-47%) for females. "The results are expressed as the percentage by packed RBCs in whole blood" (Fischbach & Dunning, 2009, p. 94). Increased levels are found in patients with polycythemia, congenital heart disease, severe dehydration, erythrocytosis, severe burns, congestive heart failure, pulmonary fibrosis, and COPD. High altitudes can also increase hematocrit levels. It is important to note that elevated levels of ~60% are associated with spontaneous clotting (Pagana & Pagana, 2011; Van Leeuwen & Poelhuis-Leth, 2009).

Decreased hematocrit levels are found in conditions associated with surgery; hematocrit value of < 30% represents severe anemia, and hematocrit of <20% can result in cardiac failure and death. Lower hematocrit levels can also be seen in patients with certain cancers (leukemia, lymphoma, Hodgkin's disease), adrenal insufficiency, chronic disease and acute/chronic blood loss, hemolytic disorders, splenomegaly, cirrhosis, acute massive blood loss, and hemodilution (Fischbach & Dunning, 2009; Pagana & Pagana, 2011; Van Leeuwen & Poelhuis-Leth, 2009). Chronic renal disease (where decreased EPO levels are excreted) can also trigger a hemocrit reduction, along with nutritional deficits and fluid retention.

Nursing considerations include knowing that values are not reliable immediately after hemorrhage (Pagana & Pagana, 2011). Critical values (18% or lower and 54% or higher) should be noted and reported immediately (Van Leeuwen & Poelhuis-Leth, 2009). It is also important to note that age and cultural variations exist: for example, after the first decade of life, individuals of Mexican and Asian descent have higher values of HCT and hemoglobin (see separate section) than Caucasians. The screener should also be aware of the normal gender differences in healthy patients. Pregnancy is another known cause for lower hemocrit levels due to plasma volume expansion and hemodilution (Pagana & Pagana, 2011). The physiological changes of pregnancy such as hydremia can affect HCT levels (Dunning & Fischbach, 2011). Finally, hydration status, red cell morphology, and high altitude will all affect hematocrit values (Van Leeuwen & Poelhuis-Leth, 2009).

Hemoglobin (HGB)

This vehicle for the transportation of oxygen, carbon dioxide, and hydrogen is a main intracellular protein in the RBC. Each protein molecule consists of heme and globulin. Heme contains iron and porphyrin molecules that have a high affinity for oxygen. The affinity of HGB molecules for oxygen is influenced by 2, 3-diphosphoglycerate (2, 3 DPG), a substance produced by anaerobic glycolysis to generate energy for RBCs. When HGB binds with 2, 3 DPG, oxygen affinity decreases. Hemoglobin serves as a buffer in maintaining acid-base balance in extracellular fluid.

The purpose of obtaining a hemoglobin level is to determine an index of the oxygen-carrying capacity of the blood. It is often used in conjunction with hematocrit to determine the need for a blood transfusion.

Normal HGB values are 14-17 g/dL for males and 12-16 g/dL for females. Increased hemoglobin levels are associated with COPD, congestive heart failure, polycythemia vera, hemoconcentration, hemolytic disorders, and dehydration. Decreased levels are associated with iron deficiency anemia, sideroblastic anemia, Cooley's anemia, hyperparathyroidism, hyperthyroidism, hemoglobininopathies, liver cirrhosis, severe hemorrhage, inherited hemoglobin defects such as sickle cell disease and thalassemia's, incompatible blood transfusion, chemical reactions such as lead or copper intoxication, Hodgkin's disease, leukemia, lymphoma, SLE, vasculitis, splenomegaly, and sarcoidosis.

Nursing considerations include knowing that higher altitudes and heavy smoking will reflect in both higher HGB and HCT. Certain medications will affect HGB levels, including many antibiotics, aspirin, and indomethacin that could result in decreased levels. The same cultural variations that influence hematocrit levels also apply here, although in addition, following "the first decade of life, the mean HGB in African Americans is 0.5g-1.0g lower than whites" (Van Leeuwen & Poelhuis-Leth, 2009). Finally, the time of day should be taken into account when assessing results, as hemoglobin levels peak ~8am and fall ~8pm.

Human Leukocyte Antigen B-27 (HLA-B27)

This complex antigen group of leukocytes (or white blood cells [WBC]; see separate section) is found in nucleated cells of tissues. The HLA system has been closely identified with tissue transplant compatibility to such a degree that some refer to HLA as histocompatibility leukocyte-A (Dunning & Fischbach, 2011); it has been found to have a relationship with various diseases. HLA-B is one of the four major subgroups of HLA and has been identified to have eight antigens, HLA-B27 being one of the eight (Van Leeuwen & Poelhuis-Leth, 2009).

HLA-B27 is used to diagnose anklyosing spondylitis; the antigen is present in 90% of these patients (Braun, 2008). Variants of rheumatoid arthritis can also be detected—such as juvenile RA (positive in more than 50% of patients) and psoriatic arthritis or Reiter's syndrome (positive in 80% of patients) (Daniels, 2010; Pagagna & Pagana, 2011). The test also detects acute anterior uveitis and Grave's disease (Dunning & Fischbach, 2011; Fischbach & Dunning, 2009; Van Leeuwen & Poelhuis-Leth, 2009). It is also used as a prime indicator in matching donor and recipient for skin and organ transplantation and for platelet and leukocyte transfusions. This test may also be used in paternity testing (Dunning & Fischbach, 2011). Unaffected patients will have a negative reaction to the test.

Nursing considerations include knowing that none of the HLA types are definitive for diagnostics. More specific tests are needed for definitive diagnosis and positive identification of disease (Dunning & Fischbach, 2011). Additionally, cultural differences exist in diagnosing ankylosing spondylitis with HLA-B27. For example, there is a higher association up to 6% of the population among Haida Indians of the Pacific Northwest of the United States (Quilon, 2010) and lower association in blacks than whites (Lozada, 2010). Finally, this test is positive more often in men than women (Lozada, 2010).

Indirect Immunofluorescence Assay (IFA)/ Lyme Antibody

One of three antibody tests, this immunofluorescence serology test detects abnormal immune complexes caused by the deer tick-borne spirochete borrelia burgdorferi, the causative organism of Lyme disease (Marques, 2010). The purpose of this test is to assess for current infection or past exposure to borrelia burgdorferi. ELISA is the preferred method/serum screening (see separate section).

In unaffected patients, the IFA test will be non-reactive. If the IFA titer is <1:256 and ELISA is non-reactive, this is considered positive. Positive test results should be confirmed by a second step, the Western Blot Method (see separate section). Elevated levels of IFA are found in 50% of patients with early Lyme disease and erythema chronicum migrans, will occur consistently with later complications of carditis, neuritis, or arthritis, and are detected in 100% patients in remission (Dunning & Fischbach, 2011).

"False positive" levels of IFA may occur with other spirochete illnesses such as syphilis; however, these patients will have a positive FTA-ABS in addition to a positive IFA. Other false positives can occur with a high rheumatoid-factor titer, as well as cross-reactivity with the Epstein-Barr virus (Van Leeuwen & Poelhuis-Leth, 2009).

Nursing considerations include the understanding that the diagnosis of Lyme disease is a clinical one and that the use of antibody testing has no role in early disease (Bratton, Whiteside, Hovan, Engle, & Edwards, 2008). IFA may be useful for negative Lyme disease work-up in symptomatic patients who live in geographic areas where deer tick-borne illnesses are common (ARUP, n.d.).

Iron (Serum Iron Concentration)

Iron is essential for hemoglobin formation, RBC evolution, oxygen transportation, and cellular respiration (Dunning & Fischbach, 2011; Fischbach & Dunning, 2009). As Van Leeuwen and Poelhuis-Leth (2009) note, iron is critical in the process of erythropoiesis. Serum iron concentration combined with TIBC (see separate section) can differentiate iron deficiency anemia, sideroblastic anemias, thalassemias, and hereditary hemochromatosis, as well as chronic illness or disorders.

The purpose of ordering this lab value is to support the diagnosis of blood loss when serum iron is decreased. This test is used to aid in the diagnosis of hemochromatosis of iron metabolism and storage. This study helps to evaluate iron absorption, iron poisoning, the body's ability to deal with infection, and possible overload in renal dialysis patients (Van Leeuwen & Poelhuis-Leth, 2009). Finally, iron levels (see Table 4.4) are used in the differentiation of hypochromic anemia when blood loss is not obviously evident.

Table 4.4. Iron Levels

Patient		Normal Values
Adult	Male	80-180 mcg/dL
	Female	60-160 mcg/dL
Child		50-120 mcg/dL
Newborn		100-250 mcg/dL

Data from Mosby's Diagnostic and Laboratory Test Reference *by K. Pagana & Pagana, 2011, St Louis, MO: Elsevier.*

Increased iron levels can be caused by conditions such as hemochromatosis, hemosiderosis, hemolytic anemias, and hepatitis. Lead poisoning, iron poisoning (in children), and high dietary iron intake also increase iron levels (Pagana & Pagana, 2011). Medications that may increase iron levels include chemotherapy, iron, methotrexate, oral contraceptives, and rifampin (Daniels, 2010).

Decreased iron levels are commonly found in patients in the postoperative state. Certain conditions trigger a decrease in iron levels, including SLE, rheumatoid arthritis, acute and chronic infection, carcinoma, and hypothyroidism. Iron levels can be lowered by inadequate dietary intake, adrenocorticotropic hormone (ACTH, a medication commonly used as adjunctive therapy for rheumatoid arthritis, ankylosing spondylitis and SLE), chronic blood loss, or recent blood donation (Pagana & Pagana, 2011; Van Leeuwen & Poelhuis-Leth, 2009). Certain chemotherapies, antibiotics, aspirin, and testosterone also decrease iron levels.

Nursing considerations include knowledge that this test is not performed within 4 days of blood transfusion or tests requiring radioactive materials. Patients must be fasting for 12 hours before the test; however, water is permitted (Van Leeuwen & Poelhuis-Leth, 2009). Supplements, including Vitamin B12, St. John's Wart, and Saw Palmetto, can interfere with results. Physiologic diurnal variation (normal or slightly higher iron levels in the morning and normally lower in the evening) should be taken into account (Fischbach & Dunning, 2009). Special considerations for women and children are that repeated pregnancies and rapid growth spurts typically lower iron levels (Van Leeuwen & Poelhuis-Leth, 2009; Pagana & Pagana, 2011).

Leukocytes/White Blood Cells (WBCs)

Another main component of the complete blood count (CBC) is the number of white blood cells in $1mm^2$ of venous blood (Pagana & Pagana, 2011). There are five types of WBCs, referred to as the "differential count" (See Table 4.5). An important distinguishing factor of WBCs is the presence of granules (Fischbach & Dunning, 2009): there are either granulocytes (polymorphonuclear cells) or agranulocytes (mononuclear cells). The five types are all derived from a multipotent cell in the bone marrow called the hemopoeitic stem cell system (Van Leeuwen & Poelhuis-Leth, 2009).

Healthy WBC counts are 5,000-10,000 cells per cubic mm. Normally, this makes between $4x10^9$ and $1.1x10^{10}$ per liter of blood, equivalent to about 1% of blood. Increased WBC count is known as leukocytosis. In general, leukocytosis occurs when one of the five types WBC increases Leukocytosis can occur with infection, age, resistance, leukemia, trauma, tissue necrosis or inflammation, and hemorrhage. A WBC decrease is known as leukopenia, which can occur with viral infections, hyperspleenism, bone marrow depression due to drugs, irradiation, heavy metal intoxication, and primary bone marrow disorders.

The purpose of obtaining a WBC count is to find or indicate the severity of disease process (Dunning & Fischbach, 2011). The results of this lab value help the health care team decide a course of treatment to fight infection, foreign material, or invading microorganisms by phagocytosis (Pagana & Pagana, 2011).

Nursing considerations associated with WBC testing include knowing that interfering factors can occur with age, exercise, pain, temperature, and anesthesia (Dunning & Fischbach, 2011). Increased levels occur with physical activity, stress (Daniels, 2010), pregnancy, history of a spleenectomy, and anticoagulant use. Common medications that lower WBC levels include antibiotics, antihistamines, chemotherapeutic agents, and diuretics. Common medications that could increase the eosinophil count include anticonvulsants such as carbamazepine/lamotrigine/clonazepam, penicillins, and sulfonamides (Pagana & Pagana, 2011).

Lupus Erythematous Cell Preparation (LE Cell Prep)

LE cells are neutrophils that contain, in their cytoplasm, large masses of depolymerized DNA from the nuclei of polymorphonuclear leukocytes (Fischbach & Dunning, 2009). LE factors are present in the gamma globulin fraction of the serum protein and have the characteristics of an antinuclear antibody.

The purpose of obtaining a LE cell prep is for the diagnosis of systemic lupus erythematous (SLE). Normal

CHAPTER 4

Table 4.5. Differential Leukocyte/WBC Count

Cell Type	Description	Normal Value	Implications of Increase	Implications of Decrease
Granulocytes				
Basophils	Function is not clearly understood but considered to be phagocytosis and to contain heparin and histamines.	0.5%-1% of differential leukocyte count	Myeloproliferative diseases, chronic inflammation, and polycythemia vera. Also seen following radiation and during the healing phase of inflamation.	Anaphylactic reaction, hyperthyroidism, stress reactions, pregnancy, aging, and ovulation. Also results following prolonged steroid therapy.
Eosinophils	Function is unknown but believed play a role in both the breakdown of protein material and phagocytizing antigen-antibody complexes. Allergens, foreign proteins, and products of protein breakdown produce the eosinophils' response and are inflammatory exudates.	14% of differential leukocyte count	Allergies, parasitic diseases, myelogenous leukemia, Hodgkin's disease, polyarteritis nodosa, and acute infection.	Infectious mononucleosis, aplastic and pernicious anemia, hypersplenisms, congestive heart failure, Cushing's syndrome, and use of certain drugs such as epinephrine and thyroxin.
Neutrophils	Most numerous important type of WBC involved in body's reaction to inflammation. Establish a defense against microbial invasion through phagocytosis activity and death in large numbers that forms "pus"/purulence.	60%-70% of differential leukocyte count	Bacterial infections, gout, uremia, acute hemorrhage and hemolysis of RBCs, myelogenous leukemia, tissue necrosis, granulocytic leukemia, myeloproliferative disorders, corticosteroids, ACTH, and sulfonamides.	Acute viral infections, blood disorders such as aplastic and pernicious anemia, agranulocytosis*, acute lymphoblastic leukemia, toxic agents, and hormonal diseases such as Addison's disease, thyrotoxicosis, and acromegaly. **Marked neutropenia – a clinical alert per Fischbach & Dunning, 2009, p.78.*
Agranulocytes (or "Non-granulocytes")				
Lymphocytes	Sub-grouped as B cells and T Cells, and closely involved in the immune response and antibody formation.	20%-40% of differential leukocyte count	Pertussis, syphilis, tuberculosis, mumps, infectious mononucleosis, German measles, ulcerative colitis, and chronic infectious states.	High level of adrenal corticosteroids, renal failure, and immunosuppressive drugs.
Monocytes	Interact with antigen-antibody complement complexes to promote phagocytosis. May be converted into large macrophages and dendritic cells in tissue with increased phagocytic capacity.	2%-6% of differential leukocyte count	Viral infections such as mononucleosis, chicken pox, and mumps; certain protozoa; ricketsial diseases such as malaria, Rocky Mountain spotted fever, and typhus; bacterial infections such as brucellosis; sub-acute bacterial endocarditis; collagen diseases; multiple myeloma; myelocytic leukemia; and lymphomas.	Can be see in HIV infection, hairy cell leukemia, prednisone therapy, massive infection, and aplastic anemia.

Data from Nurses' Quick Reference to Common Laboratory & Diagnostic Tests *by M. Dunning and F. Fischbach, 2011, New York, NY: Wolters Kluwer/Lippincott Williams & Wilkens;* A Manual of Laboratory and Diagnostic Tests *(8th ed.) by F. Fischbach & M. Dunning, 2009, New York, NY: Wolters Kluwer/Lippincott Williams & Wilkins; and* Mosby's Diagnostic and Laboratory Test Reference *by K. Pagana & Pagana, 2011, St Louis, MO: Elsevier.*

values are negative. Positive results are associated with SLE, chronic active hepatitis, rheumatoid arthritis, scleroderma, and blood sensitivity reaction (Wallace, 2006), This test is performed rarely, as it is positive with ~50%-75% of patients, including those with rheumatoid arthritis, scleroderma and drug sensitivities.

N-Telopeptide (NTx)

NTx is a "biochemical marker of bone metabolism" (Pagana & Pagana, 2011, p.187). NTx and C-telopeptides are protein fragments found in type-1 collagen that include close to 90% of the bone matrix. It is thought that serum levels correlate to urine levels of "urine measurements normalized to creatinine" (Pagana & Pagana, 2011, p. 187). Normal NTx serum findings are 5.4-24.2nm BCE for males and 6.2-19.0nm BCE for females (Pagana & Pagana, 2011).

This test is important in monitoring the treatment response for osteoporosis compared to pre-treatment levels, specifically with the use of antiresorptive medications; essentially, NTx levels in both serum and urine should decrease with anti-resorptive treatment. This test is helpful in determining subtle changes in bone metabolism. It has been shown to be prognostic in measuring bone mineral density (BMD; see separate section) and anti-fracture treatment efficiency (Pagana & Pagana, 2011). (Bone densitometry [DXA] described later in this chapter is considered the "gold standard" for diagnosing low bone density as seen in osteopenia and osteoporosis.)

Nursing indications include educating patients that body building treatments such as testosterone may cause decreased NTx levels (Pagana & Pagana, 2011). Also, being aware that that increased levels may be seen in patients with osteoporosis, Paget's disease, advanced bone tumors, acromegaly, hyperparathyroidism, and hyperthyroidism (Mayo Clinic, *81549*). Conversely, low NTx serum levels can be seen in hypoparathyroidism, hypothyroidism, cortisol therapy, and effective antiresorptive therapy (Pagana & Pagana, 2011). Finally, serum levels should be observed before treatment and 4-6 months after therapy commencement for adequate comparison.

Table 4.6. Causes for Abnormal Phosphorous Levels

Causes for Increased Levels (hyperphosphatemia)	Causes for Decreased Levels (hypophosphatemia)
■ Acromegaly ■ Addison's disease ■ Bone metastases ■ Bone tumors ■ Chronic renal failure/ renal insufficiency ■ Diabetic ketoacidosis ■ Excessive alkali intake ■ Healing fractures ■ Hypocalcaemia ■ Hypoparathryroidism ■ Severe nephritis	■ Alcoholism ■ Celiac disease and crohn's disease ■ Chronic antacid ingestion rickets (associated with malabsorption syndrome) ■ Osteomalacia ■ Gram-negative septicemia ■ High intestinal obstruction ■ Hypercalcemia ■ Hyperparathyroidism ■ Hypokalemia (inadequate dietary ingestion of phosphorus) ■ Hypothyroidism ■ Liver disease ■ Overuse of diuretics ■ Renal tubular acidosis/dystrophies ■ Severe malnutrition ■ Vomiting

Data from Delmar's Guide to Laboratory and Diagnostic Tests *by R. Daniels, 2010, Clifton Park, NY: Delmar Cengage Learning;* Diagnostic Tests Made Incredibly Easy *(2nd ed.) by J. Donofrio & D. Labus, 2009, New York, NY: Wolters Kluwer/Lippincott Williams & Wilkins;* Nurses' Quick Reference to Common Laboratory & Diagnostic Tests *(5th ed.) by M. Dunning & F. Fischbach, F., 2011, New York, NY: Wolters Kluwer/ Lippincott Williams & Wilkins;* Mosby's Diagnostic and Laboratory Test Reference *by K. Pagana & T. Pagana, 2011, St Louis, MO: Elsevier; and* Davis's Comprehensive Handbook of Laboratory and Diagnostic Tests with Nursing Implications *(3rd Ed.) by A. Van Leeuwen & D. Poelhuis-Leth, 2009, Philadelphia, PA: F.A. Davis Company.*

Phosphorus

The body uses this essential mineral (macronutrient) for storage and utilization of energy/metabolism. Distributed throughout the body in the form of phosphate (PO4) (Pagana & Pagana, 2011), this mineral is a chief intracellular anion and plays a critical function in cellular metabolism, preservation of cellular membranes, and creation of bones and teeth (Van Leeuwen & Poelhuis-Leth, 2009). Approximately 85% of the body's phosphorous (inorganic form) is stored in the bones (Pagana & Pagana, 2011). This mineral plays a major role in osmotic pressure maintenance, and it acts as a buffer to keep bodily pH at a nearly constant and equal acid-base balance (Daniels, 2010). The phosphorous-containing molecule 2,3 diphosphoglycerate (2,3 DPG) binds to hemoglobin and is important in oxygen transportation (Van Leeuwen & Poelhuis-Leth, 2009). Adequate levels of Vitamin D are necessary for their absorption.

An inverse relationship exists between calcium and phosphorus: a decrease in one mineral results in an increase in the other (Daniels, 2010). Additionally, phosphorous levels are determined by a reciprocal relationship to calcium metabolism, parathyroid hormone, and intestinal absorption (Pagana & Pagana, 2011). Urinary relationships of phosphorous increase or decrease in inverse proportion to serum calcium levels (Donofrio & Labus, 2009). The parathyroid hormone controls the concentration of phosphorous by modifying its excretion in the urine (Moore & Rosh, 2010). Normal values are 3.0-4.5 mg/dl in adults and 4.5-6.5 mg/dl in children. Abnormal levels of phosphate result from improper excretion more commonly than improper ingestion or absorption from dietary sources (see Table 4.6).

The purpose of obtaining a phosphorous level is to aid in the identification of hyperparathyroidism and/or renal failure (Van Leeuwen & Poelhuis-Leth, 2009). This test is often ordered in conjunction with calcium, PTH, and Vitamin D levels.

Nursing considerations include awareness that low levels caused by hormonal disorders cannot be prevented. Patients with low levels from dietary intake or laxative misuse/starvation should be taught careful dietary and bowel habits in attempts to reverse this process (Fischbach & Dunning, 2009). To decrease levels of hyperphosphatemia, dietary restriction may be recommended. Other interventions include administration of phosphate binders or administration of calcitriol, the active form of Vitamin D (Van Leeuwen & Poelhuis-Leth, 2009). Fasting and avoiding intravenous glucose administration may be necessary for electrolyte testing such as phosphate, as this may interfere with phosphate levels (Daniels, 2010).

The subtle role/balance between calcium and phosphorous is critical in maintaining healthy bone density and preventing osteoporosis. Nurses can educate patients that elevated phosphate levels are rarely clinically significant; however, if prolonged, they can alter bone metabolism by causing abnormal calcium phosphate deposits. Ehrlich (2009) posits that drinking popular soft drinks (500mg of phosphorous in one serving) in place of milk may contribute to osteopenia or osteoporosis. Athletes often use phosphate supplements prior to competition to prevent muscle fatigue and soreness, which could also lead to an unhealthy balance of calcium and phosphorous.

Rheumatoid Factor (RF)

This common macroglobulin-type autoantibody attaches to the fragment crystallizable (Fc) region of the human immunoglobulin G (IgG) and is important in the autoimmune response (Morehead, 2008). IgG antibodies, manufactured by lymphocytes in the synovial joints, react with other IgG or IgM to yield immune complexes, complement pathway initiation, and damage tissue (Donofrio & Labus, 2009; Van Leeuwen & Poelhuis-Leth, 2009). The IgG or IgM molecules that react with altered IgG are called rheumatoid factors (RF) (Pagana & Pagana, 2011). IgM antibody directed against the IgG molecule is the most common RF isotype, but IgG and IgA RF may also be detected in the serum (Morehead, 2008). The precise function of the RF in the pathogenesis of rheumatoid arthritis (RA) has not been clearly defined (Fischbach & Dunning, 2009); however, it is thought that these immune complexes can "migrate from the synovial fluid to other areas of the body producing vasculitis, subcutaneous nodules, or lymphadenopathy" (Donofrio & Labus, 2009, p.157).

There are currently two agglutination tests that can detect the RF. First, the sheep agglutination test involves rabbit IgG absorbed onto sheep RBCs, which is mixed with the patient's serum in serial dilutions. The second, the latex fixation test, involves latex particles coated with denatured IgG. The serum from the patient is heated and then added to the suspension of coated latex particles. If the serum contains the RF, the RF will react with the IgG fraction and cause the latex particles to agglutinate. In modern labs, the use of nephelometric techniques does provide improved quantification of the RF and may be automated. Results are typically reported in international units per ml, where a typical significant positive result might be 50 IU/ml. According to Morehead (2008), nephelometry and ELISA are capable of identifying all three isotypes. It should be noted that the anti-cyclic citrullinated peptide (anti-CCP) test has recently been included in the ACR guidelines for RA diagnostic criteria (July 2010 RA diagnosis classification criteria) (Fauci et al., 2009).

Normal RF values are 0-20 U/ml or 0-20 KU/L, based on nephelometry. Titers above 1:80 are usually considered diagnostic for RA. In patients with known RA, the RF has a sensitivity of approximately 70% (Morehead, 2008). Although present in approximately 75% of patients with RA (Daniels, 2010), the RF does not establish the diagnosis of RA. According to Tassiulas and Paget (2006) roughly, 20% of patients who meet the criteria for RA do not have RF (also called "seronegative RA"), while RF can be present in patients with no joint disease (Pagana & Pagana, 2011).

With a positive RF assay, the RF is present in a significant number of other conditions, including:

- Adult stills disease;
- Aging (up to 25% in persons older than age 60);
- Autoimmune thyroid disorders;
- Connective tissue disorders;
- Dermatomyositis;
- HIV;
- Infectious mononucleosis;
- Leukemia;
- Multiple myeloma;
- Polymyositis;
- Reynaud's phenomenon;
- Sarcoidosis;
- Scleroderma;
- SLE;
- Sjogren's syndrome; and
- Syphilis (Daniels, 2010; Morehead, 2008; Pagana & Pagana, 2011).

The RF level that is most clinically significant serological marker is the immunoglobin IgM-RF measurement, present in persons diagnosed with rheumatoid arthritis. This test can be used as one of the ACR classifications for the diagnosis of RA and can also be considered a prognostic study because very high titers of RF are associated with increased disease severity, the progression of joint/bone erosions (Fauci et al., 2009), extra-articular manifestations, rheumatoid nodules, pulmonary involvement, and greater disability. The IgA isotype has been associated with erosive disease and rheumatoid vasculitis (Morehead, 2008). The sensitivity and specificity of RF for the diagnosis of RA are ~60%-70% and 80%-90%, respectively (Mease, 2008).

Nursing considerations include awareness that, in earlier stages of the disease, the sensitivity of the RF is ~50% as patients seroconvert subsequently over weeks or months (Morehead, 2008). Additional factors include knowing that recent blood transfusions and numerous vaccinations may affect outcomes. Finally, high lipid levels may cause a false positive test and may necessitate retesting following a fat-restrictive diet (Van Leeuwen & Poelhuis-Leth, 2009). Educate patients regarding the fact that false positive RF results also limit the diagnostic specificity of this test.

Serum Glutamic-Oxalacetic Transaminase (SGOT)/Aspartate Aminotransferase (AST)

Contained within a broader group of laboratory studies known as the "liver function tests," SGOT (also referred to as AST) is defined as "enzymes that catalyze the reversible transfer of an amino group between aspartate and alpha-ketoglutarate acid" (Van Leeuwven, 2009, p. 149). It is found in the cytoplasm and mitochondria of many cells as an enzyme essential to energy production, primarily in the liver, heart, skeletal muscles, kidneys, pancreas, and to a lesser amount in RBCs (Donofrio & Labus, 2009; Van Leeuwen & Poelhuis-Leth, 2009). During acute cellular destruction, SGOT is released into the blood stream from damaged cells, with elevated levels commonly found 8 hours following injury, peaking 24-36 hours after trauma, and decreasing to normal in 4-6 days (Pagana & Pagana, 2011).

The purpose of obtaining the SGOT level is to evaluate liver, heart, and skeletal muscle injury (Fischbach & Dunning, 2009). This test is typically ordered in combination with a "liver panel" specifically with ALT levels (Pagana & Pagana, 2011). Additionally, this study is also used to compare sequentially with the enzyme alanine aminotransferase levels to monitor the progression of hepatitis and to scrutinize a patient's response to pharmacological therapy with identifiable hepatotoxic effects (Van Leeuwen & Poelhuis-Leth, 2009) such as the RA medication methotrexate.

Normal SGOT values are 8-46 U/L for males and 7-31 U/L for females. Decreased levels occur in patients with chronic liver disease, diabetic ketoacidosis, and hemodialysis (Daniels, 2010). Further categorization of elevated SGOT levels can be classified as significant, very high, high, moderate, and low (see Table 4.7).

Nursing considerations include documenting the time of blood collection and educating patients to avoid IM injections and exercise prior to testing for this lab value (Pagana & Pagana, 2011). It is important to rotate venipuncture sites to avoid false elevations. Many drugs elevate or decrease SGOT/AST levels, including anabolic steroids, amitriptyline, estrogens, erythromycin, penicillins, sulfonamides, and progesterone (Daniels, 2010).

Serum Osteocalcin

Also called Bone G1a Protein, osteocalcin is a key bone cell matrix protein that assigns itself to osteoblasts (Van Leeuwen & Poelhuis-Leth, 2009); as the osteoblastic activity increases, there is a higher level of osteocalcin in the blood. Fischbach and Dunning (2009) refer to osteocalcin as a secondary measurement marker of osteoblast activity and bone development. Produced by osteoblasts and dentin during the matrix mineralization phase of bone formation, osteocalcin is the most abundant

Table 4.7. SGOT Elevations

Significant	Very High	High	Moderate	Low/Mild
■ Hepatocellular disease ■ Shock ■ Carcinoma ■ Alcohol abuse ■ Acute pancreatitis	■ Drug-induced hepatic injury ■ Acute viral hepatitis ■ Skeletal muscle trauma ■ Extensive surgery	■ Infectious mononucleosis	■ Myocardial infarction ■ Dermatomyositis ■ Crushing injuries ■ Duchene's muscular dystrophy ■ Pulmonary embolism	■ Hemolytic anemia ■ Fatty liver ■ Lyme disease

Data from Delmar's Guide to Laboratory and Diagnostic Tests *by R. Daniels, 2010, Clifton Park, NY: Delmar Cengage Learning;* Diagnostic Tests Made Incredibly Easy *(2nd ed.) by J. Donofrio & D. Labus, 2009, New York, NY: Wolters Kluwer/Lippincott Williams & Wilkins;* Nurses' Quick Reference to Common Laboratory & Diagnostic Tests *(5th ed.) by M. Dunning & F. Fischbach, F., 2011, New York, NY: Wolters Kluwer/Lippincott Williams & Wilkins;* Mosby's Diagnostic and Laboratory Test Reference *by K. Pagana & T. Pagana, 2011, St Louis, MO: Elsevier; and* Davis's Comprehensive Handbook of Laboratory and Diagnostic Tests with Nursing Implications *(3rd Ed.) by A. Van Leeuwen & D. Poelhuis-Leth, 2009, Philadelphia, PA: F.A. Davis Company.*

Table 4.8. TIBC Levels

Normal Values: Adults: 250-460 ug/dL Children (age 2 and up): 350-450 ug/dL.	**Conventional Units:** 250-350 mcg/dL (spectrophotometry)	
TIBC Decreases:	**TIBC Increases:**	**TIBC Saturation:**
■ Anemias (anemia of chronic disease, hemolytic, megaloblastic/sideroblastic, pernicious, sickle cell) ■ Chronic infections ■ Cirrhosis / liver disease ■ Hypoproteinemia ■ Malignancies of the small intestines ■ Malnutrition ■ Neoplasms ■ Severe burns ■ Thalassemia	■ Acute hepatitis ■ Iron deficiency (70%) ■ Late pregnancy ■ Polycythemia vera	■ Hemochromatosis ■ Hemosiderosis ■ Iron overload

Data from Delmar's Guide to Laboratory and Diagnostic Tests *by R. Daniels, 2010, Clifton Park, NY: Delmar Cengage Learning; Diagnostic Tests Made Incredibly Easy (2nd ed.) by J. Donofrio & D. Labus, 2009, New York, NY: Wolters Kluwer/Lippincott Williams & Wilkins;* A Manual of Laboratory and Diagnostic Tests *(8th ed.) by F. Fischbach & M. Dunning, 2009, New York, NY: Wolters Kluwer/Lippincott Williams & Wilkins.* Mosby's Diagnostic and Laboratory Test Reference *by K. Pagana & T. Pagana, 2011, St. Louis, MO: Elsevier; and* Davis's Comprehensive Handbook of Laboratory and Diagnostic Tests with Nursing Implications *(3rd Ed.) by A. Van Leeuwen & D. Poelhuis-Leth, 2009, Philadelphia, PA: F.A. Davis Company.*

noncollagenous bone cell protein (Pagana & Pagana, 2011). Production of osteocalcin is reliant on Vitamin K (Van Leeuwen & Poelhuis-Leth, 2009). Osteocalcin serum levels correspond to alkaline phosphatase amounts.

Normal osteocalcin values are 3.0-13 ng/mL for males, 0.4-.8.2 ng/mL for premenopausal women, and 1.5-11 ng/mL for postmenopausal women. Osteocalcin levels are affected by a number of factors, including the hormone estrogen. Increased levels indicate increased bone formation in persons with hyperparathyroidism, fractures, and acromegaly. Chronic renal failure, hyperthyroidism, metastatic skeletal disease, Paget's disease, renal osteodystrophy, osteoporosis are also known causes for elevation, as are growth spurts among adolescents. Decreased levels are associated with hypoparathyroidism, growth hormone deficiency, certain medications (glucocorticosteroids, bisphosphonates, and calcitonin), pregnancy, and primary biliary cirrhosis (Fischbach & Dunning, 2009; Pagana & Pagana, 2011; Van Leeuwen & Poelhuis-Leth, 2009). Also, Lindsley (2008) notes a possible association with decreased insulin-like growth factor 1 (IGF-1) levels, although corticosteroids could play a factor as well.

The osteocalcin level is a delicate biochemical indicator of the rate of bone turnover and calcium ion homeostasis (Fischbach & Dunning, 2009; Pagana & Pagana, 2011; Van Leeuwen & Poelhuis-Leth, 2009). This test is used to monitor for treatment of osteoporosis and bone cancer (Fischbach & Dunning, 2009). It is used to observe the effectiveness of anabolic constructing treatments such as Forteo. Finally, this test monitors the efficacy of estrogen treatments (Van Leeuwen & Poelhuis-Leth, 2009).

Nursing considerations include familiarity with urinary values, as wide variations can occur (Fischbach & Dunning, 2009). While obtaining urine samples, it is important to use a double-voided specimen in the early morning to decrease any chance of inconsistency. Other issues include knowing that body-building treatments can decrease osteocalcin levels (Pagana & Pagana, 2011). Conversely, levels are typically greater in children and amplified during bed rest; however, there is no increase in bone development (Fischbach & Dunning, 2009). Radioactive scans or radiation within 1 week before the osteocalcin test can interfere with test results when radioimmunoassay is the test method (Van Leeuwen & Poelhuis-Leth, 2009).

Total Iron Binding Capacity (TIBC)

TIBC measures the capacity of serum globulin transferrin to combine with and transport iron (Fischbach & Dunning, 2009). Furthermore, this test measures iron as it appears in plasma if all the transferrin were saturated with iron (Pagana & Pagana, 2011). In general, conditions that *decrease* serum iron levels *increase* TIBC because the less iron available, the more sites for iron to bind.

The purpose of ordering TIBC levels (Table 4.8) is to distinguish iron deficiency anemias from other anemias (Fischbach & Dunning, 2009). Secondly, this study is used to screen for either an iron deficiency or overload (Van Leeuwen & Poelhuis-Leth, 2009). This test is also used in conjunction with serum iron levels (Donofrio & Labus, 2009). According to Daniels (2010), this test is the preferred method to measure liver function and iron metabolism.

Nursing considerations include interpreting studies for iron deficiency with a grouping of low serum iron, high TIBC, and high transferrin levels (Fischbach & Dunning, 2009). Nurses should understand that fluorides and oral contraceptives may increase TIBC levels, while chloramphenicol, cortisone, testosterone, and ACTH may decrease TIBC levels (Daniels, 2010). In RA patients,"serum iron may be low in the presence of adequate body stores, but TIBC may be unchanged or may drop to preserve normal saturation" (Donofrio & Labus, 2009, p.16).

Total Protein Albumin/Globulin Ratio (A/G Ratio)/Serum Electrophoresis (SEP)

The ratio of albumin and globulin concentrations in serum is usually determined by protein electrophoresis. Protein is essential to all physiological functions, as well as for the regulation of metabolic processes, immunity, and appropriate water balance (Fischbach & Dunning, 2009).

Proteins consist of amino acids, the structural blocks of blood and body tissues (Pagana & Pagana, 2011). Total protein consists of albumin and globulins (Van Leeuwen & Poelhuis-Leth, 2009) and are fractionated into five different levels: Albumin, alpha1, alpha2, beta, and gamma proteins (Fischbach & Dunning, 2009). Albumin, which makes up of more than 50% of the total serum proteins, maintains hydrostatic pressure (oncotic pressure) that fine-tunes the distribution of bodily fluid amongst blood vessels, bodily tissues, and cells. Its osmotic influence is about four times that of globulin (Van Leeuwen & Poelhuis-Leth, 2009). Albumin, the main transport protein in the body, transports substances insoluble in water alone such as bilirubin, fatty acids, hormones, and drugs (Pagana & Pagana, 2011). Globulin seems to have more diverse assignments, forming the main transport system for many substances and playing an active role in certain immunologic mechanisms (Fischbach & Dunning, 2009).

Serum electrophoresis (SEP) is the most current method for measuring serum proteins (Pagana & Pagana, 2011). Although somewhat outdated, determinations of total protein and A/G ratio are still being performed. The purpose of obtaining the A/G ratio (Table 4.9) is to determine the total protein and the albumin/globulin in the serum (Daniels, 2010). These levels can help evaluate edema (Fischbach & Dunning, 2009), as seen in patients with low total protein and low albumin levels. They can also evaluate nutritional status. Finally, after an acute infection or trauma, levels of many of the liver-derived proteins increase, whereas albumin level decreases; therefore, these conditions may not reflect an abnormal total protein determination (Pagana & Pagana, 2011).

Increased levels of total protein levels (by electrophoresis) appear in patients with multiple myeloma, RA, and osteomyelitis (Fischbach & Dunning, 2009; Daniels, 2010). Medications such as anabolic steroids, androgens, growth hormones, and insulin can cause increased levels (Pagana & Pagana, 2011). Elevated globulin levels, by electrophoresis, are noted in patients with chronic syphilis, tuberculosis, collagen diseases, SLE, and RA (Donofrio & Labus, 2009; Fischbach & Dunning, 2009; Van Leeuwen & Poelhuis-Leth, 2009).

Decreased total protein levels are seen in patients with cirrhosis, hepatitis, and other liver diseases (Dunning & Fischbach, 2011), reflecting a diminished capacity of the liver to synthesize albumin and an increase in the A/G ratio. Decreased albumin (hypoalbunminemia) is evident in collagen diseases, SLE, RA, ricketsial diseases, and malnutrition. Lower globulin levels are evident in variable neoplastic and renal diseases, hepatic dysfunction, blood dyscrasias, and prolonged immobilization such as orthopaedic surgery (Donofrio & Labus, 2009; Fischbach & Dunning, 2009)

Nursing considerations regarding SEP include knowing that prolonged use of a tourniquet during blood sample draw will increase protein fractions (Dunning & Fischbach, 2011). The blood sample should not be drawn near an IV site or after administration of large volumes of crystalloids. Finally, it is important to note that pre-test administration of a contrast agent falsely elevates protein test results (Fischbach & Dunning, 2009).

Uric Acid

This end product of protein metabolism is a class of compounds known as major end-metabolite of purine bodies (Fauci et al., 2009). The nitrogen-containing compound purines are significant elements of nucleic acids and are manufactured in the breakdown of certain

Table 4.9. Normal A/G Ratios

Normal Values: Total serum protein: 6.0-7.9 gm./100mL					
Albumin	**Globulin**	**Alpha 1-globulin**	**Alpha 2-globulin**	**Beta globulin**	**Gamma globulin**
3.2-4.5 gm/100mL	2.3-3.5 gm/100mL	0.1-0.3g/dL	0.6-1g/dL	0.7-1.4 g/dL	0.7-1.6 g/dL

Data from Diagnostic Tests Made Incredibly Easy *(2nd ed., p.44) by J. Donofrio & D. Labus, 2009, New York, NY: Wolters Kluwer/Lippincott Williams & Wilkins;* Nurses' Quick Reference to Common Laboratory & Diagnostic Tests *(5th ed., p.470) by M. Dunning & F. Fischbach, F., 2011, New York, NY: Wolters Kluwer/Lippincott Williams & Wilkins;* A Manual of Laboratory and Diagnostic Tests *(8th ed., p. 611) by F. Fischbach & M. Dunning, 2009, New York, NY: Wolters Kluwer/Lippincott Williams & Wilkins; and* Mosby's Diagnostic and Laboratory Test Reference *(p.799) by K. Pagana & T. Pagana, 2011, St Louis, MO: Elsevier.*

dietary proteins and endogenous sources (Daniels, 2010; Donofrio & Labus, 2009; Pagana & Pagana, 2011). Purine turnover occurs continuously in the body (Edwards, 2008), producing substantial amounts of uric acid even in the lack of purine consumption from nutritional sources such as legumes, yeasts, and organ meats (Van Leeuwen & Poelhuis-Leth, 2009). Uric acid is transported from the liver to the kidney (Pagana & Pagana, 2011), where it is filtered and then about 70% is excreted. The residual serum levels of uric acid are excreted into the GI tract, where they break down (Fischbach & Dunning, 2009). A lack of the enzyme uricase permits this poorly soluble substance to accumulate in bodily fluids (Pagana & Pagana, 2011; Zychowicz, Pope, & Graser, 2010).

The higher the level of uric acid, the greater risk of gout (uricosuria). Per ACR guidelines, however, this lab test is of limited value in establishing the diagnosis of gout (Kurakula & Keenen, 2010). Most patients with hyperuricemia will not develop gout (Edwards, 2008); conversely, patients with acute gouty attacks may have a normal uric acid level (Larocque, 2009). Sometimes urate levels can drop; therefore, urate levels should be repeated after an acute gouty attack. The gold standard in gout diagnosis is confirmation of MSU crystals (Edwards, 2008). Larocque (2009) further posits that all complications of gout result from hyperuricemia, while Byrd and Brasington (2010) note, "In 90% of cases, this occurs as a result of under excretion of urate, with overproduction accounting for the remainder" (p. 559).

The purpose of obtaining a uric acid level is to detect gout, renal failure, and leukemia (Dunning & Fischbach, 2011) in the face of a family history (as an autosomal dominant genetic disorder) or with signs or symptoms of gout indicated by elevated uric acid levels. Additionally, Van Leeuwen and Poelhuis-Leth (2009) note that this test is used to gauge the amount of "tissue destruction in infection, starvation, excessive exercise, malignancies, chemotherapy, or radiation therapy" and to observe the results of medications identified to modify uric acid levels, "either as a side effect or as a therapeutic effect" (p. 1186).

Normal uric acid levels range from 3.7-7.0 mg/dL for males and 2.0-6.0 mg/dL for females. In addition to gout, renal failure, and leukemia, the following conditions can increase levels of uric acid (hyperuricemia):

- Chemotherapy and radiation therapy;
- Congestive heart failure;
- Glycogen storage disease;
- Hypoparathryroidism;
- Hypothyroidism;
- Increased dietary purines;
- Lactic acidosis;
- Lead poisoning;
- Lymphoma;
- Multiple myeloma;
- Neoplasms;
- Polycythemia;
- Psoriatic arthritis;
- Sickle cell anemia; and
- Scarcoidosis (Donofrio & Labus, 2009; Fischbach & Dunning, 2009; Daniels, 2010 Pagana & Pagana, 2011; Van Leeuwen & Poelhuis-Leth, 2009).

Decreased levels of uric acid (hypouricemia) are noted with the following conditions:

- Fanconi's syndrome and Wilson's disease (inherited metabolic defects);
- Low purine diet;
- Acute hepatic atrophy; and
- Hodgkin's disease and some carcinomas (Daniels, 2010; Van Leeuwen & Poelhuis-Leth, 2009).

Nursing considerations include knowing that this test can be performed with either urine or serum. If a urine sample is used, a 24-hour collection is required to obtain all urine excreted during a 24-hour period (Pagana & Pagana, 2011). Preferably, the patient should fast 8 hours prior to the test (Fischbach & Dunning, 2009). Advise patients that alcohol use, a high-purine diet (liver, kidney, sweet breads), loop diuretics, stress, and strenuous exercise can increase uric acid levels (Daniels, 2010; Dunning & Fischbach, 2011). Additionally, aspirin, acetaminophen, ascorbic acid, levodopa, thiazide diuretics, and TB medications ethambutol and pyrazinamide may cause false elevations. Conversely, gout medication (allopurinol, probenecid, and sulfinpyrazone), azathioprine, clofibrate, corticosteroids, cyclosporine, guaifenesin, and warfarin may decrease levels (Van Leeuwen & Poelhuis-Leth, 2009). Nurses should be aware that uric acid levels must be examined throughout management of leukemia, as dangerous levels may occur following administration of cytotoxic drugs (Daniels, 2010; Fischbach & Dunning, 2009).

Vitamin D

Vitamin D is as a fat-soluble (Pagana & Pagana, 2011), organic substance with a 4-ringed cholesterol backbone. In regards to human synthesis, Vitamin D cannot be innately synthesized but needs to be obtained by outside sources, including diet, sun exposure, and supplements. There are two major forms of Vitamin D (see Table 4.10):

1. Vitamin D2: Ergocalciferol. Intestinal absorption converts this to Vitamin D 1,25-dihydroxy by the kidneys; and

2. Vitamin D3: Cholecalciferol. Sunlight absorption converts this to Vitamin D 25-dihydroxy (the most plentiful circulating form in the blood) by the liver (Van Leeuwen & Poelhuis-Leth, 2009). This is the level that therapy is based on.

Typically, Vitamin D2 and Vitamin D3 are added together and reported as a "total" 25-hydroxy Vitamin D level. The serum 1,25-dihydroxyvitamin D is the most physiologically active form. Data from Pagana and Pagana (2011) support the theory that this form of vitamin D has antitumor activities. This substance is assisted by the parathyroid hormone in maintaining calcium balance (Daniels, 2010; Van Leeuwen & Poelhuis-Leth, 2009).

The purpose of obtaining these blood tests is to assist in determining fracture risk, calcium and phosphorus maintenance, rickets, osteomalacia, hypercalcemia, and Vitamin D toxicity (Donofrio & Labus, 2009; Van Leeuwen & Poelhuis-Leth, 2009).

Table 4.10. Vitamin D Normal Levels

Type	Range
Vitamin D-2 (1,25-dihydroxy)	15-60 ng/mL
Vitamin D-3 (25-Hydroxy)	9-25 ng/mL
Total 25-Hydroxy D (D2 + D3)	25-80 ng/mL
Toxic Levels: >150.0 ng/mL	*Deficiency: <10.0 ng/mL*

Data from Nurses' Quick Reference to Common Laboratory & Diagnostic Tests *(5th ed.) by M. Dunning & F. Fischbach, F., 2011, New York, NY: Wolters Kluwer/Lippincott Williams & Wilkins;* Mosby's Diagnostic and Laboratory Test Reference *by K. Pagana & T. Pagana, 2011, St Louis, MO: Elsevier; and* Davis's Comprehensive Handbook of Laboratory and Diagnostic Tests with Nursing Implications *(3rd Ed.) by A. Van Leeuwen & D. Poelhuis-Leth, 2009, Philadelphia, PA: F.A. Davis Company.*

Increased levels of Vitamin D3 (25-OHD) could indicate excessive intake/intoxication (Van Leeuwen & Poelhuis-Leth, 2009) and may lead to renal or blood vessel injury (Dunning & Fischbach, 2011). Decreased levels of Vitamin D3 (25-OHD) are thought to be related to certain cancers, immune disorders, IBS and celiac disease, skeletal disorders (osteoporosis, osteopenia, rickets, osteomalacia) and possibly cardiovascular disease (hypertension and cardiovascular/CAD risk) (Donofrio & Labus, 2009; Dunning, 2011; Pagana & Pagana, 2011; Van Leeuwen & Poelhuis-Leth, 2009).

Nursing implications include discussing potential medication interferences such as the anti-seizure medication Dilantin that may impair Vitamin D production (Dunning & Fischbach, 2011). Secondly, a nutritional assessment of an "at-risk patient" may help reduce low levels of Vitamin D by encouraging foods rich in Vitamin D, including cod liver oil, milk products, fortified cereals, and fruit juices. The current adult Vitamin D oral daily intake advised is 2,000 IU per day (Dunning & Fischbach, 2011; Fischbach & Dunning, 2009).

Western Blot Test

Also referred to as electrophoresis separation of antigen subspecies and detection of antibodies of precise mobility, the western blot test identifies the antibodies for human T-cell lymphotrophic virus type III AIDS virus, testing for HIV-1 and HIV-2, sequentially (Daniels, 2010; Fischbach & Dunning, 2009; Van Leeuwen & Poelhuis-Leth, 2009). The separated antigens are put on an "electrophoretic sheet" using a blotting method, and the serum is incubated and then compared to two control specimens. This test permits the presence of antibodies focused against the viral protein HIV-1 and HIV-2 (Dunning & Fischbach, 2011).

The purpose of obtaining a western blot study is used as a confirmatory to the ELISA in screening serum established for the HIV protein (Donofrio & Labus, 2009). This is the most common confirmatory test for HIV-1 (Fauci et al., 2009). A positive response confirms a positive ELISA test (Donofrio & Labus, 2009). A negative response with a positive ELISA does not completely rule out the existence of HIV (Pagana & Pagana, 2011).

Nursing considerations include the understanding that informed consent is needed, and vigilant care is needed to maintain confidentiality of test results (Dunning & Fischbach, 2011). Patients should be informed that a positive western blot test means there has been an exposure to HIV but does not confirm active existence of the AIDS/disease (Pagana & Pagana, 2011). Sexual partners must be contacted and tested for the presence of the disease (Van Leeuwen & Poelhuis-Leth, 2009).

Urine Tests

Bence Jones Protein

The Bence Jones protein is considered a tumor marker for multiple myeloma (a malignancy of plasma cells) in that it detects an abnormal monoclonal globulin protein, a small cell that can easily pass through the kidney without being filtered out (Daniels, 2010). This globulin appears in the urine of patients with multiple myeloma and Waldenstrom's macroglobulinemia (Fischbach & Dunning, 2009).

The following are the three most common methods to measure Bence Jones protein:

1. "Classic" electrophoresis: heating the urine specimin to140 degrees F/60 degrees C, at which point the Bence Jones protein will precipitate and crystallize (Daniels, 2010).
2. Immunoelectrophoresis: measuring the specific low molecular weight protein in the urine from a 24-hour collection (Daniels, 2010; Pagana & Pagana, 2011).

CHAPTER 4

3. Urine immunofixation (IFE): gives a good "separation of immunoglobulins based on electrical charges" (Van Leeuwen & Poelhuis-Leth, 2009, p.731). IFE is the best method for detecting Bence Jones proteins in the urine and has largely replaced electrophoresis because it is more sensitive and easier to interpret. The purpose of the qualitative Bence Jones study is used to identify evidence of end-organ involvement in the setting of malignant bone marrow cancer, renal failure, lytic bone disease, and anemia, and to monitor treatment of multiple myeloma (Daniels, 2010; Pagana & Pagana, 2011; Van Leeuwen & Poelhuis-Leth, 2009). More recently, serum free light chain assays (Siegel, Bilotti, & van Hoeven, 2009) provide a more reliable measurement of Bence Jones protein.

In healthy individuals, the normal value is a negative test result. Positive levels will be found in 50%-80% of multiple myeloma cases. Approximately 15% of patients with myeloma excrete monoclonal light chains in the urine (Bence Jones proteinuria) in the absence of any detectable M protein in the serum. Patients with bone tumors, metastatic carcinoma to the bone, chronic lymphocytic leukemia, amyloidosis, some lymphomas, osteogenic sarcoma, macroglobulinemia, cryoglobulinemia, malignant B-cell disease, and hyperparathyroidism will also typically test positive. False positive results can occur in patients with RA, SLE, connective tissue disease, renal insufficiency, and certain cancers (Daniels, 2010; Donofrio & Labus, 2009; Pagana & Pagana, 2011).

The preferred method to test Bence Jones Protein in urine is by protein electrophoresis and quantified by immunofixation. "A light chain (lambda or kappa) in the urine is referred to as bence jones protein and is found in roughly 75% of patients with multiple myeloma and 80% patients with Waldenstroms macroglobulinuria" (Dunning, 2011, p.472). The following include reference values found by protein electrophoresis and quantified by immunofixation: Light Chain Values: Kappa total light chain: <0.68 mg/dl, Lambda total light chain: 0.40 mg/dl. Kappa/lambda ratio: 0.7-6.2 (Pagana & Pagana, 2011).

Nursing considerations include obtaining an early-morning, mid-stream urine specimen of at least 50cc (Daniels, 2010). This random urine specimen will be concentrated and electrophoresed. Discrete bands are then assayed by immunofixation to confirm that they represent intact monoclonal immunoglobulins or free light chains (Pagana & Pagana, 2011). If a Para protein is found, serial 24-hour urine collections are useful in monitoring tumor burden and response to therapy. If a 24-hour collection is needed, collect the specimins over the 24-hour period, discarding the first void and retaining the last. Additionally, this specimen should be refrigerated promptly (Daniels, 2010). Medications that can increase immunoglobins include penicillin, cimetidine, and narcotics. Conversely, medications that can decrease immunoglobulin include oral contraceptives, high doses of methyl prednisone, and phenytoin (Van Leeuwen & Poelhuis-Leth, 2009).

Urinalysis

A urinalysis is a common battery of tests on urine specimens. Urine is a fluid that contains water and metabolic products (Fischbach & Dunning, 2009) that is secreted by the kidney, stored in the bladder, and discharged via the urethra. The largest component of urine by weight is water, and the second largest is urea, followed by sodium chloride, phosphate, sulfate, and uric acid. Other normal components include potassium, calcium, magnesium, and various organic compounds.

The urinalysis primarily screens for pathology such as infection anywhere in the urinary tract or renal pathway, and helps identify metabolic and systemic disease (Donofrio & Labus, 2009; Dunning & Fischbach, 2011). The urine screening can be a part of a physical examination or pre-surgical testing. It also functions as an assessment of the kidney's capability to "selectively excrete and reabsorb substances while maintaining fluid water balance" (Van Leeuwen & Poelhuis-Leth, 2009, p.1193). In addition, systemic illnesses may be uncovered by quantitative or qualitative alterations of urine elements or by the occurrence of atypical materials, separately from their direct effects on the kidneys, including metabolic diseases not related to the urinary tract such as diabetes, thyroid dysfunction, and liver disorders (Fischbach & Dunning, 2009).

The urinalysis assesses for the following conditions (see Table 4.11):

- Atypical color, odor, and opacity;
- Specific gravity—urine weight compared to the weight of an equal volume of distilled water;
- pH—balanced hydrogen ion concentration in the blood;
- Semiquantitiative measurement of protein—evaluation of glomerular function;
- Glucose—an indicator of diabetes;
- Ketones—the products of incomplete fat metabolism in conditions (or massive fatty acid catabolism) as seen in diabetes;
- Urobilinogen—hepatic or hematopoietic conditions;
- Bilirubin—detection of liver diseases;
- Hemoglobin—presence of blood;
- Nitrites and leukocyte esterase—screening for bacteriuria;
- Crystals—urate, phosphate, and calcium oxalate; cysteine, tyrosine, and crystals of certain rugs;

Table 4.11. Urinalysis Values

Normal Values—Microscopic	Normal Values—Macroscopic/Dipstick	Causes of Increased Values	Causes of Decreased Values
	Pale yellow to amber color		
	Odor: slightly aromatic (not offensive)		
	Specific gravity: 1.005-1.035 (usually 1.010-1.025)	**Specific gravity (hypersthenuria):** acute glomerulonephritis with severe kidney damage, nephrotic syndrome, hypernatremia, dehydration, diabetes mellitus, CHF, shock.	**Specific gravity (hyposthenuria):** hyperthyroidism, pyelonephritis, diabetes insipidus, renal failure, acute tubular necrosis, diuretics, excessive fluid intake.
	PH: 4.5-8.0	**High pH:** Fanconi syndrome, UTI, metabolic acidosis, respiratory alkalosis.	**Low pH** (acidic urine): renal tuberculosis, pyrexia.
RBCs: 0-2 per high-power field	RBCs: none		
WBCs: 0-5 per high-power field	WBCs: none		
Casts: none, except 1-2 hyaline casts per low-power field	Bilirubin: none	**Bilirubin** (always abnormal): liver disease (cirrhosis).	
Epithelial cells: 0-5 per high-power field	Hemoglobin: none	**Hemoglobin/Hematuria:** obstruction, burns, infection, trauma strenuous exercise, tumors.	
Bacteria: none	Leukocyte Esterase - Nitrite (Bacteria): none	**Bacteria, yeast cells, parasites:** genitourinary tract infection, contamination of external genitalia.	
Parasites: none	Ketones: none	**Ketones:** diabetes mellitus, starvation, pregnancy.	
Yeast: none	Protein: negative	**Protein:** (benign) severe muscular exertion, multiple myeloma, hypertension, nephrotic syndrome, SLE, toxicity related to RA treatment with GOLD and Penicillinase	
Crystals: negative	Crystals: negative	**Crystals:** In acidic urine: calcium oxalate, uric acid, and urate. In alkaline urine: phosphate and carbonate. Calcium oxalate crystals: hypercalcemia. Cystine crystals: inborn error of metabolism	
	Glucose: negative	**Glucose/glycosuria:** diabetes mellitus, Cushing syndrome, impaired tubular reabsorption, advanced kidney disease.	
	Urobilinogen: normal	**Increased urobilinogen:** cirrhosis, hemolytic anemia, severe infection.	**Decreased urobilinogen:** biliary obstruction, renal insufficiency.

Data from Delmar's Guide to Laboratory and Diagnostic Tests *by R. Daniels, 2010, Clifton Park, NY: Delmar Cengage Learning;* Nurses' Quick Reference to Common Laboratory & Diagnostic Tests *(5th ed.) by M. Dunning & F. Fischbach, F., 2011, New York, NY: Wolters Kluwer/Lippincott Williams & Wilkins;* A Manual of Laboratory and Diagnostic Tests *(8th ed.) by F. Fischbach & M. Dunning, 2009, New York, NY: Wolters Kluwer/Lippincott Williams & Wilkins;* Mosby's Diagnostic and Laboratory Test Reference *by K. Pagana & T. Pagana, 2011, St Louis, MO: Elsevier; and* Davis's Comprehensive Handbook of Laboratory and Diagnostic Tests with Nursing Implications *(3rd Ed.) by A. Van Leeuwen & D. Poelhuis-Leth, 2009, Philadelphia, PA: F.A. Davis Company.*

- Casts—proteinuria and statis of the renal tubules, either hyaline or cellular; and
- Cells—renal epithelial cells, transitional epithelial cells, squamous epithelial cells, white blood cells (infection), red blood cells (tumor, glomerulonephritis) bacteria, yeast, sperm, and any other ingredients eliminated in the urine that may have clinical significance (Daniels, 2010; Donofrio & Labus, 2009; Pagana & Pagana, 2011; Van Leeuwen & Poelhuis-Leth, 2009).

Table 4.12. Abbreviated List of Common Medications Seen in the Orthopaedic Setting that Potentially Affect Urinalysis Results

Condition	Medication(s)
Urine color	Anticoagulants (orange), Iron Salts (black), sulfasalazine (orange-yellow)
Urine odor	Antibiotics, vitamins
Increased specific gravity	Radiopaque contrast media
Decreased pH	Ascorbic acid
Increased pH	Sodium bicarbonate
False results for proteinuria	Nafcillin, sodium bicarbonate
True proteinuria	Bacitracin, cephalosporins, sulfonamides
False positive for glycosuria	Ascorbic acid, salicylates in large doses
True glycosuria	Carbamazepine, corticosteroids, thiazine diuretics
False positive ketonuria	Salicylates
True ketonuria	Insulin
Increase WBC	Allopurinol, ampicillin, aspirin
Hematuria	Methicillin, sulfonamides
Drugs that cause casts	Furosemide, gentamicin, penicillin
Drugs that cause crystals	Thiazide diuretics, ascorbic acid, acetazolamide

Data from Nurses' Quick Reference to Common Laboratory & Diagnostic Tests *(5th ed.) by M. Dunning & F. Fischbach, F., 2011, New York, NY: Wolters Kluwer/Lippincott Williams & Wilkins.*

Nursing considerations include awareness that discoloration could be related to recent nutritional intake and medications (see Table 4.12). The urine sample (at least 15mL) ideally contains the first void after waking, and specimens that are not tested immediately should be refrigerated. Additionally, patients should avoid strenuous exertion before testing and review their medication list that may influence urinalysis. Patients should be instructed on methods to avoid vaginal or intestinal contamination of the specimen (Van Leeuwen & Poelhuis-Leth, 2009).

Urine Calcium

A quantitative 24-hour test determines calcium levels in the urine (Van Leeuwen & Poelhuis-Leth, 2009). Calcium homeostasis is sustained by the parathyroid hormone (Fischbach & Dunning, 2009). While the majority of calcium is eliminated in the stool, there is a lesser quantity eliminated in urine; therefore, increased calcium in the urine results from an increase in intestinal calcium absorption and a lack of renal tubular reabsorption, resorption from bone, or a blend of these mechanisms (Van Leeuwen & Poelhuis-Leth, 2009). (See Table 4.13.)

Table 4.13. Urine Calcium Levels

Normal values may vary with dietary intake: 100-300mg per 24 hours (quantitative 24 hour)	
Increased Calcium	**Decreased Calcium**
Medical Causes Hyperparathyroidism (30-80% of the time) Vitamin D intoxication Osteolytic bone metastasis (sarcoma) Paget's disease Sarcoidosis Multiple myeloma Hypercalcemia	***Medical Causes*** Vitamin D deficient rickets Metastatic carcinoma of the prostate Hypocalemia Hypoparathyroidism Renal osteodystrophy Renal insufficiency Osteomalacia
Pharmaceutical Causes Corticosteroids Calcitriol (a synthetic form of Vitamin D3) Dexamethasone Diuretics Sulfates Vitamin D	***Pharmaceutical Causes*** Thiazide diuretics Phosphate (increased ingestion) Bicarbonate Calcitonin Lithium Oral contraceptives

Data from Diagnostic Tests Made Incredibly Easy *(2nd ed.) by J. Donofrio & D. Labus, 2009, New York, NY: Wolters Kluwer/Lippincott Williams & Wilkins;* A Manual of Laboratory and Diagnostic Tests *(8th ed.) by F. Fischbach & M. Dunning, 2009, New York, NY: Wolters Kluwer/Lippincott Williams & Wilkins; and* Davis's Comprehensive Handbook of Laboratory and Diagnostic Tests with Nursing Implications *(3rd Ed.) by A. Van Leeuwen & D. Poelhuis-Leth, 2009, Philadelphia, PA: F.A. Davis Company.*

The purpose of obtaining urine calcium levels is to help estimate intestinal absorption, renal loss, and bone resorption, and to assess persistent renal nephrolithiasis (Fischbach & Dunning, 2009; Pagana & Pagana, 2011). According to Donofrio and Labus (2009), "Urine calcium generally parallel serum calcium levels " (p. 218).

Nursing considerations include knowledge that, because this procedure includes obtaining all excreted urine collected for 24 hours, specimens must be refrigerated if not tested immediately. In an emergency situation for patients suspected of potentially life-threatening hypercalcemia, a Sulkowitch test (random urine sample) can be obtained (Fischbach & Dunning, 2009). Patients should be advised to avoid contaminating the urine collection with stool or tissue (Daniels, 2010). A number of medications can increase urine calcium levels (see Table 4.13). Nurses should make a notation on the lab slip about potential medications that could affect urinary excretion of calcium (Fischbach & Dunning, 2009).

Urine Creatinine Clearance

This renal function test measures creatinine levels and a metabolite of creatinine, which is continuously formed and excreted (Donofrio & Labus, 2009). It is a final product of creatine metabolism and proportional to total muscle mass; however, if massive muscle damage has resulted from a crushing injury or degenerative muscle disease, levels will be significantly elevated (Van Leeuwen & Poelhuis-Leth, 2009). Creatinine values decrease with advancing age due to decreasing muscle mass. This test also estimates the glomerular filtration rate (GFR) that determines how efficiently the kidneys are clearing creatinine from the blood (Pagana & Pagana, 2011). The rate of clearance is expressed in the amount of blood that can be cleared of creatinine in 1 minute (Donofrio & Labus, 2009). Approximately half the nephrons must be damaged before creatinine levels become abnormal.

Urine creatinine clearance (see Table 4.14) is more precise than a spot urine creatinine level. The purpose of obtaining this level is five-fold:

1. To assess renal function, primarily glomerular function, and to evaluate the degree of nephron injury in recognized renal disease;
2. To assess diseases related to muscle damage;
3. To estimate renal function before administrating nephrotoxic drugs;
4. To gauge the precision of a 24-hour urine collection, established on the continuous amount of creatinine elimination; and
5. To monitor efficiency of management in renal disease (Daniels, 2010; Dunning & Fischbach, 2011; Fischbach & Dunning, 2009; Van Leeuwen & Poelhuis-Leth, 2009).

Nursing considerations include encouraging patients to avoid high levels of exercise and diets high in meat during testing period. The nurse should also keep in mind the medications that impact creatinine clearance (see Table 4.14.) The procedure requires specimens collected at timed intervals over a 24-hour period, usually at the 2-, 6-, 12-, and 24-hour marks (Donofrio & Labus, 2009). A venous blood sample is drawn the morning of the day that the 24-hour collection will be completed to determine plasma creatinine concentration. Additionally,

Table 4.14. Urine Creatinine Clearance Levels

Normal Values: Mean creatine clearance is measured in units of mL/min/1.73m^2. This is also referred to as the Glomuler Filtration Rate (GFR), the volume of blood (in mm) that can be cleared of creatinine in 1 minute.

Males: 94-140 mL/minute or 0.91-1.35 mL/sec/m^2

Females: 72-110 mL/minute or 0.69-1.06 mL/sec/m^2

Low Creatinine Clearance	High Creatinine Clearance
Medical Causes	***Medical Causes***
Decreased renal perfusion (such as in shock)	High cardiac output
Urinary tract obstruction (from renal calculi)	Burns
Polycystic kidney disease	Carbon monoxide poisoning
Nephritis	Acromegaly
Renal lesions	Gigantism
Acute or chronic glomerulonephritis	Diabetes mellitus
Chronic bilateral pyelonephritis	Pregnancy (substantial increase)
Muscle wasting disease	
Congestive heart failure	
Severe dehydration	
Progressive muscular dystrophy	
Muscular atrophy	
Polymyositis	
Inflammatory muscle disease	
Pharmaceutical Causes	***Pharmaceutical Causes***
Anabolic steroids	Antibiotics (cephalosporins)
Androgens	Gentamycin
Captopril	Amino glycosides
Thiazides	
Acetylsalicylic acid	
Cimetidine	
Cisplatin	
ibuprofen	
Indomethacin	
Furosemide	

Data from Delmar's Guide to Laboratory and Diagnostic Tests *by R. Daniels, 2010, Clifton Park, NY: Delmar Cengage Learning;* Diagnostic Tests Made Incredibly Easy *(2nd ed.) by J. Donofrio & D. Labus, 2009, New York, NY: Wolters Kluwer/Lippincott Williams & Wilkins;* Nurses' Quick Reference to Common Laboratory & Diagnostic Tests *(5th ed.) by M. Dunning & F. Fischbach, F., 2011, New York, NY: Wolters Kluwer/ Lippincott Williams & Wilkins;* A Manual of Laboratory and Diagnostic Tests *(8th ed.) by F. Fischbach & M. Dunning, 2009, New York, NY: Wolters Kluwer/Lippincott Williams & Wilkins;* Mosby's Diagnostic and Laboratory Test Reference *by K. Pagana & T. Pagana, 2011, St Louis, MO: Elsevier; and* Davis's Comprehensive Handbook of Laboratory and Diagnostic Tests with Nursing Implications *(3rd Ed.) by A. Van Leeuwen & D. Poelhuis-Leth, 2009, Philadelphia, PA: F.A. Davis Company.*

height and weight is needed to calculate body surface area on which the creatinine clearance values are based. Specimens are stored with preservative to prevent breakdown of creatinine and should be kept on ice or refrigerated during the collection period.

Urine Collagen-Linked N-Telopeptide (NTx)

This test is used specifically to monitor patients while being treated for osteoporosis and is considered a marker of bone resorption (Pagana & Pagana, 2011). NTx is created during bone remodeling, as collagenase and amino acids act on the bone (Van Leeuwen & Poelhuis-Leth, 2009). These NTx fragments are eliminated in the urine following bone resorption (Mayo Clinic, *81549*). A 30% decrease of NTx is desired, and a 50% decrease is sought after at approximately 12 months (Van Leeuwen & Poelhuis-Leth, 2009). According to Fauci et al. (2009), levels should be obtained prior to treatment with anti-resorptive medication and then again 4-6 months after beginning therapy.

Normal NTx levels are:

- Males: 0-85 nmol bone collagen equivalents/mmol creatinine
- Females (premenopausal): 14-76 nmol bone collagen equivalents/mmol creatinine

Elevated levels can occur in patients with hyperparathyroidism, osteomalacia, and Paget's disease (Mayo Clinic, *81549*). Conversely, as expected, lower levels are seen with appropriate osteoporosis treatment.

Nursing considerations include ongoing osteoporosis education, regardless of the results of this test. Patients may need additional dietary counseling, specifically in regards to calcium and Vitamin D intake.

Radiographic Tests

Angiography

This interventional radiology procedure of vascular structures uses radiopaque contrast medium or fluoroscopy for selective catheter placement. With this study, serial x-ray films are taken of selected vascular areas (Pagana & Pagana, 2011). The purpose of angiography is to assess peripheral vascular perfusion in the determination of amputation level, establish vessel patency, and evaluate vascularity of a known neoplasm. This test is also used to confirm vascular integrity in cases of traumatic lesions, bone tumors, orthopaedic surgery, chemotherapy, free muscle transfers, and thoracic outlet syndrome. Additionally, this test can offer pre- and postoperative assessment for vascular and tumor surgery and can assess for large or central pulmonary emboli (Fischbach & Dunning, 2009). There are three types of angiography: arteriography, venography, and digital subtraction angiography.

Arteriography examines the arterial system. This test must be performed with a sterile prep at the site. The patient is placed supine on the x-ray table, and a local anesthetic is injected at site of the catheter injection. The catheter is introduced with either a guide wire or fluoroscopy for direction to the site under examination (Dunning & Fischbach, 2011). Injection of dye is followed by serial x-ray films. Finally, the catheter is removed, and a pressure dressing is applied to site. The duration of the study is 1-2 hours.

Venography assesses the venous system, used primarily to identify deep vein thrombosis or suitable veins for arterial bypass grafting (Dunning & Fischbach, 2011). This test is the "contrast agent study of peripheral or central veins" (Fischbach & Dunning, 2009, p.787) or can assess for possible venous blockage of an existing catheter in the veinous system (Pagana & Pagana, 2011). A radiologist performs this test by injecting a radiopaque dye into the vein of the involved extremity then taking serial x-rays along the course of the extremity to view the venous structure. A positive thrombus finding will see an interruption or blockade of adequate blood flow. Patient instructions include maximal hydration following this study. It is important to assess the injection region for hematoma or infection.

Digital subtraction angiography (DSA), or transverse digital subtraction, investigates the arterial system using venous catheterization. This computer-based imaging technique has many advantages over regular arteriography: no arterial puncture necessary, reduced risk of trauma and emboli, outpatient procedure, it can obliterate bony structure from the x-ray images, and lower cost (Fischbach & Dunning, 2009; Pagana & Pagana, 2011). A local anesthetic is injected into a right antecubital or femoral area. Then the catheter is advanced over guide wire into the superior vena cava. After the catheter is advanced, dye is injected at selected time intervals via a power injector in selected amounts. Once the anesthetic is administered, pictures are taken and stored on magnetic tape or videodiscs. Finally, the catheter is removed, and the site is bandaged. The total duration of the test is 30-45 minutes.

Serious consideration with all types of angiography includes careful determination of renal function and whether the diabetic patient is taking glucophage/metformin. Patients using these medications are at danger for renal failure with lactic acidosis when contrast is used (Dunning & Fischbach, 2011). Potential complications of angiography include allergic reactions to contrast media, which can range from a mild rash to anaphylaxis (Daniels, 2010). Secondly, hemorrhage could occur at the site of arterial injection. Nursing implications for angiography are divided into pre-procedure, intra-procedure, and post-procedure sections.

Before the procedure: A consent form is necessary. Pregnancy is a contraindication (Dunning & Fischbach,

2011). It is vital to ascertain possible allergies to iodine, contrast media, or shellfish (Daniels, 2010), as well as to check labs for renal function, bleeding time, prothrombin time, and creatinine levels. The procedure is explained, including purpose, procedure, and patient's role. During the explanation, it is important to encourage any questions. It is important to let the patient know that the procedure is not painful but may cause some mild discomfort. Explain that a warm, "flushed" feeling may accompany the dye injection (Daniels, 2010), and stress the necessity to remain still during the procedure (Fischbach & Dunning, 2009). Anticoagulant therapy should be discontinued several hours to days before the procedure, and the patient must be NPO 8-12 hours prior to testing. Further procedural considerations include shaving the injection site and prep as ordered (Pagana & Pagana, 2011). Finally, the patient should void and, if applicable, remove dentures, jewelry, and metallic objects.

During the procedure: An IV infusion will be started, and glucagon will be administered if ordered for DSA, to "decrease motion artifact by stopping peristalsis" (Fischbach & Dunning, 2009, p.789). Record vital signs, premedicate with a sedative or narcotic analgesic 1 hour before the procedure or as ordered (Daniels, 2010), and prevent motion artifact as these tests can be very sensitive to physical movement.

After the procedure: For arteriography, pressure should be maintained on insertion site 5-10 minutes as either a pressure dressing or sandbag applied to the site. If a pressure device is used, reduce and remove pressure as ordered. Bed rest is maintained for 12-24 hours. It is important to restrict activities for next 24 hours. The involved extremity should be kept straight for 6-8 hours, with regular neurovascular assessment of color, motion, sensation, capillary refill time, pulse quality, and temperature. It is important to check site and vital signs frequently, including the following schedule: every 15 minutes for 1 hour; every 30 minutes for 2 hours, and every hour for 4 hours. Check temperature every 4 hours for 24-48 hours. Observe the injection site and report site swelling, bleeding, and hematoma formation. Assess peripheral pulses distal to injection site, using Doppler if necessary (Fischbach & Dunning, 2009). Finally, note temperature and color of the extremity distal to injection site. It is critical to observe for delayed allergic reactions, including tachycardia, dyspnea, skin rash, urticaria, hypotension, and decreased urine output. Finally, it is important to encourage fluid intake of at least 2,000ml unless contraindicated (Dunning & Fischbach, 2011).

Arthrography

Arthrography is defined as multiple roentgenologic examinations of an encapsulated joint cavity following injection of radiopaque dye (Daniels, 2010; Dunning & Fischbach, 2011). Contrast agents include water-soluble dye such as iodine and air; double-contrast arthrograms use both dye and air. This test outlines encapsulated synovial structures, soft tissue structures, and contour of a joint not normally visible on routine x-ray. Examples of structures evaluated with arthrogram include knee, shoulder, ankle, hip, elbow, and wrist (Daniels, 2010).

The purpose of this test is to diagnose joint damage or disease. This test can be both diagnostic and therapeutic for patients with inexplicable or continual pain in the joints. This test can also assist in identification of acute or chronic tears: if a tear exists, the contrast material will leak out of the joint and be visible on radiograph of a joint capsule or supporting ligament structures of the knee, shoulder, ankle, hips, or wrist (triangular fibrocartilage complex tears and scapholunate ligament tears). This test can assess for arthritis, dislocation, ligament tears, rotator cuff tears (particularly with patients who cannot tolerate MRI scans), synovial abnormalities such as synovitis, narrowing of joint space, and cysts such as synovial tumors (Daniels, 2010). This test allows for further characterization of chondral defects such as osteochondritis dissecans or osteochondral fractures (Van Leeuwen & Poelhuis-Leth, 2009). Knee arthrograms are very useful for assessing popliteal cysts/synovial cysts (Fischbach & Dunning, 2009), loose bodies (unless loose bodies are calcified; they will not show without contrast), and possible joint arthroplasty loosening. As far as a therapeutic arthrogram, corticosteroids can typically be injected for pain management. CT scanning (see separate section) can be added to the air-contrast arthrogram (CT arthrography), providing a better assessment of possible glenoid labrum tears. The cost of this test is less than CT and MRI and can be performed if fluoroscopy is available.

The arthrogram procedure involves the following: The patient is positioned on their back on the radiology examining table. After the skin over the affected joint is cleansed using sterile technique, a local anesthetic is injected around the puncture site. A fluoroscopically or ultrasound-guided needle is inserted into the joint space. It is important to aspirate any joint effusion, which can be sent for analysis of fluid contents. An iodinated contrast agent (gas, water, or iodine) or a negative contrast agent (such as air) is injected into the joint, which is then manipulated to disperse the agent (Dunning & Fischbach, 2011). Then an x-ray examination is made in multiple positions of soft tissue and the encapsulated joint. With CT and MR arthrogram, these studies use tomographic examination. Additionally, the following types of studies may be performed: body section radiography, planography, laminography, or stratigraphy. These types of studies allow more detail to be visualized, for example imaging structures lying in a predetermined tissue plane. Finally, the joint may be put through its range of motion under fluoroscopy while the x-ray series is made.

Nursing implications of arthrography include pre-procedure, intra-test, and post-procedure sections. Before the procedure: Although there are no physical preparations for this study, consent forms are necessary. The nurse's role includes a detailed explanation of the purpose, procedure, patient's role, and potential risks (including possible bacterial infection or reaction to the contrast material). Explain that some discomfort may be felt particularly during the joint manipulation. Rule out pregnancy and possible allergy to (iodine) contrast media (Van Leeuwen & Poelhuis-Leth, 2009). Encourage patients to bring any previous radiographs of their specific joint prior to this procedure (Fischbach & Dunning, 2009).

During the procedure: provide patient support during needle placement, as some discomfort is to be expected.

After the procedure: the joint needs to rest for 12 hours, with application of a compression (elastic bandage) dressing for 12 hours. A compressive wrap may be applied to keep joint swelling to a minimum. A mild analgesia for swelling and pain may be taken along with cool packs as needed. Clicking or cracking noises may be heard in joint for 1–2 days as dye and air are absorbed. If this "clicking sign" is persistent, the patient should notify the ordering physician (Daniels, 2010).

Complications of arthrography include persistent joint crepitus and possible infection. Precautions for this test include continuous observation for evidence of allergic reaction to dye.

Bone Scan

A bone scan (or scintigraphy) is a nuclear imaging procedure using a bone-seeking radioactive material administered intravenously (Dunning & Fischbach, 2011). A Technetium tagged to phosphate (99 mTc) is the most commonly used radionuclide. This material accumulates in areas of bone formation, abnormal metabolism, calcium deposition, and high blood flow (Donofrio & Labus, 2009). The study is interested in examining for increased osteoblast activity associated with new bone formation and, to a lesser degree, increased blood flow to an area.

The purpose of a bone scan is to evaluate conditions such as unexplained bone pain, trauma, and increased alkaline phosphate levels; frost bite; and metastatic bone disease (Dunning & Fischbach, 2011). In regards to metastatic bone disease, the following anatomical sites are targeted: breast, prostate, lung, lymph nodes, urinary tract, bladder, and thyroid (Fischbach & Dunning, 2009; Pagana & Pagana, 2011). The term "super-scan" refers to a diffuse pattern of "hot spots" associated with metastatic bone disease and other metabolic bone diseases such as Paget's disease, renal osteodystrophy, and osteomalacia (Pagana & Pagana, 2011). Interestingly, multiple myeloma is the only bone tumor that is better detected with a plain radiograph than a radionuclide bone procedure (Fischbach & Dunning, 2009).

A bone scan indicates very early (as compared to plain radiographs) bone disease and healing, including compression fractures of the spine. An example of bone healing and cancer includes the flare phenomenon that Dunning and Fischbach (2011) describe as "occurring in patients with metastatic bone disease who are receiving new cancer therapy" with breast and prostate cancers. With this phenomenom, during bone scanning, these lesions should show improvement "3 to 4 months later" (p.162). In the pediatric population, this test can be used to assess for growth plate fractures, child abuse, and stages of traumatic injuries and infections (Donofrio & Labus, 2009; Dunning & Fischbach, 2011).

Additionally, a bone scan can effectively evaluate other metabolic bone disease such as primary hyperparathyroidism, osteoporosis, and early osteonecrosis. This test can also detect stress injuries (stress fractures, shin splints, tendon avulsions, insufficiency fractures, pathologic fractures), stage cancer, and monitor degenerative bone disorders (Fischbach & Dunning, 2009; Van Leeuwen & Poelhuis-Leth, 2009). Finally, this test can detect *but not differentiate* the following: bone tumors (both benign and malignant), fibrous dysplasia, arthritis, fractures, early diagnosis of ankylosing spondylitis, secondary malignant deposits, rickets, Paget's disease, infections, synovitis, and osteomyelitis versus cellulitis (Dunning & Fischbach, 2011; Fischbach & Dunning, 2009; Pagana & Pagana, 2011).

The three-phase bone scan can also be useful in the diagnosis of complex regional pain syndrome (Gordon, 2007). Spot views or single photon imaging (SPECT) may provide more detail in diagnosing stress or traumatic spondylolysis and in detecting avascular necrosis (Dunning & Fischbach, 2011). Radionuclide imaging/scanning is most useful in screening the entire skeleton to localize the site of abnormality and also for detecting/evaluating stress fractures, osteoid osteomas, and painful prosthesis (Van Leeuwen & Poelhuis-Leth, 2009).

The bone scan procedure involves a radioactive material that is injected intravenously. Next, there is a 2-4 hour waiting period (Gordon, 2007) with no physical restrictions. During this waiting period, patients are instructed to drink at least 1 quart of liquid. Before the scan begins, the patient voids, as a full bladder masks the pelvic bones (Donofrio & Labus, 2009). Finally, the patient is placed supine on an x-ray type table, and the skeletal system is visualized by a gamma camera to produce high-resolution images (Daniels, 2010). During the study, the patient must remain still for 30-60 minutes during the scan. If necessary, a sedative may be given to maintain stillness during the procedure.

Nursing considerations for bone scans include pre-test, intra-test, and post-test implications. Before this procedure: A consent form is necessary. It is important to explain purpose, procedure, and patient's role. Furthermore, it is important to obtain a health history, including recent exposure to radionuclides, allergies, current pregnancy, and current infant breastfeeding. Additional pre-test consideration includes having the patient remove jewelry or metal objects. At this time, it is important to report any undue anxiety to the physician. Additionally, let the patient know that this test is painless and typically lasts approximately 30-60 minutes. Explain that the dose of radiation is less than a chest x-ray and that the radioactive isotope (which is harmless to patients and those with whom the patient comes in contact) is excreted from the body within 6-12 hours.

During the procedure: Blood flow and blood pool scans should be monitored, and static images should be taken 2-4 hours or more after injection of the radionuclide (Gordon, 2007).

After the procedure: There are no physical restrictions. Encourage fluid intake (Daniels, 2010), observe for allergic reaction (Dunning & Fischbach, 2011) to radionuclides, and advise patient not to schedule any other radionuclide tests for 24–48 hours (Donofrio & Labus, 2009).

Potential complications of a bone scan include an allergy to radionuclide. There are also factors affecting results, including antihypertensive medication, two radionuclide tests given in one day, movement during scan, and a distended bladder (the latter three affect the quality of images) (Van Leeuwen & Poelhuis-Leth, 2009).

Computer Tomography (CT)

A CT (or computed axial tomography [CAT]) uses a narrow beam of x-ray to scan an anatomical area in successive layers. Compared to plain radiographs, CT scans provides much greater contrast resolution (Daniels, 2010). CT diagnostic studies are extremely helpful where anatomy is difficult to view due to overlying structures that are typically obscured with conventional radiographs (Fischbach & Dunning, 2009). The CT also provides better bone definition than plain radiographs. With the mulitslice CT scanners, this provides high-resolution multi-planar (axial, coronal and sagittal) images. With these images, 3D images can be produced via a computer mathematical reconstruction (Dunning & Fischbach, 2011), providing superior views in complex fractures particularly around joints, fracture displacement, alignment, bone tumors, healing fractures, joint arthrodesis, and surgical fusion of the spine (Donofrio & Labus, 2009; Fischbach & Dunning, 2009). CT scans are routinely ordered after myelography and discography. Additionally, CT guidance for interventional procedures allows exact needle placement for bone and soft tissue biopsies, radiofrequency ablation of osteoid osteomas and other neoplasm, and spinal injections that may be difficult to perform under fluoroscopy.

In general, this routine study is noninvasive; however, CT may be ordered with contrast media to increase diagnostic accuracy. This type of CT scan characterizes certain lesions by enhancing the detection of small lesions and clarifies margins of larger lesions. A contrast study uses an iodine-based dye injected intravenously or a barium-like substance administered by mouth or by nasogastric or gastrostomy tube.

The purpose of ordering a CT scan is to evaluate head, spine, and body imaging to assess for pathology within these structures (Dunning & Fischbach, 2011). The CT scan is primarily used for visualization of bone cortex; however, an MRI (see separate section) may be the better choice for soft tissue lesions and marrow changes. Spiral or helical CT of the hip is used to evaluate size and progression of acetabular or femoral osteolytic lesions adjacent to a prosthetic implant. Flexion CT views are used to evaluate for femoroacetabular impingement of the hip joint.

During the CT procedure, X-ray beams are projected horizontally. The data is displayed on a screen (video monitor), photographed, or stored on magnetic tapes or disks. The procedure takes 45–90 minutes. New light speed technology cuts scanning time dramatically. If a contrast study is done, IV contrast medium is injected over a 2-minute period.

Head scans are used to evaluate disease, disorders, and trauma to brain, facial bones, and sinuses. This scan can evaluate headaches, loss of consciousness, and neurologic deficits. For the procedure, the patient is placed on a motorized table with the head immobilized in a cradle (Donofrio & Labus, 2009). A clicking noise may be heard as the scanner revolves around the patient's head (Fischbach & Dunning, 2009).

Spinal scans are used to assist in the diagnosis of spinal cord and peripheral nerve pathology. This study can evaluate post-fusion complications such as pseudo-arthrosis, stenosis of the central cord, and lateral recess of neural foramen. The procedure has the patient positioned supine on a table with hips and knees supported. An IV or intrathecal contrast is used (Donofrio & Labus, 2009), although not routinely used for lumbar spine studies. Typically, this type of scan is used for intra-dural processes, arachnoiditis, or postoperative fibrosis evaluation.

Body scans include the abdomen, chest, pelvis, and joints. This scan is used in the identification of soft tissue and/or bone tumors. For the procedure, the patient is placed in the supine position on a table with appropriate body part in the scanner. The patient may be asked to hold breath occasionally. As with head scans, the patient may hear a clicking noise. Patients receiving a pelvic CT will typically require a barium contrast enema.

Nursing considerations for CT scans include the understanding that radiation exposure is higher for CT scan diagnostic imaging than most other imaging studies; therefore, a careful risk-benefit analysis needs to be made before ordering this study (Brenner & Hall, 2007). Studies using barium should be scheduled after CT scans, as retained barium can obscure images. As with all diagnostic studies, explain purpose, procedure, and patient's role before the CT scan procedure. Obtain a consent form, and ascertain pregnancy status (CT is contraindicated in pregnancy). Additionally, it is critical to assess renal function before this test is performed, checking for use of metformin and iodinated contrast administration, as there is a "potential for renal failure with lactic acidosis when iodinated contrast is administered in combination with metformin" (Fischbach & Dunning, 2009, p.780). It is important to remove jewelry or metal objects. Offer emotional support to the patient and family. Showing the patient a picture of the scanner may help to allay anxiety in some patients who may experience claustrophobic fears of being in a machine as the scanner rotates about the body part. Explain the need to be still during procedure, which can last 20-90 minutes. Explain that this test is noninvasive (unless contrast used). The CT scan is considered a painless study; however, any discomfort typically comes from disease, existing trauma, or lying still.

Implications specific for contrast studies can be divided into preprocedural, intraprocedural, and postprocedural considerations. Before the procedure: Determine allergy to iodine, seafood, or other contrast media (Daniels, 2010). If there is an allergy history, the patient may be put on steroids for 3 days or antihistamines before test. The patient will be NPO for 3-12 hours before the test, if ordered. Other considerations with contrast studies include that an enema may be ordered.

During the procedure: As Donofrio and Labus (2009) note, the patient may feel a flushed and warm sensation after the dye injection, and may report a metallic or salty taste. Also, the patient may experience mild nausea or (rarely) vomiting. With this study, it is critical to have emergency drugs and equipment available for severe allergic reactions. Also, it is important to observe for nausea/vomiting and any signs of allergic reactions, and to offer verbal reassurance to patient.

After the procedure: Observe for delayed allergic reactions. These reactions include urticaria, skin rashes, nausea, vomiting, headache, and swelling of parotid glands (iodism). Administer oral antihistamines if symptoms persist. Encourage fluids to assist in the excretion of dye.

Dual Energy X-Ray Absorptiometry (DXA)

DXA, also known as bone mineral densitometry, is a method of measuring bone mineral density (BMD) using x-ray absorptiometry to test the hip and spine. This safe, non-invasive diagnostic study used in the diagnosis of osteoporosis is considered the gold standard in the quantitative measurement of bone mass (Donofrio & Labus, 2009; Pagana & Pagana, 2011). Whereas plain radiographs cannot be considered a diagnostic tool for osteoporosis because there needs to be at least a 30%-40% loss to be visible, central DXA (CDXA) allows the clinician to diagnose low bone mass before a fracture occurs (Dunning & Fischbach, 2011). This test helps stratify fracture risk, guide therapy choices, and monitor response to therapy (Pagana & Pagana, 2011).

DXA is an accurate predictor of spine and hip fractures. This test essentially compares bone mass to that of a mean young adult normal reference range (the T-score) (see Table 4.15) using a laser x-ray scanner and computer technology that records images to measure fracture risk. The computer calculates the size and thickness of the bone, as well as its volumetric density, to determine its potential resistance to mechanical stress. DXA study results are referred to as BMD values.

Table 4.15. BMD Values

Diagnosis	T-Score
Normal bone density	Between +1 and -1 SD
Osteopenia	Between -1 and -2.5 SD from peak bone mass
Osteoporosis	Below (more negative than) -2.5 SD
Severe osteoporosis	Below -2.5 SD and associated with fragility fractures
These scores are based on a population of Caucasian women and are not necessarily applicable to all ages.	

Data from Bone Mass Measurement: What the Numbers Mean *by the National Institute of Arthritis and Musculoskeletal and Skin Diseases, 2009, http://www.niams.nih.gov/Health_Info/Bone/Bone_Health/bone_mass_measure.asp.*

The DXA procedure involves positioning the patient depending on the body part being imaged. A foam block is placed under knees for spinal exam. A brace is used for leg immobilization during a femur scan or for arm immobilization during forearm scan (Van Leeuwen & Poelhuis-Leth, 2009). Total duration of the scan can take

20-55 minutes (Fischbach & Dunning, 2009), during which time the patient needs to be completely still.

Nursing implications for the DXA include the importance of explaining the purpose, procedure, and patient's role during the study. The procedure should not be scheduled within 72 hours of nuclear medicine studies or within 7-10 days of barium studies, as this may interfere with the DXA exam. Before the test, the nurse should obtain a complete medical history, including GYN history (this test is contraindicated with pregnancy) and surgical history (focused on any metal implants) (Van Leeuwen & Poelhuis-Leth, 2009; Dunning & Fischbach, 2011). The patient should be advised not to take a calcium supplement on the day of the procedure (Daniels, 2010), and all metal objects (jewelry, braces, or prosthetic devices) must be removed from the area to be scanned (Pagana & Pagana, 2011).

There are essentially no complications associated with DXA, as this is a safe, painless, non-invasive, and low-radiation study. Osteoarthritis, fractures, size of area scanned, and fat tissue distribution all influence the accuracy of the test result.

Duplex Ultrasound Imaging

This non-invasive Doppler ultrasound diagnostic study provides anatomic imaging of the major blood vessels that supply the brain and extremities in terms of blood flow and thrombosis. The purpose of obtaining this study in the orthopaedic arena includes assessment of limb swelling and pain, typically following an orthopaedic procedure such as surgery and immobilization (Daniels, 2010). Normal results show adequate blood flow, both arterially and venously (Van Leeuwen & Poelhuis-Leth, 2009).

The duplex ultrasound imaging procedure includes having the patient lie supine on an exam table. A transducer is applied to the skin with a water-based gel (Dunning & Fischbach, 2011). For upper extremities, this transducer is moved up and down the affected extremity over blood vessels from the shoulder girdle continuously to the most distal aspect of the extremity. Conversely, for lower extremities, the test moves from the pelvis to the most distal aspect of the lower extremity (Pagana & Pagana, 2011). Both extremities should be evaluated for comparison (Van Leeuwen & Poelhuis-Leth, 2009). The procedure last approximately 20-45 minutes (Fischbach & Dunning, 2009).

Nursing considerations include recommending that the patient avoid caffeinated beverages and nicotine prior to this test (Daniels, 2010). Postprocedural collaborative communication with the ordering provider and the patient is critical in terms of test results (Van Leeuwen & Poelhuis-Leth, 2009). If there is a DVT, the patient will need urgent counseling regarding potential anti-coagulation management.

Indium WBC Scan

Indium WBC scans are a method of nuclear medicine infection imaging to detect infections or abscesses in deep body cavities and/or acute abscess formation (Dunning & Fischbach, 2011). Also known as inflammatory process imaging, leukocyte imaging, or Indium- or ceretec-labeled WBC imaging, this test can locate infected sites with a "tracer" and determine if they are localized, walled off, and suitable for draining. This is an important test in the setting of sepsis, osteomyelitis, or suspected intra-abdominal abscess. According to Fischbach and Dunning (2009), this process is "90 percent *sensitive* and 90 percent *specific* for acute inflammatory disease or acute abscess formation" (p.734). Because WBCs accumulate in areas of inflammation, the Indium WBC scan uses radiolabeled WBCs (Pagana & Pagana, 2011) to determine the site of an acute infection or confirm the presence of infection/inflammation at an assumed site. The basis of this test is that any collection of radiolabeled WBCs (mostly neutrophils) "outside of the spleen, liver and a functioning bone marrow" (Dunning & Fischbach, 2011, p.734) indicates an abnormal accumulation (Pagana & Pagana, 2011).

This test is particularly useful in detecting postoperative infection sites (Van Leeuwen & Poelhuis-Leth, 2009) and in documenting lack of residual infection after a course of antimicrobial therapy. It replaces the gallium scan in patients with neoplastic lesions or non-infected healing wounds, as gallium often gives false positive for these conditions.

For the Indium WBC scan procedure, Indium-111 pentetic acid (also called In-111-DTPA) is the agent of choice for radionuclide cisternography because its half-life of 2.8 days is suitable for 24-48 hour delayed scans. A 50-80cc blood sample is obtained; granulocytes are isolated and radiolabeled pharmaceutically with Indium-111 (radioactive indium oxide) or Technetium-99 (injected intravenously) (Fischbach & Dunning, 2009). Next, the cells are re-injected intravenously. After the injection, a whole-body scan is done within 4-48 hours to assess for suspected infections (Pagana & Pagana, 2011). Finally, the results are confirmed with CT or ultrasound diagnostic studies.

Nursing implications for this test include explaining the purpose, procedure, and patient's role. First, be certain that all metallic objects be removed prior to the WBC-scan. Next, let the patient know that the radiolabeling/preparation process of the tagged WBCs can take up to 2 hours. The patient's WBC count should be at least 4.0; this is so there is enough volume of WBCs for the radionuclides to attach to. If the patient is not able to produce enough WBCs or if their WBC count is not high enough, then donor WBCs may be used (Pagana & Pagana, 2011). The nurse should be aware that radionuclide tests performed 24-48 hours after the scan and gallium scans 1 month prior to the scan will interfere with results (Fischbach & Dunning, 2009). False positive results can occur with the following conditions: GI bleeding, upper respiratory infections, pneumonitis, hemodialysis, hyperglycemia, steroid therapy, and long-term antibiotic therapy (Dunning & Fischbach, 2011; Van Leeuwen & Poelhuis-Leth, 2009).

Complications for this diagnostic study, although rare, include allergic reactions such as local skin reactions, nausea, vomiting. Precautions regarding this test include performing a "time out procedure" to verify the correct patient when injecting the radiolabeled WBCs.

Magnetic Resonance Imaging (MRI)

Also known as nuclear magnetic resonance (NMR), MRI is an imaging modality that examines interaction between (superconducting) magnetic field, radiofrequency signals waves, and tissue cells (hydrogen nuclei) to emit their own signal (Daniels, 2010). This diagnostic study helps to differentiate between healthy and diseased/damaged tissue (Pagana & Pagana, 2011). The image produced is reliant upon density of cells stimulated and the magnetic interface that differs in fat, muscle, bone, and blood. The technique obtains structural information from the density of protons in tissue and the association of these protons to their immediate environment. The image created affords rich, "sensitive tomographic images of bone and soft tissue" (Donofrio & Labus, 2009, p.374). The MRI scanner relies on atoms' magnetic properties and uses a powerful magnetic field and radiofrequency to produce images based on water content/hydrogen content of bodily tissues (Donofrio & Labus, 2009). MRI provides multi-planar images in cross-sectional, sagittal, coronal, and transverse planes without the use of ionizing radiation or the interference of bone and surrounding tissue. In regards to soft tissue differentiation, MRI is more evident than CT (Daniels, 2010).

The purpose of obtaining an MRI scan is to visualize marrow, soft tissue tumors, primary and metastatic bone tumors, and cartilage. This test is also used for anatomic delineation of muscles, ligaments, fat, nerves, blood vessels, and bones (Dunning & Fischbach, 2011). This test is very precise in diagnosing abnormalities within bones, joints, and surrounding soft tissue structures, including cartilage, synovium, ligaments, and tendons (Fischbach & Dunning, 2009).

The MRI procedure involves several steps. Prior to MRI, the patient completes a detailed medical history, including any metal implants (Fischbach & Dunning, 2009). All external metal objects and credit cards with magnetic strips must be set aside. For the procedure, the patient lies on a table that moves into a magnet scanner tube. The magnetic force is applied, and the cell nuclei respond to the force by resonating. Once the magnetic force stops, the atoms realign themselves and nuclei release energy absorbed in the form of radio waves that are received by the antenna in the MRI unit. The computer amplifies and processes these radio waves to produce a high-resolution video image (Van Leeuwen & Poelhuis-Leth, 2009). Contrast media may be used to assist in differentiating from orthopaedic postoperative scar tissue from a new musculoskeletal injury, vascular abnormalities, and distinction of metastatic from primary tumors. Contrast imaging and MRI utilizes a nonionized venous contrast agent for better characterization. The most common agent used with this study is water-soluble gadolinium 50-DTPA, gadolinium manganese, or iron, which has very low toxicity and much fewer side effects than do iodine contrast agents.

Nursing implications include an explanation of the purpose, procedure, and the patient's role. Prior to the procedure, a consent form may be necessary. A detailed health history needs to be obtained, including a detailed renal history as the use of MR gadolinium is contraindicated in chronic renal failure because of the risk of nephrogenic systemic fibrosis (Van Leeuwen & Poelhuis-Leth, 2009) and surgical history as this test is contraindicated if the patient has any metal implants such as pacemakers, prostheses, or metal braces. In regards to body habitus, the MRI scanner is a narrow tube; therefore, it is critical to know the patient's weight and abdominal girth. As such, obesity may be considered a contraindication (Pagana & Pagana, 2011).

To reduce patient anxiety, explain to the patient that this diagnostic study is noninvasive and painless. Mention that the scan will make loud clicking noises as it moves inside its scanner housing to obtain its multi-planar images. One method of allaying anxiety is to give the patient earplugs (Van Leeuwen & Poelhuis-Leth, 2009). Other methods of reducing anxiety include showing pictures of the MRI device and pointing out the two-way radio while the patient is in the MRI scan tube. Discuss the need for complete patient cooperation, including that the patient lies still during the entire procedure; therefore, consider the use of sedation for patients with extreme claustrophobia or restlessness. It is essential that emergency equipment be readily available during MRI testing. The total examination time is typically between 30-90 minutes (Dunning & Fischbach, 2011). After the MRI scan study, the patient may immediately resume normal activity and diet.

A well-documented potential complication of MRI is that metal aneurysm clips have been bent and pulled from cerebral vessels during testing (Daniels, 2010); hence the need for a thorough review of the patient's medical history. Additionally, metal instruments such as stethoscope, scissors, etc., should be kept clear of the procedural space. If MRI with Gadolinium or contrast is used, monitoring for allergic reactions is essential. If the patient is not able to tolerate a closed MRI (or high field MRI, 1-1.5 or greater Telsa), an open MRI (or low field units, 0.2-0.5 Telsa) should be considered, although the image quality of a closed scan MRI is much better with the high field unit (Fischbach & Dunning, 2009).

Musculoskeletal Ultrasound (MSKUS)

This test is defined as ultrasonography or sonography that allows the examiner to perform a non-invasive study using high-frequency sound waves to assess anatomical structures (Scott, Didie, & Fayad, 2008). MSKUS is an important diagnostic study within the fields of orthopaedics, rheumatology, and musculoskeletal (MSK) medicine that allows for non-invasive, non-claustrophobic, and painless imaging experience. More specifically, this test can allow for MSK imaging of tendon tears; muscle abnormalities; potential hemorrhaging; or fluid pockets in muscles, joints, or bursa (Schneider & Pavlov, 2006). This test allows the examiner to obtain "dynamic imaging" to view MSK anatomical structures while they are moving. This study provides significant accuracy when performing procedures such as joint injections (Jain & Samuels, 2010).

The procedure involves the patient sitting or lying comfortably with adequate exposure for the examiner. For certain upper or lower extremities conditions, the use of a gown or gym shorts may be necessary. There is no preparation for the diagnostic study. The examiner uses a transducer and a clear water-based gel to produce the high-frequency images, which will appear on a computer screen. This "real time imaging" may be saved and incorporated into the patient's medical record. Total duration of the procedure is 15-30 minutes. This test is painless, non-invasive study that can easily be performed within an office setting. Typically, results will be ready during the examination.

Nursing considerations for MSKUS include explaining that if patients are experiencing painful musculoskeletal soft tissue conditions such as painful tendinitis, there may be slight tenderness while using the transducer along the course of that tendon. Using a cool compress following this procedure may decrease this discomfort. This is a safe, non-ionizing radiation test, with little to no risk involved; however, if a joint injection is performed, the usual aseptic technique and "time out" procedure should be performed. Finally, allay patient anxiety regarding possible tendon tears or other soft tissue abnormalities by providing adequate collaborative explanation regarding appropriate follow-up if soft tissue abnormality is found, such as a malignant versus non-malignant tumor.

Myelography

Myelography, also referred to as myelogram or spinal cord x-ray, is a combination of fluoroscopy and x-ray following injection of contrast medium or air into the subarachnoid space of lumbar spine through a spinal puncture (Daniels, 2010). After this injection, fluoroscopic and x-ray examination are done (Pagana & Pagana, 2011). The spinal subarachnoid space is outlined, and distortion of the spinal cord or spinal dural sac is visualized. Because the contrast material is heavier than cerebrospinal fluid (CSF), it will flow through the subarachnoid space at the dependent area when the patient, lying prone on a fluoroscopic table, is tilted up or down. The fluoroscope allows visualization of the flow of the contrast medium and the outline of the subarachnoid space (Daniels, 2010). The contrast medium should move easily through the subarachnoid space, revealing no barrier or mechanical irregularities. During this procedure, radiographs are obtained and may be followed by a CT scan for further visualization of disk analysis (Donofrio & Labus, 2009).

The purpose of obtaining a myelogram is to determine tumor sites, herniated intervertebral discs, cysts, or other lesions blocking subarachnoid space (Donofrio & Labus, 2009). Typically, this test is requested before surgical treatment of ruptured vertebral disc (Fischbach & Dunning, 2009). This diagnostic tool evaluates the presence of unexplained back or leg pain and any suspected intraspinal pathology. Currently, due to a long list of the following serious potential complications, myelography is generally avoided unless there is a suspected lesion.

- Arachnoiditis (inflammation of coverings of spinal cord);
- Bleeding or leakage at injection site;
- Brain stem compression/herniation;
- Fever;
- Headache;
- Nausea and vomiting;
- Neck stiffness
- Paralysis;
- Seizure activity (most likely to occur 4-8 hours after the exam); and
- Sterile meningitis reaction (severe headache and slow EEG patterns) (Fischbach & Dunning, 2009).

The myelography procedure is always performed in an x-ray/radiology department. The procedure takes approximately 1 hour. The patient is positioned for lumbar puncture initially (Fischbach & Dunning, 2009). Then the patient is positioned prone and secured to the procedure table with straps (Daniels, 2010). In this position, shoulder and foot braces may be used. The lumbar area is shaved, prepped, and injected with a local anesthetic. The next step is the lumbar puncture, in which a hollow 22-gauge needle is introduced into the lumbar subarachnoid space at L4-5. Once the needle is in place, a contrast medium (see Table 4.16) is injected into subarachnoid space of the lumbar spine (Fischbach & Dunning, 2009). The head of examining table tilted downward so that the course of the contrast medium can be observed fluoroscopically and films made serially. The contrast material will pool in the lumbar region when the patient is in the prone position, facilitating aspiration or easily drip from the needle. If an oil-based contrast is used, it must be removed once visualization is complete. If left in the body, this material could cause inflammation or adhesive arachnoiditis. Although the contrast material can be easily removed with the patient lying on one side, removal of the contrast material may cause pain in the buttocks or leg area from nerve root irritation. Finally, the puncture site is cleaned and covered with a sterile dressing.

Nursing implications for myelography include obtaining the necessary consent forms prior to the exam and determining any allergy to iodine or contrast material (Daniels, 2010). Assess for use of metformin/glucophage because of the increased risk of renal failure and lactic acidosis (Fischbach & Dunning, 2009). Anticoagulation agents may need to be stopped approximately 7 days prior to this procedure. If the water-soluble contrast agent metrizamide is used, ascertain absence of drugs that lower the seizure threshold (tricyclic antidepressants, phenothiazides, CNS stimulants, amphetamines) (Donofrio & Labus, 2009; Pagana & Pagana, 2011). Instruct the patient to force fluids the night before procedure and maintain NPO 4-8 hours before the procedure. A cleansing enema may be ordered for this test. Premedication (sedative or narcotic analgesic and atropine) may be used. Caution the patient of a possible transient burning sensation and/or flushed/warm feeling as the contrast material is injected, as well as the need for strapping due to the required tilting of the exam table (Daniels, 2010; Pagana & Pagana, 2011). Finally, the patient should void just before the procedure.

Postprocedural considerations are divided into which agent is used. After metrizamide, keep the head of the patient's bed elevated 15-40 degrees for 8 hours to allow the contrast agent to be resorbed in spinal canal, due to the fact that the material can irritate cervical nerve roots and cranial structures (Fischbach & Dunning, 2009). Then the head is lowered to allow an adequate amount of fluid to re-enter and bathe cerebral meninges. Progress to bedrest-with-bathroom-privileges for 16 hours. It is important to continue avoidance of medications that lower the seizure threshold (tricyclic antidepressants, phenothiazides, CNS stimulants, amphetamines) for 24 hours. After iophendylate, the patient must lie flat in bed 12–24 hours. While on bedrest, the patient may turn side to side. It is important to force fluids (Pagana & Pagana, 2011), while assessing for bladder distention and the ability to void. It is essential to maintain intake and output record. Neurologic function and vital signs should be frequently assessed following this test. Administer pain medications as needed for headache or discomfort.

Precautions for myelogram diagnostic studies include knowing that the procedure is contraindicated in patients with multiple sclerosis (Fischbach & Dunning, 2009), as the edema of acute-stage myelinated areas may resemble a lesion; in later stages, areas of demyelinated (unprotected) white matter would be chemically traumatized by the

Table 4.16. Myelography Contrast Agents

Agent	Uses/Benefits	Side Effects
Air/Oxygen	Used for differential diagnosis of cervical cord lesions. For patients allergic to contrast media.	May be difficult controlling gas after introduction. Poor visualization of the examined structures; accompanying tomography or thermography (see separate section) is needed to improve visualization. Painful headache due to of the effort in monitoring the gas presented into the region.
Metrizamide (water-soluble; 5–15 mL)	Absorbed by the body and excreted by kidneys; does not require removal from spinal canal. Provides better nerve root and nerve sleeve visualization. Uses a smaller needle/smaller puncture. Allows immediate removal of needle.	Possible central nervous system (CNS) irritation, including possible seizures.
Iophendylate (oil-based iodine compound; 5–15 mL)	Was used to locate spinal tumors *(Note: has not been used since ~1980.)*	Possible tissue irritation and poor absorption subarachnoid space. Must be removed by syringe and needle aspiration after procedure; removal process can be painful in the buttocks or leg area.

Data from A Manual of Laboratory and Diagnostic Tests *(8th ed.) by F. Fischbach & M. Dunning, 2009, New York, NY: Wolters Kluwer/Lippincott Williams & Wilkins; and* Mosby's Diagnostic and Laboratory Test Reference *by K. Pagana & T. Pagana, 2011, St Louis, MO: Elsevier.*

contrast agent. Secondly, as stated above, seizures are possible with incorrect postprocedural positioning and care. Further considerations with all agents and myelograms are that gas or fecal material in gastrointestinal tract affects results. Finally, acute exacerbation of symptoms may be caused by manipulation of CSF pressure; immediate surgical intervention might be required.

Positron Emission Tomography (PET)

A PET scan is a nuclear medicine diagnostic study that uses a mixture of IV administered positron-emitting isotopes and emission-computed axial tomography to visualize physiologic tissue function (Dunning & Fischbach, 2011). This imaging includes tissue metabolism, tissue perfusion, and neuron activity (Pagana & Pagana, 2011). Normal results show normal tissue perfusion and adequate blood flow (Van Leeuwen & Poelhuis-Leth, 2009).

The purpose of obtaining this study is to evaluate a 3D image of blood flow and tissue metabolism (Dunning & Fischbach, 2011; Pagana & Pagana, 2011). In terms of orthopaedic oncology, this diagnostic study can be useful in further characterization and tissue evaluation of tumors, particularly in staging tumors (Van Leeuwen & Poelhuis-Leth, 2009). This test can help distinguish between recurrent orthopaedic tumors, including active tumors and necrotic masses inside tumors (Dunning & Fischbach, 2011; Van Leeuwen & Poelhuis-Leth, 2009). Finally, this test can help guide effective treatment strategies for musculoskeletal tumors (Pagana & Pagana, 2011).

The PET scan procedure uses the radiopharmaceutical agent F-18 fluorodeoxyglucose (FDG) or fluorine injected intravenously (Van Leeuwen & Poelhuis-Leth, 2009) with the patient positioned supine on the examining table. It takes 30-45 minutes before the interested anatomic region can be investigated. A gamma camera then produces images on a computer (Pagana & Pagana, 2011). Additionally, this test can use a superimposed CT scan to allow for very accurate multi-planar images to improve the scan's accuracy. The total procedure time is approximately 1-2 hours.

Nursing considerations for a PET scan include pre-test, intra-test, and post-test implications. Before the test: Pregnancy is a contraindication for this test study because of the use of ionizing radiation and the risk for ionizing radiation exposure. (Daniels, 2010). The patient should avoid high-glucose foods a few hours before the test, as these may affect the imaging results due to elevated glucose and/or serum insulin levels. Explain that this test is often combined with a CT scan for maximum efficacy (Fischbach & Dunning, 2009). Allay any patient anxiety while waiting for the test to begin and again after the IV administration.

During the test: Continue frequent monitoring for potential allergic reaction to the FDG. Also, the patient's blood pressure and serum glucose will need to be monitored. "If blood glucose levels are too high, insulin may need to be ordered as it suppresses FDG tissue uptake" and can "affect the quality" of the imaging results of the scan (Dunning & Fischbach, 2011, p.455).

After the test: The patient must understand the importance of appropriate follow-up with the ordering provider (Van Leeuwen & Poelhuis-Leth, 2009). The test results will be reviewed by the ordering provider, and discussion can take place regarding appropriate treatment (Dunning & Fischbach, 2011).

Thermography

Also referred to as medical digital infrared thermal imaging (DITI), thermography is a noninvasive measurement of skin surface temperature distribution used to detect abnormalities due to myofascial disorders, spinal nerve dysfunction, peripheral nerve dysfunction, and scleratogenous (nondermatome pain) dysfunction (Daniels, 2010). This tool is often used in the differential diagnosis of myofascial, neurologic, and articular sources of pain, as well as temporomandibular joint disorder (TMJ) and reflex sympathy dystrophy (RSD).

The purpose of thermography is to investigate inflamed, infectious, traumatic, and neoplastic diseases of spine and extremities (Daniels, 2010). It is an objective method for documenting remissions or relapses of certain conditions. It can diagnose peripheral neuropathies. Thermography is also used in assessing and monitoring treatment results and anti-inflammatory medications, and augments or complements the diagnostic studies of myelography (see separate section) (Blue Cross of Idaho, 2011).

According to the International Association of Certified Thermographers (IACT) (2007), "high resolution infrared imaging" requires a high level of operator and interpreter competency and an adherence to established and consistent protocol. The thermography procedure requires that the patient is taken to a draft-free, ambient-temperature room (ideally 69 degrees) with essentially low humidity. Nonreflective walls are recommended. A high-definition/high-resolution camera is used to record thermograms (Hildebrandt, Raschner, & Ammer, 2010). No heat source, other than the patient's own body heat, should be in the optical path of the imaging instrument (although the imaging camera should be able to adjust to fluctuations in the room temperature). The total duration of this test is approximately 5-10 minutes.

There are two different thermography techniques. The first type, a contact thermography, uses an inflated "air pillow." The second technique is a non-contact, liquid crystal thermography that uses cholesterol derivatives

CHAPTER 4

that selectively reflect polarized light. There are certain advantages of using the non-contact method. Because contact with patient's body is unnecessary, it is adaptable to any part of the body. The larger body areas can be encompassed on each view. The simplicity of the apparatus is also an advantage. Finally, high color contrast is achievable. During the procedure, if an abnormal image is seen, photography is repeated at least three times in succession for confirmation.

There are essentially no precautions associated with thermography. Nursing considerations include emphasizing to the patient that this is a noninvasive and painless study, with no radiation involved. Review with patient that there is no smoking allowed on the day of procedure. Mechanical stimulation of the patient's nervous system must be minimized; therefore, there should be no physical therapy, no use of transcutaneous electrical nerve stimulation (TENS, a nerve impulse from a machine for therapeutic reasons), or testing such as EMG/EMNG conduction (see separate section on Neurophysiology Testing) on the day of testing. The patient should not wear braces or splints, should avoid powders or lotions, and should not have a sunburn. The patient should also limit caffeine and avoid nicotine and medications that influence vasoactive substances in amounts sufficient to curb autonomic skin responses (IACT, 2007).

Table 4.17. X-Ray Views Commonly Used in Orthopaedics

View	Description
Anteroposterior (AP)	X-ray passes from front to back.
Apical lordotic	X-ray of chest with apices of the lungs and clavicle.
Breuerton	X-ray of hand specifically to view early joint changes.
Carter Rowe	X-ray of hip from a 45-degree oblique angle.
False Profile of Lequesne	Standing x-ray with the pelvis at a 60-degree angle; assesses anterior femoral head coverage in dysplasia and focal areas of osteoarthritis.
Frog Lateral (modified Lauenstein)	Taken supine with knees flexed and feet in contact; often used in osteonecrosis to assess sphericity of femoral head.
Hughston	X-ray of knee in 60 degrees of flexion at a 55-degree angle.
Lateral	X-ray beam passes from side to side (left to right or right to left).
Mortise	X-ray of ankle rotated with lateral and medial malleoli parallel to the x-ray beam.
Oblique	X-ray beam passes at an angle.
Posteroanterior (PA)	X-ray beam passes from back to front.
Scanography	X-ray of hips, knees, and ankles using a ruler to determine leg lengths.
Sunset or Tangential	X-ray of patella with knee flexed and a profile view of the knee.
Tunnel	X-ray of tibia, fibula, and femur with patella defected and PA view of knee.
Von Rosen	X-ray of hips in abduction and internal rotation.

Data from Primer on the Rheumatic Diseases *(13th ed., p. 37) by J. Klippel et al, New York, NY: Springer;* Mosby's Diagnostic and Laboratory Test Reference *by K. Pagana & T. Pagana, 2011, St Louis, MO: Elsevier; and* Essentials of Musculoskeletal Care *(4th ed.) by J. Sarwark et al, 2010, Rosemont, IL: American Academy of Orthopaedic Surgeons.*

Intra-test considerations include ensuring even temperatures in procedure room. The patient should change into a gown and remain in the "thermoregulation" room for at least 15-20 minutes prior to the thermogram study (Daniels, 2010). The area to be examined may require cooling with a water sponge bath for 10 minutes before the procedure, and skin equilibrium must be maintained throughout the procedure. During this test, the rate of change in skin temperature to room temperature should come to a relatively stable state before the final imaging.

X-Ray

An x-ray, also referred to as a conventional radiograph and formerly Roentgenogram, is a study using beams of ionizing electromagnetic radiation to create images by penetrating bone and various bodily tissues based on their density (Daniels, 2010; Donofrio & Labus, 2009). Structures in human body are comprised of air, water, fat, and bone. Air has less density and produces dark or black images on an x-ray. Organs are denser than air but not as dense as bone and appear as shades of gray (Van Leeuwen & Poelhuis-Leth, 2009). Bone has high density and produces light (radiopaque) or white images. It is the calcium in bone that increases density and thereby produces lightness. Foreign bodies absorb x-ray and will display as white on radiographs (Fischbach & Dunning, 2009; Van Leeuwen & Poelhuis-Leth, 2009).

Images that are produced via x-ray are recorded on photographic film, as digital images, or imaged on a video screen (Fischbach & Dunning, 2009). Digital imaging allows for expedited review for the ordering provider and radiologist (Scott et al., 2008). X-ray is relatively low in cost and provides high "spatial resolution" (Scott et al., 2008, p.28), allowing good visualization of bony detail, in particular trabecular bone (Schneider & Pavlov, 2006).

Bone images help to determine the integrity, density, texture, erosion, and changes in relationship to other bones and tissue. Bone cortex x-rays reveal widening, narrowing, and irregularity, while joint x-rays can detect presence of fluid, spur formation, arthritis, foreign bodies, or tumors. Plain x-rays can evaluate for fractures, fracture healing, and dislocations (Pagana & Pagana, 2011; Schneider & Pavlov, 2006). It is important to note that x-rays of long bones should include the joint above and below to determine if there is a dislocation associated with a fracture (Sarwark et al., 2010). In the pediatric population, x-rays can help to assess for child abuse and growth plate injuries and/or pattern (Van Leeuwen & Poelhuis-Leth, 2009). The advantages of ordering radiographs include the fact that this diagnostic study is rapidly and readily available in most institutions, it has the ability to survey and/or screen a large anatomic area, and it is a useful screening procedure for decision-making regarding further diagnostic tests.

For the x-ray procedure, the patient is positioned dependent upon x-ray view ordered. The patient may be standing, sitting, prone, supine, or side-lying. At times, the examiner may need to reposition or manipulate an extremity to obtain an accurate image (Fischbach & Dunning, 2009). The patient should avoid excess motion during x-ray exposure. Finally, the duration of the x-ray study is dependent upon views ordered; this diagnostic study can take approximately 5-10 minutes for a routine procedure (Pagana & Pagana, 2011). Orthopaedic x-rays (see Table 4.17) are generally described in terms of anatomic regions:

- Thorax—chest, clavicle, ribs (anterior and posterior), scapula, shoulder, and sternum.
- Upper extremity—shoulder girdles, proximal humerus, elbow, forearm, wrist, hands, and fingers.
- Lower extremity—hip, femur, knee, patella, tibia and fibula, ankle, foot, calcaneus, and toes.
- Spine/spinal area—cervical, thoracic, and lumbar spine, coccyx, pelvis, sacroiliac joints, and sacrum (Fischbach & Dunning, 2009).

Precautions with x-rays include knowledge that patients in reproductive years should have their genital areas protected during this procedure. In regards to potential genetic alteration and x-rays, mutation of reproductive cells might occur with exposure of genital organs to radiation (Fischbach & Dunning, 2009). X-rays are contraindicated during pregnancy (Pagana & Pagana, 2011). Women in the first trimester of pregnancy are at risk for developing fetal abnormalities; therefore, during this time, only emergency films are taken. With this emergency situation, a lead apron is used to shield abdominal and pelvic areas during radiation exposure. It is important to note that films for obstetric reasons are not to be repeated. Because the effects of radiation exposure are cumulative, personnel and physicians should wear lead apron, gloves, and goggles in radiology laboratory and operative room suite (Ronckers, Doody, Lonstein, Stovall, & Land, 2008; Van Leeuwen & Poelhuis-Leth, 2009). Changes might occur in tissue in other parts of the body following excessive or repeated exposure to radiation. The patient's medical records should be appraised to determine frequency and dosage of radiologic studies (Fischbach & Dunning, 2009). Extremity imaging uses less exposure (Scott et al., 2008), therefore providing little risk of overexposure, but imaging of the thorax region (lumbar spine and pelvis) requires additional exposure and increases the risk of excessive radiation exposure (Ronckers et al., 2008).

As a critical member of the health care team, the nurse is in a position to assist in recording accurate information on an x-ray requisition. This will assist the radiology technician and radiologist in performing and interpreting radiographs more accurately. To allow for accurate interpretation from the radiologist, it is critical to write the *"clinical indication"* on the requisition. Patients who are elderly, traumatized, have deformities, or are debilitated may not be able to assume required positions over periods of time necessary for radiographic procedures. This information should be included in the requisition. Safety measures should be taken with casts, immobilization devices, or surgical apparatus (Pagana & Pagana, 2011). The radiology technician will perform an x-ray procedure with the knowledge given from the ordering provider as to whether orthopaedic appliances can be removed safely or must remain during the imaging process (Fischbach & Dunning, 2009).

Further nursing considerations include the need to explain the purpose, procedure, and patient's role, and to ascertain the patient's understanding. The provider may order withholding food and drink. The nurse should encourage questions and expressions of fear or anxiety before, during, and after the exam. Explain that several images may be taken (typically, the minimum x-ray order includes two views) and that the patient may be asked to wait following exposure to be certain that films are readable and that the views capture the correct angles; if not, additional images may be required (Dunning & Fischbach, 2011). In regards to patient comfort, it is important to allow rest time between images and to administer an analgesic or anti-anxiety medication if needed (Pagana & Pagana, 2011). Analgesics, local heat, or ice applications may be necessary for pain relief following a lengthy procedure or painful positioning.

Potential complications of x-rays include a host of interfering conditions. Obesity and abdominal ascites (accumulation of fluid in the peritoneal cavity) might interfere with the clarity of some views. Improper positioning of patient may result in the need to repeat the exam, which puts an extra burden on the patient in terms of potential discomfort and excess radiation exposure. Excessive movement during imaging could also impede the views (Pagana & Pagana, 2011); therefore, the patient should be reminded to limit movement during the exposure period.

CHAPTER 4

Special Diagnostic Studies

Arthrometer Testing

An arthrometer is a device for measuring and documenting cruciate ligament laxity of the knee, both actively and passively (Figure 4.1). These types of ligament injuries may be acute or chronic. In terms of mechanism of injury, anterior cruciate ligament (ACL) trauma usually occurs following a twisting or cutting knee injury. Alternatively, a posterior cruciate ligament (PCL) injury typically results from a blow to the front of the knee. Other methods of assessing cruciate ligaments include a clinical examination using provocative maneuvers called the Lachman test and the pivot shift test (Walsh, McCarty, & Madden, 2010). The purpose of using this test is to diagnose ACL and PCL tears. It can also be used to evaluate ligament stability intraoperatively. Finally, this test can be used to confirm ligament stability during and after a rehabilitation program (Arneja & Leith, 2009).

Figure 4.1. Arthrometer in Use

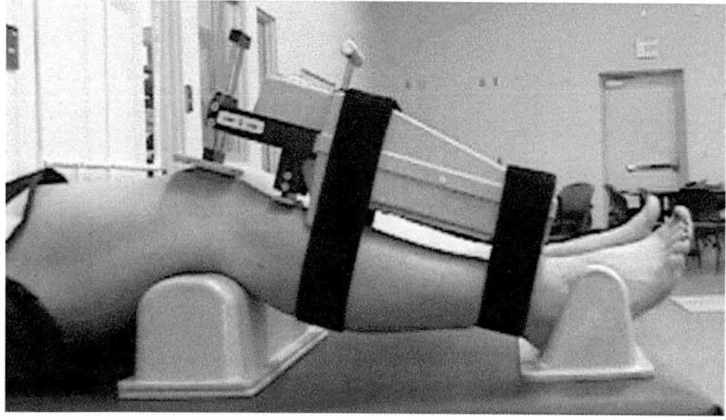

From "Comparison of Factors Influencing ACL Injury in Male and Female Athletes and Non-athletes" by S. Bowerman, D. Smith, M. Carlson, & G. King, 2006, Physical Therapy in Sport, *7(3), p.147. Reproduced with permission.*

The arthrometer procedure is typically performed in a physician's office after the physician's exam, x-rays, and arthrocentesis (joint aspiration; see separate section) if necessary. The operating instructions for the specific brand of arthrometer are followed. The patient is placed in a supine position on the exam table. The arthrometer is placed on the unaffected leg, and measurements are made using distraction forces on the knee passively, actively, and manually. Next, the arthrometer is placed on the injured leg and measurements are taken. Finally, positioning parameters and arthrometer measurements are documented in the patient's record (MEDmetric Corporation, n.d.).

Nursing implications include counseling the patient that the test is not painful and that they may return to pretest activities immediately. It is important that x-rays have been fully evaluated before the test. The date and method of reconstruction or injury should be documented on the arthrometer testing request form (MEDmetric Corporation, n.d.). The patient should be able to achieve full extension of the injured knee comfortably before the test. During this test, it is critical that the patient's quadriceps and hamstring muscles are completely relaxed.

Arthrometer diagnostic testing includes a number of complications. First, disruption or fracture near and/or involving the proximal tibia and fibula, distal femur, or patella are a possibility. Secondly, a disruption of the ACL graft can occur if the testing is done with too much force early in rehabilitation phase. Finally, it is important to note that a locked and swollen knee can abnormally restrict knee motion and result in a false negative test outcome.

Arthroscopy

This outpatient surgical procedure enables the surgeon to directly visualize the inside of joints via a fiberoptic endoscope. This procedure is most commonly used in knee diagnosis; however, this technique is now being used to explore a number of other joints, including shoulders, ankles, hips, elbow, wrist, and metacarpophalangeal joints (Fischbach & Dunning, 2009; Katz & Gomoll, 2007; McCarthy & Jibodh, 2009). Arthroscopy is often referred to as a triangulation examination as it allows for simultaneous safe (non-open) exploration, versus arthrotomy surgery or biopsy in which a cannula passes through separate instruments (Donofrio & Labus, 2009; Pagana & Pagana, 2011).

The purpose of arthroscopy is both diagnostic and therapeutic. This procedure assists in the differential diagnosis and treatment of synovial, ligament, meniscal, capsular, and articular cartilage tears. It is also extremely helpful in treatment of inflammatory processes in terms of synovial biopsy and therapeutic synovectomy. Articular cartilage disorders such as osteochondritis dissecans, osteochondral injuries, and or loose bodies commonly referred to as "joint mice" are also effectively treated by joint arthroscopy. Current literature suggests, however, that arthroscopic knee surgery is not indicated in osteoarthritis (Kirkley et al., 2008).

The arthroscopic procedure is performed in an operating suite under local, regional, or general anesthesia. The patient is positioned to facilitate the surgeon's access to the affected joint, and the operative site is shaved and prepped (as ordered) and draped in a sterile fashion. An IV is started and typically a tourniquet is applied to the extremity. According to Fischbach and Dunning (2009), surgeons may prefer to "not inflate a tourniquet, unless bleeding cannot be controlled by irrigation" (p. 899). The arthroscopic instrumentation is inserted into the joint through a portal to visually and dynamically examine the joint with the arthroscope and probe. At this point, any of the following pathology is addressed when applicable: a synovial biopsy or removal, meniscal repair or removal, articular cartilage repair or reconstruction, fracture reduction or fixation, scar tissue debridement, and foreign body and loose body removal. Arthroscopic pictures and videotaping are typically obtained sequentially while performing this procedure (Fischbach & Dunning, 2009). After the arthroscopic procedure, a sterile compression dressing is applied. A brace, sling, or cast may be used following some procedures.

Nursing considerations for arthroscopy prior to the procedure include obtaining a surgical consent form, determining drug and anesthesia allergies, recording vital signs and pertinent medical history including DVT, and assessing for anticoagulation or aspirin use. A detailed explanation of types of anesthesia (local, regional, or general) can help allay anxiety and fear regarding this procedure. General anesthesia routinely requires NPO status for 8-12 hours (Pagana & Pagana, 2011). The patient must remove jewelry, contact lenses, or glasses, and may premedicate if ordered.

After the arthroscopic procedure, the patient will go to the recovery room. Because of the use of a tourniquet during the procedure, the patient may feel tightness in the region postoperatively. Continuous monitoring of the operative site for bleeding, as well as circulation and sensation distal to operative site, must be performed (Pagana & Pagana, 2011). Nurses in the recovery room can educate patients on resuming normal diet and medications as tolerated. Aspirin may be used postoperatively per the discretion of the operating surgeon. Detailed education prior to discharge from the hospital include ambulatory status, pain management, DVT prevention, and signs and symptoms of infection. Postprocedural activity level and potential rehabilitation orders will depend on provider preference. A follow-up is typically performed on an outpatient basis to remove sutures, assess postoperative status, and develop of a rehabilitation program (Daniels, 2010). Physical therapy (PT) orders are typically discussed during the first postoperative appointment in the surgeon's office.

It is important to note that there are limiting factors to arthroscopy, including anklysosis, fibrosis, and sepsis. Fischbach and Dunning (2009) point out that recent arthrography (see separate section) can impede arthroscopy because chemical synovitis can occur from the contrast agents, which limits the visual examination; if arthroscopy is indicated after the arthrogram due to severe pain, the practitioner should be sure to irrigate the joint thoroughly to remove all contrast material. Finally, the same authors state that arthroscopy via the posterior method is not used due to risk of neurovascular structures. Other complications of arthroscopy include hemorrhage, infection, thrombophlebitis, neurovascular compromise, compartment syndrome, ligament/tendon rupture, and bone fracture (Daniels, 2010; Donofrio & Labus, 2009; Dunning, 2011).

Bone Marrow Aspiration and Biopsy

Bone marrow, the soft tissue contained in medial medullary canals of the long bones and in interstices of cancellous bone, is removed by aspiration, needle biopsy, or drilled core for a complete hematologic analysis. The purpose of this diagnostic study is used to determine cause of infection or infectious diseases by isolating bacteria or other pathogenic agents by culture. It can identify type of tumor (both primary and metastatic), anemia, osteoporosis, and certain granulomas (Fischbach & Dunning, 2009; Pagana & Pagana, 2011). It can also evaluate the response to treatment and the effectiveness of chemotherapy. It is used to further assess blood cell development (hematopoiesis), hemolytic disorders (by examining cell number appearance), insufficient stores of nutrients (vitamin B12, folic acid, iron, and pyridoxine), and the process of solid malignancies and leukemias (Dunning & Fischbach, 2011).

Bone marrow studies may be performed under a local anesthetic in a patient's hospital room, special procedure room, or radiology department, or under regional/general anesthesia in an operating room. Common anatomical sites for bone biopsy or aspiration include the posterior superior iliac spine (preferred site; Dunning & Fischbach, 2011), midsternum, spinous process of vertebral body, body of vertebra, and proximal tibia.

The *bone marrow aspiration procedure* includes obtaining a specimen through the following steps: The skin is prepped and draped, and a local anesthetic (typically lidocaine or procaine) is administered. Once local anesthesia is achieved, an aspiration needle is inserted into bone cortex through the periosteum (Van Leeuwen & Poelhuis-Leth, 2009) into the marrow cavity, followed by a stylet that is removed and a syringe is attached. A 0.1-3.0mL specimen of bone marrow fluid is aspirated. A needle may have to be repositioned if no specimen is obtained. The *bone marrow biopsy procedure* involves removing a core of marrow, and cells—not fluid—are removed. The preparation is the same as for bone marrow aspiration. Next, a biopsy needle or drill is inserted into bone at biopsy site to obtain the specimen. A sterile compression dressing is applied at the end of either procedure (Daniels, 2010).

Nursing implications for bone marrow aspiration and biopsy include need for the patient to be NPO. A consent form is necessary for this procedure (Pagana & Pagana, 2011). It is not uncommon to simultaneously obtain peripheral serum labs, including a complete blood count and a differential leukocyte count. It is important to determine sensitivity to local anesthetic and latex. During this procedure, the patient should understand that it is common to feel pressure on insertion and pulling sensation on removal of marrow. The patient may go to the recovery room if general anesthesia is used. During this time, monitor vital signs closely following procedure, check the biopsy site for bleeding and hemorrhage, and be certain to have properly labeled specimens (Dunning & Fischbach, 2011). Explain to patient that it is okay to resume diet, routine medications, and activity as tolerated. Postprocedural instruction should also include educating the patient to routinely check the procedure site for infection (Pagana & Pagana, 2011).

Potential complications of this procedure include hematoma, hemorrhage, infection, and sternal fractures if the sternum is the selected site (Daniels, 2010). Furthermore, precautions with this procedure include that the tissue specimen should be sent to the lab immediately. Severe bleeding disorders are considered a contraindication for this procedure. Additional nursing considerations include knowing that recent blood transfusions, iron therapy, and cytotoxic agents may alter biopsy results.

Discography

Discography injects radiopaque dye under low pressure into the center of several intervertebral lumbar discs (Thiyagarajah, Hord, & Vallejo, 2009). This test identifies internal derangement of a vertebral disc (RadiologyInfo.org, 2010).

The discography procedure is performed by a radiologist or surgeon in a radiology or surgical department under sterile conditions using a local anesthetic. The skin is prepped and draped in the usual sterile fashion, and a local anesthetic is infiltrated. Once the anesthetic takes effect, a long needle is inserted into the center of the selected vertebral disc using a posterior-lateral approach under fluoroscopy (Mayo Foundation for Medical Education and Research, 2009). At this point, a radiopaque dye is injected. If the patient is allergic to dye, an "air acceptance test" is done in which air is injected and resistance determined. There will be more resistance exerted with an intact disc than a herniated disc. At the end of this test, appropriate x-rays are taken (Thiyagarajah et al., 2009). A discogram is evaluated by the configuration of the dye pattern. Leakage of the dye can indicate a herniated disc. A normal/healthy disc will accept 1mL of dye with strong residual pressure; an abnormal disc will accept a greater amount of dye with minimal residual pressure.

Nursing implications include discussion about the need for NPO status 1-2 hours before procedure. The discogram test requires a consent form. Determine possible allergies to local anesthetic, seafood, iodine, and radiopaque dye. Consider administering an analgesic prior to this test. During the procedure, observe the patient for signs of anaphylaxis. Monitor the patient's pain response, and report of any radicular pain. Following the procedure, conduct regular neurological assessments and delayed anaphylaxis or allergy until the patient is stable (RadiologyInfo.org, 2010).

Potential complications of discography include nerve root damage, injection into the wrong space, a dural tear, and infection (discitis) (Thiyagarajah et al., 2009).

Joint Aspiration

Also known as arthrocentesis, this diagnostic procedure is carried out by inserting a needle into the synovial capsule of a joint to withdraw fluid for analysis (Van Leeuwen & Poelhuis-Leth, 2009). Although primarily a diagnostic study, arthrocentesis also provides pain relief when joint swelling and effusion are present (Collyott & Brooks, 2008). Synovial fluid analysis is of particular interest in diagnosing acute monoarticular arthritis or gout, differentiating inflammatory versus noninflammatory arthritis, and ruling out infection (Fye, 2008; Ma, Cranney,

Table 4.18. Synovial Fluid Analysis

	Viscosity	Appearance	RBCs per cubic micro-liter or cubic millimeter	WBCs uL/ mmm3	Polymorpho-nuclear (PMN) cells	Glucose Concentration, mg/dL	Protein Concentration, g/dL
Normal	High	Clear	<2000	<150	<0.25	Serum Glucose	1.3-1.8
Non-Inflammatory	High	Clear		<3000	<0.25	Serum Glucose	2-3.5
Inflammatory	Variable	Cloudy		>3000	<0.75	<25	>4
Purulent/Septic	Low	Cloudy		>50,000	>0.9	<25	>4
Hemorrhagic	N/A	Bloody		>2000	~0.3	Serum Glucose	....

Data from Delmar's Guide to Laboratory and Diagnostic Tests *by R. Daniels, 2010, Clifton Park, NY: Delmar Cengage Learning;* Primer on the Rheumatic Diseases *(13th ed., pp. 23). New York, NY: Springer; and "Knee Arthrocentesis Technique" by G. Shlamovitz, 2011, http://emedicine.medscape.com/article/79994-overview.*

& Holroyd-Leduc, 2009). Synovial effusions can be related to joint conditions such as noninflammatory conditions, inflammatory conditions, septic conditions, crystal-induced conditions (to distinguish between gout and pseudogout), and hemorrhagic conditions (Pagana & Pagana, 2011; Van Leeuwen & Poelhuis-Leth, 2009). This procedure is safe and should be considered in any acutely painful swollen joint particularly monoarthritis. The knee is the most common joint aspirated (Van Leeuwen & Poelhuis-Leth, 2009).

The joint aspiration procedure is performed by a physician using aseptic technique in an office or hospital setting. The site is cleansed with an antiseptic solution. A local anesthetic is infiltrated and an aspiration site indicated. Using a large sterile syringe, a sterile needle long enough with a gauge large enough to withdraw fluid is inserted into the joint capsule. The fluid is withdrawn and prepared for microscopic evaluation. Finally, the puncture site cleansed and a pressure dressing applied.

Symptomatic indication of joint pathology is increased with joint fluid (Fye, 2008). The normal characteristics of synovial fluid include the following: straw colored and clear; a cell count less than 200; glucose equivalent to ~50% of serum (Pagana & Pagana, 2011); no crystals present; and negative cultures (both aerobic and anaerobic). (See Table 4.18.)

Nursing implications include a thorough explanation of the procedure and a caution that it may have to be repeated, as indicated, if swelling recurs. Before beginning the procedure, perform a "time out" to confirm the correct extremity for the procedure. Preparation for this procedure includes a full history about joint swelling, anti-coagulation use, and hemarthrosis (bleeding into the joint). The use of anticoagulation medication may need to be limited or withheld depending on provider preference. Further, history questions should focus on any history of infection, inflammatory arthritis, injury, or exposure to insect bites. If measurement of synovial glucose is important, the patient should fast after midnight the night before the procedure (Van Leeuwen & Poelhuis-Leth, 2009).

Continual explanation of the steps of procedure is important to support the patient and decrease anxiety. The patient should be educated about the use of both a topical and a local anesthetic (Daniels, 2010). If indicated, anti-anxiety medication may be considered during this procedure. A consent form should be obtained per the provider's institution policy.

Apply a pressure dressing to the puncture site once the procedure is complete, along with an elastic wrap/bandage, to assist with pain management (Pagana & Pagana, 2011). It is important to monitor the patient for any signs of allergy. Educate the patient about expectations for possible allergic reaction to any substance used during this procedure, including the anesthetic and corticosteroid, as well as what to do for severe pain. The use of analgesic medication post joint aspiration can be considered (Daniels, 2010). Cool packs can help with pain management as well.

The patient may resume previous activity immediately, as tolerated (Daniels, 2010), although patients with recurrent effusions should rest for a few days to allow for joint swelling resolution (Van Leeuwen & Poelhuis-Leth, 2009). Contact information should be given in case of escalating pain, which could indicate an infection. Assess for increased swelling and bleeding into the joint after any joint aspiration technique (Daniels, 2010).

Infection is a potential complication of a joint aspiration, although this is a very rare outcome (Fye, 2008). Absolute contraindication for arthrocentesis includes overlying skin or soft tissue infection (Pagana & Pagana, 2011).

Neurophysiology Testing

Nerve conduction studies combine both electromyography (EMG - muscles) and electromyoneurography (EMNG - nerves) to help diagnose or detect neuromuscular disorders, measure nerve conduction, and determine electrical properties of skeletal muscles. It is important to note that this test should only be performed after a complete medical history and dedicated pertinent review of symptoms of chief complaint, coupled with a detailed analysis of range of motion, motor power, sensory deficits, and reflexes (Fischbach & Dunning, 2009).

EMG measures electrical activity that occurs across muscle membranes by way of needle electrodes (Pagana & Pagana, 2011). The electrodes record electrical activity of selected skeletal muscle groups both at rest and during contraction (Daniels, 2010). This test specifically measures the site and cause of motor neuron disorders at the "anterior horn of the spinal cord and of the peripheral nerves" (Dunning & Fischbach, 2011, p. 264). EMG can help differentiate between myopathy and neuropathy (Daniels, 2010). The purpose of this study is to diagnose both neuromuscular and spinal nerve disorders and to determine disc disease characterized by central nerve degeneration (Dunning & Fischbach, 2011). For a typical EMG procedure, the patient sits or lies quietly in the EMG lab, often a copper-lined room (Fischbach & Dunning, 2009), with the extremity positioned at rest. A 24-gauge needle electrode attached to wires is inserted into select muscles (Pagana & Pagana, 2011), and a lead strap is applied to the ankle or wrist for grounding (Dunning & Fischbach, 2011). After this, stimulation of muscles results in an electrical signal that is recorded during rest and contraction, and viewed on an oscilloscope or recorded on graphs and often audio-amplified (Donofrio & Labus, 2009).

EMNG assesses peripheral nerve disorders or trauma (Van Leeuwen & Poelhuis-Leth, 2009; Pagana & Pagana, 2011). This test is useful in detecting, locating and/or diagnosing disorders such as carpal tunnel syndrome, diabetic neuropathy, or gullian barre syndrome (Dunning & Fischbach, 2011). This test is also helpful for distinguishing between nerve and muscle disorders. Finally, this test is useful to investigate nerve disorders or nerve damage by "toxicity of substances, such as antimicrobials, heavy metals, and solvents" (Daniels, 2010, p. 307). This test can also monitor, over time, nerve injury and recovery. It is important to measure contralateral extremities, as nerve conduction from nerve to nerve can vary (Pagana & Pagana, 2011). This test is usually performed in conjunction with EMG. The procedure uses a flat metal electrode that creates a stimulus through an electrode, with the time measured simultaneously by knowing the time between stimulation of the nerve and a detected response (Daniels, 2010). The speed is then determined by dividing the distance between the point of stimulation and the recording electrode by the time between stimulation and response (Pagana & Pagana, 2011).

The entire procedure for either EMG or EMNG can last from 30 minutes to 2 hours. With today's technologically advanced computers, the results can be interpreted immediately.

Nursing considerations of neurophysiology testing include the need to obtain a consent form and to restrict nicotine and caffeine 2-3 hours prior to the procedure (Donofrio & Labus, 2009). Alert the patient of potential discomfort of the test electrode (Fischbach & Dunning, 2009). Allay pre-test anxiety by explaining the procedure, who will be performing the test (usually a neurologist), and the patient's role. Reassure the patient that there is no danger of an electrical shock. Review the patient's medical history and medication list particularly looking for muscle relaxants, anti-cholinergics, and cholinergics that may interfere with the results (Daniels, 2010; Van Leeuwen & Poelhuis-Leth, 2009). Finally, peripheral labs such as enzyme levels that reflect muscle activity (aspartate aminotransferase, lactate dehydrogenase, creatine phosphokinase) are often requested prior to the EMG study because the EMG study could elevate these levels for approximately 5-10 days after this study (Pagana & Pagana, 2011). After the procedure, apply warm compresses to painful sites if residual pain exists. The patient may resume previous medications (such as anticoagulants) (Van Leeuwen & Poelhuis-Leth, 2009) and activity immediately as tolerated.

Complications of this study are extremely rare; however, hematomas could occur if the patient is anticoagulated or using aspirin like products (Pagana & Pagana, 2011). This diagnostic test is contraindicated for patients with bleeding disorders (Fischbach & Dunning, 2009).

Pulmonary Function Tests

The pulmonary function tests (PFT) objectively assesses pulmonary function, including lung volume, capacity, and flow rate patterns of airflow involved in the respiratory function (Donofrio & Labus, 2009). The purpose of the PFT is to identify obstructive and/or restrictive defects in the respiratory system to better understand the nature and extent of the pulmonary disease (Dunning & Fischbach, 2011; Fischbach & Dunning, 2009). It is used postoperatively in the prevention of respiratory complications and the evaluation of respiratory function preoperatively. For example, PFT provides a preoperative evaluation for patients undergoing corrective surgical procedures for scoliosis (restrictive ventilator impairments) (Donofrio & Labus, 2009; Fischbach & Dunning, 2009). It evaluates patients with known obstructive respiratory disease (asthma, emphysema, COPD) or smoking history (Van Leeuwen & Poelhuis-Leth, 2009).

The PFT procedure is usually performed in a pulmonary function lab (Daniels, 2010). The patient is positioned for comfort, which is usually sitting. The patient breathes (through the mouth only) as directed for each phase of the test: air flow rates, lung volume, and diffusion.

Air Flow Rate. The patient maximally inhales and then forcibly exhales, rapidly and completely, into a spirometer, a device for measuring the volume of air inspired and expired by the lungs over a specified period (Dunning & Fischbach, 2011). This determines two main components:

1. Forced vital capacity (FVC): the maximum of amount of air that can be exhaled forcibly and completely after a maximal inspiration. This is used to evaluate restrictive defects (Donofrio & Labus, 2009); and
2. Forced expiratory volume (FEV): the volume of air exhaled at a specific time intervals of 1-3 seconds (a minimum of three times), expressed as the volume of air (in liters) expired during each second of the FVC maneuver (Donofrio & Labus, 2009). This evaluates the severity of obstruction, assesses the effectiveness of bronchodilators, and quantifies the extent and severity of airway obstruction. The results are a measure of airway function and patency. In regards to preoperative clearance or risk stratification, if the FEV1 is greater than 2L or 50% of predicted, complications are rare (Yoder, 2011).

Lung Volume. The patient either sits in a tightly closed box called a plethysmograph or inhales the gas helium, which is not absorbed systemically. This test evaluates for restrictive or obstructive defects using the following screens:

- Restrictive: The vital capacity (VC) is the maximum volume of air that can be expired after maximal inspiration (Donofrio & Labus, 2009).

- Obstructive: The volume exhaled (VE) is the volume of air exhaled at rest in 1 minute. Maximum voluntary ventilation (MVV) or maximum breathing capacity (MBC) is the maximum volume of air (in liters) a patient can breathe per minute by a voluntary effort after the patient breathes as deeply and rapidly as possible. Forced expiratory flows (FEF) is the average volume of air that a patient can exhale. This test is usually measured in 25% of lung volume, 50% of lung volume and 75% of lung volume respectively.

Diffusion (Gas Exchange) Capacity. This is the rate of transfer of carbon monoxide through the alveolar and capillary membrane in 1 minute (Van Leeuwen & Poelhuis-Leth, 2009). This test is helpful in diagnosing pulmonary vascular disease, emphysema, and pulmonary fibrosis, and evaluates the efficacy of the pulmonary capillary in contact with the functional alveoli (Donofrio & Labus, 2009). With this procedure, nose clips are applied to the patient, who is coached to "exhale maximally and then inspire maximally a diffusion gas mixture through a mouthpiece and filter combination is attached to the pulmonary function analyzer" (Dunning & Fischbach, 2011, p. 476). Following a 10-15 second breath-hold, the patient exhales, and a sample of alveolar gas is captured for analysis (Donofrio & Labus, 2009).

Nursing considerations for pulmonary function survey tests include encouraging the patient to rest before testing to ensure that the respiratory system can function at its full capacity. Patients may, however, return to pretest activities immediately following the procedure. Bronchodilators, caffeine, smoking, and narcotics/opioids affect the true functional capacity of the respiratory system (Donofrio & Labus, 2009). Patients with a history of COPD who will undergo shoulder surgery using an intrascalene block as anesthesia should have pulmonary function tests prior to surgery, as the block on the ipsilateral side may "transiently paralyze the ipsilateral diaphragm and reduce the FVC by 25-30% (Beecroft & Coventry, 2008, p.194). Riazi and colleagues (2008) even state that an intrascalene block should be avoided altogether for patients with a FEV1 <1L.

Precautions for this diagnostic study include the contraindication for patients with recent cardiovascular events such as a myocardial infarction: they should not undergo this study during the acute rehabilitation phase (Van Leeuwen & Poelhuis-Leth, 2009). Additionally, there is a small risk of developing a collapsed lung or pneumothorax during this study.

Somatosensory Evoked Potential (SSEP)

SSEP is a measurement of time, in meters per second, from the stimulation of a peripheral nerve through the response (Chawla, 2010). This test measures conduction along nerve pathways not accessible with EMG/EMNG. This diagnostic study documents axonal continuity when sensory nerve potential cannot be measured due to nerve trauma.

The purpose of SSEP is to evaluate radiculopathies of the central nervous system and peripheral nerve function. This study is indicated in spinal cord lesions/injury to help measure functional outcome, multiple sclerosis, and cervical myelopathy after an accident (Chawla, 2010; Fischbach & Dunning, 2009; Pagana & Pagana, 2011). SSEP can detect sensorimotor neuropathies and cervical pathology (Van Leeuwen & Poelhuis-Leth, 2009). It is appropriately ordered for diagnostic work-up of Charcot-Marie-Tooth disease (an inherited neurological disorder including both motor and sensory neuropathy), diabetic neuropathy (associated with diabetes mellitus that affects all peripheral nerves), and Friedreich's ataxia (an inheritable nerve disorder that affects primarily the sensory neurons in the spinal cord affecting gait). This test is also used in the preoperative evaluation and intraoperative monitoring of spinal nerves during spinal instrumentation and stabilization (Chawla, 2010; Hart & Grottkau, 2009).

For the SSEP procedure, the patient sits in a recliner or lies supine quietly. Transcutaneous or percutaneous electrodes are applied to the skin, usually along median or peroneal nerve distributions (Chawla, 2010; Fischbach & Dunning, 2009). The stimulus is applied to electrodes, and intervals are calculated by the monitoring device (Van Leeuwen & Poelhuis-Leth, 2009).

Nursing considerations for SSEP include assessing the patient for bleeding tendencies prior to the procedure; the transcutaneous electrode method must be used for such patients. Alert the patient to mild discomfort that may accompany electrode placement and stimulation. There are no restrictions for food or fluids before testing (Pagana & Pagana, 2011).

References

American College of Rheumatology (ACR). (2009, February). *Position Statement: Methodology of Testing for Antinuclear Antibodies.* Retrieved June 11, 2011, from http://www.rheumatology.org/practice/clinical/position/ana_position_stmt.pdf

ARUP Consult. (n.d.) Borrelia burgdorferi - Lyme Disease. *The Physician's Guide to Laboratory Test Selection and Interpretation.* Retrieved June 21, 2011, from http://www.arupconsult.com/Topics/LymeDisease.html#tabs=2

Arneja, S. & Leith, J. (2009). Validity of the KT-1000 knee ligament arthrometer. *Journal of Orthopaedic Surgery, 17*(1), 77-79. Retrieved February 12, 2012, www.josonline.org/pdf/v17i1p77.pdf

Baer, A.N. (2008). Metabolic myopathies. In J. Klippel, J. Stone, L. Crofford, & P. White (Eds.), *Primer on the Rheumatic Diseases* (13th ed., p. 385). New York, NY: Springer.

Beecroft, C. & Coventry, D. (2008). Anaesthesia for shoulder surgery. *Continuing Education in Anaesthesia, Critical Care & Pain, 8*(6), 193-198. Retrieved from http://ceaccp.oxfordjournals.org/content/8/6/193.full

Berbari, E., Mabry, T., Tsaras, G., Spangehl, M., Erwin, P. Murad, M... Osmon, D. (2010). Inflammatory blood laboratory levels as markers of prosthetic joint infection: A systemic review and meta-analysis. *The Journal of Bone and Joint Surgery, 92*(11), 2102-2109.

Blanchard, M. (2010). Men's health. In T.M. De Fer, M.A. Brisco, & R.S. Mullur (Eds.), *The Washington Manual for Outpatient Internal Medicine* (p. 812). New York, NY: Lippincott Williams & Wilkins.

Blue Cross of Idaho. (2011, May). *Thermography*. Retrieved July 15, 2011, from https://www.bcidaho.com/providers/medical_policies/rad/mp_60112.asp

Bockenstedt, L.K. (2008). Infectious disorders: Lyme disease. In J. Klippel, J. Stone, L. Crofford, & P. White (Eds.), *Primer on the Rheumatic Diseases* (13th ed., p. 286). New York, NY: Springer.

Brancaccio, P., Maffulli, N., & Limongelli, F. (2007). Creatinine kinase monitoring in sport medicine. *British Medical Bulletin*, 81-82. Retrieved May 30, 2011, from http://bmb.oxfordjournals.org/content/81-82/1/209.abstract

Bratton, R.L., Whiteside, J.W., Hovan, M.J., Engle, R.L., & Edwards, F.D. (2008). Diagnosis and treatment of lyme disease. *Mayo Clinic Proceedings, 83*(5), 566-571.

Braun, J.M. (2008). Ankylosing spondylitis: Pathology and pathogenesis. In J. Klippel, J. Stone, L. Crofford, & P. White (Eds.), *Primer on the Rheumatic Diseases* (13th Ed., p. 201). New York, NY: Springer.

Brenner, D.J. & Hall, E.J. (2007). Computed tomography: An increasing source of radiation exposure. *The New England Journal of Medicine, 357*, 2277-2284.

Byrd, C.J. & Brasington, R.D. (2010). Rheumatologic diseases. In T.M. De Fer, M.A. Brisco, & R.S. Mullur (Eds.), *The Washington Manual of Outpatient Internal Medicine* (pp. 556-587). New York, NY: Wolters Kluwer/Lippincott Williams & Wilkins.

Carey, W.D. (2010). *Approach to the Patient with Liver Disease: A Guide to Commonly Used Liver Tests*. Retrieved May 20, 2011, from http://www.clevelandclinicmeded.com/medicalpubs/diseasemanagement/hepatology/guide-to-common-liver-tests/

Chawla, J. (2012). *Somatosensory Evoked Potentials, Clinical Applications*. Retrieved July 16, 2011, from http://emedicine.medscape.com/article/1139393-overview

Chen, Y.R., Rachakonda, V., & Caballon, M.C.L. (2010). Laboratory assessment of kidney and urinary tract disorders. In T.M. De Fer, M.A. Brisco, & R.S. Mullur (Eds.), *The Washington Manual of Outpatient Internal Medicine* (pp. 390-391). New York, NY: Wolters Kluwer/Lippincott Williams & Wilkins.

Collyott, C.L. & Brooks, M.V. (2008). Evaluation and management of joint pain. *Orthopaedic Nursing, 27*(4), 246-250.

Couto, J.M.C., de Castilho, E.A., & Menezes, P.R. (2007). Chemonucleolysis in lumbar disc herniation: A meta-anaylsis. *CLINICS, 62*(2), 175-180. Retrieved February 12, 2012, from http://www.scielo.br/scielo.php?script=sci_arttext&pid=S1807-59322007000200013&lng=en&nrm=iso&tlng=en

Daniels, R.R. (2010). *Delmar's Guide to Laboratory and Diagnostic Tests*. Clifton Park, NY: Delmar Cengage Learning.

den Elzen, W.P., Willems, J.M., Westendorp, R.G.J., de Craen, A.J.M., Blauw, G.J., Ferrucci, L.,... Gussekloo, J. (2010). Effect of erythropoietin levels on mortality in old age: The Leiden 85-Plus Study. *Canadian Medical Association Journal, 182*(18), 1-6. doi: 10.1503/cmaj.100347

Donofrio, J. & Labus, D. (2009). *Diagnostic Tests Made Incredibly Easy* (2nd ed.). New York, NY: Wolters Kluwer/Lippincott Williams & Wilkins.

Dunning, M. & Fischbach, F. (2011). *Nurses' Quick Reference to Common Laboratory & Diagnostic Tests* (5th ed.). New York, NY: Wolters Kluwer/Lippincott Williams & Wilkens.

Eamonn, M., Koening, C., & Hoffman, G. (2010). *Polymyalgia Rheumatica and Giant Cell Arteritis*. Retrieved June 19, 2011, from https://www.clevelandclinicmeded.com/medicalpubs/diseasemanagement/rheumatology/polymyalgia-rheumatica-and-giant-cell-arteritis/

Edwards, L.N. (2008). Gout: Clinical features. In J. Klippel, J. Stone, L. Crofford, & P. White (Eds.). *Primer on the Rheumatic Diseases* (13th ed., pp. 248-249). New York, NY: Springer.

Ehrlich, S.D. (2011). *Phosphorous*. Retrieved July 3, 2011, from http://www.umm.edu/altmed/articles/phosphorus-000319.htm

Fauci, A., Braunwald, E., Kasper, D., Hauser, S., Longo, D., Jameson, J., & Loscalzo, J. (Eds.), (2009). *Harrison's Manual of Medicine* (17th ed.). New York, NY: McGraw Hill Medical.

Fischbach F. & Dunning, M. (2009). *A Manual of Laboratory and Diagnostic Tests* (8th ed.). New York, NY: Wolters Kluwer/Lippincott Williams & Wilkins.

Fye, K.H. (2008). Evaluation of the patient: Arthrocentesis, synovial fluid analysis, and synovial biopsy. In J. Klippel, J. Stone, L. Crofford, & P. White (Eds.), *Primer on the Rheumatic Diseases* (13th ed., pp. 21-27). New York, NY: Springer.

Gay, S. (2010). An inside view of venous thromboembolism. *The Nurse Practitioner, 35*(9), 32-39.

Gordon, L.M. (2012). ACR practice guideline for the performance of adult and pediatric skeletal scintigraphy (bone scan). *Skeletal Scintigraphy/PRACTICE GUIDELINE*, 1-5.

Green, G.A., Frankel, D.Z. & Puffer, J.C. (2010). Drugs and doping in athletes. In C. Madden, M. Putukian, C. Young, & E. McCarty (Eds.), *Netter's Sports Medicine* (1st ed., p. 179). Philadelphia, PA: Saunders Elselvier.

Greidanus, N., Masri, D., Barbuz S., Wilson, D., McAlinden, G., Xu, M., & Duncan, C. (2007). Use of erythrocyte sedimentation rate and C-reactive protein level to diagnose infection before revision total knee arthroplasty: A prospective evaluation. *The Journal of Bone & Joint Surgery, 89*(7), 1409-1416.

Hart, E.S. & Grottkau, B.E. (2009). Intraoperative neuromonitoring in pediatric spinal deformity surgery. *Orthopaedic Nursing, 28*(6), 286-294.

Hildebrandt, C., Raschner, C., & Ammer, K. (2010). An overview of recent application of medical infrared thermography in sports medicine in Austria. *Sensors, 10*, 4700-4715. Retrieved February 12, 2012, from http://www.mdpi.com/1424-8220/10/5/4700/

International Association of Certified Thermographers (IACT). (2007, January). *Quality Assurance Guidelines: Standards and Protocols for Medical Infrared Imaging*. Retrieved from http://s3imaging.com/sites/all/files/resources/IACT_Medical_Standards_and_Guidelines_for_IRT.pdf

Jain, M. &. Samuels, J. (2010). Musculoskeletal ultrasound in the diagnosis of rheumatic disease. *Bulletin of the NYU Hospital for Joint Diseases, 68*(3), 183-190.

Jones, R. (2007). Primary Hyperparathyroidism. *CLINICAL REVIEWS, 17*(7), 27-34.

Joy, T.R. & Hegele, R.A. (2009). Narrative review: Statin-related myopathy. *Annals of Internal Medicine, 150*(12), 858-868.

Katz, J.N. & Gomoll, A.H. (2007). Advances in arthroscopic surgery: Indications and Outcomes. *Current Opinion in Rheumatology, 19*, 106-110.

Kirkley, A.M., Birmingham, T., Litchfield, R.B., Giffin, R., Willits, D.R., Wong, C.J., …Fowler, P.J. (2008). A randomized trial of arthroscopic surgery for osteoarthritis of the knee. *The New England Journal of Medicine, 359*(11), 1097-1107.

Kruer, M.C. & Steiner, R.D. (2011). *Lysosomal Storage Disease.* Retrieved May 29, 2011, http://emedicine.medscape.com/article/1182830-overview

Kurakula, P.C. & Keenan, R.T. (2010, October). Diagnosis and management of gout: An update. *The Journal of Musuloskeletal Medicine*, S13-S19.

Kurlander, R. & Schechter, G. (2010). Interpretation of standard hematologic tests. In G. Rodgers & N.Young (Eds.), *Bethesda Handbook of Clinical Hematology* (2nd ed., p. 391). New York, NY: Wolters Kluwer/Lippincott Williams & Wilkins.

Leitman, S. & Bolan, D. (2010). Hemochromatosis. In G. Rodgers & N.Young (Eds.), *Bethesda Handbook of Clinical Hematology* (2nd ed., p. 355). New York, NY: Wolters Kluwer/Lippincott Williams & Wilkins.

Levine, B. & Stray-Gundersen, J. (2010). High-altitude training and competition. In C. Madden, M. Putukian, C.Young, & E. McCarty (Eds.), *Netter's Sports Medicine* (1st ed., p. 160). Philadelphia, PA: Saunders Elselvier.

Lindsley, C.B. (2008). Juvenile idiopathic arthritis: Special considerations. In J. Klippel, J. Stone, L. Crofford, & P. White (Eds.), *Primer on the Rheumatic Diseases* (13th ed., p. 165). New York, NY: Springer.

Ma, L., Cranney, A., & Holroyd-Leduc, J. (2009, January). Acute monoarthritis: What is the cause of my patient's painful swollen joint? *Canadian Medical Association Journal, 180*(1), 59-65. Retrieved from http://www.cmaj.ca/content/180/1/59.full.pdf+html

Margaretten, M.E., Kohlwes, J., Moore, D., & Bent, S. (2007). Does this adult patient have septic arthritis? *Journal of the American Medical Association, 297*(13), 1478-1488.

Marques, A.R. (2010, January 8). Lyme disease: A review. *Current Allergy and Asthma Reports, 10*, 13-20. Retrieved February 12, 2012, from http://www.springerlink.com/content/j708837847p73387/

Mayo Clinic/Mayo Medical Laboratories. (n.d.). *81549 Overview: NTX-Telopeptide, Urine.* Retrieved June 18, 2011, from http://www.mayomedicallaboratories.com/test-catalog/Overview/81549

Mayo Clinic/Mayo Medical Laboratories. (n.d.). *82609 Overview: Chymopapain, IgE.* Retrieved June 18, 2011, from http://www.mayomedicallaboratories.com/test-catalog/Overview/82609

Mayo Foundation for Medical Education and Research. (2009). *Discogram.* Retrieved July 16, 2011, from http://www.mayoclinic.com/health/discogram/MY01038

MEDmetric Corporation. (n.d.). *Tests Performed Using the Knee Ligament Arthrometer.* Retrieved July 15, 2011, http://www.medmetric.com/kttests.htm

McCarthy, J.C. & Jibodh, S.R. (2009). The role of arthroscopy in evaluation of painful hip. *Clinical Orthopaedics and Related Research, 467*(1), 174-180.

Mease, P.J. (2008). Current clinical strategies for rheumatoid arthritis. *A Supplement to Rheumatology News Nurse Practitioner*, 3-5.

Mobley, A.M. (2009). Slowing the progression of chronic kidney disease. *The Journal of Nurse Practitioners, 5*(2), 188-194.

Moore, D.J. & Rosh, A.J. (2010). *Hypophosphatemia in Emergency Medicine.* Retrieved July 3, 2011, from http://emedicine.medscape.com/article/767955-overview

Morehead, K. (2008). Evaluation of the patient: Laboratory assessment. In J. Klippel, J. Stone, L. Crofford, & P. White (Eds.), *Primer on the Rheumatic Diseases* (13th ed.). New York, NY: Springer.

Moses, S.M. (2007). *Serum Ferritin.* Retrieved June 19, 2011, from http://www.fpnotebook.com/Hemeonc/Lab/SrmFrtn.htm

National Institute of Arthritis and Musculoskeletal and Skin Diseases. (2009). *Bone Mass Measurement: What the Numbers Mean.* Retrieved June 18, 2011, from http://www.niams.nih.gov/Health_Info/Bone/Bone_Health/bone_mass_measure.asp

Oddis, C.V. (2008). Idiopathic inflammatory myopathies: Treatment and assessment. In J. Klippel, J. Stone, L. Crofford, & P. White (Eds.), *Primer on the Rheumatic Diseases* (13th ed., p. 375). New York, NY: Springer.

Oneal, P., Schechter, G., Griffin, R., & Miller, J. (2010). Hemolytic anemia: General overview with special consideration of membrane and enzyme defects. In G. Rodgers & N.Young (Eds.), *Bethesda Handbook of Clinical Hematology* (2nd ed., p. 29). New York, NY: Wolters Kluwer/Lippincott Williams & Wilkins.

Pagana, K.D. & Pagana, T.J. (2011). *Mosby's Diagnostic and Laboratory Test Reference.* St Louis, MO: Elsevier.

Patsnap. (n.d.). *Chymopapain and Method for its Use - US4439423.* Retrieved June 18, 2011, from http://www.patsnap.com/patents/view/US4439423.html

Peterson, J.J. (2006). Postoperative infection. *Radiologic Clinics of North America, 44*(3), 439-450.

Platt, A. & Eckman, J. (2006). Continuing education: Diagnosing anemia. *Clinician Reviews, 16*(12), 44-50.

Pozza, R. (2008). Clinical management of HIV/hepatitis C virus coinfection. *Journal of the American Academy of Nurse Practitioners, 20*(10), 496-505.

RadiologyInfo.org. (2010). *Discography.* Retrieved July 16, 2011, from http://www.radiologyinfo.org/en/pdf/discography.pdf

Riazi, S., Carmichael, N., Awad, I., Holtby, R. & McCartney, C. (2008). Effect of local anaesthetic volume (20 vs 5 ml) on the efficacy and respiratory consequences of ultrasound-guided interscalene brachial plexus block. *British Journal of Anaesthesia, 101*(4), 549–56. Retrieved from http://www.bja.oxfordjournals.org/content/101/4/549.full.pdf

Ronckers, C., Doody, M., Lonstein, J., Stovall, M., & Land, C.E. (2008). Multiple diagnostic X-rays for spine deformities and risk of breast cancer. *Cancer Epidemiology Biomarkers & Prevention, 17*(3), 605-613.

Sambrook, P. (2008). Osteoporosis: Pathology and pathophysiology. In J. Klippel, J. Stone, L. Crofford, & P. White (Eds.), *Primer on the Rheumatic Diseases* (13th ed., pp. 584-591). New York, NY: Springer.

Sarwark, J., Armstrong, A., Bevavides, J., Clanton, T., Della Vella, C., Galatz, L.....Weber, K. (Eds.). (2010). *Essentials of Musculoskeletal Care* (4th ed.) Rosemont, IL: American Academy of Orthopaedic Surgeons.

Savely, V. (2007). Controversy continues to fuel the "Lyme War." *The Clinical Advisor*, 52-61.

Savely, V. (2010). Lyme disease: A diagnostic Dilemma. *The Nurse Practitioner, 35*(7), 44-50.

Schneider, R. & Pavlov, H. (2006). Diagnostic imaging techniques. In S. Paget, A. Gibofsky, J. Beary, T. Sculco (Eds.), *Manual of Rheumatology and Outpatient Orthopaedic Disorders* (5th ed., p. 46). New York, NY: Wolters Kluwer/Lippincott Williams & Wilkins.

Schwartzman, J., Gross, R., & Putterman, C. (2010). Management of lupus in 2010: How close are the biologics? *The Journal of Musculoskeletal Medicine, 27*(11), 427-435.

Scott, W.W., Didie, W.J., & Fayad, L.M. (2008). Evaluation of the patient: Imaging of rheumatologic disease. In J. Klippel, J. Stone, L. Crofford, & P. White (Eds.), *Primer on the Rheumatic Diseases* (13th ed., p. 37). New York, NY: Springer.

Sena, A.C., White, B.L., & Sparling, F.P. (2010). Novel treponema pallidum serologic tests: A paradigm shift in syphilis screening for the 21st century. *Clinical Infectious Diseases, 51*(6), 700-708.

Sherwood, A. (2008). Diagnosis & management of paget disease of the bone. *The Journal for Nurse Practitioners, 4*(1) 54-60.

Shlamovitz, G.Z. (2011). *Knee Arthrocentesis Technique.* Retrieved April 28, 2012, from http://emedicine.medscape.com/article/79994-overview

Siegel, D., Bilotti, E., & van Hoeven, K. (2009). Serum free light chain analysis for diagnosis, monitoring, and prognosis of monoclonal gammopathies. *LabMedicine, 40*, 363-366. doi:10.1309/LMPHODC7R1L0MEWW

Slin'ko, E.I.-Q. & Al-Qashqish, I.I. (2006). Surgical treatment of lumbar epidural varices. *Journal of Neurosurgery, 5*(5), 414-23.

Stewart, L.K., Earnest, C.P, Blair, S.N., & Church, T.S. (2010). Effects of different doses of physical activity on C-reactive protein among women. *Medicine & Science in Sports & Exercise, 42*(4), 701-707.

Stolker, J. (2010). Ischemic heart disease. In T.M. De Fer, M.A. Brisco, & R.S. Mullur (Eds.), *The Washington Manual of Outpatient Internal Medicine* (p. 72). New York, NY: Wolters Kluwer/Lippincott Williams & Wilkins.

Straub, D. (2007). Calcium supplementation in clinical practice: A review of forms, doses, and indications. *Nutrition in Clinical Practice, 22*(3), 286-296.

Tassiulas, I.A. & Paget, S.A. (2006). Rheumatoid arthritis. In S. Paget, A. Gibofsky, J. Beary, & T. Sculco (Eds.), *Manual of Rheumatology and Outpatient Orthopaedic Disorders* (5th ed., p. 207 & 212). New York, NY: Wolters Kluwer/Lippincott Williams & Wilkins.

Thiyagarajah, A.R., Hord, E.D., & Vallejo, R. (2009). *Discography.* Retrieved July 16, 2011, from http://emedicine.medscape.com/article/1145703-overview

Vahabzadeh, B. &. Early, D. (2010). Common gastrointestinal complaints. In T.M. De Fer, M.A. Brisco, & R.S. Mullur (Eds.), *The Washington Manual of Outpatient Internal Medicine* (pp. 510-511). New York, NY: Wolters Kluwer/Lippincott Williams & Wilkins.

Van Leeuwen, A.M. & Poelhuis-Leth, D.J. (2009). *Davis's Comprehensive Handbook of Laboratory and Diagnostic Tests with Nursing Implications* (3rd Ed.). Philadelphia, PA: F.A. Davis Company.

Wallace, D.J. (2006). New antinuclear antibody testing: Does it cut costs and corners without jeopardizing clinical reliability? *Nature Clinical Practice Rheumatology, 2*(8), 410-411.

Walsh, W., McCarty, E., & Madden, C. (2010). Knee injuries. In C. Madden, M. Putukian, C. Young, & E. McCarty (Eds.), *Netter's Sports Medicine* (1st ed., pp. 418-419). Philadelphia, PA: Saunders Elsevier.

West, S. (2008). Musculoskeletal signs and symptoms. In J. Klippel, J. Stone, L. Crofford, & P. White (Eds.), *Primer on the Rheumatic Diseases* (13th ed., p. 53). New York, NY: Springer.

Whyte, M.P. (2006). Paget's disease of bone. *New England Journal of Medicine, 355*(6), 593-600.

Yoder, M. (2011). *Perioperative Pulmonary Management.* Retrieved October 5, 2012, from http://emedicine.medscape.com/article/284983-overview#aw2aab6b2

Yusen, R.D. & Gage, B.F. (2010). Venous thromboembolism and anticoagulation therapy. In T.M. De Fer, M.A. Brisco, & R.S. Mullur (Eds.), *The Washington Manual of Outpatient Internal Medicine* (p. 207). New York, NY: Wolters Kluwer/Lippincott Williams & Wilkins.

Zychowicz, M.E., Pope, R.S., & Graser, E. (2010). The current state of care in gout: Addressing the need for better understanding of an ancient disease. In C. Pierson (Ed.), *Supplement to the Journal of the American Academy of Nurse Practitioners, 22*(11), 623-636.

Chapter 5

Perioperative Patient Care

Patricia A. Krieger, MSN, RN, ONC, CNOR

Objectives

- List the six components of the surgical process.
- Describe nursing care during the preoperative, intraoperative, and postoperative periods.
- List examples of collaboration among agencies and organizations that ensure safety for the surgical patient.
- Identify common practices used in the operating room to prevent infection.

Perioperative care for the elective orthopaedic patient begins as soon as the patient decides to have surgery. Most orthopaedic patients have tried various treatment modalities, including nonsteroidal anti-inflammatory drugs (NSAIDs), injections, specific exercises, and/or physical therapy (PT), before opting for surgery. The decision to have surgery starts an organized, six-component process that begins in the clinic or surgeon's office and continues through Preadmission Testing (PAT), Same Day Surgery (SDS), Operating Room (OR), Post-Anesthesia Care Unit (PACU), and discharge to home or inpatient status (as shown in Figure 5.1). The steps of the surgical process are defined by the patient's insurance company requirements (inpatient vs. outpatient) and the state regulatory agencies (individual state Departments of Health), accreditation agencies of the particular hospital or ambulatory surgery center such as The Joint Commission (TJC), and are continually modified to ensure a safe surgical experience.

Figure 5.1.
The Surgical Process

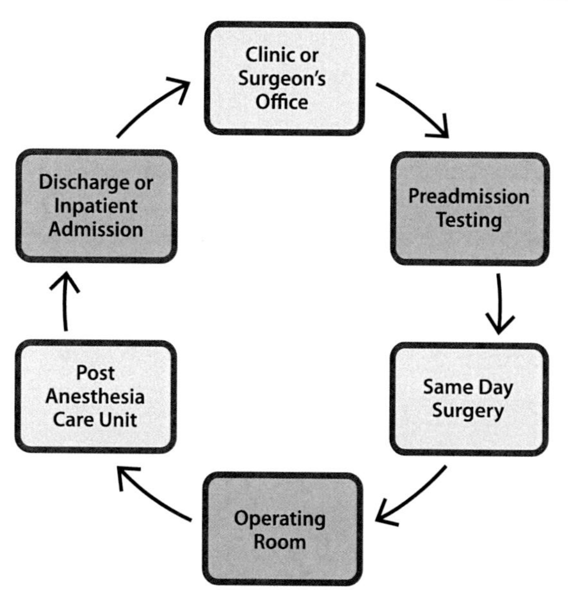

Author creation. Reproduced with permission.

Patient Safety in the Operating Room

Fung (2011) summarized several research reports on medical mistakes in the United States, including the 2008 finding that there were more than 252,000 postoperative infections at a cost of $3.36 billion. Pressure ulcers were found to be the most common preventable event, with nearly 375,000 cases at a cost of $3.27 billion. TJC (2011) reported that every week in the U.S., 40 patients undergo a procedure meant for someone else or on the wrong body part, fires occur during surgeries, patients acquire infections during routine processes, and medication errors occur. As the patient advocate, the perioperative nurse must be oriented to and knowledgeable of the most effective and up-to-date guidelines to protect the patient during the surgical process.

Perioperative nursing has its own national organization, the Association of periOperative Registered Nurses (AORN), whose purpose is to promote safe patient care. AORN is recognized as an authority for safe OR practices, a definitive source for information and guiding principles that support day-to-day perioperative practice. AORN's *Perioperative Standards and Recommended Practices* (2010) guides the perioperative nurse in providing an optimal level of patient care within the surgical and invasive procedure settings.

Collaborative Efforts

Several organizations and associations have published safety guidelines specific to OR practice. Examples of collaboration among agencies and organizations can be seen with the National Patient Safety Goals, The Universal Protocol, and The Surgical Care Improvement Project.

National Patient Safety Goals. TJC established its National Patient Safety Goals (NPSGs) in 2002 "to help accredited organizations address specific areas of concern in regards to patient safety" (TJC, 2012, p. 2). (See Table 5.1.) The Patient Safety Advisory Group—comprised of patient safety experts, nurses, physicians, pharmacists, risk managers, and other professionals with hands-on experience in addressing patient safety issues—does an annual systematic review of the literature and available databases to identify new NPSGs. These suggestions are presented to TJC along with the evidence for, validity of, and practicality/cost of implementation. If approved,

Table 5.1. The Joint Commission's 2012 National Patient Safety Goals: Hospitals
Goal 1: Improve the accuracy of patient identification.
Goal 2: Improve the effectiveness of communication among caregivers.
Goal 3: Improve the safety of using medications.
Goal 7: Reduce the risk of health care–associated infections
Goal 15: The organization identifies safety risks inherent in its patient population
* Goals are deleted as they are attained.

From Joint Commission Resources *by The Joint Commission (TJC), 2012,. http://www.jcrinc.com/Other-Resources/NPSGHLP12/4021/.pdf. Reproduced with permission.*

these recommendations are implemented the following year. All TJC-accredited health care organizations are surveyed for implementation of the NPSGs as appropriate to the services the organization provides (TJC, 2009).

Universal Protocol. The Universal Protocol is one of the most important safety issues for perioperative patient care. "The Joint Commission Board of Commissioners originally approved The Universal Protocol for Preventing Wrong Site, Wrong Procedure and Wrong Person Surgery in July 2002. It became effective July 1, 2004, for all accredited hospitals and ambulatory care and office-based facilities. The Universal Protocol was created to address the continuing occurrence of wrong site, wrong procedure, and wrong person surgery in Joint Commission accredited organizations" (TJC, 2009). It drew upon the 2003 and 2004 NPSGs and has since been updated. The three principal components of the Universal Protocol continue to be included in the TJC's 2012 NPSGs: conduct a preprocedure verification process, mark the procedure site, and perform a time-out before the procedure. Figure 5.2 shows an example of a comprehensive checklist used by many facilities.

Surgical Care Improvement Project (SCIP). Bratzler (2006) describes another collaborative project of the regulatory agencies that started in 2002. The Centers for Medicare and Medicaid Services (CMS) in collaboration with the Centers for Disease Control and Prevention (CDC) implemented the National Surgical Infection Prevention Project (SIP). The goal of this project was to decrease the morbidity and mortality associated with postoperative surgical site infections (SSIs) by promoting the appropriate selection and timing of prophylactic antimicrobials.

Figure 5.2.
Comprehensive Surgical Checklist

COMPREHENSIVE SURGICAL CHECKLIST

Blue = World Health Organization (WHO) Green = The Joint Commission – Universal Protocol (JC) 10 National Patient Safety Goals Orange = JC and WHO

PREPROCEDURE CHECK-IN	SIGN-IN	TIME-OUT	SIGN-OUT
In Holding Area	**Before Induction of Anesthesia**	**Before Skin Incision**	**Before the Patient Leaves the Operating Room**
Patient/patient representative actively confirms with Registered Nurse (RN):	**RN and anesthesia care provider confirm:**	**Initiated by designated team member** **All other activities to be suspended (unless a life-threatening emergency)**	**RN confirms:**
Identity □ Yes Procedure and procedure site □ Yes Consent(s) □ Yes Site marked □ Yes □ N/A by person performing the procedure **RN confirms presence of:** History and physical □ Yes Preanesthesia assessment □ Yes Diagnostic and radiologic test results □ Yes □ N/A Blood products □ Yes □ N/A Any special equipment, devices, implants □ Yes □ N/A Include in Preprocedure check-in as per institutional custom: Beta blocker medication given (SCIP) □ Yes □ N/A Venous thromboembolism prophylaxis ordered (SCIP) □ Yes □ N/A Normothermia measures (SCIP) □ Yes □ N/A	Confirmation of: Identity, procedure, procedure site and consent(s) □ Yes Site marked □ Yes □ N/A by person performing the procedure Patient allergies □ Yes □ N/A Difficult airway or aspiration risk? □ No □ Yes (preparation confirmed) Risk of blood loss (>500 ml) □ Yes □ N/A # of units available _____ Anesthesia safety check completed □ Yes **Briefing:** All members of the team have discussed care plan and addressed concerns □ Yes	Introduction of team members □ Yes **All:** Confirmation of the following: Identity, procedure, incision site, consent(s) □ Yes Site is marked and visible □ Yes □ N/A Relevant images properly labeled and displayed □ Yes □ N/A Any equipment concerns? **Anticipated Critical Events Surgeon:** States the following: □ critical or nonroutine steps □ case duration □ anticipated blood loss **Anesthesia Provider** □ Antibiotic prophylaxis within one hour before incision □ Yes □ N/A □ Additional concerns? **Scrub and circulating nurse:** □ Sterilization indicators have been confirmed □ Additional concerns?	Name of operative procedure Completion of sponge, sharp, and instrument counts □ Yes □ N/A Specimens identified and labeled □ Yes □ N/A Any equipment problems to be addressed? □ Yes □ N/A **To all team members:** What are the key concerns for recovery and management of this patient? _____ _____ _____ _____ _____ _____ _____ April 2010 AORN

The JC does not stipulate which team member initiates any section of the checklist except for site marking.
The Joint Commission also does not stipulate where these activities occur. See the Universal Protocol for details on the Joint Commission requirements.

From Association of periOperative Registered Nurses (AORN), (n.d.), Comprehensive Checklist, http://www.aorn.org/ClinicalPractice/ToolKits/CorrectSiteSurgeryToolKit/Comprehensive_checklist.aspx. Reproduced with permission.

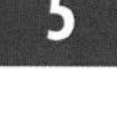

A panel of experts in SSI prevention developed three performance measures for national surveillance and quality improvement:

1. The proportion of patients who have parenteral antimicrobial prophylaxis initiated within 1 hour before incision (2 hours for vancomycin or fluoroquinolones);
2. The proportion of patients who are given a prophylactic antimicrobial regimen consistent with published guidelines; and
3. The proportion of patients whose prophylactic antimicrobial is discontinued within 24 hours after surgery end time.

These measures were used on a national sample of Medicare inpatients undergoing five types of major surgery: cardiac surgery, vascular surgery, general abdominal colorectal surgery, hip and knee total joint arthroplasty, and abdominal and vaginal hysterectomy. Because of the success of the national SIP initiative, which showed tremendous improvement in surgical morbidity and mortality, the program was expanded into the SCIP in 2003.

The SCIP is a national quality partnership of organizations committed to improving the safety of surgical care through the reduction of postoperative complications. It was formed by representatives of the CMS, CDC, Veterans Administration, the American College of Surgeons, the American Society of Anesthesiologists, the Agency for Healthcare Research and Quality, the American Hospital Association, and the Institute for Healthcare Improvement. More than 30 other organizations have committed to be supporting partners for the project. It is the first, and largest, movement to measure the quality of care delivered for surgical patients in the U.S. The SCIP partnership focused the measurement of quality on several broad areas where the incidence and cost of complications in surgery is high, and there is a significant opportunity for prevention (see Table 5.2).

Table 5.2. SCIP Measures
Infection Prevention
■ Patients who received antibiotic within 1 hour prior to surgery
■ Patients who received the appropriate antibiotic for their specific procedure
■ Patients whose antibiotics were discontinued within 24 hours after surgery
■ Cardiac surgery patients with a controlled postoperative blood glucose level
■ Surgery patients with appropriate surgical site hair removal
■ Colorectal surgery patients with immediate postoperative normothermia

From Study Examines Relationship Between SCIP Measures and Postoperative Infection *by the Case Western Reserve University School of Medicine, 2010, http://www.news-medical.net/news/20100624/Study-examines-relationship-between-SCIP-measures-and-postoperative-infection.aspx. Reprinted with permission.*

Due to the Value-Based Purchasing incentives under the Health Care Reform Act passed in March 2010 (Case Western Reserve University School of Medicine, 2010), Medicare reimbursement will be tied to hospitals' adherence to SCIP measures. Although SCIP prevention measures give a strong indication of postoperative infection complication rates, other aspects influencing surgical patient outcomes include the skill and knowledge of the surgical team, a safe and clean working environment, and a general culture of quality surrounding patient care. The perioperative nurse can make a difference in each patient's surgery and outcome by ensuring that all prevention measures are in place and all safety precautions have been taken.

Preoperative Assessment and Planning

Preoperative assessment of the patient and planning for surgery begin at the clinic or surgeon's office, continue through Preadmission Testing and Same Day Surgery, and end when the patient enters the OR.

Clinic or Surgeon's Office

Once the patient decides to have surgery, the surgeon explains the surgical procedure to the patient (and caregivers, if applicable) in terms that the patient can understand, including the nature of the problem, type of treatment, risks and benefits, consequences, alternatives to treatment, and expected outcome if surgery is not performed. The surgeon answers any questions the patient and caregivers may have and obtains a voluntary informed consent for surgery. The surgeon, physician assistant, or nurse practitioner completes a thorough medical history on the patient, paying particular attention to any preexisting conditions and family anesthetic history of malignant hyperthermia. An allergy history is obtained, including medications, foods, and latex or metal sensitivity. A medical examination accompanies the patient's medical history. The patient's current height and weight are obtained for correct computation of medications and for proper size of positioning supplies and OR equipment. A social history should be obtained to assess the patient's home situation, availability of assistance upon discharge, and financial burdens that may impact postoperative care and medication procurement; this information should be relayed to the surgical facility's Social Services Department.

The surgeon's office coordinator completes a surgical procedure form for each surgery and faxes or emails it to the OR scheduler to reserve the date and time for surgery in the OR for that particular surgeon and patient. This booking form assists the OR in preoperative planning for the specific surgical procedure. It lists the surgeon's and patient's names, operative procedure, type of admission (inpatient, same day surgery, 23-hour observation), patient's diagnosis, age, allergy to latex (which may alter the preparation of the patient's OR), allergies to medications, special positioning devices if needed, the specific vendor and type of implants and/or bone graft, intraoperative x-ray, and any other specific requests.

A Preadmission Testing form is given to the patient to take to the appointment with the Preadmission Testing department of the surgical facility. In elective surgery, this appointment is scheduled from several days to several weeks in advance of the surgical procedure. This form includes laboratory studies ordered preoperatively by the health care provider in a cost-effective manner. Hemoglobin and hematocrit is recommended for all patients. Type and Screen for blood may be ordered if blood loss is anticipated. If the patient has a history of cardiac problems, kidney or liver disease, or other conditions, it may include orders for preoperative clearance by a Medical Specialist who may order additional diagnostic tests (electrolytes, urinalysis, chest x-ray, and electrocardiogram). The orthopaedic surgeon usually orders x-rays of the operative site. A healthy patient having a procedure with local anesthesia may not have any laboratory studies ordered.

Preadmission Testing (PAT). During the scheduled PAT visit, the patient is assessed by a member of the nursing staff who obtains vital signs, interviews the patient, reviews the patient's medical history and physical, and enters the data into the hospital's electronic medical record.

For a patient with a history of nickel or other metal allergies who is having implant surgery, definitive preoperative testing may be ordered. Up to 13% of people are sensitive to nickel, cobalt, or chromium metals. Specific blood tests used to diagnose metal hypersensitivity include the lymphocyte transformation test (LTT) and the lymphokine migration inhibition factor (MIF) test. Blood tests results have more validity than previously performed dermal patch testing. Sensitization to implanted metals is still debated in the literature; however, with a positive test result, the orthopaedic surgeon may decide to order a different implant to avoid possible consequences of poor wound healing and joint failure (Rabin & Hopkinson, 2011).

If the surgery is anticipated to cause blood loss and the patient is able to donate blood preoperatively, the patient is referred to a blood collection facility. Appropriate indicators are patients having elective surgery that can be scheduled at least several weeks in advance, a surgical procedure for which blood is usually crossmatched, a hemoglobin count of > 110 g/L (hematocrit 0.33), and no medical contraindications to the donation or storage of blood. After the patient is evaluated for autologous donation, blood may be collected as frequently as every 3 days, although once a week is more common (bloodindex, n.d.). Oral iron supplementation is often ordered for the donating patient. The optimal donation period begins 4 to 6 weeks before surgery in order for a sufficient number of units to be donated and to enable more complete red blood cell regeneration. The last blood donation should not be collected later than 72 hours before surgery to allow for restoration of intravascular volume. After the units are collected and processed, they are sent to the surgical facility (bloodindex, n.d.).

CHAPTER 5

The PAT nurse answers any questions that the patient/caregivers may have about the upcoming surgery and reviews preoperative education, including to stop eating or drinking before surgery at the assigned time; to not smoke, chew gum, or suck on candy or cough drops because these will stimulate the secretions of gastric acid in the stomach; to stop all herbal medications when directed; to remove and leave any jewelry or other valuables at home; to practice coughing and deep breathing; to bring along clothes for PT if applicable; and to bathe with an antimicrobial soap before surgery per directions.

For patients in reasonably good health, preoperative telephone interviews may take the place of a PAT visit. Questions relate to pulmonary and cardiac disease; medication and alcohol use; medication, latex, or anesthetic allergies; pregnancy; and personal or family history or anesthetic reactions. The patient also receives patient education as it relates to the specific surgery (Rothrock, 2011).

Recently, various institutions have implemented a program to prevent postoperative SSIs from methicillin-sensitive *Staphylococcus Aureus* (MSSA) and methicillin-resistant *Staphylococcus Aureus* (MRSA) in their elective orthopaedic patients. During the PAT visit, the patient receives a nasal swabbing for MSSA and MRSA. If results are positive for either microorganism, the patient receives a prescription for intranasal mupirocin ointment to be used twice daily for 5 days prior to surgery. In addition, all screened patients, whether positive or negative, receive a bottle of 4% chlorhexidine gluconate to be used during their daily shower for 5 days prior to surgery (see Figure 5.3). Results have been promising and have shown a decrease in postoperative SSIs in those individuals who were carriers of MSSA or MRSA (Kim, 2010).

Patients undergoing total joint replacement surgery may have an interview with a physical therapist who previews the PT regimen that the patient will have postoperatively in the hospital. The therapist may also discuss devices to obtain for the home (long-handled grasper, raised toilet seat, shower chair, walker, crutches, wheelchair, etc.) and safety tips for the home (remove scatter rugs, have clear pathways for walking through the home, etc.). If preoperative total joint classes are offered by the surgical facility, the patient will be scheduled for them

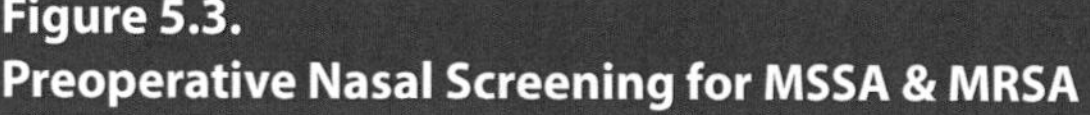
Figure 5.3.
Preoperative Nasal Screening for MSSA & MRSA

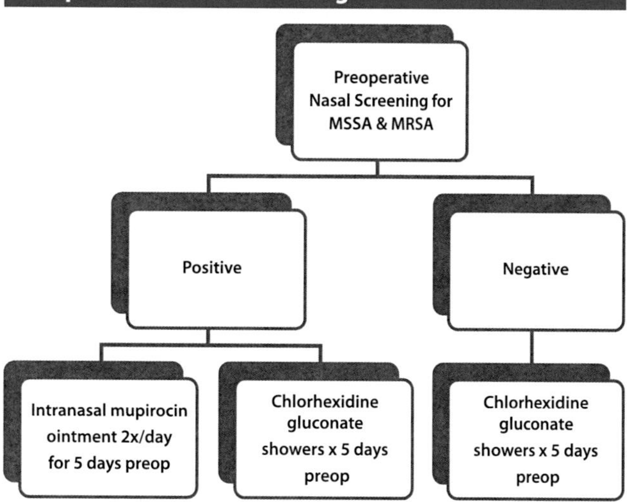

Author creation. Reproduced with permission.

Table 5.3. Home Assessment Following Orthopaedic Surgery
Exterior Assessment
■ Steps and sidewalks in good repair ■ Handrails on the stairs ■ Nonskid treads on outside steps
Interior Assessment
■ Adequate lighting ■ Uncluttered rooms and hallways for easy mobility ■ Electrical/telephone cords removed from traffic path ■ Area rugs removed or anchored to floor ■ Stairway railings present and stable ■ Doors wide enough; adequate turnaround space ■ Commonly used supplies stored in waist-high cabinets or drawers to avoid excessive bending or reaching ■ Toilet has elevated seat available ■ Grab bars by the toilet or in the bathtub ■ Safety strips or rubber mat in bath/shower ■ Tub seat/bench of appropriate height secured ■ Hand-held shower available ■ Area of rest (chair or sofa) easily accessible ■ Pillows available to support and position extremity ■ Pets maintained so that they do not become a fall hazard

Data from "Perioperative Patient Care" by S. Barnett & L. Strickland, 2007, NAON Core Curriculum for Orthopaedic Nursing *(6th ed.), Boston, MA: Pearson.*

at this time. Table 5.3 lists considerations for a home assessment, both interior and exterior, for an orthopaedic patient following surgery (Barnett & Strickland, 2007).

An anesthesiologist may meet with the patient during the preadmission appointment or in Same Day Surgery the morning of surgery where he assesses the patient's airway, condition of the teeth, ability to open the mouth, degree of neck flexion and extension, and history of sleep apnea. A potentially difficult intubation may be anticipated if the patient has a small mouth opening, large protuberant teeth, limited neck mobility, jaw deformity, obesity, or a short stocky neck. The anesthesiologist will note on the patient's chart to obtain "difficult intubation supplies," including laryngeal masks, a fiberoptic bronchoscope, or a video laryngoscope before induction of anesthesia (Rothrock, 2011). Depending upon the type of anesthesia given, the patient with diagnosed sleep apnea may use a continuous positive airway pressure machine (CPAP) during and after surgery, and may be asked to bring his own CPAP mask to the hospital.

Same Day Surgery (SDS). On the day of surgery, the patient may take a sip of water with any regular oral medications that were ordered by the anesthesiologist or surgeon during PAT and showers with an antimicrobial soap before arriving for surgery. The patient arrives 1 to 2 hours prior to surgery and is greeted by the SDS secretary, who identifies the patient by two identifiers (name and date of birth) before placing a hospital bracelet on the patient's wrist. The patient reviews and signs the hospital consents for treatment and blood transfusion before being taken to the SDS room. After changing into a hospital gown and settling onto the SDS stretcher, the patient is greeted by the SDS nurse, who verifies the name, date of birth, food or drug allergies, latex sensitivity, surgeon's name, type of surgery, and side and site of surgery. A red allergy bracelet is placed on the patient's wrist with any stated allergies written in permanent marker. The patient is assessed for:

- communication patterns, language, and comprehension;
- sensory deficits;
- level of consciousness;
- height and weight;
- vital signs;
- neurovascular, circulatory, and respiratory status;
- skin integrity;
- physical/musculoskeletal limitations, casts, or external fixation devices; and
- emotional status, anxiety, and fear.

The medical history is reviewed with the patient (including previous surgical procedures, medications, prostheses, substance abuse, and infectious diseases such as hepatitis and HIV), and the electronic medical record is updated as necessary. Any pertinent change in information is forwarded to the OR for modifications in procedure set-up. If there are any laboratory tests or studies to be done before surgery, they are ordered at this time. For female patients, testing for pregnancy may be done on the day of surgery per facility policy. In some facilities, this preparation is performed in SDS; in other facilities, the patient is moved to the surgical holding area. An intravenous (IV) solution is started in one of the patient's extremities for the administration of medications and fluids. If a "shave and prep" is ordered, the site is cleansed with chlorhexidine gluconate solution before the hair is clipped using an electric clipper with disposable cartridge. No hair is shaved with a razor as per SCIP-Inf 6 Measure (Hall, 2006); small cuts or abrasions on the skin from a razor provide an entryway for microorganisms.

If the anesthesiologist did not interview the patient during the PAT visit, the anesthesiologist now visits the patient and reviews the medical record, results of any tests or medical consults, and previous anesthetic or surgical experiences. Once the assessment is complete, the types of anesthesia available for the designated surgery are explained, any questions that the patient and family may have are answered, and an informed consent for anesthesia is obtained. The choice of anesthesia for a given surgical procedure is made by the patient, anesthesia provider, and surgeon (Rothrock, 2011). The anesthesiologist assigns a physical status classification to the patient, based on the patient's physiologic condition independent of the proposed surgical procedure (see Table 5.4).

Table 5.4. Anesthesia Risk Classes

ASA Physical (P) Status Classification	
P1	Normal healthy patient: No physiologic, psychologic, biochemical, or organic disturbance.
P2	Patient with mild systemic disease: Cardiovascular disease with minimal restriction of activity; hypertension, asthma, chronic bronchitis, obesity, diabetes mellitus, or tobacco abuse
P3	Patient with a severe systemic disease that limits activity, but is not incapacitating: Cardiovascular or pulmonary disease that limits activity; severe diabetes with systemic complications: history of myocardial infarction, angina pectoris, poorly controlled hypertension, or morbid obesity
P4	Patient with a severe systemic disease that is a constant threat to life: Severe cardiac, pulmonary, renal, hepatic, or endocrine dysfunction
P5	Moribund patient who is not expected to survive 24 hr with or without operation: Surgery is done as last recourse or resuscitative effort; major multisystem or cerebral trauma, ruptured aneurysm, or large pulmonary embolus
P6	Patient declared brain dead whose organs are being removed for donor purposes

From Alexander's Care of the Patient in Surgery *(p. 116), by J. Rothrock, 2011, St. Louis, MO: Elsevier Mosby. Reproduced with permission.*

Preoperative medications may be administered to the patient for any of the following: anxiety relief, sedation, amnesia, analgesia, drying of airway secretions, reduction of gastric fluid volume, increase pH of gastrointestinal secretions, reduction in anesthetic requirement, facilitation of induction of anesthesia, antiemetic effect, and/or prophylaxis against allergic reactions. The prophylactic antibiotic may be started in SDS or in the OR; however, it must be given within one hour prior to surgical incision per SCIP Measure INF 1 (Hall, 2006). Vancomycin must be given within 2 hours of incision.

Before proceeding to the OR, the surgeon greets the patient in SDS and answers any last-minute questions the patient or family may have. After confirming the correct procedure and surgical site with the patient, the surgeon signs the operative site with a "yes" or the surgeon's initials using a semi-permanent marking pen. No mark should appear on the non-operative side. Individual hospital policy dictates whether site marking must be done by the person performing the surgery or if it may be delegated to another member of the surgical team. The OR circulating registered nurse greets the patient and uses two identifiers for patient safety. After interviewing the patient and examining the patient's record for consents, history and physical, allergies, availability of blood (if ordered), and results of diagnostic tests, the perioperative nurse verifies the correct surgical procedure and views the "signed" surgical site with the patient. A surgical cap is placed on the patient's head to contain the hair, and the patient is transferred to the OR.

Intraoperative Implementation

Before the patient is ever brought into the OR, much planning and preparation have taken place to ensure a safe environment for the patient.

Infection Prevention and Control

The skin and mucous membranes are the patient's first line of defense to combat infection. Any break in this external barrier increases the possibility for infection. When surgery includes any type of bone, it is even more imperative to be knowledgeable of practices to protect the patient. If a microorganism finds its way into the lacy bony network, a superficial infection may develop into osteomyelitis, which is difficult to eradicate. The OR employs many practices to prevent infection. These include engineering practices, sterilization, aseptic practices, traffic patterns, surgical attire, surgical skin preparation, standard precautions, and OR sanitation.

Engineering Practices. The surgical suite should be designed to minimize and control the spread of infectious organisms. It may be built using a central-core racetrack or a single corridor design. Each design has its own specific features to separate sterile and contaminated items. All of the surfaces of the OR should be constructed of hard materials to withstand the use of heavy surgical equipment and must be able to be easily cleaned. This includes all floors, walls, doors, and cabinets.

"Air in the perioperative environment contains microbial-laden lint, dust, skin squames, and respiratory droplets. The number of microorganisms in the air in an operating room is directly proportional to the number of personnel moving in and around the room" (AORN, 2010, p. 220). It is imperative to have heating, ventilation, and air conditioning systems that function properly to remove those contaminants. The ventilated air delivered from vents in the ceiling is sequentially filtered through two filters and continues to flow in a downward direction toward the exhaust vents located on the walls near the floor. The minimum rate of total number of air exchanges is 15 per hour, with a recommended range of 20 to 25 air exchanges. A minimum of 20% of the incoming air should be from the outdoors to minimize the recirculation of indoor contaminants within the perioperative area. The relative humidity in the OR should be maintained between 20% and 60%. The decrease from 30% to 20% was recommended by the American National Standards Institute (ANSI), the American Society of Healthcare Engineers (ASHE), and the American Society of Heating, Refrigerating and Air Conditioning Engineers (ASHRAE), and became effective June 2010 (ASHRAE, 2010). The previous range was established when flammable anesthetic agents were commonly used, and there was a concern that low humidity levels could allow a static spark to ignite the flammable anesthetic agent (Stanton, 2010). The temperature should be maintained between 68 degrees F and 73 degrees F. Doors to the OR should remain closed except when patients, equipment, supplies, or personnel move into or out of the room. This assists in maintaining "positive pressure" in the room; air pressure in the room is greater than in the surrounding corridor to minimize the corridor's "less clean" air from entering the OR's "more clean" air (Rothrock, 2011).

Sterilization. The perioperative nurse is the patient's advocate; one of the major responsibilities is preventing SSIs. Ensuring that the instruments are sterile and other items are free of contamination is the first step in prevention. Rothrock (2011) defines sterilization as "the complete elimination or destruction of all forms of microbial life" (p. 67). Before an item can be sterilized, however, it must first be free of bioburden (organic debris). During surgery, the scrub person should keep the instruments as clean as possible by wiping them with a sterile wet sponge or by rinsing them in sterile water to prevent the drying of blood and fluids. When the procedure is finished, instruments may be sprayed with an enzymatic cleaner before they are sent to central sterile supply (CSS). Here they are cleaned and decontaminated, using an approved cleaning agent, by hand or mechanical cleaning methods: washer-sterilizers, washer-disinfectors/washer-decontaminators, or ultrasonic cleaners. Once instruments are clean, they are assembled into sets and placed into trays. They may be wrapped with woven or nonwoven, reusable or disposable materials; placed in sterilization packaging systems; or placed into sterilization pouches. Sterilization-specific chemical indicator tapes and chemical and/or biological indicators or integrators are placed inside and on the packages. While preparing for the surgical procedure, the surgical team checks for a change in color on the tape or indicator that ensures that the package has met specific parameters for the sterilization process, meaning that the contents are safe to use. Sterile items are also inspected for damage to the packaging, broken seals, and expiration dates, if any, and to verify that the integrity of the wrapper is intact and secure (AORN, 2010). There are many methods of sterilization. The most common include steam and chemical (ethylene oxide, low-temperature hydrogen peroxide gas plasma, and peracetic acid).

Saturated steam under pressure is the preferred method of sterilization. It permeates lumens of instruments, cannulated drills, and areas between items. It is effective, inexpensive, and a relatively rapid sterilization method for most porous and nonporous materials. Instruments are sterilized-wrapped in instrument sterilization packages or sterilization pouches. An "immediate use" sterilization cycle may be used in the OR for sterilizing urgently needed unwrapped instruments; however, these instruments must be used immediately and cannot be stored.

Ethylene oxide (EO) sterilization is a low-temperature process that is appropriate for heat- and moisture-sensitive surgical items such as fiberoptic scopes, delicate instrumentation, or electrical instruments. EO is a known human carcinogen and has the potential to cause adverse reproductive effects in humans. EO sterilization takes several hours after which the items must be aerated from 8-16 hours in a mechanical aerator to remove all traces of EO. Because of the health hazard that EO presents to patients and healthcare workers, the Occupational Safety and Health Administration (OSHA) has strict regulations for the monitoring of personnel, maintenance of equipment, and record keeping. Many smaller facilities have discontinued the use of EO with the advent of newer technology.

Low-temperature hydrogen peroxide gas plasma sterilization uses a combination of hydrogen peroxide vapor and low-temperature hydrogen peroxide gas plasma. This method sterilizes within 50 to 75 minutes, requires no aeration because the residuals and by-products are oxygen and water in the form of humidity, and is a much safer process for patients and health care workers. It has replaced EO sterilization in many facilities and can be used for items such as rigid endoscopes, camera heads, light cables, and video adapters that require lower temperatures.

Peracetic acid sterilization is a system that uses a chemical formulation of 35% peracetic acid and water. It is an oxidizing agent that is effective at low temperatures and in the presence of organic matters, and can be used on lensed instruments such as flexible endoscopes and cystoscopes. Peracetic acid is used in commercially available sterilization systems, and their relatively short cycles enable the items to be ready for use quickly. The container in which the items are processed is not sealed; thus, the items cannot be stored and must be used immediately. On May 15, 2008, the U.S. Food and Drug Administration (FDA) issued a Warning Letter to a main manufacturer of the liquid chemical sterilizer for making various unapproved changes to the original device launched in 1988 (FDA, 2009). After a 2-year dispute with the FDA, the manufacturer finally received approval on April 5, 2010, for its next-generation liquid chemical sterilizer (Vanac, 2010).

Aseptic Practices. Asepsis is defined as the absence of infectious organisms. Many of the practices in the OR appear merely ritualistic; however, these aseptic practices are based on the premise that most infections are caused by organisms exogenous to the surgical patient's body (Rothrock, 2011). By applying the same, consistent approach to surgical procedures, the risk of infection to the patient is minimized. These include opening sterile supplies as close to the time of their use as possible, using sterile drapes to create a sterile field around the incision site, using sterile instruments for the sterile procedure, and placing the operative team in sterile attire after their hands and arms have been cleansed of surface bacteria. Because perioperative personnel are the patient's advocate, they must develop a strong "Surgical Conscience" by consistently applying these practices to protect the patient from infection. In addition to the aseptic techniques, the OR staff must adhere to the following basic aseptic principles set forth by Rothrock (2011):

- Only sterile items are used within the sterile field.
- Items of doubtful sterility must be considered unsterile: "When in doubt, throw it out!"
- Whenever a sterile barrier is permeated, it must be considered contaminated.
- Sterile gowns are considered sterile in front from shoulder to level of sterile field and at the sleeves from 2 inches above the elbow to the cuff.
- Tables are sterile only at table level.
- The edges of a sterile enclosure are considered unsterile.
- Sterile individuals touch only sterile items or areas; unsterile individuals touch only unsterile items or areas.
- Movement within or around a sterile field must not contaminate the field.

Traffic Patterns. AORN recommends three designated areas within the Surgical Suite to control the movement of personnel, patients, supplies, and equipment; to provide for protection from potential sources of cross-contamination; to safeguard the privacy of patients; and to provide security. The *unrestricted area* includes a central control point where street clothes are permitted and traffic is not limited. The *semirestricted area* includes the support areas of the surgical suite: storage areas, work areas, scrub sink areas, and corridors leading to the restricted areas of the surgical suite. Personnel are required to wear surgical attire and cover all head and facial hair. The *restricted area* includes ORs, procedure rooms, and the clean core areas. Surgical attire and hair coverings are required. Masks are required where open sterile supplies or scrubbed persons are located. Persons who enter the semirestricted or restricted areas for a specific purpose and a brief time (parents of young children, biomedical engineers, law enforcement officers) should cover all head and facial hair and may don clean OR scrubs or use a single-use coverall suit (jumpsuit) that covers the outside apparel. The movement of clean and sterile supplies and equipment should be separated from contaminated supplies, equipment, and waste by space, time, and traffic patterns (AORN, 2010).

Surgical Attire. People are a major source of bacteria in the surgical setting. Outside clothing may contain dirt, bacteria, pet hair, allergens, and other contaminants. The oil in a person's hair attracts bacteria. The skin on one's arms sloughs thousands of cells per minute. Good personal hygiene is a must for perioperative personnel. OR personnel must refrain from wearing heavily scented perfumes, lotions, or deodorants because these may affect patients who have allergies, a heightened sense of smell, or are nauseated.

Surgical attire decreases and contains bacterial shedding. It consists of a two-piece pantsuit, head cover, shoe covers, and mask. All persons entering the semirestricted and restricted areas of the OR must wear clean, facility-laundered surgical attire, also known as scrub attire. Shoe covers are required if there is a chance of blood or body fluid contamination. Nonscrubbed personnel should wear long-sleeved jackets that are snapped close to help decrease bacterial and skin shedding from bare arms. A single, high-filtration surgical mask is worn in the OR to filter microbial droplets expelled from the mouth and nasopharynx of personnel and to protect health care workers from aerosolized pathogenic organisms and particles from the surgical environment.

Scrubbed personnel wear sterile gowns and gloves to provide a protective barrier between the patient and the surgical team to decrease the probability of exposing the patient to exogenous organisms resulting in a surgical site infection (Rothrock, 2010). Facilities may use either reusable cloth or disposable gowns, each having advantages and disadvantages. Sterile gloves also decrease the chance of the health care provider being exposed to blood or other potentially infectious material. The practice of double-gloving reduces the risk of infection by providing an additional barrier. With orthopaedic surgery, the risk for perforation is high; thus, the team members usually opt to wear double gloves. The inside glove is colored so the wearer can easily recognize perforations to the outer glove, which is then changed.

Body exhaust systems, also called personal protection systems, are used in many hospitals during total joint arthroplasty surgeries for "high levels of protection against contamination, exposure to infectious bodily fluids, and transfer of microorganisms and particulate matter" (Stryker *Flyte*, n.d.). The system includes a helmet with fan and battery hook-up, sterile toga with hood and clear plastic shield, and battery.

Surgical Skin Preparation. To reduce the risk of postoperative surgical site infection, skin preparation for the patient begins at home prior to surgery. The goals include removing soil and transient microorganisms from the skin, reducing the resident microbial count in a short period of time and with the least amount of tissue, and inhibiting the rapid rebound growth of microorganisms (AORN, 2010).

Patients undergoing clean, elective procedures (Class I) should have at least two preoperative showers with 4% chlorhexidine gluconate (CHG) before surgery (AORN, 2010). Recent studies have shown CHG to be more effective than povidone-iodine as a preoperative skin antisepsis for preventing SSIs (Lee, Agarwal, Lee, Fishman, & Umscheid, 2010). More than one shower is necessary to achieve maximum antiseptic effectiveness in reducing microbial counts. *Staphylococcus aureus*, from the patient's own flora, is the most common organism-causing surgical site infections. The act of washing and rinsing removes microorganisms from the skin. Care must be exercised to avoid CHG contact with the eyes, inside of the ears, the meninges, or other mucous membranes. Following each preoperative shower, the skin should be thoroughly rinsed to prevent irritation from residual CHG then dried with a fresh, clean, dry towel; the patient should don clean clothing (AORN, 2010).

Surgical skin preparation in the OR usually includes a preoperative washing or "scrub" of the site with an antimicrobial agent to remove superficial soil, oils, and transient microbes. After drying the area with a sterile towel, the antiseptic agent should be applied to the skin over the surgical site and surrounding area, progressing from the incision site (the cleanest area) to the periphery of the surgical site (less clean area). This prevents the reintroduction of microorganisms from the peripheral areas to the incision site. If a tourniquet cuff is used on an extremity, care must be taken not to allow the antiseptic agent to pool under the cuff; this could cause a chemical burn to the patient's skin. The prep agent should be allowed to dry so that any vapors completely dissipate before application of surgical drapes or use of electrosurgery; the prep agent remains flammable until completely dry. Traumatic orthopaedic injuries with exposed bone may be cleansed using low-pressure pulse lavage with sterile normal saline irrigation, being careful to use a protective shield to avoid aerosolization (a fine mist or spray containing minute particles) of wound contaminants onto the sterile field during irrigation (AORN, 2010).

Standard Precautions and OR Sanitation. Standard precautions, designed to reduce the transmission risk of bloodborne and other pathogens, should be applied to all patients receiving care regardless of their diagnosis or presumed infection status (Rothrock, 2011). These precautions apply to blood, all body fluids, secretions, and excretions (except sweat) regardless of whether they contain visible blood, mucous membranes, and nonintact skin (Rothrock, 2011). See Table 5.5 for the list of standard precautions.

All patients should be provided a clean, safe surgical environment. Contamination in the OR can occur from the patient, health care workers, and inanimate objects. Cleaning procedures are needed before, during, and after surgical procedures and at the end of each day. Sanitation of OR equipment and furniture is performed using an EPA-approved hospital disinfectant, followed by cleaning of the floor. To ensure patient and personnel safety, cleaning procedures should be uniform throughout the OR and for all patients; this eliminates the need for special cleaning procedures for "dirty cases." Terminal cleaning and disinfection of the OR should be performed after scheduled procedures are completed or at the end of each regular 24-hour period. Washing of the walls and ceiling should be completed on a regular, scheduled basis.

Table 5.6. Standard Precautions
Hand Hygiene: Most important factor in preventing spread of infection ■ Handwashing □ After contact with blood, body fluids, secretions, excretions, & contaminated items. □ After glove removal, between patients, tasks, & procedures ■ Alcohol-based hand rubs - on clean hands
Gloves ■ Clean, nonsterile gloves when touching body fluids & contaminated items ■ Change gloves between tasks & patients
Masks, eye protection, face shields ■ Protection for nose, mouth, & eyes from sprays or splashes of blood or body fluids
Gown ■ Clean, nonsterile gowns when patient care activities are likely to generate sprays or splashes of body fluids
Sharps ■ Place in puncture-resistant containers ■ Do not recap if possible; or use one-handed scoop technique
Patient care equipment ■ Discard single-use items after use ■ Clean & reprocess reusable equipment
Linens ■ Avoid skin & mucous membrane exposure with soiled linens ■ Avoid transfer of microorganisms to other patients, personnel, & environment
Environmental control ■ Monitor procedures used for routine care & cleaning of environmental surfaces, beds, & equipment
Patient placement ■ Private room, if possible ■ Cohort with patients with similar infectious organisms

From Alexander's Care of the Patient in Surgery *(p. 63), by J. Rothrock, 2011, St. Louis, MO: Elsevier Mosby. Reproduced with permission.*

For patients with a documented infection or a suspected highly transmissible pathogen, transmission-based precautions are used: airborne, droplet, and contact. The hospital's infection control policies, based on CDC guidelines, should be followed.

Wound Classification

The CDC *Guideline for Prevention of Surgical Wound Infections*, first published in 1982, is still the standard used today (Garner, 1985). Wounds are classified according to the likelihood and degree of wound contamination at the time of operation. This classification scheme has been shown in numerous studies to predict the relative probability that a wound will become infected (Garner, 1985). In addition, surgeons may use this scheme to compare their own infection rates with those of other surgeons for a given operation. This classification is also used by hospital-based infection prevention practitioners when researching infection rates that they report to their state agencies.

Clean wounds are uninfected operative wounds in which no inflammation is encountered and the respiratory, alimentary, genital, or uninfected urinary tracts are not entered. In addition, clean wounds are primarily closed, and if necessary, drained with closed drainage. Operative incisional wounds that follow nonpenetrating (blunt) trauma should be included in this category if they meet the criteria. Clean wounds have a 1% - 5% risk of infection (Garner, 1985).

Clean-contaminated wounds are operative wounds in which the respiratory, alimentary, genital, or urinary tract is entered under controlled conditions and without unusual contamination. Specifically, operations involving the biliary tract, appendix, vagina, and oropharynx are included in this category, provided no evidence of infection or major break in technique is encountered. Clean-contaminated wounds have a 3% - 11% risk of infection (Garner, 1985).

Contaminated wounds include open, fresh, accidental wounds, operations with major breaks in sterile technique or gross spillage from the gastrointestinal tract, and incisions in which acute, nonpurulent inflammation is encountered. Contaminated wounds have a 10% - 17% risk of infection (Garner, 1985).

Dirty or infected wounds include old traumatic wounds with retained devitalized tissue and those that involve existing clinical infection or perforated viscera. This definition suggests that the organisms causing postoperative infection were present in the operative field before the operation. Dirty wounds have greater than a 27% risk of infection (Garner, 1985).

Anesthesia

In the United States, anesthesia providers include anesthesiologists, certified registered nurse anesthetists (CRNA), and anesthesiologist assistants (AA). The CRNA works in collaboration with or under the direction of an anesthesiologist or physician; the AA works under the direct supervision of an anesthesiologist (Rothrock, 2011). The patient is brought to the OR by the anesthesia provider and/or the perioperative registered nurse. While introducing the patient to the surgical team, the nurse performs a preprocedure verification involving the patient by stating the patient's name (correct patient), surgeon, and surgical procedure (correct site and side). After the patient is moved to the OR bed, the nurse or anesthesia technician assists the anesthesia provider with placement of monitoring devices (Table 5.6). Critical patients or those having extensive or emergency surgery may also have a central venous pressure line (CVP), an arterial line (A-line), and/or additional intravenous lines inserted at this time if they were not previously inserted in SDS or holding area, as well as additional monitoring devices. For descriptions of the major types of anesthesia care, see Table 5.7.

Table 5.6. Basic Intraoperative Monitoring Devices
EKG leads ■ Provides continuous electrocardiogram display ■ Ensures adequacy of the patient's circulatory system
Blood pressure cuff ■ Measures blood pressure and pulse ■ Ensures adequacy of the patient's circulatory system
Pulse oximetry ■ Measures oxygen saturation in a pulsating vessel (SpO2) ■ Ensures adequate oxygen concentration in the inspired gas and the blood
Capnography ■ Measures end-tidal carbon dioxide level ■ Ensures adequate ventilation of the patient
Temperature Monitor ■ Aids in the maintenance of appropriate body temperature during surgery

From Alexander's Care of the Patient in Surgery (p. 118), by J. Rothrock, 2011, St. Louis, MO: Elsevier Mosby. Reproduced with permission.

Temperature Control. Routine monitoring of the patient's intraoperative temperature is an important part of anesthesia monitoring. SCIP expanded the normothermia measure effective October 2009 "for all patients undergoing surgical procedures under general or neuraxial anesthesia for 60 minutes or more" (Gunn, 2009, p. 1). Previously, the measure applied only to colorectal surgery patients. Normothermia is described as body temperature equal to or greater than 96.8 degrees F/36 degrees C. Risk factors for developing hypothermia include age extreme (pediatric or elderly patients), co-morbidity, length of surgical procedure, cachexia, fluid shifts, cold irrigating fluids, and general and regional anesthesia. Some anesthetic agents can interfere with the body's shivering mechanisms, autoregulation of body temperature, and vasodilation. Unintentional hypothermia can cause patient discomfort, untoward cardiac events, adrenergic stimulation, impaired platelet function, altered drug metabolism, delayed emergence from anesthesia, and impaired wound healing (Rothrock, 2011).

There are many ways that perioperative personnel can prevent hypothermia. Warm blankets are applied to the patient upon entering the OR. For pediatric patients, the room temperature is often increased, and infrared warming lamps may be used. Anesthetic gases may be humidified. A variety of IV warmers warm IV fluids or refrigerated blood products. A forced-air warming unit blows heated air onto the upper or lower body surface through a disposable warming blanket. Exposure of the patient's body during prepping and surgery should be limited. Irrigation fluids may be warmed in warming cabinets before administration to the sterile field, or may be poured into a portable warming unit that is covered with a sterile drape.

Malignant Hyperthermia. Malignant hyperthermia (MH) is a rare, hereditary, life-threatening, hypermetabolic syndrome. It is triggered by a halogenated inhalation anesthetic agent — sevoflurane (Ultane), isoflurane (Forane), or desflurane — or by the neuromuscular blocking agent succinylcholine. The incidence of MH is increased in patients with central core disease (an inherited myopathy) and some muscular dystrophies. The hypermetabolic condition begins in the skeletal muscle cells and involves altered mechanisms of calcium function at the cellular level (Rothrock, 2011). This cellular hypermetabolism can cause the following signs and symptoms, in order of occurrence:

- Hypercarbia;
- Tachycardia;
- Tachypnea;
- Muscle stiffness or rigidity;
- Hypoxia and dark blood in operative field;
- Unstable or elevated blood pressure;
- Cardiac dysrhythmias;
- Changes in CO_2 absorbent (temperature, color);
- Metabolic and respiratory acidosis;
- Peripheral mottling, cyanosis, and sweating;
- Rising body temperature (1 to 2 degrees C every 5 minutes);
- Myoglobinuria;
- Hyperkalemia, hypercalcemia, lactic acidemia; and
- Pronounced elevation in creatine kinase level (Rothrock, 2011).

Once MH is diagnosed, immediate initiating of treatment is critical. The anesthesia provider immediately discontinues all triggering agents and ventilates with 100% oxygen at the highest flow rate. If possible, surgery should be terminated or continued with safe anesthetic drugs. The MH protocol includes immediate intravenous infusion of dantrolene (Dantrium), a skeletal muscle relaxant that also has effects on vascular and heart muscle. Additional treatment includes cooling the patient with ice packs and cold IV solutions, administering diuretics, treating cardiac dysrhythmias,

Table 5.7. Major Types of Anesthesia	
Types of Anesthesia	**Nursing Implications**
General Anesthesia ■ Reversible, unconscious state with amnesia, analgesia, depression of reflexes, and muscle relaxation ■ Divided into 3 phases: induction, maintenance, and emergence ■ Wide variety of agents used: □ Inhalation agents □ Opioid analgesics □ Muscle relaxants □ Intravenous anesthetics ■ To maintain airway, may use: □ Endotracheal tube □ Laryngeal mask airway (LMA) □ Mask anesthesia	■ During induction and emergence, keep noise to a minimum; hearing is the last sense to leave and the first sense to return ■ During intubation, the circulating nurse may be asked to apply cricoid pressure (downward pressure on the cricoid cartilage, with the thumb and index finger) to occlude the esophagus and prevent aspiration ■ If difficult intubation, the nurse needs to be familiar with and assist with the equipment on the difficult intubation cart
Regional Anesthesia ■ Reversible loss of sensation in a special region of the body ■ Local anesthetic is injected to block or anesthetize nerve fibers □ Spinal: Lidocaine, tetracaine, or bupivacaine	■ Assess for sensory and motor function before and after block ■ Assist anesthesia provider in placing appropriate monitoring devices (EKG, blood pressure, oximeter), supplemental oxygen if necessary, reassuring patient, and assisting with properly positioning the patient for the block
■ Regional Anesthesia includes: □ **Spinal anesthesia** – injected into the cerebrospinal fluid in the subarachnoid space	■ Spinal responses: □ Hypotension □ High spinal block □ Positioning problems □ "Spinal headache"
□ **Epidural anesthesia** – injected through the intervertebral spaces into the epidural space • May be a "single shot epidural" or a small catheter may be left in the epidural space • May be used for post-operative pain control □ **Caudal anesthesia** – injected through the caudal canal in the sacrum into the epidural space	■ Epidural complications: □ Inadvertent dural puncture □ Subarachnoid injection □ Vascular injection
□ **Major peripheral nerve blocks (PNBs)** • Portable ultrasound guidance assists in accurate needle placement for peripheral nerve and plexus blocks • Upper extremity brachial plexus – Interscalene, supraclavicular, and infraclavicular used for shoulder surgery – Axillary site for hand surgery • Lower extremity – Femoral nerve block for knee procedures – Ankle block for foot/toe surgery	■ May be done in a preoperative holding area to allow time for the local anesthetic to penetrate the peripheral nerve before taking the patient to the OR ■ Inter scalene block may cause Horner syndrome (miosis, ptosis, and increased salivation) and a unilateral phrenic nerve paralysis that causes breathing difficulty ■ With PNBs, patient has lost pain sensation □ Watch patient positioning, pad pressure points □ Post-op: inform patient of risk of burns or falls until sensation returns
□ **Intravenous regional block:** "Bier Block" is used mostly on upper extremity • A small IV catheter is inserted as distal as possible • A double-cuffed tourniquet is placed on the extremity • The limb is raised, exsanguinated using an Esmarch bandage, and the proximal cuff of the tourniquet is inflated • Local anesthetic is injected	■ To deflate tourniquet; □ If tourniquet time is < 20 minutes, deflate the cuff for a few seconds at a time for several cycles when surgery is finished to prevent a toxic reaction or overdose from the lidocaine □ If > 20 minutes, tourniquet may be deflated as usual

Table continued on next page.

Table 5.7. Major Types of Anesthesia (continued)	
Types of Anesthesia	**Nursing Implications**
Monitored Anesthesia Care (MAC) ■ Infiltration of the surgical site with a local anesthetic by the surgeon AND ■ Supplemented by IV drugs by the anesthesia provider to provide sedation, amnesia, and systemic analgesia □ Monitors patient's vital functions □ May give supplemental oxygen ■ Used for healthy patients having minor surgical procedures ■ May be used for critically ill patients who may not tolerate a general anesthetic	■ Depending on the clinical situation, the anesthesia provider may have to induce general anesthesia or use one of the regional techniques
Conscious Sedation/Analgesia ■ Administered for specific, short-term surgical, diagnostic, and therapeutic procedures in a hospital or ambulatory center ■ Patient has IV line established to administer drugs and IV fluids if necessary ■ Patient has patent airway and spontaneous ventilation ■ May be given by RNs who have additional training in administering these medications and monitoring these patients	■ The nurse who administers the conscious sedation/ analgesia: □ Should have no other duties than monitoring the patient □ Be clinically competent in the use of monitoring equipment and oxygen-delivery systems □ Should be knowledgeable of all aspects of the medications she administers to the patient □ Document on the intraoperative nursing record
Local Anesthesia ■ Administration of an anesthetic agent to a part of the body by local infiltration or topical application usually by the surgeon □ Topical agents include: cocaine hydrochloride, tetracaine, or lidocaine □ Injected agents include: Lidocaine 0.5% - 2% with or without epinephrine; Marcaine (bupivacaine) may also be used □ Epinephrine may be added to the local anesthetic • Used for vasoconstriction properties • Slows the rate of absorption • Lowers rate of toxicity • Allows longer duration of action of the anesthetic agent by reducing blood flow to the area • Use with caution in patients with hypertension, diabetes, or heart disease ■ Used for minor procedures when a patient's cooperation is needed, or if patient's physical condition warrants ■ No anesthesia provider is involved ■ All syringes and containers must be clearly labeled with the name and strength of the local anesthetic	■ The perioperative nurse: □ Reviews the patient's chart and checks for allergies □ Monitors the patient for heart rate, respiratory rate, and mental status; may include blood pressure and oxygen saturation if patient's condition warrants □ Provides support to the patient □ Documents dosage, route, and times of medication administration □ Gives a "hand-off" report to the SDS area with transfer of patient

correcting acid-base and electrolyte imbalances, and monitoring fluid intake and output and body temperature. The patient is transferred to the intensive care unit (ICU) when stable, and monitored for at least 24 hours for recurrence of MH and for late complications. Following this protocol has dramatically decreased mortality from 80% to 7%. Many hospitals have an emergency MH cart or kit that contains the medications, laboratory tubes, other supplies, location of chilled saline, and instructions in or near the OR area. A 24-hour hotline sponsored by the Malignant Hyperthermia Association of the United States (MHAUS; www.mhaus.org) is available for medical professionals (Smith, 2010).

Positioning

Proper patient positioning is essential for safe, successful surgery and is the responsibility of every surgical team member. Many institutions include confirmation of the correct patient position during the time-out that occurs before the surgical incision is made. Rothrock (2011) acknowledges the following goals of surgical positioning:

- Providing optimal exposure and access to the surgical site;
- Maintaining body alignment;
- Supporting circulatory and respiratory function;
- Protecting neuromuscular and skin integrity;
- Allowing access to intravenous sites and anesthesia support devices; and
- Maintaining patient comfort and safety.

The perioperative nurse must be knowledgeable of the anatomic and physiologic changes that occur when positioning the patient. Factors that affect these changes include the particular surgical position; length of time the patient is in that position; OR bed, padding, and positioning devices used; anesthesia given; and operative procedure (Rothrock, 2011). The changes may involve the skin and underlying tissue, musculoskeletal system, nervous system, cardiovascular system, and respiratory system.

Skin and underlying tissue may be injured by the physical forces used to establish and maintain a surgical position, including pressure, shear, and friction. OR conditions such as moisture, heat, cold, and excess layers of sheets or blankets placed over the OR mattress increase vulnerability of the skin and underlying tissues to injury (Rothrock, 2011). Pressure ulcers were found to be the most common preventable event, with nearly 375,000 cases in 2008 at a cost of $3.27 billion (Fung, 2011). The National Pressure Ulcer Advisory Panel (NPUAP, 2007) defines a pressure ulcer as a "localized injury to the skin and/or underlying tissue usually over a bony prominence, as a result of pressure, or pressure in combination with shear and/or friction." Pressure ulcers have also been referred to as pressure sores, bed sores, and decubitus ulcers. In 2008, CMS decided to halt reimbursement to hospitals for many preventable hospital-acquired conditions that they called "never events." These included stage III and IV pressure ulcers that develop after admission (Rothrock, 2011). Research has shown that both extrinsic and intrinsic factors listed on Table 5.8 interact to contribute to the development of pressure ulcers. The perioperative nurse should assess integrity of the patient's skin preoperatively, especially over bony prominences. Any fragile skin areas or those in contact with hard surfaces should be padded. After surgery is completed, the skin should be reassessed; any findings should be documented on the intraoperative record with any changes reported to appropriate personnel.

Table 5.8. Factors That Contribute to Pressure Ulcers

Extrinsic Factors = physical forces & conditions the patient experiences

- Pressure
  - Intensity
  - Duration
- Effects of anesthesia given
  - Hypotension
    - Reduced tissue perfusion
    - Reduced exchange of oxygen & carbon dioxide
  - Hypothermia
- Type of surgery
  - Blood loss
  - Extracorporeal circulation
- Patient's position & positioning devices
- Safety measures

Intrinsic Factors = health & body structure of the patient

- Respiratory disorders
- Diabetes mellitus
- Anemia
- Malnutrition
- Advanced age
- Body size
- Body temperature
- Impaired mobility
- Smoking

From Alexander's Care of the Patient in Surgery *(p. 146), by J. Rothrock, 2011, St. Louis, MO: Elsevier Mosby. Reproduced with permission.*

During operative positioning, the patient's musculoskeletal system may be subjected to unusual stress. The goal of safe positioning is to maintain the body in natural alignment as much as possible, while providing adequate access to the surgical site. After anesthetic drugs and muscle relaxants have been given, normal defense mechanisms cannot guard against joint damage or muscle stretch and strain. The perioperative nurse must be aware of normal range of motion (ROM) and not extend a joint beyond what is absolutely necessary (Rothrock, 2011).

The administration of anesthetic agents and other drugs causes depression of the *nervous system*. Peripheral nerves can be injured during positioning, resulting in impaired sensory function, motor function, or both. The principle factors in position-induced nerve injuries are stretching and compression. Upper extremity neuropathies arise from injury to the brachial plexus, which contains four nerves: musculocutaneous, radial, median, and ulnar. The surgical team must be aware of positioning techniques to prevent injury to the brachial plexus. The armboard must be level with the OR bed. When placing the arms on the armboards, they must not extend beyond a 90-degree angle to the body. Surgical team members must be aware not to lean on the patient or against the shoulder or arm if it is tucked against the body. In lateral position, the dependent shoulder and arm must not be compressed under the rib cage. Eliminate pressure on the medial aspect of the elbow to protect the ulnar nerve by padding above or below the elbow.

Lower extremity neuropathies result from injuries to the common peroneal, sciatic, and femoral nerves. Soft padding under the dependent knee should be used to protect the peroneal nerve when the patient is in lateral position. With the patient in supine position, pillows or soft padding should be used to protect the peroneal and tibial nerves that pass behind the knees. With the patient in stirrups in lithotomy position, the femoral and obturator nerves may be injured due to excessive stretching. The position of the patient, positioning devices, and any measures to prevent injury should be documented on the patient's intraoperative record.

The *cardiovascular system* is affected by anesthesia and changes in position, especially in patients with cardiovascular disease, hypovolemia, and obesity. Hypotension can result from both general and regional anesthesia, and is treated with pharmacologic agents and increased intravenous infusion. Position changes should be delayed until blood pressure stabilizes (Rothrock, 2011). Venous thromboembolism (VTE) can be a serious complication of surgical positioning, resulting from compression on deep and peripheral vessels or when legs are in a dependent position causing slowed venous return and possibly thrombosis. The use of sequential compression devices (SCDs) or antiembolic stockings can reduce this risk.

The *respiratory system* can be compromised when the body is placed in surgical positions where abdominal viscera are shifted upward toward the diaphragm, thus reducing tidal volume. If a patient experiences dyspnea, the head of the bed should be elevated during transport and surgery if possible. In some orthopaedic surgeries, the arms may be placed across the chest, which further restricts chest movement and lung function. The elbow should be padded to protect the ulnar nerve, and the time in this position should be limited. The anesthesia provider always uses pulse oximetry to monitor respiratory status.

Surgical Positions used for Orthopaedic Procedures. Rothrock (2011) describes five positions for patients undergoing orthopaedic surgery. The *supine position* is the most commonly used position, with the patient usually anesthetized in this position. It is used for most extremity and anterior cervical spine procedures, closed reduction of fractures, and some total hip arthroplasty procedures. The patient lies on the OR bed with his back flat on the bed; a pillow may be placed under the calves to free the popliteal areas and heels from pressure and to reduce back strain. Arms may be placed on padded armboards equal to the level of the OR bed or tucked at the sides of the patient; ankles are uncrossed. The head rests on a small pillow or head cushion to support cervical alignment, reduce occipital pressure, and reduce strain on the neck muscles. The patient is covered with warm blankets followed by a safety strap placed approximately 2 inches above the knees.

The *fracture bed position* is used on a special OR bed called the "fracture bed" or "fracture table," as seen in Figure 5.3. Usually used for the patient with a hip fracture, this bed also has attachments for positioning for a femoral or tibial fracture. The patient is transferred to the OR in the hospital bed with traction applied to the extremity and is usually anesthetized before transfer to the fracture table. The patient is positioned supine; the pelvis is stabilized against a well-padded vertical perineal post. Traction of the injured leg is achieved by placing the foot of the affected side in a well-padded, boot-like device connected to the traction bar. This bar enables the leg to be rotated, pulled into traction, or released as surgery requires. The unaffected leg rests on a well-padded, elevated leg holder or is secured in a well-padded, boot-like device; it is abducted well out of the field so that the orthopaedic surgeon can use C-Arm fluoroscopy during the surgery. The arm on the operative side is usually positioned and secured on a padded sling or post-supported arm holder that goes over the patient's body. The elbow should be padded and positioned in such a way that prevents injury to the ulnar nerve.

Figure 5.4.
Fracture Table

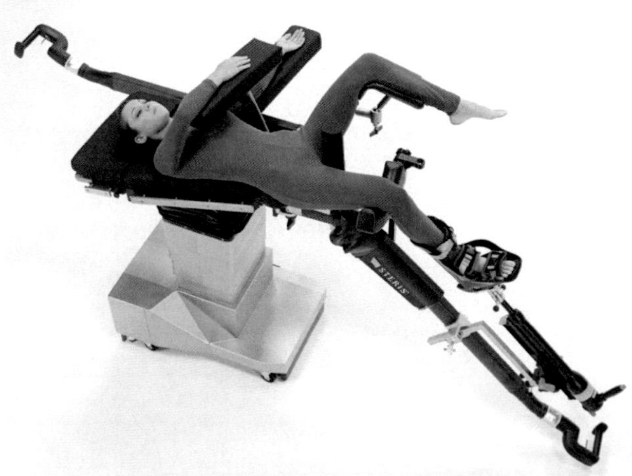

From STERIS Corporation, Mentor, OH. Reproduced with permission.

Semi-Fowler position (or beach chair) may be used for shoulder and humeral surgeries. After the patient is anesthetized in supine position, the upper body section of the bed is flexed 45 degrees, and the leg section is lowered slightly, flexing the knees. Legs are uncrossed, and a pillow may be placed under the knees to relieve pressure and ensure that the heels are not resting on the bed. A shoulder chair attachment, seen in Figure 5.5, allows for vertical torso support. It has drop-away shoulder panels that can be removed on the affected side during shoulder procedures to allow full access to the shoulder. This attachment also includes arm supports and a padded head restraint to prevent the head from forward and lateral movement while the patient is in semi-fowler position. A side brace is applied to keep the patient's torso in place during the surgery. Eye shields are often placed over the patient's eyes for protection from pressure placed on the head or eyes inadvertently by the assistant, retractors, or instrumentation.

Figure 5.5.
Shoulder Chair Attachment

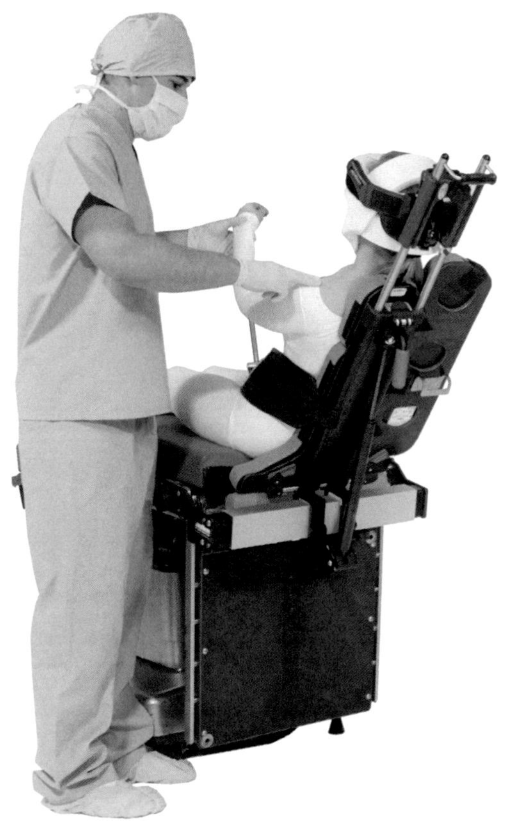

From Allen Medical, (n.d.), www.allenmedical.com/allen-orthopaedics.html. Reproduced with permission.

In the *prone position*, the patient lies with the abdomen on the surface of the OR bed mattress or spinal frame. This position is used for posterior cervical, thoracic and lumbar spine surgeries, as well as some lower extremity procedures. Anesthesia is induced with the patient in supine position. The anesthesia provider secures the endotracheal tube in place with tape, applies ointment to each eye, and tapes the eyelids closed to prevent corneal abrasions. The patient's bed or stretcher is aligned with the OR bed and locked into place. Using the "log roll" technique, four people turn the supine patient to prone position in a safe, smooth, and gentle manner. The anesthesia provider supports the head and neck during the turn. A second person stands at the side of the stretcher/bed with hands at the patient's shoulders and buttocks to initiate the roll of the patient. A third person stands on the opposite side of the OR bed, with arms extended to support the chest and lower abdomen as the patient is log-rolled laterally onto his or her abdomen. The fourth person stands at the foot of the stretcher/bed to support and turn the legs. When the arms are placed on armboards, they are brought down and forward slowly, with minimal abduction to prevent shoulder dislocation and brachial plexus injury. Armboards are at the same height as the OR bed or at a lower parallel line to the OR bed; the arms should rest with elbows flexed (not beyond 90 degrees) and hands pronated. Pads should be placed distal and proximal to the elbow so the ulnar nerve is not in contact with the armboard. Pads are placed under the knees with a pillow under the ankles when using the regular OR bed. Eyes should be checked to ensure that no direct pressure is being applied to the globe of the eye because this may result in temporary or permanent blindness. Female breasts are checked for compression on the chest supports; soft ventral supports on the lateral sides of the breasts divert the breast toward the midline and are better tolerated. Male genitalia must hang free and not be compressed between the pelvis and the spinal frame, which could cause a crush injury.

The *lateral position (lateral recumbent, lateral decubitus, or Sims)* may be used for shoulder arthroscopy, elbow, anterior spine, femur, or hip procedures. When referencing right or left lateral position, the side relates to the side on which the patient lies; in left lateral position, the patient is positioned with the left side down. The patient lies supine on the bed for induction of anesthesia. A four-person team uses a draw sheet that is under the patient to facilitate the turn that places the nonoperative side down. A pillow or cushion is placed under the patient's head to maintain good alignment with the cervical spine and thoracic vertebrae. The upper arm is placed on an elevated armboard or rests on a pillow in front of the patient. Shoulder arthroscopy requires a shoulder positioner device with traction for the upper arm. The lower arm is flexed and rests on an armboard. The lower shoulder is brought slightly forward, and an axillary roll is placed under the rib cage, posterior to the axilla, to prevent injury to the brachial plexus. The bottom leg is flexed at the knee and hip to stabilize the patient on the bed. The top leg is straight or slightly flexed. A pillow is placed lengthwise between the patient's legs. Padding is placed under the lateral aspect of the bottom knee to prevent pressure on the common peroneal nerve located superficially at the head of the fibula. Various positioning devices may be used to stabilize the patient, including pillows, rolled blankets, padded kidney braces, or a Vac-Pac (beanbag).

Electrosurgery

Electrosurgery, using high-frequency (radio frequency) electrical current, is used routinely in orthopaedic surgery to cut, coagulate, dissect, ablate, and shrink body tissue (AORN, 2010). Electrosurgical units (ESUs) are high-risk equipment with the potential for injuries to the patient or user, for fires in the OR, or for electromagnetic interference with other medical equipment and internal electronic devices (such as pacemakers). ESUs have two modes of electrosurgical cutting or coagulation: monopolar and bipolar. In the *monopolar system*, electrical energy flows from the generator through an active electrode (pencil) to the patient, where controlled heat is generated to provide cutting or coagulation of the tissue. The electrical energy then passes through the patient to a dispersive electrode pad placed on the patient's body. Energy is then returned to the generator to complete the circuit. The dispersive electrode should be placed on the patient over an area on the surgical side that is well-vascularized, such as muscle mass, as close as possible to the surgical site. Avoid using excessively hairy sites, bony prominences, excessively dry skin, adipose tissue, scar tissue, and previously implanted sites, which may impede return of the electrical current and could cause a tissue burn (AORN, 2010).

An advanced technology uses a capacitive "gatekeeper" design in either a large (20"x 46") pad for adults and a smaller (12"x 26") pad for infants, which is placed on the OR bed (Megadyne, 2007). The principles of "bulk resistivity" and "capacitive coupling" allow the patient's weight on the pad to complete the circuit (Rothrock, 2011). The reusable pad also serves as a pressure reduction pad; in addition, it eliminates the need to shave excessively hairy sites.

A *bipolar system* does not need a dispersive electrode; electrical energy flows from one tine (prong) of the blade, through the tissue, to the other tine of the instrument. The flow of energy directly returns to the generator, and current does not flow through the patient. Bipolar forceps are used in delicate areas such as the spine and hand because of the lack of stray current.

Tourniquet Use

Pneumatic tourniquets (Figure 5.6) are used to maintain a bloodless surgical field in procedures involving the extremities and to confine a bolus of anesthetic in an extremity for intravenous regional anesthesia (Bier Block). The newest tourniquet technologies include microprocessor controls, self-check calibration, a 4- or 5-hour battery back-up, a "Limb Occlusion Pressure" (LOP) feature (Zimmer, n.d.), and tourniquet report summary to a printer or an interface to the electronic intraoperative record (Stryker *Tourniquet*, n.d.). The tourniquet cuff is a fabric-covered cylindrical bladder that is inflated by compressed gas or ambient air, comes in a variety of shapes and sizes, and may be single-use or reusable. When inflated, it applies circumferential pressure to the arterial and venous circulation, which results in the bloodless surgical field. Prior to inflation, it is necessary to exsanguinate the limb by elevating it to allow venous blood to exit the limb by gravity, or by elevating the limb and wrapping an Ace or Esmarch rubber bandage around the limb, distally to proximally (Rothrock, 2011).

Figure 5.6.
Pneumatic Tourniquet

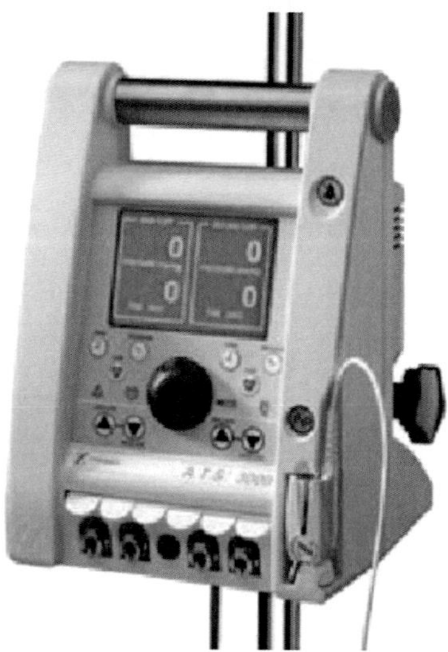

From Zimmer, 2008, www.zimmer.com/z/ctl/op/global/action/1/id/9371/template/MP/prcat/M8/prod/y. Reproduced with permission.

Perioperative personnel must check the tourniquet equipment for proper functioning and set the inflation pressures. Actual inflation pressures are based on the patient's systolic blood pressure, age of the patient, and circumference of the extremity, although common pressure ranges are 250-300 mm Hg for the arm or lower leg, and 300-350 mm Hg for the thigh. Prior to use, the perioperative nurse must assess the patient for location of tourniquet ("correct site"), size and shape of extremity, condition of skin under and distal to the cuff site, and peripheral pulses distal to the cuff. The nurse must also assess for the following relative contraindications for tourniquet use:

- Extremity infection;
- Open fracture;
- Tumor distal to the tourniquet;
- Sickle cell anemia;
- Impaired circulation;
- Previous revascularization of the extremity;

- Extremities with dialysis access (AV shunts or fistulas);
- VTE;
- Increased intracranial pressure; and
- Acidosis (AORN, 2010).

Any prophylactic antibiotics ordered must be completely infused before inflation of the tourniquet for optimum efficacy. The skin beneath the tourniquet is protected with stockinette or soft padding. The tourniquet cuff is sized to wrap around the extremity with a 3-6 inch overlap and is positioned as high as possible on the extremity without pinching the skin or wrinkling the padding. A too-short tourniquet can loosen after inflation; a too-long tourniquet may not allow enough compression for a bloodless surgical field.

Tourniquet inflation time should be kept to a minimum, although safe tourniquet inflation time has not been precisely determined (AORN, 2010). There is general agreement that the tourniquet time for the upper extremity should not exceed 60 minutes and the lower extremity 90 minutes. AORN (2010) states, "When prolonged tourniquet time is desired, the tourniquet should be released for reperfusion of the limb every hour. The reperfusion time should be 15 minutes, after which the tourniquet may be reinflated for another full period… Reperfusion allows oxygenation and continued viability of the tissue" (p. 180). The perioperative nurse should inform the surgeon of the duration of the tourniquet time at regular, established intervals. The anesthesia care provider should be alerted before wrapping the extremity, inflating the tourniquet cuff, and deflating the cuff in order to be aware of and manage any physiologic changes that may occur to the patient.

To ensure patient safety, AORN (2010) urges the perioperative nurse to fully document the following when using a pneumatic tourniquet:

- Identification serial number;
- Calibrations;
- Cuff pressure;
- Skin protection;
- Location of tourniquet cuff;
- Skin integrity under the cuff before and after use;
- Person placing the tourniquet cuff;
- Time of inflation and deflation; and
- Assessment and evaluation of entire extremity.

Surgical Counts

Surgical counts, performed as a patient safety measure in the OR, help to prevent injury to the patient as a result of a retained foreign body. All members of the surgical team can be held liable in litigation for retained foreign bodies and can likewise prevent this occurrence. Surgical counts include the counting of sponges, sharps, and the following instruments:

- Needles;
- Scalpel blades;
- Hypodermic needles;
- Bovie tips;
- Vessel clip bars;
- Vascular inserts;
- Cautery scratch pads;
- Vessel loops;
- Umbilical/hernia tapes; and
- Trocar sealing caps (Rothrock, 2011).

Institutions that follow AORN Standards count sharps and miscellaneous items for all procedures (Rothrock, 2011). Sponges and instruments are counted on procedures where there is a possibility that a sponge or instrument could be retained. Counts are performed before the procedure to establish a baseline, before closure of a cavity within a cavity, before wound closure, at skin closure or end of procedure, and at the time of permanent relief of the scrub person and/or circulating nurse. Once the initial count occurs, no counted item may leave the OR. Items are counted audibly and viewed concurrently by the two individuals who are counting, one of whom should be a registered nurse circulator. When additional items are added to the field, they are also counted and recorded on the "count sheet." Broken items (sharps or instruments) must be accounted for in their entirety. All sponges used during a surgical procedure should be x-ray detectable and should not be cut into pieces or used for dressings. Whenever possible, sharps must be handed to and from the surgeon on an exchange basis using a "neutral zone" or a hands-free technique to prevent injury to the surgical team members at the sterile field. If a discrepancy in the count is identified, the surgical team is responsible for following the hospital's policy, which should include the following steps to locate the missing item:

- Count discrepancy reported to surgeon and surgical team;
- Procedure suspended, if patient's condition permits;
- Manual inspection of the operative site;
- Visual inspection of the area surrounding the surgical field, including floor, kick buckets, and linen and trash receptacles;
- If the patient's condition permits, an intraoperative x-ray should be taken and read before the patient leaves the OR or, if the patient's condition is unstable, an x-ray should be taken as soon as possible;

1. Documentation of all measures taken and outcomes on patient's record;
2. Reporting of incident following organization policy; and
3. Review of incident or near miss for cause, effect, and prevention (AORN, 2010).

Accurate documentation of surgical counts should appear on the patient's perioperative record, including the following items recommended by AORN (2010):

- Types of counts (sponges, sharps, instruments);
- Names and titles of personnel performing the counts;
- Results of surgical item counts;
- Notification of the surgeon;
- Instruments intentionally remaining with the patient or sponges intentionally retained as packing;
- Actions taken if count discrepancies occur;
- Outcome of actions taken; and
- Rationale if counts are not performed or completed as prescribed by policy.

Medications

Many types of medications are used during surgeries, including antibiotics, irrigation solutions, hemostatic agents, local anesthetics, steroids, antispasmodics, and antibacterial agents. *Preoperative antibiotics* are given intravenously within 1 hour of incision time. Cefazolin is the orthopaedic antibiotic of choice; if the patient has a true allergy to penicillin , clindamycin or vancomycin may be substituted (Hall, 2006). Sterile normal saline solution or lactated ringers solution are used for irrigation by bulb syringe or pulse lavage. Antibiotics such as bacitracin, polymixin B, or gentamicin may be added to the irrigation fluids.

Hemostatic agents are used on bone or in soft tissue. Bone wax is processed beeswax that is applied directly to the ends of cut bone to seal the interstices. Thrombin is a topically applied liquid that catalyzes the conversion of fibrinogen to fibrin for clot formation. Avitene is a powdered microfibrillar collagen agent used to aggregate platelets during conversion of prothrombin to thrombin. Gelfoam is an absorbable gelatin sponge that absorbs up to 45 times its weight in blood and fluid. Surgicel is an oxidized cellulose product that absorbs up to 10 times its weight in blood and fluids (Barnett & Strickland, 2007).

Local anesthetics, both short- and long-acting, may be injected subcutaneously in local or monitored anesthesia care (MAC) procedures to anesthetize the skin and underlying tissues. Epinephrine may be added to the local anesthetic to increase the duration of the medication, to cause vasoconstriction, and to decrease bleeding at the surgical site. Traditionally, local anesthetic with epinephrine was not injected into the finger for fear of digital infarction caused by irreversible vasospasm. This theory remains controversial (Lalonde, 2005). Long-acting local anesthetics such as bupivacaine may be injected at the end of surgery to minimize postoperative pain. Steroids may be mixed with a local anesthetic and injected intraarticularly to decrease inflammation and pain.

Antispasmodics may be used during microsurgery to control and/or limit spasm of the vessels. Gauze dressings may be impregnated with *antibacteriostatic* ointments (xeroform dressing) from the manufacturer or may be preapplied before application of the dressing (bacitracin ointment).

Fluid Balance

The anesthesia provider maintains the patient's fluid and electrolyte balance during surgery, including careful monitoring of blood loss. Some anesthesia providers prefer to estimate blood loss by visual inspection of the drapes, suction canisters, and used sponges. In the surgical management of critically ill or elderly orthopaedic patients undergoing complex spine or total hip procedures, trauma patients, or patients with abnormal bleeding or clotting time, the perioperative nurse assists by weighing sponges to calculate a more accurate estimated blood loss (EBL). Using a gram scale, the nurse weighs a clean sponge in a plastic bag and zeroes the scale. Succeeding bloody sponges are weighed (1 gram equals 1 ml of blood loss) and documented as a running total. At specified intervals, the nurse calculates the weight of the sponges, plus the amount of fluid the suction containers, minus the amount of irrigation used, and informs the anesthesia provider (Rothrock, 2011).

With complex surgeries, the surgeon may have ordered intraoperative blood salvage (IBS), more commonly known as "cell saver." "The procedure starts with the surgeon aspirating blood from the surgical field through a suction wand attached to dual-channel tubing; this allows anticoagulant and blood to be mixed as the blood is aspirated. The aspirated blood is collected in a reservoir until there is sufficient blood for processing. The salvaged blood is pumped into the centrifuge bowl, where it is concentrated and then washed with an isotonic electrolyte solution, most often saline. The processed red cell suspension is then pumped from the centrifuge bowl into an infusion bag. Modern cell salvage instruments can process a full reservoir of blood, and provide 225 ml of washed, saline-suspended red cells with a hematocrit of 50 percent or more in approximately three minutes" (Silvergleid, n.d.). The anesthesia provider administers the salvaged blood to the patient in the OR. IBS is often accepted by patients who refuse blood based on religious beliefs (Rothrock, 2011).

Postoperative blood salvage is also used in orthopaedic surgeries such as total hip replacements, total knee replacements, and spine fusions with instrumentation (bloodindex, n.d.). A drain is inserted into the operative site at the end of the surgical procedure, and the tubing is attached to a closed blood recovery system. The system collects, filters, and allows for reinfusion of the autologous blood collected from the operative site. The drainage chamber is marked with the time that the unit was connected and started in the OR; any collected blood must be reinfused to the patient within 6 hours (Stryker *Blood Products*, n.d.).

Depending on the patient's intraoperative condition and hemodynamic status, the anesthesia provider may draw blood samples during surgery to be analyzed for hematocrit, electrolytes, and blood gases. In addition, the patient with a urinary catheter is observed for the amount, color, and character of urine, as well as the patency of the catheter (Barnett & Strickland, 2007).

Implants

Depending on the amount of orthopaedic procedures performed in the particular institution, most ORs have an extensive inventory of implants, including plates and screws (hardware), intramedullary nails and rods, total joint implants, bone cement, and bone grafts. Stock items are selected by surgeon preference, patient population, and implant cost. The inventory is organized according to manufacturers, type of implants, and sizes. Implants may be purchased or stocked on a consignment or loaner basis.

Many different alloys are used in the manufacturing of implants; most frequently used are stainless steel, cobalt-chromium, and titanium-vanadium-aluminum (Rothrock, 2011). Other materials used for implants include ceramic and polyethylene. It is important for the surgical team to have a working knowledge of the general types and sizes of implants that are in the OR's inventory and that may be used. All devices implanted in the patient—including the screws, plates, and any additional hardware—must be of the same metallic composition to prevent galvanic corrosion. Screws and plates should be of the same metal. Screws and plates used for internal fixation must not be reused; abrasions, scratches, or bending from previous use weakens the implant, increasing the chance of corrosion and breakage of the hardware.

Most implants are received from the manufacturer in sterilized packaging. Some plates and screws are received unsterile and are stored until needed. It is important to handle implants with care so that they are not damaged. When sterilizing the implants and instrumentation, it is necessary to follow the manufacturer's instructions.

Strict guidelines are required by the FDA when documenting and tracking implant devices. Many manufacturers enclose pre-printed labels with the implants that may be placed on the patient's permanent record, the operative record, and the implant registry maintained by the OR. Otherwise, the perioperative nurse must record the lot and serial numbers of the implants used, as well as the manufacturer, size, type, and anatomic location of the implants.

Bone Cement

Polymethylmethacrylate (PMMA), or "bone cement," is not really a cement or glue but acts as a grout (Webb & Spender, 2007). This acrylic, cement-like substance is composed of a liquid monomer (methylmethacrylate) and a powder polymer (methylmethacrylatestyrene) that contains 10% barium sulfate to provide radiopacity to the finished product (Rothrock, 2011). PMMA had early applications in dentistry; however, the major breakthrough in the use of PMMA was the work of Sir John Charnley in the 1960s, who used it to secure the acetabular and femoral components of total hip replacement and to transfer loads to bone (Webb & Spencer, 2007).

The liquid and powder components are mixed together in a bowl or syringe/cartridge, using a vacuum device that suctions the acrid fumes of the monomer and prevents excessive exposure to the OR personnel. This exposure may cause irritation of the respiratory tract and eyes, and OR personnel working in these rooms should not wear soft contact lenses. Manufacturers produce bone cement of varying viscosities (low, medium, and high) for different clinical applications. Bone cement goes through three phases (sticky phase, working phase, and hardening phase) until polymerization is complete. Polymerization is an exothermic reaction and produces heat. The anesthesia provider should be alerted before using bone cement. Adverse reactions to the patient from PMMA may include transitory hypotension, cardiac arrest, cerebrovascular accident, pulmonary embolus, thrombophlebitis, and hypersensitivity reaction (Rothrock, 2011).

Antibiotic laden cement (ABLC) has been used for more than 30 years to deliver antibiotics in the treatment of infected total joint arthroplasty (TJA). The antibiotic of choice is added to the powder polymer of the PMMA. Antibiotics used include tobramycin, gentamycin, and vancomycin. The ABLC is mixed using "poor mixing technique" by whipping the mixture to increase the leaching rate of the antibiotic into the joint (Clyburn & Cui, 2007). Commercially premixed ABLCs with gentamycin or tobramycin have been available since 2005 (medcompare, 2005).

Bone Grafts

Bone grafts have various applications in orthopaedic surgery. If a substantial amount of bone must be removed, bone graft may be used to fill the resulting bony cavity to prevent instability. It may also be used to fill bony defects and to promote the union of fractures at the time of open reduction. Bone grafts may also be used in revision joint surgeries if there has been significant resorption of bone around the prosthesis or mechanical destruction of bone when removing the previous implant and bone cement (Rothrock, 2011).

There are two types of bone graft: autograft and allograft. *Autograft* refers to the patient's own bone because it is autogenous in origin. It may be harvested from the iliac crest or from the site of injury. *Allograft* is obtained from a tissue bank and is homogeneous in origin. It is used when the patient lacks sufficient quantity or quality of bone, if a second procedure for harvesting the bone graft is undesirable for the patient, or if a musculoskeletal allograft is needed. Both types of bone graft may be harvested as cortical struts to provide structural strength, or cortical or cancellous bone chips to fill in bony defects.

Tissue banks that comply with guidelines and regulations of the American Association of Tissue Banks (AATB), the FDA, and other state health department regulations use strict processing procedures that ensure quality and safe tissue grafts for transplantation. Packaged grafts are prepared as freeze-dried (lyophilized) or frozen tissue and may be sterilized using gamma irradiation. *Lyophilized musculoskeletal tissue* may be stored at room temperature for up to 3 years. *Frozen musculoskeletal tissue* may be stored at -40 degrees C or colder for 5 years or -20 degrees for temporary storage of up to 6 months (Community Tissue Services, n.d.). Tissue is reconstituted or thawed according to the manufacturer's directions. Usually sterile normal saline or lactated ringers solution is used for reconstitution for a specified amount of time prior to cutting, shaping, or implanting the graft. Documentation must include the type of allograft tissue, name of the tissue bank, identification or access number of the graft, implanting surgeon's name, location of the graft, and expiration date of the graft.

Radiographic Safety

Preoperative radiographic studies are widely used for diagnosing an orthopaedic problem in the patient. During orthopaedic surgery, radiographic intervention in the form of portable x-ray or fluoroscopy is frequently used. Also known as image intensification or C-Arm, fluoroscopy allows the surgical team to view the progression of the surgery in "real time." Fluoroscopy shows reduction of the fracture; reaming of the intermedullary canal; and correct placement of bone plates, screws, and other hardware as the surgery is being performed. Other procedures may only require an x-ray at the end of the procedure.

An x-ray technician operates the radiographic equipment. The perioperative circulating nurse supplies sterile plastic covers to the scrub nurse to drape over the C-Arm or enclose the x-ray cassettes. The circulating nurse also observes movement of the equipment around the sterile field to prevent contamination. Radiation exposure is minimized by time, distance, and shielding. Each member of the surgical team should wear a lead apron and lead thyroid shield for protection from radiation, as well as a radiation monitoring device clipped to the neckline on the outside of the lead apron to monitor the amount of radiation received. The patient should be protected from unnecessary radiation exposure; care should be taken to keep extraneous body parts out of the radiation beam. If possible, protective lead shielding should be placed between the patient and the source of radiation (AORN, 2010). Individuals not at the sterile field should maintain a distance of 6 feet from the radiation source. Lead aprons should be protected from damage by storing in a vertical position. Documentation on the patient's intraoperative record should include the amount of fluoroscopy time used during the procedure (Rothrock, 2011).

Many of today's ORs are equipped with electronic Picture Archiving and Communication Systems (PACS) that are integrated with their computers. These systems enable images captured on x-rays and scans to be stored electronically and viewed on a computer screen, creating a near-filmless process and improved diagnostic methods (NHS Connecting for Health, 2011). Many surgeons who previously used x-ray films to template the surgical site for sizes of implants for joint replacement, fracture treatment, or deformity correction now use computer software to perform these measurements. These computerized aids enable the surgeon to plan ahead for surgery at any computer equipped with these programs and ensures that the correct sized implant is available for the surgery (Voyant Health, 2009).

Dressing and Casting

At the completion of surgery, the scrub nurse cleans the surgical site with sterile water and dries it before applying a dressing. Many orthopaedic surgeries require some type of immobilization device such as a cast, splint, immobilizer, or an abduction pillow during healing. (Also see Chapter 10—Therapeutic Modalities.)

Casts may be either plaster or synthetic. Plaster is less expensive and requires a greater weight of plaster to produce the same strength of synthetic material (weight/strength ratio); this may make the cast too heavy and burdensome. Usually, plaster casts are used as the primary cast after surgery because they are more moldable and are replaced later with a lighter synthetic cast to promote patient mobility (Rothrock, 2011). After the initial dressing is applied, stockinette and soft padding are applied to the extremity before the cast is applied; this protects the skin from thermal injury while the plaster sets and protects the skin from pressure and abrasion afterward.

Splints may be used instead of casting. Because they are not applied circumferentially, they allow for swelling and closer observation of the surgical site. Splints are held in place with elastic bandages.

There are several types of shoulder *immobilizers* used after shoulder surgeries and knee immobilizers or braces used after knee surgeries. An *abduction pillow* is used after a total hip replacement to prevent the patient's leg from adducting or rotating internally, and the hip from flexing, which could result in dislocation of the hip.

Postoperative Care and Evaluation

The postoperative phase of care begins as soon as the surgical procedure concludes, and the patient is transferred to the Post-Anesthesia Care Unit (PACU). Also called Level 1 PACU or Phase 1 PACU, this unit actually serves as a short-term critical care unit and is staffed by specially trained perianesthesia nurses.

In most institutions, the OR circulating nurse calls PACU to give a preliminary status report on the patient's condition before transporting the patient to PACU. This report includes the surgical procedure performed, type of anesthesia provided, any special equipment required (ventilator, T-piece, arterial pressure monitor, etc.), and information specific to the patient's preoperative diagnosis and subsequent outcome related to intraoperative intervention (Rothrock, 2011). Before exiting the OR, the patient is assessed for needs during transport, including bed vs. stretcher, supplemental oxygen, or manual positive-pressure device (Katz, 2008).

The perioperative nurse accompanies the patient and anesthesia provider to PACU, and identifies the patient with the PACU nurse. During the initial assessment, the airway is assessed for patency, humidified oxygen is applied, and respirations are counted. The quality of the patient's breath sounds is determined as pulse oximetry is initiated. The patient is connected to the cardiac monitor to evaluate heart rate and rhythm. Blood pressure is measured with a manual or automatic cuff. If the patient has an arterial line, it is connected to the monitor (Rothrock, 2011).

After the initial assessment of "ABCs" (airway, breathing, and circulation), the PACU nurse receives a comprehensive hand-off report on the status of the patient from the perioperative nurse and anesthesia provider. The 2009 TJC *National Patient Safety Goals* emphasizes "a standardized approach to hand-off communications, including an opportunity to ask and respond to questions" (TJC, 2008, p.12). The American Society of PeriAnesthesia Nurses (ASPAN, 2008) recommends that the hand-off report contain the following elements:

- Relevant preoperative status;
- Anesthesia/sedation technique and agent;
- Length of time anesthesia/sedation administered, time reversal agents given;
- Pain and comfort management interventions and plan;
- Medications administered;
- Type of procedure;
- Estimated fluid/blood loss and replacement;
- Complications occurring during anesthesia course, treatment initiated, response; and
- Emotional status on arrival to the OR or procedure room.

After the hand-off report, the PACU nurse begins a more thorough postanesthesia assessment of the patient, using a head-to-toe or "major body systems" approach, but paying careful attention to the operative procedure performed. Drains are checked for patency, as well as type, color, and amount of body fluids. Dressings, splints, and/or casts are checked for break-through bleeding; any areas of bleeding are outlined with a marker, including the time noticed. Patients are more likely to have medical difficulties as they emerge from anesthesia; therefore, for the first 15 minutes, there is a 1:1 ratio of nurse to patient.

Patients are admitted to PACU after three classes of anesthesia, all of which have been monitored by an anesthesia provider: general anesthesia, regional anesthesia, or monitored anesthesia care. To prevent hypoxemia, all patients recovering from general anesthesia should receive 30%-40% oxygen during their emergence.

Most patients who have had general anesthesia take 15-30 minutes to become fully awake, breathe normally, and be physiologically stable. Vital signs and blood oxygen saturation are recorded every 5 minutes until the patient is awake and stable. Subsequently, vital signs, blood oxygen saturation, level of consciousness, independence of breathing, and ability to make voluntary movements are measured every 15 minutes; the patient's temperature is measure and recorded at least once early in the PACU stay (Katz, 2008). Postoperative patients take time to regain effective muscular control and are regularly assessed to see if they are able to lift their head off the bed and hold it up for 5 seconds.

Postoperative Complications

Respiratory Concerns. A patent airway is the first priority in the care of the postanesthesia patient. Airway obstruction can be caused by the tongue, which is relaxed from the anesthetic agents and muscle relaxants used during surgery. The patient may show signs of snoring, little or no movement of air on auscultation of the lungs, retraction of intercostal muscles, and a decreased oxygen saturation level. Initial nursing actions include stimulating the patient to breathe, positioning the patient on the right side (recovery position), or providing supplemental oxygen. With an unresponsive patient, the nurse may need to open the airway by using the chin tilt or jaw thrust, or insert an oral or nasal airway.

Laryngospasm is a serious PACU complication caused by sudden contraction of the muscles of the larynx. The patient can become hypoxemic quickly; an awake patient will be terrified and need reassurance. Interventions include removing the irritating stimulus, suctioning any secretions, hyperextending the patient's neck, oxygenating the patient, and using positive-pressure ventilation delivered by mask and bag. If symptoms last longer than 1 minute, administration of a muscle relaxant such as succinylcholine is required to relax the muscles of the larynx.

Bronchospasm, a lower airway obstruction, is caused by spasms of the bronchial tubes that can cause complete airway closure. Clinical signs include wheezing, dyspnea, use of accessory muscles, and tachypnea. Bronchospasm may be caused by aspiration, pharyngeal suctioning, and histamine release from an allergic reaction. Treatment includes bronchodilators and steroids for an allergic reaction.

Cardiovascular Concerns. Hypotension is defined as a blood pressure reading that is 20% less than baseline or preoperative blood pressure measurement, and usually indicates hypovolemia (Rothrock, 2011). Clinical signs include a rapid, thready pulse; disorientation; restlessness; oliguria; and cold, pale skin. Initial intervention is the administration of IV fluids at a maximum rate while making a specific diagnosis. Hypovolemia may be caused by hemorrhage, dehydration, or increased positive end-expiratory pressure, medications, general or regional anesthesia, or anaphylaxis.

Hypertension is defined as a 20%-30% increase above baseline blood pressure measurement. Clinical signs and symptoms are the most important indicators of the severity of the hypertension and may include headache, mental status changes, and substernal pain. Causes include end-organ damage, volume overload or pulmonary edema, pain, anxiety, reflex vasoconstriction from hypothermia, hypoxemia, hypercapnia, and viscus distention. Treatment is specific to the cause.

Dysrhythmias seen in PACU are usually unrelated to myocardial injury. Sinus tachycardia (rate >100 beats/min in an adult), sinus bradycardia (rate <60 beats/min in an adult), and premature ventricular contractions (PVCs) are most commonly seen. Treatment of dysrhythmias begins with determining and removing any source of the problem.

Temperature Regulation. Hypothermia is defined as a core body temperature less than 36 degrees C or 96.8 degrees F (ASPAN, 2008). Postoperative hypothermia can prolong recovery time and contribute to postoperative morbidity. Signs and symptoms include shivering, piloerection, and /or cold extremities from peripheral vasoconstriction. Shivering can increase the need for oxygen by 300%-400%, which may cause morbid cardiac incidents and ventricular tachycardia. Other problems seen with hypothermia include hypovolemia, depressed central nervous system (CNS), longer wake-up time, impaired wound healing, surgical site infections, decreased metabolism, and decreased platelet activity (Rothrock, 2011). For hypothermic patients, PACU should initiate the active warming measures listed on Table 5.9.

Table 5.9. Active Warming Measures for Hypothermia
Apply forced air warming system
Apply passive insulation: ■ Warm blankets ■ Socks ■ Head covering ■ Limited skin exposure
Increase ambient room temperature
Warm fluids: Intravenous
Humidify and warm gases: Oxygen
Assess temperature and patient's thermal comfort ■ Every 30 minutes ■ Until normothermia is reached

Data from 2008-2010 Standards of Perianesthesia Nursing Practice *by the American Society of PeriAnesthesia Nurses (ASPAN), 2008, Cherry Hill, NJ: ASPAN.*

Nausea and Vomiting. Postoperative nausea and vomiting (PONV) affect approximately 30% of PACU patients. Risk factors of PONV are female gender, nonsmoker, history of PONV or motion sickness, use of volatile anesthetics, use of nitrous oxide, postoperative use of opioids, duration of surgery, and type of surgery (Rothrock, 2011). Management of patients at high risk for PONV starts with assessment preoperatively and treatment with medication in SDS and the OR.

Pain. "Pain is a subjective experience and may or may not be verbalized" (Rothrock, 2011, p. 280). The guiding principle in pain management is that pain is whatever the patient says it is. All patients should be assessed for pain on admission to PACU and at frequent intervals, using a verbal descriptor rating scale, numeric rating scale, or a visual analogue scale. A common form of opioid-delivery system is patient-controlled analgesia (PCA), which allows the patient to control delivery of analgesia medication by pressing a button. The machine is programmed with the dosage, minimum time between doses, and the maximum dosage that can be administered. Other forms of postoperative pain control include spinal or epidural anesthesia and use of a long-acting local anesthetic at the surgical site at the conclusion of the surgical procedure.

Table 5.10. Modified Aldrete Scoring System

Criterion	Score (Maximum Score: 10)	
Consciousness	Fully awake	2
	Aroused by verbal stimulus	1
	Not aroused by verbal stimulus	0
Breathing	Takes full breaths and can cough	2
	Takes only shallow breaths or has dyspnea	1
	Cannot breath without assistance (apnea)	0
Blood Pressure	Within 20 mm Hg of pre-op value	2
	20- 50 mm Hg different from pre -op value	1
	≥50 mm Hg different from pre-op value	0
Oxygenation	>92% blood oxygen saturation (SpO2) on room air	2
	Needs supplemental O2 to maintain SpO2 >90%	1
	SpO2≥90% on supplemental O2	0
Motor Function	Can move all 4 extremities on request	2
	Can move 2 extremities on request	1
	Cannot move any extremities on request	0

From "The Postanaesthesia Recovery Score Revisited [letter]" by J.A. Aldrete, 1995, Journal of Clinical Anesthesia, *7:89–91. Reprinted with permission.*

PACU Discharge Criteria. Patients stay in PACU until they have become awake and alert with stable vital signs; this recovery normally takes 30-70 minutes. When all signs have returned to preadmission level and have remained there for 30 minutes, the perianesthesia nurse checks to see if the patient meets the discharge criteria on a standardized scale such as the Aldrete Score seen on Table 5.10. When the patient attains the PACU discharge criteria and receives discharge approval from the anesthesiologist, the patient may be admitted to one of several areas, depending on the surgery performed and the patient's response to the surgery: a critical care unit (surgical intensive care unit), an inpatient unit, a 23-hour observation unit (outpatient in a bed), or SDS.

Discharge

The patient is admitted to Same Day Surgery (SDS) for Phase 2 of Recovery with the goal of preparing the patient for discharge to home. The SDS nurse receives a hand-off report from the PACU nurse, then assesses the patient's state of consciousness and takes vital signs. The operative site is assessed, with careful attention to any bleeding, swelling, or discoloration. If the patient has a cast, the extremity is assessed for neurovascular compromise, using the "6 Ps" method as described as described in Table 8.5 in Chapter 8—Orthopaedic Complications. If a problem is noted, the surgeon is notified and correction may include changing the compression wrap, bi-valving (cutting) the cast, or an emergency fasciotomy for compartment syndrome.

The patient should have minimal nausea and vomiting, and be able to tolerate liquids and a light snack such as juice or crackers. When vital signs are stable, the patient is assisted with ambulation and encouraged to urinate. Any surgical pain should be controlled with oral medication; no IV sedation or analgesia should be given within 1 hour prior to discharge. An escort should be present to drive the patient home.

Prescriptions may be emailed or faxed to the patient's pharmacy, or may be given to the patient. Written discharge instructions are reviewed with the patient/ escort, and a copy is given to them. They include specific instructions for activity, diet, medications, bathing, wound care, and follow-up care.

The SDS nurse should emphasize the importance of rest in assisting the healing process and allowing the effects of any anesthetic to decrease. If the surgery involved an extremity, it should be elevated on pillows to decrease swelling and pain. The surgeon may order application of ice to the surgical site to decrease swelling and pain, and place limitations on the amount of ambulation. If assistive devices such as crutches are ordered, the patient will be assessed for the ability to use them. If this was not done preoperatively, a physical therapist may instruct the patient in the proper use before discharge. The patient is advised not to drive, operate machinery, or make important decisions for 24 hours, due to the side effects of the anesthesia and/or pain medication.

The patient may resume a preoperative diet as tolerated but should not drink any alcoholic beverages for at least 24 hours. Preoperative medications are resumed as directed by the surgeon or consulting medical provider. The patient should be encouraged to take pain medication as directed but before the pain is severe. The surgeon gives instructions for when the patient may shower or bathe, when the dressings may be removed, and the type of care for the wound. The patient should be instructed about neurovascular checks; care of splints, cast, or other device; and signs and symptoms of infection. If any complications occur (such as fever, difficulty voiding, persistent pain, nausea, vomiting, headache, or excessive bleeding), the patient should call the surgeon. The patient should schedule an appointment with the surgeon for follow-up care as directed on the discharge instruction sheet. The patient can also expect a follow-up telephone call from the SDS or ambulatory surgery center nurse for postoperative assessment of any complications, to reinforce discharge instructions, and to evaluate care given by the facility.

References

Aldrete, J.A. (1995). The postanaesthesia recovery score revisited [letter]. *Journal of Clinical Anesthesia*, 7, 89–91.

Allen Medical. (2012). *Allen Orthopaedic: Products*. Retrieved January 11, 2012, from http://www.allenmedical.com/product/orthopaedics-products/A-91500.html

American Society of Heating, Refrigerating and Air-Conditioning Engineers, Inc. (ASHRAE). (2010). *ANSI/ASHRAE/ASHE Addendum d to ANSI/ASHERAE/ASHE Standard 170-2008: Ventilation of Health Care Facilities*. Retrieved November 25, 2010, from http://www.fgiguidelines.org/pdfs/ASHRAE170ad_d.pdf

American Society of PeriAnesthesia Nurses (ASPAN). (2008). *2008-2010 Standards of Perianesthesia Nursing Practice*. Cherry Hill, NJ: Author.

Association of periOperative Registered Nurses (AORN). (2010). *Perioperative Standards and Recommended Practices*. Denver: Author.

Association of periOperative Registered Nurses (AORN). (n.d.). *Comprehensive Checklist*. Retrieved January 14, 2012, from http://www.aorn.org/ClinicalPractice/ToolKits/CorrectSiteSurgeryToolKit/Comprehensive_Checklist.aspx

Barnett, S. & Strickland, L. (2007). Perioperative patient care. In National Association of Orthopaedic Nurses, *Core Curriculum for Orthopaedic Nursing* (6th ed, pp. 99-126). Boston: Pearson.

bloodindex. (n.d.). *Autologous Blood Transfusion*. Retrieved October 20, 2010 http://www.bloodindex.org/autologous_blood_transfusion.php

Bratzler, D. (2006, November). The surgical infection prevention and surgical care improvement projects: Promises & pitfalls. *General Surgery News, Supplement to November 2006*. Retrieved January 29, 2011, from http://generalsurgerynews.com/download/037gsnse2006.pdf

Case Western Reserve University School of Medicine. (2010). Study examines relationship between SCIP measures and postoperative infection. *The Medical News*. Retrieved January 30, 2011, from http://www.news-medical.net/news/20100624/Study-examines-relationship-between-SCIP-measures-and-onpostoperative-infection.aspx

Clyburn, T. & Cui, Q. (2007). Antibiotic laden cement: Current state of the art. *AAOS Now, 1:5*. Retrieved December 15, 2010, from http://www.aaos.org/news/bulletin/may07/clinical7.asp

Community Tissue Services. (n.d.). *Processing Tissue Grafts*. Retrieved December 15, 2010, from http://www.communitytissue.org/processing/index.html

Fung, A. (2011). Healthcare: Medical errors cost health care system billions. *National Journal*. Retrieved April 10, 2011, from http://www.nationaljournal.com/healthcare/medical-errors-cost-health-care-system-billions-20110407?mrefid+site_search/

Garner, J. (1985). *Guideline for Prevention of Surgical Wound Infections, 1985*. Retrieved December 5, 2010, from http://wonder.cdc.gov/wonder/prevguid/p0000420/p0000420.asp

Gunn, M. (2009). SCIP expanded normothermia measure to go into effect for all surgical patients in October. *AORN Management Connections, July 2009*. Retrieved March 26, 2011, from http://www.aorn.org/News/Managers/July2009Issue/Normothermia/

Hall, M. (2006), Surgical care improvement project (SCIP) module 1: Infection prevention. *Medscape Orthopaedics, 2006*. Retrieved January 15, 2012, from http://www.medscape.org/viewarticle/531895_print

Katz, M. (2008). *Postanesthesia Care of Adults*. Retrieved October 19, 2010, from http://www.nursingceu.com/courses/249/index_nceu.html

Kim, D.S. (2010). Institutional prescreening for detection and eradication of methicillin-resistant staphylococcus aureus in patients undergoing elective orthopaedic surgery. *Journal of Bone and Joint Surgery, 92*(9), 1820-1826.

Lalonde, D.B. (2005). A multicenter prospective study of 3,110 consecutive cases of elective epinephrine use in the fingers and hand: The Dalhousie Project clinical phase. *The Journal of Hand Surgery, 30*(5), 1061-1067.

Lee, I., Agarwal, R.K., Lee, B.Y., Fishman, N.O., & Umscheid, C.A. (2010). *Systematic review and cost analysis comparing use of chlorhexidine with use of iodine for preoperative skin antisepsis to prevent surgical site infection*. Retrieved March 5, 2011, from http://www.ncbi.nlm.nih.gov/pubmed/20969449

medcompare. (n.d.). *Bone Cement Now Comes Pre-mixed with Antibiotic*. Retrieved December 15, 2010, from http://www.medcompare.com/spotlight.asp?spotlightid=70

Megadyne. (n.d.). *Patient Return Electrodes*. Retrieved December 12, 2010, from http://www.megadyne.com/return_electrodes.php

National Pressure Ulcer Advisory Panel (NPUAP). (2007). *Pressure Ulcer Stages Revised by NPUAP*. Retrieved May 1, 2011, from http://www.npuap.org/pr2.htm

NHS Connecting for Health. (2011). *Picture Archiving and Communications System (PACS)*. Retrieved March 20, 2011, from http://www.connectingforhealth.nhs.uk/systemsandservices/pacs

Rabin, S. & Hopkinson, W. (2011). *Immune Response to Implants*. Retrieved October 9, 2011, from http://emedicine.medscape.com/article/1230696-overview

Rothrock, J. (2011). *Alexander's Care of the Patient in Surgery*. St. Louis: Elsevier Mosby.

Silvergleid, A. (n.d.). *Intraoperative and Postoperative Blood Salvage*. Retrieved April 9, 2011, http://www.uptodate.com/contents/intraoperative-and-postoperative-blood-salvage

Smith, C. (2010). Malignant hyperthermia. *OR Today, 10*(8), 26-33.

Stanton, C. (2010). New rules for humidity in the OR. *AORN Management Connections May 2010*. Retrieved November 25, 2010, from http://www.aorn.org/News/Managers/May2010Issue/HUMIDITY

Stryker. (n.d). *Stryker Flyte*. Retrieved October 9, 2011, from http://www.stryker.com/en-us/products/OREquipmentConnectivity/GeneralMultiSpecialtyEquipment/AccessoriesandDisposables/SterishieldHoods/Flyte/058203

Stryker. (n.d.). *Stryker Blood Products*. Retrieved April 10, 2011, from http://www.stryker.com/en-us/products/OREquipmentConnectivity/GeneralMultiSpecialtyEquipment/BloodProducts/index.htm

Stryker. (n.d.). *Stryker Tourniquet*. Retrieved December 15, 2010, from http://www.stryker.com/en-us/products/OREquipmentConnectivity/GeneralMultiSpecialtyEquipment/Tourniquet/index.htm

The Joint Commission (TJC). (2011). *Facts About Patient Safety*. Retrieved January 15, 2012, from http://www.jointcommission.org/PatientSafety/NationalPatientSafetyGoals/

The Joint Commission Resources. (2012). *National Patient Safety Goals: Hospital*. Retrieved January 11, 2012, from http://www.jcrinc.com/Other-Resources/NPSGHLP12/4021/

U.S. Food and Drug Administration (FDA). (2009). *Questions and Answers About the Steris System 1 Processor for Healthcare Facilities*. Retrieved November 26, 2010, from http://www.fda.gov/MedicalDevices/Safety/AlertsandNotices/ucm192685.htm

Vanac, M. (2010). STERIS settles system 1 dispute with FDA; plans customer rebates. *MedCity News*. Retrieved November 27, 2010, from http://www.medcitynews.com/2010/04/steris-settles-system-1-dispute-with-fda-plans-customer-rebates

Voyant Health. (2009). *TraumaCad*. Retrieved December 14, 2010, from http://www.voyanthealth.com/traumacad.jsp

Webb, J. & Spencer, R. (2007). The role of polymethylmethacrylate bone cement in modern orthopaedic surgery. *Journal of Bone and Joint Surgery*, 89(7), 851-7. Retrieved December 14, 2010, from http://www.totaljoinnts.info/bone_cement_reference.htm

Zimmer. (n.d). *Zimmer A.T.S. 3000 Automatic Tourniquet System*. Retrieved December 15, 2010, from http://www.zimmer.com/z/ctl/op/global/action/1/id/9371/template/MP/prcat/M8/prod/y

Chapter 6

Orthopaedic Effects of Immobility

Elizabeth Turcotte, MSN, RN-BC, ONC

Objectives

- Define immobility.
- Classify causes of immobility that orthopaedic patients might experience.
- Explain potential pathologic outcomes of immobility.
- Identify appropriate nursing interventions for selected diagnoses for immobilized orthopaedic patients.

Immobility affects individuals through varying avenues. A patient may suffer a traumatic event in which a fracture occurs that renders him immobile either temporarily or permanently. A medical condition may also compound immobility in a patient who would otherwise have been mobile. Immobility has a pathophysiologic affect on all systems of a patient's body. This chapter will discuss the impact on each of those systems along with assessment, common therapeutic modalities, and nursing considerations for the care of immobile patient.

Immobility is defined as a state that either prevents or limits movement necessary to complete tasks within the environment. Mobility restriction may be generalized to the entire body or limited to an isolated area or areas. The extent and duration of immobilization contribute to the degree that physiologic body systems are affected. Causes of mobility impairment are varied, classified by either gradual or immediate immobility (see Table 6.1). There are two rationales for the etiology of immobility, as follows:

1. Environmental restriction: This occurs when physical activity is limited due to external forces. Bodily movement is restricted due to either confinement to a specific area (such as when an individual is on bed rest) or application of restrictive devices (such as casts, traction, or other external devices).
2. Physical or cognitive restriction: This occurs when physical activity is limited due to internal forces. Movement is restricted by factors within the person such as pain, impaired or lost motor function, critical illness, and cognitive, social, or emotional instability.

Table 6.1. Causes of Mobility Impairment

Gradual Immobility	Immediate Immobility
Reduced motor skills (secondary to disease process)	Fractures
Cardiovascular disease	Fear of pain
Pain – arthritis/osteoporosis, etc.	Sudden trauma/fall
Ineffective foot care	Stroke
Reduced cognitive function	Heart attack
Depression & anxiety	Change in life style / surroundings
Failing eye sight	Lack of choices
Weight gain / loss – fatigue	Hypostatic pneumonia / chest infections
Respiratory impairment (secondary to chronic diseases)	Urinary tract infections – confusion
Decreased muscle tone	Pressure ulcers – sacral and foot
Neuropathy	Sudden onset of conditions requiring bed rest

Data from "Providing Excellent Service for Those with Mobility Impairment" by M. Chadwick, 2010, Nursing & Residential Care, *12(6), 278-282.*

Integumentary Issues

Overview

Pathophysiology (see Table 6.2). Immobility has a great impact on the human integumentary system. It fosters muscle disuse and decreased circulation in soft tissues. Prolonged pressure on a body area leads to disrupted nerve impulses and decreased circulation, all leading to skin breakdown (Institute for Clinical Systems Improvement [ICSI], 2010). Ultimately, prolonged pressure from immobility may result in dermal pressure ulcers. With the immobile patient, bony pressure points will need attention in an effort to increase prevention of pressure sores. The integument of the occiput, scapula, spinous processes, lower sacrum, coccyx, ischial tuberosities, iliac crests, greater trochanter, patella, tibial tuberosity, fibular head, malleoli, heels, head of humerus, and elbows are all at high risk for pressure sore development when the patient is immobile. This occurrence increases in these areas because the prominences are covered with skin and only a small amount of subcutaneous tissue. The immobile patient is at risk of sustaining prolonged pressures greater than normal over these prominences. Capillary pressures of 30-32 mm Hg (arterial) and 12 mm Hg (venous) may lead to circulatory compromise, deep tissue injury (DTI), and tissue necrosis (Wound, Ostomy, and Continence Nurses Society [WOCN], 2010). An indication that an area of pressure is developing is when redness remains at the site of pressure for greater than 30 minutes after the area has been relieved of pressure (WOCN, 2010).

Table 6.2. Overview of Integumentary Issues

Assessment	■ Assess skin for breakdown and/or erythema every 2 hours ■ Observe for sensory loss at every skin check ■ Review CBC, protein, and albumin levels ■ Monitor for signs of infection
Interventions	■ Identify patients at risk for skin breakdown ■ Turn & reposition at least every 2 hours ■ Keep skin clean and dry ■ Use therapeutic mattresses and treat pressure ulcers ■ Encourage high protein intake and adequate hydration
Summary	■ Increased risk of skin breakdown ■ Increased risk of pressure ulcers

There are several contributing factors that affect the integumentary system of the immobile patient. The first of these factors are sensory and neurological deficits. The immobile patient who suffers from sensory deficits experiences interrupted vasomotor pathways that can be related to shock, spinal shock, and flaccid paraplegia.

Patients with neurological deficits experiencing an impaired level of consciousness may be unaware of the discomfort of prolonged cutaneous pressure and/or may be unable to reposition themselves to relieve that pressure. Impaired blood circulation and edema in the immobile patient should also be considered as risks for compromising the integumentary system in the immobile patient. This could include artherosclerosis and diabetes, causing peripheral arterial occlusion. Venous engorgement related to edema, which effects oxygenation and nutritional support to the tissues, is also included in this category. Tissue ischemia most often occurs in patients with low hemoglobin. Assurance of hemodynamic stability is imperative to counteract this contributing factor.

Nutritional support is of the utmost importance, as it becomes a contributing factor in preserving the health of the integumentary system in immobile patients. During illness or after trauma or surgery, alterations in the body's metabolic demands have implications for maintaining skin integrity. Most of these changes are initiated by the immune system, which, when stimulated, causes the body to undergo a series of physiologic and metabolic changes known as the acute phase response. The liver reacts to the acute phase response by increasing protein uptake, which can be broken down and resynthesized into acute phase proteins or used for energy. The source of this protein is serum albumin, muscles, skin, and the gastrointestinal tract. A decrease in serum albumin will be seen even if nutritional intake is adequate because the body produces proteins in the acute phase instead of albumin (Kline, 2008).

Circulation is affected by hypoabluminemia, which is an imbalance of nitrogen, sulfur, phosphorus, and calcium; therefore, it is critical that these levels be monitored and maintained within normal values. Infection and elevation in body temperature will increase the patient's metabolic rate (as with any healthy individual), which can lead to cellular metabolic deficiencies. Hypothermia in lower extremities of spinal cord patients may promote pressure ulcers. As with any open wound, if an immobile patient sustains an infected pressure ulcer, the patient is at risk for systemic infection.

The body becomes hypermetabolic as the need for energy increases. The demand for glucose increases, although hyperglycemia is a common response to stress and injury. Insulin levels increase, but hyperglycemia often persists due to increased insulin resistance in peripheral tissues. An increase in the breakdown of triglycerides is seen during illness. The fatty acids are used to produce ketones, and the glycerol is used for glucose. There may be a build-up of fats in the blood until the internal hormonal environment returns to normal (Kline, 2008). When an injury or illness renders a patient immobile and at risk for integumentary compromise, there is an increased need for calories and energy. Every nutrient is important to maintain skin integrity and promote the healing process, although some are more important in efficient healing.

Linens and incontinence pads / diapers should be frequently assessed and changed, as trapped moisture in these areas predisposes skin to maceration, breakdown, and subsequent microorganism invasion. Excretory waste and radiation treatment can also damage skin. Other instances of potential skin breakdown can be caused from shearing forces and friction that can result in skin abrasion. The sacrum and heels are most susceptible to the effects of shear (WOCN, 2010). Sensitive skin areas at high risk for skin breakdown are scar tissue, skin grafts, areas of hematoma, and existing dermatologic problems such as dermatitis psoriasis or seborrhea.

Medications can contribute to skin compromise. Anticoagulants and corticosteroids are often responsible for hemorrhage into soft tissue, as well as easy bruising and skin eruptions. Central nervous system depressants decrease a patient's movement during sleep, which in turn increases pressure ulcer development in prone areas. Diuretics can increase loss of fluid in cutaneous and subcutaneous tissue.

Age and trauma are also factors affecting the integumentary system in the immobile patient. Skin loses elasticity as a part of the normal aging process, resulting in degeneration of elastic fibers, reduced thickness, and vascularity of dermis. Loss of adipose tissue and decreased peripheral circulation increase elderly patients' risks for pressure sores, especially when there is prolonged immobility and pressure. While elderly and post-trauma patients present the highest risk for pressure ulcers, compromised children can exhibit the same problems as adults because the effects of immobility on the body possesses the same characteristics.

Assessment

All vulnerable skin surfaces should be assessed every 2 hours, usually during patient repositioning. When noted, assessment of skin breakdown should include location, size of breakdown, presence of sinus tracts, undermining, tunneling, exudates, necrotic tissue, and epithelialization. Pressure ulcers are staged I-IV according to degree of severity or tissue involvement, as follows:

- Stage I is intact skin with nonblanchable redness of a localized area, usually over a bony prominence. Darkly pigmented skin may not have visible blanching; the skin color may differ from the surrounding area.
- Stage II is partial-thickness-loss dermis presenting as a shallow open ulcer with a red pink wound bed without slough, defined as dead tissue that is shed from the wound (Mosby's Medical

Table 6.3. The Braden Scale

SENSORY PERCEPTION Ability to respond meaningfully to pressure related discomfort	**1. Completely Limited** Unresponsive (does not moan, flinch, or grasp) to painful stimuli, due to diminished level of consciousness or sedation OR limited ability to feel pain over most of body.	**2. Very Limited** Responds only to painful stimuli. Cannot communicate discomfort except by moaning or restlessness OR has a sensory impairment that limits the ability to feel pain or discomfort over 1/2 of body.	**3. Slightly Limited** Responds to verbal commands but cannot always communicate discomfort or the need to be turned OR has some sensory impairment which limits ability to feel pain or discomfort in 1 or 2 extremities.	**4. No Impairment** Responds to verbal commands. Has no sensory deficit that would limit ability to feel or voice pain or discomfort.
MOISTURE Degree to which skin is exposed to moisture	**1. Constantly Moist** Skin is kept moist almost constantly by urine, perspiration, etc. Dampness is detected every time patient is moved or turned.	**2. Very Moist** Skin is often, but not always moist. Linen must be changed at least once a shift.	**3. Occasionally Moist** Skin is occasionally moist, requiring an extra linen change approximately once a day.	**4. Rarely Moist** Skin is usually dry, linen only requires changing at routine intervals.
ACTIVITY Degree of physical activity	**1. Bedfast** Confined to bed.	**2. Chairfast** Ability to walk severely limited or non-existent. Cannot bear own weight and/or must be assisted into chair or wheelchair.	**3. Walks Occasionally** Walks occasionally during day, but for very short distances, with or without assistance. Spends majority of each shift in bed/chair.	**4. Walks Frequently** Walks outside room at least twice a day and inside room at least once every 2 hours during waking hours.
MOBILITY Ability to change and control body position	**1. Completely Immobile** Does not make even slight changes in body or extremity position without assistance.	**2. Very Limited** Makes occasional slight changes in body or extremity position but unable to make frequent or significant changes independently.	**3. Slightly Limited** Makes frequent though slight changes in body or extremity position independently.	**4. No Limitation** Makes major and frequent changes in position without assistance.
NUTRITION Usual food intake pattern	**1. Very Poor** Never eats a complete meal. Rarely eats more than 1/3 of any food offered. Eats 2 servings or less of protein (meat or dairy products) per day. Takes fluids poorly. Does not take a liquid dietary supplement OR is NPO and/or maintained on clear liquids or IVs for more than 5 days.	**2. Probably Inadequate** Rarely eats a complete meal and generally eats only about 1/2 of any food offered. Protein intake includes only 3 servings of meat or dairy products per day. Occasionally will take a dietary supplement OR receives less than optimum amount of liquid diet or tube feeding.	**3. Adequate** Eats over half of most meals. Eats a total of 4 servings of protein (meat, dairy products) per day. Occasionally will refuse a meal, but will usually take a supplement when offered OR is on a tube feeding or TPN regimen which probably meets most of nutritional needs.	**4. Excellent** Eats most of every meal. Never refuses a meal. Usually eats a total of 4 or more servings of meat and dairy products. Occasionally eats between meals. Does not require supplementation.
FRICTION & SHEAR Force applied to patients skin when repositioned	**1. Problem** Requires moderate to maximum assistance in moving. Complete lifting without sliding against sheets is impossible. Frequently slides down in bed or chair, requiring frequent repositioning with maximum assistance. Spasticity, contractures or agitation leads to almost constant friction.	**2. Potential Problem** Moves feebly or requires minimum assistance. During a move skin probably slides to some extent against sheets, chair, restraints or other devices. Maintains relatively good position in chair or bed most of the time but occasionally slides down.	**3. No Apparent Problem** Moves in bed and in chair independently and has sufficient muscle strength to lift up completely during move. Maintains good position in bed or chair	

From "The Braden Scale" by B. Braden & N. Bergstrom, 1988, KCI Licensing, Inc. Reproduced with permission.

Dictionary, 2009). Stage II may also present as an intact or open / ruptured serum-filled blister.

- Stage III is a full-thickness skin loss. Subcutaneous fat may be visible but bone, tendon, or muscle is not exposed. Slough may be present but does not obscure the depth of tissue loss. Stage III may include undermining and tunneling.
- Stage IV ulcers are classified as full-thickness skin loss with exposed bone, tendon or muscle. Slough or eschar, defined as a scab or dry crust that results from trauma, such as a thermal or chemical burn, infection, or excoriating skin disease (Mosby's Medical Dictionary, 2009), may be present on some parts of the wound bed. Stage IV often includes undermining and tunneling.

Unstageable ulcers are full-thickness tissue loss in which the bed of the ulcer is covered by slough (yellow, tan, gray, brown, or black) in the wound bed. Wounds can also be classified as suspected deep tissue injury and unstageable. Suspected deep tissue injury (DTI) is visualized as a purple or maroon localized area of discolored intact skin or a blood-filled blister due to damage of underlying soft tissue from pressure and / or shear. The area may be preceded by tissue that is painful, firm, mushy, feels fluid-filled ("boggy") warmer, or cooler as compared to adjacent tissue.

The most common tool used to assess the patient's level of risk for development of pressure ulcers is the Braden Scale (See Table 6.3). A lower Braden Scale score indicates a lower level of functioning and, therefore, a higher level of risk for pressure ulcer development. A score of 18 or higher, for instance, would indicate that the patient is at low risk, with no need for treatment at this time.

The National Pressure Ulcer Advisory Panel (NPUAP) recommends the assessing for the following as part of a Wound Assessment Checklist:

- Location
- Size
- Dressing used
- Stage
- Pressure redistribution
- Nutritional assessment
- Drainage (amount, color, odor)
- Viable tissue in wound
- Undermining/tunneling (NPUAP, 2007).

Common Therapeutic Modalities

The below interventions for integumentary concerns derivate from treatment guideline recommendations developed by WOCN (http://www.wocn.org/) and ICSI (http://www.icsi.org/). They address the following areas: assessment, prevention, treatment, infection management, documentation, and education and quality improvement by way of communication.

Pressure Ulcer Risk Assessment. Risk assessment should be performed in both the outpatient and the inpatient settings. For outpatient considerations, a set of yes-or-no questions should be used. ICSI (2010) recommends a list of questions that should be considered to assess patient risk for impaired skin integrity when entering an outpatient setting (see Table 6.4)

Table 6.4. Outpatient Ulcer Prevention Assessment Questions

Adult Assessment Is the patient:	Pediatric Assessment Is the baby or child:
Bed- or wheelchair-bound?	Moving extremities or body inappropriately for developmental age?
Immobile for more than 2 hours?	Responding to discomfort inappropriately for developmental age?
Incontinent?	Demonstrating inadequate tissue perfusion?
In poor nutritional status?	
Hemodynamic-stable?	
Presenting with co-morbidities?	

Data from Pressure Ulcer Prevention and Treatment. Health Care Protocol *by the Institute for Clinical Systems Improvement (ICSI), 2010. Bloomington, MN: ICSI.*

For inpatient considerations, ICSI (2010) recommends the use of a standardized risk assessment tool such as the Braden Scale (see Table 6.3) or Braden Q (a modified Braden Scale for integumentary risk assessment for those patients under the age of 16). Risk assessment should be completed on a regularly scheduled basis, based upon individual organizational policy or when there is significant change in the patient's condition.

Pressure Ulcer Prevention. Factors that increase risk for integumentary breakdown in the immobilized patient are advanced age, incontinence, sources of friction and shear, diminished nutritional status, an altered level of consciousness, and presence of immobilization devices such as braces and casts. Prevention of integumentary breakdown with the presence of the above can be assisted through minimizing or eliminating friction and shear, minimizing pressure by off-loading or removing the pressure on the skin over bony prominences, managing moisture, and maintaining adequate nutrition and hydration. Pressure ulcer prevention should be provided for all patients at risk of pressure ulcer development and those individuals who have a pressure ulcer (WOCN, 2010).

Prevention and treatment via off-loading: Immobility is the most significant risk factor for pressure ulcer development. Passive range of motion (ROM) should be considered for prevention and treatment of joint contractures, and a referral should be sought for physical therapy (PT)/rehabilitation services to provide additional treatment. Patients who have any degree of immobility should be closely monitored for pressure ulcer development.

Patients have greater intensity of pressure over the bony prominences such as their sacrum and ischial tuberosities when sitting in a chair because there is less distribution of weight. Along with increased weight over the bony prominences, there is a tendency for the body to slide in a downward motion, causing shearing and destruction of the soft tissue over the bony prominences. A sitting position includes sitting in bed with head elevation greater than 30 degrees, as well as in a recliner or wheelchair. When in this position, it is important for the patient to shift weight every 15 minutes if he/she is able to do so independently. If unable to shift weight independently, his/her position should be changed by care providers on an hourly basis. It is important to utilize chair cushions when the patient is upright and placing pressure on the ischial tuberosities to help distribute the weight evenly (ICSI, 2010).

While in bed, the patient should not be positioned on a pressure ulcer or other bony prominences. The head of the bed should remain low to prevent shearing and to increase support of the body surface area. Pressure-reducing mattresses should be used to prevent initial or further development of pressure ulcers in the immobile patient (McInnes, Dumville, Jammali-Blasi & Bell-Syer, 2011). Care providers should take into consideration the height and weight of the patient when selecting a pressure-relieving surface. Static support surfaces such as high-density foam, air, or liquid mattress overlays are recommended if the patient can assume various positions. Otherwise, dynamic support should be used such as air-fluidized, oscillating, or kinetic beds. If the patient has stage III or stage IV ulcers on numerous sites, a low-air-loss mattress should be used. The number of linen layers between the support surface and the patient should be limited (McInnes et al., 2011). Free-float the patient's heels by elevating calves on pillows and keeping heels free of all surfaces. At minimum, nursing should turn the patient every 2 hours.

Pressure Ulcer Treatment. Debridement, the removal of necrotic tissue or contaminated foreign matter, is typically used in the treatment of stage III and stage IV ulcers.. The goals of debridement are to remove obstructive tissue, decrease risk of infection, accelerate wound healing, and prevent further complications by reducing tissue destruction. ICSI (2010) categorizes five types of debridement as sharp debridement, chemical/enzymatic debridement, mechanical debridement, autolytic debridement, and bio-surgical debridement. Surgical debridement is preferred for larger or deeper pressure ulcers to quickly shift the state of the wound from burdened, infected or chronic healing to free to proliferate in a normal or acute healing process.

Operative repair can be required for stage III or stage IV pressure ulcers. Operative procedures are dependent upon degree of ulcer and characteristics. They include direct closure, skin grafting, skin flaps, musculocutaneous flaps, and free flaps. Vigilant postoperative care includes proper positioning to ensure adequate perfusion and provision of nutrition to enhance healing.

Adjunct therapies can augment the healing process for pressure ulcers in any phase of wound healing, as long as the standard of care is implemented at the same time. Biophysical agents or modalities such as electrical stimulation, induced electrical stimulation, photo therapy (i.e. infrared and ultraviolet), negative pressure wound therapy, hyperbaric oxygen, and noncontact/nonthermal ultrasound all add energy to the wound bed to enhance the healing process, especially in the compromised tissues of immobilized patients. Biological applications are products that donate physiological constituents in wound healing to the wound bed. They can donate extracellular matrices, cells of repair, cellular communicators, and growth factors. They take the form of gels and sheets placed in the wound bed that is prepared free of necrosis and bacterial bioburden. Categories are platelet gels, platelet-derived growth factor therapy, biological skin substitutes, and extracellular matrix sheets. Should a biological application be desired to treat an ulcer, a wound specialist should select the type of application.

Infection Management. Wound healing is optimized and risk of infection is reduced when all necrotic tissue, exudates, metabolic wastes, and residue of wound care products are removed from the wound. Routine wound cleansing is used for both necrotic and clean wounds. The goals of wound cleansing are to remove nonviable tissue, bacteria, and bacterial toxins from the wound surface; protect the healing wound; and facilitate wound assessment by optimizing visualization of the wound bed. The general points of wound cleansing are to clean the wound initially and at each dressing change; use universal precautions to reduce the risk of cross-contamination; and minimize mechanical force when cleansing ulcers with gauze, cloth, or sponges.

All chronic wounds—including pressure—ulcers have bacteria. The clinician needs to determine if the bacterial load in the wound is balanced or has critical colonization or infection. Because bacteria reside in nonviable tissue, debridement of this tissue and wound cleansing are important to reduce bacteria and avoid adverse outcomes such as sepsis.

Wound Documentation. Documentation of factors that increase risk for integumentary breakdown in the immobilized patient using a validated risk assessment tool. Should the patient be at risk for integumentary breakdown, documentation should also include prevention measures put into place. These prevention measures should include minimizing or eliminating friction and shear, minimizing pressure (off-loading), managing moisture, supporting surfaces, maintaining adequate nutrition/hydration, and educating patient/caregivers (ICSI, 2012).

Skin inspection should be documented on assessment and reassessment. It should include notation of alteration in skin moisture, texture, tugor, temperature, color, or consistency. Wound description/staging documentation should occur when the wound is identified, with dressing changes, and prior to any transition to another health care facility (ICSI, 2012). According to the ICSI (2012), accurate documentation of wound assessment should consider the following list:

- Anatomic location of the wound(s);
- Size and shape of the wound(s);
- Staging (if the wound is a pressure ulcer);
- Characteristics of exudates;
- Appearance of surrounding skin;
- Presence and degree of tunneling in the wound;
- Appearance of wound margins;
- Appearance of wound edges;
- Any smell noted from the wound; and
- Characteristics of tissue in wound base.

Integumentary Education and Quality Improvement. Education and continued quality improvement efforts should always be included in the therapeutic modalities of integumentary assessment and treatment in the immobile patient. Prevention, treatment, and education regarding pressure ulcers should all be part of continuous quality improvement monitoring. The patient and/or caregivers should know how to assess for integumentary issues. If the patient is at risk, an educational program for the patient and family or caregivers should be implemented regarding prevention and treatment course.

Nursing Considerations

Nursing Diagnoses. Nursing diagnoses for this condition are expanded upon in the Appendix.

- Skin integrity, impaired.
- Skin integrity, risk for impairment.

Nursing Interventions. The desired outcome is that skin remains intact. The key to maintaining skin integrity is to prevent complications. Interventions to support the above nursing diagnosis will be relative to inspection and positioning of patient, moisture management, pressure ulcer risk assessment, and prevention of complications. Skin should be inspected minimally (once every shift or as needed) with specific attention to bony prominences. Findings should be documented. The care provider should turn and reposition the patient often, inspecting skin over bony prominences with each turn. Positioning should be done assuring that body weight is evenly distributed, body alignment is neutral with as little stress as possible on bony prominences, and circulation is not compromised by supportive devices such as pillows, splints, casts, or drains. Oscillating beds and alternating pressure mattresses or overlays should be considered in skin integrity maintenance in the immobile patient. Linens should be dry and wrinkle-free. An individualized toileting schedule can help minimize incontinence. Risk assessment for development of pressure ulcers should be performed with the patient, including assessment of level of sensory perception, consciousness, and cognitive functioning. Other considerations for pressure ulcer risk assessment with the immobile patient are an assessment of prolonged exposure to moisture, activity and mobility level, nutritional status, and potential for friction or shear.

If a pressure ulcer is present on an immobile patient, the pressure should be removed immediately from the site of the ulcer by repositioning the patient, bridging, support devices, and specialized beds. A high-protein diet should be encouraged to compensate for the loss of serum protein that will occur with most pressure ulcers. Carbohydrates and fats should also be included in the diet of a patient with a pressure ulcer, as these nutrients maximize mobilization of proteins. Debridement could be considered depending on the severity of the ulcer, as should wound cleansing, dressings, and infection control. Frequent monitoring and assessment of the treatments that are implemented is essential.

Respiratory Issues

Overview

Pathophysiology (see Table 6.5). The immobile patient may experience change in metabolic processes. After 3 weeks of bed rest, muscles work less efficiently and require 26% less oxygen (Behroozi, Brennan & Bellantonio, 2007). Cells that require less oxygen produce less carbon dioxide, causing respirations to become slower and shallower in accordance with less demand for oxygen.

Decreased respiratory movement can be caused by a variety of factors. A supine position causes the diaphragm to move toward the head, resulting in decreased thoracic size. Quiet breathing while supine is due to abdominal muscle involvement rather than rib cage involvement as when upright. Decreased

Table 6.5. Respiratory Overview	
Assessment	■ Assess respirations every 2 hours ■ Check movements of the chest wall ■ Check capillary refill every 2-4 hours ■ Observe for any respiratory difficulties
Interventions	■ Change patient's position every 2 hours ■ Encourage coughing and deep breathing every 2 hours ■ Encourage incentive spirometry, if ordered ■ Maintain a patent airway ■ Encourage fluids to keep secretions thin (100-200mL every 2 hours) if not contraindicated (goal of 3L/day)
Summary	■ Decreased respiratory muscle tone ■ Decreased depth of respiration ■ Decreased rate of respiration ■ Pooling of secretions ■ Impaired gas exchange

compliance of the immobile patient's thoracic cage can be related to the aging process. Diminished strength in respiratory muscles with age can possibly be related to a decrease in elastic recoil, an increase in residual volume, and changes in the skeletal muscle (Behroozi et al., 2007). Because the immobile patient is either chair- or bed-bound, the counter-resistance of these diminish chest expansion. Abdominal distention due to an accumulation of feces, flatus, and fluid also compromises the respiratory status in these patients. The immobile patient may also be on narcotics, sedatives, or other medications affecting the central nervous system, which can impact the rate and depth of respirations. Decreased respiratory movement in the immobile patient can also be attributed to a decrease in overall muscle strength.

Position changes (from upright to supine) also change lung volume. With the immobile patient, thoracic size decreases, which contributes to the development of atelectasis. Loss of the lung's elastic recoil in the elderly also increases the risk of atelectasis in this population. Tissues become hypoxic due to changes in respiratory movement and retention of secretions. Increased carbon dioxide in the blood is due to the failure to expel it from the body, a condition known as hypercapnia. This condition initially stimulates respirations by way of the respiratory centers in the pons and medulla, but this stimulus gradually weakens and carbon dioxide narcosis occurs. A decrease in oxygen concentration initially stimulates respirations by way of the aortic and carotid bodies, but this stimulus also becomes depressed. Finally, increased arterial and venous concentrations of carbon dioxide (as carbonic acid) create respiratory acidosis that can lead to respiratory or cardiac failure or death in the immobile patient (Dean, 2008).

Other existing medical problems and age also play a role in respiratory compromise in the immobile patient. Children exhibit respiratory problems related to immobility similar to that of adults. Age-related changes in lung tissue can be accelerated by such things as frequent pulmonary infections, smoking, and exposure to second-hand smoke and environmental pollutants.

Assessment

Proper patient positioning is essential for an appropriate respiratory assessment (Massey & Meredith, 2010). This may not always be easy to accomplish in the immobile patient. Respiratory assessment should include inspection of the thoracic region, both anterior and posterior, including abnormalities of respiration, posture, respiratory muscles, and neck veins (Massey & Meredith, 2010). Palpation should also be part of the respiratory assessment to confirm, reject, or supplement information previously gathered through inspection such as the expansion and symmetry of chest rise and fall and the presence of crepitus. Capillary refill should be assessed on upper and lower extremities. Finally, auscultation of the patient's lungs to assure appropriate movement of air (with or without evidenced abnormal lung sounds) should be documented and reported.

Common Therapeutic Modalities

The immobilized patient will need care focused on the prevention and treatment of atelectasis and secretion stasis. A hyperinflation device such as an incentive spirometer should be utilized, along with coughing, deep breathing, and repositioning every 1-2 hours to promote this prevention and treatment.

Nursing Considerations

Nursing Diagnoses. Nursing diagnoses for this condition are expanded upon in the Appendix.

- Airway clearance, ineffective.
- Breathing pattern, ineffective.

Nursing Interventions. Ideally, the patient will be afebrile without respiratory congestion or distress. In an effort to maintain breathing patterns and airway clearance in the immobile patient, assessment, mobilization, and promotion of respiratory exercises are recommended interventions. Lungs should be auscultated every 8 hours. The patient should use an incentive spirometer at least 10 times every hour until the patient's activity increases and they are out of bed. The patient should be encouraged to turn, breathe deeply, and cough every 2 hours. Early ambulation should be promoted as tolerated in the immobile individual to positively affect respiratory status. Consider placing the patient on a rotational bed if unable to mobilize as readily as desired (Goldhill, Imhoff, McLean, & Waldmann, 2007). Oral fluids should be encouraged to decrease the viscosity of secretions produced. An increase in oral fluid intake will also assist in avoiding dehydration. Anticholinergic drugs should be avoided whenever possible as they cause bronchodilation and decreased respiratory tract secretions. Promote regular bowel and bladder practices per the patient's usual schedule, and assess for abdominal distention every 8 hours. Oversedation should be avoided in the immobile patient, as this will further compromise respiratory status.

Cardiovascular Issues

Overview

Pathophysiology (see Table 6.6). Orthostatic intolerance (or postural hypotension) is defined as a drop in blood pressure of more than 20mm Hg or a rise in heart rate to more than 120bpm, or 20bpm above the patient's resting heart rate in those patients receiving beta blocker therapy (Romero-Ortuno, Cogan, Foran, Kenny, & Wei Fan, 2011). This is the most common sign of cardiac deconditioning related to bed rest (Behroozi, et al., 2007). Immediately after standing, there is gravitationally mediated redistribution of the blood volume and a pooling of blood in the lower extremities. This reduces the ability to maintain cerebral perfusion. If the immobile patient is in a horizontal position, this can result in a short-term increase in circulating blood volume by causing extracellular fluid to shift to the venous system. This increased venous volume increases the blood pressure (BP), cardiac output (CO), stroke volume (SV), and heart rate (HR) (Freeman et al., 2011).

As the patient on bed rest assumes an upright position, HR increases as a result of decreased SV and CO. Similar to remaining on bed rest, maintaining an upright position can also lead to cardiovascular compromise in the immobile patient. Syncope, tachycardia, nausea, and diaphoresis may all be experienced by the immobile patient when remaining in an upright position. Health status, including existing major trauma and/or disease processes, contribute to how well a patient's cardiovascular system will tolerate major position changes. The elderly patient is at higher risk for postural hypotension, as are patients who take medications that dispose them to hypotension. Patients with coronary artery disease (CAD) may experience angina when getting out of bed due to reduced diastolic filling, causing an inadequate coronary blood supply (Freeman et al., 2011).

Incidence of thrombus formation is thought to increase with duration of bed rest, although the risk of thrombosis drops dramatically after 3-4 months of immobilization in the spinal cord injured patients (McKinney, 2011). Bed rest results in compression of veins, promoting venous stasis in these patients. Loss of normal muscle contraction will also occur if the patient is immobilized by casting or bed rest. Decreased contractions of the lower extremity muscles contribute to venous pooling. Venous pooling and dehydration, which often accompany immobility, cause blood to become more viscous and contribute to thrombus formation. External pressure on veins restricts circulation and may also damage vein walls, thus placing the patient at a greater risk for the formation of a deep vein thrombus (DVT). Thrombi development may lead to thrombophlebitis or thromboembolism in these cases (Oschman & Kuhn, 2010).

The Valsalva maneuver is applied when a patient uses the upper extremities and trunk to move in bed. When this movement occurs, the thorax becomes fixed when the patient holds their breath. The breath is forced against the glottis, and the intrathoracic pressure rises ad interferes with the entry of venous blood into the large veins. When the patient releases their breath, a surge of blood is delivered to the heart, causing tachycardia and changes in systolic blood pressure. Cardiac arrest may result in these cases if the heart is not at an optimal level of function. A case report by Tawashy, Eng, Krassioukov, Miller, and Sproule (2010) revealed that arterial oxygen concentration was lower after bed rest, resulting in reduced oxygen delivery due to a reduction in hemoglobin and a down-regulation of the oxygen transport system that follows bed rest.

Table 6.6. Overview of Cardiovascular Concerns

Assessment	■ Measure blood pressure ■ Check peripheral and apical pulses ■ Check temperature of extremities ■ Check for edema ■ Measure circumference of calves and thighs ■ Check for Homan's sign
Interventions	■ Mobilize patient as soon as possible with orders ■ Dangle at bedside first ■ Discourage Valsalva maneuver ■ Active and passive ROM ■ Leg and ankle exercises ■ Intermittent compression stockings / devices ■ Low-dose heparin therapy or other anticoagulant therapy ■ Encourage fluids
Summary	■ Increase in cardiac workload ■ Increased risk of orthostatic hypotension ■ Increased risk of venous thrombosis

Exercise in an upright position or use of a sequential compression device that reduces venous pooling and simulates standing may prevent or reduce a decline in VO2 max (also known as maximal oxygen consumption, maximal oxygen uptake, peak oxygen uptake, or maximal aerobic capacity). Immobility or the total interruption of activity is associated with reduced arterial dispensability. Daily activities are essential for maintaining arterial mechanical properties. The degree of deconditioning syndrome that can occur with patients on bed rest can be minimized by the duration and intensity of certain isotonic exercises (a contracting muscle shortening against a constant load) and isokinetic exercises (performed with a specialized apparatus that provides variable resistance to a movement, so that no matter how much effort is exerted, the movement takes place at a constant speed) (Gay, Hamilton, Heiskell, & Sparks, 2009). Examples of isotonic exercises include utilization of free weights or resistance bands, while an isokinetic exercise example would be the use of a stationary bike.

Assessment

In an effort to assure proper cardiac assessment, prior patient cardiac history should first be obtained and reviewed. Current vital signs should be taken and documented, as well as any cardiac symptoms that the patient may be experiencing. According to Scott & MacInnes (2006), assessment data that reflects the patient's cardiac status would include:

- Chest pain
- Dyspnea
- Edema
- Palpitations
- Poor peripheral circulation
- Syncope
- Vital signs

Common Therapeutic Modalities

Hemodynamic function must be monitored with the immobilized patient. Elastic support and/or sequential compression devices should be applied to lower extremities. PT should be involved in the patient's care for active and passive extremity exercise, unless contraindicated by other existing conditions. Change of position should be considered to stimulate the autonomic nervous system such as elevating the head of the bed or placing the patient in reverse Trendelenburg, in which the head is low and the body and legs are on an inclined plane. Reverse Trendelenburg is sometimes used in pelvic surgery to displace the abdominal organs upward, out of the pelvis, or to increase the blood flow to the brain in hypotension and shock (Mosby's Medical Dictionary, 2009). The physician may consider fluid-challenging a patient who is hypovolemic.

Nursing Considerations

Nursing Diagnoses. Nursing diagnoses for this condition are expanded upon in the Appendix.

- Fluid volume, deficient; Fluid volume, risk for deficient.
- Fluid volume, excess; Fluid volume, risk for excess.
- Tissue perfusion: peripheral, ineffective.

Nursing Interventions. The desired outcome is that patient experiences no evidence of venous thrombus formation or pulmonary embolus. The patient's fluid balance is maintained, and there is an absence of acute orthostatic hypotension. Maintaining the cardiovascular status of an immobile patient begins with assessment of vital signs. This should occur at a minimum of every 8 hours. Orthostatic blood pressure readings should be taken and recorded prior to ambulation as needed, every morning if possible. When vital signs are assessed and recorded, the patient can also be assessed for thrombophlebitis. Fluid volume changes that increase the risk of orthostatic hypotension should be taken into consideration such as diuresis, diaphoresis, and vasodilator therapy. Active and passive ROM should be performed, as well as isometric and isotonic exercises such as ankle dorsi/plantar flexion and ankle rotation. Self-care practices should be promoted in the immobile patient to assist with cardiovascular status. Immobile patients should don elastic support hose and/or sequential compression devices to the lower extremities. Assist the patient to change positions frequently to alter intravascular pressure, stimulate neural reflexes of blood vessels, and help prevent hypotension. When changing positions, alternate from horizontal to nearly vertical by raising the head of the bed, reverse Trendelenburg, or by sitting a patient up in a chair unless contraindicated. While the patient is immobile, static and dynamic exercises should be stressed to limit the degree of deconditioning that the patient experiences that ultimately affects cardiovascular health. When the patient is moving or defecating, they should be encouraged to exhale rather than holding their breath. All actions performed with the patient should be done with the intent of avoiding patient fatigue.

Musculoskeletal Issues

Overview

Pathophysiology (See Table 6.7). Muscles generally experience disuse atrophy secondary to decreased muscle load and activity (Behroozi et al., 2007). Skeletal muscle fiber size, diameter and the number of capillaries are all decreased in disuse atrophy. Immobility decreases muscle load, activity, and protein synthesis and also increases protein breakdown, resulting in muscle disuse atrophy.

Decreased muscle mass and strength are due to a loss as a result of inactivity.

Table 6.7. Overview of Musculoskeletal Concerns

Assessment	■ Muscle tone ■ Muscle mass ■ Contractures ■ ROM ■ Urine and blood for calcium levels
Interventions	■ ROM ■ Turning ■ Exercises and assisted ambulation ■ Crutch walking ■ Wheelchair and adaptive devices
Summary	■ Decreased muscle size, tone and strength ■ Decreased joint mobility and flexibility ■ Decreased endurance ■ Decreased stability ■ Increased bone demineralization ■ Increased risk of contracture formation

Tension of one third of the maximal capacity is required to maintain a muscle's mass. Muscle contraction of 20%-30% of maximal strength is required to maintain muscles strength. The number of contractions during immobilization is the overall determinant of muscle loss. Immobilized muscles lose about 5% of their original strength per day (Puthucheary, Montgomery, Moxham, Harridge, & Hart, 2010). This varies with degree of immobility. Muscles immobilized by casting decrease linearly, with the greatest change in muscle occurring during week 1 of immobilization. Immobilization for 1-2 months can cause a decrease of muscle size by one half. Immobilization longer than 4 months can cause degeneration of nerve fibers to the degree that full recovery of muscle function is unlikely.

When muscle is immobilized in shortened positions, specific changes are exhibited. The muscle becomes contracted, fibrous tissue eventually replaces this muscle, and the normal function is lost. The muscle experiences a decrease in weight. Muscle immobilized in a shortened position atrophies more rapidly than muscles that are held in the stretched position.

Pre-immobilization of muscle mass presents possible prognosis for the postimmobilization state of the muscle. Poor muscle mass will probably worsen, and good muscle mass will recover at a better rate. Age, gender, and duration are contributing factors to postimmobilization muscle state (Dean, 2008). The length of stretch at which muscle was immobilized will have effect on outcomes, as will the type of muscle and muscle fiber. Fever and trauma cause an increase in metabolic needs, which results in a rapid decline in muscle strength and endurance by accelerating protein catabolism.

Disuse osteoporosis generally occurs with loss of bone matrix and bone mineralization in the immobilized patient. Loss of bone matrix is due to the decrease of longitudinal stress on long bones of the legs. Osteoblasts form the osseous matrix of bone and require the stress of mobility and weight-bearing. With prolonged bed rest, osteoclasts break down bone faster than osteoclasts can build it. Bone density is decreased as a result. Thirty percent of bone loss must be present to be visualized by x-ray. Complications can include fractures, renal calculi, calcium depletion, and increased secretion of phosphorous and nitrogen. Disuse osteoporosis is believed to be self-limiting. A balance between bone formation and resorption is regained when bone mass has been reduced to a critical level. Disuse accelerates bone resorption, especially of cancellous bone, and the bone becomes atrophic and fragile. Osteocytes embedded in the bone matrix respond to the mechanical load and changes of bone metabolism. Contributing factors to disuse osteoporosis are poor premobility degree of bone density, cessation of menses, pre-existing metabolic, endocrine, and hormonal imbalances, and certain medications and medical conditions such as poor nutritional status, disordered vasoregulation, hypercortisolism (either therapeutic or stress-related), alterations in gonadal function, and other endocrine disorders. Because disuse osteoporosis is most visible in cancellous bone, it can be seen in metaphysis and epiphysis, with first signs being in the epiphyseal and subchondral area, commonly distal to fracture sites. An increased prevalence of this is seen in the paralyzed patient (Jiang, Dai, & Liang, 2006).

In immobile children, bone becomes osteopenic from disuse and lack of stress across the osseous tissue. The process is accelerated with neuromuscular diseases and osteogenesis imperfecta. Gradual return to activity is important. Treatment may be modified to avoid the vicious cycle of increase fragility followed by recurrent immobilizing device (Day, 2004). Osteoporosis in the elderly, augmented by immobility, places the patient at greater risk for stress fractures. The cycle of increased fragility, followed by recurrent fracture upon removal of immobilizing device, may occur with the elderly patient.

Hypercalcemia occurs when the kidneys fail to excrete enough calcium. Immobility causes negative bone calcium due to the mobilization of calcium from bone. Calcium loss in the immobile patient is probably due to the lack of longitudinal pressure on weight-bearing bones rather than to inactivity. Calcium loss most frequently occurs in adolescent males who are physically active and in an active bone growth phase just prior to incidence of immobilization. The predisposing factor is rapid bone turnover prior to injury. Adults with Paget's disease and primary hyperthyroidism are also at risk. Symptoms include headache, nausea, lethargy, weakness, neurological compromise, and a decreased glomerular filtration rate. Anorexia, nausea, and vomiting can all lead to dehydration, at which point the kidneys cannot excrete enough calcium. Calcium levels normalize 5 weeks after resuming full activity. Crystalluria or ureteral stones are seldom found in these cases. Calcium depletion in the elderly, with low bone mass prior to injury, presents an increased risk of fracture. Even short-term immobilization can be detrimental.

Joints generally experience alterations in synovial fluid with intraarticular degeneration, shortening of ligaments and tendons, and connective tissues changes resulting in some degree of joint contracture or decreased joint mobility, as a result of immobility. A superficial layer of cartilage nourished by synovial fluid clings to cartilage. Joint motion promotes an interchange of fluid between surface layers of articular cartilage and synovial fluid. Immobility prevents fluid diffusion into and out of cartilage, in addition to compression and distention of cartilage. Cartilage, extracellular fluid, and nutrition stagnate, and degenerative changes become permanent.

Contracture of joint capsule and periarticular muscle also presents itself in the immobile patient (Clavet, Hébert, Fergusson, Doucette, & Trudel, 2011). The joint capsule thickens, and the synovia become hyperemic, resulting in fibro-fatty proliferation of connective tissue in the joint space. Inside the joint cavity, connective tissue becomes abundant and causes adhesions that in turn limit joint motion. The increased density of the connective tissue around the joint is due to failure to keep the latticework of tissue stretched open. Normal flexion and extension of the muscles aid in keeping this latticework open. Muscles bridging the immobilized joint shorten. This process is cyclic: with more contracture, there is more guarding of the joint and subsequently less movement, which results in further contracture. A contracture occurs when there is lack of full passive ROM of the joint due to abnormalities with the joint, muscle, or soft tissue. Aging causes tissues to become stiffer, thereby decreasing joint mobility and increasing the risk of contracture in the elderly. The reverse is true for joints that have increased mobility or instability of the joint related to lax ligaments. Stretching of the muscle or decreased muscle tone causes laxity. Joints are held together in alignment by ligaments pulled tight by muscle tension. A joint not maintained in proper alignment may become unstable and painful.

Assessment

When assessing the musculoskeletal system of the immobile patient, the priority consideration is the nature of the immobility. Inspect for overall body build, posture, and gait. Inspect and palpate joints for swelling, deformity, masses, movement, tenderness, and crepitation. Inspect and palpate muscles for size, symmetry, tone, and strength. Assess the patient's pain level at rest. From here, the nurse can assess active and passive ROM of all capable joints and, if possible, the weight-bearing abilities of the patient to determine degree of immobility.

Common Therapeutic Modalities

To maintain bone mass, the intake of Vitamin D and minerals should be optimized. For the immobile patient, PT for muscle strengthening will promote maintenance of muscle mass and joint ROM. Splints or other support will maintain functional alignment and maintain joint mobility.

Nursing Considerations

Nursing Diagnoses. Nursing diagnoses for this condition are expanded upon in the Appendix.

- Disuse syndrome, risk for.
- Mobility: physical, impaired.

Nursing Interventions. The immobilized patient should exhibit no evidence of joint stiffness, joint contracture, joint laxity, or fracture, and should maintain muscle tone and strength. In an effort to prevent and maintain the above musculoskeletal outcomes for the immobilized patient, assessment of baseline should first occur and be documented. Assess active and passive ROM every 8 hours, including ROM against resistance in all affected and adjacent joints. Mobilize the patient as feasible, with weight-bearing and activity as prescribed. Regardless of mobility status, patient should change positions minimally every 2 hours. Isotonic exercise should be performed. This is also known as dynamic or static exercise, where the muscle is moved beyond its normal level of activity to restore muscle bulk and strength. Isometric exercises should be used if the joint is inflamed. Progressive resistive exercises should be used. Throughout the exercise regimen, the patient should be educated on the importance of exercise. Maintain proper body alignment at all times, paying special attention to joint support to prevent contractures. If one limb is affected and the other is not, encourage use of the unaffected limb as much as possible. A foot support should be considered for the prevention of foot drop. Hands should be supported in a position of function. If able, the patient should ambulate as much as possible. A whirlpool or warm bath may be used during exercise, if appropriate, to promote comfort and decrease joint stiffness. Finally, the family and caretakers of the patient should be encouraged to participate in the patient's exercise and activity plans.

Neurosensory Issues

Overview

Pathophysiology (see Table 6.8). Peripheral nerves do not degenerate with disuse but can be damaged by pressure or disruption of blood supply. Improper positioning of casts or restraints can put undue pressure on nerves and blood vessels. Frequent sites of nerve compression are the peroneal and radial nerves. Pressure can cause pain in the immobile patient, leading to sensory changes (such as tingling and then numbness) if the patient is not repositioned. Other changes that can occur when immobility affects the neurosensory system of a patient are sensation awareness, vision problems, poor pain perception, and impaired coordination.

Table 6.8. Overview of Neurosensory Issues

Assessment	■ Mental status and level of consciousness ■ Cerebellar function: posture, gait, balance ■ Reflexes ■ Contractures ■ Urine and blood for calcium levels
Interventions	■ Maintain body temperature ■ Monitor electrolyte levels ■ Maintain fluid and nutritional intake ■ Consult dietary
Summary	■ Decrease in peripheral nerve function ■ Increase in pain ■ Change in sensation ■ Change in vision ■ Change in perception / coordination

Assessment

The nurse should be diligent to assess mental and thought status, along with the patient's level of consciousness, general appearance, and behavior. As the patient tolerates, cerebellar function should be assessed, including posture, gait, balance, and coordination. Motor and sensory function can be determined through muscle size and tone, strength, abnormal or involuntary movements, light touch, superficial pain, temperature, vibration, and position sense. Deep tendon, superficial, and pathologic reflexes should be considered when assessing the immobile patient. The immobile patient should be assessed for contractures. Labs should include urine and blood levels of calcium.

Common Therapeutic Modalities

Patient should be positioned for protection of desensitized areas. Neurosensory function should be assessed every 4 hours in the immobilized patient. Reorient patient frequently as needed.

Nursing Considerations

Nursing Diagnoses. Nursing diagnoses for this condition are expanded upon in the Appendix.

- Body temperature, risk for imbalance.
- Fluid volume, deficient.
- Peripheral neurovascular dysfunction, risk for.
- Thermoregulation, ineffective.

Nursing Interventions. The desired outcome is to maintain the patient's body temperature within normal limits, as well as fluid and electrolyte balance. Body temperature should be monitored and documented every 8 hours. When in bed, lightweight bed clothing and bed coverings should be used to allow for loss of body heat by radiation. Daily fluid and nutritional intake and output should be maintained. Monitor serum electrolyte values. Consultation with a dietician, when appropriate, should be considered, as the immobile patient will benefit from a well-balanced diet with adequate nutritive intake.

Metabolic/Gastrointestinal Issues

Overview

Pathophysiology (see Table 6.9). The immobile patient experiences a decrease in metabolic rate related to decreased energy requirement of cells. This causes an imbalance in the metabolic processes of the body. A negative nitrogen balance due to atrophy of muscle begins between day 6-10 of immobilization. Anabolic processes decrease and catabolic processes increase with nitrogen excreted in the urine. Loss of nitrogen exceeds nitrogen intake, resulting in insufficient protein needed for muscle building and wound healing. Decreased nutritional intake is a contributing factor of this in the immobilized patient, which often leads to a decreased metabolic rate and a negative nitrogen balance associated with catabolism and a high calcium level. Individuals in negative nitrogen balance may feel sluggish, be anorexic, have a poor appetite for protein, and become malnourished (Dean, 2008).

Thermoregulation of the immobile patient should also be taken into consideration. Body temperature can be elevated due to prevention of loss of body heat by way of conduction and radiation in relation to restrictive bed coverings. To lower body temperature, the blood vessels dilate and the person perspires, contributing to a loss of sodium, potassium, and chloride (Dean, 2008).

Endocrine imbalances also occur in the immobile patient. Supine position fosters the production of adrenocortical hormones. Glucocorticoids affect fat, carbohydrate, and protein metabolism. Mineralocorticoids affect electrolyte imbalances such as sodium, potassium, and chloride.

Table 6.9. Overview of Metabolic / Gastrointestinal Issues

Assessment	■ Check bowel sounds every shift ■ Check bowel movement frequency with patient ■ Check intake and output every 8 hours ■ Check percent of meals taken—assess appetite ■ Assess protein and albumin levels in the labs
Interventions	■ Record appetite at each meal—% eaten ■ Record intake every 8 hours and compare to output ■ Be sure to include patient's likes and dislikes ■ Observe for diarrhea ■ Daily weights ■ Monitor daily labs for protein, albumin, and WBC ■ Monitor urine for protein ■ Check muscle mass and strength
Summary	■ Disturbance in appetite ■ Altered protein metabolism ■ Altered digestion and utilization of nutrients ■ Decreased peristalsis resulting in constipation, poor defecation reflex, and an inability to expel flatus

Activity of the pancreas declines, as does the patient's ability to tolerate glucose, as the patient's insulin tolerance is increased (Dean, 2008). Endogenous insulin loses its ability to lower serum glucose as the patient's insulin tolerance is increased (Dean, 2008). These effects are often seen within 3 days of immobility.

When a patient is immobile, less energy is expended. Gastrointestinal functions of ingestion, digestion, and elimination are all affected; however, the alterations in ingestion and elimination are the most prominent. Taking ingestion into consideration, negative nitrogen balance occurs 6-10 days after immobilization from increased catabolic activity related to muscle atrophy. Prolonged negative nitrogen balance stimulates anorexia and decreased intake of nutrients. A high-protein diet is required for the patient who is rendered immobile, coupled with a need to meet basal metabolic requirements. Because the stress of immobility stimulates the parasympathetic nerves, dyspepsia, gastroparesis, distention, anorexia, diarrhea, or constipation may develop. GI elimination is also affected by immobility (Dean, 2008). Abdominal muscles, the diaphragm, and levatorani muscles all experience atrophy and contribute to the difficulty with defecation. Lack of exercise promotes general muscle weakness. Inactivity slows the movement of feces into ascending colon and sigmoid. Suppression of defecation may lead to complete absence of defecation sensation, and constipation may result. Positioning assumed during the use of a bedpan while recumbent is not conducive to defecation. Fecal impactions and fecalomas may develop after feces have been retained for a long period. The patient will experience passage of liquid stool around the impaction as a symptom. Cardiovascular accidents, hemorrhoids, ulcers, rectal prolapse, and a heart block may occur as a person strains to pass the impacted stool. Mechanical bowel obstruction may be due to fecal impaction, accompanied by abdominal distention, dehydration, and fluid and electrolyte imbalance. Dyspnea is related to abdominal distention, interfering with movement of the diaphragm.

Assessment

Appetite and caloric intake should be assessed in the immobile patient. Pain and irritability can be a sign of constipation, and diarrhea can result from impaction. Auscultation of bowel sounds and abdomen palpation should be assessed each shift and as needed with changes. Bowel patterns should be documented and reviewed shift to shift and with care providers. Nurses should also assess intake and output amounts throughout each shift, as well as the percentage of meals that the patient has consumed. Protein and albumin levels should be considered with lab review.

Common Therapeutic Modalities

In an effort to assure that metabolic needs are being met, vital signs and serum electrolytes should be monitored. The key to treating most patients with constipation is correction of dietary deficiencies, so a consideration should be taken in obtaining a dietary consult. A proper diet for the immobilized patient would include high protein and an adequate fluid intake in an effort to maintain the changing metabolic needs of the body.

A prophylactic high-fiber diet should be considered for the immobile patient, coupled with increased fluid intake and stool softeners as needed. The immobile patient is at a high risk for constipation, and this is stressed even more when opioid analgesic therapy is added to the patient's medication regimen. Should the immobile patient suffer a bowel obstruction, the goal is conservative treatment. This would include maintaining an NPO status, administering intravenous fluids, utilizing nasogastric suction (to rest the bowel), administering an enema, inserting a rectal tube, and obtaining x-rays to assess progress of the decompression of distended colon. Should the conservative treatment modalities be ineffective, surgical intervention may be necessary.

Nursing Considerations

Nursing Diagnoses. Nursing diagnoses for this condition are expanded upon in the Appendix.

- Constipation, risk for.
- Nutrition, imbalanced: risk for less than body requirements.
- Nutrition, imbalanced: risk for more than body requirements.

Nursing Interventions. The immobile patient will ideally experience a positive or neutral nitrogen balance and maintain weight, without incidence of constipation or bowel obstruction. To reach these desired outcomes, diet should consist of small, well-balanced meals that are high in carbohydrates and moderate in protein. A daily bowel program should be reviewed with the patient in an effort to provide adequate timing and privacy. High fiber should also be promoted in the diet of an immobilized patient. Fluid intake should be at a minimum of 3 liters per day. Stool softeners and laxative can be provided as needed. Bowel sounds should be assessed and documented at a minimum of every 8 hours. While bowel sounds are being auscultated, the abdomen can also be assessed for distention. Should a fecal impaction be present, it should be assessed and removed digitally as needed.

Genitourinary Issues

Overview

Pathophysiology (see Table 6.10). Immobilization in the supine position is not conducive to optimal function of the genitourinary system. In the supine position, urine must be passed to the ureters against gravity. Because peristalsis may not be strong enough to overcome gravity, the renal pelvis may not empty completely into the ureters. Decreased muscle tone as a result of immobility may compromise the patient's ability to empty the bladder. Urinary stasis may precipitate renal calculi or infection. Excessive stretching of the bladder may also prevent the sensation to void. With bladder distention, overflow may occur. Males with prostate hypertrophy may experience an exacerbation of symptom when immobile.

Table 6.10. Overview of Genitourinary Issues

Assessment	■ Monitor intake and output every shift ■ Monitor vital signs every 4 hours ■ Monitor WBC count daily for sign of infection ■ Assess urine for color, odor, clarity, and amount every shift
Interventions	■ Encourage fluids ■ Measure and monitor each void ■ Encourage patient to drink fluids such as cranberry juice effort to keep urine acidic
Summary	■ Increased urinary stasis ■ Increased risk of urinary calculi ■ Increased risk of urinary tract infection ■ Decreased bladder muscle tone ■ Decreased urinary output

Assessment

Careful attention should be taken to monitor, document, and report intake and output every shift. Vital signs should be taken every 4 hours. A WBC count should be drawn daily to monitor the patient for signs and symptoms of infection, and the patient's urine should be assessed for color, odor, clarity, and amount throughout each shift.

Common Therapeutic Modalities

Fluid challenges and/or PO or SC cholinergic agents may be indicated if the immobile patient produces little to no urine. In the event that renal calculi form, they may need to be removed by surgical techniques if the patient's body is unable to pass the stone voluntarily. Antibiotics should be considered if a urinary tract infection develops in the immobile patient.

Nursing Considerations

Nursing Diagnoses. Nursing diagnoses for this condition are expanded upon in the Appendix.

- Urinary elimination, impaired.

Nursing Interventions. In an effort to maintain the desired balance of intake and output, daily assessment, monitoring, and documenting occur with the patient. Frequency and amount of urination will be part of the output aspect of monitoring. Utilize a bladder scanner as necessary to monitor for bladder distension and urine retention. If the patient is unable to void, consulting with the primary care provider regarding cholinergic medication or placement of an indwelling catheter. Fluids should be strongly encouraged; the immobile patient requires 3 liters a day of fluid unless contraindicated. Also notable with intake is that the intake of acidifying juices may be helpful to prevent renal calcium calculi. As with all other interventions, repositioning in bed, ambulating, and frequent turning will assist with the urinary functions of the body. Patient should be educated on the cause and prevention of calculi formation at this time.

Psychosocial / Mental Status

Overview

Pathophysiology (see Table 6.11). Immobility affects patients differently at different ages. Pediatric, adult, and elderly patients will all have special care considerations in working through psychosocial issues when immobile.

Table 6.11. Overview of Psychosocial / Mental Status

Assessment	■ Assess emotional state ■ Observe for changes in behavior
Interventions	■ Attempt to determine causes of behavior changes ■ Document and report changes
Summary	■ Increased stress and anxiety ■ Feelings of isolation and boredom ■ Potential developmental delays in children ■ Increased potential for depression and cognitive changes in the adult

Immobile Children. Forced inactivity in the form of immobility deprives a child of the means to deal with stress. Sensory deprivation in children leads to feelings of isolation, boredom, and being forgotten. When children experience prolonged sensory deprivation, behavioral changes are noted such as greater-than-normal anxiety, restlessness, difficulty problem-solving, inability to concentrate, egocentrism, and sluggish intellectual and psychomotor functions (Judd & Wright, 2008). Sensory and perceptual deprivation may lead to developmental delays in the immobile child. In children, physical activity is an instrument for communication and a means of learning. Learning, motivation, drives, expectancies, and emotions are all affected by immobility. Play is necessary for a child to cope successfully with hospitalization. When children are able to see the reason for restraint, such as a cast or an IV, they are less likely to be resistant than when the reason is less obvious (Judd & Wright, 2008).

Immobile Adults. As with children, adults' physical activity is an instrument for communication and a means of learning. As such, learning, motivation, drives, expectancies, and emotions are all negatively impacted by immobility. An individual's roles and activities are altered with immobility, leading to depression, noncompliance, and confusion. Perceptual behaviors are altered due to the patient's decreased interaction with the environment. Interaction with the environment is essential for ego identity formation, and this is limited under these circumstances.

Immobile Elderly. The elderly immobilized individual may exhibit anxiety, fear, depression, and rapid mood swings. The elderly patient may express difficulty concentrating, noncompliant behavior, and somatic complaints in the realm of cognitive changes secondary to immobility. Perceptions may change, and they may daydream, hallucinate, or lose sense of time.

Assessment

Assess and document mood and behavioral changes. Report abnormal findings. Engage the patient in conversation and interaction with others (family, friends, staff, other patients), and assess patient's ability to interact with others.

Common Therapeutic Modalities

Assess the patient's environmental sensory stimulation as needed. In an effort to maintain normalcy for the patient, duplicate normal prehospital routine as much as possible such as timing of meals, medications, and activities of daily living (ADLs). Assure that appropriate referrals are made. Institute play therapy for the immobilized child. Encourage and provide socialization with peers, and change the environment as much as possible. Place the patient in a specialty chair, or wheel the bed into the hallway or outside of the hospital. Allow for personalization of the environment. Encourage family to bring in pictures, own clothes, and food from home.

Nursing Considerations

Nursing Diagnoses. Nursing diagnoses for this condition are expanded upon in the Appendix.

- Diversional activity, deficient.
- Social interaction, impaired.

Nursing Interventions. The immobile patient will ideally maintain interaction with significant others and the environment. In an effort to move forward with interventions, a baseline state of orientation and cognition is needed. Visits by friends, family, and significant others are strongly encouraged. The patient should be mobilized as much as possible. Group activities should be sought out to maintain the patient's social interaction. Positive reinforcement to the patient about progress in care and learning self-care procedures assist the patient's positive outlook. If the patient has hearing aids, glasses, or other assistive devices that they normally use, assure that these items are available to them to enhance self-care. Reorient the patient as needed, and provide a clock and a calendar to assist with orientation. The care environment should be as normal as possible and to the patient's liking. Such things in the environment as lighting and activity should be taken into consideration. The patient should be encouraged to continue communication with family, friends, coworkers, and the like. Problem-solving should be performed as part of the care plan, with the patient involved in selecting appropriate coping mechanisms. Consider an occupational therapy (OT) consult as needed. Consider palliative care consult if status of immobility is permanent. Diversional activities should be encouraged such as crafts, reading, music according to the patient's preferences, and play therapy should be considered for the immobilized child. At all points of care planning, the patient, family, and significant other should be involved with the process.

General Home Care Considerations

When preparing to send the immobilized patient home, special considerations should be made regarding specialized equipment and caregiver needs (Oliveira, Campos, Padilha, Pereira, & Sousa, 2011).

Home Care Equipment. Special hospital beds to promote optimal positioning of the patient should be considered for the home environment. Assistive devices such as slide boards, lifts, and overbed trapezes will help the patient – as well as the caregiver – to foster safety in the environment for the immobile patient. If the patient is able to be out of bed to a chair, a wheelchair should be considered as well. A commode or bedpan should be accessible by the patient or the caregiver to promote safe and proper toileting schedules.

Caregiver Considerations. To prevent unnecessary personal injury, the caregiver of the immobilized patient will need to learn safe body mechanics for him- or herself when moving or repositioning the patient. Resources should be made available to the caregiver regarding support groups, meal delivery services, and home health agencies (Oliveira et al., 2011). It is also important to ensure that the caregiver is educated on and able to recognize any signs in the patient of complications due to immobility, as well as how to deal with these complications.

References

Behroozi, S., Brennan, M., & Bellantonio, S. (2007). Recognizing common problems in hospitalized older adults. *Family Practice Recertification, 29*(8) 39-45.

Braden, B. & Bergstrom, N. (1988). Braden Scale. KCI Licensing, Inc.

Chadwick, M. (2010). Providing excellent service for those with mobility impairment. *Nursing & Residential Care, 12*(6), 278-282.

Clavet, H., Hébert, P., Fergusson, D., Doucette, S. & Trudel, G. (2011). Joint contractures in the intensive care unit: Association with resource utilization and ambulatory status at discharge. *Disability & Rehabilitation, 33*(2), 105-112.

Day, H. (2004). Preventing bone fractures in immobile children. *Pediatric Nursing, 16*(2), 31-33.

Dean, E. (2008). Mobilizing patients in the ICU: Evidence and principles of practice. *Acute Care Perspectives, 17*(1) 2-9, 23.

Enguidanos, S., Kogan, A., Keefe, B., Geron, S. & Katz, L. (2011). Patient centered approach to building problem solving skills among older primary care patients: Problems identified and resolved. *Journal of Gernontologic Social Work, 54*(3), 276-291.

Freeman, R., Wieling, W., Axelrod, F., Benditt, D., Benarroch, E., Biaggioni, I.… Gert van Dijk, J. (2011). Consensus statement on the definition of orthostatic hypotension, neurally mediated syncope and the postural tachycardia syndrome. Retrieved 9, 2012, from http://web.ebscohost.com.ezp.waldenulibrary.org/ehost/pdfviewer/pdfviewer?sid=9c86aaab-ef43-4e5c-8d53-81eb54dc7c15%40sessionmgr12&vid=20&hid=14

Gay, V., Hamilton, R., Heiskell, S., & Sparks, A. (2009). Influence of bedrest or ambulation in the clinical treatment of acute deep vein thrombosis on patient outcomes: A review and synthesis of the literature. *MEDSURG Nursing, 18*(5), 293-299.

Goldhill, D., Imhoff, M., McLean, B. & Waldmann, C. (2007). Rotational bed therapy to prevent and treat respiratory complications: A review and meta-analysis. *American Journal of Critical Care, 16*(1), 50-62.

Guidelines for Staging of Pressure Ulcers. (2007) *National Pressure Ulcer Advisory Panel (NPUAP)* Retrieved from http://www.npuap.org/resources/educational-and-clinical-resources/npuap-pressure-ulcer-stagescategories/.

Institute for Clinical Systems Improvement (ICSI). (2012). *Pressure ulcer prevention and treatment: Health care protocol* (3rd ed.). Bloomington, MN: ICSI.

Jiang, S., Dai, L. & Liang, L. (2006).Osteoporosis after spinal cord injury. *Osteoporosis International, 17*(2), 180-192.

Judd, J. & Wright, E. (2008). Benchmarks for children's orthopaedic nursing. *Pediatric Nursing, 20*(5), 34-36.

Kline, D.A. (2008). Healing from the inside out. *Today's Dietician, 10*(7), 12.

Massey, D. & Meredith, T. (2010). Respiratory assessment 1: Why do it and how to do it? *British Journal of Cardiac Nursing, 5*(11), 537-541.

McInnes, E., Dumville, J., Jammali-Blasi, A. & Bell-Syer, S. (2011). Support surfaces for treating pressure ulcers. *Cochrane Database of Systematic Reviews, 7*(12). doi:10.1002/146511858.CD009490

McKinney, D. (2011). Prevention of thromboembolism in spinal cord injury. *Medscape Reference.* Retrieved from http://emedicine.medscape.com/article/322897-overview#aw2aab6b5

Mosby's Medical Dictionary (8th ed.). (2009). St. Louis, MO: Elsevier, Mosby, Inc.

Oliveira, M., Campos, M., Padilha, J., Pereira, F. & Sousa, P. (2011). Exploring the family caregiving phenomenon in nursing documentation. *Online Journal of Nursing Informatics, 15*(1).

Oschman, A. & Kuhn, R.J. (2010). Pharmacology update. Venous thromboembolism in the pediatric patient. *Orthopedics, 33*(3), 180-184.

Puthucheary, Z., Montgomery, H., Moxham, J., Harridge, S., & Hart, N. (2010). Structure to function: Muscle failure in critically ill patients. *The Journal Of Physiology, 588*(23), 4641-4648.

Romero-Ortuno, R., Cogan, L., Foran, T., Kenny, R. & Wei Fan, C. (2011). Continuous noninvasive orthostatic blood pressure measurements and their relationship with orthostatic intolerance, falls, and frailty in older people. *Journal of the American Geriatrics Society, 59*(4), 655-665.

Scott, C. & MacInnes, J. (2006). Cardiac patient assessment: Putting the patient first. *British Journal of Nursing, 15*(9), 502-508.

Tawashy, A., Eng, J., Krassioukov, A., Miller, W. & Sproule, S. (2010). Aerobic exercise during early rehabilitation for cervical spinal cord injury. *Physical Therapy, 90*(3), 427-437.

Wound, Ostomy, and Continence Nurses Society (WOCN). (2010). *Guidelines for Prevention and Management of Pressure Ulcers.* Mount Laurel, NJ: WOCN.

Chapter 7
Orthopaedic Pain

Donna M. Barker, APRN, ANP-BC, ONC, RN-C & Patti A. Murray, DNP, RN-C

Objectives

- Differentiate types of pain.
- Identify key components of a comprehensive pain assessment.
- Identify appropriate pain assessment tools for different populations.
- Describe common pain myths and their correlation related to pain management.
- Explain the difference between opioid tolerance, dependence and addiction.
- Identify appropriate pain relief interventions for selected groups of patients

The Institute of Medicine (2011) estimates that chronic pain affects 116 million American adults – more than the combined total affected by heart disease, cancer, and diabetes. Aside from its health implications, pain has significant financial effects: Americans annually spend as much as $635 billion on chronic pain (Gaskin & Richard, 2012) and $849 billion on bone and joint health (American Academy of Orthopaedic Surgeons, 2011). In addition, the economic ramifications of uncontrolled pain can be seen in the millions of Americans missing work and the subsequent substantial loss in businesses' productivity. The annual corporate loss due to poorly controlled pain could exceed $100 billion (American Medical Association [AMA], 2010).

The consumption of health care resources used to evaluate, diagnose, and treat patients in pain, including both prescription and nonprescription treatments, have exploded in the past several years. With the continued aging of the U.S. population, there will be more people living with diseases affecting bones and joints than ever before. The prevalence of doctor-diagnosed arthritis, for example, is expected to increase in the coming decades. By 2030, the Centers for Disease Control and Prevention (2010) conservatively estimate that 67 million (or 25% of) adults ages 18 and older will have doctor-diagnosed arthritis, compared with today's 50 million sufferers, and that two thirds of these will be women.

It is anticipated that the number of joint replacement surgeries will explode as the "Baby Boomer" generation experiences arthritis, fails conservative management, and seeks surgical interventions to manage pain and preserve their quality of life. The aging workforce will place increasingly more challenges and demands on our health care system, as people delaying retirement will be forced to obtain care to remain competetive in the workplace.

Orthopaedic issues such as arthritis of hips and knees, diseases of the spine, trauma, and oncologic involvement will further drain the system. As technology and medical advances continue to grow, more of those with a disease process involving joints will look to the orthopaedic team to keep them active and maintaining a productive lifestyle. This will require health care providers and patients to possess greater knowledge of pain management to ensure adequate and timely diagnosis and treatment of these painful orthopaedic conditions.

Definitions of Pain

The International Association for the Study of Pain defines pain as "an unpleasant sensory and emotional experience associated with actual or potential tissue damage or described in terms of such damage" (Merskey & Bogduk, 1994, p. 209-214). This definition emphasizes that, because pain is physical and emotional in its presentation, both of these dimensions must be included in the evaluation of pain. The patient's report of pain is often validated through both radiographic testing and laboratory results; however, describing pain only in terms of damage can be limiting. The absence of disease or the amount of damage represented on computed axial tomography (CAT) or magnetic resonance imaging (MRI) is not always representative of the pain reported by the patient. An example would be the pain associated with nerve compression: the amount of pain from a "pinched nerve" cannot be seen on any x-ray film.

To date, there is no definitive test or instrument that identifies the presence of pain or accurately measures the degree to which the patient is experiencing pain. The commonality of all definitions of pain is that they have been created in an attempt to speak to the subjective, multidimensional, diverse nature of the specific pain and the individual patient experiencing it. There is no universally accepted definition that encompasses all pain for all people. McCaffery (1968) provided the classic definition of pain, that still stands today, as "whatever the experiencing person says it is, existing whenever the experiencing person says it does" (p. 95). Patient expression and subjectivity to direct his or her care speaks to the fact that pain is a personal experience and that each person will have an individual response to a painful experience. That response is based on multiple factors, including previous experience with pain, age, gender, culture, and social mores. Health care providers get the most accurate assessment of pain or discomfort from the patient experiencing it.

Physical effects of pain include multisystem involvement. These physical sequale of uncontrolled pain ultimately contribute to a potential for increased mortality and morbidity in the orthopaedic patient. The endocrine effects of uncontrolled pain produce an increased stress response from multiple hormones that result in a weakening of the immune response. Coupled with impaired pulmonary function due to inability to effectively cough and deep-breathe, this response may lead to atelectasis that predisposes the patient to a pulmonary infection or even pneumonia (Pasero & Portenoy, 2011). The pain-stress response causes the pituitary gland to release vasopressin, antidiuretic hormone (ADH), and other hormones and enzymes, which results in the retention of sodium and water and subsequent urinary retention. Wound healing is also compromised in the patient with uncontrolled pain.

Early mobilization and ambulation, in addition to adequate pain management, will modulate the fluid shift and muscle spasm in the postoperative patient. Immobility due to uncontrolled pain makes the necessary tasks of getting out of bed difficult, predisposing the patient to skin breakdown and potential for deep vein thrombosis (DVT). In the orthopaedic population, delay in mobilization leads to poor postoperative rehabilitation and potential development of chronic pain syndromes (Ballantyne, 2002).

Psychological or emotional effects of pain can be related to lack of control and the subsequent effects of that pain. Uncontrolled pain often elicits fear and anxiety. When pain lacks a physiologic diagnosis and no longer has the same meaning for the patient or family, the patient's fear may progress and launch a negative cycle. Depression may develop, related to multiple losses due to the feeling of hopelessness and perceived suffering of chronic pain. Quality of life is impaired, as performing activities of daily living (ADLs) becomes difficult and reliance on family or strangers takes its toll on relationships.

The heath care provider acts as a support system and patient advocate, providing adequate education for patients and their families/caregivers to help everyone involved in the care to fully understand the disease trajectory, treatment options, and therapy goals. Education may help to minimize the potential development of the negative impact of pain such as chronic pain syndromes and associated maladaptive behaviors.

The consequences of uncontrolled pain can have long-lasting ramifications. These potential effects can and should be prevented whenever possible by preemptive management. When they cannot be prevented, a team of trained and educated health care professionals who possess knowledge of pain management treatments should attempt to manage and modulate the course of pain.

Typical Pain Process

The neuroscience of the pain experience is broken down into neurophysiologic steps or sequences, beginning with the pain insult. Simply put, there is a pain insult, and a chemical soup develops. The chemical soup allows for the conversion of the physical incident of pain to change into a traveling electrical pain experience. The pain chemical event travels up the spinal cord to the brain, where it is processed and interpreted, then back down the opposite side of the spinal cord to the pain site. This circuit happens within moments as the body responds to the painful event. There are four steps of the normal physiologic pain process (Polomano, Dunwoody, Krenzischek, & Rathmell, 2008).

Transduction is the initial step, in which the patient experiences the sensation of pain, or nociception. The stimuli may be from the release of chemicals due to mechanical injury such as surgery, chemical injury as chemotherapy, or thermal injury such as heat. Whenever there is damage, chemical mediators are released from the injured tissues that cause a cascade of chemical reactions as seen with acute pain. The chemicals histamine, serotonin, prostaglandins bradykinin, substance P, Mast cells, inflammatory cells and nerve growth factor (Polomano et al., 2008) are released from the cells and converted to an electrical pain signal.

Transmission is the second step in the coordination of pain. From the chemical soup at the site of pain, the impulse is transmitted to the spinal cord. The transmission is dependent on which type of nerve fiber is stimulated at the site of pain and how it is stimulated, as different fibers transmit different electrical signals. The signal that goes fast is transmitted by the large-diameter, mylinated high-intensity A-fibers. A-fibers are usually stimulated by thermal and mechanical injury. That type of pain is perceived as sharp, stabbing, or shooting. The smaller, unmylinated C-fibers transmit the slower electrical pain signal to the dorsal horn of the spinal cord. The character of this pain is a steady, slow, poorly localized, and constant type of pain. In addition to thermal and mechanical injury, C-fibers also respond to chemical injury. The chemical impulse enters the dorsal horn of the spinal cord, where it is integrated and modulated by a complex neurobiological and chemical reaction within the spinal neuroanatomy before it is sent on to higher centers by a complex neuroregulatory pathway (AMA, 2010). The impulse is transmitted up to the brain, but the exact mechanisms that occur at this level are still poorly understood. Aberrant neurophysiology or abnormal pain impulses at this level are thought to play an important role in the development of the abnormal biochemical process of central sensitization, in which the acute pain mechanism becomes confused neurobiochemically and is misinterpreted. An example of this is the development of hyperalgesia, an exaggerated heightened abnormal response to a painful stimulus (Polomano et al, 2008).

In the third step of perception, the pain is transmitted from the spinal cord to the cerebral cortex. There it is perceived, localized, and interpreted (Miaskowski, Payne, & Jones, 2005). The person's individual subjective and cognitive response to pain is processed here. Pain perception occurs in the cerebral cortex. This pain experience involves multiple levels within the cortex, where it is interpreted based on past physical and emotional experiences (Berry et al., 2006).

The fourth and final step in the pain process is modulation. The pain is modulated as it is processed down the descending pathways. Multiple substances that include opioids, antidepressants, and treatments such as biofeedback may provide an attenuation of the conscious perception of pain.

This complex coordination of pain impulses helps to explain why there is such wide variation in the patient's response to pain, even when the cause and treatment are the same. When there is a repeated or ongoing stimulation of this process, sensitization may occur either (a) in the periphery, resulting in hyperalgesia (an increase or exaggerated response to a painful stimuli) and allodynia (pain due to a stimuli that normally does not cause pain); or (b) centrally, where the spinal cord neurons are hyperexcited (Fishman, Ballantyne, & Rathmell, 2010).

Classifications and Causes of Pain

Duration

There are many ways to classify pain to better understand and manage it. Pain can be classified by the duration of the pain: acute pain is considered to have duration of less than 3 months, and chronic pain lasts longer than 3 months. *Acute pain* is an immediate pain in which the onset, trigger or precipitating event is known and could be a short-term illness, accident, injury, trauma or surgery. The course is usually predictable and of short duration of days to weeks. The cause of acute pain is usually associated with tissue damage and an inflammatory process. Acute pain acts as a warning to the body. It indicates that something is wrong for which the person should seek help (Fishman, Ballantyne, & Rathmell, 2010; Miaskowski, Payne, & Jones, 2005). Untreated or inadequately treated acute pain can lead to a chronic pain syndrome (Pasero &McCaffery, 2011).

Chronic pain, also known as persistent or nonmalignant pain, is one in which the pain extends beyond the expected period of healing (Fishman et al., 2010). This definition is very relative while the actual insult may or may not be known or easily identified. In addition, each of us may heal at a different rate. Pain such as that after a healed traumatic fracture may continue months to years after all clinical healing has occurred. This definition also includes pain associated with ongoing chronic diseases such as arthritis, gout, back pain, or headaches. Chronic pain serves no protective function or purpose for the body. It ultimately interferes with normal activities of daily living and quality of life, and often limits functionality (Miaskowski et al., 2005).

Type of Management

Pain may also be grouped by those who are managing it such as oncologic pain (managed by the oncologist), postoperative pain (managed by the surgical service), and palliative pain (managed by the palliative care services). Another way to label pain is by the presence of progressive disease such as malignant (cancer pain) vs. nonmalignant (peripheral neuropathy).

Cancer, oncologic, or malignant pain is caused by an oncologic disease process, chemotherapy-related pain, and radiation-induced pain. The patient may also experience pain that remains after a surgical intervention. Improvement in the management of oncologic disease and associated pain has resulted in an increase in the "cumulative incidence of tumor-related pain syndromes" (Scholz & Woolf, 2002, p. 1062). Patients are living longer with their oncologic disease or may be in recovery from the disease. This lends to cancer being classified as a chronic disease with a chronic pain syndrome associated with the disease.

Palliative pain services are provided at any point in the disease process. Pain management in the hospice population is for patients who are no longer seeking a cure for the disease and are treating pain for the purpose of providing comfort. (Kaplan, 2010) The goals of hospice therapy have changed to comfort rather than cure, to provide control of symptoms and provide for quality of life. An example of this would be a patient with metastatic lung cancer to the spine that has been diagnosed as inoperable. While the disease eradication has failed, comfort is a priority to live out the remainder of life.

Damage Noted

Alternatively, the pain can be classified by noting damage either to the central or the peripheral nervous system. The presence of nerve and tissue destruction points to nociceptive pain, while its absence is indicative of neuropathic pain.

Nociceptive pain results from ongoing pathology or damage. This type of pain is caused by noxious or painful stimuli. There is damage or progressive disease, which can explain the cause of the pain. Pain can be somatic (well-localized) or visceral (vague). Somatic pain involves well-defined pain from a surgical intervention such as an arthroscopy. Visceral pain is vague and often associated with discomfort from internal organs. An example would be a splenic hematoma after a trauma. It is difficult to localize the cause of visceral pain described as vague, gnawing, achy, sore, or cramp-like.

Neuropathic pain may or may not have clear signs of ongoing tissue damage (Gilron, Watson, Cahill, & Moulin, 2006; Pasero, 2004). It is thought to arise from abnormal central or peripheral nerve damage. As this pain serves no purpose, it is often called "pathologic pain" (Berry et al., 2006). It is seen more frequently in patients with other chronic diseases such as diabetes. An example of this would be persistent shooting, lancinating, tingling, itching, or burning pain after spine surgery (Wilkie, Huang, Reilly, & Cain, 2001). The health care system spends millions of dollars each year treating this type of pain.

Terminology

There are several terms that are confusing when caring for patients and treating all types of pain. Some are used, incorrectly, in an interchangeable manner. "Tolerance" explains the state of the body's normal adjustment when exposed to a pain medication that results in the decrease of one or more of the medication's effects over time (Pasero, Quinn, Portenoy, McCaffery, & Rizos, 2011). An example of this is the patient who experiences nausea with the first dose of an opioid that resolves with subsequent doses.

"Physical dependence" is a state of adaptation by the body to a medication. When the medication is abruptly stopped, rapidly reduced, or reversed, the body will experience withdrawal or abstinence syndrome. Symptoms include nausea, vomiting, diarrhea, abdominal pain, restlessness, muscle aches, tachycardia, and hypertension (Gordon & Dahl, n.d.). An example of this occurs when a sedate patient is given a large amount of an opioid reversal agent. The body will suddenly respond with signs and symptoms of withdrawal as the opioid is abruptly reversed. This is also seen with a rapid dose reduction or when the conversion from IV opioid to oral is insufficient.

"Pseudoaddiction" is a phenomenon associated with the undertreatment of pain. It is manifested by the display of drug-seeking behaviors such as anger, clock-watching, or escalating demands for more or different pain medication. The behaviors resolve when the pain is adequately controlled. An example is the patient who reports back pain that has failed to be controlled with an opioid, despite titration. Pain becomes controlled when an adjunctive medication for neuropathic pain is added. Another example is the patient who requests pain medication for a headache. Upon further work-up, a tumor is found to cause the pain. Unfortunately, pseudoaddiction is usually diagnosed retrospectively – after the pain is controlled or a cause for new pain is identified (McCaffery, Herr, & Pasero, 2011).

"Addiction"is a chronic, relapsing, treatable neurobiological disease with genetic, psychosocial, and environmental factors that influence its development and manifestations. It is characterized by the four C's as reported by D'Arcy (2010): lack of Control, Compulsivity of use, Craving for the substance, and Continued use despite harm. While addiction is always a concern when using opioids to treat pain, this concern should not necessarily prevent pharmacologic treatment of a patient's pain. The stress of unrelieved pain may contribute to relapse in the patient who has been in recovery or increase the aberrant use of those still using the medication. The management of this small patient population requires thorough assessment, documentation, and care by an interdisciplinary team for the best patient outcomes.

Myths and Ethics in Pain Management

Many ill-conceived notions serve as barriers to pain management. These myths interfere with the proper management of the patient in pain across the life span (see Table 7.1). These may come from the patients and families, as well as health care team or the health care system itself.

Myths are often deeply rooted in personal and cultural beliefs that dictate how we respond to the response to pain. People learn the culturally acceptable response to pain at a very early age by watching the verbal and nonverbal cues of the family. Some cultures are very emotive about the pain, while others are very stoic.

The patient's cultural response to pain becomes a barrier to assessment and treatment. It may be difficult to assess the pain due to the culture because of the cultural values in the expression of pain and judgments in seeking treatment. An example is the young athlete who is taught to "act tough" and not give into pain. The Drug Abuse Resistance Education (DARE) project's call to "Just say no to drugs!" may not support the adequate treatment of a child in pain due the misunderstanding of the difference between medication needed for pain and elicit use of drugs. It remains the young and old, who cannot advocate for themselves, who are at the greatest risk for the undertreatment of pain.

A health care professional can act as a barrier to adequate pain management and often perpetuates myths related to pain. Some of the myths are related to what the patient looks like or how they present, leading to questions of believability of the extent of the pain. Professionals have doubts about the validity and intensity of the patient's pain, and this may lead to underassessment and undertreatment of pain. An example is the person with back pain, well-known to the provider, who reports the "worst pain ever." The care provider may not believe the patient's claim until an MRI reveals a new compression fracture as the cause of the pain. Generally, barriers from the health care professional come from lack of knowledge and education related to assessment and management of the patient in pain. Poor assessment, coupled with inadequate of knowledge related to pain management, are key barriers to pain management. Staff caring for the patients should understand the medications and other treatment modalities used to treat painful orthopaedic conditions. Management of low back pain, for example, has changed in recent years with the development and publication of new guidelines for this specific patient population. In 2007, The American Pain Society and the American College of Physicians jointly published comprehensive guidelines for diagnosis and treatment of patients with low back pain (Chou et al., 2007). The health care team uses these guidelines to direct patient care from the emergency room through rehabilitation. As more guidelines are developed, health care providers need to stay current in their knowledge about evidenced-based practice related to care of unique patient populations.

Table 7.1. Pain Myths Across the Life Span			
Age	**Misconception**	**Fact**	**Other Thoughts**
Neonates/ Preterm Infants	*Nervous system is too immature to experience pain.*	There is no evidence to confirm this; observation of neonates undergoing painful procedures or with known painful processes indicates this is not true.	Physiologic, paraverbal, and behavioral assessment is primary (e.g., facial expression, motor rigidity, crying).
	Infants cannot safely be given centrally acting analgesics.	Until about 1 month of age, clearance is delayed. Weight-calibrated doses are necessary.	Frequently monitor vital signs. Use neonatal pain scales.
Children	*Children can tolerate more discomfort than adults.*	Children younger than age 4 have lower levels of endorphins, suggesting the younger the child, the more pain is felt. Children may deny pain to avoid injections, be allowed privileges (playroom or going home), or calm anxious parents.	Assessment as above plus: Preverbal child: Use family's word for pain ("ouchie", "boo-boo", etc.). Assessment tools useful (drawing of happy to screaming faces or cyinders "Empty to Full" with pain as tools. Children can point to be descriptor of pain).
	Active children are not in pain.	A change in activity is frequently a sign of pain.	Observe changes in daily activity. Verbal child: Encourage verbalization by suggesting words to child. Consult with parents about child's usual activity level.
Adolescents	*This age group cannot be trusted to report pain accurately.*	May see medical or nursing personnel as authority figures and be reluctant to communicate for fear of being misunderstood. May need information about availability and appropriate use of pain management strategies.	Use standard pain assessment tools to observe inappropriate behavior (irritability, withdrawal, regression), and consult with parent about child's characteristic behavior, as these may be signs of pain.
Adults	*People often become addicted to narcotics while in the hospital.*	Undertreatment of acute pain is a most common error. Tolerance and/or physical dependence may occur but can be managed by gradual withdrawal when painful process is alleviated. Addiction is a psychological need for CNS active agents, which predates an acute episode but is not caused by analgesics when opioids are administered for acute pain in the acute setting.	"Clock-watching" is an indication of ineffective pain management.
	Escalating doses will cause tolerance and eventual increase in side effects and can be dangerous.	Development of tolerance (side effects to the medication disappear over time) and side effects (nausea, vomiting, itching, sedation, constipation) are widely individual. Respiratory depression is easily reversible with naloxone. Sedation may occur with elevation of dose but is usually transient, lasting a few days.	Monitor respiratory rate. Reaction to first doses of a narcotic is predictive of individual's pattern of response.
	Placebo responders do not have pain.	The fear of pain is a large component of the total pain experience. Patient trust/ confidence in the health care system and individual care provider is used inappropriately in placebo use.	The patient's report of pain is to be accepted.
Elderly	*Older people must expect aches and pains.*	Painful conditions are not necessarily part of the normal aging process; many common nonmalignant processes are very painful but manageable. Use of trusted home remedies is often helpful.	Elderly are often reluctant to report pain because of cultural factors such as those encouraging stoicism or fear of rejection by youth-oriented society, or fear of drugs and addiction.

Table 7.1. Pain Myths Across the Life Span (continued)			
Age	**Misconception**	**Fact**	**Other Thoughts**
Elderly (continued)	*The elderly have less pain sensitivity.*	This unproven belief can increase anxiety and feelings of helplessness and loneliness.	Change in activity patterns (giving up favorite activities, social occasions, etc.) are often most accurate indicators of pain in this group.
	The elderly cannot tolerate centrally acting opioids.	Same principles apply through adulthood into very old age. Major difference: duration of analgesia (in the elderly, clearance may be delayed).	Dose must be titrated to effect. "Start low and go slow": Usual starting dose 1/4 to 1/3 of the suggested starting doses.
	Confusion postoperatively is due to the pain medication.	Confusion can be due to unrelieved pain.	Assume pain and trial pain relief measures.
	Persons who can be distracted or can sleep do not have pain.	Distraction and sleep are coping mechanisms for some people. Pain can be exhausting.	Accept the patient's pain report and medicate around the clock.
	Morphine is to be kept as a "last resort"—use should be avoided until later, and it has a toxic, lethal limited dosage.	Morphine can and SHOULD be used early in treatment. No dose ceiling for morphine exits.	"Start low and go slow": Titrate dose to effectively relieve pain with the least side effects.
	It's best to wait as long as possible to get/take pain medication.	The longer the interval between doses, the more uncontrolled the pain.	Use around-the-clock dosages for best management. Long-acting opioids for chronic pain in the elderly are most effective.

Data from Pain: Clinical Manual *(2nd ed., p. 455) by M. McCaffery & C. Pasero, 1999(b), St. Louis, MO: Mosby; and* Pain Assessment and Pharmacologic Management *by C. Pasero & M. McCaffery, 2011, St. Louis, MO: Mosby*

An attempt to manage all orthopaedic pain by algorithm creates another barrier to pain management, as care providers seek ways to standardize care of the orthopaedic patient. The use of a standard implies that all pain is the same in all patients with the same diagnosis or condition. It also makes the assumption that the same medication and same treatment should work on all patients all the time without variability. Yet we know that the very nature of pain makes it a unique and subjective experience. Each patient pain experience may have individual response to medications that are different from the norm. Care of the patient needs to be individualized; if one medication does not work, another medication should be trialed. For some people, Morphine works well for some, but hydromorphone works better for others with the same disease process. People metabolize medication differently based on age, genetics, and previous exposure to the medication. The person who has been on opioids for years will respond differently than the patient who has never taken any. Thus, it is imperative that the health care team assess the individual response to any pain treatment plan. The plan should be made and evaluated, and medication titrated up or down (or changed) based on the unique response of the individual patient and subsequent reassessment.

Another barrier to the adequate management of pain is labeling a patient who presents with either a history of substance abuse or is currently on pain medication prescribed by a provider. These patients with a chronic pain syndrome are often labeled as "drug-seeking" as opposed to "comfort-seeking." Those who have a history of substance abuse can pose a difficult challenge. If the patient is honest about previous abuse, he or she may not receive the usual care. On the other hand, if he or she does not tell the healthcare provider, there is danger of undermedication due to bias related to previous use. In addition, there is the inappropriate fear by the health care provider that by administering opioids they may cause an addiction. This scenario presents a dilemma for the patient and the team trying to manage pain. An adverse drug event such as respiratory sedation and/or respiratory arrest from overmedication is a real fear of health care providers. These events require the use of reversal agents and the knowledge to deliver the medication correctly.

The health care system can pose a barrier to the care of the patient in pain. According to the National Cancer Institute (n.d.), system barriers prevent the patient from getting medications or treatments. Difficulties in accessing medications or limited pharmacy formulary options can negatively impact the care of patients. One medication may be substituted with another medication that may or may not adequately control the patient's pain. Some other system barriers are related to support services and nurse-patient ratios: patients are sicker, but nurses are pulled in many other directions. The use of computers and the training, education, and time constraints present yet other potential barriers to adequate patient pain management (Elcigil, Maltepe, Esrefgil, & Mutafoglu, 2011).

Despite these myths and barriers, health care professionals are obligated to provide adequate care to the patients in their care. The right of the patient to have pain addressed and treated with their input is validated in The Joint Commission Standard of Care (The Joint Commission, 2008). The "Code of Ethics for Nurses" (American Nurses Association, 2001) supports the following four main ethical tenets that direct and shape nursing care, so that all nurses provide compassionate and unrestricted appropriate care while they advocate for patients who cannot speak for themselves:

1. Autonomy: All patients have the right to self-determination. This is achieved by including the patient in all discussions related to his or her own care and treatments, with full knowledge of the possible outcomes.
2. Beneficence: This is the ethical principle of "the duty to benefit another". Pain management is for the benefit of the patient, and care providers have a duty to provide safe and adequate pain management.
3. Nonmaleficence. It is "the duty to do no harm" that guides nursing practices and encourages monitoring for side effects of treatments.
4. Justice: All patients have equal right to pain management and access to pain care, independent of the patient's ability to pay (Herr et al., 2006; Pasero, Eksterowicz, Primeau, & Cowley, 2007; Whedon & Ferrell, 1991).

Pain Treatment

Pain Assessment

Although all medical disciplines agree that pain must be assessed, the subjectivity of pain makes objective measurement difficult. While all patients deserve prompt and appropriate treatment of discomfort, pain must be assessed before it can be treated. A comprehensive pain assessment is the cornerstone from which treatment will be based and evaluated by the health care team, as well as the patient.

History and Physical Exam. The assessment of the patient in pain begins with a review of past medical history, past surgical history, and past psychiatric history. An assessment of previous treatments for pain should be included in the review of the patient's history. An example would be the patient with back pain and the review of interventional procedures, as well as their effectiveness. The patient will need to disclose current medications, both prescription and over-the-counter, including an open discussion as to how the patient is actually taking the medication, i.e. taking a medication every 4 hours instead of every 6 six hours as ordered. A conversation with the patient and/or family should include the effectiveness of past medication or treatments. The comprehensive assessment will give a clear understanding of the patient's perception of the effectiveness of previous and current treatment plans. This insight to the patient's perception will aid in the discussion, re-education, and development of a new pain management plan.

A comprehensive physical exam should be performed at the patient's initial visit and at regular intervals thereafter. All radiographic results and laboratory reports are reviewed to support the diagnosis and treatment plan. The medication plan may need to be modified, based on hepatic and renal disease. Some medications such as nonsteroidal anti-inflammatory medications are dependent on kidney function, while acetaminophen will require a review of liver function.

The assessment of the orthopaedic patient in pain must include an understanding of the anatomy and physiology of the affected area. The musculoskeletal system is a complex integrated system made of muscles, bones, tendons, ligaments, and cartilage. Muscles respond to stretch and inflammation, as seen with sprains and strains, and different receptors within the periosteum respond to pressure. Nerve pain may be related to a tumor within the bone or the fracture of a bone that impinges or compresses on nerve roots. An understanding of normal anatomy will drive care when a pathological state exists. This knowledge will assist in the appropriate treatment and management of care for the patient in pain.

Self-Reporting. It is widely accepted that the patient's self-report of pain is the most reliable method of evaluating pain (Herr et al., 2006). The components of the pain assessment include the exact words the patient uses to describe the pain experience such as "throbbing," "aching," "stabbing," "shooting," "cramping," or "burning." Because pain is a personal experience, the patient should be encouraged to explain the pain in his or her own personal words. The intensity of the pain should be assessed initially and after any intervention to determine the effect of the selected pain treatment. Pain assessment should be put in terms that the patient can relate to: "On a scale of 0-10, with 0 being no pain and 10 being the most intense pain imaginable, what number would you place on your pain?" This Numeric Rating Scale (NRS) has been translated into multiple languages to universally assess verbal patients' pain and individualize their care. The Wong-Baker FACES Pain Rating Scale is another pain assessment tool in which faces are paired with numbers to assist the patient in quantifying the amount of pain or discomfort experienced (McCaffery, Herr, & Pasero, 2011).

Other components of the assessment include the location of the pain and the presence of radiation. The location of the pain is important because a patient may be experiencing more than one site of pain simultaneously. Each site may have different types of pain and thus require different types of treatment, as in the case of a patient with a joint replacement who has a migraine headache. When the location and type of each pain are identified, the cause and the possible treatment options become clearer. The duration of the pain is equally important, to know if it is old or new pain in addition to what improves or exacerbates the pain. When interviewing the patient about the pain, ask about what has made the pain better or worse in the past. This information is key to planning future pain treatment. Multiple acronyms (Table 7.2) are used to remind the health care team about all of the necessary components of comprehensive pain assessment.

Table 7.2. Pain Assessment Acronyms

OLD CART	PQRST	WILDA
Onset	Provoking	Words
Location	Quality	Intensity
Duration	Radiating	Location
Characteristics	Severity	Duration
Aggravates	Timing	Aggravating, Alleviating Associated
Timing		

Treatment Goals

Health care providers strive for pain-free orthopaedic patients, but this is not always possible. While not all pain can be relieved, the goal is to provide the patient with tolerable and acceptable expectations of pain. When pain treatment goals are unmet (Table 7.3), patient outcomes suffer through loss of appetite, decreased mobility, and/or gait disturbances that may translate to more patient falls.

The goals of pain management need to be negotiated individually with each patient, especially postoperatively, including what level of pain can still allow the patient to participate in activities that are necessary to achieve the highest level of function possible. The documentation of the intensity of the pain assists in evaluating the pain plan and guiding modification of nursing care, as well

Table 7.3. Negative Effects of Unrelieved or Uncontrolled Pain

Domains Affected	Specific Responses to Pain
Endocrine	↑ Adrenocorticotrophic hormone (ACTH), ↑ cortisol, ↑ antidiuretic hormone (ADH), ↑ epinephrine, ↑ norepinephrine, ↑ growth hormone (GH), ↑ catecholamines, ↑ renin, ↑ angiotensin II, ↑ aldosterone, ↑ glucagon, ↑ interleukin-1, ↓ insulin, ↓ testosterone
Metabolic	Gluconeogenesis, hepatic glycogenolysis, hyperglycemia, glucose intolerance, insulin resistance, muscle protein catabolism, ↑ lipolysis
Cardiovascular	↑ Heart rate, ↑ cardiac workload, ↑ peripheral vascular resistance, ↑ systemic vascular resistance, hypertension, ↑ coronary vascular resistance, ↑ myocardial oxygen consumption, hypercoagulation, deep vein thrombosis
Respiratory	↓ Flows and volumes, atelectasis, shunting, hypoxemia, ↓ cough, sputum retention, infection
Genitourinary	↓ Urinary output, urinary retention, fluid overload, hypokalemia
Gastrointestinal	↓ Gastric and bowel motility
Musculoskeletal	Muscle spasm, impaired muscle function, fatigue, immobility
Cognitive	Reduction in cognitive function, mental confusion
Immune	Depression of immune response
Developmental	↑ Behavioral and physiologic responses to pain, altered temperaments, higher somatization, infant distress behavior, possible altered development of the pain system, ↑ vulnerability to stress disorders, addictive behavior, anxiety states
Future Pain	Debilitating chronic pain syndromes: postmastectomy pain, postthoracotomy pain, phantom pain, postherpetic neuralgia
Quality of Life	Sleeplessness, anxiety, fear, hopelessness, ↑ thoughts of suicide
↓ Decreased; ↑ Increased	

From Pain Assessment and Pharmacologic Management (p.11) by C. Pasero and M. McCaffery, 2011, St. Louis, MO: Mosby, Inc. Reprinted with permission.

as the overall patient plan of care toward achieving the agreed goal.

Other key aspects of pain treatment goals relate to how the pain is interfering with ADLs. Key activity functions will require evaluation within the context of pain, the causative disease process, and goals of therapy. When a patient presents with acute pain caused by surgery, the goals of pulmonary function and mobility are paramount. In the acute care setting, the goal would be to control the pain well enough to cough, deep-breathe, and participate in physical therapy (PT).

If the pain is chronic, the immediate goals of therapy may be less important than sleep and social interaction. Someone with an oncologic disease will have different goals of therapy as it relates to the underlying disease and treatment plan. The patient's functionality and goals of therapy are key components in the evaluation of the patient comfort goals and treatment plan. Is the amount or type of pain preventing the patient from putting shoes on or getting dressed? Can the patient brush teeth, comb hair, or fix meals? Is the patient able to cough, deep-breathe, and perform postoperative PT? The answers to these questions are important to direct treatment and discuss the goals of therapy with the health care team, the patient, and family.

Nonverbal Patients. Patients who are unable to verbally describe their pain pose a unique challenge for the health care team, both from an assessment standpoint and in deciding what should be used to treat the pain as safely as possible. The American Society for Pain Management Nursing position statement (2010) outlines clinical practice recommendation for the nonverbal patient. Multiple pain behavior assessment tools (Table 7.4) have been developed to identify the presence of pain or discomfort in patients who cannot self-report. Many behavioral tools assess and screen for the presence of pain and or discomfort, and no single tool is superior to another for all populations all of the time. The best choice is reliable and valid for the particular population being assessed, easy to use for the entire health care team and patient's family/caregivers.

The patient who cannot self-report and presents no behavioral signs of pain requires assessment and subsequent treatment based on the current disease process or procedure(s) performed on the patient. An example is the patient who has experienced multiple traumas: because pain is likely present based on mechanism of trauma, surgical treatment, and underlying chronic diseases, it is best to "assume pain present" (APP).

Table 7.4. Pain Assessment Tools for Patients Unable to Self-Report

Patient	Name of Tool	Abbreviation	Setting Used
Elderly	Assessment of Discomfort in the Dementia Protocol	ADD	Tested in long-term care
	Checklist of Nonverbal Pain Indicators	CNPI	Acute care and long-term care
	Nursing Assistant-Administered Instrument to Assess Pain in the Demented Individual	NOPPAIN	Long-term care
	Pain Assessment Scale for Seniors with Severe Dementia Scale	PACSLAC	Long-term care
	The Pain Assessment in Advanced Dementia Scale	PAINAD	Long-term care
Infant / Toddler	Children's Hospital of Eastern Ontario Pain Scale	CHEOPS	Ages 1-5
	Children's Project on Palliative/Hospice Services	CHIPPS	Newborn and infant acute care
	COMFORT – alertness, calmness,	COMFORT	Child and cognitively impaired adult chronic care
	CRIES– Crying, Requires (Oxygen), Increase vital signs, Expression and Sleepless	CRIES	Neonatal acute care
	Distress Scale for Ventilated Newborn Infants	DSVNI	Neonatal ICU
	Faces, Legs, Activity, Cry, Consolability Observational Tool	FLACC	Ages 2-7 (Also for adult)
	Douleur Enfant Gustave Roussy	DEGR Scale	
	Neonatal Pain, Agitation, & Sedation Scale	NPASS	Newborn to 2 months
	Premature Infant Pain Profile	PIPP	Neonatal ICU
	Riley Infant Pain Scale	RIPS	Preverbal postoperative infants and children
Adult	Behavior Pain Scale	BPS	
	Critical Care Pain Observational Tool	CPOT	

Data from "Pain Assessment in the Nonverbal Patient: Position Statement with Clinical Practice Recommendations" by K. Herr et al., 2006, Pain Management Nursing, *7(2), 44-52; and Pain Assessment and Pharmacologic Management (p. 123-161) by C. Pasero and M. McCaffery, 2011, St Louis, MO: Mosby.*

Pain Reassessment

Once a pain treatment has been implemented, it must be reassessed to evaluate the outcome of the intervention. Pain should be reassessed within a reasonable time after a treatment, usually no more than 1 hour, to evaluate the efficacy. For continuity of care, the same tool should be used for both assessment and reassessment to show change over time, unless the status of the patient has changed. This reassessment should be done in concert with assessment of goals of therapy, with a focus on a patient's functionality. Pain should be decreased to the level where the patient is comfortable enough to cough and deep-breathe, participate in PT, and perform ADLs to ensure quality-of-life and therapy goals. If the pain score is unchanged, the pain management plan needs to be modified. A pain behavior tool (Table 7.4) will assist a patient who cannot self-report. Just like with the verbal patient, reassessment with the same pain behavior tool is imperative to determine a change in the patient's perceived discomfort.

The reassessment should also evaluate any side effects related to the current treatment. It is critical to document how well the patient tolerated any analgesic trial or if he/she developed transient side effects such as nausea, vomiting, itching, and sedation. Nausea and vomiting are usually self-limiting and become tolerable with the administration of an antiemetic. Itching is transient and self-limiting, typically resolving quickly. Sedation always precedes respiratory depression. Unfortunately, the individual patient response to medication prevents an accurate prediction of who will develop sedation. All patients are screened using a scale such as the Pasero Opioid Sedation Scale (POSS) for the development of progressive sedation that requires the administration of a reversal agent such as naloxone (Narcan®) (Pasero & McCaffery, 2011). After such medications are administered, these bothersome side effects usually resolve as tolerance occurs. Constipation is a side effect that can be persistent and needs constant surveillance. Prevention of constipation is preferred over aggressive treatment when the patient has become uncomfortable and possibly develops an ileus or obstruction. The elderly are at the greatest risk for the development of constipation, as the older body processes medications differently due to hepato-renal slowing thus necessitating a lower dosage of medication. Side effects may last longer in the elderly and are dependent on a longer time to metabolize and excrete medication.

Nursing Diagnosis, Outcomes, Interventions

Gulanick and Myers (2010) defined the nursing diagnosis of pain as an alteration in comfort, impaired, related to both acute and chronic pain. The patient in pain has lost the ability to independently control his or her internal and external environment to maintain a level of comfort due to disease, treatment, or procedures. Subjective data comes from the patient's verbal report of pain or through the use of pain behavior tools to assess pain. Objective data is observed such as grimacing, posturing, crying, or moaning that is sometimes seen with acute pain. Chronic pain may be associated with muscle atrophy, irritability, changes in ADL abilities, altered sleep patterns, fatigue, weight changes, change in appetite, and decreased interaction with people, but rarely are there changes in vital signs.

Nursing outcomes related to acute and chronic pain interventions include patient expression of pain relief, understanding of and agreement to the plan of care, and performance of activities that are required to maintain health and quality of life. The ongoing assessment of pain allows for individualization of care and education of the patient and the family. The nursing care plan can then be modified based on the patient's response to treatment to achieve the best patient outcomes.

For some patients, pain is secondary to the acute, chronic, oncologic, and palliative disease process. Pain affects all domains of life. Some of the nursing diagnoses related to pain may include anxiety, impaired mobility with an associated increase in fall risk, ineffective body image, disturbance in role performance, self-care deficit, constipation: actual or risk for, and sleep pattern, disturbed.

Nonpharmacologic and Pharmacologic Pain Management

It is often assumed that medication is the best treatment option for the patient in pain. There are, however, many other treatments that provide comfort to the patient and should be used to support the analgesic treatment plan.

Nonpharmacologic Alternatives

In the orthopaedic population, options such as ice (decreases inflammation), elevation (decreases edema) and ace wrapping (decreases pooling of blood) successfully provide comfort to the postoperative patient. Trans Electrical Nerve Stimulation (TENS) and massage therapy apply a different sensation to be sent to the spinal cord, and thus not all of the painful stimuli get through to the brain.

Cognitive behavioral therapies with the use of relaxation therapy (reduces tension), biofeedback, and aromatherapy (produces a pleasing smell for distraction) can often produce a decrease in anxiety. By decreasing anxiety, the patient may be able to manage the pain with less medication. Distraction therapy with music, touch, or deep-breathing allows the patient to concentrate on something other than the pain (Kopf & Patel, 2010).

Pharmacologic Principles

The principles of pharmacologic pain management are based on the World Health Organization (WHO) analgesic ladder for acute/chronic/cancer pain relief (WHO, 1996). This ladder has three steps that range from mild to severe pain (Vargas-Schaffer, 2010). Step one addresses mild pain. Usually, a non-opioid analgesic plus or minus an adjuvant analgesic non-steroid anti-inflammatory drug (NSAID) will successfully manage pain.

Step two of the ladder is management of mild-to-moderate pain that is not relieved by a non-opioid alone. On this step, one of the following is used: an opioid analgesic for mild-to-moderate pain such as hydrocodone with acetaminophen (Norco®, Vicodin®), acetaminophen with codeine (Tylenol No. 3®), or acetaminophen with oxycodone (Percocet®) plus or minus a non-opioid analgesic and or adjuvant. An adjuvant medication (also known as co-analgesia) has a primary indication other than pain management but is often used in the treatment of pain. An example of an adjuvant is anti-seizure medication such as gabapentin (Neurontin®). If opioids are prescribed, a stool softener/stimulant is often needed to prevent constipation, as this opioid side effect does not resolve on its own (Pasero & McCaffery, 2011).

Step three on the WHO analgesic ladder is that of moderate-to-severe pain management. This step requires stronger opioids such as hydromorphone, morphine sulfate, fentanyl, or oxycodone, plus or minus an adjuvant. For pain that is present 24 hours a day such as immediate postoperative or oncologic pain, the use of extended/continuous release opioids is recommended. This ensures that there is a convenient continuous delivery of pain medication that covers the constant pain. Extended/continuous relief preparations are prescribed at evenly spaced intervals usually administered every 8, 12, or 24 hours/around-the-clock. An important teaching point for use of continuous/extended release opioids is that the patient should not chew, crush, or open a capsule because this may cause rapid absorption of the drug that can cause respiratory depression, severe nausea, or death from an opioid overdose.

A short-acting opioid can be added for the incident or for any breakthrough pain. Immediate-release or short-acting opioids are used in combination with extended/continuous-release opioids for breakthrough pain. A short-acting medication is used as rescue dosing for activity. It can be used as a preventative, anticipatory, or preemptive intervention before an activity. An example is a dose prior to PT, with the intent of providing pain control during exercise and thus eliciting better performance and compliance from the patient. Sometimes the long-acting medication does not last the full time. An example is a long-acting medication ordered every 12 hours that does not provide adequate relief for that full time frame. The patient may experience a pattern of pain before the next does is due, called end-dose failure, and may need a short-acting medication to control the pain. A full evaluation of the patient's pain history can assist in deciding if the pain medication plan needed to be modified.

The recommended immediate relief dosage for breakthrough pain is 10%-25% of the 24-hour sustained/continuous release dose. Exceeding 2-4 doses of an immediate-release opioid in a 24-hour period indicates the need to reassess the patient's pain, with a probable need to increase the 24-hour sustained/continuous-relief opioid dosing. A clinical example is a patient receiving extended-release 100mg of morphine every 8 hours. To find the 24-hour dosing, multiply three times 100mg, equaling 300mg for 24 hours. To calculate the short-acting dose of the medication, take 10% of 300mg (30mg) or 25% of 300mg (75 mg). The short-acting medication dosage is then 75mg every 4-6 hours PRN.

Administration Routes

Routes of medication administration include oral, intravenous, transdermal, rectal, buccal, epidural, intrathecal (spinal), local anesthetic nerve block or continuous local nerve infusions, and subcutaneous and intramuscular (IM). See Table 7.5 for abbreviations commonly used in practice related to medication routes and administration timing.

Table 7.5. Abbreviations for Dosage Routes and Timing

Abbreviation	Definition
ATC	around-the-clock
CR	oral controlled-release
H	hour
IM	intramuscular
IV	intravenous
ug	microgram
mg	milligram
min	minute
NR	not recommended
NS	nasal spray
OT	oral transmucosal
PO	oral
R	rectal
SC	subcutaneous
SL	sublingual
TD	transdermal
UK	unknown

Oral. Oral administration (per os, Latin for "by mouth," otherwise known as PO) is the most frequent and preferred route of medication administration. This route is convenient, easily titratable to the requirements of the patient, and provides steady blood levels of analgesia when used properly. Another way of defining the oral route per Pasero and McCaffery (2011) is patient-controlled analgesia by mouth. This is seen in some areas where over-the-counter medication such as acetaminophen and ibuprophen may be left at the bedside for the patient to self-administer. The patient should be educated about pain and the medication, and notify the nurse when taking the medication. This is common practice by the healthy post-partum patient on a mother-baby unit.

Rectal. Rectal administration is an alternative method of opioid administration that may be used in the case of nausea, vomiting, or inability to swallow. Opioid dosage varies, as does absorption time for the drug to become bioavailable. Sustained/continuous opioids can be used rectally at the same dosage as oral opioids. This may be an option for the patient who was taking an oral medication, transitioned to hospice, and objected to IV medication. Providing medication by the rectal route would prevent opioid withdrawal and provide adequate pain management. The rectal route is contraindicated in thrombocytopenic patients secondary to risk of infection related to potential bleeding from insertion of the suppository (Pasero & McCaffery, 2011).

Transmucosal. The transmucosal/buccal and sublingual routes for opioid administration are not often considered, but these are good alternative administrative routes of opioid analgesics for the patient who cannot swallow or needs rapid onset of pain relief for a short period of time. These routes have approval from the Federal Drug Administration (FDA) for cancer breakthrough pain and black box contraindicated in the pediatric population and the narcotic-/opioid-naïve patient.

Transmucosal fentanyl citrate (Actiq®) looks like a "candy" sucker, and is absorbed thru the buccal and oral mucosa. Fentanyl buccal (Fentora®) is a fentanyl lozenge that also absorbs through the oral mucosa. Fentanyl buccal soluble film (Onsolis®) is applied directly to the inside of the cheek and absorbs into the oral mucosa. All of these products are available at different dosage strengths and can be titrated as needed for greater control of breakthrough pain. Disposal of these products in a safe manner is key, along with close usage monitoring in opioid-naïve patients.

Transdermal. The transdermal Fentanyl (Duragesic®) patch is used for the alleviation of chronic pain. It has a slow onset of action of 12-24 hours to provide adequate analgesia. This method of opioid administration is difficult to titrate, and the use of a short-acting opioid for breakthrough pain is recommended. Tips to remember about this drug:

- Do not use to treat acute, severe, increasing pain.
- Do not use for patients with fevers, which may increase absorption of the drug.
- Do not use with heating pads or other heat sources, which also increase absorption.
- Do not use in cachectic, anorexic patients with little or no subcutaneous fat, as fentanyl absorbs through the fat.

Intramuscular. Intramuscular (IM) injections should be avoided. They can be painful, and the absorption rates vary person to person. There wide distribution in dose absorption makes them ineffective for either acute or chronic pain management. They can also cause sterile abscesses of the muscle and soft tissue or damage to nerves if improperly administered. In acute care settings, most patients have IV (intravenous) access, so IM route is rarely given and hopefully will disappear as an acceptable route of administration. The subcutaneous route is preferred to IM when vascular access is interrupted or not available.

Intravenous. Intravenous (IV) administration provides a very fast onset of action for any drug, as it reliably enters the bloodstream. This route bypasses the stomach, omitting the second pass effect or the dilution/digestion of the drug, which slows onset of analgesic effects. Candidates for this route are:

- NPO patients;
- Patients experiencing nausea/vomiting;
- Patients who are unable to swallow;
- Preoperative, intraoperative, and postoperative patients; and
- Unconscious or cognitively impaired uncooperative patients.

The most frequently used method of opioid administration is IV push (IVP), small amounts of an opioid given through a port in the IV tubing. An example is 1-2mg morphine sulfate IVP every 3 hours as needed for pain. Another frequently used method is patient-controlled analgesia (PCA). PCA may be ordered by two different methods. With bolus delivery, the patient pushes the PCA button to receive the drug (example: 1 mg morphine every 6 minutes on demand, once every 6 minutes as needed with a 1-hour lockout 6 mg). With bolus delivery + continuous (basal) infusion, the basal rate is given whether or not the demand (bolus dose) is used (example: 1 mg morphine every 6 minutes on demand, basal rate 0.5 mg, 1 hour lockout of 6.5 mg). The last method of IV opioid delivery is a continuous infusion with no demand dose (example: PCA morphine, 1 mg basal rate, 1 hour lockout of 2 mg). The patient receiving this type is unable to push the button on demand, such as an unconscious or cognitively impaired patient. In this case, is the nurse's responsibility to assess if the pain is well-controlled and administer an IVP extra dose if needed.

Patient-Controlled. Patient-controlled analgesia (PCA) is effective for acute and chronic/cancer pain when a consistent serum analgesic concentration is needed, the parenteral route is necessary, and the patient benefits from being in control. PCA may need to be modified in patients with sleep apnea, cognitive inability to follow instructions to use PCA, and physical inability to access the patient-administered dosing device. Advantages to PCA include the ability to titrate the drug quickly, maintenance of analgesic serum concentration with supplemental continuous infusion, predictable absorption rate, and patient control.

The first step in PCA use is choosing a patient based on patient history, disease process, and goals of therapy. The most commonly used PCA analgesic medications are morphine sulfate, fentanyl, and hydromorphone. Meperidine (Demerol®) use is limited in PCAs, not recommended because its active metabolite, normeperidine, can lower the seizure threshold and precipitate seizures even in those patients with no seizure history. Meperidine is not recommended for more than 48 hours due to the ongoing accumulation of normeperidine that has delayed excretion in the renal system.

The second step in a prescription order for PCA is an optional loading dose or bolus. If the patient is not comfortable, the dose can be titrated to comfort. Selection of the mode is next. PCA allows several modes of administration; the most common mode is patient bolus with a lockout interval. PCA can also be programmed to give a continuous basal rate with a demand dose and lockout, or just a basal rate without a demand dose.

The next step is to determine the patient demand dose amount and lockout interval (when the patient is unable to administer the analgesic). The last step is to determine an optional 1- to 4-hour lockout for the amount of analgesic to be administered. A sample order would look like this:

Morphine sulfate 1:1 concentration, 1mg every 6 minutes, 0.5mg basal rate, 1 hour lockout = 10.5mg

Loading doses must be adequate to achieve analgesia. A smaller dose given every 5 minutes is more effective than one large bolus dose. Addition of a baseline (basal) rate promotes a steady state of analgesia during sleep and allows the patient to achieve analgesia more quickly when awakened by pain. Use of baseline/basal infusion requires more frequent assessment/reassessment, however, and should be used with extreme caution. According to the Institute for Safe Medical Practices (ISMP) (2009), basal infusions require extreme caution for those with obstructive sleep apnea and are not recommended for opioid-naïve patients.

Tolerance to opioids must be considered when determining analgesic dosage. Assess the patient's recent opioid use history (i.e., opioid-naïve or opioid-tolerant.) If the patient is scheduled for surgery, this history must be elicited during the pre-admitting or admitting process to help determine patient opioid dosage requirements.

Assessment and reassessment are keys to effective use of PCA therapy. Assessment and reassessment determine an effective lockout interval for effective analgesia. The pharmacologic half-life of the opioid in use can also be used to aid in determining the lockout interval. Hourly and 4-hour limits of analgesic administration are encouraged as safety measures. These time limits may artificially limit the patient's ability to achieve or maintain analgesia when doses have been inadequately prescribed. When the lockout interval is being reached consistently and analgesia is inadequate, consider increasing the patient administered dose and increasing or eliminating the hourly or 4-hour limit.

Nurse- or family-administered PCA is a controversial topic. The American Society of Pain Management Nursing (2010) supports this practice for a nurse or specially trained family member to push the PCA button if the patient is unable to do so. Hospitals or other institutions using PCA should have a policy and procedure stating their support or non-support of this practice.

Education for PCA use should include the patient and family in the teaching, stressing the patient's right to have pain adequately controlled. The fact that addiction to opioids occurs in less than 1% of patients using opioids should be shared to allay patient/family fears of addiction. If the patient is able to press the button, no one except the patient should press it unless "PCA by proxy" (nurse or specially taught family member) is to be used. If the proxy or designated person were unable to understand and administer the PCA, the traditional method of nurse-delivered IVP opioid would be a better choice for safety reasons.

PCA teaching should ensure that the patient knows how the PCA works, why it is effective, how to access doses, when to administer them, and side effects to report. The patient needs to be taught to report any "new" or unrelieved pain or change in the pain to the RN. Children who have attained the developmental level to operate the button and understand its use can use PCA. Pasero and McCaffery (2011) recommend the following patient assessment parameters when using PCA:

- Vital signs, especially respiratory rate and quality;
- Use of a 0-10 pain scale or other age/developmentally appropriate scale;
- Use of a sedation scale such as the Pasero Opioid Sedation Scale;

- Frequent assessment/reassessment of pain level, and pain relief versus side effects;
- Level of sedation and respiratory status monitored every 1 hour for 12 hours; every 2 hours for 12 hours; then every 4 hours if stable;

Consider increased frequency of assessment during the first 24 hours postoperatively due to variability of patient response to opioid medications. Institutional policy and procedure for assessment intervals should be used as a reference guide.

PCA safety issues require that two RNs set up and program the PCA to verify ordered dosage and parameters. Some institutions may require yearly recertification to validate the ability of the RN to safely set up and accurately program the PCA. Subcutaneous or interosseous (IO) are two other routes that can be used when IV access is not available. Absorption is slower in either of these two methods, but the dosage of opioid remains the same. Subcutaneous dosing places the needle under the skin of the patient for absorption, while interosseous places the needle directly into a long bone, such as the femur, for absorption. This route, used infrequently, may be used in the very old or the very young.

Regional Analgesia

Regional anesthesia includes epidural steroid injection, nerve block, Bier or other anesthetic blocks, and peripheral catheter local anesthetic infusion primarily for acute pain and some limited chronic pain. It also includes implantable long-term analgesia pumps for chronic and oncologic pain management.

Epidurals. Epidural analgesia is defined as the administration of opioids and/or local anesthetic agents through a catheter into the epidural space for acute/chronic/oncologic pain when oral and parenteral routes are anticipated to be inappropriate or ineffective. Physician orders for epidurals should include the names and concentrations of the opioids and local anesthetics to be used in the epidural solutions. The anesthesiologist most often orders the solution to be used and inserts the epidural. Analgesia occurs downward from the catheter insertion site. An example is an epidural catheter inserted at T8 that gives excellent abdominal wound analgesia.

Epidural advantages include quick and effective titration, long duration of analgesia, and selective numbing effect. Epidurals have a low side effect profile and are minimally sedating if properly titrated. Cough reflex is retained, and patients ambulate more quickly due to better pain control. DVT incidence is decreased because the patient is ambulating more quickly. Gastrointestinal motility is increased, allowing patients to eat earlier with less likelihood of bowel ileus (Whiteman & Stephens, 2010).

Contraindications to the use of epidural analgesia are:

- Coagulopathy (use of blood thinners such as warfarin [Coumadin®], clopidogrel [Plavix®], heparin, or low molecular weight heparin [LMWH]);
- Infection or high white blood cell count;
- Positive blood, urine, and/or sputum cultures;
- Use of antibiotic therapy;
- Immunosuppression (thrombocytopenia, pancytopenia);
- Institutional restrictions;
- Difficulty inserting due to deviated anatomy (spinal stenosis, cysts, spinal fusions) or patient reluctance/resistance; and
- Lack of family/patient willingness or resources to continue self-care at home if this route requires long-term analgesia.

The most catastrophic epidural complication is an epidural hematoma. This is most likely to occur following catheter insertion or removal. Epidural hematoma requires emergency decompression to prevent permanent deficits of bowel and bladder dysfunction or paraplegia. Symptoms of epidural hematoma include unexplained increasing constant back pain coupled with sensory and motor deficits. Other complications include neurologic impairment, which can occur if the epidural catheter migrates to the cerebrospinal fluid (also called intrathecal or spinal). This can result in hypotension, paraplegia, or respiratory depression. An epidural catheter site infection is rare, and the incidence decreases when strict aseptic technique is used during insertion and administration of medications by anesthesia (Pasero & McCaffery, 2011).

Urinary retention is common with lumbar epidurals. Most surgical epidural patients have a urinary catheter, but those who do not may need intermittent or foley catheterization. A decrease in the local anesthetic in the epidural solution to lessen blockade of motor and sensory bladder nerves can reduce urinary retention. Nausea and/or vomiting are less common for those with epidurals than other administration routes. Decreasing the concentration of the opioid in the epidural solution usually is the remedy for this problem (Pasero & McCaffery, 2011).

Hypotension/orthostatic hypotension may occur with epidural use due to the sympathetic nerve blockade by the epidural solution with local anesthetics and or opioids. If this occurs, an intravenous fluid bolus can be administered (Whiteman & Stephens, 2010). Keep ephedrine or any other institution approved blood pressure stabilization medication in the unit's crash cart.

Commonly used epidural opioids include morphine sulfate, fentanyl (Sublimaze®), the stronger medication sufentanyl, and hydromorphone (Dilaudid®). Local anesthetics include lidocaine, bupivacaine, and ropivicaine. Clonidine or baclofen may be used to target different types of pain. Administration methods include continuous, patient-controlled epidural analgesia, or both. The epidural catheter may also be bolused intermittently. With intermittent dosing, a time interval must be determined and programmed into the epidural pump or administered manually by anesthesia providers or acute pain service personnel. This may be done either when starting therapy, or when the pain is uncontrolled and the patient needs to be "topped off" or needs a bolus. Patient-administered dosage is also called patient-controlled epidural administration (PCEA).

Proper monitoring and assessment for epidural analgesia includes detailed documentation of the:

- Pain scale used and patient rating of pain;
- Sedation scale use;
- Respiratory rate;
- Intermittent or continuous pulse oximetry or capnography;
- Blood pressure;
- Management of side effects (nausea/vomiting/itching) related to opioids;
- Insertion site for redness, swelling, tenderness, drainage, and intactness of the dressing; anesthesia provider should be notified if there are any abnormal findings; and
- Catheter–tubing connection and review of the medication prescription.

In addition, motor function must be documented if local and sensory when local anesthetic is used in the epidural solution due to impaired motor function as local anesthetic blocks nerve fibers. Assess moving feet and bending legs to determine motor function, and evaluate discrimination between dull vs. sharp or change in temperature in areas covered by local anesthetic to determine the spread of local anesthetic pain coverage. Local anesthetic toxicity must be assessed, which is seen if a catheter migrates out of the epidural space and goes intravascular. The patient might sense metallic taste in the mouth, ringing of the ears, and/or numbness around the lips. The infusion should be stopped immediately and anesthesia notified stat.

The epidural catheter is inserted using aseptic technique percutaneously into the epidural space. Correct placement is determined by the anesthesia care provider, who covers the insertion site with a transparent dressing such as Tegaderm® and tapes the catheter securely to the patient's back. When preemptive analgesia is used, an opioid is administered as the surgery begins, and the catheter may be used to provide spinal anesthesia during surgery. A continuous infusion is optimally initiated in the operating room or the post-anesthesia recovery unit (PACU). Because the epidural catheter is not sutured into place, frequent inspection of the dressing is necessary with assessment of the insertion site for redness, swelling, drainage, tenderness, or leakage of fluid around the insertion site.

If long-term continuous analgesia is necessary such as in the oncology patient, the epidural catheter can be implanted by subcutaneous tunneling to the anterior lower abdomen for easy access. This route provides a refillable reservoir as the method of analgesia for chronic pain relief. The delivery of a single medication or multiple medications is another option for patients who need long-term pain relief. When determining the analgesic dose, patient tolerance to opioids must be considered.

For safety reasons, epidural analgesia requires two nurses to program the pump, check the dosage, and verify the parameters. One provider should be identified as the responsible health care provider for epidural orders on a patient. Standing orders should be written per institutional policy and procedure following best practice guidelines. No other analgesics, hypnotics, or sedatives in addition to the epidural dosage are to be administered unless written by the provider responsible for the infusion. The hospital system needs to have external pumps that are dedicated to epidural infusions to avoid errors. If another all-purpose pump is used for epidural infusion, it must be labeled clearly to avoid errors (Oruntа, Cairns, & Greene, 2005).

Education for epidural analgesic infusions must include the patient and family/caregivers. The nurse should explain how the epidural analgesia works, why it is effective, and how to the patient may access intermittent self-administered bolus like a PCA. Extra clinician-administered boluses may be dosed by the anesthesiologist, nurse practitioner, clinical specialist, nurse if extra pain medication is required. Patients should be taught to report the following epidural side effects so they may be effectively safely treated:

- Itching;
- Urinary retention;
- Nausea and vomiting;
- Headache;
- Constipation;
- Local anesthetic toxicity (numbness around lips, ringing in ears, metallic taste in mouth);
- Oversedation;
- Ineffective analgesia;
- Any new pain; or
- Severe low back pain.

Lumbar epidural steroid injection (LESI), most often administered by an anesthesiologist, is usually used for pain treatment in patients with lower back and leg pain. Sterile preparation of the posterior lumbar spine is required, and a local anesthetic is used to numb the injection site. An epidural needle is placed into the epidural space under fluoroscopy. A corticosteroid/local anesthetic solution is then injected. This solution bathes the spinal nerves and nerve roots to try and decrease swelling and inflammation. Patient response to this method of analgesia varies. Some patients need only one injection for relief; others need as many as three injections in 2-week intervals; and for some patients, LESI does not work at all. A limit of three injections per year is the usual rule of thumb. Nursing considerations include teaching the patient to report any new pain, swelling, fever, or other signs of infection. Patients should be taught to ice the injection site on and off for the first 24 hours after injection to decrease swelling and pain. Blood sugars for those with diabetes may increase due to steroid use, and they may need sliding-scale insulin coverage to manage higher blood glucose levels. Steroids can cross the placenta, so LESI is contraindicated during pregnancy. Any postinjection changes in motor or sensory function need to be reported immediately (Pasero & McCaffery, 2011).

Nerve Blocks. Peripheral nerve block (PNB) involves the strategic placement of local anesthetic solution under ultrasound guidance or with the use of a nerve stimulator around a major nerve trunk. This produces both sensory and motor blockade of nerve impulses. The deposition of local anesthetic works by blocking the sodium channels so the nerve impulse cannot be transmitted. The patient may have a single nerve block and or a continuous nerve catheter. Common types are upper extremity brachial plexus blocks (interscalene, supraclavicular, and axillary) and lower extremity lumbar plexus blocks (fascia iliaca, femoral, saphenous, sciatic, and ankle blockade). All patients with blocks must be assessed for pain; block resolution; local anesthetic toxicity; and injection site bleeding, redness, drainage, or swelling.

Upper extremity blocks involve the clavicle and can be used for shoulder, elbow, or wrist surgery. The most superior approach to the brachial plexus is the interscalene block at C5-C7 distribution. It can be used for the shoulder, arm, and forearm. The next block for the upper extremity is the supraclavicular block that covers a surgical approach to the upper arm, forearm, and hand. Lastly, the infraclavicular block is used for the upper arm, forearm, and hand.

Monitoring of patients with a brachial plexus block include evaluation of low oxygen saturation, heaviness in the chest, drooping of the eyes, and hoarseness of the voice. This constellation called Horner's Syndrome is a perfectly normal – and temporary – finding after a block and indicates an appropriate sympathetic block. Supportive management, oxygen as needed, and elevating the head of the bed at 45 degrees will facilitate breathing. Assess carefully for breath sounds post-procedure due to proximity of the injection site to the lungs that may result in a unilateral pneumothorax or hemothorax. This block should not be used in a patient with severe pulmonary disease such as COPD due to phrenic nerve paralysis that can further impair pulmonary function (Moos, 2011).

Axillary blocks have the same indications as the supraclavicular block. Monitor patients with supraclavicular/axillary blocks for hematoma formation by checking the axillary insertion site frequently for swelling, bleeding and pain. For all upper extremity blocks, apply a sling to the affected arm when the patient is out of bed, apply ice as necessary to decrease swelling, and elevate the arm on a pillow when the patient is in bed.

Lower extremity blocks include facia iliaca, femoral, sciatic, popliteal, saphenous, and ankle. Facia iliaca is a single injection block or catheter that is inserted for hip surgery. Femoral blocks, affecting the femoral nerve as the largest lumbar plexus nerve branch covering L2-to L4, are used for procedures of the knee or for chronic pain. More than one block is frequently done to assure adequate anesthetic deposition over the entire surgical field. The femoral nerve block covers the thigh and anterior knee. The patient may experience quadriceps motor weakness, so care must be used when ambulating to prevent falls. Sciatic blocks may be used alone or with the femoral block for better coverage of the lower extremity. The sciatic nerve is composed of L4-S3 nerve roots (Moos, 2011). This block is often used for knee or ankle surgery.

Popliteal block of the lower extremity is used is ankle, Achilles tendon, and foot surgeries. It blocks the sciatic nerve at the popliteal fossa. The saphenous nerve block is an adjunctive block for the femoral, popliteal, or sciatic blocks when surgery is being done below the knee. Another block of the lower extremity used in ankle surgeries is the ankle blockade. The surgeon in the operating room usually does this block during surgery on the foot or toes.

The patient should be educated about expectations related to the nerve block. A lower extremity block will only cover the anterior, medial, and lateral aspects of the knee; the posterior aspect may still have pain because these blocks do not cover that area. If a block were done to cover both the anterior and posterior knee, the patient would not be able to ambulate because the quadriceps and hamstrings would both be affected. Patients should be administered pain medications as needed to control any pain not covered by the blocks. It is important to keep the immobilizer on while ambulating. The patient should walk with assistance and a walker.

Bier Blocks. Bier block anesthesia is less common in orthopaedic procedures due to the development of safer techniques. It has been used for procedures below the knee or elbow. To perform this block, a tourniquet is applied to the extremity being operated on, at pressure greater than arterial flow rate, to force blood out of the extremity. Local anesthetic is then injected into the extremity and allowed to dwell while it numbs up the affected limb. Tourniquet time must be greater than 30-40 minutes to allow local anesthetic to be metabolized prior to being released into systemic circulation (toxic reactions can result) but no more than 90 minutes to prevent ischemic damage to the limb. Assess the patients carefully for return of normal color, sensation, and capillary refill time (American Society of Regional Anesthesia & Pain Medication [ASRA], 2012).

Care of any patient with a block involves starting oral breakthrough pain medications prior to the block wearing off. This allows for a smoother transition from the block to oral medication for pain management. A "pins and needles" sensation is common as the block wears off. Pregabalin (Lyrica®) or gabapentin (Neurontin®) may be used to modulate or prevent this sensation. Because the extremity is numb, the patient must be taught to protect it and keep it in anatomic alignment.

Watch for signs of local toxicity from local anesthetics: tachycardia, metallic taste in the mouth, ringing of the ears, numbness of the lips, twitching of the eyes or lips, and confusion (especially in the elderly). If any of these side effects occur, discontinue the medication and notify anesthesia staff immediately.

Nursing care includes assessment for pain at the surgical site as well as other sites. The goal of the PNB is sensory loss without loss of motor function. The patient should be assessed for ability to move the distal extremity (toes/fingers). The extremity must be maintained in anatomical position and secured with pillows, immobilizer, or sling because of the limb's decreased functionality. The block site should be assessed for bleeding or drainage. If a catheter is in place, the site must be assessed for the intactness of the dressing, redness, swelling, drainage, or tenderness. If any of these should occur, notify anesthesia immediately (Turjanica, 2007).

Local Anesthetic Infusions. Also known as peripheral catheters, local anesthetic infusions such as the On-Q ball® or Stryker® pain pump are disposable spring-loaded syringes or bulb syringes (usual size is 100ml). These devices are filled with local anesthesia that is set to infuse from 0.5ml to 2ml an hour into the postoperative surgical site to assist in pain management. Nursing considerations follow those of other regional blocks.

Intrathecal Pumps. Long-term analgesia pumps are implanted in subcutaneous pockets in the abdomen or side to provide continuous or intermittent infusion of preservative-free (PF) opioid or opioid/local anesthetic. Adjuvant pump medications are clonidine and Prialt®. Prialt® is derived from sea snail venom. The exact mechanism of action remains unknown, but it is thought to bind to N-Type calcium channels on primary nociceptive afferent nerves in the dorsal horn of the spinal cord (Epocrates, 2012). Many variations of solutions (off label) can be individualized for the patient's pain relief. The pump will be used for continuous, long-term relief, but the patient may still require an immediate release opioid for breakthrough pain.

Candidates for an implanted pump include patients with:

- Chronic pain unsuccessfully treated with oral or IV analgesic therapy;
- Conditions with pain that are not appropriate for neurosurgical procedures;
- Pain mid-thoracic and lower in the body; and
- Life expectancy greater than a few months.

Drawbacks to this procedure include the costs of the procedure, the pump, and the drug(s) needed to refill it at intervals. Another drawback is the ability of the patient and/or the facility to take on the responsibility of care.

One safety recommendation related to implanted pumps is to notify the radiology department, prior to any MRI, CAT scan, or any other test, that the pump is in place. The patient must be taught to identify when the pump needs to be refilled. The nurse serves as a resource for the patient and family in learning how to manage the pump and troubleshoot problems. From the perspective of safety, it is best for a nurse to be credentialed in working with implanted pumps. The risk of this high-tech procedure related to access and pump refill is decreased when the nurse has been educated. The nurse may also alter the pump parameters with orders from the prescribing physician. If the patient expires, the pump needs to be removed if the patient is to be cremated.

Conscious Sedation

The purpose of conscious sedation is to provide safe and effective analgesia during painful diagnostic/therapeutic procedures. The definition of conscious sedation is the combinations of pharmacologic agents (Versed®), an amnesic drug given with fentanyl (Sublimaze®) or other opioid drug, given by one or more routes to minimally depress consciousness. This sedation method provides satisfactory analgesia, allows the patient to maintain his/her airway, and allows the patient to respond to verbal commands and physical stimulation (Kost, 1998). Goals of conscious sedation include that the patient:

- Maintains consciousness;
- Maintains own airway;
- Can swallow and gag;
- Responds to commands or stimulus;
- Has a decrease in anxiety and fear;
- Has acceptable pain relief;

- Has stable vital signs;
- Is able to cooperate through procedure;
- Has amnesia through procedure; and
- Recovers safely.

The most common medications used in conscious sedation are opioid analgesics (morphine sulfate, hydromorphone [Dilaudid®], fentanyl [Sublimaze®] and meperidine [Demerol®], and anti-anxiety/amnesic/muscle relaxants such as midazolam (Versed ®), lorazepam (Ativan®), and diazepam (Valium®) (Kost, 1998). During administration of conscious sedation, the nurse should continuously observe and document patient response, blood pressure, respiratory rate and O2 saturation according to institutional guidelines. Assess level of consciousness and mental status, skin color and condition, and pain status frequently per institutional policy. Observe institutional conscious sedation protocol, and maintain IV access, and a 1:1 nurse/patient ratio for safety (Pascarelli, 1996).

Post-procedure, continue to monitor vital signs, level of consciousness, and pain level every 10-15 minutes for at least 1 hour after the last drug is given. Report any changes in vital signs or adverse reactions. As part of the discharge criteria, the nurse should ensure that at least 1 hour has passed since the last dose of sedative or analgesic, that the patient is alert and oriented, that vital signs are stable, that O2 saturation is 95% or above, and that pain is controlled. The patient should be able to move and ambulate. A responsible adult should drive the patient home and stay with the patient for 24 hours, if possible. Review any/all discharge instructions per physician with the patient and family/caregiver. Make sure the patient has instructions for follow-up care and telephone contact numbers, and reinforce that the patient should make no major decisions for 24 hours (Pascarelli, 1996).

Administration of Medication

Analgesics are titrated to effect while balancing adequate analgesia and unwanted side effects. When administering pain medication, the onset is key to knowing when the patient will expect some relief from the pain. The peak effect of the analgesic is important when assessing for side effects, especially sedation. The duration of the medication is important in knowing when to administer a subsequent dose of pain medication. The goal is to use the smallest dose of opioid that relieves the pain with the fewest side effects.

There is a ceiling on analgesia provided by nonopioids and adjuvant medications. Acetaminophen (Tylenol®) dosage limit for the healthy adult is 4 grams (4,000mg) in a 24-hour period to avoid hepatic issues; however, there is NO ceiling on the analgesia provided by pure mu-agonist opioids. Optimizing administration of opioids includes staying ahead of the pain and using preemptive analgesia, as indicated, to give the next dose of analgesia before the last dose wears off and/or give a dose prior to PT or activities that cause pain to increase.

Around-the-clock (ATC) dosing is recommended for acute or chronic pain, which is present more than 12 hours per day. Consider waking patients at night for ATC scheduled analgesic dosages to diminish the potential for decreased blood levels of the medication. The ATC route decreases the anxiety and consequences of unrelieved pain. Supplemental analgesia may be needed for escalating or breakthrough pain relief. An immediate release (IR) analgesic should be available. A common dosing method is known as PRN (pro re nata, Latin for "according to" or "as necessary"). This is the least effective method due to the delay in the patient actually receiving the dose. Medications given PRN should be given when the pain is intermittent. The patient notifies the nurse that a dose is needed (pain is increasing or worsening), the nurse must sign it out, administer it to the patient, and then wait for the analgesia to take effect. The delayed effect can lead to patient dissatisfaction and nurse frustration. Instead, PRN analgesics can be administered ATC if assessment of pain reflects this need. As pain decreases, assessment will reflect a need for "as necessary" dosing.

Classification of Analgesics

Nonsteroidal Anti-inflammatories & Acetaminophen

The most basic analgesics are peripherally acting medications such as nonsteroidal anti-inflammatory drugs (NSAIDs) and acetaminophen (Tylenol®), which are nonopioid-based analgesics. These preparations are anti-inflammatory, analgesic, or antipyretic in varying combinations. NSAIDs relieve pain by blocking the production of prostaglandins, which are released from damaged cells and sensitize nociceptors to transmit pain impulses (Portenoy, 2007). Acetaminophen and NSAIDs are effective for pain in the musculoskeletal system or pre- or postoperatively. Most are available over the counter (examples are ibuprofen, indomethiacin, naproxen, and piroxicam), although some such as Ketorolac (Toradol®) are only available by prescription.

Ketorolac is the one NSAID that can be given orally, IV, or IM. It is used frequently as a preemptive (pre-surgery) analgesia prior to orthopaedic procedures. Although used for a maximum of 5 days, around-the-clock (ATC) doses every 6 hours is the most effective dosage schedule. As with all NSAIDs, renal function and platelets must be reviewed prior to administration. The maximum dosage of Toradol per day is 40 mg orally, and 120 mg IV/IM. According to Epocrates (2012), the usual IV/IM dose is less than 30 mg.

A trial period at least 7 days is recommended, as individual patient response to NSAIDs varies. Cox2 inhibitors, a subset of NSAIDS, have little or no effect on platelet aggregation. Cox2-specific drugs block the pain mediating prostaglandins at the Cox2 receptor sites but spare the Cox1 inhibitors to release prostaglandins that protect the mucosal lining of the stomach (Portenoy, 2007). Celecoxib (Celebrex®) is the only Cox2 inhibitor currently on the market. Its use is contraindicated in a patient with an allergy to sulfa drugs (Pasero, Portenoy, & McCaffery, 2011). (Brand name alert: Celecoxib (Celebrex®) sounds like the antidepressant citalopram (Celexa®) and the anticonvulsant fosphentoin sodium (Cerebyx®).

Physical side effects of NSAIDs include nausea, anorexia, gastritis, and gastrointestinal (GI) bleeding. Major GI bleeds are known to occur without any GI symptoms. NSAIDs can affect platelet aggregation that, in turn, can cause prolonged bleeding time and moderate elevation of partial pro-thrombin time (PTT). NSAIDs are contraindicated for patients with chronic renal failure, aspirin allergy, asthma, or a prior history of GI bleeds (Pasero, Portenoy, & McCaffery, 2011).

It is important to note that up to 4 grams (4,000 milligrams) of acetaminophen can be administered in a 24-hour period to healthy adults. Higher amounts can result in hepatic failure for healthy adults, and much less than that amount can result in hepatic failure in those with co-morbidities. Careful monitoring of acetaminophen amounts is very important.

Opioids

Central acting mu-agonist opioid drugs block pain at the central nervous system level at the dorsal horn of the spinal cord. Morphine sulfate is the "gold standard" to which all mu-agonists are compared. Morphine, derived from the opium poppy, is one of the oldest analgesics used since ancient times to relieve pain. Mu-agonists come in multiple formulations such as topical, long-acting, short-acting, liquids, IV, rectal, and sublingual. Mu-agonist opioids are the strongest drugs currently available for moderate or severe pain of acute or chronic origin. Examples of central-acting pure mu-agonist opioid medications are morphine sulfate, hydromorphone HCL, codeine sulfate, fentanyl (Sublimaze®), meperidine HCL (Demerol®), and oxymorphone (Opana®). Common receptor sites for analgesia are reviewed in Table 7.6.

Table 7.6. Receptor Sites for Analgesia

Drug	Activity	Receptor Site
Codeine Fentanyl Hydromorphone Meperidine Methadone Morphine	Analgesia, respiratory depression, constipation, euphoria, tolerance	Mu receptors
Buprenorphine Butorphanol Nalbuphine Pentazocine	Analgesia, sedation	Kappa receptors
Butorphanol Pentazocine	Vasomotor stimulation, psychotomimetic effects	Sigma receptors

Principal side effects of central acting mu-agonist opiods are:

- Sedation;
- Respiratory depression (rare with chronic user);
- Pruritis;
- Urinary retention;
- Nausea and/or vomiting;
- Confusion/disorientation;
- Tolerance to opioid side effects develops before tolerance to opioids; and
- Constipation.

Morphine sulfate comes in immediate release or extended release forms. Morphine IV, either IV push or PCA, oral morphine such as Morphine IR (MSIR® morphine immediate release oral), and Roxinol® liquid morphine deliver pain relief immediately.

Extended release morphine exists in many forms and release formats. Long-acting MS Contin® morphine may be given every 12 or 8 hours. Kadian® extended release morphine is every 12-24 hours dosing. Avinza® is once daily extended-release dosing. Oxycodone extended-release (OxyContin®) may be titrated every 8 or 12 hours. Immediate release Oxycodone is the active ingredient in Percocet® (oxycodone + acetaminophen) and in oxycodone (Oxy IR®) as the immediate release formulation. Oxymorphone extended release (Opana ER®) is a newer pain reliever that comes in 5mg, 7.5mg, 10mg, 15mg, 20mg, 30mg and 40mg tablets for dosing every 12 hours on an empty stomach. The immediate release preparation, Opana®, is available in 5mg and 10mg tablets for breakthrough pain. Hydromorphone (Dilaudid®) extended release hydromorphone HCL (Exalgo®) is available for once-daily dosage for opioid-tolerant patients only. Extended release hydromorphone HCL (Exalgo®) is available in 8mg, 12mg, and 16mg tablets. Hydromorphone also is formulated as a short acting IV and PO. Hydromorphone is approximately seven times stronger than morphine.

Two new buccal preparations of fentanyl (Sublimaze®) are available. Buccal fentanyl (Actiq®) lozenges are used for immediate-release relief of severe breakthrough pain. The buccal fentanyl preparation (Fentora®) is also a lozenge and is given at 4-hour intervals. It is available in 100mg, 200mg, 400mg, 600mg, and 800mg lozenges. Another buccal version of fentanyl (Onsolis®) is a thin soluble film applied to the buccal membrane and dissolves. It is available in 200mg, 400mg, 800mg, and 1200mg film patches. The long-acting Fentanyl (Duragesic®) patch, available in 12mcg, 25mcg, 50mcg, 75mcg, and 100mcg, can be applied once every 48 or 72 hours for chronic pain.

Combination opioids are usually an opioid plus acetaminophen. Examples are

- Hydrocodone bitartrate with acetaminophen (Vicodin®);
- Hydrocodone with a smaller amount of acetaminophen (Narco®);
- Oxycodone with aspirin (Percodan®);
- Oxycodone with acetaminophen (Percocet®); and
- Tramadol hydrochloride with acetaminophen (Ultracet®).

The one side effect of all opioids that does not go away is constipation. Constipation is preventable and should not be tolerated. It is good practice to prescribe an accompanying stool softener/stimulant when opioids are used to manage pain. All prescribers should follow this clinical pearl: The hand that prescribes the opioid should also prescribe the stool softener/stimulant; otherwise, a hand will be needed for the disimpaction of the resulting constipation (Woelk, 2007).

Some mu-agonists will have side effects that can discourage their usage. Meperidine (Demerol®) has a dangerous metabolite, normeperidine, that accumulates in the body and causes side effects such as a lowering of the seizure threshold resulting in seizures, confusion, anxiety, and hallucinations. Use of meperidine for greater than 72 hours or more than 300-mg in 24 hours is not recommended, especially in elders with slower metabolisms, or for patients with liver/kidney disease.

Antidepressants

Antidepressants can be used as adjuvant analgesics for chronic pain. Analgesic effect/response may be seen before the antidepressant effect is noted. The effective dose for pain management is usually less that the dose used for depression. Use of amytriptyline (Elavil®) or nortriptyline (Pamelor®) may require serum levels to evaluate effective dosing. These medications should be started at low doses and titrated slowly for best effect.

Antidepressants have three classifications: tricyclic antidepressants (TCA), serotonin and norephinephrine reuptake inhibitors (SNRI), and selective serotonin reuptake inhibitors (SSRI). TCAs increase levels of both serotonin and norephinephrine, and block the action of acetylcholine, which enhances neurotransmission and improves mood. The FDA approved TCAs in 1964 for the treatment of pain. TCAs are composed of two classes: secondary amines such as desipramine (Norpramin®) and nortriptyline (Pamelor® or Aventyl®) and tertiary amines such as amytriptyline (Elavil®), clomipramine (Anafranil®), doxepin (Sinequan®), and imipramine (Tofranil®). Severe dry mouth is one of the side effects of this drug. These antidepressants can be sedating, so the dosing is usually at bedtime to promote sleep. (See Table 7.7 for known side effects of all three antidepressant classifications.)

CHAPTER 7

Table 7.7. Known Side Effects of Antidepressants

TCAs	SNRIs	SSRIs
■ Blurred vision ■ Dizziness ■ Dry mouth ■ Hypoglycemia ■ Sedation/ sleepiness ■ Seizures ■ Tachycardia	■ Abnormal dreams ■ Agitation ■ Anxiety ■ Blurred or double vision ■ Constipation ■ Dizziness ■ Dry mouth ■ Insomnia ■ Gas ■ Headache ■ Nausea ■ Sexual dysfunction ■ Sleepiness ■ Sweating ■ Tremors ■ Vomiting	■ Agitation ■ Diarrhea ■ Drowsiness ■ Dry mouth ■ Headache ■ Insomnia ■ Nausea ■ Nervousness ■ Rash ■ Restlessness ■ Sexual dysfunction ■ Sweating/ increased sweating ■ Weight gain

SNRIs increase the levels of both serotonin and norepinephrine by inhibiting their reabsorption into the brain. The mechanism of action isn't clear, but SNRIs enhance neurotransmission and thus improve/elevate mood. Medications in this group of antidepressants are sometimes called dual reuptake inhibitors. Examples are duloxetine (Cymbalta®) and venlafaxine (Effexor® and Effexor XR®). A newer SNRI on the market indicated for fibromyalgia is milnacipran HCL (Savella®). It is available in 12.5mg, 25mg and 50mg tablets. The dosage is titrated upwards with the goal of 50mg twice daily.

SSRIs first came on the market in 1987, with the introduction of fluoxetine (Prozac®). Exactly how SSRIs help with pain and depression isn't clear, but SSRIs seem to relieve symptoms of depression by blocking reabsorption (reuptake) of serotonin by certain nerve cells in the brain. This leaves more serotonin in the brain, which enhances neurotransmission (the sending of nerve impulses) and improves mood. Some SSRIs are available in controlled release form, providing once-a-day or once-a-week dosing. Examples are fluoxetine (Prozac®, Prozac Weekly), citalopram (Celexa®), escitaprolam (Lexapro®), paroxetine (Paxil®, Paxil CR®, and Pexeva®), and sertraline (Zoloft®). A new drug, which is a combination of olanzapine and fluoxetine (Symbyax®), recently received FDA approval for treating bipolar depression. Symbyax® is classed as both an SSRI and an atypical antipsychotic. SSRIs are the least effective for pain of the three antidepressants (Sansone & Sansone, 2008).

The concomitant use of SNRIs and SSRIs must be done with caution due to the potential for drug interaction. These drugs cannot be stopped suddenly and must be weaned slowly. A rare but life-threatening side effect is serotonin syndrome, characterized by dangerously high levels of serotonin in the brain, that requires immediate medical treatment. Serotonin syndrome can occur with taking antidepressants monoamine oxidase inhibitors (MAOI) and within 2 weeks of starting SSRIs (PubMed Health, 2012). Patients who are concomitantly taking SSRIs or SNRIs taken with tramadol (Ultram®), sumatriptan (Imitrex®) and rizatriptan (Maxalt®), or supplements such as St. John's Wart that affect serotonin levels need to be monitored for the increased risk of serotonin syndrome. Signs and symptoms include:

- Confusion;
- Restlessness;
- Hallucinations;
- Extreme agitation;
- Fluctuations in blood pressure;
- Increased heart rate;
- Nausea and vomiting;
- Fever;
- Seizures; and
- Coma (PubMed Health, 2012).

Corticosteroids

Corticosteroids decrease edema of damaged tissues and therefore decrease pressure on pain noiciceptors. Examples are prednisone and dexamethasone (Decadron®). Various routes of steroid administration are used to treat multiple conditions. Steroids are used in epidural injections to decrease pressure on spinal nerves. They can be administered IV or oral to decrease intracranial pressure, lymphadema, control metastatic bone pain, and neuropathic pain caused by infiltration or compression of peripheral nerves.

Steroids have some risks that go along with their administration. These include weight gain, blood pressure increases, osteoporosis, increased risk of infection (depresses the immune system), hyperglycemia, confusion, and nausea and vomiting. Abrupt cessation of steroid therapy may cause an increase pain severity.

Alpha2 Adrenergic Agonists

Alpha2 adrenergic agonists such as clonidine (Catapres®) are used to treat chronic headaches, reflex sympathetic dystrophy (Chronic Regional Pain Syndromes I and II), chronic low back pain, neuropathic cancer pain, diabetic neuropathy, and other neuropathic pain syndromes.

Side effects include increased sedation and decreased blood pressure. Routes of administration include oral, transdermal, and epidural. Clonidine may also be used off-label as therapy for withdrawal from opioids. Tizanidine (Zanaflex®) is frequently used for muscle spasms or spasticity.

Anticonvulsants

Anticonvulsant drugs were originally used off-label for chronic neuropathic lancinating, shooting, burning, stabbing pain. Examples are carbamazine (Tegretol®), tiagabine (Gabitril®), gabapentin (Neurontin®), pregabalin Lyrica®), phenytoin (Dilantin®), clonazepam (Klonopin®), valproic acid (Depakene®), and lioresal (Baclofen®). The most commonly prescribed drugs in this category are gabapentin (Neurontin®), pregabalin (Lyrica®), carbamazine (Tegretol®), clonazepan (Klonopin®), and tiagabine (Gabitril®). Other anticonvulsants include Lamotrigine (Lamictal), oxycarbizepine (Trileptal), and topiramate (Topamax) for chronic headache management.

The efficacy of anticonvulsant drugs in the management of persistant neuropathic pain has been demonstrated in a number of systematic research reviews (Dworkin et al., 2007; Moulin et al., 2007). In addition, the preoperative use of gabapentin and pregabalin has been found to decrease anxiety, decrease postoperative pain, and improve function in the postoperative knee surgical patient (Menigaux, Adam, Guignard, Sessler, & Chauvin, 2005).

The most common side effects of this class are dizziness, peripheral edema, and somnolence. A current FDA black box warning for tiagabine discourages its off label use due to paradoxical occurrence of seizures in patients without epilepsy. Additionally, patients who require concomitant treatment with morphine may experience increases in gabapentin concentrations and should be observed for signs of CNS depression. Close patient observation and titration of gabapentin or morphine should be adjusted appropriately.

Calcium Regulators

Calcium regulators have been found to provide reduction of pain for some patients with bone pain from osteoporosis or progressive cancers (Pasero, Polomano, Portenoy & McCaffery, 2011). Calcitonin (Miacalcin®)

nasal spray can be used as an adjuvant medication to decrease bone pain, as it decreases the rate of bone absorption/reabsorption (especially in osteoporosis). Calcitonin is available in subcutaneous, intramuscular, and nasal spray routes. Gallium nitrate (Ganite®), which is available only in intramuscular injection form, is an osteoclast inhibitor that may be used for malignant (oncological) bone pain. Further studies are needed to prove its effectiveness and side effects.

Radiopharmaceuticals

Radiopharmaceuticals are used primarily for pain caused by metastatic bone disease. The first radionuclide introduced into clinical practice was phosphorus-32 orthophosphate, which was found to be as effective for metastatic bone pain as external-beam radiotherapy (Pasero, Polomano, Portenoy & McCaffery, 2011).

Bone marrow suppression is the main toxicity attributed to radiopharmaceuticals. Newer radionuclides such as phosphorus-32, strontium-89 (Metastron®) and samarium-153 (Quadramet®) that are usually are administered intravenously are considered to be less toxic to the bone marrow.

Benzodiazepines

Benzodiazepines have limited usage in pain management but have seen some use in the management of musculoskeletal and neuropathic pain, particularly muscle spasm (Pasero, Polomano, Portenoy & McCaffery, 2011). Diazepam (Valium®) is widely used benzodiazepine for muscle relaxation. It can reduce myotonic activity in acute cases of muscle spasms. Clonazepam (Klonopin®) is classified as an anticonvulsant and anxiolytic. It also produces muscle relaxation in low doses (0.5mg PO every 8 hours). Other drugs in this category are lorazepam (Ativan®) and aprazolam (Xanax®).

Because of the sedating effects of benzodiazipines, their use as muscle relaxants should be limited to short courses of 10 days or less. Longer duration can lead to dependence and require dose tapering if discontinued. In addition, the elderly have an increased sensitivity to the effects of this drug class, and added caution is needed when administering to this age group (Pasero, Polomano, Portenoy & McCaffery, 2011).

Muscle Relaxants

Muscle relaxants are said to relieve musculoskeletal pain by decreasing spasticity and relaxing skeletal muscle. However, evidence is lacking as to whether these drugs actually relax skeletal muscle (Pasero, Polomano, Portenoy & McCaffery, 2011). They inhibit polysynaptic myogenic reflexes in animals, but the relationship between this action and similar actions in humans is unknown. These drugs are usually administered orally. Examples are orphenadrine (Norflex®) and tricyclic compounds structurally similar to the tricyclic antidepressants such as cyclobenzeprine (Flexeril®). Other drugs in this category are carisoprodol (Soma®), chlorzoxazone (Parafon Forte DSC®), and methocarbomol (Robaxin®).

Muscle relaxants are best used as adjuvants to be used with opioid and nonopioid analgesics. Use is short-term only, 10-14 days. Side effects include sedation, nausea, vomiting, dizziness, hallucinations, and headache. Because these drugs can cause sedation, patients should be instructed on fall precautions.

Promethazine (Phenergan®) and hydroxyzine (Vistaril®) are often given erroneously in combination with opioid analgesics with the belief that they "potentiate" or make the opioid more effective, but there is no evidence to support this (Atkinson, Kremer, & Gabfin, 1985). Studies show that Phenergan actually increases both pain sensitivity and the amount of opioid needed to relieve pain (Pasero & McCaffery, 2011). The effects of higher doses of Vistaril® needed to produce analgesia increase the risk of respiratory depression that is not reversible by naloxone (as it is not an opioid). Because of the extreme irritation to tissue, producing a "burning" sensation, when administered parentally, Phenergan should be IV, diluted with normal saline and pushed slowly only after making sure of proper venous access. Phenergan was recently given a black box warning by the FDA, as it can cause extreme pain and sloughing of the skin if the IV catheter is not securely in the vein.

Topical Agents

Topical local anesthetics and analgesics are often used in painful neuropathy syndromes (post-herpetic neuralgia, diabetic neuropathies, and rheumatoid or osteoarthritis). Examples are capsaicin 8% patch (Zostrix®, Qutenza®), lidocaine 5% patch (Lidoderm®), diclofenac epolamine patch (Flector®), and diclofenac sodium topical solution 1.5% (Pennsaid®). Topical creams used for venipunctures and accessing implanted ports are lidocaine 2.5% and prilocaine 2.5% (EMLA®). Each topical patch has different indications and numbers of patches that can be applied for a specific duration of time. It is recommended that manufactures directions be followed for each patch.

Capsaicin is a natural substance obtained from hot peppers. It is thought that capsaicin decreases pain (especially that of post-herpetic neuralgia and diabetic neuropathy) by reducing the concentrations of small peptides in the primary afferent neurons. These peptides include substance P, which may activate the noiciceptive systems in the dorsal horn of the spinal cord, and reduce transmission of pain impulses. The topical medications need to be applied regularly for best benefit; however, some patients do not tolerate the burning sensation and may even develop redness after application.

The Flector patch and the Pennsaid solution have shown good results for patients with rheumatoid or osteoarthritis. They also help patients who are unable to take systemic NSAIDs, such as those with previous GI bleeds, those at risk for a GI bleed, or those who are anticoagulated. Many OTC creams and gels that contain aspirin or acetaminophen with menthol are available for topical use. These provide a soothing sensation and decrease inflammation at the site of application.

Special Pharmacologic Considerations

Multimodal Balanced Analgesia

Balanced analgesia is defined as the simultaneous use of more than one pharmacologic pain control agent. This allows for more effective management of pain over time. This multimodal continuous analgesia uses a continuous delivery of combined analgesic regimens, including more than one drug and more than one route of administration. Multimodal balanced analgesia is usually implemented for acute pain, but the concept applies equally well to all other types of pain. Table 7.8 provides examples of clinical application of the balanced analgesia concept. Table 7.9 gives examples of analgesic combining options to support multimodal balanced analgesia.

Equianalgesia

"Equianalgesic" means approximately the same pain relief. Two doses of different drugs can provide approximately the same level of pain relief. This technique of equianalgesia can best be explained by understanding the concept of potency and the fact that medications provide similar pain relief (Pasero, Quinn, Portenoy, McCaffery, & Rizos, 2011; Rapp & Gordon, 2000). Potency is the intensity of the analgesic effect of the drug. For example, hydromorphone is more potent than morphine, as it takes only 1.5mg of parenteral hydromorphone to produce the same level of analgesia as 10mg of parenteral morphine (see Table 7.9). Describing one drug as more potent than the other does not mean that it is more effective, just that the patient may require less medication to attain pain relief. It is a fallacy that IV dosing is more potent than oral dosing, as 10mg of IV morphine provides the same pain relief as 30mg of oral morphine (see Table 7.9).

Due to patient variability, conversion from one opioid to another is not an absolute but an estimate of the amount of medication a patient may require. When switching between opioids, the nurse should start at a low dosage and longer intervals between doses and titrate to the patient's individual response. The longer a patient has been receiving an opioid, the more conservative the starting dose of a new opioid should be. When converting from one opioid to another, the new opioid must be decreased by 25%-50% to allow for new opioid side effects such as sedation, also known as incomplete cross-tolerance (American College of Physicians [ACP], n.d.).

Using a table for conversion from one drug or another with equianalgesic dosage units increases the probability that dose route or drug changes will be accomplished without loss of pain control (see Table 7.10). A conversion table is helpful when switching from one drug to another or switching from one route of administration to another. This guideline for selecting doses for opioid-naïve patients suggest a ratio for comparing the analgesic effects of one drug to those of another.

When switching routes of drug delivery or changing to another opioid, the nurse should consider the following questions:

- Is the current medication the best choice for the patient at this time?
- Is the current dose adequate such as 1 mg of morphine as opposed to 2 mg?
- Is the current frequency appropriate should the medication be given every 1 hour or every 4 hours?
- Is the current medication route appropriate?

Managing Pain in Special Orthopaedic Populations

Individuals in special populations historically are at risk for the undertreatment of pain. These populations include cognitively impaired patients and individuals with impaired ability to communicate (such as the deaf, the blind, and nonverbal individuals such as stroke patients or those in critical care), as well as those who are non-English speaking. A patient with a history of mental health issues, substance abuse and previous opioid use (tolerant), bipolar disease, or traumatic brain injury (TBI) poses a different type of challenge to the orthopaedic nurse. Patients at the extremes of the age distribution (young children and elderly) also fall into the at-risk category for undertreatment of pain (Pasero & McCaffery, 2011).

Assessment of special populations at risk is possible with specific behavior tools (see Table 7.4). If the report of pain from a verbal cognitively intact patient with an orthopaedic diagnosis is accepted, so should the reports of pain in the cognitively impaired patient. More than one attempt should be made to obtain a pain assessment with a tool that fits the patient's physical and mental

Table 7.8. Clinical Application of Multimodal Balanced Analgesia	
Clinical examples of balanced analgesia	■ Systemic NSAID = systemic opioid (ibuprofen PO + morphine PQ). ■ Systemic NSAID + epidural opioid and local anesthetic (ketorolac IV + fentanyl/bupivacaine epidurally). ■ Local infiltration of anesthetic + systemic NSAID + systemic opioid (lidocaine infiltration of surgical site + ketorolac IV + IV PCA morphine). ■ Regional block + systemic NSAID + epidural opioid and local anesthetic (epidural anesthetic during surgery; postoperatively epidural fentanyl/bupivacaine + ketorolac IV).
Examples of improved outcomes for the patient with acute pain (postoperative pain or trauma)	■ Early ambulation. ■ Early enteral feeding. ■ Increased participation in recovery activities (coughing, physical therapy). ■ Early discharge.

Data from Pain: Clinical Manual *(2nd ed.) by M. McCaffery & C. Pasero, 1999, St. Louis, MO: Mosby; and* Pain Assessment and Pharmacologic Management *by C. Pasero & M. McCaffery, 2001, St. Louis, MO: Mosby.*

CHAPTER 7

Table 7.9. Combining Analgesics

Medications	Status
Acetaminophen + Any Other Analgesic	Acceptable Common Practice Acetaminophen may be given along with any of the NSAIDs, opioids, or adjuvants.
Acetaminophen + NSAID	Acceptable Common Practice Acetaminophen may be given with any of the NSAIDs, including acetaminophen. Usually adds analgesia without increasing side effects.
NSAID + NSAID	Not Recommended The additional pain relief is minimal, and the risk of side effects is considerable.
Corticosteroid + NSAID	Caution Prolonged administration of this combination increases the risk of side effects such as peptic ulcer.
Opioid (mu agonist or agonist-antagonist) + Nonopioid (acetaminophen and/or NSAID)	Highly Recommended For all analgesic regimens, consider including a nonopioid, even if pain is severe enough to require an opioid. Many opioids given orally for mild to moderate pain (codeine, oxycodone) are compounded with a nonopioid (aspirin, acetaminophen).
Mu Agonist + Agonist-Antagonist	Rarely Appropriate Very few situations exist when use of a mu agonist should be followed by an agonist-antagonist. This sequence may reverse analgesia of the mu agonist or precipitate withdrawal in a physically dependent patient. A opioid-naïve patient experiencing side effects such as itching or sedation from spinal opioids may, however, receive nalbuphine to reverse these supraspinal side effects.
Mu Agonist + Mu Agonist	Usually Not Necessary Few situations exist when more than one mu agonist should be administered to a patient; however, any or all of the mu agonists may be combined or given to the same patient. Side effects and analgesia simply will be addictive.
Adjuvant + Opioid + Acetamiophen/NSAID	Often Appropriate for Chronic Pain / Sometimes Appropriate for Acute Pain This combination may be very appropriate for a patient with chronic pain. If the adjuvant analgesics provide a reasonably rapid onset of analgesia, this combination may be appropriate for acute pain.
Adjuvant + Adjuvant	Sometimes Appropriate for Chronic Pain An adjuvant from one group of drugs may be combined with an adjuvant from another group and is sometimes helpful in relieving chronic cancer pain or chronic noncancer pain. There might be a patient who would benefit from a combination of all of the following: dexamethasone (Decadron®), a corticosteroid; dextroamphetamine (Dexedrine®), a psychostimulant; amitriptyline (Elavil®), a tricyclic antidepressant; and clonazepam (Klonopin®), an anticonvulsant.

Data from Pain: Clinical Manual (2nd ed.) by M. McCaffery & C. Pasero, 1999, St. Louis, MO: Mosby; and Pain Assessment and Pharmacologic Management by C. Pasero & M. McCaffery, 2001, St. Louis, MO: Mosby.

Table 7.10. Equianalgesic Dose Chart[1]

This table provides equianalgesic doses and pharmacokinetic information about selected opioid drugs. *ATC*, around-the-clock; *h*, hour; *IM*, intramuscular; *IV*, intravenous; *MR*, oral modified release; *ND*, no data; *NR*, not recommended; *NS*, nasal spray; *OT*, oral transmucosal; *PO*, oral; *R*, rectal; *SC*, subcutaneous; *St*, sublingual; *TD*, transdermal.

Opioid	Oral (PO) (over ~4 h)	Parenteral (IM/SC/IV) (over ~4 h)	Onset (min)	Peak (min)	Duration (h)[2]	Half-life (h)
Mu Agonists						
Morphine	30 mg	10 mg	30-60 (PO) 30-60 (MR)[3] 30-60 (R) 5-10 (IV) 10-20 (SC) 10-20 (IM)	60-90 (PO) 90-180 (MR)[3] 60-90 (R) 15-30 (IV) 30-60 (SC) 30-60 (IM)	3-6 (PO) 8-24 (MR)[3] 4-5 (R) 3-4 (IV)[2,4] 3-4 (SC) 3-4 (IM)	2-4
Codeine	200 mg *NR*	130 mg	30-60 (PO) 10-20 (SC) 10-20 (IM)	60-90 (PO) ND (SC) 30-60 (IM)	3-4 (PO) 3-4 (SC) 3-4 (IM)	2-4
Fentanyl		100mg IV 100 mcg/h of transdermal fentanyl is approximately equal to 4 mg/h of IV morphine[5]; 1 mcg/h of transdermal fentanyl is approximately equal to 2 mg/24 h of oral morphine[5]	5 (OT)[6] 5 (B)[6] 3-5 (IV) 10-15 (IM) 12-16 h (TD)	15 (OT)[6] 15 (B)[6] 15-30 (IV) 30-60 (IM) 24 h (TD)	2-5 (OT)[6] 2-5 (B)[6] 2 (IV)[2,4] 2-3 (IM) 48-72 (TD)	3-47 >24 (TD)
Hydrocodone (as in Vicodin, Lortab)	30 mg[8] *NR*	--	30-60 (PO)	60-90 (PO)	4-6 (PO)	4
Hydromorphone (Dilaudid)	7.5 mg	1.5 mg[9]	15-30 (PO) 15-30(R) 5 (IV) 10-20 (SC) 10-20 (IM)	30-90 (PO) 30-90 (R) 10-20 (IV) 30-90 (SC) 30-90 (IM)	3-4 (PO) 3-4 (R) 3-4 (IV)[2,4] 3-4 (SC) 3-4 (IM)	2-3
Levorphanol (Levo-Dromoran)	4 mg	2 mg	30-60 (PO) 10 (IV) 10-20 (SC) 10-20 (IM)	60-90 (PO) 15-30 (IV) 4-6 (IV)[1,3] 60-90 (SC) 60-90 (IM)	4-6 (PO) 4-6 (SC) 4-6 (IM)	12-15
Meperidine (Demerol)	300 mg NR	75 mg	30-60 (PO) 5-10 (IV) 10-20 (SC) 10-20 (IM)	60-90 (PO) 10-15 (IV) 15-30 (SC) 15-30 (IM)	2-4 (PO) 2-4 (IV)[2,4] 2-4 (SC) 2-4 (IM)	2-3
Oxycodone (as in Percocet, Tylox)	20 mg	--	30-60 (PO) 30-60 (MR)[10] 30-60 (R)	60-90 (PO) 90-180(MR)[10] 30-60 (R)	3-4 (PO) 8-12 (MR)[10] 3-6 (R)	2-3 45 (MR)[10]
Oxymorphone	10 mg (10 mg R)	1 mg	30-45 (PO) 15-30 (R) 5-10 (IV) 10-20 (SC) 10-20 (IM)	30-90 (PO) 60 (MR)[11] 120 (R) 15-30 (IV) ND (SC) 30-90 (IM)	4-6 (PO) 12 (MR)[11] 3-6 (R) 3-4 (IV)[2,4] 3-6 (SC) 3-6 (IM)	7-11 2(parenteral)
Propoxyphene[12] (Darvon)	--	--	30-60 (PO)	60-90 (PO)	4-6 (PO)	6-12

Table 7.10. Equianalgesic Dose Chart[1] (continued)

Opioid	Oral (PO) (over ~4 h)	Parenteral (IM/SC/IV) (over ~4 h)	Onset (min)	Peak (min)	Duration (h)[2]	Half-life (h)
Agonist-Antagonists						
Buprenorphine[13] (Buprenex)	--	0.4 mg	5(SL) 5(IV) 10-20 (IM)	30-60 (SL) 10-20 (IV) 30-60 (IM)	3 (SL) 3-4 (IV)[2,4] 3-6 (IM)	2-3 5-6
Burtorphanol[13] (Stadol)	--	2mg	5-15 (NS)[14] 5 (IV) 10-20 (IM)	60-90 (NS) 10-20 (IV) 30-60 (IM)	3-4 (NS) 3-4 (IV)[2,4] 3-4 (IM)	3-4
Dezocine (Dalgan)	--	10 mg	5 (IV) 10-20 (IM)	ND (V) 30-60 (IM)	3-4 (IV)[2,4] 3-4 (IM)	2-3
Nalbuphine[13] (Nubain)	--	10 mg	5 (IV) <15 (SC) <15 (IM)	10-20 (IV) ND (SC) 30-60 (IM)	4-6 (IV)[2,4] 4-6 (SC) 4-6 (IM)	5
Pentazocine[13] (Talwin)	50 mg	30 mg	15-30 (PO) 5 (IV) 15-20 (SC) 15-20 (IM)	60-180 (PO) 15 (IV) 60 (SC) 60 (IM)	3-4 (PO) 3-4 (IV)[2,4] 3-4 (SC) 3-4 (IM)	2-3

[1] An expert panel was convened for the purpose of establishing a new guideline for opioid rotation and proposed a two-step approach (Fine, Portenoy, & Ad Hoc Expert Panel on Evidence Review and Guidelines for Opioid Rotation, 2009). The approach presented in the text for calculating the dose of a new opioid can be conceptualized as the panel's Step One, which directs clinicians to calculate the equianalgesic dose of the new opioid based on the equianalgesic table. Step Two suggests that clinicians perform a second assessment of patients to evaluate the current pain severity (perhaps suggesting that the calculated dose be increased or decreased) and to develop strategies for assessing and titrating the dose as well as to determine the need for breakthrough doses and calculate those doses.

[2] Duration of analgesia is dose-dependent: the higher the dose, usually the longer the duration.

[3] e.g., MS Contin and Oramorph (8-12 hours) and Avinza and Kadian (12-24 hours).

[4] IV boluses may produce analgesia that lasts nearly as long as IM or SC doses; however, of all routes of administration, IV produces the highest peak concentration of the drug, and the peak concentration is associated with the highest level of toxicity (e.g. sedation). To decrease peak effect and lower toxicity, IV boluses may be administered more slowly (e.g. 10mg of morphine over a 15-minute period), or smaller doses may be administered more often (e.g., 5 mg of morphine every 1-1.5 hours).

[5] This is the ratio that is used clinically.

[6] The delivery system for transmucosal fentanyl influences potency, e.g., buccal fentanyl is approximately twice as potent as oral transmucosal fentanyl.

[7] At steady state, slow release of fentanyl from storage in tissues can result in a prolonged half-life (e.g., 4-5 times longer).

[8] Equianalgesic data are not available.

[9] The recommendation that 1.5mg of parenteral hydromorphone is approximately equal to 10mg of parenteral morphine is based on single-dose studies. With repeated dosing of hydromorphone (as during PCA), it is more likely that 2-3mg of parenteral hydromorphone is equal to 10mg of parenteral morphine.

[10] As in, e.g. OxyContin

[11] As in Opana ER

[12] 65 to 130mg= approximately 1/6 of all doses listed on this chart.

[13] Used in combination with mu agonist opioids, this drug may reverse analgesia and precipitate withdrawal in opioid-dependent patients.

[14] In opioid-naïve patients taking occasional mu agonist opioids such as hydrocodone or oxycodone, the addition of butorphanol nasal spray may provide additive analgesia. In opioid-tolerant patients such as those receiving ATC morphine, the addition of butorphanol nasal spray should be avoided because it may reverse analgesia and precipitate withdrawal.

From Pain Assessment and Pharmacologic Management *(pp. 444-446) by C. Pasero and M. McCaffery, 2011, St. Louis, MO: Mosby. Reprinted with permission.*

needs. The same tool must be used for consistency and continuity when reassessing the patient for the presence of pain and the effects of treatment.

Pain in Cognitively Impaired Patients

According to the ASPMN (2010) guidelines, the self-report is the most reliable and should always be attempted first. If the patient is unable to self-report, potential causes of distress or discomfort should be sought. A behavioral tool should be used next to assess for the presence of pain. Surrogate reporting is next in the guidelines for pain assessment, followed by an analgesic trial. Cognitively impaired patients are unable to give a reliable self-report of pain (Pasero & McCaffery, 2011). They may be comatose, nonverbal, mentally challenged (dementia, Alzheimer's disease, delirium), mentally retarded, or victims of a cerebral vascular accident (CVA). These patients must be assessed for pain with behavioral observations using a validated and reliable nonverbal scale (see Table 7.4).

Behavioral assessment of the cognitively impaired includes observation of the patient's facial expressions: frowns, sad expression, grimacing, or a fearful expression. Vocalizations are also included, such as crying, moaning, groaning, noisy breathing, and sighing. Physical movements are a large part of pain assessment. Patient restlessness, fidgeting, confusion, guarding of body parts, tension, rigid muscles, and beckoning motions (trying to get attention) are all indicators of pain or discomfort. These behaviors summarized in Table 7.11 should be assessed at rest and with movement to get an adequate, concise pain picture. The patient's family or caregivers can also help interpret patient behavior, as they spend much time caring for and observing the patient. These patients should be treated as a noncognitively impaired patient is treated.

Table 7.11. Behaviors Indicative of Pain

Behavior	Indication
Facial Expression	Wrinkled forehead, grimace, fearful, sad, muscle contraction around mouth and eyes.
Physical Movement	Restlessness, fidgeting, absence of movement, slow movements, cautious movements, guarding, rigidity, generalized tension (not relaxed), trying to get attention (beckoning someone).
Vocalization	Groaning, moaning, crying, noisy breathing.
This is a simple guide to behavioral assessment of pain in patients who are unable to provide a self-report of pain. It is NOT an exhaustive list.	

From Pain Assessment and Pharmacologic Management (p.127) by C. Pasero and M. McCaffery, 2011, St. Louis, MO: Mosby. Reprinted with permission.

The nurse should use term "Assume Pain Present" (APP) to guide interventions after the assessment has been accomplished to the fullest extent possible, given the unresponsive patient's clinical picture and the inadequacy of any available pain tools (Pasero & McCaffery, 2011). It is reasonable to surmise that an alert patient in this situation would be experiencing pain, and care should be based on that assumption. APP would be expected during illness, trauma, surgery, an extended stay in a critical care setting, with patient history of a painful condition, or accompanying any invasive or noninvasive procedure. The nurse should document exactly how the APP conclusion was reached and any interventions planned. The usual conclusion to APP is that an "analgesic trial" is in order.

Nonspecific behaviors such as withdrawal and agitation, lack of appetite, and other behavioral changes can indicate pain in the very young, elders, or those with dementia. APP is important while the work-up is in progress. If other sources of distress have been ruled out or pain can't be ruled out, APP can be considered. Analgesic trials are easier to justify in the very ill, comatose, or chemically paralyzed patient. As long as there are conditions that could cause pain, APP should be used and the pain should be treated. Attempts to minimize pain are ethically required as long as APP is determined (Herr et al., 2006).

Pain in Children

Insufficient treatment of pain in infants and children results from misconceptions and inadequate knowledge of medical and nursing staff. Many myths exist, the prime example being the fallacy that infants and neonates are incapable of feeling pain. Infants have the capacity to feel pain at birth, yet the International Association for the Study of Pain (IASP) estimates that more than 120 million untreated painful procedures are performed on neonates annually (IASP, 2011). Another myth is that infants can't remember pain. Studies support that past pain experiences influence present and future pain responses, thus emphasizing the need for adequate pain management throughout the life span (Pasero & McCaffery, 2011). Data also supports the fact that premature infants, who have experienced pain, develop an increased sensitivity to pain (Johnston & Stevens, 1996).

An infant communicates pain and distress via inconsolable crying and screaming, and through changes in facial expressions and behaviors. This is supported by many neonate and infant/pediatric pain behavior tools (see Table 7.4) that allow the nurse to safely monitor the infant for changes in behavior/facial expression/body movement. The knowledge of pain in infants will assist the pediatric orthopaedic nurse when caring for with infants who may be born with genetic defects related to painful bone and connective tissues, such as osteogenesis imperfecta.

Opioid analgesics and anesthetics were thought to be unsafe for infants due to the infant inability to metabolize and eliminate drugs, and their sensitivity to respiratory depression due to their small size and immature organs (Pasero & McCaffery, 2011). If the pharmacodynamics of these drugs are understood by the health professional, however, and the infant is closely monitored in a setting where resuscitation is immediately available, analgesics can safely be administered for infant pain relief. Monitoring and assessing for behavior changes is key to evaluating the analgesic effectiveness and screening for safety.

Pain in Elders

Pain in elders is a growing concern in society today as the "Baby Boomer" generations are approaching the age of Social Security eligibility. A thorough understanding of the body changes during the aging process will assist the nurse when caring for the older adult. Aging leads to loss of lean muscle, decrease of total body water, and an overall increased percentage of adipose tissue. This change in the redistribution results in fat-soluble medications remaining in the system longer and water-soluble medications being more concentrated (Robeck, 2012). Other pathophysiology changes that are unique to the older adult include the decreased surface area of the small bowel, resulting in constipation and decreased liver metabolism, thus causing slower metabolism of medication. Renal insufficiency results in a slower clearance of the water-soluble medication.

The cumulative effect of cognitive changes in the older adult with memory and sensory impairment (seeing, hearing), coupled with the number of different health care providers they may see, poses a unique challenge. The greater the number of consultants the patient sees, the higher the risk of medication interaction and possible medication duplication with generic and trade name medication. An example of this is the hidden acetaminophen listed as different names in OTC and prescription medications that may lead to unintended acetaminophen toxicity. Older adult medication guidelines include carrying a complete list of their medications. When dosage adjustments are necessary, titrate analgesia to effect. "Start low and go slow" at a third to half the usual adult dosage. A simple drug regimen should be used for pain relief, and potential side effects of medication should be evaluated.

Summary

Pain is a phenomenon that occurs across the lifespan, from the newborn to the end of life. The pain of the orthopaedic patient is complex and dynamic, whether acute or chronic. The combination of acute and chronic pain arises from multiple pain generators. If not treated aggressively with a multimodal interdisciplinary approach, this may result in a life-long pain issue.

As the bridge between the patient and physician, pharmacist, physical therapist, and any other member of the health care team, the nurse is an advocate for every patient in pain. Pain assessment, intervention, and reassessment are the keys to all pain treatment plans. The nurse assists in the alleviation of pain through thorough knowledge of pain management, both pharmacologic and nonpharmacologic. Nonpharmacologic methods are well-known to the bedside nurse, such as use of heat, cold, and repositioning techniques to provide comfort. Pharmacologic knowledge, including dosage and routes of medication administration, and basic math skills are essential tools that the nurse needs to adequately care for patients.

Special populations, including the cognitively impaired, the elderly, addicted patients, and children, each have their own special requirements. The nurse's knowledge of pharmacologic, metabolic, and developmental changes provides the basis for developing and implementing the patient's individualized treatment plan.

Pain Resources

Agency for Healthcare Research and Quality: www.guidelines.gov

American Academy of Pain Medicine: www.painmed.org

American Cancer Society: www.cancer.org

American Chronic Pain Association: www.theacpa.org

American Pain Society: www.ampainsoc.org

American Pain Foundation: www.painfoundation.org

American Society of Addiction Medicine: www.asam.org

American Pain Society: www.ampainsoc.org

American Society of Pain Management Nursing: www.aspmn.org

American Society of Perianesthesia Nurses: www.aspan.org

American Society of Regional Anesthesia & Pain Medication: www.asra.com

Arthritis Foundation: www.arthritis.org

Behavioral Pain Tools – City of Hope Pain Resource Center: http://prc.coh.org/

End of Life/Palliative Education Resource Center (EPERC): www.eperc.mcw.edu

M. D. Anderson Cancer Center's Complementary/Integrative Medicine Education Resources: www.mdanderson.org

Neuropathy Association: www.neuropathy.org

National Cancer Institute at the National Institutes of Health: www.cancer.gov/cancertopics

Reflex Sympathetic Dystrophy Syndrome Association: www.rsds.org

Wisconsin Pain Initiative: www.wisc.edu/wcpi

References

American Academy of Orthopaedic Surgeons (AAOS). (2011). *The Burden of Musculoskeletal Diseases in the United States* (2nd ed.). Rosemont, IL: American Academy of Orthopaedic Surgeons. Retrieved from http://www.boneandjointburden.org/

American College of Physicians (ACP). (n.d.). *Chronic Pain Management Charts.* Retrieved from http://www.acpinternist.org/archives/2008/01/extra/pain_charts.pdf

American Medical Association (AMA). (2010). *Module 1 Pain Management: Pathophysiology of Pain and Pain Assessment.* Retrieved from http://www.ama-cmeonline.com/pain_mgmt/printversion/ama_painmgmt_m1.pdf

American Pain Society (APS). (2003). *Principles of Analgesic Use in the Treatment of Acute and Cancer Pain* (5th ed). Glenview, IL: APS.

American Society of Pain Management Nurses (ASPMN). (2010). *ASPMN Position Statement: Use of Placebos for Pain Management.* Pensacola, FL: ASPMN. Retrieved from http://www.aspmn.org/Organization/documents/Placebo_Position_FINAL.pdf

American Society of Regional Anesthesia and Pain Medicine (ASRA). (2010). *Anticoagulation* (3rd ed.) Retrieved from http://www.asra.com/publications-anticoagulation-3rd-edition-2010.php

American Nurses Association (ANA). (2001). *Code of Ethics for Nurses with Interpretive Statements.* Silver Springs, MD: Americian Nurses Publishing.

Atkinson, J.H., Kremer, E.F., & Garfin, S.R. (1985). Psychopharmacological agents in the treatment of pain. *The Journal of Bone & Joint Surgery, 67*(2), 337-342.

Ballantyne, J. (Ed.). (2002). *The Massachusetts General Hospital Handbook of Pain Management* (2nd ed.). Philadelphia, PA: Lippincott Williams & Wilkins.

Berry, P.H., Chapman, C.R., Covington, E.C., Dahl, J.L., Katz, J.A., Miaskowski, C. & McLean, M.J. (Eds.). (2006). *Pain: Current Understanding of Assessment, Management and Treatments.* Retrieved from http://www.npcnow.org/App_Themes/Public/pdf/Issues/pub_related_research/pub_quality_care/Pain-Current-Understanding-of-Assessment-Management-and-Treatments.pdf

Cassileth, B., & Gubili, J. (2010). Complementary therapies for pain management. In A. Kofp & N.B. Patel (Eds.), *Guide to Pain Management in Low Resource Settings* (pp. 59-64). Seattle, WA: IASP Press.

Centers for Disease Control and Prevention (CDC). (2010). *NHIS Arthritis Surveillance.* Retrieved from http://www.cdc.gov/arthritis/data_statistics/national_nhis.htm#future

Chou, R., Quaseem, A., Snow, V., Casey, D., Cross, T., Shekelle, P., & Owens, D. (2007). Diagnosis and treatment of low back pain: A joint clinical practice guideline from the Americian College of Physicians and the American Pain Society. *Annals of Internal Medicine, 147*(7), 478-491.

D'Arcy, Y. (2010). Treating pain in addicted patients. *Advance for Nurse Practitioners, 18*(5), 20-25.

Dworkin, R.H., O'Connor, A.B., Backonja, M., Farrar, J.T., Finnerup, N.B., Jensen, T.S., …Wallace, M.S. (2007). Pharmacologic management of neuropathic pain: Evidence-based recommendations. *Pain, 132*(3), 237-251.

Elcigil, A., Maltepe, H., Esrefgil, G., & Mutafoglu, K., (2011). Nurses' perceived barriers to assessment and management of pain in a university hospital. *Journal of Pediatric Hematology/Oncology, 33,* S33-S38.

Fine, P.G., Portenoy, R.K., & Ad Hoc Expert Panel on Evidence Review and Guidelines for Opioid Rotation. (2009). Establishing best practices for opioid rotation: Conclusions of an expert panel. *Journal of Pain Symptom Management, 38*(3), 418-425.

Fishman, S.M., Ballantyne, J.C., & Rathmell, J.P. (Eds.). (2010). *Bonica's Management of Pain* (4th ed.). Philadelphia, PA: Lippincott Williams and Wilkins.

Gaskin, D. & Richard, P. (2012). The economic costs of pain in the United States. *Journal of Pain, 13*(8), 715-724. Retrieved from http://www.jpain.org/article/S1526-5900(12)00559-7/fulltext

Gilron, I.C., Watson, P.N., Cahill, C.M., & Moulin, D.E. (2006). Neuropathic pain: A practical guide for the clinician. *Canadian Medical Association Journal, 175*(3), 1-20.

Gordon, D.B. & Dahl, J.L. (n.d.). *#095 Opioid Withdrawal* (2nd ed.). Retrieved from http://www.eperc.mcw.edu/EPERC/FastFactsIndex/ff_095.htm

Gulanick, M. & Myers, J. (2010). *Nursing Care Plans: Nursing Diagnosis and Intervention.* St. Louis, MO: Mosby.

Herr, K., Coyne, P., Key, T., Manworren, R., McCaffery, M., Merkel, S.,...Wild, L. (2006). Pain assessment in the nonverbal patient: Position statement with clinical practice recommendations. *Pain Management Nursing, 7*(2), 44-52.

Institute for Safe Medical Practices (ISMP). (2009). *ISMP Medication Safety Alert!* Retrieved from http://www.ismp.org/newsletters/acutecare/archives/Mar09.asp

Institute of Medicine. (2011). *Relieving Pain in America: A Blueprint for Transforming Prevention, Care, Education, and Research.* Retrieved from http://www.iom.edu/Reports/2011/Relieving-Pain-in-America-A-Blueprint-for-Transforming-Prevention-Care-Education-Research.aspx

International Association for the Study of Pain (IASP). (2011). Acute pain management in newborn infants. *Pain Clinical Updates, 19*(6), 1. Retrieved from http://www.iasp-pain.org/AM/AMTemplate.cfm?Section=2005_2006_Pain_in_Children1&SECTION=2005_2006_Pain_in_Children1&CONTENTID=15068&TEMPLATE=/CM/ContentDisplay.cfm

Johnston, C.C. & Stevens, B.J. (1996). Experience in a neonatal intensive care unit affects pain response. *Pediatrics, 98*(5), 925-930.

Kaplan, B. (2010). Hospice versus palliative care: Understanding the distinction. *Oncology Nurse Advisor*. Retrieved from http://www.oncologynurseadvisor.com/hospice-versus-palliative-care-understanding-the-distinction/article/168852/

Kost, M. (1998). *Manual of Conscious Sedation.* Philadelphia, PA: W.B. Saunders Company.

McCaffery, M. (1968). *Nursing Practice Theories Related to Cognition, Bodily Pain, and Man-Environment Interactions.* Los Angeles, CA: UCLA Students' Store.

McCaffery, M. & Beebe, A. (1993). *Pain: Clinical Manual for Nursing Practice.* Baltimore, MD: V.V. Mosby Company.

McCaffery, M., Herr, K., & Pasero, C. (2011). Assessment. In C. Pasero & M. McCaffery, *Pain Assessment and Pharmacologic Management.* St. Louis, MO: Mosby, Inc.

McCaffery, M. & Pasero, C. (1999). *Pain: Clinical Manual* (2nd ed.). St. Louis, MO: Mosby, Inc.

Menigaux, C., Adam, F., Guignard, B., Sessler, D., & Chauvin, M. (2005). Preoperative gabapentin decreases anxiety and improves early functional recovery from knee surgery. *Anesthesia & Analgesia, 100*(5), 1394-1399.

Merskey, H. & Bogduk, N. (1994). *Classification of Chronic Pain, International Association for the Study of Pain Task Force on Taxonomy* (2nd ed.). Seattle, WA: IASP Press.

Miaskowski, C.A., Payne, R., & Jones, W.K. (2005). *Breakthroughs and Challenges in the Management of Common Chronic Pain Conditions: Focus on Neuropathic Pain.* Califon, NJ: IMED Communications.

Moos, D. (2011). Understanding peripheral nerve blocks. *OR Nurse, 5*(5), 24-32.

Moulin, D., Clark, A., Gilron, I., Ware, M., Watson, C., Sessle, B.,… Velly, A. (2007). Pharmacological management of chronic neuropathic pain: Consensus statement and guidelines from the Canadian Pain Society. *Pain Research & Management, 12*(1), 13-21.

National Cancer Institute. (n.d.) *Pain (PDQ@) Overview.* Retrieved from http://www.cancer.gov/cancertopics/pdq/supportivecare/pain/HealthProfessional.

Orunta, I., Cairns, C., & Greene, R. (2005). Improving the safety of epidural analgesia. *The Pharmacological Journal, 275*(7363), 228-231.

Pascarelli, P. (1996). The role of the nurse during intravenous conscious sedation. *Orthopaedic Nursing, 15*(6), 23-25.

Pasero, C. (2004). Pathophysiology of neuropathic pain. *Pain Management Nursing, 5*(4), 3-8.

Pasero, C., Eksterowicz, N., Primeau, M., & Cowley, C. (2007). Registered Nurse management and monitoring of analgesia by catheter techniques: Position statement. *Pain Management Nursing, 8*(2), 48-54.

Pasero, C. & McCaffery, M. (2011). *Pain Assessment and Pharmacologic Management.* St. Louis, MO: Mosby, Inc.

Pasero, C., Polomano, R. C., Portenoy, R.K., McCaffery, M. (2011). Adjuvant analgesics. In C. Pasero & M. McCaffery, *Pain Assessment and Pharmacologic Management* (pp. 623-818). St. Louis, MO: Mosby, Inc.

Pasero, C. & Portenoy, R.K. (2011). Neurophysiology of pain and analgesia and the pathophysiology of neuropathic pain. In C. Pasero & M. McCaffery, *Pain Assessment and Pharmacologic Management* (pp. 1-12). St. Louis, MO: Mosby, Inc.

Pasero, C., Portenoy, R.K., & McCaffery, M. (2011). Nonopioid analgesics. In C. Pasero & M. McCaffery, *Pain Assessment and Pharmacologic Management* (pp. 177-276). St. Louis, MO: Mosby, Inc.

Pasero, C., Quinn, T.E., Portenoy, R.K., McCaffery, M., & Rizos, A. (2011). Opioid analgesics. In C. Pasero & M. McCaffery, *Pain Assessment and Pharmacologic Management* (pp. 277-622). St. Louis, MO: Mosby, Inc.

Polomano, R.C., Dunwoody, C.J., Krenzischek, D.A., & Rathmell, J.P. (2008). Perspective on pain management in the 21st century. *Pain Management Nursing, 23*(1 Suppl), S4-14.

Portenoy, R.K. (2007) Treatment of pain. *The Merck Manual Home Health Handbook.* Retrieved from http://www.merckmanuals.com/home/brain_spinal_cord_and_nerve_disorders/pain/treatment_of_pain.html

PubMed Health. (2012). *Serotonin Syndrome: Hyperserotonemia; Serotonergic Syndrome.* Retrieved from http://www.ncbi.nlm.nih.gov/pubmedhealth/PMH0004531/

Rapp, C.J. & Gordon, D.B. (2000). Understanding equianalgesic dosing. *Orthopaedic Nursing, 19*(3), 65-71.

Robeck, I. (2012). Chronic pain in the elderly: Special challenges. *Practical Pain Management, 12*(2), 30-43.

Sansone, R.A. & Sansone, L.A. (2008). Pain, pain, go away: Antidepressants and pain management. *Psychiatry (Edgmont), 5*(12), 16–19.

Scholz, J. & Woolf, C. (2002). Can we conquer pain? *Nature Neuroscience, 5,* 1062-1067.

Turjanica, M., (2007). Postoperative continuous peripheral nerve blockade in the lower extremity total joint arthroplasty population. *MEDSURG Nursing, 16*(3), 151-154.

The Joint Commission. (2008). *What You Should Know About Pain Management.* Retrieved from www.jointcommission.org.

Vargas-Schaffer, G. (2010). Is the WHO ladder still valid? *Canadian Family Physician, 56*(6), 514-517.

Warden, V., Hurley, A., & Volicer, L. (2003). Development and psychometric evaluation of the Pain Assessment in Advanced Dementia (PAINAD) Scale. *Journal of the American Medical Directors Association, 4*(1), 9-15.

Whedon, M. & Ferrell, B. (1991). Professional and ethical considerations in the use of high-tech pain management. *Oncology Nursing Forum, 18*(7), 1135-1143.

Whiteman, A. & Stephens, R.C. (2010). Epidurals and their care on a surgical ward. *British Journal of Hospital Medicine, 71*(3), M41-3.

Wilkie, D., Huang, H., Reilly, N., & Cain, K. (2001). Nociceptive and neuropathic pain in patients with lung cancer. *Journal of Pain and Symptom Management, 22*(5), 899-910.

Woelk, C.J. (2007). The hand that writes the opioid… *Canadian Family Physician, 53*(6), 1015–1017.

World Health Organization (WHO). (1996). *Cancer Pain Relief* (2nd ed.). Retrieved from http://whqlibdoc.who.int/publications/9241544821.pdf

CHAPTER
7

Chapter 8
Orthopaedic Complications

Rebecca Parker, MSN, RN, CNL, ONC

CHAPTER 8

Objectives

- Explain the importance of preventing orthopaedic complications.
- Outline assessment techniques for orthopaedic complications.
- Relate the pathophysiology to the clinical manifestations of orthopaedic complications.
- Describe nursing interventions to enhance patient outcomes.
- Determine patients at risk for specific complications and apply strategies to prevent complications from occurring.
- Explain recommended treatment plans for complications from orthopaedic injury or surgery.
- Highlight discharge education needs of the patient for constipation, VTE, SSI, pneumonia, nonunion, and pressure ulcer.

Complications of orthopaedic injury or surgery can lead to disability, loss of limb, or, on rare occasion, loss of life. Some are avoidable, while others are not. Knowing about various complications and interventions for prevention helps the orthopaedic nurse provide the best care possible. Patients most at risk for complications are older adults and those with comorbid conditions such that they have an American Society of Anesthesiologists (ASA) classification of 3 or greater. The ASA classification defines the physical status of a patient from healthy (1) to dying (5). A classification of 3 signifies that the patient has a severe systemic disease (Unbeck, Dalen, Muren, Lillkrona, & Harenstam, 2010). A patient's home medications, poor nutritional status, and the type of injury also influence the incidence of complication. Developing a complication means a longer length of hospital stay and delayed healing (Unbeck et al., 2010). Awareness of possible complications, with the knowledge of what to do if a complication arises, will improve patient outcomes, relieve patient anxiety, and enhance patient comfort.

Delirium

Overview

Delirium is defined by an abrupt onset of a cluster of fluctuating, transient changes, coupled with disturbances in consciousness, cognition, and perception in medically ill patients. Delirium is also referred to as a hyperkinetic confusional state, which is further delineated as a type of acute confusional state. During states of delirium, there is an association with the right middle temporal gyrus or left temporo-occiptal junction disruption within the brain. These areas receive extensive input from the limbic areas to modulate motivational and affective aspects of attention. A disruption of the cholinergic pathways, critical for attention and arousal, also occurs within the brain (Boss, 2010). Despite this knowledge, the overall pathophysiology of delirium in poorly understood (Juliebo et al., 2009; Inouye, 2006).

Delirium can have an abrupt onset over 2-3 days. Early manifestations include difficulty concentrating, restlessness, irritability, insomnia, tremulousness, and poor appetite. Patients suffering from delirium may often present with incoherent conversation and appear perplexed or distressed. In a very small percentage of patients, seizures and even unpleasant or terrifying dreams may be experienced. In fully developed delirium states, there is complete inattentiveness and grossly altered perceptions and interpretations, with the possible presence of hallucinations. The duration of delirium is generally short but can vary patient to patient; however, for some patients, delirium may persist over several weeks. Generally, resolution will begin to occur gradually over 2-3 days and up to 10-12 days. Resolution may occur more quickly with early identification and addressing of causative factors (Boss, 2010; Inouye, 2006; Neitzel, Sendelbach, & Larson, 2007).

Incidences of delirium vary greatly within the literature. It mainly occurs in the elderly; very rarely does it occur in children and young adults. Overall postoperative delirium is estimated to occur in about 20% of patients ages 65 and older (Inouye, 2006). The incidence rate of delirium for patients who sustain a hip fracture is greater than 35% postoperatively (Juliebo et al., 2009). Neitzel, Sendelbach, and Larson (2007) determined a range of incidence from 5.1% to 61% in the orthopaedic patient. Regardless of the incidence of delirium, it is often under-recognized by health care professionals.

The cause and risk factors for delirium are often multifactorial. Risk factors can be delineated by predisposing (or preoperative) causes and precipitating (or intraoperative/postoperative) causes (see Table 8.1). Interplay between predisposing factors and precipitating factors increases the patient's chances of developing delirium (Inouye, 2006). In the preoperative category, preexisting cognitive impairment such as underlying dementia is a strong risk factor for delirium (Juliebo et al., 2009; Monk & Price, 2011).

Complications of delirium may include longer lengths of stay in the hospital and the associated increased health care costs. During hospitalization, patients who experience delirium are at an increased mortality risk. Due to the confusional state associated with delirium, patients are at a much higher risk for falls and injury related to falls. A patient being treated for a fracture is less likely to recover prefracture levels of function and ambulation, which could lead to long-term care placement. Patients may experience long-term cognitive impairment, in addition to the functional impairment, further requiring the need for extended long-term or skilled care placement (Neitzel, Sendelbach, & Larson, 2007).

One of the main prevention strategies for delirium is early identification of the modifiable risk factors—and the elimination or minimization of those risk factors. Strategies may include continued orientation of the at-risk patient, early mobilization, use of visual and hearing aids, prevention of dehydration, uninterrupted sleep time, and reduction of the use of psychoactive drugs. Correction of fluid and electrolyte imbalances, proper pain management, correction of hypoxia, regulation of bowel and bladder function, nonpharmacological approaches to sleep and anxiety management, and nutrition maintenance are also beneficial with the prevention of delirium (Young & Inouye, 2007; Tullman, Mion, Flectcher, & Foreman, 2008; Sendelbach & Guthrie, 2009; Inouye, 2006; Evans & Kurlowicz, 2007).

Assessment

History. When assessing patients who may be suffering from delirium, it is important to determine the cause of the acute medical problem with a full evaluation. By obtaining a thorough clinical history, physical examination, and laboratory studies, a more accurate diagnosis of delirium can be made versus other causes of confusion (Evans & Kurlowicz, 2007). Obtaining an accurate baseline of the patient's mental status from family members and nursing staff who have cared for the patient is helpful in determining the presence of delirium.

Physical Exam. By performing exams that test the mental status of the patient, the presence of delirium can be determined. The Mini-Mental Status Examination (MMSE) is a screening test to assess cognition and may be completed on patients with suspected delirium; however, MMSE is a more time-consuming exam that requires specific expertise. Two other informal behavior observation instruments can be performed prior to this formalized testing: the Confusion Assessment Scale (CAS) and the Confusion Assessment Method (CAM) diagnostic algorithm can be effectively done by health care providers using observation techniques with a high degree of sensitivity and specificity for accurately determining the presence of delirium. For rapid evaluation of acute confusion, the Neelon and Champagne (NEECHAM) Confusion Scale can be completed at the bedside by the nurse during the routine assessment and overall patient interaction (Neitzel et al., 2007; Evans & Kurlowicz, 2007).

Diagnostic Tests. Depending upon the results of the history and physical, various diagnostic tests may be completed to determine if there are any other underlying causes of delirium. Diagnostic tests may include a complete blood count (CBC), serum albumin, liver enzyme levels, thyroid function tests, comprehensive metabolic profile (specifically looking for hyponatremia and potassium imbalances), and urinalysis to rule out urinary tract infection (Evans & Kurlowicz, 2007; Boss, 2010). Chest radiographs and electrocardiography are usually performed to determine if underlying respiratory infections or arrhythmias exist. Depending on the severity of delirium, practitioners may order radiologic studies such as computerized tomography (CT) scans of the brain and evaluation of cerebral spinal fluid. Electroencephalography may also be used if there is difficulty differentiating between delirium and other acute psychotic states (Neitzel et al., 2007; Evans, & Kurlowicz, 2007)

CHAPTER 8

Table 8.1. Delirium Risk Factors

Predisposing Risk Factors (Preoperative)	Precipitating Risk Factors (Intraoperative or Postoperative)
■ Age of 65 or older ■ Alcohol abuse ■ BMI<20 kg/m2 ■ Coexisting medical conditions (i.e. chronic renal/hepatic disease, neurological disease, history of stroke, HIV, severe or terminal illness) ■ Fracture upon admission to hospital ■ Injury occurred indoors ■ Male ■ Polypharmacy ■ Underlying cognitive impairment (i.e. dementia, history of delirium, depression) ■ Underlying poor functional status ■ Underlying visual/hearing impairment	■ Alcohol withdrawal ■ American Society of Anesthesiologists group 3, 4, or 5 ■ Anesthesia ■ Bladder catheterization ■ Dehydration ■ Electrolyte derangements (i.e. hypoglycemia, hypercalcemia, hyponatremia, hypokalemia) ■ Environment ■ Hemoglobin <12.9 g/dl ■ Hypoxia ■ Immobilization ■ Infection (particularly urinary tract and respiratory) ■ Metabolic disturbances (i.e. azotemia, pH alterations, malnutrition, dehydration) ■ Pain ■ Polypharmacy ■ Restraint use ■ Sedative/hypnotic withdrawal ■ Sleep deprivation ■ Use of high-dose opioids, anticholinergic drugs, and benzodiazepines

Data from "Complex Care Needs in Older Adults with Common Cognitive Disorders" by L. Evans & L. Kurlowicz, http://www.ngna.org; "Delirium in Older Persons" by S. Inouye, 2006, New England Journal of Medicine, *354, 1157-1165; "Risk Factors for Preoperative and Postoperative Delirium in Elderly Patients with Hip Fracture" by V. Juliebo et al., 2009,* Journal of the American Geriatrics Society, *57(8), 1354-1361; "Postoperative Cognitive Disorders" by T. Monk & C. Price, 2011,* Current Opinion in Critical Care, *17(4), 376-381; "Delirium in the Orthopaedic Patient" by Neitzel et al., 2007,* Orthopaedic Nursing, *26(6), 354-363; and "Delirium in Older People" by J. Young, & S. Inouye, 2007,* British Medical Journal, *334(7598), 842-846.*

Common Therapeutic Modalities

Once the diagnosis of delirium is made, immediate identification and treatment of precipitating factors is the most critical approach to the management (Young & Inouye, 2007). It is important to discontinue medications that may be causing delirium unless issues may occur due to the withdrawal of the medication (Boss, 2010; Young & Inouye, 2007). It is important to manage hypoxia, provide adequate hydration and nutrition, mobilize the patient, and provide supportive measures to keep the patient safe during this time (Boss, 2010). Any underlying infections should be managed with prompt identification and appropriate treatment (Tullman, Mion, Fletcher, & Foreman, 2008).

The use of low-dose haloperidol may be effective on limiting duration and severity of postoperative delirium (Young & Inouye, 2007; Sendelbach & Guthrie, 2009; Evans & Kurlowicz, 2007). Haloperidol can also be effective for patients who are distressed or are considered a risk to themselves or others (National Collaborating Centre for Acute and Chronic Conditions, 2010).

Nursing Considerations

Nursing Diagnoses. Nursing diagnoses for this condition are expanded upon in the Appendix.

- Confusion, acute.
- Falls, risk for.
- Injury, risk for.
- Memory, impaired.
- Sensory perception, disturbed.
- Sleep pattern, disturbed.

Interventions. Overall, the interventions that should be employed with delirium include assessment of predisposing or precipitating risk factors, assessment for delirium with a valid exam, and multicomponents if the patient is suffering from delirium. Pharmacological interventions such as haloperidol may be needed if the patient is extremely anxious, agitated, or a potential risk to others. Ideally, primary prevention is the goal if the patient is identified as at-risk (Sendelbach, & Guthrie, 2009).

Patient Teaching. Patient teaching is not likely to be effective when a patient is experiencing delirium; however, education for family members/caregivers regarding the patient's status and interventions that they can provide may be helpful. Family can be encouraged to stay with the patient to enhance an environment of familiarity. Reassuring the family is also important, as the situation can be unknown to them (Inouye, 2006; Tullman et al., 2008).

Practice Setting Considerations. Due to the abrupt onset and acute nature of delirium, practice considerations are generally focused within the acute inpatient care setting. Prior to discharge from the hospital, patients should have had a thorough physical and diagnostic assessment to rule out other causes and have a resolution of symptoms prior to the discharge.

Pressure Ulcers

Overview

A pressure ulcer is an area of injury to the skin and underlying tissue. It usually occurs over a bony prominence and is the result of pressure, with or without the combination of shear or friction. Pressure ulcers occur when soft tissue is compressed between bony prominences and the support surface below. As pressure builds, the capillaries are unable to handle the pressure. This results in occluded blood flow, interstitial fluid flow, ischemia, pain, necrosis, and sloughing of dead tissue. Pressure over 32mm Hg exceeds the tolerated threshold and leads to collapse of vessels. The results are a deprivation of oxygen and nutrients and a build-up of waste. The resulting toxic metabolites cause edema,

Table 8.2. Pressure Ulcer Prevention and Management: Questions to Ask
Beds and aids ■ Suitable mattress for present clinical condition?
Assessment and documentation ■ Turn chart? ■ Skin assessment documented on care plan? ■ Risk assessment (Braden or Nelson) score up to date?
Nutrition ■ Dietician referral? ■ Nutritional supplement drinks given as appropriate?
Patient education ■ Patient information given? ■ Explanation given?
Mobility ■ How does patient transfer? ■ Patient sat out of bed as appropriate? ■ Turned every 2 hours as needed?
Continence ■ Incontinence aids in use? ■ Toileting schedule
Pressure ulcer development ■ Wound, Ostomy, and Continence Nurse (WOCN) referral? ■ Skin care products in use?

From "Reducing Pressure Ulcers in Hip Fracture Patients" by M. Thompson, 2011, British Journal of Nursing, *20(15), S10-S18, doi:10.1016/j.injury.2007.08.030.*

increased tissue perfusion, acidosis, and eventual cell death. While the healthy individual would receive a signal to the brain to change position, independent position change is not possible for the at-risk patient (Remaley & Jaeblon, 2010).

Pressure ulcers are staged from I-IV, as follows:

- Stage I: an area of reddened intact skin that is nonblanchable.
- Stage II: partially open skin with a red or pink wound bed. There is loss of dermis. This stage can also be serum-filled blisters that are intact or open.
- Stage III: full thickness skin loss. Subcutaneous fat may be visible, but bone, tendon, and/or muscle are not exposed.
- Stage IV: full thickness skin loss with exposed bone, tendon, or muscle (National Pressure Ulcer Advisory Panel [NPUAP], 2007).

Pressure ulcers can develop at any point in a hospitalization—preoperatively, intraoperatively, or postoperatively (Haleem, Heinert, & Parker, 2008). The literature has shown that surgical patients have an incidence of pressure ulcers of as high as 45% (Remaley & Jaeblon, 2010). Risk factors for developing a pressure ulcer are increased age, history of diabetes mellitus, anemia, malnourishment, low mental test scores, and impaired mobility. Surgical patients are at high risk for sensory loss from anesthesia, and surgical duration exceeding 2 hours places patients at higher risk. Orthopaedic risk factors include cast or brace immobilization, traction use, weight-bearing restrictions, and immobility (Remaley & Jaeblon, 2010).

Patients who develop pressure ulcers have higher morbidity and mortality rates. They have an increased infection risk that can lead to septicemia and osteomyelitis, with the possible need for surgical intervention. Osteomyelitis develops in 17% to 32% of pressure ulcers that become infected (Bluestein & Javaheri, 2008). Pressure ulcers increase the need for nursing care, and often delay discharge and postoperative rehabilitation (Remaley & Jaeblon, 2010).

Pressure ulcer prevention and management takes many forms; see Table 8.2. The first step in preventing pressure ulcers is to know if any are present on admission. Comprehensive skin assessment is a head-to-toe skin evaluation with particular emphasis over bony prominences. The goals of the comprehensive skin assessment are to identify any existing pressure ulcers and determine other skin conditions or factors that would predispose the patient to pressure ulcer development. The skin assessment is repeated on a regular basis to determine whether any changes in skin condition have occurred, typically once every shift.

The next prevention strategy is to identify patients at high risk of developing a pressure ulcer. The Norton Scale (see Table 8.3) and the Braden Scale (see Table 6.3 in Chapter 6—Orthopaedic Effects of Immobility) are widely used to determine this risk, with established reliability and validity. With both scales, a lower number indicates a higher risk of pressure ulcer development. A daily risk assessment with one of these scales provides a standardized process to identify patients at risk for developing pressure ulcer in order to implement plans for preventive care (Agency for Healthcare Research and Quality, n.d.). Risk assessment is information gathering about specific factors that place the patient at risk for pressure ulcer development such as immobility, decreased activity, and nutritional status (Magnan & Maklebust, 2009). Frequent repositioning moves

CHAPTER 8

Table 8.3. Norton Scale of Pressure Ulcer Risk

Physical Condition	Good	4	
	Fair	3	
	Poor	2	
	Very Bad	1	
Mental Condition	Alert	4	
	Apathetic	3	
	Confused	2	
	Stuporous	1	
Activity	Ambulant	4	
	Walks with help	3	
	Chair bound	2	
	Bedfast	1	
Mobility	Full	4	
	Slightly Impaired	3	
	Very Limited	2	
	Immobile	1	
Incontinence	None	4	
	Occasional	3	
	Usually Urinary	2	
	Urinary and Fecal	1	

Generally, the risk factor is coded this way:

Greater than 18	Low Risk
Between 18 and 14	Medium Risk
Between 14 and 10	High Risk
Lesser than 10	Very High Risk

From Nutrition 411, http://www.rd411.com/wrc/pdf/w0513_norton_presure_sore_risk_assessment_scale_scoring_system.pdf. Reprinted with permission.

the pressure spots around. To reduce pressure over bony prominences when a patient is sitting or lying, repositioning must be done at least every 2 hours. Minimize the amount of friction and shear the patient experiences during repositioning. Do not elevate the head of the bed greater than 30 degrees unless contraindicated. Prompt surgical intervention and early mobilization are other prevention strategies (Institute for Clinical Systems Improvement [ICSI], 2010). Nutrition status must be assessed to ensure that the patient's needs are being met (Remaley & Jaeblon, 2010).

Assessment

History. Scores from the risk assessment screening help the health care team identify if a patient is at risk of developing a pressure ulcer (Remaley & Jaeblon, 2010). Obtain information to determine the age and level of consciousness of the patient. Assess the patient's activity level, especially related to bedrest, immobility, and the ability to turn independently. Verify nutritional status because poor nutrition can alter wound healing. Determine if the patient has undergone recent surgery or trauma, experiences incontinence, or has decreased awareness of sensation (Mantik-Lewis, 2004).

Physical Exam. A comprehensive head-to-toe skin assessment is necessary for identification of pressure ulcer. After the initial skin assessment is completed, reassessments are done to monitor the skin to prevent pressure ulcer development. ICSI (2010) recommends that the initial skin assessment be completed within 6 hours of the patient's arrival, with reassessment to monitor for changes completed every 8-24 hours based on the patient's status. Skin assessment includes palpation, especially over bony prominences; changes in skin moisture, texture, or turgor; temperature that is different than the surrounding tissue; color changes; and consistency changes (ICSI, 2010). Any area of concern is documented, monitored, and addressed. Photography may be helpful in some circumstances to monitor progression (Remaley & Jaeblon, 2010).

Diagnostic Tests. Laboratory values, including albumin, pre-albumin, and total protein, monitor nutritional status for wound healing (Remaley & Jaeblon, 2010). CBC with specific monitoring of white blood cells is monitored for leukocytosis and indication of infection (Mantik-Lewis, 2004). X-ray may be ordered as needed. If osteomyelitis is suspected, magnetic resonance imaging (MRI) will assist to locate the infection within the bone, but recommendations are for a needle biopsy of the bone in order for antibiotic therapy (Bluestein & Javaheri, 2008).

Common Therapeutic Modalities

If a pressure ulcer develops, the ultimate goal is wound healing. This will be achieved in different ways, depending on the stage of the wound. In general, stage I wounds require a protective dressing. Stage II wounds need to be cleaned and covered with a moist dressing such as transparent film. Stage III and IV wounds need moist or absorbent dressings such as hydrogel, foam, or alginate. A surgical consult might be necessary if the wound is not healing as expected. A consult with a Wound, Ostomy, and Continence Nurse (WOCN) is appropriate for any patient with a pressure ulcer or with a high risk based on the score from the risk assessment. All wounds require appropriate cleansing initially and prior to any dressing change (Bluestein & Javaheri, 2008). Debridement is a possibility and might be surgical. Topical treatment and dressing changes will depend on the wound itself, and the rule to follow is to keep the wound bed and surrounding tissue moist. Adjunct therapies are sometimes appropriate, including electrical stimulation for Stage II, III, and IV pressure ulcers or negative pressure wound therapy for Stage III and IV pressure ulcers. It is important to remember to manage pain from the wound and to monitor the patient's nutritional status to ensure sufficient oral intake of fluids, protein, calories, Vitamin C, and zinc to help the wound heal. There are circumstances when the wound will require surgical repair by a plastic surgeon (ICSI, 2010).

Nursing Considerations

Nursing Diagnoses. Nursing diagnoses for this condition are expanded upon in the Appendix.

- Infection, risk for.
- Skin integrity, impaired.
- Tissue integrity, impaired.

Interventions. Because pressure ulcers are often avoidable, most nursing interventions are related to prevention. Turning and position changes should occur frequently because pressure ulcers can occur in as little as 2 hours of immobility (Remaley & Jaeblon, 2010). Minimize and eliminate friction and shear by using lift sheets to move the patient, elevate the head of the bed to 30 degrees, use transfer devices, avoid skin-to-skin or skin-to-equipment contact with padding, protect bony prominences with transparent film, and protect skin from moisture. Minimize pressure by encouraging the patient to shift weight if able to do so independently, or providing frequent position changes for them (every 2 hours while in bed and every 1 hour when up in a chair). Support surface interventions include reducing the layers of linen under the patient, floating the heels off the bed, positioning with pillows and wedges, turning every 2 hours, and using pressure redistribution mattresses. Manage moisture for the patient by eliminating incontinence with a toileting schedule or bowel/bladder program. Clean the skin after every incontinence episode, and use a moisture protectant barrier and absorbent pads to wick moisture. Monitor the patient's weight, laboratory values and oral intake, encouraging protein, calories, and fluids to maintain adequate nutrition (ICSI, 2010).

Patient Teaching. Families and caregivers outside of the hospital setting should be involved in education for patients with pressure ulcers. Explain the causes and prevention of pressure ulcers to help avoid new issues. Patients and families should also be taught dietary needs and signs of infection (ICSI, 2010). Provide education regarding proper positioning, the need for turning every 2 hours, and how to position to avoid pressure directly on the ulcer (Remaley & Jaeblon, 2010). Caregivers who will be inspecting the skin at home need to know about normal and abnormal tissue colors in order to recognize problem areas. If a pressure ulcer has already developed and dressing changes are needed, demonstrate exactly how to perform the dressing change, and explain the purpose for the dressing. Infection control and the importance of hand-washing are of utmost importance to prevent further complications (ICSI, 2010).

Practice Setting Considerations. Because pressure ulcers can develop at any point during or after a hospitalization, it is necessary to continue to complete thorough skin assessments after discharge, whether the patient is at home or a rehabilitation facility. Home care nurses will provide ongoing education to family members caring for the patient at home to ensure proper turning and wound care.

Constipation

Overview

The American Gastroenterology Association (2000) defines constipation as two or fewer stools per week, often accompanied by straining, hard stools, and feelings of incomplete evacuation. Constipation is a complaint of millions of people annually and one of the most common symptoms in postoperative patients (Ho, Kuhn, & Smith, 2008). Orthopaedic patients are often prescribed opioids for pain management. These medications have a well-known adverse effect of constipation (Ho et al., 2008). This uncomfortable side effect can also be due to diet changes, changes in daily routines, environmental constraints, ignoring the urge to defecate, chronic laxative use, depression, and stress (Zimmaro-Bliss & Sawchuk, 2004). While it is a common symptom among both genders and all age groups, constipation affects women more often than men; the rate increases with age for both genders (Ho et al., 2008; Dosh, 2002).

The symptoms of constipation can lead to extended hospital stays and patient discomfort (Behm & Stollman, 2003). It is possible for a paralytic, or postoperative, ileus to develop (Linari, Schofield, & Horrom, 2011; Behm & Stollman, 2003). An ileus is a temporary malfunction in the motility of the GI tract. In postoperative patients, ileus is usually associated with the use of opiates. Morphine has been shown to lessen peristalsis, slow stool passage, and increase water absorption in the lumen, which results in hard and dry stool (Behm & Stollman, 2003). Straining with the Valsalva maneuver can lead to feelings of dizziness and blacking out, as well as hemorrhoids and rectal prolapse (Zimmaro-Bliss & Sawchuk, 2004, National Digestive Diseases Informational Clearinghouse [NDDIC], 2007). Preventing constipation can begin with increasing fluid and fiber in the diet (Ho et al., 2008). Increased fiber requires increased fluid because water adds fluid to the colon that can be retained by the stool, adding bulk (NDDIC, 2007). When possible, avoid the use of medications that cause constipation. A number of medications are available to help treat the symptom of constipation and work to retain water, limit the absorption of water, and stimulate contractions in the colon (Ho et al., 2008). Mobilization and exercise help to prevent constipation. It is beneficial for the patient to be able to stimulate a home routine.

Assessment

History. Patients need ongoing assessment of their bowel elimination patterns while hospitalized. Descriptions of constipation symptoms, stool consistency, and normal bowel habits should be obtained (NDDIC, 2007). A history that includes normal elimination pattern, medication use, and any recent changes in diet, activity, lifestyle, routine, and mood will determine baseline data to compare elimination patterns in the hospital (Zimmaro-Bliss & Sawchuk, 2004).

Physical Exam. Assessment of the patient could present a number of clinical signs. These will include abdominal distention and pain, nausea, headache, anorexia, urinary retention, dizziness, stool with blood, stool that is hard and dry, increased flatulence, a palpable mass, and straining (Zimmaro-Bliss & Sawchuk, 2004).

Diagnostic Tests. While chronic constipation without a secondary cause requires a full examination to determine the cause, this is usually not necessary for the orthopaedic population. In some cases, abdominal radiography will be necessary identify if a mechanical blockage is present (Johnson & Walsh, 2009).

Common Therapeutic Modalities

When normal elimination pattern is not being reached, patients should be encouraged to increase fluid, fiber, and mobilization (Ho et al., 2008). Several different types of agents help treat constipation (see Table 8.4). Short-term use of laxatives can help reestablish normal pattern. Bulking agents such as psyllium and methylcellulose work to retain water in the stool. While they are the most

Table 8.4. Agents for Treatment of Constipation				
	Mechanism of Action	Example	Side Effects	Other
Bulking Agents	Retains water in the stool	Psyllium (Metamucil®), methylcellulose (Citricel®), wheat bran	Bloating, slow to work	Require liquids to work, safe and natural, first line for chronic constipation
Osmotic	Creates an osmotic gradient to retain water in intestinal lumen	Magnesium hydroxide (Milk of Magnesia®), polyethylene glycol (MiraLax®)	Diarrhea, hypovolemia, electrolyte imbalance	Appropriate for chronic constipation
Stool Softeners	Softened stool is formed by an interaction between stool and water	Docusate sodium/calcium	Minimal	Appropriate for occasional constipation
Stimulating Laxatives	Inhibits water absorption and stimulates colon mucosal sensory nerve endings	Senna (Senokot®), bisacodyl (Dulcolax®)	Abdominal discomfort, electrolyte imbalance, hepatotoxicity, cathertic colon	Appropriate for occasional constipation, not for chronic use

Data from "Evaluation and Treatment of Constipation" by S. Dosh, 2002, Journal of Family Practice, 51*(6), p. 555-9; and "Update on Treatment Options for Constipation" by J. Ho, R. Kuhn, & K. Smith, 2008,* Orthopedics, 31*(6), 570-4.*

effective and natural agent, bloating can occur with the use of bulking agents, and they are slow to begin working. Patients must ingest liquid as directed for bulking agents to work effectively. Osmotic laxatives such as milk of magnesia and polyethylene glycol cause water retention in the intestinal lumen. Stool softeners such as docusate sodium and docusate calcium soften stool with interaction between water and stool. Stimulating laxatives should be limited to short-term use and work by inhibiting water absorption and stimulating colon mucosal sensory nerve endings (Ho et al., 2008; Dosh, 2002). Peripherally selective opioid antagonists, which reverse the GI slowing without reversing the effect of the opioid analgesia, are being studied for the treatment of opioid-induced bowel dysfunction and postoperative ileus (Ho et al., 2008).

Nursing Considerations

Nursing Diagnoses. Nursing diagnoses for this condition are expanded upon in the Appendix.

- Constipation, risk for.
- Gastrointestinal motility, dysfunctional.
- Pain, acute.

Interventions. Encourage adequate fluids and a diet high in fiber. Constipation can be overcome by helping patients to follow their same strategies and routines as at home (NDDIC, 2007). Providing privacy for the patient will help promote defecation, as will proper positioning. If using a bedpan, positioning the patient with the head of the bed elevated as high as possible will increase success (Zimmaro-Bliss & Sawchuk, 2004). Encourage physical activity and mobility by assisting the patient out of bed as allowed.

Patient Teaching. Educate patients that everyone has different bowel habits. Defecation can occur as often as multiple times daily or as few as 3 times a week. Constipation is an adverse effect of many pain medications. Ensure that patients understand why they need to mobilize and how much fluid and fiber to consume on a daily basis. Fiber will only be successful with fluid as assistance. Use medication as needed at home to promote defecation, but do not use laxatives chronically. Because the reflexes that assist in peristalsis in the colon are most active after the morning meal, encourage patients to attempt defecation at this time of the day.

Practice Setting Considerations. Orthopaedic patients are often discharged with opioid medication to manage pain, leading to constipation. Home care and follow-up office appointments must ascertain the patient's bowel habits and if they differ from the patient's norm. Encourage the patient to increase fiber and fluid intake. If the patient is using opioids, encourage adding a stool softener to their home medications while on the opioid.

Hemorrhage/Significant Blood Loss

Overview

Hemorrhage is acute blood loss. It can be caused by trauma, surgical complications, or interrupted vascular integrity. Management of hemorrhage depends on whether the blood loss is sudden or gradual. When loss is sudden, hypovolemic shock can occur because of the reduction in the total blood volume. When the loss is gradual, the number of red blood cells (RBCs) that are available to carry oxygen to the body is reduced, although blood volume is maintained with an increase in plasma volume (Jones, 2004). Total joint replacement surgeries can have estimated blood loss of 500-1500cc, and it is common for hemoglobin to fall 1-3g/dL postoperatively

(Krebs, Higuera, Barsoum, & Helfand, 2006). Surgical procedures account for two thirds of blood transfusions (Keating & Meding, 2002).

Patients at higher risk of blood loss have a history of bleeding or pathologic conditions. Anticoagulants, aspirin, and non-steroidal anti-inflammatory drugs increase the risk of bleeding. Abnormal bleeding time or platelet count can also increase risk of blood loss (Halpern & Manion, 2009). Blood loss has been found to be greater in men. A study by Prasad, Padmanabhan, and Mullaji (2007) showed that longer tourniquet use during surgery correlated to higher blood loss after surgery. Intraoperative blood management is influenced by surgical technique. The use of antifibrinolytic agents such as Tranexamic acid and aminocaproic acid have shown benefits in decreasing intraoperative blood loss by boosting the clotting mechanism (Friedman, 2010). Kagoma (2009) showed that, in total knee arthroplasty and total hip arthroplasty, the antifibrinolytic agents reduced bleeding by at least 300cc and reduced transfusion need by 50%. Complications from hemorrhage include increased length of stay after elective surgery and decreased postoperative strength that can delay therapy, as well as shock and death (Keating & Meding, 2002).

Assessment

History. Knowledge about recent blood loss or trauma is an important part of assessment. Any recent surgery that the patient has undergone should also be known. The patient's use of medications, including aspirin, anticoagulants, and NSAIDs, can lead to increased bleeding risk (Coyer & Lash, 2008). Guidelines from American Society of Anesthesiologists, Inc. (ASA) require preoperative knowledge of the patient's medication history, medication history, preoperative labs, and a discussion regarding autologous blood transfusions (2006). A number of herbal supplements and vitamins can affect blood loss, including fish oil, flax seed oil, garlic, ginger, gingko biloba, chamomile, Vitamin E, and Vitamin K. Anticoagulants must be addressed prior to surgery to eliminate the risk of blood loss (ASA, 2006).

Physical Exam. The patient will experience different symptoms, depending on the amount of blood loss experienced. Patients can have pale skin and pale mucous membranes with poor skin turgor. Tachypnea, ankle edema, confusion, irritability, and unsteady gait can also be present. Tachycardia and postural hypotension are likely to be present (Coyer & Lash, 2008; Jones, 2004). Fatigue is a common complaint, and the patient may experience lightheadedness when standing (Coyer & Lash, 2008). Hypovolemic shock can occur with a direct loss of blood. Symptoms in the early signs of shock include low urine output, tachycardia and tachypnea, a change in pulse pressure, and cool and pale extremities. Symptoms in the late stage of shock include hypotension, altered level of consciousness, confusion, and oliguria (Mulryan, 2009).

Diagnostic Tests. Laboratory values will reflect lower RBCs in CBC, hemoglobin, and hematocrit values. The ASA (2006) support autologous transfusion when hemoglobin is less than 6g/dL and holding transfusion for hemoglobin greater than 10g/dL. A transfusion for hemoglobin results between these ranges needs to take into account organ ischemia, potential for bleeding, and patient risk factors (ASA, 2006). Labs to be expecting are CBC, PTT, PT, thrombin time, type and cross, chemistry profile, and ABGs (Stainsby, MacLennan, Thomas, Isaac, & Hamilton, 2006). When the bleeding is unable to be visibly located, radiography, ultrasound, or CT scan will be helpful to discover the location (Halpern & Manion, 2009). Anticipate blood typing for blood transfusion (Halpern & Manion, 2009). Follow hemoglobin and hematacrit levels after a procedure or transfusion (Jones, 2004).

Common Therapeutic Modalities

With any sudden blood loss, health care personnel must locate the hemorrhage and terminate the bleeding (Jones, 2004). Once the source is located, halting the bleeding is achieved through early surgical intervention or interventional radiology procedures (Stainsby et al., 2006). Treatment of hemorrhage is aimed at replacing blood volume to prevent shock. This can be done with IV fluids or blood transfusion. Warmed crystalloid or colloid is used as needed, as are saline, dextran, albumin, and plasma (Stainsby et al., 2006; Coyer & Lash, 2008). Blood transfusion can be either allogenic or autologous. Allogenic is the mainstay but carries with it risks such as infection, hemolysis, immunosuppression, and contraction of disease (Keating & Meding, 2002; Habler, 2006). A positive correlation exists between wound infection and the number of blood products used (Habler, 2006). Providers must have a rational focus on the use of blood in order to use it most effectively and benevolently (Krebs et al., 2006). Preoperative autologous donation allows patients to donate their own blood prior to surgery. While the benefit of safety can be enticing, patients may experience preoperative anemia, and it has been shown that overcollection occurs with preoperative autologous donation because the donation is not always used postoperatively (Keating & Meding, 2002). Acute normovolemic hemodilation (ANH) and acute hypervolemic hemodilation (AHH) are other autologous blood options. In ANH, whole blood is exchanged for cell-free crystalloid of colloid solution immediately prior to surgery. The whole blood is held at the bedside through the surgery and can be reintroduced. In AHH, extra crystalloid of colloid solution is introduced to the patient immediately prior to surgery. The goal with ANH and AHH is to dilute the blood to decrease the number of RBCs lost during surgery (Habler, 2006).

Intraoperative and postoperative cell salvage are other options for using autologous blood. With cell salvage, blood is collected, washed, and transfused to the patient (Habler, 2006). Its use has been shown to decrease the use of allogenic transfusion. Intraoperative cell salvage is not often used in orthopaedic surgery due to the need for large blood loss during surgery. Postoperative cell salvage, however, can appropriately be used for orthopaedic procedures. Postoperative cell salvage requires blood to be collected during the first 6 hours postoperative and reinfused. At least 1 unit must be collected to be cost-effective (Munoz et al., 2006).

Some patients refuse to receive blood products. This may be due to religious reasons such as affiliation with Jehovah's Witnesses or for nonreligious reasons such as fear of disease transmission, transfusion reactions, or medical errors. In these cases, patients need to be educated in alternatives to transfusions and must be given the treatment options, including risks and benefits of treatments. A bloodless care program at a facility can assist with referrals, consent forms, advanced directives, education, and follow-up care in patients who refuse blood products (Yhlen, 2006).

Nursing Considerations

Nursing Diagnoses. Nursing diagnoses for this condition are expanded upon in the Appendix.

- Activity intolerance.
- Tissue perfusion: peripheral, ineffective.

Interventions. Nursing interventions during hemorrhage are aimed at keeping the patient stable. Monitoring vital signs and oxygen saturation is necessary for patient safety and stabilization during blood transfusion. Laboratory value monitoring will assist the nurse to recognize when transfusion could be appropriate (Coyer & Lash, 2008). Monitoring for blood loss from tubes, drains, and dressings will aid in identifying how much blood loss a patient is sustaining (Jones, 2004). When sudden blood loss is seen, Stainsby et al. (2006) support contacting key personnel such as the clinician in charge and anesthesia to arrange appropriate placement for the patient. Blood loss monitoring is completed visually through assessment of the wound and quantitatively with drains or sponges (ASA, 2006). Continual reassessment is critical to prevent shock (Mamaril, Childs, & Sortman, 2007).

Interventions of the circulating nurse will include reporting the estimated blood loss at the end of the case, as well as assisting to transfuse blood products as needed. Sponges, sutures, and other equipment are provided by the circulating nurse when hemorrhage is occurring (Girard, 2009).

Blood transfusion is the mainstay treatment for acute blood loss. Large-bore IV access (larger than a 19-gauge needle) is typically required for transfusion of blood products. Blood must be hung based on each organization's policy, which will include Y-type tubing with a filter and normal saline to prevent hemolysis. Proper patient identification is done in order to prevent hemolytic transfusion reactions. The care provider should remain with the patient for at least the first 15 minutes of a transfusion, as this is the most likely time for a reaction to occur (Jones, 2004). Transfusion risks include immunological reactions, transmission of disease, intravascular hemolysis, transfusion-induced coagulopathy, renal failure, admission to ICU, and death (Sukeik, Alshryda, Haddad, & Mason, 2011).

Patient Teaching. Prior to surgery, patients will require education regarding medications, herbal supplements, and vitamins that should be stopped. An explanation of blood transfusion is provided to the patient, who is given to chance to make an educated decision about preoperative autologous donation or allogenic transfusion (ASA, 2006). The causes and symptoms of anemia are explained to the patient in order for them to know what they might experience. Those patients who have any type of a drain after surgery should understand the purpose of the drain, the length of time to anticipate the drain, and what to expect to see in the drain. Patients should be told preoperatively that they can expect some blood loss. Medications being used for treatment of hemorrhage are explained. The care provider should outline the treatment options, including alternatives and what the patient can expect with the treatment (Krebs et al., 2006), as well as any laboratory testing that is being done to the patient should be explained. If a patient receives a blood transfusion, patients are educated about adverse effects and the importance of immediately reporting adverse events in order to prevent or minimize transfusion reactions.

Venous Thromboembolism

Overview

Venous thromboembolic events (VTE), including deep vein thrombosis (DVT) and pulmonary embolism (PE), are the most common preventable causes of hospital death (Harvey & Runner, 2011). DVT is a thrombus in a deep vein, most commonly in the calf or thigh. PE is a thrombus in the lung. VTE develops when RBCs, fibrin, and platelets form a blood clot mass within an intact vein. The pathophysiology of VTE is explained by Virchow's Triad of venous stasis, trauma, and hypercoagulability state (Meetoo, 2010) (see Figure 8.1). Venous stasis is caused by immobility and leads to blood pooling. Trauma is through venous wall injury and is caused by injury or surgery. The injury stimulates the release of tissue factor to activate clotting. Hypercoagulability causes blood clots to form more easily (Rowswell & Law, 2011). It has been the belief that PE is a thrombus that breaks free from DVT and travels through the veins to the lung, but one new theory is that PE develops de novo in the lung (Welle, 2011).

Figure 8.1.
Virchow's Triad

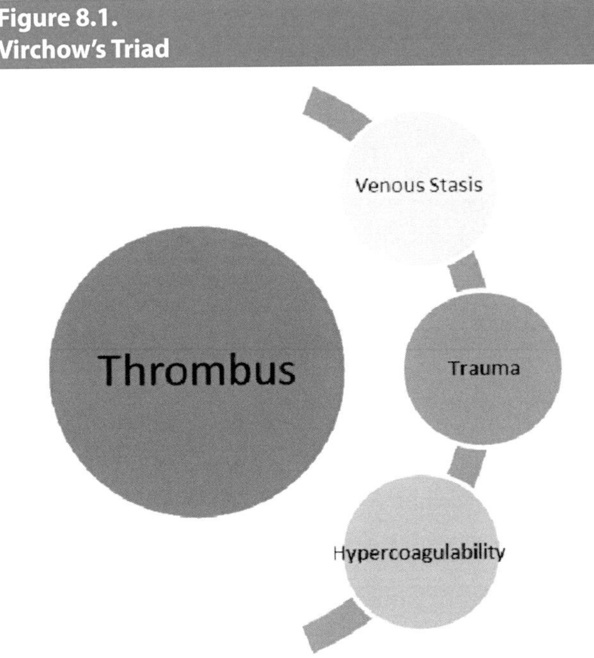

Author creation. Reproduced with permission.

VTE is estimated to affect 300,000-650,000 Americans each year and may cause up to 100,000 deaths (Harvey & Runner, 2011). Without prophylaxis, 50% to 60% of patients undergoing elective total hip replacement, total knee replacement, and hip fracture repair would develop DVT within 7-14 days following surgery (Geerts et al., 2008). Risk factors for VTE development are age, history of past DVT or PE, vein disease, pregnancy, and genetics. Use of estrogen, as with oral contraceptives or hormone replacement therapy, puts patients at increased risk of VTE. A patient who has recently undergone surgery or trauma, is obese, smokes, or is immobile is also at higher risk (Meetoo, 2010). VTE is linked to longer length of hospital stays, are more costly, and result in higher mortality rates (Meetoo, 2010). Postthrombotic syndrome can develop after DVT with symptoms of chronic swelling and discomfort, as well as venous leg ulcers in the severely affected (Rowswell & Law, 2011). Chronic pain can occur, as well as dermatitis and cellulitis (Harvey & Runner, 2011).

VTE risk assessment is the best prevention method. By recognizing those patients who are most likely to suffer VTE, appropriate thromboprophylaxis can be provided. Estimates are that the risk of developing VTE can be reduced by two thirds through the use of risk assessment and prophylaxis (Rowswell & Law, 2011). Risk assessments and recommendations for prevention are group-specific. Patients undergoing orthopaedic surgery are a group with an increased risk for VTE (Geerts et al., 2008). Prevention strategies are mechanical, physical, and pharmacological. Examples of mechanical prophylaxis are antiembolic stockings and pneumatic compression devices. Physically, the formation of clots can be prevented with early ambulation, bed exercises such as ankle pumps, and anticoagulation (Harvey & Runner, 2011). The recommended medications for anticoagulation are dependent on procedure and include low-molecular-weight heparin, unfractionated heparin, fondaparinex, and Vitamin K antagonists such as warfarin. Aspirin is not recommended as a sole anticoagulant for any orthopaedic procedure. It is also recommended that patients be ambulated frequently to prevent VTE (Geerts et al., 2008). PE prevention with inferior vena caval interruption was first introduced in 1893, but current evidence is inconclusive for the placement of inferior vena cava filters (AAOS, 2011).

Assessment

History. Patient history might include recent surgery or trauma. The patient has likely been immobile. A patient with DVT complains of sharp, throbbing pain that becomes constant, which is accompanied by a red, warm, swollen extremity (Harvey & Runner, 2011). A patient with PE will complain of rapid onset chest pain, shortness of breath, and syncope (Rowswell & Law, 2011). The patient might feel restless or agitated from hypoxia or might experience apprehension that could include feelings of distress, fear, and impending disaster (Peate, 2008).

Physical Exam. VTE is clinically silent in 10% to 50% of patients. Because of this, recognizing signs of DVT or PE during exam will assist in further testing for definitive diagnosis. In a patient with suspected DVT, unilateral swelling of the suspected extremity, induration, redness, edema, and warmth could be present (Harvey & Runner, 2011). If a PE is suspected, hypotension, tachypenea, and tachycardia could be present (Rowswell & Law, 2011). Cyanosis, productive cough with hemoptysis, and a low-grade fever might also occur in a patient with a PE (Peate, 2008).

Diagnostic Tests. Ultrasonography, venogram, impedance plethysmography, computerized strain gauze, and spiral CT and MRI can be used to confirm DVT, while the venogram is still considered the gold standard (Meetoo, 2010). Due to the invasive nature of venogram, however, ultrasonography is preferred for diagnosis. Venous Doppler ultrasonography is also referred to as venous duplex ultrasonography, or Doppler flow studies (Harvey & Runner, 2011). Routine screening with ultrasound for all patients is not recommended (Geerts et al., 2008). The best choice for PE diagnosis is with a CT pulmonary angiography (Roberts & Arya, 2011). D-dimer is the product that is present in the blood by fibrin degredation after a clot is broken down. While not diagnostic by itself, a negative d-dimer can exclude a clot. A positive d-dimer requires further testing for VTE (Carter, 2009).

Common Therapeutic Modalities

If VTE occurs despite prevention strategies, the goal of treatment is to prevent recurrent thrombus, clot propagation, and embolus. To achieve this goal, patients are placed on anticoagulation medications. Unfractionated heparin or low-molecular-weight heparin and warfarin are administered together until warfarin is therapeutic. Warfarin is administered to prevent recurrent embolus and is used long-term (Meetoo, 2010). The AAOS (2011) recommends that the duration of anticoagulant use be determined by the physician for each individual patient, and Geerts et al. (2008) recommend duration of 10-35 days postoperatively. Elevation of the extremity affected by DVT, along with warm moist compresses, will assist with pain control (Harvey & Runner, 2011). IVC filters can be placed to reduce the risk of DVT advancing to PE (Harvey & Runner, 2011).

Nursing Considerations

Nursing Diagnoses. Nursing diagnoses for this condition are expanded upon in the Appendix.

- Anxiety.
- Gas exchange, impaired.
- Mobility: physical, impaired.
- Pain, acute.
- Peripheral neurovascular dysfunction, risk for.
- Tissue perfusion: peripheral, ineffective.

Interventions. It is the responsibility of the bedside nurse to be aware of the signs and symptoms of DVT. Nurses need to know the clinical symptoms of DVT to assess in the hospitalized patient. Because DVT prevention is of utmost importance to decreasing the incidences of this complication, assigning a risk level to each patient is a proven way to take proper prophylactic measures.

The nurse is responsible for ensuring that thromboprophylactic measures are ordered and carried out. Mechanical prophylaxis requires measurement of legs for proper fit of stockings. Make certain medications are administered as ordered and on schedule. Mobilize the patient and encourage leg exercises such as ankle pumps and circles through collaboration with physical therapy (Rowswell & Law, 2011). Monitor lab values, especially clotting factors if the patient is on warfarin (Harvey & Runner, 2011).

Patient Teaching. Prior to surgery, patients are taught how to reduce the risk of VTE through mobilization, bed exercises, and use of prophylaxis. Smokers are provided smoking cessation to help minimize risk factors of VTE occurrence (Meetoo, 2010).

During an inpatient stay, education focuses around adherence to use of prophylactic measures, both chemical and mechanical. Leg exercises, antithrombotic stockings, and/or pneumatic compression devices are encouraged. Teaching related to medications must include self-administration of injection for patients using low-molecular-weight heparin. Patients who will be discharged on warfarin need to know about the risk of bleeding, as well as signs and symptoms of bleeding, interaction with other medications, interaction with Vitamin K in the diet, importance of taking the medication at the same time, and lab draws with INR range (Harvey & Runner, 2011; Morris, 2004). Techniques for bleeding prevention include avoiding blade razors or sharp tools. Signs of bleeding can be evident in the nose, gums, or stool, and patients will bruise more easily (Harvey & Runner, 2011).

Upon discharge, education continues to reinforce teaching about medication regimen and the importance of maintaining leg exercises (Meetoo, 2010). Patients need to know the signs and symptoms of DVT and PE, as well as the importance of seeking medical attention if signs and symptoms are present (Rowswell & Law, 2011).

Practice Setting Considerations. Patients continue to be at risk for development of VTE at discharge. Assess for signs and symptoms during home visits and at follow-up office appointments. The patient discharged on anticoagulation must understand the purpose and duration of the medication, as well as interactions with medications, interactions with foods, and bleeding risks. These patients must be continually monitored for administration knowledge and reminded of the need for follow-up labs.

Fat Embolism Syndrome

Overview

Fat embolism syndrome (FES) occurs when fat globules from bone marrow and disrupted tissue enter the bloodstream (Carlson & Pfadt, 2010). While the exact pathophysiology is unknown, two theories exist. Mechanical theory is the belief that fat globules are released from the bone marrow after a fracture. The biochemical or metabolic theory is the belief that trauma leads to the release of stored fatty acids and neutral fats (Galway, Tetzlaff, & Helfand, 2009). The formation of fatty globules and platelet aggregation then occur. The deposit of fat leads to the onset of a disorder that is clinically similar to acute respiratory distress syndrome (ARDS). The fatty acids that are released by impacted fat droplets cause endothelial injury, which leads to fluid leaking into interstitial space. With increased perfusion pressure and engorged pulmonary vessels, there is an increase in the workload of the right side of the heart and failure ensues. Fat globules occluding the pulmonary circulation are hydrolyzed into free fatty acids that increase capillary permeability and activate lung surfactant. The resulting pulmonary edema and collapse of alveoli leads to severe hypoxia (Roberts, 2009).

FES most often occurs 24-48 hours after long bone fractures or fracture repairs and usually manifests itself within 72 hours of the injury (Walls, 2002). Long bone fractures account for 90% of FES (Roberts, 2009). FES is most likely to affect males ages 20-40 who are involved in motor-vehicle crashes with sustained trauma and older adults who sustain hip fractures (Gore & Lacey, 2005). Total joint replacements, especially bilateral replacements, also place patients at higher risk of developing FES (Carlson & Pfadt, 2010).

Complications of FES include respiratory failure, loss of consciousness and unresponsiveness, and fluid overload (Walls, 2002) Health care personnel can assist with prevention of FES by carefully handling the fracture and with appropriate and early splinting. Because manipulation increases FES incidence in trauma patients, movement of the fracture should be as minimal as possible to avoid the release of fat globules. The reaming technique is a surgeon-specific surgical technique that has been shown to prevent FES (Galway et al., 2009). It has been proposed that using corticosteroids to prevent elevated free fatty acid levels and blunt inflammatory response aids in the prevention of FES. While an analysis found that corticosteroids prevented FES without an increased risk of mortality or infection, this continues to be controversial and warrants further studies (Bederman, Bhandari, McKee, & Schemitsch, 2009).

Assessment

History. Obtain a thorough history of the injury or surgery, including what bone was involved in the fracture and when the injury occurred. Knowledge of the stabilization time and what happened up to that point assists in proper diagnosis of FES (White, Petrisor, & Bhandari, 2006).

Physical Exam. The classic triad of symptoms of FES is neurological abnormalities, respiratory distress, and petechial rash (Carlson & Pfadt, 2010). The neurological symptoms are likely in response to hypoxia and will include apprehension, anxiety, confusion, irritability, lethargy, and change in consciousness. Respiratory symptoms include hypoxia, dyspnea, tachypnea, and increasing distress with use of accessory muscles. A petechial rash is present in 25% to 50% of FES cases and is most likely to occur on the head, neck, anterior thorax, axillae, and conjunctiva. A fever is also present (Roberts, 2009).

Diagnostic Tests. FES diagnosis is done by exclusion and is based on clinical criteria. In 1974, Gurd and Wilson proposed that diagnosis is made with the presence of at least 1 major symptom, 4 minor symptoms, and fat macroglobulaemia. Major symptoms are petechial rash, respiratory insufficiency, and cerebral involvement. Minor symptoms are tachycardia, fever, retinal changes, jaundice, and renal signs (Gurd & Wilson, 1974). This inclusion criteria is still used today (Gore, 2005). A chest CT to rule out a pulmonary embolism may be completed. Chest x-ray will show bilateral infiltrates (Galway et al., 2009). An electrocardiogram (EKG) will show tachycardia and ST and T-wave changes. Atrial blood gases will show PaO2 of less than 60% with no other obvious cause. Anemia, thrombocytopenia, increased lipase, and elevated ESR are labs that accompany FES. Fat in the blood and urine are unspecific tests. A T2-weighted MRI could show starfield pattern, acute cerebral microinfarcts (Galway et al., 2009).

Common Therapeutic Modalities

FES is treated with supportive therapy. Patients often require intubation and intensive care. Prevention of hypovolemia and hypoxia are necessary and are achieved with administration of blood products as needed and oxygen therapy (Galway et al., 2009).

Nursing Considerations

Nursing Diagnoses. Nursing diagnoses for this condition are expanded upon in the Appendix.

- Anxiety.
- Breathing pattern, ineffective.
- Gas exchange, impaired.
- Tissue perfusion: cardiac, risk for decrease.

Interventions. Nursing interventions for FES are supportive. Supportive oxygen is administered when respiratory function deteriorates. Continue to monitor oxygenation and ABGs with further respiratory assessment. Blood product administration, including platelets and RBCs, may occur for anemia and thrombocytopenia. Administer fluids and monitor the patient's response to fluid resuscitation. All of this is done while also ensuring stabilization of the fracture (Gore & Lacey, 2005). As interventions are being performed, be sure to educate the patient and family about the disease process and supportive therapies being provided.

Compartment Syndrome

Overview

Compartment syndrome occurs when pressure increases within the closed fascia space that houses muscle, blood vessels, and nerves (Altizer, 2004; Walls, 2002). Compromised tissue viability results because areas are unable to receive necessary blood. Compartment syndrome can be categorized as acute, chronic, or crush syndrome. There are 46 compartments in the body that can be affected by compartment syndrome, with the 36 compartments of the extremities most likely to be affected (Walls, 2002). Acute compartment syndrome is seen most frequently in the lower leg and forearm but can also be present in the upper arm, shoulder, thigh, lumbar spine, extraocular area, gluteal muscles, and feet (Malik, Khan, Chaudhry, Insan, & Cullen, 2009; Altizer, 2004).

Acute compartment syndrome may be the result of a specific injury or from external factors that increase the pressure in a muscle compartment. The inflammatory response leads to decreased blood flow distal to the injury and tissue hypoxia. As the inflammatory mediators are released, the capillary loses its integrity. Colloid proteins seep into the soft tissue and draw in more fluid. This increases edema, and the cycle is repeated. Eventually, blood flow to the affected extremity is obstructed. Pressure increases and causes muscle ischemia. Normal pressure in a compartment is less than 8mm Hg. In acute compartment syndrome, the pressure exceeds 30mm Hg (Walls, 2002). Acute compartment syndrome is caused by external and internal factors. External factors include pressure from application of a tight dressing, cast, or tourniquet. It can also be caused by pressure from poor positioning of limbs in the operating room. Internal factors include increased volume within the compartment from bleeding, swelling, or venous obstruction (Malik et al., 2009). Acute compartment syndrome occurs within hours to days after fracture or its surgical repair. Injuries that place individuals at increased risk for developing acute compartment syndrome are crush injury, fracture, and reduction of a long-bone fracture (Walls, 2002).

Younger patients (ages 18-30) seem to have a greater risk of developing acute compartment syndrome (Shadgan, 2010). Complications of acute compartment syndrome are irreversible muscle damage, foot drop, nonfunctioning extremities, joint contracture, and amputation (Walls, 2002). The limb deformity Volkmann's Contracture can result from untreated compartment syndrome.

Chronic compartment syndrome is caused by a gradual increase in pressure, often from exercise or stretching. The pathophysiology of chronic compartment syndrome is not well understood, although some feel that the increased pressure could be the accumulation of metabolic waste during exercise. The increased pressure causes pain and ischemia. It is usually resolved with rest but can develop into acute compartment syndrome if the exertion of the muscle continues (Altizer, 2004). Exercise or overexertion places individuals at risk for developing chronic compartment syndrome (Altizer, 2004).

Crush syndrome, also called rhabdomyolosis, occurs from an injury with prolonged compression of the compartment and subsequently results in a systemic breakdown of the body. Crush syndrome is systemic breakdown caused by a cascade of chemical events, starting with the depletion of adenosine triphosphate (ATP) in the muscle. ATP depletion results in failure of calcium and sodium/potassium pumps, leading to eventual skeletal muscle necrosis and release of muscle contents into the systemic circulation. As muscle cells die, isoenzymes such as creatine kinase (CK) are released. Myoglobic is released and contributes to the cola-colored urine the patient develops and resulting renal failure associated with rhabdomyolosis (Criner, Appelt, Coker, Conrad, & Holliday, 2002). There are numerous causes of rhabdomyolosis, including genetic and metabolic disorders, heat-related syndrome, excessive exercise, certain medications, infection, and burns. Common causes of crush syndrome are from muscle injury and compromised vascular supply such as being struck by a heavy object or getting thrown or dragged from a vehicle (Criner et al., 2002; Walls, 2002). Trauma, dehydration, renal insufficiency, and certain medications can place certain people at risk for rhabdomyolosis (Criner et al., 2002). Complications that can occur with crush syndrome are hyperkalemia and acute renal failure from myoglobinuria (Altizer, 2004, Criner et al., 2002).

Early identification and treatment is necessary to prevent complications (Bongiovanni, Bradley, & Kelley, 2005). Compartment syndrome usually occurs 6-8 hours after injury but can happen up to 2 days after the injury or fracture repair occurred (Altizer, 2004). Prevention of acute compartment syndrome requires vigilant assessment of the patient's neurovascular status by the bedside nurse. The attentive nurse will see early signs of acute compartment syndrome and is in a position to communicate concerns and assessment findings. Monitoring for proper positioning will assist in preventing compartment syndrome (Johnston-Walker & Hardcastle, 2011). As external pressure contributes to compartment syndrome development, avoid placing a cast or heavy dressing too early on a fracture. If appropriate, a splint can maintain proper alignment and immobilization of a fracture prior to surgical stabilization (Walls, 2002).

Assessment

History. With acute compartment syndrome, identify the mechanism of injury, the energy involved in the injury, if a fracture is present and where it is, if there was injury to vascular system, and any coagulopathies (Malik et al., 2009). The patient will complain of pain that might be described as deep, localized, and/or throbbing. Chronic compartment sufferers will have tenderness at the muscle compartment. In crush syndrome, identify what was crushed, the position of the patient when found, what was compressed and how, and the time frame of the injury (Altizer, 2004). Patient complaints might include muscle pain and tenderness, swelling, bruising, weakness, fever, malaise, and nausea (Walls, 2002; Criner et al., 2002).

Physical Exam. Use "the 6 Ps" to assess for acute compartment syndrome (see Table 8.5). Pain will not be relieved by analgesia, will increase with passive motion, and is out of proportion to the injury. Paresthesia, an abnormal sensation such as burning, might be present because nerves are sensitive to pressure. Pressure with palpation might be present, and the affected area could be firm to the touch and appear taut. Pallor from pressure injuring the artery in the compartment and paralysis from nerve compression or muscle damage are late signs. Pulselessness is a very late sign and signals death of tissue. In patients at risk, compare the extremities during routine neurovascular assessments completed every 1-2 hours (Walls, 2002; Bongiovanni et al., 2005). The exam in crush syndrome could reveal decreased response to deep tendon reflexes, muscles that feel "doughy," discoloration at affected muscles, agitation, or delirium. Crush syndrome might show decreased urine output or anuria with urine that is a dark cola color (Walls, 2002; Criner et al., 2002).

Table 8.5. The 6 Ps Defined

Pain	Unrelieved pain, increases with passive stretch, disproportionate to injury
Paresthesias	Numbness or tingling
Pressure	Tense or tight compartment, edematous, shiny skin
Pallor	Sluggish or absent capillary refill/pale skin tone. Late sign.
Paralysis	Inability to dorsiflex/plantarflex.
Pulselessness	Weak or absent peripheral pulses

Data from "Compartment Syndrome" by L. Altizer, 2004, Orthopaedic Nursing. *23(6), p.391-6; and "Orthopedic Trauma!" by M. Walls, 2002,* RN.*:65(7), p.53-6.*

Diagnostic Tests. Acute compartment syndrome is initially diagnosed based on clinical symptoms (Shadgan, 2010). Presence of any or all of the 6 Ps can lead to diagnosis. Further testing is done with compartment pressure monitoring, where a needle is injected into the affected compartment and the pressure is measured (Altizer, 2004). Types of monitoring devices are needle manometer, wick catheter, or slit catheter (Johnstone & Hardcastle, 2011). Unfortunately, the current devices are invasive, and accuracy is dependent on the skill of the person using it. With the advances in technology, use of a near-infrared spectroscopy may soon be available to measure and monitor compartment pressure by using muscle oxygenation (Shuler, 2010). Crush syndrome will show many altered lab values, including BUN and creatinine, hemoglobin and hematocrit, myoglobin, potassium, phosphorus, calcium, and sodium. The patient's creatine phosphokinase (CK) value will be extremely elevated, up to 5 times the normal value (Altizer, 2004; Walls, 2002; Criner et al., 2002).

Common Therapeutic Modalities

The goal of acute compartment syndrome management is to relieve pressure by releasing dressings or splints or bivalving casts. Maintain the limb no higher than heart level because elevating above the heart will decrease blood flow to the limb (Malik et al., 2009). Neutral position keeps the compartment pressure from changing and lessens the risk for aggravating the condition (Newton, 2007). A fasciotomy, an incision into the skin and fascia over the compartment, is necessary with elevated compartmental pressure (Altizer, 2004). The goals of a fasciotomy are to decrease tissue pressure, restore blood flow, and minimize tissue damage and functional loss (Johnstone & Hardcastle, 2011). A fasciotomy is left open for 2-3 days to decompress the compartment (Mamaril, Childs, & Sortman, 2007). The goals of treatment for crush syndrome are to resolve pressure and manage life-threatening systemic effects (Altizer, 2004). Treatment is with aggressive fluid replacement, requiring 12-15 liters (Criner et al., 2002).

Nursing Considerations

Nursing Diagnoses. Nursing diagnoses for this condition are expanded upon in the Appendix.

- Infection, risk for.
- Pain, acute.
- Peripheral neurovascular dysfunction, risk for.

Interventions. Assessment and documentation of the 6 Ps needs to be done on schedule (Bongiovanni et al., 2005). Monitoring the pressure that is present at the extremity and loosening any constricting devices helps to reduce the progress of compartment syndrome. Because the outcomes of compartment syndrome are time-dependent, communicating abnormal assessment findings to the physician is of utmost importance (Mamaril et al., 2007). Pain control is necessary before and after fasciotomy (Criner et al., 2002). After fasciotomy, monitor for infection, perform neurovascular checks, and assess capillary refill every hour. Pack and dress the wound until closure is completed (Walls, 2002). Position the limb properly at heart level to optimize blood flow to the extremity, maintain normotension, and manage hypovolemia (Malik et al., 2009). In crush syndrome, monitor intake and output, as well as urine color and fluid overload. Assess daily weights and lab values (Criner et al., 2002).

Patient Teaching. Because acute compartment syndrome can occur up to 2 days after the initial injury, the patient who is discharged to home needs to know the signs to monitor, especially the 6 Ps (Altizer, 2004). If a fasciotomy was performed, educate the patient in wound care and signs/symptoms of infection. Patients with chronic compartment syndrome should be taught to rest if they experience tenderness after strenuous exercise. Those who have experienced crush syndrome need education on staying hydrated. Education about the changes in urine color and watching for cola-colored urine or decreased urine output is critical for the patient to monitor for improvement. Due to the many causes of rhabdomyolosis, education about the condition itself will depend on the etiology of the disease. Patients might need education about how to take their medications, or how to obtain rehabilitation services for drug or alcohol abuse (Newton, 2007).

Delayed Union/Nonunion

Overview

A nonunion is the failure of bone ends to grow together after a fracture, and a delayed union is when union does not occur for 8-9 months (Crowther & McCance, 2006). Incidence rates are at 5% to 10%, depending on the injury, the host factors, and the site of the injury (Harwood, Newman, & Michael, 2010). In order for proper fracture healing to occur, osteogenic cells, growth factors, stable osteoconductive scaffold, and mechanical stability are all necessary. If one of these factors is out of place, nonunion or delayed union is more likely to occur (Harwood et al., 2010).

Risk factors for nonunion are patient-specific and injury-related. Patient-specific risk factors include a history of diabetes, malnourishment, anemia, older age, and poor soft tissue. Medications, including steroids, anticoagulants, and non-steroidal anti-inflammatories, also contribute to nonunion. Nicotine use doubles the amount of time that a fracture takes to grow together. Injury-related risk factors include the degree of damage, multiple injuries, irradiation of the bone, interruption to the blood supply, nerve injuries, an open fracture, and compartment syndrome. An unstable fixation device can also contribute to nonunion (Moulder & Sharma, 2008).

Assessment

History. Patients exhibiting a nonunion or delayed union will present complaining of activity-related pain. Obtaining a thorough history about the pain, which is the most common complaint, will help dictate whether treatment is necessary. Obtaining history about the patient's functional requirements and current impairments is necessary, as well as information about the initial mechanism of injury and treatment. Having original documentation about the initial history is crucial to effective treatment of this complication (Harwood, et al., 2010). Comorbidities, current medications, and social history will also play a role in the management of the nonunion.

Physical Exam. On exam, the patient will likely have local tenderness and pain when stressing the fracture site (Moulder & Sharma, 2008). The pain at the fracture site can be either constant or just when the appendage is used (American Association of Orthopaedic Surgeons [AAOS], 2007). Examination of both the affected limb and the neighboring joints is necessary. Immobility, warmth, range of motion (ROM), segments that are shortened or lengthened, and functional impairment should all be assessed on examination (Harwood et al., 2010).

Diagnostic Tests. The orthopaedic surgeon will assess nonunion in follow-up appointments (Miller & Askew, 2007). Nonunion is diagnosed with imaging studies such as x-rays, CT, or MRI. Healing over time is followed through these studies. The radiology studies will show a gap with no bone over the fracture site, no progress in bone healing with repeated imaging over several months, or inadequate healing over a time that is usually long enough for normal healing (AAOS, 2007). Nonunion should be followed through radiology for 6 months, usually with x-ray although CT or MRI can be used as needed (Moulder & Sharma, 2008). Laboratory tests may be used to find a cause for nonunion such as infection, anemia, or diabetes (AAOS, 2007).

Common Therapeutic Modalities

The goal of treatment in delayed union or nonunion is to heal the fracture with the fullest function possible. Surgical and nonsurgical treatment options are available, dependent on the patient and the fracture site. Internal fixation is used to stabilize the nonunion. External fixation is used to stabilize injured bone but is lengthy and inconvenient (AAOS, 2007). When lengthening on the bone is needed, internal and external treatments can be combined, although this increases the risk for infection compared to either one individually. Bone grafting is another way to treat nonunion, and it provides a latticework for new bone growth after normal healing has failed. Grafting material can be allograft, autograft, or bone graft substitute. Autogenous bone is the best grafting material (AAOS, 2007; Rodriguez-Merchan & Forriol, 2004).

Nonsurgical treatment uses a bone stimulator that produces electromagnetic waves to stimulate healing. Ultrasound stimulation quickens healing of function of both upper and lower extremities and has influence at all phases of fracture healing (Rodriguez-Merchan & Forriol, 2004). The bone stimulator, applied over the site of the nonunion, is worn daily for 20 minutes to hours. It must be used every day to be successful (AAOS, 2007).

Nursing Considerations

Nursing Diagnoses. Nursing diagnoses for this condition are expanded upon in the Appendix.

- Body image, disturbed.
- Knowledge deficit.
- Mobility: physical, impaired.

Interventions. The patient's weight-bearing status is identified, and the patient made aware of how to maintain the restrictions. Explain that bone healing cannot occur efficiently in the presence of nicotine. Provide the smoking patient with resources to assist in cessation, as smokers are more likely to suffer from nonunion (Miller & Askew, 2007).

Patient Teaching. To prevent nonunion, patients need to be given information about activity limitations and weight-bearing restrictions. Information about the possible options for treatment must be covered in depth so that the patient can make an informed decision about the treatment plan. Explain that the bone stimulator must be worn as directed in order for it to be effective (AAOS, 2007).

Nosocomial Surgical Site Infection

Overview

A surgical site infection (SSI) is defined as an infection developing near an incision within 30 days of a procedure or within one year if a prosthesis is in place. The Centers for Disease Control (CDC) estimate that approximately 500,000 SSIs develop annually (Salkind & Rao, 2011). There are different classifications of SSIs: superficial SSI is infection in the skin and subcutaneous tissue; deep incisional infection involves the fascia and muscle layers; and infection can also invade the organ space (Anderson et al., 2008). It is estimated that SSIs make up 22% of hospital acquired infections and that 84% of SSIs are diagnosed following discharge from the hospital (AAOS, 2007; Cowman, 2007).

Infection occurs as a result of pathogens invading a host. When pathogens enter through the external barriers of defense, such as skin and the cells and biochemical of immunity, they begin to injure cells through the production of exotoxins (destructive enzymes) and endotoxins. The exotoxins damage the membranes of the host cells and prevent phagocytosis, while the endotoxins activate the inflammatory response and produce fever (Rote & Huether, 2006). Infections develop in four stages:

1. Colonization occurs when pathogens are present on or in the body without tissue invasion.
2. During invasion, the pathogen attaches to the host cells through receptors and adhesion
3. Multiplication allows the pathogen to use the nutrients and environment of the host for reproduction.
4. In the last stage, spread, the pathogen can migrate either locally or through the bloodstream (called bacteremia or septicemia) (Rote & Huether, 2006).

There are many known risk factors for SSI development. Old age, history of diabetes mellitus, smoking, obesity, immune system condition (such as cancer or HIV), malnourishment, and paralysis or other limited mobility make some people more susceptible to postoperative infections. Operative risk factors include emergency procedures, long operative time, and hypothermia at any point in the surgical process. Hospitalization can also increase a patient's risk for SSI development, as there is a higher risk of contracting a multi-drug-resistant organism at a health care facility (Torpy, Burke, & Glass, 2005).

Complications of SSI are numerous. If tissue necrosis is present, patients can require surgical debridement for the infection. Infection can spread to the bloodstream and cause septic shock (Torpy et al., 2005). SSI also impact patients by reducing quality of life, adding hospital days, increasing the cost of the procedure up to 3-fold, readmission, increased ICU days, and death (Salkind & Rao, 2011).

Prevention strategies for SSI are well-documented. The Surgical Care Improvement Project (SCIP) measures were implemented in 2006 with the goal to reduce morbidity and mortality rates associated with SSI (Fitzgerald, 2010). Prevention with appropriate antibiotic selection and timing, as well as hair removal with clippers rather than razors, are the measures that affect orthopaedic patients the most. Other ways to prevent SSI include decreasing modifiable patient risk factors, appropriate cleaning and disinfection of the environment and equipment, proper preparation and disinfection of the operative site and hands of the surgical team, practicing correct hand hygiene, and controlling traffic in the operating room. Education must be provided to surgeons and operating room personnel about risk factors, outcomes with SSI, local epidemiology provided by surveillance surveys about SSI rates by procedure and the rate of MRSA in the facility, and basic prevention strategies (Anderson et al., 2008).

Assessment

History. Patients with suspected SSI will have had recent surgery. Patients might complain of a recent history of fever malaise, fatigue, weakness, loss of concentration, generalized aching, and loss of appetite (Rote & Huether, 2006).

Physical Exam. The exam will likely reveal a red incision that is warm and tender. There could be pus present with foul-smelling whitish-yellow fluid. The hallmark sign for infection is a fever (Torpy et al., 2005).

Diagnostic Tests. The primary diagnostic tests for suspected infection are erythrocyte sedimentation rate (ESR) and c-reactive protein (CRP) (Garino, 2011). A CBC shows how the body is reacting systemically. It has recently been determined that a positive interleukin 6 is a more appropriate marker for detecting a periprosthetic infection (Garino, 2011). When an infection is suspected, fluid is obtained and sensitivity-tested for microbiology. The aspirated fluid will be checked for white blood cells (WBCs) and cultured (Garino, 2011). This must be done prior to administration of antibiotics to ensure that the proper organism is isolated (Mantik-Lewis, 2004).

Common Therapeutic Modalities

Therapy will depend on the nature of the wound, the degree of infection, and the type of bacteria that is present. Antibiotics might be prescribed and could be administered either intravenously or orally (Torpy et al., 2005). Antibiotics will often be necessary for 4-6 weeks to combat the infection appropriately (Garino, 2011). Acute infections can usually be treated with aggressive debridement and component retention. Spacer exchanges are done when possible in order to eliminate previously contaminated prosthetic parts. Chronic infections require removal of the infected components and replacement with antibiotic impregnated spacers to deliver localized antibiotics, preserve mobility, and facilitate reconstruction (Garino, 2011).

Nursing Considerations

Nursing Diagnoses. Nursing diagnoses for this condition are expanded upon in the Appendix.

- Pain, acute.
- Pain, chronic.
- Surgery recovery, delayed.

Interventions. Cleanse the wound if it is contaminated. Cover with appropriate dressing as needed. Administer appropriate antibiotics on schedule to kill microorganisms. Encourage intake of fluid for fever. Nutrition will promote healing, especially with intake of protein, carbohydrates, and vitamins (Mantik-Lewis, 2004).

Patient Teaching. Before surgery, patients and their care providers should receive instructions and information about how to reduce SSI risk. Preprinted materials are available for patients from a number of Web sites (Anderson et al., 2008). Teach hand hygiene to prevent infection and its spread. Explain that the patient must take antibiotics as prescribed and until the course is completed in order to prevent resistant organisms. Teach that antibiotics cannot be stopped early, even if the patient feels better. Because a patient will likely be discharged before the wound is completely healed, caregivers need to be able to care for the wound and complete dressing changes (Mantik-Lewis, 2004).

Hospital Acquired Pneumonia

Overview

Hospital acquired pneumonia (HAP) is pneumonia that develops more than 48 hours after a patient is admitted without preceding signs of pneumonia on admission (Kieninger & Lipsett, 2009). It is the third-most common postoperative infection – and the deadliest, with 20% to 30% of cases resulting in death (Wren, Martin, Yoon, & Bech, 2010; Goss, 2009). The microbiology and organism causing the pneumonia is what differentiates HAP from community acquired pneumonia (CAP). The most common pathogens in HAP are *Enterobacteraciea, Haemophilus influenzae, Streptococcus pneumonia*, and methicillin-sensitive *Staphyloccous aureus*. When HAP develops in patients who have a recent history of antibiotic use, there is higher risk of contracting a multi-drug resistant pathogen, including *Pseudomonas aeruginosa, Acinetobacter baumannii*, and methicillin-resistant *Staphylococcus aureus* (MRSA) (Kieninger & Lipsett, 2009).

HAP develops when microorganisms bypass the upper airway defense mechanisms of the cough and mucocilliary clearance. A full-body defense mechanism is activated if the microorganism is virulent or numerous enough to reach the lower respiratory tract and overwhelm the host. Release of inflammatory mediators, cellular infiltration, and immune activation damage bronchial mucous membranes and alveolocapillar membranes, causing alveoli to fill with infectious debris and exudate (Brashers, 2006). Aspiration plays a large role in the development of HAP.

Many risk factors can predispose patients to developing pneumonia. Patients who are older than age 60 with a history of chronic obstructive pulmonary disease (COPD) or congestive heart failure (CHF) are at high risk. A patient who is dependent or partially dependent on caregivers to perform activities of daily living (ADLs) and requires assistive equipment or devices is at higher risk for developing pneumonia. Smokers are also at risk for poor pulmonary outcomes postoperatively (Qaseem, 2006). Other patient factors include prolonged immobilization, aspiration history, compromised immunity, malnutrition, and dehydration (Goss, 2009). Supine positioning is another risk factor (Kieninger & Lipsett, 2009). Risk factors related to the procedure include length of operation (with 3-4 hours being highest risk), general anesthesia, and emergent surgery. It has been found that obesity and mild or moderate asthma are not risk factors for pneumonia development (Qaseem, 2006). Complications from HAP include longer lengths of stay for the hospitalized patient, up to $40,000 in additional health care costs, possible ICU admission with the need for mechanical ventilation, and increased morbidity and mortality (Kieninger & Lipsett, 2009; Goss, 2009).

There are strategies to prevent HAP. All health care workers must perform proper hand hygiene before and after every patient contact to decrease microorganism spread. To prevent aspiration leading to HAP, elevate the head of the patient's bed to 30-45 degrees. Perform oral care to decrease microorganisms breeding in the mouth. Encourage deep breathing, ambulation, and use of incentive spirometry to maximize lung volume and promote coughing (Goss, 2009). Managing pain will help patients participate in many of the lung expansion techniques. Patient education with demonstration must occur in order for patients to understand how to perform the techniques (Wren et al., 2010). Assess smoking status with supportive cessation available early in preparation for nonemergency surgery. The best outcomes have been connected to preoperative smoking cessation 6-8 weeks prior to surgery and lasting at least 10 days after surgery (Qaseem, 2006).

Assessment

History. Knowing the patient's risk factors and baseline will assist in assessment. Patients may complain of a cough, dyspnea, chest pain, weakness, fever, and headache. The older patient might experience a dry cough, while younger patients can have a productive cough. Due to hypoxia, patients can experience agitation, confusion, and restlessness (Goss, 2009).

Physical Exam. The exam of a patient with HAP will reveal fever, chills, sweats, fatigue, cough, and dyspnea. Hypoxia is sometimes present. Inspiratory and expiratory rhonchi and crackles may be present (Goss, 2009).

Diagnostic Tests. Chest x-ray is used to diagnose HAP. Leukocytosis is likely to be present as the body works to fight a foreign organism. Specimen collection to isolate the organism will be necessary to ensure proper antibiotic therapy and will sometimes be obtained with a bronchoscopy (Kieninger & Lipsett, 2009; Goss, 2009). Blood cultures could be indicated (Goss, 2009) Serum albumin of less than 35g/L has been linked to postoperative pulmonary complications. It has been recommended that serum albumin is measured in all patient suspected of having hypoalbuminemia, and measurement is considered in patients with one or more risk factors for HAP development (Qaseem, 2006).

Common Therapeutic Modalities

Antibiotic therapy is necessary to treat pneumonia in order to destroy the organism that is present. Broad-spectrum antibiotics are used until a specific organism is isolated (Brashers, 2006). Antibiotics should be prescribed and administered for the shortest amount of time possible and no more than 8 days (Goss, 2009). Respiratory support will include oxygen administration and bronchodilators as needed. Nutritional support and ensuring the patient is receiving appropriate nutrition as well as managing fluids and electrolytes will promote healing.

Nursing Considerations

Nursing Diagnoses. Nursing diagnoses for this condition are expanded upon in the Appendix.

- Airway clearance, ineffective.
- Aspiration, risk for.
- Gas exchange, impaired.

Interventions. All members of the health care team who will have contact with the patient must practice hand hygiene and universal precautions for infection control. Ambulate the patient, and allow rest during the activity. Proper patient positioning, with the head of the bed at least 30 degrees, will promote effective breathing and decrease aspiration risk. Encourage oral intake by learning and providing what the patient likes to eat. Maintain venous access for antibiotic administration. Oxygen therapy is administered to maintain oxygen saturation, and the patient must tolerate the administration route (Goss, 2009). Encourage pulmonary hygiene exercises with use of the incentive spirometer, coughing exercises, and deep breathing. Confirm that the patient can perform the exercises and document the frequency with which they are being performed (Kieninger & Lipsett, 2009).

Patient Teaching. Teach patients how to perform coughing and deep breathing exercises, and explain that use of the incentive spirometer helps clear the airway and promote cough. The inability (or unwillingness) to perform pulmonary hygiene is related to the development of HAP. Urge the patient to continue the pulmonary exercises after discharge (Kieninger & Lipsett, 2009; Goss, 2009). Encourage good oral care to inhibit colonization of organisms in the mouth. Monitor the patient's nutritional status, and explain that nutrition promotes healing. Explain how to prevent aspiration by elevating the head of the bed. With administration of medications, explain the purpose of the medication and when it will be administered (Goss, 2009). Explain to patients and families that handwashing is the best way to prevent the spread of infection, and demonstrate proper techniques (Kieninger & Lipsett, 2009).

Postoperative Nausea and Vomiting

Overview

Postoperative nausea and vomiting (PONV) is nausea and vomiting that occurs within the first 24 hours after surgery or any time an individual is an inpatient (Wender, 2009). Nausea is epigastric discomfort with the desire to vomit, while vomiting is partially digested food ejected forcefully from the upper GI tract (McLean-Heitkemper, 2004). The brainstem contains a vomiting center that coordinates the components that are involved in vomiting. Input from visceral receptors in the GI tract, kidneys, heart, and uterus is received by the vomiting center from afferent pathways of the autonomic nervous system. The vomiting center initiates the vomiting reflex when these receptors are stimulated. The vomiting center can also receive impulses from the chemoreceptor trigger zone in the fourth ventricle of the brain, which responds to the stimuli of drugs and toxins, as well as labyrinthine stimulation such as motion sickness (McLean-Heitkemper, 2004).

PONV is the most common postsurgical complication and occurs in one third of patients who receive general anesthesia and causes more surgical anxiety than postoperative pain (Wender, 2009). There are four primary risk factors for adults: female gender, nonsmoker, history of PONV or motion sickness, and use of opioids intraoperatively or postoperatively (Craig, Flynn, & Hatton, 2011). PONV is also affected by the type and length of anesthetic used, duration of surgery, and type of surgery—ENT, neurosurgery, plastic surgery, breast surgery, and laparoscopy have the highest incidences (Gan et al., 2003). Vomiting occurs twice as frequently in children as in adults, and the risk of PONV in children increases as young children age and then decreases after puberty (Gan et al., 2003). Because vomiting occurs more than nausea in children, medication for children should focus on treating vomiting rather than nausea.

Dehydration and electrolyte imbalance are complications from PONV. If vomiting occurs several times, a cause must be ruled out (McLean-Heitkemper, 2004). PONV can cause increased discomfort and further anxiety for the hospitalized patient. It can also result in increased length of stay if it is not appropriately controlled (Gan et al., 2003).

Prevention is possible by identifying high-risk patients and decreasing baseline risk factors when able. Using regional rather than general anesthesia helps in PONV prevention. Prophylactic medications are used in high-risk patients and should be considered for use in moderate-risk patients (Gan et al., 2003). Prevention is cost-effective. Treatment of vomiting costs 3 times as much as treating nausea due to the cost of medications (Gan et al., 2003). Not all patients will require prophylaxis for PONV. Due to the risk of side effects from medications, only patients at moderate or high risk for PONV should be treated with prophylaxis. Serotonin receptor antagonists such as ondansetron are the most effective antiemetic and are most effective when used prophylactically at the end of surgery. Other medications that might be used include promethazine, haloperidol, prochlorperazine, transdermal scopolamine, and IM ephedrine. Combination therapy should be used for patients assessed at moderate or high risk of developing PONV, and a combination of 2-3 medications in different classes will best optimize the effectiveness of the medications (Craig et al., 2011; Gan et al., 2003).

Assessment

History. Identify moderate and high PONV risk in all patients prior to surgery. When able, elimination of risk factors before and during surgery will result in less PONV. If PONV occurs, assess for precipitating factors and document a description of the contents. Assess the patient for opiate use, recent surgeries, and abdominal pain or tenderness for feelings of nausea (McLean-Heitkemper, 2004).

Physical Exam. Prior to vomiting, the patient may be tachycardic, tachypnic, diaphoretic, and have an increase in salivation. Patients experiencing PONV may complain of lethargy and pallor. Nausea is accompanied by anorexia that is caused by unpleasant stimulation by any of the five senses (McLean-Heitkemper, 2004).

Diagnostic Tests. There are no diagnostic tests for PONV.

Common Therapeutic Modalities

PONV can occur in those who did not receive prophylaxis or those in whom prophylaxis failed. Administration of antiemetics for prophylaxis and rescue is necessary for patients experiencing PONV. Along with medications, minimizing the contributing factors such as patient-controlled analgesia, blood draining in the throat, or abdominal obstruction help with this symptom (Gan et al., 2003). Because strong smells or tastes can cause nausea and vomiting, eliminating the cause will benefit the patient (Bennett, 2009). Nonpharmacological approaches to PONV include acupuncture, acupressure, and hypnosis (Gan et al., 2003). Intravenous fluids administered per physician orders will help decrease any complications from PONV (Smith, 2004).

Nursing Considerations

Nursing Diagnoses. Nursing diagnoses for this condition are expanded upon in the Appendix.

- Fluid volume, risk for deficient
- Fluid volume, risk for imbalanced
- Nausea

Interventions. Administration of prophylactic and rescue medication to treat PONV will result in better patient outcomes. If vomiting occurs, nursing interventions focus on safety and patient comfort. Prophylactic and rescue medications are administered to prevent and control PONV. Elevation of the head of the bed helps prevent aspiration, as well as position changes and suction as needed. Assist the patient to take slow, deep breaths to calm down. Provide oral care after vomiting. A cool cloth to the face and hands is another therapeutic intervention for those experiencing PONV (Smith, 2004).

Patient Teaching. Focusing on how to deal with and prevent PONV will benefit the patient experiencing the nausea and vomiting. Teach the patient that a quiet, well-ventilated, odor-free environment, along with avoiding or limiting position changes will best eliminate nausea feelings. Instruct the patient in the use of relaxation techniques, rest, and distraction when experiencing PONV (McLean-Heitkemper, 2004).

Practice Setting Considerations. Post-discharge nausea and vomiting can occur in patients who discharge to home following ambulatory surgery and experience nausea and vomiting without medical supervision. High-risk patients are treated with oral ondansetron, scopolamine patches, and acupressure (Wender, 2009). Inpatients should have PONV resolved prior to discharge.

Postoperative Urinary Retention

Overview

Postoperative urinary retention (POUR) is being unable to void following surgery despite having a full bladder (Buckley & Lapitan, 2010). In orthopaedic surgeries, POUR incidence has been reported between 10% and 84% (Baldini, Bagry, Aprikian, Carli, & Phil 2009). A component of the urinary system, the bladder consists of the detrusor muscle and a funnel-shaped neck. Parasympathetic fibers contract the detrusor muscle and relax the bladder neck, allowing micturition. Sympathetic fibers relax the detrusor muscle and close the internal urethral sphincter. Together, these fibers aid the bladder in the storage and emptying of urine. Bladder volume is usually 400-600mL, with bladder stretching usually felt with about 300mL (Darrah, Griebling, & Silverstein, 2009).

POUR is caused by dysfunction within the urinary system. One dysfunction, bladder outlet obstruction, is often caused by an enlarged prostate gland. Another dysfunction causing POUR is when the detrusor muscle is unable to contract with enough force to empty the bladder, leading to altered detrusor contraction strength (Baldini et al., 2009). Because opioids, used generously in postoperative pain relief, decrease parasympathetic and detrusor tone, they permit passive filling of the bladder and can impair the perception of bladder fullness and urge to void (Darrah et al., 2009).

Age and gender are both risk factors, with older men being most at risk of developing POUR. Having a medical history that includes stroke, polio, cerebral palsy, or diabetes increases a patient's chance of suffering from POUR. Anticholinergic medication, beta-blockers, and certain anesthesia types can place patients at higher risk. Prolonged surgery places patients at increased risk, and it has been found that more than 750cc of intravenous fluids in the perioperative period makes patients less able to void postoperatively (Baldini et al., 2009). Postoperative analgesia and epidural also cause higher rates of POUR (Buckley & Lapitan, 2010; Lingaraj, Ruben, Chan, & Das, 2007).

A number of complications can result from POUR. One of these is infection, specifically urinary tract infection (UTI). If a UTI develops, it has the potential to lead to bacteremia or a deep infection, which can affect prosthesis and require removal (Darrah et al., 2009). POUR can also lead to bladder overdistension, detrusor muscle damage, or long-term bladder dysfunction with the potential for hydronephrosis and kidney damage, especially in the elderly (Buckley & Lapitan, 2010). All of these complications can lead to an increased length of stay for the hospitalized patient (Darrah et al., 2009).

Assessment

History. Identify any risk factors the patient might have that could increase susceptibility to POUR (Ringdal, Borg, & Hellstrom, 2003). Urine color, clarity, amount, and frequency should be assessed if the patient has successfully voided. Patients should be assessed for urinary function, mobility, and cognitive function (Gray, 2004).

Physical Exam. Patients will often complain of pain and discomfort in the lower abdomen when POUR is present; however, the sensation is often masked postoperatively by anesthesia. Palpation and percussion can aid in discovering POUR, but is difficult to know how much urine is actually present. Deep palpation should be avoided because it can cause discomfort for the patient and could elicit a vagal response (Baldini et al., 2009).

Diagnostic Tests. POUR can best be determined by use of a portable bladder ultrasound to determine the volume of urine in the bladder (Darrah et al., 2009). Because the volumes measured by ultrasound and the volumes measured by catheterization have been found to be very close, the nurse can be reassured of the bladder volume (Baldini et al., 2009). A recent study by Cutright (2011) showed that use of a portable ultrasound, along with a protocol for when to catheterize, decreased the need for catheterization by 80% in postoperative orthopaedic patients.

Common Therapeutic Modalities

The goal of treatment with POUR is to reestablish the patient's normal voiding pattern (Buckley & Lapitan, 2010). Intermittent catheterization is the current best practice. Duration and bladder volume for catheterization has not been determined, although it has been recommended to catheterize high-risk patients with more than 600cc in the bladder for more than 2 hours (Baldini et al., 2009). No specific medications are currently recommended for the reestablishment of normal voiding, although cholienergics, acetylcholine, muscle relaxants, anxiolytics, and alpha-adrengergic blockers all appear to have some effectiveness (Buckley & Lapitan, 2010).

Nursing Considerations

Nursing Diagnoses. Nursing diagnoses for this condition are expanded upon in the Appendix.

- Infection, risk for.
- Pain, acute.
- Urinary retention, acute.

Interventions. Provide bladder ultrasound to assess the volume of the bladder, and catheterize when necessary. Intermittent catheterization is preferred to indwelling catheter due to cost and lower risk of infection (Baldini et al., 2009). Determine the high-risk patient to use appropriate interventions for POUR.

Patient Teaching. Reassure the patient to alleviate anxiety about any inability to void. Explain the interventions that will be taking place. If patient is discharged to home with a catheter, explain how to clean around and empty the catheter, and help schedule follow-up visits with a urologist.

Practice Setting Considerations. Ambulatory surgical cases are appropriate to discharge to home with instructions to monitor voiding habits. As the number of ambulatory orthopaedic surgeries increases, standards about voiding prior to discharge are being studied. According to Darrah et al. (2009), it is appropriate to discharge patients to home with instructions to return to the hospital if they are unable to void in 6-8 hours. This education will help with patient flow in the hospital, decrease length of hospital stay, and improve patient satisfaction. Inpatient POUR should resolve prior to discharge.

Summary

Many complications of orthopaedic injury or surgery can be prevented. Use risk assessment tools when appropriate to identify the patients who are more likely to suffer from any of these complications. Understanding which patients are at highest risk for specific complications will allow the nurse to prioritize the workload and provide the best patient care. Strong nursing assessment skills direct the nurse to intervene early and appropriately. Nursing interventions are done preoperatively, intraoperatively, and postoperatively to minimize complications. Understanding the role of the nurse at each stage will aid in seamless care for the patient. It is necessary to ensure that an appropriate follow-up plan is formulated for all orthopaedic patients, but especially for those who have experienced any of the aforementioned complications, in order to ensure proper and appropriate healing.

References

Agency for Healthcare Research and Quality. (n.d.). Preventing pressure ulcers in hospitals: A toolkit for improving quality of care. Retrieved October 18, 2011, from http://www.ahrq.gov/research/ltc/pressureulcertoolkit/putool3.htm

Altizer, L. (2004). Compartment syndrome. *Orthopaedic Nursing, 23*(6), 391-6.

American Association of Orthopaedic Surgeons (AAOS). (2007). *Nonunions*. Retrieved October 21, 2011, from http://orthoinfo.aaos.org/topic.cfm?topic=A00374

American Association of Orthopaedic Surgeons (AAOS). (2011). Preventing venous thromboembolic disease in patients undergoing elective hip and knee arthroplasty. Retrieved October 16, 2011, from http://www.aaos.org/research/guidelines/VTE/VTE_full_guideline.pdf

American Gastroenterological Association. (2000). American Gastroenterological Association medical position statement: Guidelines on constipation. *Gastroenterology, 119*, 1761–1778. doi:10.1053/gast.2000.20390

American Society of Anesthesiologists, Inc. (2006). Practice guidelines for perioperative blood transfusion and adjuvant therapies. *Anesthesiology, 105*(1), 198-208.

Anderson, D.J., Kay, K.S., Classen, D., Arias, K., Podgorny, K., Burstin, H...Yokoe, D.S. (2008). Strategies to prevent surgical site infections in acute care hospitals. *Infection Control and Hospital Epidemiology, 29*(S1), S51-S61. doi:10.1086/591064

Baldini, G., Bagry, H., Aprikian, A, & Carli, F. (2009). Postoperative urinary retention: Anesthetic and perioperative considerations. *Anesthesiology, 110*(5), 1139-57.

Bederman, S.S., Bhandari, M., McKee, M.D., & Schemitsch, E.H. (2009). Do corticosteroids reduce the risk of fat embolism syndrome in patients with long-bone fractures? A meta-analysis. *Canadian Journal of Surgery, 52*(5), 386-93.

Behm, B. & Stollman, N. (2003). Postoperative ileus: Etiologies and interventions. *Clinical Gastroenterology and Hepatology, 1*, 71–80. doi:10.1053/jcgh.2003.50012

Bennett, S. (2009). Antiemetics: Uses, mode of action, and prescribing rationale. *Nurse Prescribing, 7*(2), 63-70.

Bluestein, D. & Javaheri, A. (2008). Pressure ulcers: Prevention, evaluation, and management. *American Family Physician, 78*(10), 1186-1194.

Bongiovanni, M.S., Bradley, S.L., & Kelley, D.M. (2005). Orthopedic trauma: Critical care nursing issues. *Critical Care Nursing Quarterly, 28*(1), 60-71.

Boss, B.J. (2010). Alterations in cognitive systems, cerebral hemodynamics, and motor function. In K.L. McCance, S.E. Huether, V.L. Brashers, & N.S. Rote (Eds.) *Pathophysiology: The Biologic Basis for Disease in Adults and Children* (6th ed., pp. 525-582), Maryland Heights, MI: Mosby Elsevier.

Brashers, V.L. (2006). Alterations of pulmonary function. In K. McCance & S. Huether (Eds.), *Pathophysiology*. (pp. 1205-1248). Philadelphia, PA: Mosby.

Buckley, B.S. & Lapitan, M.C.M. (2010). Drugs for treatment of urinary retention after surgery in adults. *Cochrane Database of Systematic Reviews 2010*, 10. doi:10.1002/14651858.CD008023.pub2

Carlson, D.S. & Pfadt, E. (2011). Fat embolism syndrome. *Nursing2011, 41*(4), 72. doi:10.1097/01.NURSE.0000395312.91409.7f

Carter, K. (2009). Identifying and managing deep vein thrombosis. *Primary Health Care, 20*(1), 30-38.

Coyer, S.M. & Lash, A.A. (2008). Pathophysiology of anemia and nursing care implications. *MEDSURG Nursing, 17*(2), 77-83, 91.

Craig, J., Flynn, J., & Hatton, K. (2011). Managing postoperative nausea and vomiting: Current controversy. *Orthopedics, 34*(1), 28. doi:10.3928/01477447-20101123-16

Crowther, C.L. & McCance, K.L. (2006). Alterations of musculoskeletal function. In K. McCance & S. Huether (Eds.), *Pathophysiology* (pp. 1573-1607). Philadelphia: Mosby.

Cutright, J. (2011). The effect of the bladder scanner policy on the number of urinary catheters inserted. *Journal of Wound Ostomy Continence Nurses, 38*(1), 71-6. doi:10.1097/WON.0b013e318202b495

Darrah, D.M., Griebling, T.L., & Silverstein, J.H. (2009). Postoperative urinary retention. *Anesthesiology Clinics, 27*(3), 465-84. doi:10.1016/j.anclin.2009.07.010

Dosh, S.A. (2002). Evaluation and treatment of constipation. *Journal of Family Practice, 51*(6), 555-9.

Evans, L.K. & Kurlowicz, L.H. (2007). Complex care needs in older adults with common cognitive disorders. Section B: Assessment and management of delirium. Retrieved from http://www.ngna.org

Fitzgerald, J. (2010). *Venous thrombosis: Have we made headway? Orthopaedic Nursing, 24(4)*, 226-234.

Friedman, R.J. (2010). Limit the bleeding, limit the pain in total hip and knee arthroplasty. *Orthopedics, 33*(9 Supp), 11-3. doi:10.3928/01477447-20100722-62

Galway, U., Tetzlaff, J.E., & Helfand, R. (2009). Acute fatal fat embolism syndrome in bilateral total knee arthroplasty: A review of the fat embolism syndrome. *The Internet Journal of Anesthesiology, 19*(2) 1-14.

Gan T.J., Meyer, T., Apfel, C.C., Chung, F., Davis, P., Eubanks, S...Temo, J. (2003). Consensus guidelines for managing postoperative nausea and vomiting. *Anesthesia and Analgesia, 97*(1), 62-71. doi:10.1213/01.ANE.0000068580.00245.95

Garino, J. (2011). Current concepts in diagnosis and management of periprosthetic infection. *American Journal of Orthopedics, 40*(12suppl), 10-12.

Geerts, W.H., Bergqvist, D., Pineo, G.F., Heit, J.A., Samama, C.M., Lassen, M.R., & Colwell, C.W. (2008). Prevention of venous thromboembolism: American College of Chest Physicians evidence-based clinical practice guidelines (8th Edition). *Chest, 133*(6), 381S-453S. doi:10.1378/chest.08-0656

Girard, N.J. (2009). Clients having surgery: Promoting positive outcomes. In J. Black & J. Hokanson Hawks (Eds.), *Medical-Surgical Nursing: Clinical Management for Positive Outcomes* (8th ed., pp. 183-228). St. Louis: Saunders.

Gore, T. & Lacey, S. (2005). Bone up on fat embolism syndrome. *Nursing2005, 35*(8), 32hn1-4.

Goss, L.K., Coty, M.B., & Myers, J.A. (2011). A review of documented oral care practices in an intensive care unit. *Clinical Nursing Research, 20*(2), 181-96.

Gray, M. (2004). Renal and urologic problems. In S. Mantic Lewis, M. McLean Heitkemper, S. Ruff Dirksen (Eds.), *Medical-Surgical Nursing: Assessment and Management of Clinical Problems* (6th ed., pp. 1172-1209). St. Louis: Mosby.

Gurd, A.R. & Wilson, R.I. (1974). The fat embolism syndrome. *The Journal of Bone and Joint Surgery, 56B*(3), 408-416.

Habler, O. (2006). Indications for perioperative blood transfusion in orthopedic surgery. *Transfusion Alternatives in Transfusion Medicine, 8*(1), 17–28. doi: 10.1111/j.1778-428X.2006.00005.x

Haleem, S., Heinert, G., & Parker, M.J. (2008). Pressure sores and hip fractures. *Injury, 39*(2), 219-223. doi:10.1016/j.injury.2007.08.030

Halpern, J.S. & Manion, P.A. (2009). Management of clients in the emergency department. In J. Black & J. Hokanson Hawks (Eds.), *Medical-Surgical Nursing: Clinical Management for Positive Outcomes* (8th ed., 2189-2217). St. Louis, MO: Saunders.

Harvey, C.V. & Runner, M. (2011). Venous thromboembolism after fibula fracture: A patient's perspective. *Orthopedic Nursing, 30*(3), 182-91. doi:0.10971NOR.0b013e318219ae94

Harwood, P.J., Newman, J.B., & Michael, A.L. (2010). An update on fracture healing and non-union. *Orthopaedics and Trauma, 24*(1), 9-23.

Ho, J., Kuhn, R.J., & Smith, K.M. (2008). Update on treatment options for constipation. *Orthopedics, 31*(6), 570-4.

Inouye, S.K. (2006). Delirium in older persons. *New England Journal of Medicine*, 354, 1157-1165.

Institute for Clinical Systems Improvement (ICSI). (2010). Pressure ulcer prevention and treatment: Health care protocol. Retrieved October 16, 2011, from http://guidelines.gov/content.aspx?id=16004&search=pressure+ulcer+prevention

Johnson M.D. & Walsh, R.M. (2009). Current therapies to shorten postoperative ileus. *Cleveland Clinic Journal of Medicine, 76*(11), 641-648. doi:10.3949/ccjm.76a.09051

Johnston-Walker, E. & Hardcastle, J. (2011). Neurovascular assessment in the critically ill patient. *Nursing in Critical Care, 16*(4), 170-7. doi:10.1111/j.1478-5153.2011.00431.x

Jones, K.J. (2004). Hematologic problems. In S. Mantic Lewis, M. McLean Heitkemper, S. Ruff Dirksen (Eds.), *Medical-Surgical Nursing: Assessment and Management of Clinical Problems* (6th ed., pp. 705-755). St. Louis: Mosby.

Juliebo, V., Bjoro, K., Krogseth, M., Skovlund, E., Ranhoff, A.H., Wyller, T.B. (2009). Risk factors for preoperative and postoperative delirium in elderly patients with hip fracture. *Journal of the American Geriatrics Society, 57*(8), 1354-1361.

Kagoma, Y.K., Crowther, M.A., Douketis, J., Bhandari, M., Eikelboom, J., & Lim, W. (2009). Use of antifibrinolytic therapy to reduce transfusion in patients undergoing orthopedic surgery: A systematic review of randomized trials. *Thrombosis Research, 123*(5), 687–696. doi:10.1016/j.thromres.2008.09.015

Keating, E.M. & Meding, J.B. (2002) Perioperative blood management practices in elective orthopaedic surgery. *The Journal of the American Academy of Orthopaedic Surgeons, 10*(6), 393-400.

Kieninger, A.N. & Lipsett, P.A. (2009). Hospital-acquired pneumonia: Pathophysiology, diagnosis, and treatment. *Chest Surgery Clinics of North America, 89*(2), 439-61. doi:10.1016/j.suc.2008.11.001

Krebs, V.E., Higuera, C., Barsoum, W.K., & Helfand, R. (2006). Blood management in joint replacement surgery: What's in and what's out. *Orthopedics, 29*(9), 801-3.

Linari, L.R., Schofield, L.C., & Horrom, K.A. (2011). Implementing a bowel program: Is a bowel program an effective way of preventing constipation and ileus following elective hip and knee arthroplasty surgery? *Orthopedic Nursing, 30*(5), 317-21. doi:10.1097/NOR.0b013e31822c5c10

Lingaraj, K., Ruben, M., Chan, Y.H., & Das, S.D. (2007). Identification of risk factors for urinary retention following total knee arthroplasty: A Singapore hospital experience. *Singapore Medicine Journal, 48*(3), 213-6.

Magnan, M.A. & Maklebust, J. (2009). The nursing process and pressure ulcer prevention: Making the connection. *Advanced Skin Wound Care, 22*(2), 83-92.

Malik, A.A., Khan, W.S., Chaudhry, A., Ihsan, M., & Cullen, N.P. (2009). Acute compartment syndrome: A life and limb threatening surgical emergency. *Journal of Perioperative Practice, 19*(5), 137-42.

Mamaril, M.E., Childs, S.G., & Sortman, S. (2007). Care of the orthopaedic trauma patient. *Journal of PeriAnesthesia Nursing, 22*(3), 184-194. doi:10.1016/j.jopan.2007.03.008

Mantik Lewis, S. (2004). Inflammation, infection, and healing. In S. Mantic Lewis, M. McLean Heitkemper, S. Ruff Dirksen (Eds.), *Medical-Surgical Nursing: Assessment and Management of Clinical Problems* (6th ed., pp. 204-233). St. Louis, MO: Mosby.

McLean Heitkemper, M. (2004). Upper gastrointestinal problems. In S. Mantic Lewis, M. McLean Heitkemper, S. Ruff Dirksen (Eds.), *Medical-Surgical Nursing: Assessment and Management of Clinical Problems* (6th ed., pp. 1003-1051). St. Louis, MO: Mosby.

Meetoo, D. (2010). In too deep: Understanding, detecting and managing DVT. *British Journal of Nursing, 19*(16), 1021-7.

Miller, N.C. & Askew, A.E. (2007). Tibia fractures: An overview of evaluation and treatment. *Orthopaedic Nursing, 26*(4), 216-223.

Monk, T.G., & Price, C.C. (2011). Postoperative cognitive disorders. *Current Opinion in Critical Care, 17*(4), 376-381.

Moore, Z. & Cowman, S. (2007). Effective wound management: Identifying criteria for infection. *Nursing Standard, 21*(24), 68-76.

Morris, B. (2004). Nursing initiatives for deep vein thrombosis prophylaxis: Pragmatic timing of administration. *Orthopaedic Nursing, 23*(2), 142-7.

Moulder, E. & Sharma, H.K. (2008). Tibial non-union: A review of current practice. *Current Orthopaedics*, 22, 434-441. doi:10.1016/j.cuor.2008.07.005

Mulryan, C. (2009). An introduction to shock. *British Journal of Healthcare Assistants, 31*(1), 21-24.

Munoz, M., Campos, A., Munoz, E., Carrero, A., Cuenca, J., & Garcia-Erce, J.A. (2006). Red cell salvage in orthopedic surgery. *Transfusion Alternatives in Transfusion Medicine, 8*(1), 41-51. DOI: 10.1111/j.1778-428X.2006.00007.x

National Collaborating Centre for Acute and Chronic Conditions. (2010). *Clinical Guideline no. 103: Delirium: Diagnosis, Prevention and Management*. London, England, UK: National Institute for Health and Clinical Excellence (NICE).

National Digestive Diseases Informational Clearinghouse (NDDIC). (2007). Constipation. Retrieved November 26, 2011, from http://digestive.niddk.nih.gov/ddiseases/pubs/constipation/#serious

National Pressure Ulcer Advisory Panel (NPUAP). (2007). Pressure ulcer stages revised by NPUAP. Retrieved October 15, 2011, from http://www.npuap.org/pr2.htm

Neitzel, J., Sendelbach, S., & Larson, L.R. (2007). Delirium in the orthopaedic patient. *Orthopaedic Nursing, 26*(6), 354-363.

Newton, E. (2007). Acute complications of extremity trauma. *Emergency Medicine Clinics of North America, 25*(3), 751-61. doi:10.1016/j.emc.2007.06.003

Nutrition 411. The Norton Pressure Sore Risk-Assessment Scale Scoring System. Retrieved from http://www.rd411.com/wrc/pdf/w0513_norton_presure_sore_risk_assessment_scale_scoring_system.pdf

Peate, I. (2008). Caring for the person with a pulmonary embolism. *British Journal of Healthcare Assistants, 2*(7), 318-322.

Prasad, N., Padmanabhan, V., & Mullaji, A. (2007). Blood loss in total knee arthroplasty: An analysis of risk factors. *International Orthopedics, 31*(1), 39-44. doi:10.1007/s00264-006-0096-9

Qaseem, A., Snow, V., Fitterman, N., Hornbake, E.R., Lawrence, V.A. Smetana, G.W…Owens, D.K. (2006). Clinical Efficacy Assessment Subcommittee of the American College of Physicians. Risk assessment for and strategies to reduce perioperative pulmonary complications for patients undergoing noncardiothoracic surgery: A guideline from the American College of Physicians. *Annals of Internal Medicine, 144*(8), 575-80.

Remaley, D.T. & Jaeblon, T. (2010). Pressure ulcers in orthopaedics. *The Journal of the American Academy of Orthopaedic Surgeons, 18*(9), 568-75.

Ringdal, M., Borg, B., & Hellstrom, A. (2003). A survey on incidence and factors that may influence first postoperative urination. *Urologic Nursing, 23*(5), 341-354.

Roberts, D. (2009). Management of clients with musculoskeletal trauma or overuse. In J. Black & J. Hokanson Hawks (Eds.), *Medical-Surgical Nursing: Clinical Management for Positive Outcomes* (8th ed., pp. 507-540). St. Louis: Saunders.

Roberts, L.N. & Arya, R. (2011). Deep vein thrombosis and pulmonary embolism: Diagnosis, treatment and prevention. *Clinical Medicine 2011, 11*(5), 465–6.

Rodriguez-Merchan, E.C. & Forriol, F. (2004). Nonunion: General principles and experimental data. *Clinical Orthopaedics*, 419, 4–12. doi:10.1097/01.blo.0000118182.32042.1a

Rote, N.S. & Huether, S.E. (2006). Infection. In K. McCance & S. Huether (Eds.), *Pathophysiology* (pp. 293-309). Philadelphia, PA: Mosby.

Rowswell, H. & Law, C. (2011). Reducing patients' risk of venous thromboembolism. *Nursing Times, 107*(14), 12-14.

Salkind, A.R. & Rao, K.C. (2011). Antibiotic prophylaxis to prevent surgical site infections. *American Family Physician, 83*(5), 585-590.

Sendelbach S. & Guthrie, P.F. (2009). Acute confusion/ delirium. Retrieved from http://www.guideline.gov/content.aspx?id=14340%20

Shadgan, B., Menon, M., Sanders, D., Berry, G., Martin, C., Duffy, P… O'Brien, P. (2010). Current thinking about acute compartment syndrome of the lower extremity. *Canadian Journal of Surgery, 53*(5), 329-334.

Shuler, M.S., Reisman, W.M., Kinsey, T., Whitesides, T.E., Hammerberg, E.M., Davila, M.G., & Moore, T.J. (2010). Correlation between muscle oxygenation and compartment pressures in acute compartment syndrome of the leg. *The Journal of Bone and Joint Surgery, 92*(4), 863-70. doi:10.2106/JBJS.I.00816

Smith, D.J. (2004). Postoperative care. In S. Mantic Lewis, M. McLean Heitkemper, S. Ruff Dirksen (Eds.), *Medical-Surgical Nursing: Assessment and Management of Clinical Problems* (6th ed., pp. 393-415). St. Louis, MO: Mosby.

Stainsby, D., MacLennan, S., Thomas, D., Isaac, J., & Hamilton, P.J. (2006). Guidelines on the management of massive blood loss. *British Journal of Haematology, 135*(5), 634-41.

Sukeik, M., Alshryda, S., Haddad, F.S., & Mason, J.M. (2011). Systematic review and metaanalysis of the use of tranexamic acid in total hip replacement. *Journal of Bone and Joint Surgery British Volume, 93*(1), 39-46. doi:10.1302/0301-620X.93B1.24984

Thompson, M. (2011). Reducing pressure ulcers in hip fracture patients. *British Journal of Nursing, 20*(15), S10-S18. doi:10.1016/j.injury.2007.08.030

Torpy, J.M., Burke, A., & Glass, R.M. (2005). Wound Infections. *JAMA*, 294(16). Retrieved October 15, 2011, from http://jama.ama-assn.org/content/294/16/2122.full.pdf

Tullmann, D.F., Mion, L.C., Fletcher, K., & Foreman, M.D. (2008). Delirium: prevention, early recognition, and treatment. In E. Capezuti, D. Zwicker, M. Mezey, & T. Fulmer (Eds.) *Evidence-Based Geriatric Nursing Protocols for Best Practice* (3rd ed., pp. 111-25). New York, NY: Springer Publishing Company.

Unbeck, M., Dalen, N., Muren, O., Lillkrona, U., & Harenstam, K.P. (2010). Healthcare processes must be improved to reduce the occurrence of orthopaedic adverse events. *Scandinavian Journal of Caring Sciences, 24*(4), 671-677. doi: 10.1111/j.1471-6712.2009.00760.x

Walls, M. (2002). Orthopedic trauma! *RN, 65*(7), 53-6.

Welle, M.K. (2011). Inferior vena cava filter use as pulmonary embolism prophylaxis in trauma. *Orthopaedic Nursing, 30*(2), 98-114. doi:10.10971NOR.0b013e31820f5128

Wender, R.H. (2009). Do current antiemetic practices result in positive patient outcomes? Results of a new study. *American Journal of Health-System Pharmacy, 1*(66), S3-10. doi:10.2146/ajhp080465

White, T., Petrisor, B.A., & Bhandari, M. (2006). Prevention of fat embolism syndrome. *Injury*, Suppl4:S59-67. doi:10.1016/j.injury.2006.08.041

Wren, S.M., Martin, M., Yoon, J.K., & Bech, F. (2010). Postoperative pneumonia prevention program for the inpatient surgical ward. *Journal of the American College of Surgeons, 210*(4), 491-495. doi:10.1016/j.jamcollsurg.2010.01.009

Yhlen, K. & Ashton, K. (2006). Bloodless care: When blood transfusion is not an option. *Journal of Legal Nurse Consulting, 17*(2), 3-5.

Young, J. & Inouye, S.K. (2007). Delirium in older people. *British Medical Journal, 334*(7598), 842-846.

Zimmaro Bliss, D. & Sawchuk, L. (2004). Lower gastrointestinal problems. In S. Mantic Lewis, M. McLean Heitkemper, S. Ruff Dirksen (Eds.), *Medical-Surgical Nursing: Assessment and Management of Clinical Problems* (6th ed., pp. 1052-1103). St. Louis, MO: Mosby.

Chapter 9
Orthopaedic Infections

Linda R. Greene, RN, MPS, CIC

Objectives

- Identify common infections encountered in orthopaedic practice.
- Describe the epidemiology of orthopaedic infections.
- List microorganisms commonly associated with orthopaedic infections and explain virulence factors associated with these organisms.
- Describe host characteristics and procedures that place the patient at risk for developing infections.
- Discuss common diagnostic and therapeutic modalities used to treat infections in orthopaedic patients.

Orthopaedic infections are associated with significant morbidity and mortality. Infections of skin and soft tissue can lead to infection of bones (osteomyelitis) and infection of joints (septic arthritis). Orthopaedic infections may be associated with a variety of bacteria and fungi that can enter the body as a result of trauma or surgery, destroying healthy tissue and spreading through the blood. The specific organism causing an orthopaedic infection has an impact on the severity, onset, and even the outcome of an infection due to rates of growth, ability to survive in the host environment, and virulence (Greene, Mills, Moss, Sposato, & Vignari, 2010). Without prompt identification and treatment, orthopaedic infections can become chronic. Nursing plays a pivotal role in the assessment, treatment, and prevention of these costly and often debilitating infections. This chapter will review common orthopaedic infections and nursing strategies related to care, treatment, and prevention of these infections.

Osteomyelitis

Overview

Definition. Osteomyelitis is an inflammatory disorder of bone caused by infection. It can lead to necrosis and destruction of the bone. The infection may be acute or chronic. *Acute osteomyelitis* is often described as infection that occurs prior to necrosis or bone destruction. *Chronic osteomyelitis* refers to cases in which symptoms have been present for longer than 3 months or in which initial therapeutic regimens to treat acute osteomyelitis have failed. The main types of osteomyelitis that are commonly seen in the hospital setting are contiguous spread from soft tissues and joints via decubitus or diabetic ulcers, hematogenous seeding such as in vertebral or long bone metaphyses, direct inoculation of a microorganism into the bone as a result of trauma or surgery, and infections associated with a prosthetic joint (Berbari, Steckelenberg, & Osmon, 2010; Howell & Goulston, 2011).

There are two major osteomyelitis classification schemes that are used today. Lew and Waldvogel (2004) classified osteomyelitis based on the duration of illness (acute versus chronic) and the mechanism of infection (hematogenous or secondary to a contiguous focus of infection). The more recent Cierny, Mader, and Penninck (2003) classification is based on the affected portion of the bone. This classification system, summarized in Table 9.1, stages osteomyelitis according to anatomic structure, physiologic class status of the host, and local environment. This classification system lends itself to treatment and prognosis.

Table 9.1. Cierny, Mader, and Penninck Osteomyelitis Classification System
Host Characteristics
Class A: Denotes a normal host
Class B: Denotes a host with either systemic or localized infection
Class C: Denotes a host who has a poor prognosis for cure.
Anatomic
Stage 1: Medullary osteomyelitis: Denotes infection confined to the intramedullary surfaces of the bone. Hematogenous osteomyelitis and infected intramedullary rods are examples of this anatomic type.
Stage 2: Superficial osteomyelitis: A true contiguous focus infection of bone; it occurs when an exposed infected necrotic surface of bone lies at the base of a soft-tissue wound
Stage 3: Localized osteomyelitis: Usually characterized by a full thickness, cortical sequestration which can be removed surgically without compromising bony stability
Stage 4: Diffuse osteomyelitis: A through-and-through process that usually requires an intercalary resection of the bone to arrest the disease process. Diffuse osteomyelitis includes those infections with a loss of bony stability either before or after debridement surgery.
Systemic or Local Factors
Systemic factors include malnutrition, hepatic disease, diabetes, immune disease, malignancy, extremes of age and immunosuppression
Local factors may include tobacco abuse, vessel disease, venous stasis, scarring, radiation fibrosis, and neuropathies

Data from "Osteomyelitis" by E. Berbari, J. Steckelenberg, J., & Osmon, D. (2010). In G. Mandell, J. Bennett & R. Dolin (Eds.) Principles and Practice of Infectious Diseases *(7th ed., pp. 1457-1467). Philadelphia, PA: Churchill Livingston.*

Pathophysiology. Although bone is normally resistant to bacterial colonization, events such as trauma, surgery, introduction of foreign bodies, or presence of prosthesis may disrupt bony integrity and lead to the onset of bone infection. Bone has unique physiological and anatomical characteristics that are affected when it is infected. When an organism causes acute inflammation of the bone, various inflammatory factors and leukocytes contribute to necrosis and destruction of the bone. Vascular channels are compressed and obliterated by the inflammatory process, and this ischemia leads to bone necrosis (Chihara & Segreti, 2010).

Osteomyelitis can also result from hematogenous spread after bacteremia. Biofilm plays a significant role in the pathogenesis of prosthetic orthopaedic infections. Once microorganisms have made contact and formed an attachment with a living host or nonliving surface or object, development of a biofilm can take place. Foreign bodies such as prosthetic devices and methylmethacrylate (bone cement) allow small inocula of bacteria to flourish out of the reach of the body's normal defenses and develop into a sticky matrix called glycocalyx, or biofilm. In the presence of foreign bodies, certain bacteria such as *Staphylococcus* and *Pseudomonas* produce biofilm that further protects the bacteria from the host defenses. Once microorganisms have made contact and formed an attachment with a living host or nonliving surface or object, development of a biofilm can take place. Bacteria living in a biofilm can have significantly different properties from free-floating bacteria, as the dense extracellular matrix of biofilm and the outer layer of cells may protect the bacteria from antibiotics and normal host defense mechanisms of the white blood cells such as phagocytosis (Greene et al., 2010).

Incidence. Acute hematogenous osteomyelitis is rare. It occurs mainly in children, IV drug abusers, and patients with indwelling catheters. Acute osteomyelitis is generally initiated by the spread of microorganisms through the vascular system and into the medullary cavity. In children, the infection generally occurs due to characteristics unique to the immature anatomy. Capillary ends of the nutrient artery make sharp ends under the pediatric growth plate, which feeds into large venous sinusoids where the blood flow becomes slow and turbulent. An obstruction of this blood flow can lead to an area of avascular necrosis. Because these capillaries lack phagocytic lining cells, any minor trauma can lead to a hematoma, vascular obstruction, and subsequent bone necrosis. This area can also be seeded from a transient bacteremia (Berbari et al., 2010). The most common organisms isolated in hematogenous osteomyelitis are *Staphylococcus aureus* and *Streptococcus pneumoniae*. In neonates, common pathogens include those that cause neonatal sepsis such as Group B *Streptococci* and *Escherichia coli. Candida and Pseudomonas aeruginosa* are more commonly encountered with IV drug abusers and patients with indwelling central catheters.

Age-related incidence of acute osteomyelitis is approximately 1:5,000 in children younger than age 13. Neonatal prevalence is approximately 1 case per 1,000 infants. Femur and tibia sites account for approximately 50% of childhood cases of osteomyelitis (Krogstad, 2012). In adults, the most common sites are the spine, pelvis, and small bones (Berbari et al., 2010). The incidence of osteomyelitis after fracture is reported to be between 2%-16% depending on the degree of trauma. The prevalence of osteomyelitis after foot puncture may be as high as 16% in the general population and 30%-40% in patients with diabetes. The incidence of vertebral osteomyelitis is rare: approximately 2.4 cases per year in a population of 100,000. It is most common following open fracture with direct contamination of the wound; however, it can occur in any bone. The most common site is in the long bones, especially the tibia, which is the most common site of open fracture (Chihara & Segreti, 2010).

Risk Factors. Risk for developing osteomyelitis varies, depending upon the type and cause of the infection. Young age is a risk factor for acute hematogenous osteomyelitis. Factors that favor the development of acute bone infection are those that predispose the patient to bacteremia, including indwelling intravascular catheters, distant foci of infection, and intravenous drug abuse. The distant sites of infection that are most commonly associated with acute osteomyelitis include the skin, urinary tract, and respiratory tract. Two patient groups with a susceptibility to acute skeletal infections are those with sickle cell anemia and chronic granulomatous disease. The second major mechanism for the development of acute osteomyelitis is by direct inoculation. Injuries due to penetrating bites and puncture wounds of the foot may infect bone directly. Diagnostic procedures (lumbar puncture, fetal monitoring electrodes, suprapubic aspiration, and heel sticks) may result in inadvertent inoculation of a neighboring osseous structure (Krogstad, 2010). Surgical procedures such as internal fixation of long bone fractures and skeletal traction may also cause an infection of the bone. Patients with open fractures of bones are at high risk for osteomyelitis (Chihara & Segreti, 2010). Osteomyelitis may also develop as a consequence of contiguous spread of infection from adjacent soft tissue, particularly if vascular insufficiency complicates the clinical picture. Infection of the mandible, maxilla, and frontal or mastoid bones may result from persistent or neglected infection of the teeth, paranasal sinuses, or middle ear cavity, respectively (Berbari et al., 2010). Diabetic foot ulcers and decubitus ulcers are also risk factors for osteomylelitis (Chihara & Segreti, 2010). Osteomyelitis affects up to a third of patients with stage IV pressure ulcers, predominantly in elderly patients with limited mobility (Rao, Ziran, & Lipsky, 2010). The major risk factor for chronic infection of bone is inadequate or delayed management of acute osteomyelitis or completely unrecognized bone infection (Chihara & Segreti, 2010).

Complications. In the absence of appropriate therapy, acute osteomyelitis can be associated with morbidity and mortality. Suppurative infection may involve adjacent structures such as the joints and soft tissues, leading to sinus tract formation associated with malignancies especially in patients with long-standing osteomyelitis When an organism causes acute inflammation of the bone, various inflammatory factors and leukocytes contribute to necrosis and destruction of the bone. Vascular channels are compressed by the inflammatory process, and this ischemia leads to bone necrosis, creating regions of the bone where there is insufficient antibiotic penetration (sequestra). In these cases, surgical intervention is needed for debridement of necrotic tissue. This can lead to bone loss and localized osteoporosis, resulting in further weakening of the bone.

Osteolysis and pathologic fractures may occur, although such complications are rare with early recognition and treatment. Occasionally, hematogenous spread and sepsis can occur (Chihara & Segreti, 2010).

Preventive Strategies. Early care of injuries that break the skin and aseptic care of surgical wounds are essential to prevent the development of infection. Osteomyelitis often presents as a draining wound or sinus tract. Absorbent wound care products or dressings such as calcium alginates can be helpful in managing the drainage. Adherence to and compliance with antibiotic treatment regimens are extremely important to prevent acute conditions from becoming chronic. Inadequate or incomplete antibiotic regimens have also been associated with the development of drug resistant bacteria.

Special Considerations. Osteomyelitis is two times more frequent in boys than in girls – probably secondary to active play and resultant minor trauma. About 40% of cases occur in children younger than age 20, and around 35% occur in adults older than age 50. If growth plates are involved, the osteomyelitis may lead to progressive limb-length discrepancies and deformities (Krogstad 2010). Another problem is that recurrences are possible even years after initial treatment. Because osteomyelitis affects up to 33% of patients with stage IV pressure ulcers, the elderly and those with limited mobility are at risk (Rao et al., 2010). Osteomyelitis may affect patients with sickle cell disease due to their compromised immune status and poor circulation of blood in the bone. Patients undergoing dialysis may develop vertebral osteomyelitis due to infections resulting from the repetitive access of the arteriovenous fistula or the dialysis catheter Osteomyelitis is rarely seen in patients with human immunodeficiency virus (HIV), despite their immunocompromised state; however, patients with systemic lupus erythematosus (SLE) on steroid therapy have a significant increase in risk of acquiring tuberculosis with subsequent skeletal mycobacterium infection (Chihara & Segreti, 2010).

Assessment

History. Presenting symptoms of acute osteomyelitis are often dependent on age. Infants may have minimal symptoms secondary to a poor inflammatory response by the immature immune system. The presenting symptoms in infants may range from irritability when the affected limb is touched to pseudoparalysis or signs of sepsis. Young children usually present with localized pain or refusal to use the affected limb. As the infection progresses, signs of inflammation are present. Effusions in adjacent joints can occur. Older children and adolescents usually present with significant localized pain and tenderness, coupled with fever and chills (Krogstad, 2010). In adults, acute osteomyelitis typically displays a gradual onset of symptoms over several days. Patients usually present with dull pain at the involved site, with or without movement. Local findings (tenderness, warmth, erythema, and swelling) and systemic symptoms (fever and rigors) may also be present. Patients with osteomyelitis involving sites such as the hip, vertebrae, or pelvis, however, tend to manifest few signs or symptoms other than pain (Lalani, 2011). Subacute osteomyelitis generally presents with mild pain over several weeks, with minimal fever and few constitutional symptoms. Chronic osteomyelitis may present with pain, erythema, or swelling, sometimes in association with a draining sinus tract. The presence of a sinus tract is characteristic of chronic ostomyelitis. The medical history associated with acute osteomyelitis may include recent history of systemic bacterial or viral infection. This can be following a throat infection, abscessed tooth, skin or soft tissue infection, and urinary tract infection (Chihara & Segreti, 2010). Another important fact would be a recent history of mild trauma (bruising) and puncture wounds. Adults may have also a history of immunodeficiency, providing an opportunity for bacteria or viruses to seed bone. A classic history for chronic osteomyelitis is described as cyclical pain increasing to severe deep tense pain with fever that subsides when pus breaks through the fistula. Another important fact would be a previous history of acute osteomyelitis treated or not treated with continuous or intermittent symptoms (Berbari et al., 2010).

Table 9.2. Findings on Physical Examination
Hematogenous Long-Bone Osteomyelitis
Abrupt onset of high fever (only present in 50% of neonates with osteomyelitis)
Fatigue
Irritability
Malaise
Restriction of movement (pseudoparalysis of limb in neonates)
Local edema, erythema, and tenderness
Hematogenous Vertebral Osteomyelitis
Insidious onset
History of an acute bacteremic episode
May be associated with contiguous vascular insufficiency
Local edema, erythema, and tenderness
Failure of a young child to sit up normally
Chronic Osteomyelitis
Nonhealing ulcer
Sinus tract drainage

Data from "Osteomyelitis" by S. Chihara and J. Segreti, 2010, Disease-A-Month, *56(1), 5-31.*

Physical Exam. In addition to a complete physical examination, the assessment should include a health history and a review of symptoms. It is important to look for signs or symptoms of soft tissue and bone tenderness, as well as possible swelling and redness. In patients with diabetes, the classic signs and symptoms of infection may be absent or masked due to vascular disease and neuropathy (Chihara & Segreti, 2010). Patients should be asked to describe their symptoms. Table 9.2 describes findings on physical examination that help differentiate osteomyelitis.

Diagnostic Tests. Tools for diagnosing osteomyelitis include imaging studies, laboratory tests, joint aspiration, and tissue biopsy. When a prosthetic joint infection is suspected, analysis of joint fluid (with cell count, gram stain, and culture) or tissue (with biopsy and culture) is required to establish the diagnosis, identify the causative organism, and guide choice of antimicrobial therapy.

Imaging studies: Imaging studies may be helpful but are not diagnostic because changes are not specific for infection and may represent noninfectious processes as well. Routine x-rays generally show no changes in the early phase. It can take from 10-14 days after the start of infection for x-rays to detect bone lysis. Computed tomography (CT) and magnetic resonance imaging (MRI) are considered the standard of care for radiologic diagnosis of osteomyelitis (Ratliff, 2007). CT scans can assess bone integrity of the suspected osteomyelitis and help guide needle bone biopsies to diagnose the infection. CT can also show abnormal thickening of the bone with sclerotic changes and illuminate draining sinuses (Pineda, Vargas, & Rodriguez, 2006). MRI is considered helpful for diagnosing suspected osteomyelitis, especially in the pelvis; however MRI cannot distinguish between osteomyleitis and tumors or other postoperative changes (Prandini et al., 2006).

Laboratory studies: Laboratory studies such as white blood cell count, erythrocyte sedimentation rates, and C-reactive protein may be elevated in the patient with osteomyelitis, but these tests are not specific for osteomyelitis because they can be elevated in the presence of any type of inflammatory process. Blood cultures may be positive especially in hematogenous osteomyelitis. In vertebral osteomyelitis, blood cultures are positive in 20%-50% of cases (Chihara & Segreti, 2010).

Other studies: Probing to the bone may be a helpful diagnostic tool especially in diabetic patients. The palpation of bone with a metal probe to detect infection is based on the concept that if the probe can reach bone, so can bacteria. A bone biopsy is one of the most specific diagnostic tools; however, it requires special considerations because it is an invasive procedure. The identification of the causative organism, crucial from both a diagnostic and therapeutic perspective, can be accomplished surgically or by needle aspiration with radiologic guidance to obtain tissue samples for histological examination and bacterial cultures (Berbari et al., 2010).

Common Therapeutic Modalities

Nonsurgical treatment for osteomyelitis starts with improving host deficiencies (e.g., correcting anemia, hypoxemia, hyperglycemia, or other metabolic derangements). The most common therapeutic modality is antibiotic treatment. Clinicians must select an appropriate initial antibiotic regimen, which should then be reviewed and modified (if needed) based on the patient's clinical response, culture, and susceptibility data. Initial antibiotic therapy is usually systemic and most often is administered parenterally. Some patients are treated with locally delivered antibiotics, calcium sulfate beads, or biodegradable cement, either alone or combined with systemic therapy. Acute hematogenous osteomyelitis may often respond favorably to a course of antibiotics alone. More complex cases may require extensive surgical debridement and possibly reconstructive surgery such as tissue flaps and bone grafts. Even with standardized treatment, therapeutic failures and recurrences are common, often in the range 20%-30% (Rao et al., 2010).

Adjunctive therapies for osteomyelitis include hyperbaric oxygen (HBO) and negative pressure wound therapy (NPWT), also called vacuum-assisted closure. HBO has been used as an adjunct to surgery and antibiotics to treat chronic osteomyelitis. HBO has been shown to improve available oxygen at the bone site, enhancing the ability of white blood cells to phagocytize the bacteria and promote osteogenesis. More studies are needed on the role of HBO in chronic osteomyelitis, however, as early studies are inconclusive (Fang & Galiano 2009).

Nursing Considerations

Nursing Diagnoses. Nursing diagnoses for this condition are expanded upon in the Appendix.

- Activity intolerance, risk for.
- Infection, risk for.
- Mobility, impaired physical.
- Pain, acute.
- Skin integrity, risk for impaired.

Nursing Interventions. Nursing interventions span the continuum of care. In the acute care setting, the pain assessment is very important. It is helpful to assess and, whenever possible, treat pain prior to activity to allow the patient to ambulate more freely. Activity intolerance can also lead to pressure ulcers. Turning/positioning the patient and assessing skin integrity are important interventions. After discharge, patients seen in the physician's office will need reinforcement of discharge instructions. Promotion of appropriate physical therapy (PT) is important during this time. The role of the nurse in the home care setting is to reinforce activity and PT instructions. The nurse should assess progress toward goals and communicate with other members of the health care team when identifying a lack of progress. It is also important to assess the home environment for factors that precipitate decreased activity tolerance.

Patient Teaching. Patients with osteomyelitis will be on long-term antibiotic therapy and will need reminders on the importance of taking antibiotics as prescribed and for the entire course as ordered. Instruction should include proper catheter site wound care, dressing change technique, importance of hand washing, and pin care as needed. The patient must also know the important signs and symptoms to report, including fever, chills, increased drainage, changes in tissue surrounding the area, and side effects of antibiotic therapy. It is important for the nurse in the practice setting to teach appropriate use of mobility aids and appropriate limitations of weight-bearing prior to discharge.

Septic Arthritis

Overview

Definition. Septic arthritis refers to an infection of the synovium and joint space by microorganisms, leading to an inflammatory response. Septic arthritis may be either acute or chronic. The clinical manifestations, severity, treatment, and prognosis are dependent upon the nature and virulence of the infecting organism and the immune status of the host (Ohl, 2010). Septic arthritis usually is divided into gonococcal and nongonococcal varieties. Clinical manifestations and treatment differ for the two types. Patients at risk for septic arthritis have abnormal joints because of arthritis (including rheumatoid arthritis, osteoarthritis, or injury-induced arthritis) and subsequently develop an infection that reaches the bloodstream.

Etiology. Septic arthritis most commonly occurs when bacteria or microorganisms spread through the bloodstream to a joint. It can be spread by direct inoculation into the joint through puncture wounds from either trauma or surgical intervention. An extension into the joint from a contiguous site of infection, such as in childhood acute osteomyelitis, can also lead to septic arthritis. Any microorganism can cause septic arthritis, but the most common organisms are gram-positive bacteria such as *Staphylococcus aureus* and Beta *Streptococcus*. Septic arthritis is generally not polymicrobial unless caused by a puncture wound or animal bite. In the immunocompromised patient, bacteria that are usually not pathogenic frequently cause the infection. *Staphylococcus aureus* is the most common organism isolated, followed by *Streptococcus* species. *Haemophilus influenzae* is the most common organism in young children but is rare in immunized children. *Neisseria gonorrhea* is most common in sexually active young adults. Chronic septic arthritis (which is less common) is caused by organisms such as *Mycobacterium tuberculosis* and *Candida albicans* (Espinoza, 2007).

Pathophysiology. The microorganisms invade the joint through hematogenous, contiguous, or direct extension routes. Once the microorganism is present, it causes intense local reactions of hyperemia, vascular congestion, and synovial proliferation. Symptoms usually develop quickly, including fever, joint swelling, and joint pain. As the infection progresses, destruction of the cartilage occurs due to inhibition of cells that form cartilage, pressure necrosis, and the release of proteolytic enzymes from the breakdown of the bacteria. As the organism proliferates in the synovium, it also causes enzymatic digestion of the articular cartilage.

Incidence. The annual incidence of septic arthritis in the general population is 2-5 per 100,000 (Kherani & Shojania, 2007). The most commonly involved joint in septic arthritis is the knee (50% of cases), followed by the hip (20%), shoulder (8%), ankle (7%), and wrists (7%). Other joints each make up 1-4% of cases (Brusch, 2011). In adults, septic arthritis most commonly affects the knee; in children, infection into the hip joint predominates. Septic arthritis usually involves only one joint. Polyarticular involvement occurs about 9% of the time (Mathews et al., 2007), is usually in elderly patients or those undergoing steroid treatment for rheumatoid arthritis. Gonococcal infection generally occurs in young, healthy, sexually active adults.

Considerations Across the Life Span. A patient who suffers from septic arthritis may develop arthritis or bony ankylosis secondary to loss of cartilage. Children may develop limb-length deformities or other local discrepancies. Patients with septic arthritis of the hip may develop later avascular necrosis of the femoral head.

Complications. The most common complication of the septic joint is the failure to resolve the infection and progression of articular cartilage damage, severe degenerative changes, and profound functional loss. These changes often result in arthroplasty or arthrodesis and, in rare cases, amputation. Irreversible destruction of the joint occurs in a large percentage of patients, despite proper treatment. In the elderly, complications may include renal failure, cardiac or respiratory failure, disseminated infection, and premature death. In patients with compromised immune systems or debilitating diseases, infections from open wounds may spread into soft tissues and tissue planes. One study evaluated 121 adults and 31 children with bacterial arthritis. A poor joint outcome (as described by the need for amputation, arthrodesis, prosthetic surgery, or severe dyfunction) was identified in one third of these cases. Mortality rates range from 10%-15 % overall and as high as 50% in patients in patients who have polyatricular septic arthritis, especially when virulent pathogens such as *Staphylococcus aureus* are the predominant pathogen (Goldberg & Sexton, 2011).

Preventive Strategies. Preventing septic arthritis focuses on appropriate, timely and complete treatment for infections and avoidance of high-risk behaviors associated with diseases such as gonorrhea.

Assessment

History. The most common presenting symptoms include joint pain (often exaggerated with motion), swelling, erythema, and heat in the involved joint. In the early stages of the condition, these symptoms may be minimal. Newborns and infants may experience symptoms of fever, irritability, and the inability to move the limb with the infected joint. In children and adults, these symptoms may be accompanied by joint swelling and joint redness. The medical history of a child will include any recent infection at another site, including upper respiratory infection, impetigo, otitis media, or recent history of trauma to the involved joint. The adult history may include a family or patient history of rheumatoid arthritis; recent history of uninvolved joint sepsis; and recent history of acute illness such as gonorrhea, hepatitis, or rubella.

Physical Exam. A thorough inspection of all joints for signs of erythema, warmth, and tenderness is essential in diagnosing the infection. Infected joints usually exhibit effusion, which is associated with marked limitation of both active and passive ranges of motion (ROM). If the septic arthritis is in the lower extremity, of the patient may exhibit an antalgic gait or inability to walk. If an upper extremity is involved, the patient may exhibit guarding of the affected extremity.

Diagnostic Tests. The physician will order x-rays that may show joint effusion, soft tissue swelling, and synovial thickening. A synovial fluid aspirate often shows elevated leukocytes. The differential white blood cell (WBC) count will usually indicate an increase in neutrophils. Neutrophils usually comprise approximately 70% of the total leukocytes; in patients with septic arthritis, neutrophils may account for approximately 90% of the total WBC. Elevated neutrophils usually indicate an acute infection associated with a bacterial origin. The joint aspirate fluid culture will generally grow out the causative pathogen, other than gonococcus bacteria, which are difficult to grow. A sedimentation rate and C-reactive protein are generally elevated with septic arthritis. Blood cultures are frequently ordered because septic arthritis may be due to hematogenous spread.

Common Therapeutic Modalities

The most important intervention is immediate antibiotic therapy based on the culture results. Empiric therapy is usually started prior to culture results if suspicion is high. Drainage of the purulence—by aspiration, arthroscopic, or open surgical drainage—is necessary to promote healing and resolution of the infection. Rest and immobilization of the affected extremity are important measures to assist with the body's immune and defense response until the acute symptoms resolve, and post-resolution rehabilitation of the joint may involve physical therapy.

Nursing Considerations

Nursing Diagnosis. Nursing diagnoses for this condition are expanded upon in the Appendix.

- Activity intolerance, risk for.
- Infection, risk for.
- Mobility, impaired physical.
- Pain, acute.
- Skin integrity, risk for impaired.

Nursing Interventions. Nursing interventions in the acute setting are aimed at assessment for worsening infection. This includes temperature and vital signs, as well as changes in mental status or increased pain. Interventions also include measures to prevent further infection, including adherence to hand hygiene, maintenance of sterile technique during invasive procedures, and care of urinary and intravenous catheters according to evidence-based practices and organizational policy. In the office and home care setting, the nurse should observe carefully for any signs or symptoms of extended infection and assess the patient's response to antibiotic therapy. Review treatment modalities with the patient, and assess for any changes in the individual treatment plan.

It is important that the orthopaedic nurse also offer emotional support. Parents of pediatric patients may experience a high degree of anxiety. Thorough explanation of the treatment regime and expected outcomes can help lessen the anxiety. Providing adult patients the opportunity to verbalize fears and apprehension can also help with adherence to the treatment plan.

Patient Teaching. One of the most important aspects of the educational plan is adherence and compliance with antibiotic treatment regimens. Inadequate or incomplete antibiotic regimens have also been associated with the development of drug-resistant bacteria. It is also important t once symptoms have improved, to reinforce active ROM exercises and the necessity for the patient to follow the established, individualized PT regime. Effective nursing management requires attention to position, exercise, and rehabilitation. Initial therapy consists of maintaining the joint in its functional position and providing passive ROM exercises as inflammation begins to resolve, in order to preserve joint function. The nurse should assure that the joint bears no weight until symptoms have resolved.

Prosthetic Joint Infections

Overview

Definition. A prosthetic joint is one in which the arthritic or dysfunctional joint surface is replaced with an orthopaedic prosthesis. A prosthetic joint infection is an infection surrounding a prosthetic joint. These infections can be classified into early, delayed, and late onset infections (Table 9.3).

Etiology. Prosthetic joints can facilitate infection by either locally introduced contamination or hematogenous spread of microorganisms. Locally introduced contamination usually occurs during the perioperative period. Infections that arise due to local contamination are the result of an infection adjacent to the prosthesis or to contamination during the surgical procedure (Brause, 2010).

Hematogenous spread of microorganisms, an event that typically happens following the perioperative period, is associated with primary bacteremia or infection at a distant site with secondary bacteremia, leading to microbial seeding of the prosthetic joint. Hematogenous spread from transient bacteremia may occur from obvious sources of infection such as intravascular catheters, pneumonia, urinary tract infections (UTIs), dental caries, gum disease, and skin conditions. Transient bacteremia may occur during invasive procedures such as colonoscopy, urinary catheterization, and dental cleaning. Commonly isolated organisms at fault are *Staphylococcus aureus, Staphylococcus epidermidis, Streptococcus, Pseudomonas aeruginosa*, and *Escherichia coli* (Brause, 2010).

Compromising factors that increase the risk of prosthetic joint infection include prior surgery at the site, soft tissue loss, prior radiation to the surgical area, fistula formation, or other active infection present longer than 3-4 months. Compromise secondary to malnutrition, cardiac or pulmonary insufficiency, renal failure, diabetes, immune compromise, systemic inflammatory disease, alcoholism, smoking, or chronic indwelling catheters are also risk factors for the development of prosthetic joint infection (Baddour & Sexton, 2011).

Pathophysiology. Prosthetic joint infection develops once the causative pathogen is introduced into viable tissue and then creates local edema, necrosis, and inflammation reducing local circulation. The bacterial toxins accumulate and increase the local acidity. As the acidity increases, the phagocytes die, releasing enzymes and creating further tissue destruction. Microorganisms may contain or produce toxins and other substances that increase their ability to invade a host, produce damage within the host, or survive on or in host tissue. Characteristics of the specific infecting microorganism, particularly related to virulence and the ability to adhere to a foreign object such as an implantable device, play a role in the presentation of infection (Greene et al., 2010).

Incidence. The rate of prosthetic joint infection ranges from 0.5%-1.0% for hip replacements, 0.5%-2% for knee replacements, and less than 1% for shoulder replacements (Baddour & Sexton, 2011). In a study of 69,000 patients undergoing elective total knee replacement (TKR) followed longitudinally from 1997 to 2006, the rate of infection was highest during the first 2 years following surgery (incidence 1.5%). The rate of infection 2-10 years after joint replacement was 0.5% (Kurtz, 2010).

Preventive Measures. Surgical site infections (SSIs) following joint replacements have decreased since evidence-based practices related to skin preparation,

Table 9.3. Classifications Based on Differences Among Onset of Infection

Early Onset	Delayed Onset	Late Onset
Occurs within 30 days of surgery.	Occurs more than 30 days postoperatively. Up to 1 year postoperatively is considered health care-associated.	More than 1 year after surgery.
Usually acquired during implantation.	Usually acquired during implantation but can also be acquired in postoperative period.	Frequently develop hematogenously in the setting of infection at another site (vascular catheter, urinary tract, or soft tissue infection).
Often due to virulent organisms such as Staphylococcus aureus or gram-negative bacteria.	Often associated with less virulent or indolent organisms such as coagulase negative staphylococcus.	Can be associated with Streptococci, Staphylococci, and gram-negative bacilli.
Present with acute onset pain, fever, drainage.	Present with indolent course and progressive pain.	Presentation similar to acute onset in previously well-functioning joint.

Data from Principles and Practice of Infectious Diseases *(7th ed., p.1469-1484), by B. Brause, 2010, Philadelphia, PA: Churchill Livingston.*

surgical technique, and antibiotic prophylaxis have become the accepted standard of care in orthopaedic surgery. The adverse outcome of SSIs related to a prosthetic joint infection, however, continues to be associated with significant morbidity, cost, and even mortality (Brause, 2010). The patient's functional status may also be adversely affected by an orthopaedic SSI. Prevention measures used to reduce the likelihood of prosthetic joint infection include preoperative showers with chlorhexidine, surgical antibiotic prophylaxis, chlorhexidine/alcohol surgical skin preparation, laminar flow air or body exhaust suits, antimicrobial sutures, incisional adhesives, antibiotic-impregnated cements, and antimicrobial gauze dressings (Moucha, Clyburn, Evans, & Prokuski, 2011). Measures that have not been shown to reduce prosthetic joint infection include routine use of bacitracin/polymixin irrigation and antimicrobial-impregnated incise drapes.

Recent evidence also points to the process of screening patients for Staphylococcus carriage and administering nasal mupirocin to eliminate carriage preoperatively. In a randomized, double-blind, placebo-controlled, multicenter trial, rapid identification of *Staphylococcus aureus* nasal carriers followed by treatment with mupirocin nasal ointment and chlorhexidine soap reduced the risk of hospital-associated infection with this organism (Bode et al., 2010).

Complications. Each prosthetic revision increases the chance of subsequent sepsis and generally increases bone loss. These infections, and their resulting complications, can be costly and devastating for both the patient and the surgeon Prosthetic joint infections are both costly and disabling, usually requiring either 1.) removal of the prosthesis followed by a disabling arthrodesis; or 2.) removal of the materials, stabilization of the joint, administration of intravenous antibiotics for several weeks, and implantation of a new joint. Reinfection is a major problem. In the case of TKR, progressive infections can lead to amputation.

Assessment

History. The most common presentation is pain with or without other signs of infection. Some patients will have fever, night sweats, chills, local erythema, drainage, wound sinus, and secondary bacteremia. Risk factors often include revision joint surgery, diabetes, obesity, immunosuppressive therapy, recent dental surgery, local skin conditions, blood transfusions, presence of a postoperative hematoma, and intravascular or invasive procedures.

Physical Exam. The physical manifestations of a prosthetic join infection will depend on the virulence of the organism and host factors. Pain in the region of the prosthesis may be present, particularly with compression. Often the patient will have decreased ROM in the affected joint, coupled with erythema, swelling, edema, and increased warmth. Wound drainage may be serous, serosanguinous, seropurulent, or purulent. A local cellulitis may also be the presenting symptom.

Diagnostic Tests. The surgeon will generally perform an arthrocentesis to obtain joint fluid prior to the initiation of antibiotic therapy. This procedure is generally conducted under fluoroscopy. The joint fluid is sent for gram stain, culture, and cell count. Joint fluid is culture-positive in approximately 60%-70% of infected joints, and gram stain may just show polymorphonuclear cells. Surgical biopsy obtained during irrigation and debridement is necessary for definitive diagnosis, with specimens sent for culture and pathology examination. An elevated sedimentation rate and C-reactive protein are generally present with prosthetic joint infection. X-rays of the joint may show loosening or cyst formation if the infection is long-term. A bone scan can rule out infection if negative. A gallium scan may identify an increased uptake in mechanical loosening or infection.

Common Therapeutic Modalities

Therapeutic modalities include a variety of options from medical treatment to surgical intervention. Acute infections can often be treated with antibiotics if diagnosed early. Arthroscopic drainage and long-term intravenous antibiotic therapy can be used in patients with early onset prosthetic joint infection. Late onset infections usually require surgical intervention. Debridement may be necessary. In the case of total knee replacements, a two-stage exchange arthroplasty are often successful (Kalore, Gioe, & Singh, 2007). Arthrodesis (fusion of the joint) is sometimes the treatment of choice for patients who have poor skin coverage and inadequate tissue. Elderly patients who have contraindications to general anesthesia are occasionally treated with long-term suppressive therapy (Baddour & Sexton, 2011).

Nursing Considerations

Nursing Diagnoses. Nursing diagnoses for this condition are expanded upon in the Appendix.

- Activity intolerance, risk for.
- Infection, risk for.
- Pain, acute.
- Mobility, impaired physical.
- Skin integrity, risk for impaired.

Nursing Interventions. See "Osteomyelitis / Septic Arthritis."

Bone and Joint/Extrapulmonary Tuberculosis

Overview

Definition. Bone and joint tuberculosis (TB) is an infectious process from the hematogenous spread of *Mycobacterium tuberculosis*, causing destruction of the bones and joints. It is an extrapulmonary form of TB that occurs after hematogenous spread from a primary lung lesion. This form of musculoskeletal TB is not communicable to others.

Etiology. *Mycobacterium tuberculosis* is transmitted through the airborne route, and the infection develops in the lungs after inhaling the tubercule bacilli. A positive tuberculin test indicates latent TB infection as the body exhibits an immune response to the presence of the organism in the lung. As it progresses, the infection develops into TB disease, and the *Mycobacterium tuberculosis* can spread hematogenously through the bloodstream to the bones or synovial lining of joints.

Pathophysiology. The onset is usually insidious, with a long history of mild or moderate joint or bone pain. Only 50% of patients with bone or joint TB have active pulmonary TB. The *Mycobacterium tuberculosis* causes an inflammatory reaction, followed by the formation of granulation tissue. The organism does not produce enzymes to destroy the cartilage, but rather the granulation tissue eventually erodes the cartilage and the bone. In advanced disease, abscesses may form around the joint, eventually draining through the skin and producing secondary bacterial contamination. In spinal TB, the disc space quickly narrows, followed by destruction of the vertebral bodies. The anterior body generally collapses, producing gibbous deformities and significant kyphosis of multiple vertebrae (Bozkurt, Dogan, Sesen, Turanli, & Basbozkurt, 2005).

Incidence. The incidence of extrapulmonary TB in the United States has increased consistent with the prevalence of HIV, which alters the cell-mediated immune system. The Centers for Disease Control and Prevention (CDC) estimate that persons with HIV are 20-30 times more likely to develop TB than those without HIV (Jensen, 2005). Pott's disease is a presentation of extrapulmonary TB that affects the spine. It is a form of tuberculous arthritis of the intervertebral joints. The lower thoracic and upper lumbar lesions are more common in adults, while the upper thoracic is more common in children. In order, spine, hip, knee, ankle, sacroiliac joint, shoulder, and wrist are the most commonly affected joints (McDonald & Sexton, 2010). One third of skeletal TB cases involve the spine. This is primarily a result of past hematigenous foci, contiguous disease, or lymphatic spread from pleural disease (Fitzgerald, Sterling, & Hass, 2010). According to the CDC 2010 report on tuberculosis in the United States, bone and joint TB accounts for approximately 10% of extrapulmonary TB cases and 1%-2% of total cases (CDC, 2010). It is more common in individuals of Asian, African, and Latin American descent.

Considerations Across the Life Span. The risk of developing TB and subsequent skeletal TB are increased with extremes of age (very old and very young), immunosuppression, and malnutrition. Infants and children are at increased risk for developing skeletal TB due to the vascularity of immature pediatric bone, allowing easier hematogenous spread. Spinal and bone deformities can occur following skeletal TB in both children and adults.

Complications. Some of the complication associated with bone and joint TB include loss of joint function, fractures secondary to osteoporosis, and bone and joint deformities. Patients may also develop chronic pain and possible paralysis from untreated spinal TB.

Assessment

History. The common presenting symptoms include mild to moderate joint or bone pain, joint effusions, systemic symptoms such as night sweats or weight loss, and spinal deformity. The medical history should include questions about country of birth, as well as inquiries into pulmonary TB or household exposure to TB. Experiences of night sweats, weight loss, immune compromise, and joint effusions also point toward bone and joint TB.

Physical Exam. On physical examination, the synovium may be thickened and possible joint effusion may be noted. The joint may have increased warmth, severe muscle atrophy surrounding the joint, and limited motion—especially in later infection. Alterations in posture, gibbous deformities, or kyphosis of the spine may be present.

Diagnostic Tests. The diagnostic work-up for bone and joint TB will include X-rays. Severe osteoporosis of the surrounding bones is often found, even early in the infection. There may also be soft tissue swelling but preservation of the cartilage until late in the disease process. CT and MRI may be useful in diagnosing skeletal TB. A tuberculin skin test will usually be positive, unless the patient is immunocompromised. The sedimentation rate may be elevated, and the complete blood count might show a normal or slightly elevated WBC count. Culture of synovial fluid is usually positive for *Mycobacterium tuberculosis*, but the culture results may take 6-8 weeks because it is a slow-growing bacterium. Needle aspiration and biopsy are recommended for confirming spinal disease (McDonald & Sexton, 2010)

Common Therapeutic Modalities

The antibiotic therapy for TB includes a multidrug regimen. Because of the slow-growing nature of the TB and its ability to mutate, treatment is a combination of drugs that is effective against TB in all phases of its life span and is adjusted based on culture and sensitivity. Compliance with a full course of treatment is necessary to gain cure, prevent the emergence of drug resistance, and stop the transmission of disease. The earlier the diagnosis is made and treatment initiated, the better the outcome. The tubercle bacilli tend to mutate into drug-resistant forms if they are exposed to drugs but not initially killed. The same drugs used to treat pulmonary TB are effective for bone and joint TB. Current recommendations are to treat spinal TB with a 6- to 9-month regime that includes Isoniazid (INH) and Rifampin combined with pyrazinamide (PZA) and ethambutol for 2 months (Fitzgerald et al., 2010).

Surgical intervention may be used to establish diagnosis, drain abscesses, or stabilize joints. With spinal TB, surgical fusion may be necessary if spontaneous fusion does not occur. Synovectomy is sometimes done to remove a large site of infection.

Nursing Considerations

Nursing Diagnoses. Nursing diagnoses for this condition are expanded upon in the Appendix.

- Activity intolerance, risk for.
- Infection, risk for.
- Mobility, impaired physical.
- Pain, chronic.

Nursing Interventions. Nursing interventions should focus on drug management and tolerance to medications. Patients who take their medications in an irregular way are at greatly increased risk of treatment failure, relapse, and the development of drug-resistant TB strains. A major side effect of TB treatment is drug-induced hepatitis. Liver function tests should be checked at the start of treatment, and the patient should be advised of the symptoms of hepatitis that must be reported immediately.

Patient Teaching. Because antituberculosis drugs may be associated with hepatic dysfunction, patients are advised not to consume alcohol.

Practice Setting Considerations. Cases of TB must be reported to state agencies in accordance with public health law. Drug resistance is almost always secondary to inadequate or inappropriate drug therapy. Patients must be monitored for toxic side effects of medications. Directly observed therapy is beneficial for those at risk for noncompliance or drug-resistant TB.

Skin and Soft Tissue Infections

Overview

Definition. Skin and soft tissue infections are common and are usually uncomplicated; however, these infections can worsen if not recognized and treated promptly.

- Impetigo (or pyoderma) is a superficial localized infection of the skin characterized by pustules. It usually occurs on exposed areas such as the face or extremity, but it may also cause local and regional lymphadenopathy.
- Folliculitis is a minor infection of the hair follicle that can progress to inflammatory nodules called furuncles that may become infected.
- Cellulitis is an extensive inflammation of the skin and subcutaneous tissue infections, but a multitude of organisms can be responsible and it may occur secondary to a local trauma, a break in the skin, or a surgical wound (Eron, 2009). Occasionally, it occurs without a preceding incident. Infection usually is caused by *Streptococcus* but can be related to abrasions or eczematous lesions. Facial cellulitis may develop following an upper respiratory tract strep infection.
- Pyomyositis is an acute bacterial infection of skeletal muscle.
- Clostridial myonecrosis (or gas gangrene) is an acute infection of the soft tissue and muscle, with clostridium quickly causing muscle necrosis. It can quickly become life-threatening.
- Necrotizing fasciitis is an acute infection of the fascia and surrounding muscle that can quickly become life-threatening.

Etiology. *Staphylococcus* and *Streptococcus* are the most common infections, but a multitude of organisms can be responsible. Impetigo is generally caused by streptococcal organisms at the site of previous abrasions or insect bites. Folliculitis is generally caused by normal skin flora bacteria such as *Staphylococcus* in areas of friction and sweat gland activity. Cellulitis, usually found in areas of venous stasis or areas where lymphatic drainage is blocked, is often caused by *Streptococcus* organisms but may be caused by multiple organisms. Erysipelas, a type of cellulitis that frequently occurs at the site of free tissue transfers (especially in the leg), is due to the lack of lymphatic drainage in the flap and thus inability to clear transient streptococcus organisms. Pyomyositis is generally caused by *Staphylococcus aureus* (about 95% of the time) after deep nonpenetrating trauma to the involved muscle. Clostridial myositis, caused by gas-forming anaerobic bacteria (usually *Clostridium perfringens*), frequently occurs secondary to puncture wounds. The gram stain will show gram-positive rods. (Other organisms can produce myonecrosis, but they generally do not advance as rapidly or produce the toxins.) Necrotizing fasciitis is generally caused by *Streptococcus* (but can be caused by other organisms) that causes infection at the site and then quickly spreads to the surrounding fascia, producing putrification of the fascia.

Pathophysiology. Skin lesions such as minor abrasions, burns, IV sites, and decubitis ulcers may become secondarily infected. Infections can be mild or life-threatening, depending on the virulence of the organisms, portal of entry, and condition of the host.

Incidence. Skin and soft tissue infections affect 1.1%-6% of the general population. The annual incidence of cellulitis is about 200 cases per 100,000 patients (McNamara et al., 2007). Cellulitis is observed most frequently among middle-aged and elderly individuals, while erysipelas occurs in young children and the elderly. Infections range from very mild requiring little (if any) treatment to those with life-threatening consequences. Group A strep infections occur at an estimated 3.5 cases per 100,000 persons (Stevens, 2011). Methicillin-resistant *Staphylococcus* (MRSA) soft tissue infections can occur in anyone but are most common in athletes, students, military recruits, men who have sex with men, incarcerated individuals, and anyone who shares a common shower area or dormitory. An estimated 126,000 hospitalized patients are infected with MRSA each year (Eron, 2009).

Preventive Strategies. Wounds should be thoroughly cleaned with soap and water. Crush injuries and open fractures require extensive irrigation and surgical debridement as necessary. Diabetic patients should receive appropriate foot care and seek prompt treatment for any signs of infection or injury.

Assessment

History. Patients with skin and soft tissue infections should be assessed for poor nutrition and recent trauma—including surgery—to the involved area. In cellulitis and infections of the muscle and fascia, fever, chills, and general malaise may also be present. Localized muscle pain may progress quickly to swelling and induration (sclerosis or hardening). Soft tissue infection due to gas gangrene exhibit toxins that necrotize the muscle and release gas, producing the classic symptoms of swelling with purple or bronze discoloration. Bullae, watery discharge, and (in later stage) crepitation may be present due to the gas within the tissues. In deep muscle infections and necrotizing fasciitis, the skin may not indicate the true extent of the infection. Patients can quickly become toxic, and pain is usually severe.

Physical Exam. Common findings on physical examination include pain, erythema, edema, fluctuance, or drainage. It is important to observe for breaks or abnormalities in the skin such as cuts, scrapes, bruises, and ulcers. Patients with necrotizing fasciitis may have skin discoloration, blisters, skin drainage, and crepitus, as well as swollen glands near the affected site.

Diagnostic Tests. Culture of drainage from the affected areas (if it is present) and blood cultures may be ordered as indicated. An aspiration for culture of deep abscesses should be obtained to determine the causative agent and direct appropriate antimicrobial therapy. A CT scan or MRI should be ordered to visualize the extent of muscle and fascia involvement. Lab tests include a complete blood count (CBC) and WBC count that will often be elevated, significantly with myonecrosis. Radiological exams may be helpful to detect gas in tissue or underlying fracture, foreign body, or osteomyelitis.

Common Therapeutic Modalities

Local or oral antibiotics are indicated for mild infections. More severe infections require systemic antibiotics that are started empirically, based on the organisms that commonly cause the diagnosis, and then adjusted to the specific organism once culture and sensitivities are available.

Surgical exploration is often required to define the nature of the infection, assess the degree of tissue involvement, and begin necessary debridement. Serial surgical debridements are often necessary to remove all nonviable tissue, followed by gradual closure once no further necrosis is present. Clostridial myonecrosis requires extensive surgical excision and possibly fasciotomy to drain the watery discharge and relieve swelling. Fasciotomy as necessary to reduce compartment pressures caused by deep abscesses within the muscle. HBO therapy inhibits toxins present in the tissues and aids in maintaining viable tissue. The patient will need general supportive nursing care and may need mechanical ventilation and total parenteral nutrition.

Nursing Considerations

Nursing Diagnoses: Nursing diagnoses for this condition are expanded upon in the Appendix.

- Activity intolerance, risk for.
- Infection, risk for.
- Mobility, impaired physical.
- Pain, acute.

Nursing Interventions and Patient Teaching: See "Osteomyelitis."

Practice Setting Considerations. *Hospital:* The nurse will have to instruct the patient in proper wound care and dressing changes. Another important aspect of patient education will be the need to regain or maintain adequate nutritional intake.

Office: In the office setting, the patient should be reinforced to follow the instructions for care given in the hospital. The importance of ambulation and mobility should be stressed.

Home: The nurse should explain, and ask the patient to reiterate, the importance of proper wound care and the importance of maintaining proper nutrition. Both the patient and the family/caregivers must be instructed on the importance of compliance with the antibiotic regimen. The patient and family must be instructed to assess skin regularly and report any signs of onset of infection.

Healthcare-Associated Infections

Overview

Definition. A healthcare-associated infection (HAI) is acquired within a hospital or health care institution, including ambulatory surgery centers and extended care facilities. The source of most HAIs is from endogenous sources from the patient's own bacterial flora. Other sources are exogenous from the hands of health care workers, contaminated medical equipment, and cross-contamination from other patients (Yoeke, 2008). Common HAIs include the following:

- Catheter-associated urinary tract infection (CAUTI)
- Surgical site infection (SSI);
- Ventilator-associated pneumonia (VAP); and
- Central line associated bloodstream infection (CLABSI).

Common HAI Pathogens. *Escherichia coli*, gram-negative rods, and Group D *Enterococci* are most common in UTI. They colonize the gastrointestinal tract and distal meatus and can therefore ascend around the catheter into the bladder. *Pseudomonas aeruginosa* and *Staphylococcus aureus* are most common in VAP. Gram-negative rods can easily colonize respiratory equipment due to the moisture in the equipment. *Staphylococcus aureus* also colonizes the upper respiratory tract, and the excretions around the endotracheal tube aspirate into the lungs. *Staphylococcus aureus* and coagulase-negative *Staphylococcus* are the two most common bacteria responsible for CLABSI and septic phlebitis. These organisms are skin colonizers and produce biofilm that can adhere to catheters and ascend into the bloodstream. Another pathogen common with the use of total parenteral nutrition is *Candida albicans* that can grow in the higher glucose concentration. An increasing number of pathogens associated with HAIs are becoming resistant to conventional antibiotics secondary to the overuse and misuse of antibiotics, such as MRSA, Methicillin-resistant *Staphylococcus epidermidis* (MRSE), Vancomycin-resistant *enterococci* (VRE), multidrug resistant *Acinetobacter*, and Carbapenem-resistant *Klebsiella pneumoniae* (CRKP).

Pathophysiology. UTI is the most common HAI. Bacterial infections develop in 2%-4% of these cases. Risk factors are urinary catheterizations, keeping the catheter is in place for an extended duration, being female due to the short length of the urethra, and breakage of the closed urinary system.

SSI may be superficial, deep, or extend into organ space. Risk factors include extended preoperative hospitalization, long surgical operative time, high operating room traffic, poor nutritional status, and inappropriate antibiotic prophylaxis. Routes of bacterial entry can be direct contamination or hematogenous spread.

VAP is associated with significant morbidity and mortality. Risk factors include age >70 years, chronic lung disease, contamination of mechanical ventilation equipment, immunosuppression, recent surgery, and fall/winter seasons. Routes of bacterial entry can be by aspiration of gastric contents, inhalation of contaminated solutions in nebulizers, and direct introduction of pathogens by suction catheters and endotracheal tubes.

CLABSI is commonly associated with sepsis and bacteremia introduced via central and peripheral venous catheters. Risk factors include the type and location of venous catheter, the length of time catheter is in place, and immunosuppression. Routes of entry can be intraluminal by contaminated solutions or extraluminal by bacteria that colonize the catheter entry site.

The ever-increasing antibiotic-resistant bacteria are associated with longer or more frequent hospitalizations, prolonged illness, immunosuppression, and use of more toxic antibiotics. Risk factors include prior antibiotic therapy; intensive care unit (ICU) stay; and the presence of invasive devices such as IVs, catheters, and endotracheal tubes.

Incidence. Approximately 5% of all hospital admissions will develop HAIs (Scott, 2009), which result in excess length of stay, higher mortality rates, and increasing health care costs. An estimated 1.7 million HAIs occurred in the United States, resulting in 99,000 deaths (Klevens, 2007).

Complications. HAIs can lead to morbidity, mortality, excess length of stay, and increased cost. CLABSI may lead to secondary seeding of valves, resulting in endocarditis. The patient who develops a CAUTI may develop a secondary bloodstream infection. Treatment of CAUTI may result in excess use of antibiotics and emergence of antibiotic resistance.

Prevention. Patients with orthopaedic infections often require acute care, rehabilitation, or long-term care. These patients may also be discharged to their home with invasive devices such as urinary catheters or peripherally inserted central catheter (PICC) lines. Each facility should establish strategies to avoid these preventable infections (see Table 9.4).

Table 9.4. HAI Prevention Strategies

Infection Type	Prevention Strategies
Catheter Associated Urinary Tract Infections (CAUTI)	■ Follow appropriate indications for insertion. ■ Remove as soon as possible. ■ Aseptic technique during insertion. ■ Keep drainage bag below the level of the bladder.
Surgical Site Infections (SSI)	■ Appropriate and timely surgical prophylaxis. ■ Appropriate surgical skin prep. ■ Maintain sterile field during surgery. ■ Pre-op surgical hand scrub.
Ventilator Associated Pneumonia (VAP)	■ Keep head of bed 30-45 degrees. ■ Routine mouth care. ■ Sedation vacation and weaning. ■ Aseptic technique. ■ Hand hygiene.
Central Line Blood Stream infections (CLABSI)	*Central line insertion bundle* ■ Hand hygiene. ■ Maximum barrier precautions. ■ Avoid femoral site. ■ Assess daily for need for line. ■ Chlorohexidine skin prep. *Central line maintenance* ■ Scrub the hub prior to access. ■ Aseptic technique. ■ Hand hygiene.
Drug-Resistant Organisms and ***Clostridium difficile***	■ Isolate patient and don appropriate protective attire as indicated per organizational policy. ■ Target antibiotics based upon the organism. ■ Do not treat colonization. ■ Hand hygiene. ■ Environmental disinfection. ■ Clean equipment between patients.

Data from "Compendium of Strategies to Prevent Healthcare-Associated Infections in Acute Care Hospitals" by D. Yoeke et al., 2008, Infection Control and Hospital Epidemiology, *29(Suppl 1), S12-S21.*

Assessment

History. Patients who develop HAIs may have a history of recent hospitalization or surgical intervention.

Certain host specific risk factors may be associated with increased risk of infection such as diabetes, history of smoking or chronic pulmonary disease, obesity cancer, and prior colonization with a resistant organism (Greene et al., 2010)

Physical Exam. Findings on the physical examination are consistent with the type of HAI. For example, CAUTIs are often associated with fever, urgency, dysuria, and suprapubic tenderness. Patients with a suspected SSI will often have purulent drainage from the surgical incisional area, as well as pain and tenderness. Patients with a suspected CLABSI often have unexplained fever and elevated WBC counts.

Diagnostic Tests. Cultures are obtained based upon the suspected site of infection. For example, a urine culture is obtained if a CAUTI is expected or blood cultures if a CLABSI is suspected. Physicians may order cultures from various sources if the potential source of the infection is unclear. Cultures are usually positive. Sedimentation rate and C-reactive protein may be elevated. X-rays are useful to confirm a pneumonia diagnosis.

Common Therapeutic Modalities

Infections are treated with antibiotics targeted at the source of infection. Although broad-spectrum antibiotics may be started initially, the antibiotic is narrowed or changed based upon culture and sensitivity data. SSIs may require drainage or debridement. In the case of CLABSI, removal of the infected line may be required. Patients with CAUTIs should have the catheter removed and replaced if needed.

Nursing Considerations

Nursing Diagnoses. Nursing diagnoses for this condition are expanded upon in the Appendix.

- Gas exchange, impaired.
- Infection, risk for.
- Ventilation, impaired spontaneous.

Nursing Interventions. Because these infections can quickly become life-threatening, it is vital for the orthopaedic nurse to work with the entire health care team in preventing or minimizing complications. Infection-prevention measures for sepsis include general infection control practices, hand-washing principles, and measures to prevent HAIs (oral care and proper positioning to prevent pneumonia, care of invasive catheters, skin care, wound care, identifying patients at risk for infection, prioritizing cultures for patients with suspected infection, and providing astute clinical assessment for early detection of sepsis). It cannot be stressed enough that hand hygiene is an essential element in reducing the spread of infection.

Nursing-related care aimed at preventing UTSs includes thorough assessment to determine need for indwelling catheter use, aseptic insertion technique, indwelling catheter care to minimize infection risk, and astute monitoring of patients with urinary catheters for signs of infection. Measures to reduce the incidence of CLABSI include ensuring maximal barrier precautions during line insertion, maintenance of the central line site to minimize infection risk, prevention of contamination of central line ports during blood sampling, and maintenance of sterile techniques for dressing changes.

Patient Teaching. Patient teaching is important across the continuum of care. In the acute care setting, patients should be instructed to report increased pain, chills, or rigors. Deep breathing exercises to prevent pneumonia and proper catheter care are important. Patients who are discharged with an invasive device (such as a urinary catheter or an intravenous catheter for the administration of medications) must be instructed on aseptic technique, as well as know the signs and symptoms of infection to report immediately.

Summary

Orthopaedic infections can be associated with significant morbidity and mortality. Disease-carrying bacteria, viruses, and parasites that get into the body can destroy healthy tissue, multiply quickly, and spread through blood. Infection of skin and other soft tissue can lead to infection of bones (osteomyelitis) and joints (septic arthritis). Without prompt treatment, orthopaedic infections can become chronic. Fortunately, early diagnosis, appropriate antibiotic therapy, and surgical intervention when required can cure most infections and prevent permanent problems. Nursing plays a pivotal role in both prevention of these infection and health restoration.

References

Baddour, L. & Sexton, D. (2011). *Prevention of Prosthetic Joint Infections.* Retrieved August 18, 2011, from http://www.uptodate.com/contents/prevention-of-prosthetic-joint-infections

Berbari, E., Steckelenberg, J., & Osmon, D. (2010). Osteomyelitis. In G. Mandell, J. Bennett & R. Dolin (Eds.) *Principles and Practice of Infectious Diseases* (7th ed., pp. 1457-1467). Philadelphia, PA: Churchill Livingston.

Bode, L.G., Kluytmans, J.A., Wertheim, H.F., Bogaers, D., Vandenbroucke-Grauls, C.M., Roosendaal, R., … Vos, M.C. (2010). Preventing surgical-site infections in nasal carriers of staphylococcus aureus. *New England Journal of Medicine*, 362(1), 9-17.

Bozkurt, M., Dogan, M., Sesen, H., Turanli, S., & Basbozkurt, M. (2005). Isolated medial cuneiform tuberculosis: A case report. *Journal of Foot & Ankle Surgery*, 44(1), 60-63.

Brause, B. (2010). Infections with prosthesis in bones and joints. In G. Mandell, J. Bennett & R. Dolin (Eds.) *Principles and Practice of Infectious Diseases* (7th ed., pp. 1469-1484). Philadelphia, PA: Churchill Livingston.

Brusch, J. (2011). *Septic Arthritis of Native Joints Organism-Specific Therapy.* Retrieved September 2, 2011, from http://emedicine.medscape.com/article/2018439-overview

Centers for Disease Control and Prevention (CDC). (2010). *Reported Tuberculosis in the US.* Retrieved March 2012, from http://www.cdc.gov/statistics/reports/2010

Cierny, G., Mader, J., & Penninck, J. (2003). A clinical staging system for adult osteomyelitis. *Clinical Orthopedics and Related Research*, 414, 7-24.

Chihara, S. & Segreti, J. (2010). Osteomyelitis. *Disease-A-Month, 56*(1), 5-31.

Eron, L. (2009). Cellulitis and soft tissue infections. *Annals of Internal Medicine, 150*(1), ITC11.

Espinoza, L.R. (2007). Infections of bursae, joint, and bones. In L. Goldman & D. Ausiello (Eds.) *Cecil Medicine* (23rd ed., pp.20161-2069). Philadelphia, PA: Saunders.

Fang, R.C. & Galiano, R.D. (2009). Adjunctive therapies in the treatment of osteomyelitis. *Seminars in Plastic Surgery, 23*(2), 141-147. doi:10.1055/s-0029-1214166

Fitzgerald, D., Sterling, T., Hass, D. (2010.) Mycobacterium tuberculosis. In G. Mandell, J. Bennett & R. Dolin (Eds.) *Principles and Practice of Infectious Diseases* (7th ed., pp. 3129-3263). Philadelphia, PA: Churchill Livingston.

Goldberg, D. & Sexton, D. (2011). *Septic Arthritis in Adults.* Retrieved February 18, 2012, from http://www.uptodate.com/contents/septic-arthritis-inadults?source=search_result&search=septic+arthritis&selectedTitle=1%7E150

Greene, L., Mills, R., Moss, R., Sposato, K., & Vignari, M. (2010). *Guide to Elimination of Orthopedic Surgical Site Infections.* Retrieved August 1, 2011, from http://www.apic.org/Resource_/EliminationGuideForm/34e03612-d1e6-4214-a76b-e532c6fc3898/File/APIC-Ortho-Guide.pdf

Howell, W. & Goulston, C. (2011). Osteomyelitis: An update for hospitalists. *Hospital Practice, 39*(1), 153; Feb-160.

Jensen, P., Lambert, L., Iademarco, M., & Ridzon, R. (2005). *Guidelines for Preventing the Transmission of Mycobacterium Tuberculosis in Health Care Settings: 2005 Morbidity and Mortality Report.* Retrieved from http://www.cdc.gov/mmwr/pdf/rr/rr5417.pdf.

Kalore, N.V., Gioe, T.J., & Singh, J.A. (2011). Diagnosis and management of infected total knee arthroplasty. *Open Orthopedics Journal, 5*, 86-91. doi:10.2174/1874325001105010086

Kherani, R.B. & Shojania, K. (2007). Septic arthritis in patients with pre-existing inflammatory arthritis. *Canadian Medical Association Journal, 176*(11), 1605-1608.

Klevens, M. (2007). Estimating health care-associated infections and deaths in U.S. hospitals. *PublicHealth Reports, 122*(2), 160–166.

Krogstad, P. (2012). *Epidemiology, Pathogenesis, and Microbiology of Hematogenous Osteomyelitis in Children.* Retrieved February 28, 2012, from http://www.uptodate.com/contents/epidemiology-pathogenesis-and-microbiology-of-hematogenous-osteomyelitisinchildren

Lalani, T. (2011.) *Overview of Osteomyelitis in Adults.* Retrieved February 21, 2012, from http://www.uptodate.com/contents/overview-of-osteomyelitis-in-adults

Lew, D.P. & Waldvogel, F.A. (2004). Osteomyelitis. *Lancet.* 364:369–379.

Mathews, C.J., Kingsley, G., Field, M., Jones, A., Weston, V.C., Phillips, M., . .Coakley, G. (2007). Management of septic arthritis: A systematic review. *Annals of the Rheumatic Diseases,* 66(4), 440-445.

McDonald, M. & Sexton D. (2010). *Spinal Tuberculosis.* Retrieved February 21, 2012, from athttp://www.uptodate.com/contents/skeletal-tuberculosis

McNamara, D.R., Tleyjeh, I.M., Berbari, E.F., Lahr, B.D., Martinez, J.W., Mirzoyev, S.A., & Baddour, L.M. (2007). Incidence of lower-extremity cellulitis: A population-based study in Olmsted County, Minnesota. *Mayo Clinic Proceedings, 82*(7), 817-821.

Moucha, C.S., Clyburn, T., Evans, R.P., & Prokuski, L. (2011). Modifiable risk factors for surgical site infection. *Journal of Bone & Joint Surgery - American Volume, 93*(4), 398-404.

Ohl, C.A. (2010). Infectious arthritis native joints. In G. Mandell, J. Bennett & R. Dolin (Eds.) *Principles and Practice of Infectious Diseases* (7th ed., pp. 1443-1456). Philadelphia, PA: Churchill Livingston.

Pineda, C., Vargas, A., & Rodriguez, A. (2006). Imaging of osteomyelitis: Current concepts. *Infectious Disease Clinics of North America, 20*(4), 789-825.

Prandini, N., Lazzeri, E., Rossi, B., Erba, P., Parisella, M. G., & Signore, A. (2006). Nuclear medicine imaging of bone infections. *Nuclear Medicine Communications, 27*(8), 633-644.

Rao, N., Ziran, B., & Lipsky, B. (2011). Treating osteomyelitis: Antibiotics and surgery. *Plastic & Reconstructive Surgery, 127*(Suppl 1), 177S-187S.

Ratliff, C.R. (2007). Osteomyelitis: Principles to guide prevention, diagnosis and treatment. *Advance for Nurse Practitioners, 15*(7), 25-29.

Scott, R.D. (2009). *The Direct Costs of Healthcare-Associated Infections in U.S. Hospitals and the Benefits of Prevention.* Retrieved September 2, 2010, from http://www.cdc.gov/HAI/pdfs/hai/Scott_CostPaper.pdf

Stevens, D. (2011). *Necrotizing Infections of the Skin and Fascia.* Retrieved September 1, 2011, from http://www.uptodate.com/contents/necrotizing-infections-of-the-skin-and-fascia

Yoeke, D., Mermel, L., Anderson, D., Arias, K., Burstin, H., Calfee, D., … Classen D. (2008). Compendium of strategies to prevent healthcare-associated infections in acute care hospitals. *Infection Control and Hospital Epidemiology, 29*(Suppl 1), S12-S21.

Chapter 10

Therapeutic Modalities

Cathleen E. Kunkler, MSN, RN, ONC, CNE

Objectives

- Describe the purpose and indications for use of a treatment modality.
- Explain key nursing care considerations for each therapeutic modality.
- Summarize a comprehensive neurovascular assessment for specific modalities.
- List potential complications associated with each specific modality.
- Verbalize practice setting considerations for both inpatient and outpatient settings.

The individual with musculoskeletal compromise or injury will often require a therapeutic modality. While some of these modalities will be of short-term duration, others will aid the patient in their activities of daily living (ADLs) for a lifetime. Each modality can improve the recovery of the individual or help him or her live with a postrecovery disability, yet each has potential complications that the nurse must assess and educate the individual/support persons. Ambulatory devices such as canes, crutches, walkers, braces, splints, and other orthotic devices are used by many individuals. The correct technique of use is imperative to prevent further injury or unsafe use. The use of a wheelchair, for example, would appear straightforward; however, the user must be aware of the many safety issues, and caregivers of younger children and adolescents must be aware of the need to upgrade the size of the wheelchair as growth occurs. Significant musculoskeletal injury may require the use of a cast, traction, or external fixation. Postoperative individuals may benefit from the use of continuous passive motion (CPM). Whatever modality is indicated, the nurse must have the knowledge to assess, implement, educate, evaluate, and adapt for each individual in a variety of practice settings.

Ambulatory Devices and Techniques

Overview

Individuals may require assistance to ambulate and can use a variety of devices to assist in weight-bearing. Indications to use an assistive devices and techniques for using them are selected on the basis of multiple factors. The amount of weight-bearing allowed (see Table 10.1), as well as the specific muscle and joints involved in their musculoskeletal injury, is coupled with the patient's overall strength to be able to properly and safely use an assistive device to achieve locomotion. It is also important to consider the patient's cognitive function, judgment, vision, strength, physical endurance, and living environment. In general, individuals use an assistive device (crutches/walker/cane) with conditions affecting the hips, pelvis, or lower extremities.

Table 10.1. Weight-Bearing Status
1. Non-weight-bearing (NWB): no weight is borne by affected extremity.
2. Touch-down weight bearing (TDWB): foot (toe touch) makes contact with floor, but no weight is supported.
3. Partial weight-bearing (PWB): 25–50% of patient's weight is borne on affected extremity.
4. Weight-bearing as tolerated (WBAT): amount of weight borne is dictated by patient's pain and tolerance.
5. Full weight-bearing (FWB): no limitations, full weight is borne by affected extremity.

Assessment

The history focuses on acute injury, or chronic, developmental, or congenital conditions requiring an ambulatory devices. Effects of the use of an ambulatory device on the patient's lifestyle and environment must be assessed. A thorough evalutation of the patient's prior ambulatory status is vital.

During the physical examination, the major emphasis is placed on assessment of the musculoskeletal and neurologic systems. The patient's overall physical strength, stability, and balance are carefully evaluated. Pain, stiffness, motion of the joints (especially the knees, elbows, wrists, hands, and fingers), and the strength of the quadriceps and triceps will determine the most appropriate assistive device for the patient.

Common Therapeutic Modalities

Per the physician order for weight-bearing to be permitted, and in consultation with physical and occupational therapy, evaluate the type of assistive device that is most appropriate for the patient. Once determined, discuss the device with the patient and his or her support system to begin the education of how to use the device as well as gaining compliance with use and adherence to weight-bearing restrictions.

Whatever transfer technique is used, the focus is to frame the potential benefits within a goal-directed approach to mobility rather than focus on the transfer technique itself. The patient who is independent with transfers requires no assistance, and his or her transfer and ambulation performance is safe. A standby assist of one requires only verbal cuing or direct visual observation, with the clinician ready to assist if the need arises. With contact guard of one, the patient has poor balance and judgment; therefore, the clinician places a hand on the patient and provides support if needed. Some patients will require more physical assistance (minimal to maximal) of one or more clinicians who will utilize support devices (such as transfer belts) or mechanical devices (electric or hydraulic lifts). The patient requiring total/complete assistance needs two or more clinicians and will require a mechanical device to complete transfers.

Considerations across the life span begin with safety considerations that vary with the age of the patient. School-age children and adolescents may tend to "overdo it" or avoid using assistive devices, while the elderly patient may have visual impairments that make them unable to see potential hazards. Age also affects the choice of assistive device because older adults may not have sufficient upper body strength and balance to use crutches. Additionally, the social stigma of aging finds many elderly not using an assistive device, as it is an obvious outward sign of declining health. The elderly may hide their need to use a mobility aid/ device and withdraw from society. The perception of "temporary" versus "permanent" affects compliance of use, and women tend to use an assistive device before men. The nurse's approach as a "tool for living" can facilitate compliance, as well as a physician "order." Walkers are more likely to be used before a cane as a walker is used after hip fracture or total joint arthroplasty (TJA) and is associated with the healing/rehabilitation process, not old age and frailty.

Crutches. Crutches are a commonly used assistive device and may be axillary, forearm Lofstrand, or forearm crutches with an attached platform. Axillary crutches, made of adjustable wood or metal, are most commonly used. The patient's weight is borne on the hands and wrists, so an assessment of the patient's upper body strength is essential. Axillary crutches are usable for all five crutch walking gaits, which will be discussed in detail later in this chapter.

Forearm crutches have a platform for the forearm, instead of an axillary bar, with a strap to keep the forearm in place and a handgrip for the hands. The elbows are kept at a constant 90-degree angle while using the crutches. The platform permits weight-bearing to be distributed over the forearm rather than on the wrist and hands. The patient may need assistance in attaching the arm straps. The 2-point or 4-point gait is traditionally used with this device.

Forearm Lofstrand, sometimes called Canadian crutches, also have no axillary bars; cuffs/bands fit around the forearms, allowing the person to release the handgrips without dropping the crutches. The cuffs should fit comfortably around the forearms below the elbows and permit weight-bearing on the wrists and hands. While providing less stability, Lofstrand crutches are less cumbersome and easier to use than axillary crutches, especially on stairs without a railing. A 2-point or 4-point gait is safely used with Lofstrand crutches.

Measurement for correct crutch height is extremely important to achieve the desired weight-bearing limitations and to maintain safety for the patient. One method is to determine the patient's height and subtract 40 cm (16 inches). Should the patient need to be measured in bed, have the patient lie supine (wearing the actual shoes to be used for ambulation), measure from the anterior fold of the axilla to the sole of the foot, and then add 5 cm (2 inches). If the patient is able to sit without back support, have the patient sit up and abduct both arms straight out from the body. Then have the patient flex one arm at the elbow, and measure across the patient's back from the fingertip on the one hand to the elbow on the other. Be cautious that the back is not bowed or flexed. If the patient can stand, measure 3.75 to 5 cm (1½ to 2 inches) below the axillary fold to a point on the floor 10 cm (4 inches) in front of the patient and 15 cm (6 inches) laterally from the small toe. Then adjust the handgrips to allow the elbows to be flexed 15-30 degrees when the patient is standing. When the patient is using crutches, the tops should be 1 to 1½ inches below the axilla (two fingers can be inserted between the crutch and the axilla). An improper fit may result in crutch palsy or back strain.

Crutch walking gaits have two, three, or four points, depending upon the patient's injury, strength, and stamina, or their endurance when considering chronic musculoskeletal diseases. The 2-point gait (Figure 10.1)

**Figure 10.1.
2-Point Gait**

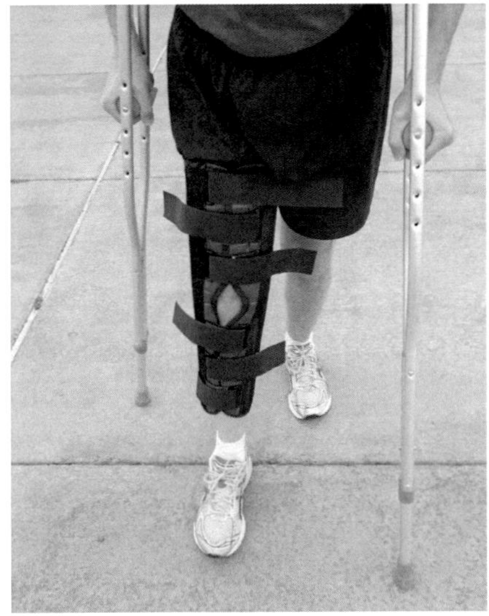
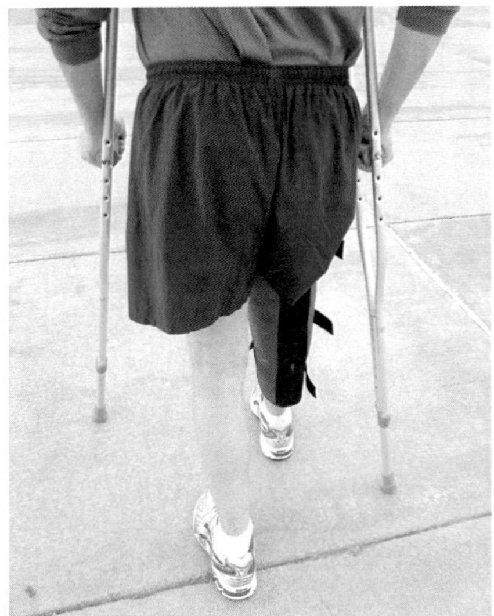
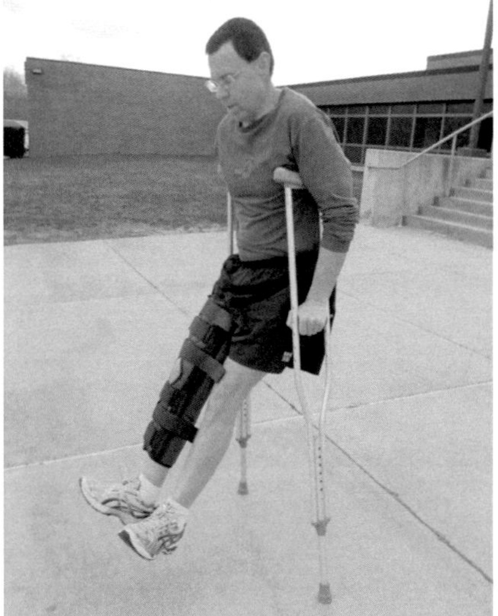

Author-created image. Reproduced with permission.

Figure 10.2.
3-Point Gait

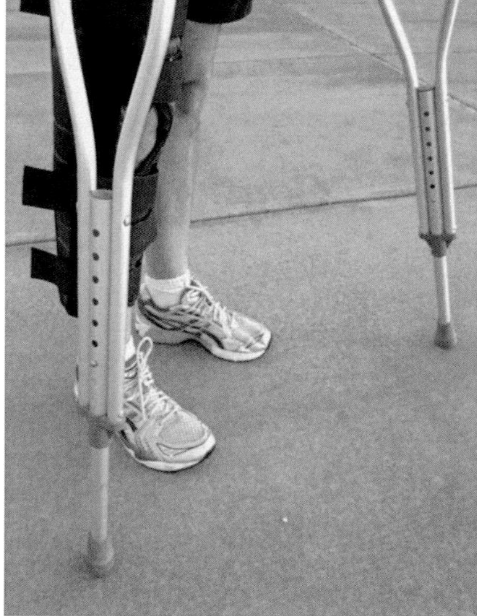
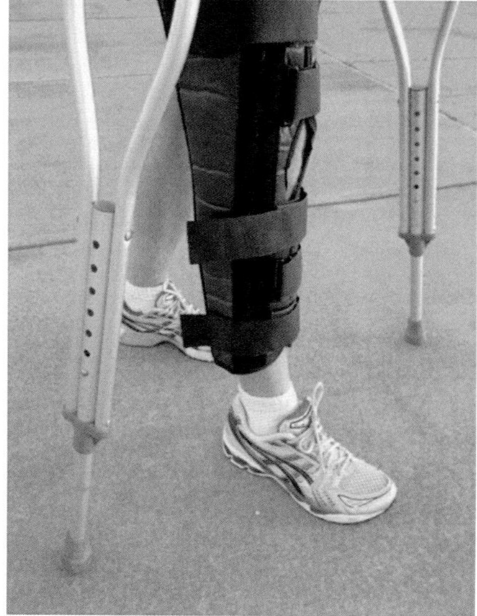
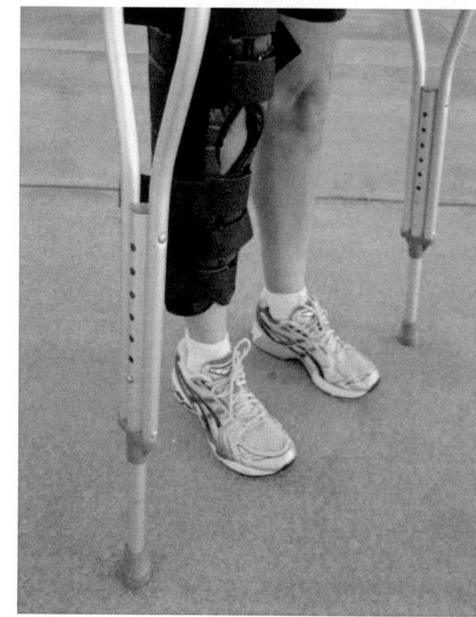

Author-created image. Reproduced with permission.

is faster than the 4-point gait because there are only two points of contact with the floor at one time. For the 2-point gait, partial bilateral weight-bearing is permitted on both legs, and the crutch and foot advance together. The right leg and left crutch move forward simultaneously, followed by the left leg and right crutch.

The 3-point gait (Figure 10.2) is advised for non-weight-bearing to partial weight-bearing on the affected leg. The patient must be able to support the entire body weight on the arms, as this is a fast gait that requires the most strength and balance. The weakest foot (non-weight-bearing or toe-touch weight-bearing) and both crutches move forward simultaneously. The stronger leg then moves forward, while the person's body weight is supported on the crutches (the affected leg may be used for balance if partial weight bearing is allowed).

The swing-to gait and swing-through gait are usually used when both of the patient's lower extremities are weak or paralyzed. The patient may or may not be wearing long leg braces. Additionally, the swing-to gait is used by patients who not only have weakened leg muscles but also have poor abdominal and back muscles, which make it more difficult to regain and maintain balance once they have moved forward. Starting with the feet together and crutches at their side, both crutches are moved forward at the same time. The patient then lifts the body by transferring weight to the crutches. The swing-to gait swings the body weight up to the crutches,

Figure 10.3.
4-Point Gait

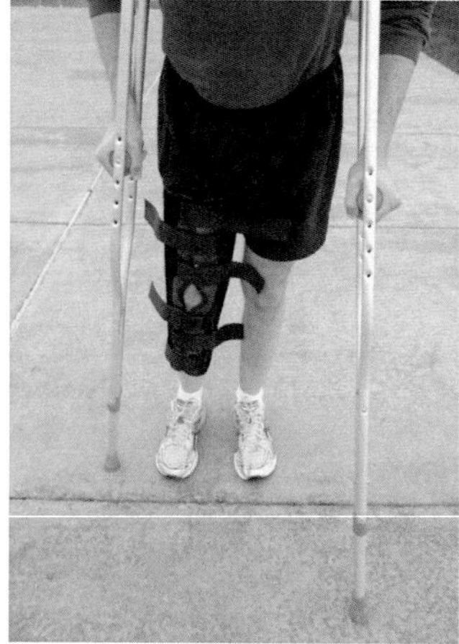
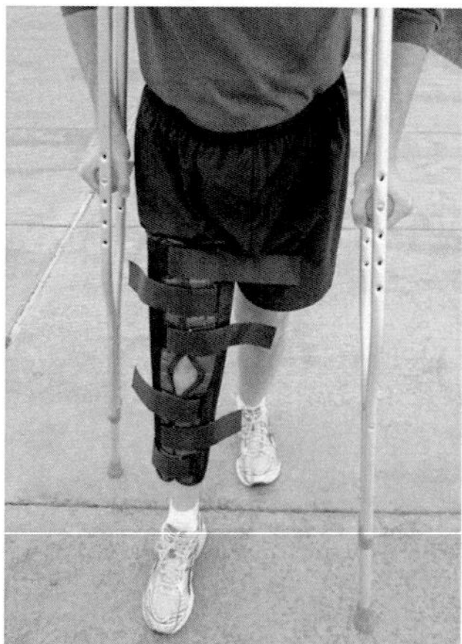
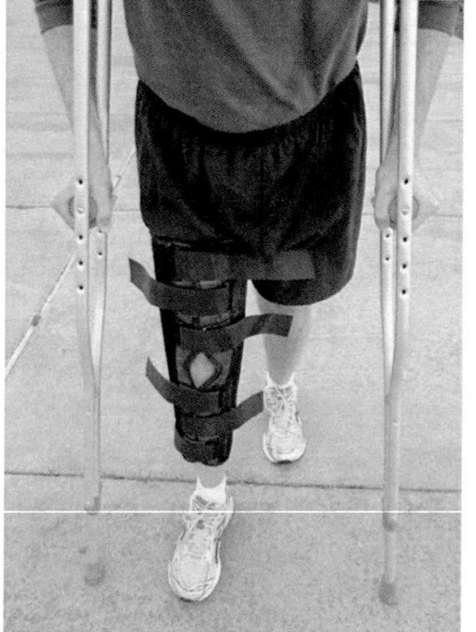
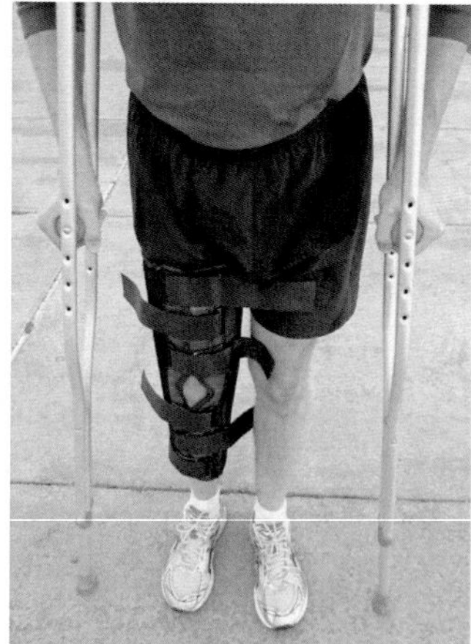

Author-created image. Reproduced with permission.

Figure 10.4.
Ascending and Descending Stairs

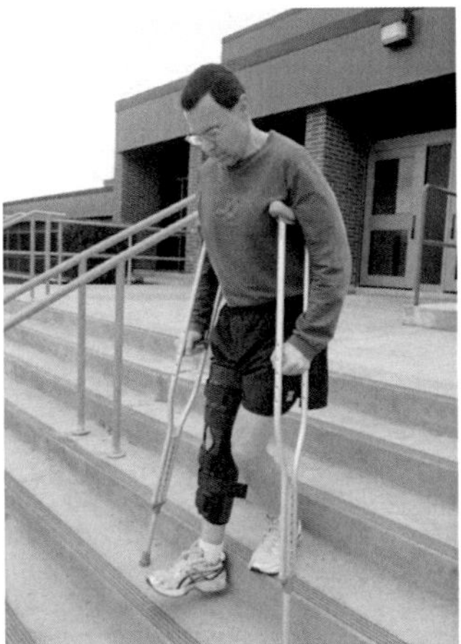

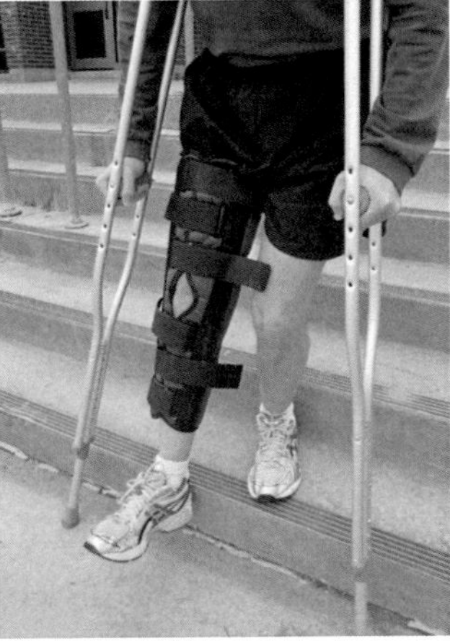

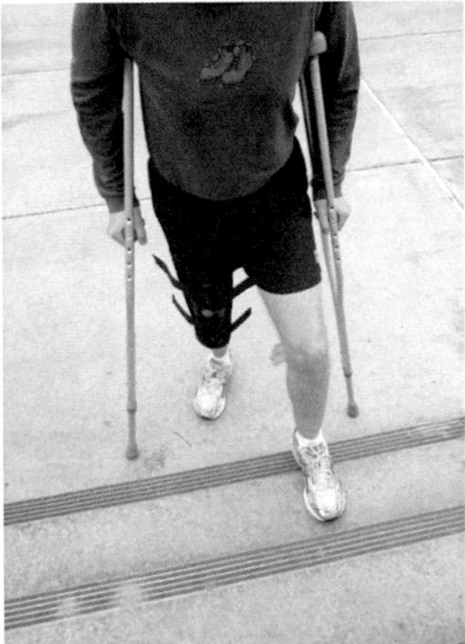

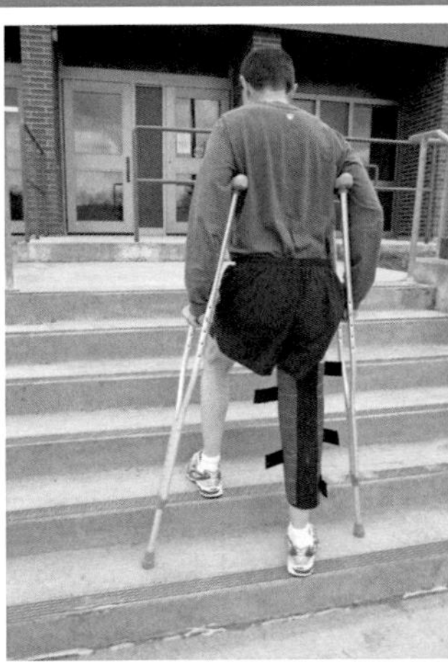

Author-created image. Reproduced with permission.

whereas the swing-through gait swings the body weight through and past the crutches. With either gait, the patient must straighten and stabilize the body before moving the crutches forward.

The 4-point gait (Figure 10.3), supporting partial weight-bearing on both legs, is considered the safest gait because it promotes maximal balance as there are always three points of contact with the floor. The 4-point gait is considered a slow gait because it requires constant shifting of weight, as the crutches and feet move in alternately sequence: right crutch (most right-handed people start with the right), left foot, left crutch, right foot. This alternating sequence is continually repeated during the ambulation process.

An alternate 4-point sweep-through gait may be used by patients with concurrent visual and neuromuscular disability, and provides exploration of upcoming terrain by the crutches before they are placed in traditional reciprocal position. Both crutches are placed just lateral to the foot. The patient then advances the left crutch obliquely to the right, just above the ground, and places the crutch in front of right foot. The left crutch is swept horizontally along the ground, from right to left, until located in front of the left foot. The patient advances the right foot until opposite the left crutch. Then the patient advances the right crutch obliquely to the right, just above the ground, and places it in front of the left foot. The right crutch sweeps horizontally along the ground, from right to left, until located in front of the right foot. The left foot is then advanced until opposite the right crutch.

Ascending and descending stairs using crutches takes practice (Figure 10.4). Two memory devices help the patient remember the sequence. The first is that the strong leg goes up first and comes down last. The second and more commonly known to patients is "up with the good and down with the bad."

Going up stairs begins with the patient walking forward to about a half-step away from the stairs. The patient places weight on the hands and lifts the stronger or unaffected leg up to the next step. The patient's arms must be strong enough to support the patient's body during the move. Once the foot is safely on the next step, the affected or weaker leg and crutches are advanced. If there is a handrail, the patient places both crutches in one hand, grasps the handrail, and then follows the same sequence.

Going down stairs has the patient walk to the forward edge of the step. The patient advances the crutches and weaker or affected leg to the next lower step by tilting the pelvis and bending the unaffected leg at the knee and hip. Once the crutches are safely placed on the lower step, the stronger or unaffected leg is advanced. If there is a handrail, both crutches are held in one hand and the rail with the other while going through the described procedure.

Walkers. Walkers provide more support and stability than crutches. A walker should be high enough so that the patient does not have to bend over or lean forward to use it. For patients with decreased cardiopulmonary function, a walker facilitates partial weight-bearing or full non-weight-bearing. A walker also reduces the risk of falls as it enhances the stability of patients with poor balance. Just as with crutches, there are multiple configurations of walkers to meet the variety of patient needs. In pediatrics, a reverse walker is sometimes used for patients with cerebral palsy to encourage standing up straight. Safety is crucial. The patient should lift the walker, set it ahead, and step up to it. Neither the walker nor feet should slide, and the patient is encouraged to wear supportive footwear with good soles.

A stationary walker has four legs with rubber tips and no moveable parts, and can be safely used with 4-point, 2-point, 3-point, and swing-to gaits (Figure 10.5). The folding walker has the same basic design as the standard

Figure 10.5.
Stationary Walker Ambulation

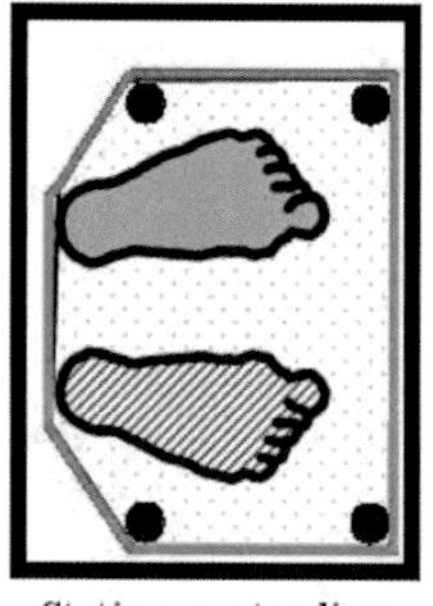
Stationary standing with walker

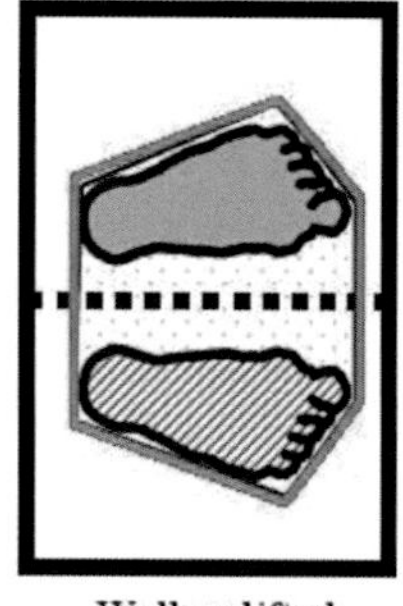
Walker lifted for advancement

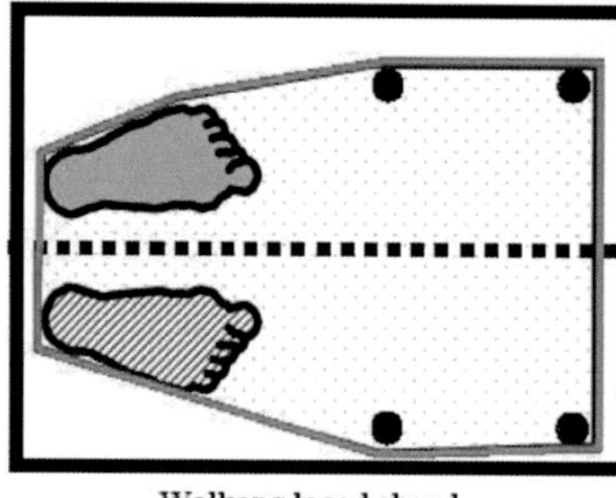
Walker placed ahead

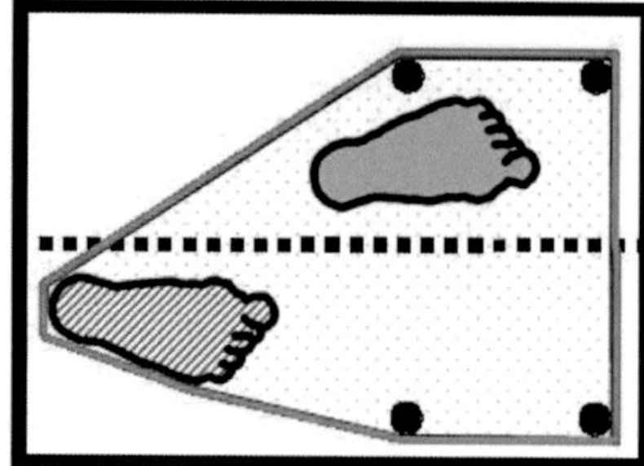
First step forward into walker

From "Assistive Devices for Balance and Mobility: Benefits, Demands, and Adverse Consequences" by H. Bateni & B. Maki, 2005, Archives of Physical Medicine and Rehabilitation, *86:1, p. 134-145. doi:10.1016/j.apmr.2004.04.023). Reproduced with permission.*

walker except that it is hinged, which allows the sides to fold when not in use. When opened, the sides swing out and lock into place, permitting the patient to use a 4-point, 2-point, 3-point, or swing-to gait. Commonly used by the elderly, a gliding walker has metal plates on the tips instead of rubber and can be pushed or slid for a 4-point, 2-point, or 3-point gait. More frail elderly often use a wheeled or rolling walker, which has wheels on the front legs that lock when pressure is applied. The 4-point, 2-point, and 3-point gaits can be used with a wheeled/rolling walker. The reciprocal walker has a hinge mechanism that allows one side to be advanced ahead of the other, thus providing more stability than a stationary walker. The reciprocal walker is used by the elderly in a 4-point or 2-point gait. The hemiwalker is designed for the patient who has the use of only one arm. It allows for maneuvering with one hand, using a step gait, as the handgrip is placed in the center front of the walker. The platform walker has elevated armrests to allow the patient to grasp the walker and advance; this can be attached to a stationary or rolling walker to accommodate the patient with a compromised upper extremity. The Winnie walker has three or four wheels, plus a seat and safety brakes.

Canes. Canes are used to provide support, aid in balance, and relieve pressure on weight-bearing joints. Canes are considered the least stable of the assistive devices for ambulation. A cane is used on the side opposite the affected leg (or on the good side) and helps support body weight as the affected/weaker leg is moved forward. Two canes may be used like crutches when both lower extremities are weakened.

Just as with the other assistive devices, there are several types of canes. A standard cane comes with a C-curve (standard crook cane) or a T-handle, is made of wood or aluminum, and has a small base of support. Quad/tripod canes provide a wide base of support through the number of legs projecting from the base of the cane. The walkane provides greater stability than a quad cane and looks like a cross between a cane and a walker. While the walkane is lighter and smaller than a walker, it is more versatile than a hemiwalker and more stable than a cane; however, the base is too large to be used on stairs. A hemicane is used synonymous with a hemiwalker.

To correctly fit a cane, the patient's elbow must be flexed to a 25-30 degree angle. The cane handle should approximate the greater trochanter for correct alignment. If the patient already has a cane, measure the distance from their wrist crease to the floor. An important safety intervention is to keep the rubber tips in good condition to prevent slippage.

Nursing Considerations

Nursing Diagnoses. Nursing diagnoses for this condition are expanded upon in the Appendix.

- Body image, disturbed.
- Falls, risk for.
- Hopelessness.
- Injury, risk for.
- Mobility: physical, impaired.
- Role performance, ineffective.
- Self-care deficit: bathing/hygiene, dressing/grooming, feeding, toileting.
- Self esteem: situational low. Risk for.
- Social interaction, impaired.

Limiting the potential for injury requires that the assistive devices are the correct height/length; that the patient demonstrates appropriate/safe gait using the device; and that the home environment is free of safety hazards. Nursing interventions require that the assistive devices—whether crutches, a walker, or a cane—be correctly fitted for the patient and properly used. Patient/family education emphasizes that when using crutches, weight-bearing is on the hands NOT through the axilla. A return demonstration of the gait recommended with the assistive device, and practice on the stairs is paramount. Make sure the patient has a sturdy, secure pair of shoes for ambulation.

Encourage the patient to dangle their legs, sitting on edge of the bed, prior to standing up. The patient (or support persons) need to replace rubber tips at first sign of wear on any assistive device. Once home, the patient should sit in chairs with armrests. To facilitate easier access, the patient may use wooden blocks to increase the height of low-positioned chairs. The patient should feel the chair at the back of the legs, and grip the hand-pieces of both crutches with one hand on the unaffected side. Using the other hand on the chair armrest, the patient should lower him- or herself into the chair. To stand, the patient will slide forward to the chair's edge and place both crutches on the unaffected (stronger) side. The patient then leans forward and pushes off with the hand on the affected (weaker) side.

Practice Setting Considerations. *Home care:* Environmental safety precautions must be discussed as the patient prepares for discharge. Whether the assistive device is for short- or long-term use, it is imperative to assess the home environment. A clear environment, free of tripping hazards, must be guaranteed. Remove furniture or cords that might cause tripping, remove scatter rugs, make sure floors are dry, etc. For long-term use, assist in planning modifications to make the home environment safe.

Braces/Orthotics/Orthoses

Overview

A brace/orthotic/orthosis is an external appliance that applies forces to or removes forces from the body in a controlled manner to enhance function and mobility, control motion, and provide pressure relief. Numerous indications may require one of these devices to maintain or correct position, improve function, or facilitate mobility. The correction or prevention of anatomic deformities, or the maintenance of a surgical correction to provide protection during the postoperative healing process, are also indications for use. Another indications is to aid in control of involuntary muscle movement, prevent increased muscle imbalance, and provide support, which in turn may facilitate normal movement patterns and assist muscles in re-education. These devices also offer relief of pain by limiting motion or weight-bearing, and can transfer strength from one joint to another. Additional indications are to reduce axial load, friction, and shear, as well as the ability to immobilize and protect weak, painful, or healing musculoskeletal segments.

Bracing/splinting is an individualized treatment modality. The patient's brace/splint may be designed by an orthotist or occupational therapist. A variety of braces, immobilizers, and splints are commercially available. There are two major types of devices: orthotics and splints. A sling can support and immobilize an injured arm, collarbone, or shoulder to in turn prevent dependent edema, promote rest, and healing, as well as hold a fractured arm in alignment (Pullen, 2007). A guideline for sling application can be found with Figure 10.6.

Figure 10.6.
Using a Sling Properly

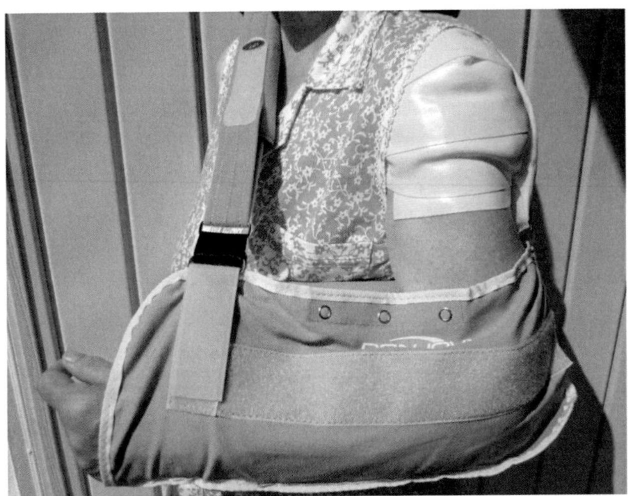

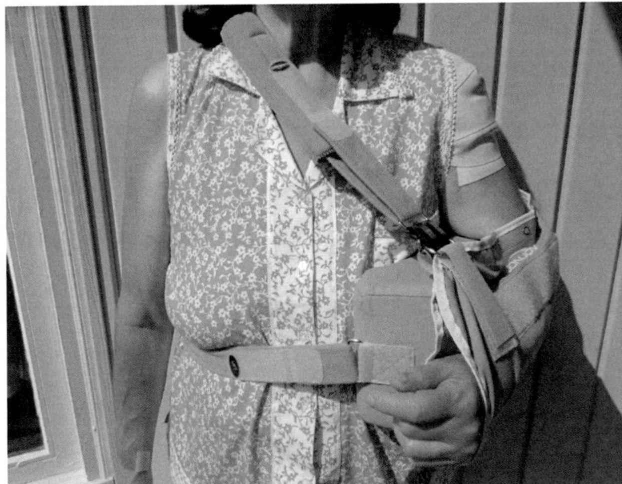

Author-created image. Reproduced with permission.

How to properly use a sling.

- Assess skin integrity & neurovascular status.
- Remove rings, watch or other jewelery from extremity.
- Position arm across chest with elbow flexed 90 degrees; bring strap around opposite shoulder and adjust to support extremity. Adjust strap around body if included as part of sling for individual's with shoulder injury or surgery.

- Sling must be proper length to support extremity including wrist. Emphasize mobility limitations ordered, including flexion-extension of joints to prevent contractures.
- Teach patient & support persons to assess neurovascular status and what changes in patient warrant contacting their healthcare provider.

Orthotics. Orthotics are created for each individual and can be used on multiple joints. An ankle foot orthosis (AFO) is a short leg brace to prevent equinus deformity with peroneal palsy or mechanical weakness, and is able to accommodate foot deformities, relieve pressure, and enhance comfort through custom shoes, shoe modifications, or inserts. The knee-ankle-foot orthosis (KAFO) is a long-leg brace used to stabilize the hip, knee, or ankle joints. The hip-knee-ankle-foot orthosis (HKAFO) is a long-leg brace with a pelvic band used to stabilize the pelvis and lower extremity joints. The cervicothoracolumbosacral (CTLSO) is commonly known as a Milwaukee brace, whereas a thoracolumbosacral (TLSO) may be referred to as a Boston brace. The Scottish Rite brace (Lovell) is used as a hip abduction orthosis. Knee immobilizers utilize de-rotation and are a hinged orthosis used to support cruciate or collateral ligament injuries. The Ilfeld splint is a hip abduction orthosis used to control selected hip motions to prevent recurrent dislocations, and is commonly seen as a Pavlik harness (Figure 10.7) used for newborn-to-3-month or as an A-frame orthosis, both used for hip abduction.

Figure 10.7. Pavkik Harness

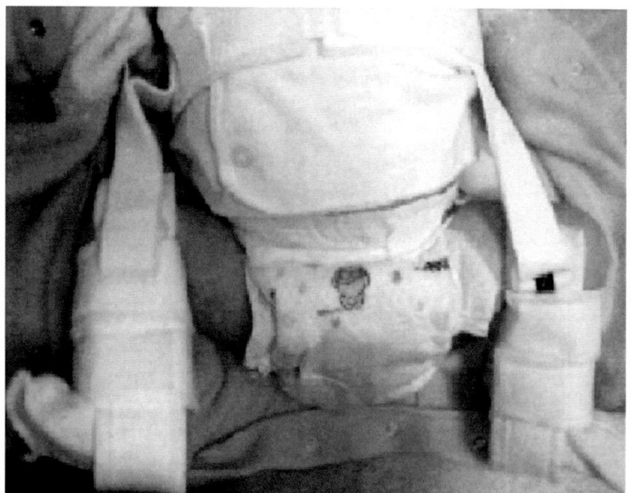

From "Developmental Dysplasia of the Hip: Nursing Implications and Anticipatory Guidance for Parents" by E. Hart, M. Albright, G. Rebello, and B. Grottkau, 2006, Orthopaedic Nursing *25(2), p. 105. Reproduced with permission.*

Splints. Splints are either static or dynamic. Static splints have no moving parts and hold a movable part in functional position. A resting pan, cock-up, or thumb spica are static splints that primarily are used to immobilize for pain management. Dynamic splints have a static base plus one or more moving parts to provide the desired mobility to the joint.

Across the life span, all patients must be assessed routinely for brace/splint fit during episodes of rapid growth. Keeping the brace/splint in good condition during active stages of childhood/adolescence is essential. The health care provider must closely monitor compliance with schedule of wear and activity limitations, particularly during the adolescent period, due to self-concept concerns. Initially, begin a patient with 1 to 2 hours of brace wear, and gradually progress to 2- to 4-hour intervals. Teach the patient to wear clean, wrinkle-free, white socks, t-shirts, or other liners beneath the brace and to avoid powders or lotions. It may be necessary to toughen sensitive skin areas with alcohol. Skin integrity and neurovascular assessment are also critically assessed in the geriatric patient. Othotics may require changes due to growth or following reconstructive surgery, or as one muscle gains strength.

The complications associated with orthotics arise from prolonged immobility of the affected body part in the brace/splint that may cause decreased ROM or contractures, skin breakdown, pressure ulcers, neurovascular compromise, calluses, and verrucae. The inappropriately applied brace/splint may, in fact, worsen a deformity.

Assessment

A comprehensive history focuses on a previous or acute injury, chronic injury, or any developmental or congenital condition that has required bracing or splinting. All prior experiences with braces or splints, as well as prior compliance, must be assessed. The patient must understand the reasons for bracing, care, application, and schedule of wear. The age/developmental considerations regarding compliance, potential for brace/splint wear or damage, and possibility of skin breakdown must all be taken into consideration.

The physical examination includes a complete musculoskeletal and neurologic examination with focus on neurovascular status, skin integrity, mental/emotional status, nutritional status, elimination status, and brace/splint fit.

Common Therapeutic Modalities

The physician, in conjunction with an occupational or physical therapist and orthotist, will determine the type of brace/splint to be used. Activity limitations, the desired position, and the amount and type of movement to be permitted will be a collaborated decision.

Nursing Considerations

Nursing Diagnoses. Nursing diagnoses for this condition are expanded upon in the Appendix.

- Activity intolerance.
- Body image, disturbed.
- Disuse syndrome, risk for.
- Health maintenance, ineffective.
- Home maintenance, impaired.
- Noncompliance.
- Powerlessness.
- Self-care deficit: bathing/hygiene, dressing/grooming, feeding, toileting.
- Skin integrity, risk for impairment.
- Tissue perfusion: peripheral, ineffective.
- Transfer ability, impaired.
- Walking, impaired.

Maintaining skin integrity for the patient utilizing a brace/splint focuses on the patient's skin remaining intact. Nursing interventions to be taught to the patient/family and/or care provider of a child begin with the correct application of the brace/splint, proper positioning, correct securement of ties and straps, and avoidance of direct skin contact. Care of the brace/splint needs to include cleaning, oiling, and drying. Vigilant assessment of the skin is imperative, and rubbing or pressure from the brace/splint or the presence of pressure areas must be reported immediately. Special attention should be given to insensate extremities. It is also important to provide a specific contact person if the brace/splint breaks or becomes unusable.

The potential for noncompliance with the use of a brace/splint also needs to be considered. Nursing outcomes focus on teaching the patient the importance of using the brace/splint as prescribed. The patient/family/caregiver must be able to verbalize (a) the prescribed schedule of wear and allowed activities; (b) the purpose of bracing/splinting and the required follow-up care; and (c) the potential problem areas and appropriate management of problems. The nursing interventions focus on teaching the patient/family/caregiver the rationale behind bracing/splinting, a prescribed schedule of wear, and the activities permitted while in the brace/splint. Brace/splint fit and condition, as well as function, mobility, and proper position in the brace/splint, must be taught.

Practice Setting Considerations. *Home care:* The age of the patient is a major factor in the compliance of using a brace/splint. For the young child, it is up to the caregiver to realize the importance to the musculoskeletal health of the child and the impact that noncompliance can have on future mobility as the child grows. For the adolescent, dominating factors in noncompliance may be peer pressure or the desire to be healed in order to get back into an athletic activity. For adults, the interference with ADLs may lead to an assumption that the brace is not really helping an injury/deformity and that it is a waste of time. The use of braces/splints takes a long time to see the effect; and in our instant-gratification society, waiting weeks or months for even small progress may not be reasonable for an adult.

Casts

Overview

A cast is a temporary circumferential immobilization device that serves to immobilize; maintain, support, and protect the realigned bone; prevent or correct deformities; and promote healing and early weight-bearing. A cast must include the joint above and the joint below a fractured long bone (Patterson & Wraa, 2010). Casts can be of a natural or synthetic material, or a hybrid of the two. The most common natural material is Plaster of Paris, powdered calcium sulfate crystals incorporated into a bandage (roll of tape). As more synthetic materials are being developed, the use of Plaster of Paris is diminishing. Occasionally a hybrid combination of Plaster of Paris beneath layers of synthetic fiberglass may be preferred.

Multiple synthetic materials are utilized to form casts. A polyester/cotton knit or a thermoplastic (open-weave polyester polymer fabric tape) are two commonly used materials. A frequently used synthetic is fiberglass. Knitted fiberglass tape, most commonly used, is permeated with a water-activated polyurethane prepolymer. With the increasing rate of latex allergy, a fiberglass-free, latex-free polymer is produced in a polyester substrate with extensible yarns incorporated into tape. This product is used with known or suspected latex allergy or with allergy-prone individuals.

In addition to the casting material, numerous supplies are required to complete the casting application process. Protection of both patient and health care provider necessitate the use of gloves, not only for infection control, but for protection of the skin of the individual applying the cast. An apron is also preferred to protect the applier's clothing. To protect the patient's skin integrity, a stockinette and webril, cast padding, or sheet wadding is applied after the patient's skin has been thoroughly cleansed. A liner, such as a Gore-Tex® barrier, for moisture absorption may also be utilized. Once the type of casting material is determined, a plastic-lined bucket or basin ¾ filled with warm water will be required. Blunt-end bandage scissors and a cast saw will aid in trimming the cast to further prevent skin integrity impairment. Once the weight-bearing status of the fracture has been established, a walking heel may be incorporated or, alternately, a cast shoe may be suggested. For alterations to the cast or during cast removal, a duckbill cast bender and a cast spreader must be available.

Casts come in a variety of configurations (Table 10.2). On the upper extremity (Table 10.3), a cast may be a short-arm, long-arm, hanging long-arm, long-arm cylinder, or thumb spica. On the lower extremity (Table 10.4), cast are either short-leg, long-leg, a leg cylinder, or a total contact cast that is a well-molded, minimally padded cast that has contact with the entire plantar aspect of the foot/toes and lower extremity. To correct deformity, lower extremity

Table 10.2. Cast Types and Common Uses

Type	Illustration	Body Part Covered	Common Uses
Short-leg cast	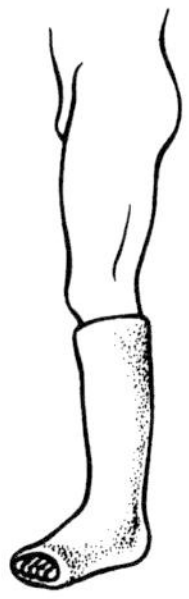	Foot to below knee	■ Fracture of the foot, ankle or distal tibia or fibula ■ Severe sprain or strain ■ Postoperative immobilization following open reduction and internal fixation ■ Correction of deformity, such as talipes equinovarus
Long-leg cast	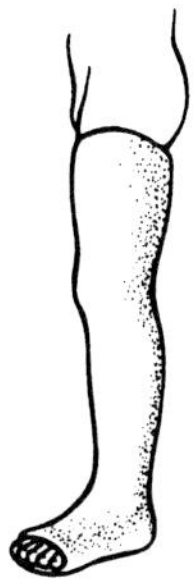	Foot to upper thigh	■ Fracture of the distal femur, knee, or lower leg ■ Soft tissue injury to the knee or knee dislocation ■ Postoperative immobilization following arthrodesis of the knee
Abduction boots	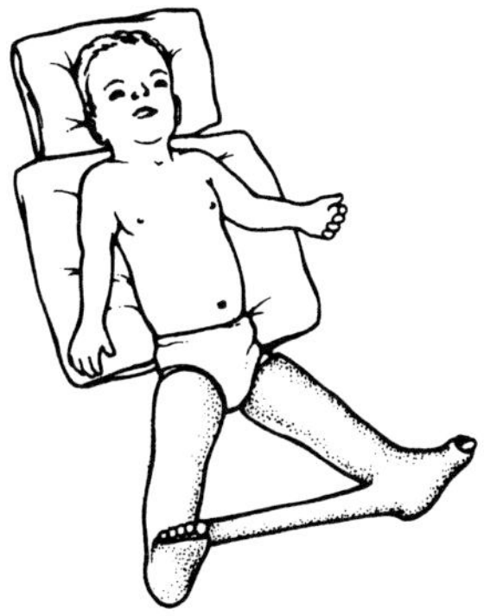	Feet to below knee or upper thigh	■ Postoperative immobilization following hip abductor release ■ Maintain abduction
Unilateral hip spica cast	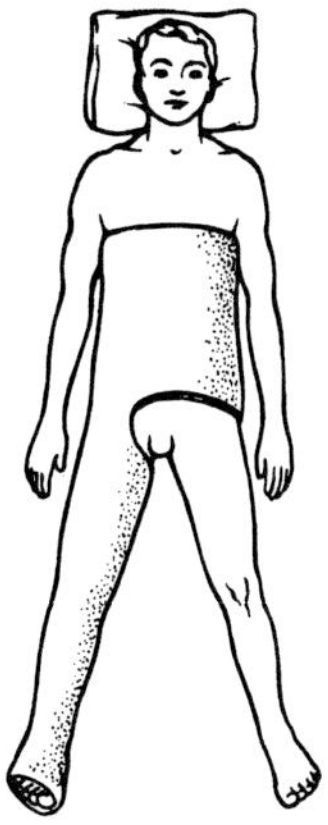	Entire leg and trunk to waist or nipple line	■ Fracture of the femur ■ Postoperative immobilization following open reduction and internal fixation ■ Correction of deformity, such as congenital soft tissue injury following dislocation of the hip

CHAPTER 10

Table 10.2. Cast Types and Common Uses (continued)			
Type	**Illustration**	**Body Part Covered**	**Common Uses**
Bilateral long-leg hip spica cast	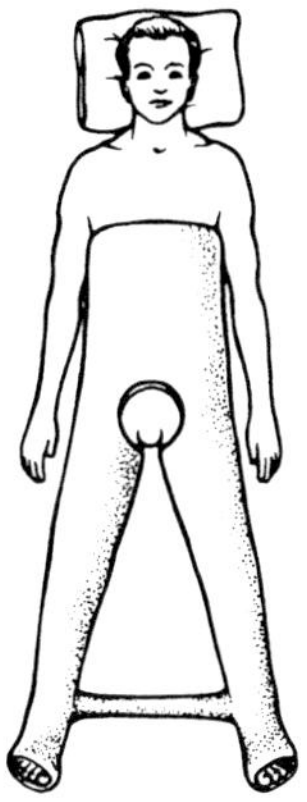	Entire leg bilaterally to waist or nipple line	■ Fractures of femur, acetabulum, or pelvis ■ Postoperative immobilization following open reduction and internal fixation
Short-leg hip spica cast	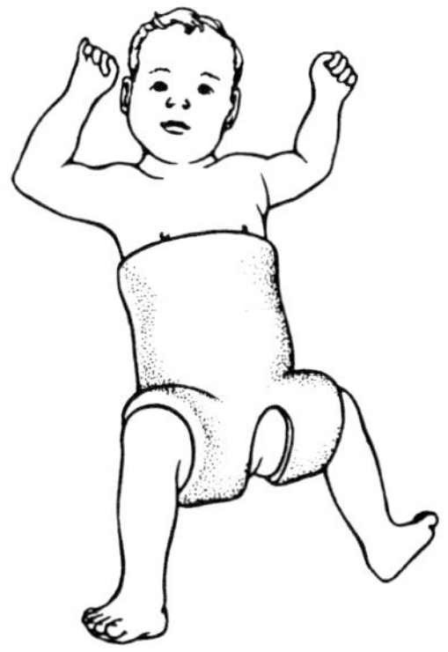	Knees or thighs bilaterally to waist or nipple line	■ Development dysplastic hip
Short-arm cast	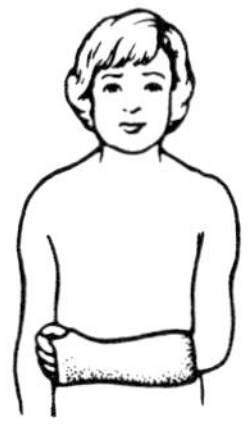	Hand to below elbow	■ Fracture of the hand or wrist ■ Postoperative immobilization following open reduction and internal fixation
Long-arm cast	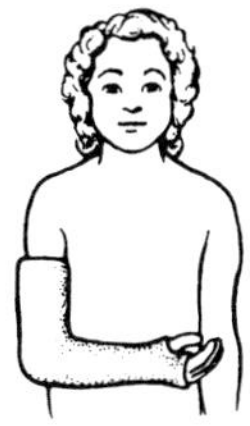	Hand to upper arm	■ Fracture of the forearm, elbow, or humerus ■ Postoperative immobilization following open reduction and internal fixation
Shoulder spica cast	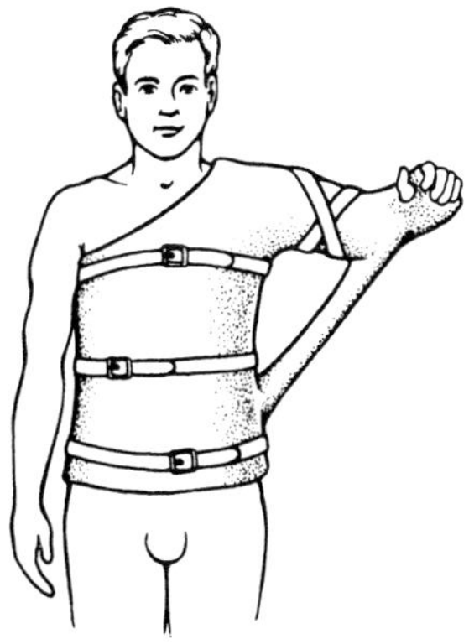	Trunk and shoulder arm and hand	■ Shoulder dislocation ■ Soft tissue injury to the shoulder, such as a rotator cuff tear ■ Postoperative immobilization following open reduction and internal fixation

From "Casting for Immobilization" by L. Altizer, 2004, Orthopaedic Nursing *23(2), p. 139. Reproduced with permission.*

Table 10.3. Upper Extremity Casting and Splinting Chart				
Region	**Type of Splint/Cast**	**Indications**	**Pearls/Pitfalls**	**Follow-up/Referral**
Ulnar side of hand	Ulnar gutter splint/ cast	Fourth and fifth proximal/ middle phalangeal shaft fractures and select metacarpal fractures	Proper positioning of MCP joints at 70-90 degrees of flexion, PIP and DIP joints at 5 to 10 degrees of flexion	One to two weeks Refer for angulated, displaced, rotated, oblique, or intra-articular fracture or failed closed reduction
Radial side of hand	Radial gutter splint/cast	Second and third proximal/ middle phalangeal shaft fractures and select metacarpal fractures	Proper positioning of MCP joints at 70 to 90 degrees of flexion, PIP, DIP joints at 5 to 10 degrees of flexion	One to two weeks Refer for angulated, displaced, rotated, oblique, or intra-articular fracture or failed closed reduction
Thumb, first metacarpal, and carpal bones	Thumb spica splint/cast	Injuries to scaphoid/trapezium Nondisplaced, nonangulated, extra-articular first metacarpal fractures Stable thumb fractures with or without closed reduction	Fracture of the middle/ proximal one third of the scaphoid treated with casting	One to two weeks Refer for angulated, displaced, intra-articular, incompletely reduced, or unstable fracture Refer displaced fracture of the scaphoid
Finger injuries	Buddy taping Aluminum U-shaped splint Dorsal extension-block splint Mallet finger splint	Nondisplaced proximal/middle phalangeal shaft fracture and sprains Distal phalangeal fracture Middle phalangeal volar plate avulsions and stable reduced PIP joint dislocations Extensor tendon avulsion from the base of the distal phalanx	Encourage active range of motion in all joints Encourage active range of motion at PIP and MCP joints Increase flexion by 15 degrees weekly, from 45 degrees to full extension Buddy taping permitted with splint use Continuous extension in the splint for six to eight weeks is essential	Two weeks Refer for angulated, displaced, rotated, oblique, or significant intra-articular fracture or failure to regain full range of motion
Wrist/hand	Volar/dorsal forearm splint Short arm cast	Soft tissue injuries to hand and wrist Acute carpal bone fractures (excluding scaphoid/trapezium) Childhood buckle fractures of the distal radius Non displaced, minimally displaced, or buckle fractures of the distal radius Carpal bone fractures other than scaphoid/trapezium	Consider splinting as definitive treatment for buckle fractures	One week Refer for displaced or unstable fractures Refer lunate fractures
Forearm	Single sugar-tong splint	Acute distal radial and ulnar fractures	Used for increased immobilization of forearm and greater stability	Less than one week Refer for displaced or unstable fractures
Elbow, proximal forearm, and skeletally immature wrist injuries	Long arm posterior splint, long arm cast Double sugar-tong splint	Distal humeral and proximal/ midshaft forearm fractures Nonbuckle wrist with fractures Acute elbow and forearm fractures, and nondisplaced, extra-articular Colles fractures	Ensure adequate padding at bony prominences Offers greater immobilization against pronation/supination	Within one week Refer for displaced or unstable fractures Less than one week Refer childhood distal humeral fractures

DIP = distal interphalangeal; MCP = metacarpophalangeal; PIP = proximal interphalangeal.

CHAPTER 10

casts may also incorporate short and long abduction boots or be an abduction cast (Petrie/A-frame). After amputation, casts may be used to shrink and mold the residual limb. Body casts have numerous variations, including a spinal body vest with or without straps, a Risser and pantaloon Risser, a Minerva jacket, an airplane spica or shoulder spica, a turnbuckle, a unilateral, one-and-a-half, and bilateral hip cast or an English walking cast.

Casting has numerous advantages for immobilization. The relative ease of application and minimal care required, combined with no need for hospitalization, rank high in terms of advantages. The ability of a cast to protect the underlying tissue, and allow the patient to generally be active and mobile, are positive for patient compliance. Casts do require skill and time to apply, however, and have a risk of complication if not applied properly (Boyd, Benjamin and Asplund, 2009). For the health care provider, the continuing advances in new quick-setting and lightweight materials expedite treatment intervention and discharge in a timely manner.

Across the life span, the health care provider must be aware of the use of casts and patient compliance, as well as the principles of fracture healing. Fractures in children usually require a shorter period of immobilization, although pediatric patients have poor pain acknowledgment that may mask potential complications; therefore, pediatric patients require more astute assessment of cast loosening and neurovascular changes due to changes in edema. For elderly patients, frail skin necessitates extra padding, especially over bony prominences. There may also be an increased fall risk in already unsteady elderly patients due to changes in the their center of gravity.

Assessment

The patient history will focus on previous acute injury and chronic, developmental, or congenital conditions that may have required casting. Inquire about any other treatments that may have utilized casting. Assess the effects of casting on the patient's lifestyle by determining hand dominance, noting the effect on ambulatory status, evaluating the home situation, and ensuring available support systems.

Physical examination must be comprehensive, with special emphasis on the extremity or area of the body requiring immobilization by casting. Ipsilateral assessment of the affected extremity with the unaffected extremity when possible is crucial. Ongoing assessments will provide vital data to compare with previous assessments.

Table 10.4. Lower Extremity Casting and Splinting

Region	Type of splint/cast	Indications	Pearls/pitfalls	Follow-up/referral
Ankle	Posterior ankle splint ("post-mold")	Severe sprains Isolated, nondisplaced malleolar fractures Acute foot fractures	Splint ends 2 inches distal to fibular head to avoid common peroneal nerve compression	Less than one week Refer for displaced or multiple fractures or significant joint instability
Ankle	Stirup splint	Ankle sprains Isolated, nondisplaced malleolar fractures	Mold to site of injury for effective compression	Less than one week
Lower leg, ankle, and foot	Short leg cast	Isolated, nondisplaced malleolar fractures Foot fractures – tarsals and metatarsals	Compartment syndrome most commonly associated with proximal mid-tibial fractures, so care is taken not to over-compress Weight-bearing status important; initially non-weight bearing with tibial injuries	Two to four weeks Refer for displaced or angulated fracture or proximal first through fourth metatarsal fractures
Knee and lower leg	Posterior knee splint	Acute soft tissue and bony injuries of the lower extremity	If ankle immobilization is necessary, as with tibial shaft injuries, the splint should extend to include the metatarsals	Days
Foot	Short leg cast with toe plate extension	Distal metatarsal and phalangeal fractures	Useful technique for the toe immobilization Often used when high-top walking boots are not available	Two weeks Refer for displaced or unstable fractures

From "Splints and Casts: Indications and Methods" by A. Boyd, H. Benjamin, and C. Asplund, 2009, American Family Physician *80(5), p. 495. Reproduced with permission.*

Prior to casting, correct anatomic alignment of the affected body part is completed, and the peripheral vascular status of the injured area is assessed. The neurovascular assessment will evaluate the color, temperature, capillary refill, and sensation of the extremity, i.e. any impairment such as burning, decreased sensation, numbness, or paresthesia. Motor ability, pain, and the presence of edema must also be assessed. An assessment of the underlying skin integrity examines for rashes, scars, open lacerations or wounds, pressure ulcers, bruises, contusions, ecchomytic areas, varicosities, and peripheral vascular disease. Atrophy of the extremity is evaluated, which determines muscle strength and tests reflexes. The patient's overall hygiene level also needs to be assessed, and jewelry and/or nail polish must be removed.

A cast impacting respiratory effort requires an assessment of respiratory rate and the quality of breath sounds. Dependent upon the location of the cast, abdominal and urologic characteristics of the area to be covered by the cast must be assessed. Bowel sounds, abdominal or bladder distention, softness upon palpation, any history of nausea and vomiting, and elimination patterns must be considered.

The use of casts for treatment requires astute assessment for the numerous complications that may occur. Incorrect fracture alignment, skin breakdown from pressure, neurovascular compromise/dysfunction, and compartment syndrome are the complications most vigilantly assessed for during treatment. Body casts are at high risk for cast syndrome, also known as superior mesenteric artery syndrome (SMAS).

The potential for SMAS must be a nursing priority for the patient with a body spica cast. SMAS is a compression of the duodenum anteriorly and the aorta and vertebral column posteriorly, causing a decrease in blood supply to the bowel, which results in hemorrhage and necrosis of the gastrointestinal tract. Contributing factors include: avoidance of lumbar lordosis during cast application of a body cast or hip spica cast; extensive supine positioning/recumbency; hyperextension of lumbar spine; or the use of spinal instrumentation and distraction. Sign and symptoms of SMAS may begin with vague abdominal pain, pressure, and distention. These symptoms can progress to nausea and projectile vomiting, and result in bowel obstruction. SMAS may occur days or weeks after cast application due to weight loss of retroperitoneal fat after immobilization.

Interventions to prevent fluid loss from SMAS for patients in body spicas entails comprehensive care. The body spica cast must have an adequate abdominal window to allow the nurse to auscultate bowel sounds, palpate the abdomen, and assess for abdominal distention and rebound tenderness. Observe the patient for prolonged nausea and projectile vomiting, which must be immediately reported to the physician. Keep the patient NPO if nausea and vomiting occur, and monitor and record any NG tube drainage. The patient will require intravenous fluid replacement therapy, and it is necessary to monitor electrolyte levels and results of any abdominal diagnostic tests. Patient positioning to the prone position may provide some relief from pressure if the patient is able to tolerate this position. Cast removal may be considered by the physician if the patient's condition does not improve. Alternately, surgical intervention to release the ligament of Treitz may be considered by the physician if the condition continues. Untreated, SMAS can be fatal.

Following casting, the patient's peripheral vascular and neurovascular status is once again assessed above and below the cast. Documentation of the shape and size of the cast is paramount to determine if the cast becomes deformed or damaged before drying/setting. Skin integrity around the cast edges, along with alignment of the casted body part, is also documented. The patient's comfort and pain management, as well as the patient's response to the presence of the cast, is assessed. While the health care provider checks for drainage on the cast and notes any odor from the injured area casted, the patient is also taught this as part of discharge instructions.

Common Therapeutic Modalities

Cast Application. In preparation for cast application, the type of cast to be applied must be determined. The patient is assessed to determine the need for premedication, which could include muscle relaxants, NSAIDs, or analgesics. General anesthesia may be indicated in some cases due to positioning, stability, spasticity, age of the patient, or fear or discomfort of the individual. Walsh (2009) identifies several types of anesthesia available for the patient requiring casting, including (a) general anesthesia, which is achieved through inhalation of various agents to produce reversible unconsciousness or paralysis; (b) monitored anesthesia care; and (c) regional anesthesia, which includes peripheral nerve blocks, central nerve blocks, spinal, epidural, and local anesthesia.

General principles of care during cast application focus on protecting the skin/bony prominences beneath the cast. Following a thorough cleansing of the skin and reduction of the fracture/deformity, stockinette, webril, sheet wadding, or felt padding is placed next to the skin. The appropriate casting material is selected, and the proper water temperature for preparation of casting material is established. Casting materials harden faster with the use of warm water compared with cold water; the faster the material sets, the greater the heat produced and the greater the risk of significant skin burns (Boyd et al., 2009). Attentive application is necessary in eliminating indentations that could impair skin integrity, and in facilitating a smooth external surface to prevent injury to the skin that may come in contact with the cast during treatment. When appropriate, an abdominal opening (window) is cut if the patient is in a body cast.

The application of a cast begins with the reduction of the fracture site by a physician, nurse practitioner, or physician assistant. The skin surfaces are covered with padding and/or stockinette, prior to applying dampened plaster rolls/synthetic cast tapes smoothly and evenly. Casting material should be applied evenly on the extremity, distal to proximal (Satryb, Wilson, & Patterson, 2011). Overlap each turn of plaster roll by approximately one half its width so that no two turns directly overlap, which could cause undue pressure in that area. Cover any joint areas while in moderate or full flexion by using partially overlapping "figure 8" turns. If additional strength is needed for support around joints, incorporate longitudinal strips of wet plaster. If the cast will not need trimming, petal the edges while casting by turning down the ends of the stockinette over the plaster, then covering the turned-down edges with plaster/synthetic casting material to hold the stockinette in place and create a smooth edge against the skin. For a cast created with cast tape, the cast tape adheres to the previous turn and is stable in approximately 15 minutes. Most casts are adequate and stable with a thickness of one-quarter inch.

Once casting is complete, elevate the casted extremity to heart level. Trim the edges of the cast to prevent roughness and tape rough edges if needed, i.e. petal the edges with transpore tape. Cleanse any residue from casting materials off the patient's skin after application is complete. Instruct the patient not to place foreign objects beneath cast. Note the amount of blood on the cast (circling may or may not be considered helpful due to porosity of cast materials), and apply ice bags to lessen bleeding. Plaster casts act like sponges and absorb drainage, whereas synthetic casts act like wicks and pull drainage away from the drainage site. For either casting material, the padding can also absorb wound drainage (Murray, 2010). In patients with a cast jacket, observe for respiratory or cardiac distress. Have a cast cutter available and be aware of the quickest method to remove a cast jacket to initiate cardiopulmonary resuscitation (CPR). An Allen wrench should also be taped to a cast jacket.

To maintain the integrity of plaster casts, leave the cast uncovered and open to air to dry. Place the cast on a firm, smooth surface with a pillow (without rubber or plastic) under joints to prevent flattening of plaster or trapping of heat. Reposition the patient, alternating from supine, prone, and lateral side-to-side when possible every 2-4 hours to promote drying. Avoid putting any pressure on toes. The drying period of a large plaster cast may be 48-72 hours, depending on humidity and temperature. Drying of a cast may be aided by the use of fans. Explain to the patient that he or she may feel warmth as plaster sets and dries. Support and move a cast with the palms of the hands instead of the fingers to prevent indentations in the plaster. Always turn the patient by supporting major joints. Do not use an abductor bar to turn the patient in a spica cast. Weight-bearing, if ordered, is not recommenced until a cast is completely dry. When turning the patient, inspect the cast for cracks, softening, or excessive flaking; report these areas to the physician, and document in the medical record. Conduct neurovascular assessment of extremities, based on institutional policy (such as every 15 minutes x 2 hours, every 30 minutes x 2 hours, every 2 hours x 4 hours, every 4 hours x 8 hours, and then every 8 hours) if the neurovascular assessment is within normal parameters. Above all, keep a plaster cast dry by covering the cast with a plastic bag securely closed at the top when showering or bathing, avoid rain or other sources of moisture (humidifiers), and prevent plaster contamination with urine or stool. Petal perineal openings to prevent soiling. If necessary, cleanse soiled plaster with a mild powdered cleanser and a slightly dampened cloth, and pat dry completely.

Synthetic casts dry completely by blotting the cast with towels and using a hand blower on a cool or warm setting to thoroughly dry the cast and lining to prevent skin maceration/burns and alterations in cast integrity. Inform the patient that the warmth felt is due to the chemical reaction from the synthetic cast curing. Thermal burns are dependent upon the water temperature and if the cast has more than ten layers (Drozd, Miles, & Davies, 2009). The patient may bear weight in 30 minutes, per order. The surface of the cast is rough, so caution needs to be taken to protect the opposite limb and furniture from scratches. Synthetic casts may be immersed in water, depending on the casting material and the physician's permission. Patients should be taught to flush out the cast well with clear fresh water after bathing or swimming to remove mild soaps or chlorine residue. The cautious use of a hair dryer on a low setting will aid in drying out the cast.

The patient and everyone involved with the patient's care need to monitor for and prevent possible ongoing complications. It is imperative to inspect the skin around the edges of cast for redness or skin irritation. Areas over bony prominences must be monitored for pressure or burning sensation. The skin may be massaged and cooled with alcohol. Perform neurovascular checks to ascertain local effects of a cast on tissues by assessing capillary refill (< 2 seconds is considered normal), the color of skin, skin temperature, the presence and amount of edema, the level of comfort/pain/sensations of the casted area, the mobility of the tissues contiguous to the encasted tissues, and any changes in function experienced. The cast should be felt for any abnormally warm areas, any smell, or any drainage, which may indicate a pressure sore or wound infection beneath the cast.

Numerous casts may create the potential for an ineffective breathing pattern by the patient. The anticipated nursing outcomes for the patient normal breath sounds in all quadrants and the ability to perform deep breathing and coughing exercises. Nursing interventions include assessing the respiratory function in patients with a body or spica cast, teaching and encouraging deep breathing and coughing exercises in immobilized patients, and aiding the patient to change position every 2 hours and PRN to increase perfusion.

Post-Casting Care. Post-casting, the patient (and/or caregiver) receives instructions on care of the cast. Pain is managed through analgesics/NSAIDs. Activity orders will follow weight-bearing limitations, and generally can include isometrics of quad sets and gluteal sets 10 times every hour. Ice, rest, and elevation are stressed to facilitate the reduction of edema and possible neurovascular compromise. The general guidelines for the amount of elevation: "Hands above the heart, and toes above the nose." Thus, the hand rests higher than elbow, the elbow higher than shoulder, the foot higher than knee, and the knee higher than hip. A thorough explanation of signs of neurovascular compromise and compartment syndrome are reinforced, such that the patient will return to have the cast bivalved, univalved, or removed should compromise occur. Any change requires the patient to notify the health care provider of possible complications. Pressure problems commonly occur at joints and bony prominences with short-arm and short-leg casts.

Upper extremity casts may require the use of a sling. The sling supports the weight of the casted hand and wrist in a slightly flexed position to prevent shoulder muscle strain. Place the upper extremity in a sling until the edema or tenderness subsides. Slings greatly reduce neck fatigue and elbow and wrist pressure. The basic design gives comfort and support by spreading the weight of the upper extremity evenly across the neck and shoulders, but should not obstruct access to check neurovascular status. Commercially made slings are available, or slings can be cut from canvas. With canvas, make a triangular sling, and pin at both sides of the back of the neck (rather than knotted over cervical spine) to prevent pressure. Remove the sling to rest the extremity and to wash the sling, if necessary.

During the treatment period, a cast may need to be changed. Reasons for cast change could be the result of poor original application or looseness due to reduced edema, which now causes the cast to slide off the extremity. Complaints of pain, tightness, excessive wetness, excessive trauma to the cast, or a foreign object in the cast warrant evaluation and probable change. An incision beneath the cast may require change if not accessible via a window.

Cast Removal. Cast removal requires support of the joints above and below the injury during the removal procedure. Caution the patient about cast saw noise, and explain that the saw cuts by vibrations (oscillates) and that the dust produced should not be inhaled. Ear and eye protection may be suggested for both the patient and health care provider.

The patient needs to be aware that the initial appearance of the skin will be dry and scaly, especially if the cast has not been changed during the treatment period. As the health care provider continues to provide support to the joints above and below the affected joint, the skin is washed gently with mild soap and water. Do not attempt to remove all of the dead skin. The skin is to be lubricated with protective emollient, lotion, cream, or ointment.

Nursing Considerations

Nursing Diagnoses. Nursing diagnoses for this condition are expanded upon in the Appendix.

- Aspiration, risk for.
- Body image, disturbed.
- Constipation, risk for.
- Disuse syndrome, risk for.
- Gastrointestinal motility, risk for dysfunctional.
- Mobility, physical, impaired.
- Pain, acute.
- Peripheral neurovascular dysfunction, risk for.
- Self-care deficit: bathing/hygiene, dressing/grooming, feeding, grooming.
- Sleep pattern, disturbed.
- Tissue perfusion: peripheral, ineffective.

The potential for injury and impaired skin integrity is critical for casted patients. Nursing outcomes focus on no evidence of skin irritation, maintenance of neurovascular integrity, and the ongoing integrity of a clean, dry cast that provides no evidence of dislocation/subluxation or refracture. Nursing interventions to prevent/monitor skin and cast complications begin even before casting occurs. During pre-casting, examine the skin for bruises, rashes, varicosities, peripheral vascular problems, poor turgor, atrophy, open wounds, or lacerations. Document any abnormalities on the patient's medical record, and assess the tetanus status and need for prophylaxis.

Following cast removal, there is the potential for injury such as refracture, dislocation or subluxation. The nursing outcomes center on patient compliance with activity restrictions, thus preventing post-cast removal injury. Nursing interventions begin by explaining to the patient that muscles and joints in a cast will be weak and sore, and that use and movements should be initiated moderately with rest periods. Patients may use analgesic/NSAIDs for soreness, pain, or inflammation. It is suggested to elevate the affected extremity frequently after cast removal to prevent edema. The nurse must discuss activity restrictions, exercises for muscle strengthening, and methods to avoid refracture and dislocation after cast removal. The patient must understand that a casted limb takes twice as long as the time spent in the cast to regain full function.

Practice Setting Considerations. *Home care:* Both the patient and caregivers require discharge teaching. Provide the patient/caregiver with information and instruction related to the signs and symptoms of complications (severe pain, burning, numbness, tingling, skin discoloration, swelling, paralysis, foul odor, warm spots, elevated temperature, soft areas and cracks, pallor and coolness of fingers and toes). Instruct the patient to keep the extremity elevated when possible, emphasizing the importance of skin care and the integrity of the cast. Patients/caregivers must be able to verbalize when to notify the physician of any abnormalities. Provide information on both pharmacologic and nonpharmacologic pain management techniques. Instruct the patient regarding the permitted activity level and use of ambulatory devices or a sling, if indicated. Explain how atrophy may occur with casting, stressing the need to continue exercises, both active and passive as permitted by the physician, in order to maintain muscle tone, reduce the potential for multiple complications, and aid in the post-cast recovery process. If appropriate, discuss sexual activities and positions.

When considering home care, carefully observe the patient's mobility. Assess the patient's ability to ambulate, climb stairs, and transfer bed-to-chair or chair-to-bed. Ascertain that safety is essential for both the patient and family/support persons. Reinforce cast care, complications to report to the health care provider, and expectations as cast removal becomes imminent.

Continuous Passive Motion Machine

Overview

Continuous passive motion (CPM) is a technique for applying continuous range of motion to a joint using a stationary electronically controlled machine. CPM has been shown to reduce the development of adhesions during healing and to stimulate healing of articular cartilage. Used in a variety of situations involving healing of articular cartilage in joints, CPM may be implemented after total joint arthroplasty, synovectomy, open meniscectomy, incision and drainage of septic joint, arthrotomy, capsulotomy, or joint debridement. Tibial plateau fractures, supracondylar fractures, or an open reduction internal fixations (ORIF) of intra-articular fractures might also benefit from CPM therapy. Procedures in the knee joint such as patellectomy, synovectomy for rheumatoid arthritis, and hemophilic arthroplasty or knee manipulation are also indications for use. Additional indications are joint contractures (in hemophiliacs), adhesive capsulitis, ligamentous repair, restricted motion secondary to adhesions, finger flexor tendon repair, or biologic resurfacing for a major defect in a joint surface.

CPM has many advantages for use in the patient with musculoskeletal injury. CPM reduces disuse atrophy and provides early mobilization to enhance healing and tissue remodeling. This therapy aids in nutrition to involved tissues, reduces capsular contracture, maintains articular cartilage, reduces joint effusions and associated pain, and lessens joint hemiarthrosis. Following total knee arthroplasty (TKA), CPM therapy reduces the postoperative hospitalization, the amount of time required to attain range of motion (ROM) goals, and the incidence of postoperative knee manipulation.

CPM is most effective when it is continuous (6–22 hours daily). Patients are permitted restricted activity and are only allowed out of the machine for limited periods. This places them at increased risk for problems related to immobility and bed rest. Additional reported complications include increased bleeding at the surgical site, and an increased incidence of knee flexion contracture after total knee arthroplasty. In some patients, CPM therapy increases pain and analgesic requirements. The only contraindications are an unstable fracture and wound dehiscence.

Assessment

The comprehensive patient history will document a description of the acute injury, chronic, developmental, or congenital deformity, any previous history of treatment with CPM, and assess hand dominance if the upper extremity is involved.

The physical examination places an emphasis on the extremity to be treated with CPM and on the body systems most affected by immobility. The general peripheral vascular status and neurovascular status of the involved extremity, as well as skin integrity including the condition of any surgical incisions, are documented. The exam must also include a thorough respiratory assessment and document elimination, nutritional, and sleep patterns.

Common Therapeutic Modalities

For the duration of CPM use, the degrees of flexion and extension, the schedule for being in and out of the machine, and documentation of the patient's compliance with time spent in the device are placed in the medical record. The proper positioning of the extremity – so that the joint is over the area of flexion and extension while using CPM therapy – aids in patient compliance. Table 10.5 identifies best practices for CPM care.

Table 10.5. Best Practice for Patient Safety & Quality Care: The Patient Using CPM

- Ensure that the machine is well padded.
- Check the cycle and range-of-motion settings at least once every 8 hours.
- Ensure that the joint being moved is properly positioned on the machine.
- If the patient is confused, place th econtrols to the machine out of his or her reach.
- Assess the patient's response to the machine.
- Turn off the machine while the patient is having a meal in bed.
- When the machine is not in use, do not store it on the floor.

Data from Medical-Surgical Nursing Patient-Centered Collaborative Care *(6th ed., pp. 322-361) by D. Ignativiticus and C. Murray, 2010, St. Louis, MO: W.B. Saunders.*

Nursing Considerations

Nursing Diagnoses. Nursing diagnoses for this condition are expanded upon in the Appendix.

- Injury, risk for.
- Knowledge deficit.
- Noncompliance.
- Peripheral neurovascular dysfunction, risk for.
- Powerlessness.
- Sleep pattern, disturbed.

For the client in CPM, the feeling of powerlessness is appropriate. Patient outcomes to overcome any resulting noncompliance will focus on the patient's participation in self-care and decision-making regarding the prescribed CPM regimen. The nursing interventions to achieve the patient outcome are to organize the environment to facilitate patient's independence while in the CPM machine. The nurse must allow the patient as much control as possible over time out of CPM therapy. Additionally, the nurse must provide information to alleviate anxiety related to purpose and understanding of CPM machine, stressing the long-term benefits of the therapy. In order to provide optimal support and guidance, the nurse should remain with the patient for one complete cycle before leaving the patient alone. It is also imperative that the nurse demonstrate the technique for immediate discontinuance of CPM for emergent situations (sharp, sudden acute pain).

Practice Setting Considerations. *Home care:* The increased use of CPM in the home requires a thorough understanding and correct application and use of the machine. Signs and symptoms of complications, including new or increased joint swelling, increased redness, tenderness or itching, or unusual pain or fever, warrant an immediate call to the physician.

External Fixators

Overview

An external fixator is a versatile method of immobilization that employs percutaneous transfixing pins/wires inserted into a bone, which are then attached to a rigid external frame. This allows a wide range of anatomic correction, both congenital and acquired. External fixation can be constructed in six basic types of frame configurations and are classified according to the design of the principle components.

1. A *unilateral (monolateral)* frame incorporates fixation on one side of limb.
2. A *bilateral* fixator has a rigid bar on both sides of the limb connected to full pins that transfix the bone, although may utilize only half.
3. A *quadrilateral* frame consists of four bars, two on each side of the limb, connected to pins that transfix the bone.
4. A *semicircular* frame utilizes bars that incompletely encircle the limb.
5. A *triangular* fixator has pins that are placed on two or more planes.
6. A *circular* frame is a modular half ring assembled to encircle the limb transfixed by small wires.

External fixators vary in appearances but have similar purposes: to anchor the frame in main bony fragments (pins/wires), provide longitudinal support (rods), and connect pins/wires to a supporting frame. The critical factors in providing stability are the number of wires, the tension in the wires, and the size of the wires, while causing minimal damage to periosteal and endosteal blood supply.

A variety of factors affects the selection of external fixation, including the patient's age, the affected bone/limb, and the existence of multi-trauma along with the severity of local soft tissue injury. The complexity of a congenital or acquired deformity/defect often plays a major role in the determination to use external fixation.

The patient's ability for self-care is also a consideration, along with his or her personal preference.

The use of external fixation is indicated with both simple fractures (open and closed) and complex fractures with extensive soft tissue injury. Common uses include correction of bony or soft tissue defects/ deformities, ligamentotaxis (comminuted epiphyseal fracture), pseudoarthroses (false joint) of a long bone (congenial and acquired) that develops at the site of a former fracture, non-/malunion, limb length discrepancies, and stabilization of a joint arthrodesis (ankylosis) or fixation of a joint. Circumstances in which urgent transport is needed and/or facilities for internal fixation are not available may necessitate the application of an external fixator.

The use of external fixation is contraindicated in patients in whom cooperation or mental competence is lacking. Fractures that will heal with more conservative treatment or that are best treated with internal fixation do not warrant this method of fracture management. Diabetic patients or those on corticosteroids are not optimal candidates due to their increased potential for pin tract infection.

There are many advantages to the use of external fixation. The skeletal stability proximal to or a distance from the site of injury and the rigid fixation with compression to ensure primary bone healing make external fixation a successful treatment option. Free access to an injured site for primary and secondary procedures facilitates vascular and soft tissue reconstruction. This affords greater versatility in treating a wide variety of bone and soft tissue lesions by the ability to access open wounds and reduce wound sepsis. This access facilitates nursing care. The ability to stabilize injuries extending across two or more adjacent limb segments limits the interference with adjacent joints. With congenital or limb lengthening procedures, the adjustability of alignment, length, and mechanical properties are vital. External fixators have the ability to be used simultaneously and/or sequentially with internal fixation and other methods of skeletal stabilization, which can help to maintain bone and muscle bulk. Less scarring may also occur than with internal fixation. Immediate fracture fixation/stabilization provides the opportunity to reduce blood loss with pelvic fixation and often enables early mobilization of the patient from non-/partial to full-weight bearing. Early mobilization reduces the occurrence or severity of the many complications associated with immobilization.

Complications associated with external fixators can be classified as clinical, mechanical, or multi-factorial. The appearance may frighten the patient or family, and body image concerns must be addressed. Clinical complications are numerous. Improper insertion of the pin/wires may cause damage to a joint space or result in iatrogenic treatment/diagnostic neurovascular injuries, muscle impingement, or cutaneous nerve injury. Compartment syndrome has less of an incidence than with ORIF. Loss of alignment or correction, joint stiffness, or contractures can occur. Pin tract infections or superficial and deep wound infection in patients with soft tissue injury can lead to delayed healing (non-union/malunion). Infections in pin sites are a major concern because of the risk of osteomyelitis, a spreading of the infection from the skin and soft tissues to the bone, which is almost impossible to eradicate (Santy & Duffield, 2009). Septic arthritis, refracture, and osteomyelitis have been documented. While use of an external fixator is generally an advantage, the fixator frame may obstruct injury access. Epiphyseal plate disturbances (where new bone forms along the plate) or the improper use of lengthening—either too quickly, resulting in early union/non-union, or too slowly, causing early consolidation/ union—must be monitored.

Mechanical complications of external fixation involve component failure from misuse. Inadequate mechanical frame properties and the malfunction or breakage of components are other common mechanical complications. Multiple factors that can result in complications include mismatch of clinical needs and the frame selection; pin problems (drainage, loosening, infection); skin excoriation and necrosis from the frame; delayed or inhibited bone consolidation or regeneration; unrealistic expectations; and lack of experience or long-term treatment planning.

Patterson (2006) examined the literature on the use of external fixation in adolescents and found that depression to the point of suicidal ideations or attempts was the most pronounced psychological effect. While temporary for some patients, the depression continued even after completion of treatment and removal of the external fixation device for others. A range of emotions, intentionally contaminating pin sites, body image (especially for adolescents treated with halos), social isolation, sleep disturbance, and a return to dependence upon others were common findings in the reviewed research. The findings indicate an interdisciplinary approach to dealing with these issues in the adolescent population, whether for limb lengthening or a traumatic need for external fixation use.

Assessment

A thorough patient history will provide a description of the mechanism of injury for the acute injury or chronic, developmental, or congenital condition that will require external fixation, as well as a baseline neurovascular assessment. The patient's normal level of function, weight-bearing status, ROM, and ability to

Table 10.6. Nursing Considerations According to Type of Traction		
Type of Traction	**Indications**	**Nursing Considerations According to Type of Traction**
Halo ■ Skeletal Tongs: Vinke Gardner-Wells Barton Crutchfield	■ Cervical and high thoracic fractures, subluxations, dislocations, fusions, scoliosis; maintain stability during surgery.	a. Provide continuous pull (20-30 pound weight). If pin loosening or penetration occurs, apply manual traction and support sides of head with sandbags or apply Philadelphia collar. Notify physician immediately. b. Incorporate signs and symptoms of cranial nerve impairment with neurovascular assessments. c. Observe for eye movements, pupillary changes, blurred vision, photosensitivity, difficulty with swallowing, speech, or tongue control. d. Administer pin care every shift. e. Log roll. f. Muscle setting exercises and active range of motion in appropriate joints. g. Provide distraction or social/recreational activities. h. Provide emotional support. i. Skin assessment beneath vest. j. Allen wrench on vest for emergency use.
Cervical head halter ■ Skin	■ Severe sprains, strains, torticollis, mild cervical trauma.	a. Observe for pain and pressure in the ears, temporomandibular joint (TMJ), chin, and occiput. b. Add a soft, thin, foam pad beneath chin. c. Perform baseline cranial nerve assessment and document baseline findings. d. Men should be clean-shaven when possible. e. May be set up so head is kept in a straight position or so that head of bed can be elevated depending on the patient's condition. As long as the patient's spinal column remains in correct alignment, patient is able to change position, with assistance. f. Use of small cervical pillow determined by patient's condition. g. Elevate HOB 20-30 degrees for correct alignment. h. Traction removed for meals if permitted by physician. i. Intermittent cervical skin traction is sometimes used, physician orders.
Side arm traction/90-90 upper extremity traction ■ Skin or skeletal	■ Supracondylar fractures of the elbow, humerus and shoulder.	a. Do not change position in bed (back-lying position) or position of the head of bed. b. Tilt patient toward affected extremity. c. Maintain 90-90 traction with shoulder and forearm flexed or shoulder abducted and elbow flexed. d. Countertraction can be applied by placing shock blocks under the traction side of the bed. e. Observe for radial, ulnar, and median nerve pressure, numbness, and tingling of one or more fingers; decreased ability to oppose thumb and fingers (sings of Volkmann's ischemic contracture). f. Patient can use his/her feet to lift buttock for bedpan, skin care, and changing the bed. g. Back and skin care for the upper portion of the body is accomplished by pressing down on the mattress. h. 2-3 weeks callus formation may be sufficient to allow for spica cast application. i. Provide emotional support and teaching about the traction and future care management. j. Provide social and recreational activities.

Table 10.6. Nursing Considerations According to Type of Traction (continued)		
Type of Traction	**Indications**	**Nursing Considerations According to Type of Traction**
Dunlop traction ■ Skin or skeletal	■ Supracondylar fractures of the elbow. ■ Humerus.	a. See side arm traction. b. Used with children. c. Check for Volkmann's ischemic contracture. d. 5-7 pounds weight for humerus. e. 3-5 pounds weight for forearm.
Pelvic sling ■ Skin (suspension)	■ Pelvic fractures.	a. Sling compresses side of pelvis. b. Provide good perineal and lower back care. c. Check for foot drop, voiding difficulties, perineal irritations, skin breakdown, correct size, fit, and application of sling. d. Maintain sling beneath lower back with cheek of buttocks elevated 1-2 inches from the bed. e. Clarify orders for lifting and turning. f. 20 to 35 pounds weight effective.
Pelvic (belt) traction ■ Skin	■ Muscle spasms associated with low back pain, ruptured disc.	a. Apply the pelvic belt across the patient's lower abdomen, making sure it is on the pelvis and that it does not go above the iliac crest or umbilicus, and directly on the patient's skin, when possible. b. Make sure of the correct size. c. Amount of weight varies from 15-40 pounds, depending on patient's size and amount of muscle spasms. d. Assure even/straight pull along thighs/knees to the spreader bar or weight attachment. e. William position (supine with 15-20 degrees elevation of the knees and 30-45 degree elevation of the head) preferred. If necessary, bed flat when side lying. f. Observe skin for irritation, heat and redness. Massage iliac crests. g. Instruct patient to ask for assistance to remove weights and belt, if allowed bathroom privileges.
Cotrel's traction ■ Skin (combination head halter and pelvic belt)	■ Preoperative treatment to help straighten spinal curvatures before insertion of skeletal rods for corrections of scoliosis.	a. Pull in opposite directions helps to overcome deforming muscle pull causing curvature. b. See cervical head halter. c. See pelvic (belt) traction. d. 1-2 hours on, 1-2 hours off for sleep. e. 5-7 pounds for head halter. f. 10-20 pounds for pelvic belt.
Bryant traction ■ Skin (Gallow's traction in UK)	■ Developmental dysplasia of the hip (DDH). ■ Femur fracture in child younger than 2-3 years of age, weighing less than 30-35 pounds.	a. Make sure patient's buttocks just clear the mattress, with hips flexed 90 degrees and knees extended. b. Assure that spreader bar keeps pressure from being applied to malleoli. c. Be sure traction is taken down daily (every shift and PRN) to provide skin care of both extremities. d. Child may be positioned either parallel or perpendicular to head and foot of bed. If positioned perpendicular, then caregiver may bring child out of bed to hold in arms and feed. e. Toddlers may need to be restrained to prevent "flipover." f. Family may be taught to provide care for home Bryant traction, a 2-4 week period with 2-4 pounds of weight, followed by hip spica cast if necessary.

Table 10.6. Nursing Considerations According to Type of Traction (continued)		
Type of Traction	**Indications**	**Nursing Considerations According to Type of Traction**
Buck extension ■ Skin	■ Fractures of the hip for short term, hip contractures, muscle spasms from surgery (hip/knee) or arthritic conditions of hip/knee.	a. Keep patient's heels off the bed. Use pillow and/or heel protectors. b. Avoid pressure on the dorsum of the foot and over the head of the fibula or malleolus. c. Assess for peroneal nerve palsy. d. 5-7 pounds weight effective. e. Countertraction may be applied by elevating the foot of bed to prevent sliding down and shearing or by slightly elevating the knee gatch. f. The leg in traction should be on the mattress without a pillow under the leg. g. Place rolled towel or padded sandbag along the external surface of knee to prevent external rotation of affected leg. h. If on an unrepaired fracture, do not release the traction. i. Teach patients to use trapeze and unaffected foot/leg to lift themselves in assisting with bedpan use, skin care, and linen changes. j. In most instances, head of bed may be elevated for meals, but not for continuous positioning.
Russell traction ■ Skin	■ Fractured hip. ■ Short-term use fractured femur not amenable to internal fixation. ■ Fracture tibia/fibula.	a. Modification of Buck with the addition of a sling under the femur, not affected knee, to provide more comfort and less rotation. b. Hips and knees slightly flexed 30 degrees or less and immobilized. c. 2 to 5 pounds weight effective. d. Make sure the sling is smooth and doesn't apply pressure in the popliteal space or the head of the fibula. Due to arrangement of the pulleys, the pull of the traction is double the amount of weight applied. e. The arrangement of the ropes, pulleys, and knee sling distributes the pull more effectively throughout the entire limb, therefore less injurious to skin. f. Back-lying position.
Adjunct to traction: balanced suspension with Thomas splint and Pearson attachment **Balanced Suspension Skeletal Traction (BSST)**	■ Device that supports the extremity and overcomes the force of gravity. ■ Used with skin or skeletal traction for femur or tibial fractures not amenable to internal fixation, for acetabular fractures, for maintaining joint space following removal of a prosthesis and for hip/knee contractures. Can be used alone for exercise, to support dependent part and/or to maintain correct alignment. ■ Steinmann pin or Kirschner wire 20 to 35 pounds weight effective.	a. Pad ischial ring; check increased pressure in groin and knee areas. b. Neurovascular assessment. c. Position the extremity in sling to keep pressure off the heel and Achilles tendon to not carry weight of lower extremity. d. Pearson attachment parallels knee. e. Prevent foot drop; use footboards. f. If bed in semi-Fowlers, lay flat at least 20 minutes every shift to prevent hip flexion contracture. g. Assure no external rotation of extremity to prevent peroneal nerve palsy. h. Perform quadriceps muscle setting exercises and heel cord exercises 10 times per hour while awake and PRN.

From Core Curriculum for Orthopaedic Nursing *(6th ed., pp. 242-244) by National Association of Orthopaedic Nurses (NAON), 2007, Boston, MA: Pearson.*

use supportive devices and adapt to the limitations of an external fixator must be evaluated. The effects of external fixation on the patient's lifestyle, as well as transportation concerns, demand inquiry. A medical/surgical history (endocrine/metabolic) concerning any comorbid conditions under treatment or a history of infections, pain management history, and coping mechanisms are included in the history and physical.

Upon physical examination, the focus is on the affected extremity for pain, pallor, paresthesia, paralysis, pulse, and leg-length discrepancy. The stability of the patient, bed position, and affected limb alignment, plus any early intervention immobilization devices, are thoroughly assessed. Should any external fixation have already been applied, the appearance and placement of pin/wires must be verified. The neurovascular status is constantly reassessed and radiologic diagnostics evaluated. Consultation with physical/occupational therapy for evaluation may be indicated.

Common Therapeutic Modalities

Treatment intervention with this therapeutic modality begins with an evaluation for the type of external fixation device to be applied, after considering the immediate and long-term treatment plans, and the application of the apparatus. When appropriate, distraction is integrated into the treatment plan at an optimal rate of 1-1.5 mm/day divided into four equal doses in children; the adult distraction rate is 3 mm/day in three divided doses. The patient's level of activity and progression with short- and long-term goals are developed in consultation with physical therapy and occupational therapy needs. Pain management, care of the device, dressing changes, ROM, pin/wire care, and instructions for immediate home care are part of a comprehensive discharge plan with ongoing outpatient follow-up care.

Nursing Considerations

Nursing Diagnoses. Nursing diagnoses for this condition are expanded upon in the Appendix.

- Body image, disturbed.
- Coping, ineffective.
- Infection, risk for.
- Knowledge deficit.
- Mobility: physical, impaired.
- Pain, acute.
- Peripheral neurovascular dysfunction, risk for.
- Self-care deficit: bathing/hygiene, dressing/ grooming, feeding, toileting.
- Self-concept, readiness for enhanced.
- Self-esteem, situational low.
- Skin integrity, impaired.

Patient outcomes for injury potential and impaired physical mobility center on the patient's adjustment to an altered gait pattern/weight-bearing status. The patient must evaluate him- or herself for safety relative to self-injury from dizziness, disturbed balance, and vertigo, which could result in a fall. Appropriate nursing interventions are to teach patients safety maneuvers to balance themselves with their frames and use assistive devices to prevent falls. The patient must be taught safe use of assistive devices and may benefit from a PT/OT referral.

Pin Care and Skin Integrity. Musculoskeletal patients are consistently evaluated for the potential of impaired skin integrity. Patient outcomes focus on pin sites with no evidence of pin necrosis or infection as evidenced by minimal serous drainage from pin sites. The primary nursing intervention centers upon observation for early signs and symptoms of pin tract infection, including pain, erythema, tenderness, and discharge (Rose, 2010). Serous drainage in a small amount is normal until "tenting" occurs. "Tenting" (migration of the skin around the pin/wire) can cause pin site infection as the skin often adheres to the pin as a result of the presence of serous exudate, which becomes sticky or dry. During patient movement, the skin moves up and down the pin; as the skin migrates up the pin, this leaves a space just under the skin adjacent to the pin, which acts as a reservoir for fluid, an ideal environment for the growth of bacteria (Santy & Duffield, 2009).

It is essential that the nurse perform and teach the patient/caregiver the importance of pin care, noting any pin-skin motion, tension on pins/wires, or loosening of the pins. Pin care is performed with a solution determined by institutional policies and physician preference. Table 10.7 outlines NAON's evidence-based pin care site recommendations. Saline should be used if chlorhexidine solution is contraindicated according to the Royal College of Nursing (2011). Any redness, swelling about pins/wires, tightness of skin around pins, or warmth of extremity are to be documented and reported. Pin care, a form of wound care, is performed as directed under sterile conditions. A culture for suspected pin tract infection determines an appropriate antibiotic regimen. Betadine solution, betadine ointment, alcohol, and peroxide should be avoided, as these agents can cause tissue damage, loosening of pins, and deterioration of the pin itself (Murray & Rawls, 2010).

Table 10.7. NAON Evidence-Based Pin Site Care Recommendations
1. Pins located in areas with considerable soft tissue should be considered at greater risk for infection.
2. At sites with mechanically stable bone-pin interfaces, pin site care should be done on a daily or weekly basis (after the first 48–72 hours).
3. Chlorhexidine 2 mg/ml solution may be the most effective cleansing solution for pin site care.
4. Patient and/or their families should be taught pin site care before discharge from the hospital. They should be required to demonstrate whatever care needs to be done and should be provided with written instructions that includes signs and symptoms of infection.

Data from "Skeletal Pin Site Care" by S. Holmes and S. Brown, 2005, Orthopaedic Nursing *24(2), 99-107.*

Teach the patient/caregiver how to perform frame integrity checks, pin/wire care, and/or wound care. Additionally, monitor for skin tears as the external fixator is adjusted to correct a deformity/defect or limb lengthening, as the pins/wires must pull through soft tissue to correct the problem. These skin tears usually heal quickly because pin/wire motion is at slow rate and rhythm.

Continuously check the integrity of the external fixator. A loose frame can cause friction and pin-skin motion, resulting in pain, infection, and an inability to do physical therapy. Mark the external fixator with nail polish, tape, or some other means (not needed if it has a clicking mechanism) to indicate where daily/weekly adjustment of the frame is necessary to achieve goals.

Practice Setting Considerations. *Home care:* Prior to discharge, the patient with external fixation has many teaching needs. The patient and any caregivers should be able to identify pin site infection, know methods for controlling swelling and pain, and what to report to clinicians. The patient should demonstrate an ability to transfer and safely use mobility aids (Patterson, 2010).

Both the patient and caregiver should be able to demonstrate prescribed pin site care. Pin site care will require the use of a new cotton tip applicator each time and for each pin. The applicator is to be saturated with a solution of chlorhexidine. Reinforce to proceed from the skin out and to remove "tenting" crusting. Within 1–2 weeks, the patient can shower daily with antibacterial, nonemollient soap.

The patient/caregiver must report any signs and symptoms of pin site infection to the physician. Loosening/movement of pins, an increase in drainage from a pin site, redness, soreness, pain, itching, compromised neurovascular status, or fever must be reported. The patient also needs to be aware of the integrity of the frame and keep vigilant with treatment goals. Distraction or compression technique, active and passive ROM including stretch breaks to prevent joint stiffness, and keeping the extremity elevated are continually monitored throughout each day. Because smoking/nicotine use causes vasoconstriction and may interfere with healing, patients should receive assistance with smoking cessation as needed. Sexual functions/needs in light of immobility and placement of external fixator need to be discussed as age-appropriate. Adaptive clothing/devices with hook-and-loop fasteners (such as Velcro®), snaps, ties, nonskid socks, and shoes can be arranged for the patient. A tub mat and shower chair, as well as other safety needs in the home, require evaluation. Children may need to have a wheelchair, or use of a wagon may be more appropriate, depending upon their level of development. School or work adaptations for prolonged absence may also need to be investigated.

Traction

Overview

Traction is the application of a pulling force to an injured or diseased body part while a countertraction pulls in the opposite direction. Traction serves to:

- reduce fractures and/or subluxations/dislocations and maintain alignment;
- decrease muscle spasm associated with low-back pain or cervical whiplash and relieve pain;
- correct, lessen, or prevent deformities/contractures;
- promote rest of a diseased or injured part or provide immobilization to prevent soft tissue damage;
- promote active and passive exercise; and
- expand a joint space during arthroscopic procedures or prior to joint reconstruction.

Traction can be delivered through a variety of mechanisms. Static traction promotes immobilization (continuous), whereas dynamic traction promotes movement (intermittent). Running traction exerts a pull in one plane (straight), while balanced suspension allows the patient movement without a change in the pull of the traction. Traction is not used as frequently today due to the advances in instrumentation for fracture repairs and new methods of trauma management (Murray & Rawls, 2010).

A set of basic principles has been established to maintain effective traction. Countertraction is achieved using part of the patient's body, bed positioning, or pull of weights in the opposite direction. It is necessary to prevent friction by not tucking in top linens, allowing the foot-plate to rest against the bed, or allowing shearing of elbows or heels against linen. Other ways to prevent friction are by avoiding clamps, hooks, etc., from resting against the bed frame, making sure weights move freely through pulleys, clearing the footboard, and suspending the weights off the floor. Traction knots are not maintained near the pulleys or at the patient attachment point. The line of pull established by the physician, usually neutral unless otherwise specified, is maintained via continuous or intermittent traction as required by the physician's order and type of traction. Patients with halo traction demand additional safety considerations due to their altered field of vision.

Classifications. The three classifications of traction (Table 10.8) are manual, skin, and skeletal. *Manual* traction is applied via the hands with a steady pull maintained. The indications to use manual traction are during an emergency, for fracture reduction, while applying a cast or a halo apparatus.

Skin traction attaches to skin and soft tissue as it provides a light pull. It may be removed and reapplied intermittently as per physician orders. A maximum weight of 5-8 pounds for adults and 1-5 pounds for children's arms and legs will prevent occlusion of small blood vessels. The weight is applied with skin adherent strips, a cervical head halter, Ace wraps, or commercial encircling devices such as foam splints, traction boots, or pelvic belts. If the weight is distributed over a larger area such as the pelvis, more weight can be used. Weight is distributed evenly over the largest possible body surface to prevent uneven pull and skin breakdown. Skin traction is maintained for relatively short periods. The primary indications for use of skin traction are the stabilization of a fracture prior to repair with surgery or skeletal traction, the relief of muscle spasms, the immobilization of joints/bones with inflammatory conditions to relieve pain, and the prevention of flexion contractures.

Skeletal traction attaches directly to the bone and provides a strong, steady, continuous pull. Skeletal pins are placed at the proximal ulna, distal femur, or proximal tibia. Weight is applied to the extremity via Steinmann's pins or Kirschner wires. Tongs attach a halo to the head. A range of 15-40 pounds of weight is commonly used, depending on the mechanism of injury/pathology, body size, and the degree of muscle spasm. Traction should not be removed without a physician's order. Skeletal traction is frequently used in conjunction with balanced weighted suspension.

On occasion, to achieve the desired line of pull, traction must be applied in more than one direction, thus one line of pull (vector of force) counteracts the other. The actual resultant pulling force is somewhere between the two lines.

Considerations across the life span relate directly to the type of traction used relative to the patient's age. For example, Bryant's traction is only used on children younger than age 3 who weigh less than 35 pounds. Teaching should be appropriate for the patient's developmental level and include the use of play therapy for children. Developmental delays may become present with prolonged treatment. An emphasis can be placed on independence/control in age groups for whom these issues are crucial, especially in adolescents. An increased risk of complications, especially complications related to immobility and acute or temporary confusion, need to be evaluated in the elderly population.

Complications associated with traction use include inadequate fracture alignment and neurovascular compromise, which can be manifested in muscle or nerve weakness, numbness or tingling, an increase in pain, muscle spasms or a loss of sensation. Inadequate fracture alignment may present as posttreatment arthritis if muscles and joints are malaligned in full extension with skin traction. Deep vein thrombosis, pulmonary emboli, or fat emboli syndrome can occur. (For further discussion on these complications, see the related chapters in this text.) Skin traction carries the risk of skin integrity impairment due to breakdown over bony

Table 10.8. Classification of Major Types of Traction

Traction	Type	Term	Duration	Other
Cervical				
Skin traction	Skin	Short-term	Intermittent	
Skeletal traction	Skeletal	Short-term or long-term	Continuous	
Halo traction	Skeletal		Continuous	Traction via halo vest
Upper Extremity				
Side-arm traction	Skin or skeletal		Continuous	Vertical suspension to forearm
Overhead/90-90			Continuous	Vertical traction to humerus; horizontal suspension to forearm
Dunlop	Skin	Short-term	Continuous	
Pelvic				
Pelvic belt	Skin	Short-term	Intermittent	
Pelvic sling	Skin	Long-term	Continuous	
Lower Extremity				
Bryant	Skin	Long-term	Continuous	Bilateral; vertical suspension
Buck	Skin	Short-term	Continuous	Unilateral or bilateral
Russell	Skin	Usually short-term	Continuous	Balanced suspension
Lower extremity 90-90	Skin or skeletal		Continuous	Suspension; unilateral (children) or bilateral (adults)
Skeletal traction with balanced suspension	Skeletal	Long-term	Continuous	Usually unilateral

From An Introduction to Orthopaedic Nursing *(4th ed., p. 96) by C. Murray and C. Rawls, 2010, Chicago, IL. Reproduced with permission.*

prominences or the loss of skin attachment (epidermis from subcutaneous tissue). Skeletal traction has a risk of pin tract infection, and the immobilization increases the risk of development of pressure ulcers (sacrum, coccyx, heels, trochanters, spine, scapulae, elbows, ears).

Assessment

The focus in the patient's history is on previous acute injury or chronic, developmental, or congenital conditions that have required treatment with traction. The complete physical examination checks for a history of diabetes or vascular disease, with a specific emphasis on the extremity or area of the body requiring treatment with traction. A comparison of the affected extremity with the unaffected extremity, when possible, establishes baseline neurovascular assessment. Subsequently, compare each assessment with previous assessments, and compare side to side. A comprehensive peripheral vascular and neurovascular assessment includes color, temperature, capillary refill, pulses, sensation, motion, pain, and edema. Skin integrity assessment will include evaluating scars, open lacerations, pressure ulcers, bruises, rashes, or other skin disorders. An overall assessment of the patient's hygiene must be completed, and GI and GU elimination patterns should be ascertained, as well as a comprehensive respiratory assessment. The most critical diagnostic tests are radiologic: during application of traction to establish injury or condition, and after application to establish realignment of the bone and progression of healing.

Common Therapeutic Modalities

Premedicate the patient, as necessary, prior to traction application. Skin traction may be applied by a nurse or orthopaedic technician. Skeletal traction is applied by an orthopaedic surgeon. General anesthesia may be used in some cases to facilitate application of traction. After application, orders are specified for the amount of traction weight, activity/exercise/positioning limitations, skeletal pin care, ice application, and pain management.

Nursing Considerations

Nursing Diagnoses. Nursing diagnoses for this condition are expanded upon in the Appendix.

- Body image, disturbed.
- Constipation, risk for.
- Coping, ineffective.
- Disuse syndrome, risk for.
- Gastrointestinal motility, risk for dysfunctional.
- Infection, risk for.
- Knowledge deficit.
- Mobility: physical, impaired.
- Pain, acute.
- Peripheral neurovascular dysfunction, risk for.
- Powerlessness.
- Self-care deficit: bathing/hygiene, dressing/grooming, feeding, toileting.
- Self-concept, readiness for enhanced.
- Self-esteem: situational low, risk for.
- Skin integrity, impaired.
- Social interaction, impaired.
- Urinary elimination, impaired.

Impaired physical integrity is an appropriate nursing diagnosis for the patient in traction. The patient outcomes to be achieved are to maintain the traction mechanism, to maintain countertraction by keeping the patient pulled up in bed, to maintain the desired position and alignment to promote healing, and to prevent skin breakdown or neurovascular impairment.

The nursing intervention to maintain the traction mechanics requires inspection of the traction apparatus each shift and PRN. All bolts and ancillary equipment on the apparatus frame should be checked and tightened regularly. There are several types of bed frames that may be used, but a "four poster" Balkan frame is most common. Only new traction cord should be used, and the cord should run freely through pulleys, unrestricted by the bed linens. All slip knots are to be secured with tape and need to be observed for fraying. Weights are to remain free-hanging and the amount of weight verified. The nurse should never add or remove weight without a physician order, nor remove or lift weights when moving the patient. Traction weights should never hang over the patient.

Nursing care for the patient with adherent skin traction begins with the application of commercial skin traction tapes, strips of moleskin, or adhesive lengthwise to either side of affected extremity. It is imperative that the skin beneath the skin traction tape be properly prepared to prevent skin breakdown. The tapes are to extend far enough on the extremity to apply the prescribed amount of weight. It is important to not go beyond the tibial tubercle to prevent pressure on the peroneal nerve. Wrap the extremity with the elastic bandage using a spiral or "figure-8" configuration. The elastic bandage should cover the longest surface possible for an even distribution of pull. The spreader bars must be wide enough to prevent pressure on any bony prominences and neurovascular compromise. Each shift, the nurse inspects the skin traction for sliding and wrinkles by palpating over the taped area. Documentation of the assessment is critical, especially noting any tenderness or skin breakdown. The patient is repositioned as permitted by the traction and per physician's orders. If the skin traction becomes nonfunctional, it must be reapplied. Removal of skin traction for skin care is ordered by the physician. Skin traction such as a Buck's boot should be removed at least daily for limb washing and skin inspection (Whiteing, 2008). The skin is inspected (note any redness, skin irritation, burning sensation, drainage, or foul odor), massaged, and lubricated with gel or ointment, especially around the edges of traction. Powder, lotion, and creams are not recommended for use. See Table 10.6 for nursing considerations for specific types of traction.

The patient in skeletal tractions has many nursing care requirements. Maintanence of the desired position and alignment to promote healing requires proper positioning for each specific type of traction. Uncooperative patients present challenges and may require the use of chemical or physical restraint to maintain the appropriate traction regimen. Frequent visualization is necessary to re-evaluate the patient's position to note continued alignment, as well as an increase or decrease in symptoms of soreness, pain, or muscle spasms. Prevention of the hazards of immobility in the respiratory, gastrointestinal, integumentary, and vascular systems require many nursing interventions. Neurovascular assessment demands astute nursing skill and complete documentation of color, temperature, pulses, edema, motor and sensory innervation, and pain. Pin insertion site care follows the ordered protocol. With skeletal traction, the weights should not be lifted or removed, as this can cause severe muscle contraction with displacement of the fracture fragments.

Teach the patient to perform ROM and muscle strengthening exercises, as isotonic and isometric exercises help to reduce complications. The patient can also be encouraged to use the overhead trapeze for repositioning in bed. Dependent upon the injury and length of time skeletal traction will be required, the patient may be at risk of foot drop. Nursing interventions to prevent foot drop include keeping the forefoot and ankle in a neutral position with or without the aid of a splint and not gatching the knees of bed. The nurse must also be alert to the many psychological issues associated with immobility, dependence, body image, and reduced self-esteem.

Practice Setting Considerations. *Home care:* Coordination of the hospital with community resources for home traction care is increasing with the move of long-term treatment into the home setting. Numerous factors promote successful home traction therapy. First, the patient/caregiver must be competent to use the traction device(s) and posses the physical and psychosocial ability. An ongoing 24-hour commitment of caregivers, and available support network, must be well-established. The patient's commitment to home traction therapy and compliance must be supported by an availability of home care services and their comfort with traction. The physical layout of the home must be able to accommodate a bed with a traction set-up. The patient/caregiver must be receptive to education and performance of special duties including set-up, application, and removal of the traction apparatus. The signs and symptoms of neurovascular complications, skin breakdown, bowel/bladder alterations, respiratory/cardiac compromise, and infection must be thoroughly understood. Telephone contact numbers of health care providers, for notification of any complications, must be conveniently posted. Age-appropriate positioning and activity limitations will vary from adult to pediatric patient. Pediatric positioning may involve being in a bed, high chair, infant seat, lap, or playpen (dependent on traction apparatus). All patients will require modifications in/assistance with ADLs, skin care, pin care, and pain management. Diversional activities will need to be varied, dependent upon the length of home traction treatment. Ongoing public health nurse and PT/OT home visits are advantageous.

Wheelchairs

Overview

A chair mounted on wheels, especially for the use of a physically challenged person is, commonly referred to as a wheelchair. There are a number of indications for the patient with musculoskeletal injury. A lack of stamina to walk or the inability to bear weight during the injury-healing process is common. Additionally, wheelchairs are used as an aid to promote independence and enhance mobility of the individual with musculoskeletal injury or a progressive disease. Wheelchairs are also used by individuals with amyotropic lateral sclerosis, multiple sclerosis, spinal cord injury, stroke, traumatic brain injury, Parkinson's disease, and COPD (Hubbard et al., 2007). Wheelchair use allows the individual to expend his/her energy to optimally perform ADLs, while still affording an ability to lead an active life. Based on physical and emotional preference and/or needs, a wheelchair is a useful adjunct in the recovery process to allow the individual's increased psychosocial participation.

Wheelchair technology has become increasingly complex due to rapid technological advances in wheeled mobility technology (Hubbard et al., 2007). Hubbard et al. (2007) also state that the increased visibility of wheelchair users due to war injuries, an aging population, and the reduced stigma as a result of the Americans with Disabilities Act and the disability rights movement are fueling wheelchair technological advances.

There are eight basic types of wheelchairs based on function, weight, and adjustability, which is essential for customizing a wheelchair to an individual patient's needs:

- Nonadjustable manual for > 36 pounds;
- Manual nonadjustable, lower seat only wheelchairs for hemiplegics > 36 pounds;

- Manual lightweight nonadjustable for > 36 pounds;
- Manual lightweight for < 34 pounds with adjustable seat/back height and some adjustability in axle;
- Manual ultra lightweight for < 30 pounds with an adjustable seat/back height/axle;
- Manual heavy duty;
- Power wheelchairs that may be nonadjustable, have nonprogrammable controls and be usable by standard weight patients, while other power wheelchairs can be highly customized for an individual's needs; and
- Scooters (Hubbard et al., 2007).

One wheelchair not noted in this listing is the geriatric wheelchair. The geriatric chair often has an attached table for placement of meals or other activities.

Common features found on wheelchairs are arm rests, which may be stationary or removable, and leg rests, which may also be removable and hopefully adjustable to swing out and elevate. The collapsibility of the chair for ease of transport is important, as are the safety locks to prevent motion during transfers. Many wheelchairs also require reclining positions for not only comfort of the patient, but also attention to the many complications associated with prolonged sitting.

Simpson, LoPresti, and Cooper (2008) state that studies have shown that both children and adults benefit substantially from access to independent mobility, as it increases vocational and educational opportunities, reduces dependence on caregivers and family members, and promotes feelings of self-reliance. Furthermore, reductions in functional mobility are linked with reduced participation and loss of social connections, which can lead to feelings of emotional loss, reduced self-esteem, isolation, stress, and fear of abandonment. With the technological research in mobility devices currently available, Simpson et al. (2008) look forward to the production of the "smart" wheelchair, which will improve the quality of life for every person who uses a wheelchair.

There are numerous considerations across the life span in the selection and use of a wheelchair. Safe use through proper instruction and routine wheelchair maintenance are essential. The selection of appropriate seating systems is a process of matching needs with available technology through clinical assessment of the patient's medical condition (Lau, Tam, & Cheng, 2008). The pediatric patient warrants particular attention to prevent skeletal deterioration while a wheelchair is being customized or re-configured due to a growth interval. Lau et al, (2008) describe how a wheelchair bank (funded by Cathay Pacific Airways and UNICEF) provides immediate intervention of postural support to not only prevent skeletal deformity but also maintain cardiopulmonary function and improve the quality of life for children with cerebral palsy, muscular dystrophy, spinal muscular atrophy, and spina bifida.

Complications of wheelchair use are directly related to immobility and include deep vein thrombosis, skin breakdown and pressure ulcers, and injury related to improper use. For adolescents or young adults, emphasize the importance of not "popping wheelies." Proper care and maintenance may also be a contributing factor.

Assessment

The patient's history is centered on the longevity of need for a wheelchair and his or her mobility requirements regarding work or school attendance that may be easier when combining use of an assistive device with a wheelchair. Determining the overall strength of the patient and the ability to independently use a wheelchair is an integral component of the type of wheelchair selected for use. The patient's social needs, and the psychological impact that wheelchair use may have on the patient, is another factor to be discussed with the patient. While the elderly may view use of a wheelchair negatively, the younger patient may look upon a wheelchair as being "really neat" and special for short-time use.

Physical examination evaluates the patient's ability to sit erect and participate in the movement of the wheelchair. If the patient is unable to roll the wheelchair manually, he or she must be able to use a motorized chair without assistance and work the available controls. There also needs to be a determination of caregiver support to push the wheelchair and maintain safety, as well as to aid the patient into and out of the chair (Table 10.9).

Table 10.9. Safe Transfer Technique to/from Chair
1. Place wheelchair parallel to bed/chair and lock.
2. Use a transfer belt to ensure additional safety, if patient cannot weight bear.
3. Patient should be wearing slippers or nonskid footwear.
4. Assist to standing position, pivot, and then sit in wheelchair.
5. For patient with a cast, one person can hold casted leg while a second individual helps patient with stand pivot transfer.
6. A lifting device can also be used to place patient in wheelchair.
7. For patients unable to weight bear, a wheelchair with removable arms placed parallel to the bed and a sliding transfer board help get them out of bed.
8. Always remember to lock the wheels and to support the patient's lower extremities.

Common Therapeutic Modalities

Dependent upon the reason for wheelchair use, it is necessary to determine the appropriateness and length of time for wheelchair use. Short-term therapy must be looked upon very differently than the long-term chronic disabled patient's need. Thus, it is imperative to investigate costs of wheelchair rental versus purchase options.

Nursing Considerations

Nursing Diagnoses. Nursing diagnoses for this condition are expanded upon in the Appendix.

- Body image, impaired.
- Comfort, impaired.
- Constipation, risk for.
- Coping, ineffective.
- Falls, risk for.
- Fatigue.
- Growth and development, delayed.
- Hopelessness.
- Injury, risk for.
- Lifestyle, sedentary.
- Loneliness, risk for.
- Mobility: wheelchair, impaired.
- Powerlessness.
- Self-care deficits: bathing/hygiene, dressing/grooming, feeding, toileting.
- Self-esteem, situational low, risk for.
- Skin integrity, risk for impaired.
- Tissue perfusion: peripheral, ineffective.
- Transfer ability, impaired.
- Urinary elimination, impaired.

The potential for injury is great for the patient using a wheelchair, especially long-term. The patient outcomes center on the proper use and safety precautions, especially the use of correct transfer techniques to/from a chair. Nursing interventions begin with determining the correct size of wheelchair for the patient. With pediatric patients in the inpatient setting, the nurse must determine the correct pediatric chair; with adults, the nurse needs to consider if a standard, wide, or geriatric chair is indicated. The nurse always teaches and reinforces to the patient/caregiver the proper use of a wheelchair and the necessary safety precautions.

Practice Setting Considerations. *Home care:* Provide the patient/caregiver with education about transfer techniques and safety as soon as the treatment modality is initiated. While some patients will require only short-term use, assist to facilitate the acquisition of a wheelchair from a loan closet, rental medical supply company, or direct purchase. Depending upon the strength and age of the patient's support system, ascertain if their caregiver's transportation can accommodate a wheelchair, and if the caregiver can physically lift the chair into the vehicle.

A thorough check of the home environment is necessary to reduce safety hazards and begins with the need for a permanent or temporary ramp to enter the dwelling. It is essential to determine where the patient is living: if he or she lives in an apartment, is there an elevator to be able to get inside? Are the doorways large enough to accommodate the width of the chair, and are countertops accessible by the patient? Smooth flooring, preferably with nonresilient hard finish, and adequate lighting help to reduce the risk of injury. For the patient who will use a wheelchair long-term, home renovations may be required.

Regular home visits by the physical and/or occupational therapist may be beneficial to maintain proper use of a wheelchair and reduce the patient's desire to abandon this important mobility aid. If the patient does not feel the wheelchair is a help and has a poor opinion of the device, he or she may decide to abandon use of the wheelchair. While the physical therapist may be looking for an outcome related to postural control, pressure relief, and sitting tolerance, the occupational therapist is seeking an outcome measured in terms of quality of life and occupational performance.

Summary

This overview of therapeutic modalities has outlined the indications for use, nursing considerations, patient teaching, and potential complications. Each of these modalities plays a vital role in the recovery from injury or in the adaptation to everyday living associated with disability or chronic musculoskeletal diseases. The nurse must be knowledgeable of the correct use of therapeutic modalities and demonstrate competency in their use. The individual and support persons will look to the nurse as the expert. Successful integration of the modality into the individual's daily life will hinge upon the nurse's ability to facilitate compliance with the care and use of the modality.

References

Boyd, A., Benjamin, H., & Asplund, C. (2009). Splints and casts: Indications and methods. *American Family Physician, 80*(5), 491-499.

Drozd, M., Miles, S., & Davies, J. (2009). Casting: Complications and after care. *Emergency Nurse, 17*(13), 26-27.

Hart, E., Albright, M. Rebello, G. and Grottkau, B. (2006). Developmental dysplasia of the hip: Nursing implications and anticipatory guidance for parents. *Orthopaedic Nursing, 25*(2), 100-109.

Hubbard, S., Fitzgerald, S., Vogel, B., Reker, D., Cooper, R., & Boninger, M. (2007). Distribution and cost of wheelchairs and scooters provided by Veterans Health Administration. *Journal of Rehabilitation Research & Development, 44*(4), 581–592.

Kunkler, C.E. (2007). Therapeutic modalities. In NAON, *Core Curriculum for Orthopaedic Nursing* (6th ed., pp. 227-257). Boston, MA: Pearson Custom Publishing.

Lau, H., Tam, E., & Cheng, J. (2008). An experience on wheelchair bank management. *Disability and Rehabilitation: Assistive Technology, 3*(6), 302-308.

Murray, C. & Rawls, C. (2010). Care of the patient with traumatic orthopaedic injuries. In C. Mosher (Ed.), *An Introduction to Orthopaedic Nursing* (4th ed., pp. 85-104). Chicago, IL: National Association of Orthopaedic Nurses.

Murray, C. (2010). Care of the patient with musculoskeletal trauma. In D. Ignativicus, & M. Workman, (Eds.), *Medical-Surgical Nursing Patient Centered Collaborative Care,* (6th ed., pp. 1178-1121). St. Louis, MO: W.B. Saunders.

National Association of Orthopadic Nurses (NAON). (2007). *Core Curriculum for Orthopaedic Nursing* (6th ed., pp.242-244). Boston, MA: Pearson.

Patterson, M. (2006). Impact of external fixation on adolescents: An integrative research review. *Orthopaedic Nursing, 25*(5), 300-308.

Patterson, M. (2010). Musculoskeletal Care Modalities. In O'Connell Smeltzer, S.C., Bare, B.G., Hinkle, J. L, & Cheever, K.H. (Eds.), *Brunner & Suddarth's Textbook of Medical-Surgical Nursing* (12th ed., pp. 2023- 2051). Philadelphia, PA: Lippincott Williams & Wilkins.

Patterson, M. & Wraa, C. (2010). Caring for the patient with musculoskeletal trauma. In K. Osborn, C. Wraa, & A. Watson (Eds.), *Medical-Surgical Nursing Preparation for Practice* (pp. 1776-1801). Upper Saddle River, NJ: Pearson.

Pullen, R. (2007). Using slings without errors. *Nursing, 37(7)*, 24.

Redemann, S. (2002), Modalities for immobilization. In Maher, A., Salmond, S., & Pellino, T. (Eds). *Orthopaedic Nursing* (3rd ed., pp. 302-323). Philadelphia, PA: W.B. Sanders.

Rose, R. (2010). Pin site care with the Ilizarov circular fixator. *The Internet Journal of Orthopedic Surgery, 16*(1).

Royal College of Nursing. (2011). *Guidance on pin site care: Report and recommendations from the 2010 consensus project on pin site care.* London, England, UK: Author.

Santy, J. & Duffield, B. (2009) The principles of caring for patients with Ilizarov external fixation. *Nursing Standard, 23*(26), 50-55.

Satryb, S., Wilson, T., & Patterson, M. (2011). Casting all wrapped up. *Orthopaedic Nursing, 30*(1), 37-41.

Simpson, R., LoPresti, E., & Cooper, R. (2008). How many people would benefit from a smart wheelchair? *Journal of Rehabilitation Research & Development, 45*(1), 53-72.

Walsh, C. (2009). Sign off on casting. *OR Nurse, 3*(5), 45-51.

Whiteing, N. (2008). Fractures: pathophysiology, treatment and nursing care. *Nursing Standard, 23*(2), 49-57.

Chapter 11
Pediatric & Congenital Disorders

Mary Jane Smalley, MSN, CRNP, CPNP-PC

Objectives

- Identify common pediatric orthopaedic conditions.
- Describe clinical signs of each condition.
- Cite examples of current treatment modalities for these conditions.
- Explain the rationale of nursing interventions for these conditions.
- Develop a nursing care plan for a child diagnosed with two of these conditions.

Pediatric orthopaedic conditions encompass a myriad of diagnoses that affect a child, either temporarily or permanently. Many of these disorders, particularly those that are chronic, present ongoing challenges for parents and other caregivers who are attempting to understand and cope with the condition while simultaneously helping the child grow and develop. One in six children in the United States has a chronic medical condition or disability, and many of these conditions seriously impair their function (Berry, Bloom, Foley, & Palfrey, 2010). Inherent in many pediatric orthopaedic diagnoses is limited, decreased, or absent mobility, which impacts a child's normal developmental progress and function. In order to foster normal growth and development, it is imperative that nurses caring for children recognize the long-lasting, and often devastating, effects that an orthopaedic condition has on the child.

Achondroplasia

Overview

Achondroplasia is a form of skeletal dysplasia, which is a disorder of the growth and remodeling of bone and its cartilaginous precursor. Although cartilage grows and develops, both at the physes and other locations, bone that is formed by endochondrial means is most underdeveloped in length, resulting in disproportionate, short stature (Sponseller & Ain, 2006).

Achondroplasia is caused by a point mutation in the gene that encodes fibroblast growth factor receptor-3 (FGFR3), and the gene for this receptor is on the short arm of chromosome 4. The mutation causes a change in a single amino acid, from arginine to glycine (Sponseller & Ain, 2006), and results in abnormal endochondral ossification (Hawk & Bailie, 2007). FGFR is expressed in cartilage and in the central nervous system (Sponseller & Ain, 2006). The defect is most apparent in fast-growing bones such as the femora and humeri, and the proximal segments are more severely affected than the middle or distal segments, resulting in rhizomelic extremities (Hawk & Bailie, 2007). The term rhizo- means "root." The trunk length is within the lower range of normal, whereas the extremities are much shorter than normal (Sponseller & Ain, 2006). Normal diameter of the bones is achieved through normal periosteal ossification.

Achondroplasia is the most common form of skeletal dysplasia, occurring in 1 of every 30,000-50,000 live births (Hawk & Bailie, 2007). The disorder is transmitted as an autosomal dominant condition, but in at least 80% of patients, the disorder is due to a spontaneous mutation. The risk of having a child with achondroplasia rises with increased paternal age (Sponseller & Ain, 2006).

The condition is usually easily recognized at birth (Staheli, 2008f) with clinical features that are uniform and predictable. The facial appearance is characterized by frontal bossing and midface hypoplasia. The hypoplasia develops because of the endochondral origin of the facial bones (Sponseller & Ain, 2006). Recurrent otitis media is common (Hawk & Bailie, 2007) and may result in hearing loss. Other ear, nose, and throat problems occur because of underdevelopment of the midfacial structure, and maxillary hypoplasia leads to dental crowding and malocclusion (Sponseller & Ain, 2006).

Enlargement of head circumference is the norm in individuals with achondroplasia (Sponseller & Ain, 2006), and the combination of cranial enlargement with poor head control increases an infant's risk for cervical extension injuries (Hawk & Bailie, 2007). Occasionally, there are patients who appear to have clinical hydrocephalus. Those patients with progressive head enlargement should be seen by a neurosurgeon familiar with skeletal dysplasia, and may benefit from treatment with a vetriculo-peritoneal shunt (Sponseller & Ain, 2006) or, more frequently now, a decompression. Since 1990, shunts have been used less due to better imaging, which ascertained the cause of clinical hydrocephalus to be compression at the foramen magnum. Ventriculomegaly is very common in children with achondroplasia and tends not to be progressive. Shunt placement in a child with achondroplasia is not straightforward, and the incidence of revisions and complications are higher than in the general patient population (King, 2009).

Intelligence and mental development is normal, but early motor development is delayed and may be due to neural compression at the foramen magnum. Children with achondroplasia meet developmental milestones later than average-stature children, and the mean age at which children with anchondroplasia walk unaided is 17 months (Sponseller & Ain, 2006).

According to Staheli (2008f), stenosis of the foramen magnum causes increased hypotonia, sleep apnea, and sudden infant death syndrome (SIDS). The most evident cause of low muscle tone in the trunk and extremities may be neural compression at the foramen magnum. Infants with achondroplasia should be closely monitored in the first 2 years of life for severe foramen magnum stenosis. These signs may include severe developmental delay, sleep apnea, persistent hypotonia, or spasticity. Sleep studies should be used for evaluating brain stem functions. If the diagnosis of foramen magnum stenosis is made and the clinical picture persists, decompression of the brain stem should be undertaken by an experienced neurosurgeon. Early decompression of the brain stem may help ventilatory potential (Sponseller & Ain, 2006).

Neural deficits that may arise from progressive spinal stenosis include disc herniation, lumbar lordosis, and anterior wedging of vertebral bodies. Symptoms may include backache, sciatica, bowel and bladder disturbances, paraplegia, and sexual dysfunction (Sponseller & Ain, 2006). Complications from a narrow chest diameter include pneumonia, cyanotic spells, and apnea (Hawk & Bailie, 2007).

The development of spinal stenosis is explained by the fact that the spinal canal forms through endochondral ossification at the neurocentral synchondroses. These obliquely oriented growth plates contribute to the length of the pedicles and to the distance between them. These dimensions are decreased at all levels of the achondroplastic spine and are most diminished in the distal lumbar spine (Sponseller & Ain, 2006).

Genu varum (bowed legs) is seen in many children with achondroplasia, and the fibula overgrows the tibia. Kyphosis and hyperlordosis at the thoracolumbar junction is common, especially in infancy, and the condition usually improves with age. Kyphosis is present in most infants with achondroplasia, presumably because of low muscle tone and ligamentous laxity (Hawk & Bailie, 2007; Sponseller & Ain, 2006).

The body habitus, or physique, of children with achondroplasia is distinctive. Affected children have shortened humeri and femurs, and fingertips reach only to the tops of the greater trochanters, which leads to difficulties in personal care. The digits of the hands have extra space between the third and fourth rays, so that the digits are separated into three groups, including the thumb—the "trident hand." There is usually a flexion contracture of the elbows, and the radial heads may be subluxed. Neither of these features causes significant functional impairment. The knees are most commonly in varus alignment, and tibial torsion is common. The joints are not directly affected by this condition to any considerable degree, and the limbs have a muscular appearance (Sponseller & Ain, 2006). Obesity is a lifelong problem for those with achondroplasia (Hawk & Bailie, 2007).

Although patients with achondroplasia are among the most stable and healthy of those with skeletal dysplasias, mortality rates are elevated in all age groups. The most common causes are SIDS in young infants, central nervous system events and respiratory problems in older children and young adults, and cardiovascular problems in older adults (Sponseller & Ain, 2006).

Assessment

When assessing a child diagnosed with achondroplasia, the presenting symptoms as well as the onset, progression, and previous treatment should be elicited. The perinatal, developmental, family history, neurologic involvement, and functional limitations should be obtained.

The child's height, weight, and head circumference should be obtained and plotted on a growth curve for children with achondroplasia. Disproportionate dwarfing will be seen, in addition to a normal trunk length. Rhizomelic short extremities will be present, and the humeri and femora will appear the most disproportionate. The child's head will be enlarged with a flattened appearance, due to early closure of the cranial ossification centers. Trident hands will be seen, along with fingertips that only reach the hip joint. Due to the shortened upper limbs, the child may not be able to reach to the top of the head, the middle of the back, or the intergluteal region. Elbow contractures of 15-30 degrees may be seen, along with subluxed radial heads. Assessment of the lower limbs may reveal externally rotated legs, genu varum, genu recurvatum, or lateral torsion of the knee. Hip flexion contractures may be seen and are associated with lordosis. An ankle varus deformity may be present, and the child will most likely have ligamentous laxity. Overdeveloped musculature will be seen, along with a waddling gait if the child is ambulatory. Depending on the child's age, kyphosis may be present, or exaggerated lumbar lordosis might be noted with associated prominent abdomen and buttocks (Hawk & Bailie, 2007).

The alterations that are seen in radiographic images involve regions in which the growth and development occur primarily through processes of endochondral ossification. In the skull, consequently, the facial bones, skull base, and foramen magnum are underdeveloped, and the cranial bones are normal in size and shape. The spine displays central and foraminal stenosis, which becomes worse at progressively caudal levels (Sponseller & Ain, 2006). Radiographics will reveal that all of the long bones are short and the flat bones are less affected (Hawk & Bailie, 2007). A metaphyseal flare with a "ball and socket" relationship of the epiphysis to the metaphysis contributes to abnormal knee alignment. The fibula typically grows more than the tibia, and this also contributes to the varus in some cases. Before walking age, kyphosis at the thoracolumbar junction may be seen. If this fails to resolve, the apical vertebrae develop a progressively round or wedge shape. Scoliosis is rare. Cervical instability is not usually seen in achondroplasia, although it is commonly seen in many other forms of skeletal dysplasia. The metacarpals and metatarsals are all of almost equal length (Sponseller & Ain, 2006).

Common Treatment Modalities

No medical treatment of the underlying defect is necessary. Early nutritional management to prevent and control obesity is essential (Hawk & Bailie, 2007).

Maintenance of an ideal body weight presents a continuous challenge, and obesity is more common in those with achondroplasia than in the general population (Sponseller & Ain, 2006).

Foramen magnum stenosis is surgically addressed with a decompression of the brain stem. The procedure consists of enlargement of the foramen magnum and, sometimes, laminectomy of the atlas (Sponseller & Ain, 2006).

Nonsurgical options to address various orthopaedic issues include pelvic tilt exercises to relieve hyperlordosis and stretching maneuvers to address hip flexion contractures (Hawk & Bailie, 2007). Bracing of a child with kyphosis with a thoracolumbosacral orthosis (TLSO) is indicated if the deformity is accompanied by significant and progressive structural changes in the anterior vertebral bodies, such as anterior beaking and wedging, if the kyphosis does not reduce below 30 degrees on prone hyperextension radiographs, or if it does not resolve by age 3. For children in whom bracing treatment has failed, a hyperextension cast can be worn for several months, until the correction is maintained. For patients in whom this therapy also fails, two options exist: prophylactic posterior spinal fusion during childhood; or observation, with stabilization or correction of kyphosis only in those who require decompression for spinal stenosis (Sponseller & Ain, 2006).

Spinal stenosis is the most common serious problem in individuals with achondroplasia. Most patients present with symptoms of neurogenic claudication, usually in the third decade of life, although it has been noted as early as age 11. Diagnosis is best made by myelography or magnetic resonance imagery (MRI). The diagnosis of stenosis is an immediate indication for spinal decompression, and the procedure should extend from several levels above the blockage seen on myelogram or MRI, down to the second sacral vertebra (Sponseller & Ain, 2006).

In cases of genu varum, no evidence shows that bracing is effective in children with achondroplasia. Varus may progress in some patients and appear to cause pain and difficulty walking. Pain originating from the knee joint should be differentiated from the leg pain of spinal stenosis. In spinal stenosis, the aching is more diffuse and is relieved by decreasing the lumbar lordosis by flexing the lumbar spine or "hunching over." Treatment of severe genu varum usually involves surgery, usually an opening or closing tibial osteotomy with internal or external fixation. The decision for surgery is not made until the child is at least 4 years old. If internal tibial torsion exceeds 10-20 degrees, that problem should be corrected at the same time. Fibular shortening alone has been advocated, but no long-term studies are available. Severe degenerative arthritis of the knee is not often seen in adults with achondroplasia.

Limb lengthening procedures for achondroplasia remain controversial, but this is gaining acceptance because the joints are normal and the musculotendinous units and nerves have excellent tolerance for stretch. The expected benefits of limb lengthening include increased function in the average-height world, improved self-image, and possibly decreased lumbar lordosis. Decreased lumbar lordosis is purported to occur if the hip flexors are lengthened and an extension osteotomy is performed at the time of femoral lengthening. If the lower extremities are lengthened significantly, the humeri should be lengthened also to facilitate personal care (Sponseller & Ain, 2006).

Proximal and distal fibular ephysiodeses can be done to stop the relative overgrowth of the fibula and to correct its growth over time (Hawk & Bailie, 2007).

Nursing Considerations

Nursing Diagnoses. Nursing diagnoses for this condition are expanded upon in the Appendix.

- Anxiety.
- Grieving.
- Nutrition, imbalanced: potential for more than body requirement.
- Self-care deficit: bathing/hygiene, feeding, dressing/grooming, toileting.
- Self-concept, readiness for enhanced.

Nursing Interventions. Develop a plan of care to minimize patient/parental anxiety, recognizing that guilt is a common parental response to which counseling/education must be targeted. Allow the patient/family to express fears and concerns related to the diagnosis and treatment. Include the patient/family in the decision-making process, and provide education regarding the underlying pathology, normal developmental progression, treatment, community resources, and genetic counseling, if indicated. An ideal outcome is a patient/family with an understanding of the diagnosis, normal progression, treatment plan, community resources, and genetic counseling, if appropriate.

To support the patient/family through the grieving process, encourage verbalization of their feelings/fears associated with their perceived losses. Support them through the diagnostic period and assist with identifying lifestyle modifications. Help the family identify sources of support, and refer them to an appropriate disease-related support group. Provide for spiritual and psychological support, as needed, and help the family recognize the child's strengths and skills while acknowledging limitations. A patient/family that is supported during the grieving process is the best outcome.

Counseling with family and caregivers about the potential for obesity should begin in early infancy and should continue throughout the child's life. The child's weight should be monitored, and a referral to a dietician should be made for an accurate assessment of the child's caloric needs and for dietary recommendations.

Promotion of a child's independence in self-care activities should be ongoing. The use of assistive devices, such as hand extensions to reach a light switch or a step stool to address a height differential should be explored. Consider methods of facilitating activities of daily living (ADLs) within the child's capabilities. An ideal outcome is a child who is able to achieve independence in self-care activities. Promoting personal strengths and skills and focusing on the child as a whole helps with the attainment of typical developmental skills consistent with the child's age. The best outcome is a positive self-concept (Hawk & Bailie, 2007).

Arthrogryposis Multiplex Congenita

Overview

Arthrogryposis multiplex congenita (AMC) is the best-known of the multiple contracture syndromes. The condition is pain-free and characterized by movement beyond a very limited range. There are three subcategories:

1. Classic arthrogryposis, in which all four extremities may be involved (Alman & Goldberg, 2006);
2. Distal arthrogryposis, seen predominantly or exclusively of the hands and feet; and
3. Pterygial syndrome, characterized by skin webs across the knees, elbows, and other joints.

Contractures are due to fibrosis of the affected muscles, with thickening and shortening of the periarticular capsular and ligamentous tissue of the joint. AMC is not progressive, but some contractures seem to worsen with age, and the joints become stiffer. The etiology of AMC is unknown (Alman & Goldberg, 2006), and it is not considered a genetic condition (Hawk & Bailie, 2007).

Classic arthrogryposis can affect only one of identical twins. The development of AMC may be influenced by an adverse intrauterine factor or the twinning process itself. Teratogens have been suggested, but none are proven, despite the multiple animal models that lend support to that theory. Some mothers of children with arthrogryposis have serum antibodies that inhibit fetal acetylcholine receptor function. One possibility is that maternal antibodies to these fetal antigens cause the disorder. The degeneration of anterior horn cells occurring in the early months of gestation (Alman & Goldberg, 2006) or a decreased number of these cells indicate that a central nervous system disorder may have some role in the cause of arthrogryposis (Hawk & Bailie, 2007). The pattern of motor neuron loss in specific spinal cord segments correlates with the peripheral deformities and the affected muscles (Alman & Goldberg, 2006).

The incidence of this condition is 0.03% in the general population, although statistics vary widely in different geographic areas (Hawk & Bailie, 2007). The condition is sporadic, with affected individuals having reproduced only normal children (Alman & Goldberg, 2006).

The pathophysiology of neuropathic or classic AMC is the reduction, degeneration, or absence of anterior horn cells. The feet are the most susceptible, due to the extrinsic muscles of the feet having the shortest anterior horn of all the columns in the lumbar spine, and the distal segments of the limbs (hands, ankles, and feet) are the most affected joints. The muscles may be normal but small, or absent and replaced by fat or fibrous tissue. A muscle biopsy reveals de-enervation atrophy. In affected joints there may be destruction of articulating surfaces with degenerative changes and capsular thickening occurring later.

Myopathic arthrogryposis is characterized by fibrous, fatty alterations in the muscles. There are no central nervous system alterations, but there is destruction of the muscle fibers in the fetus. Clinically apparent changes include partial fixation of the joints, as well as the development of shortened and restrictive ligaments and periarticular tissues.

In mixed arthrogryposis, findings of both the neuropathic and myopathic types are present (Hawk & Bailie, 2007). In two thirds of patients, all four limbs are affected equally; but in one third, lower-limb deformities predominate. On rare occasions, the upper extremities predominate, and these deformities tend to be more severe and more rigid distally (Alman & Goldberg, 2006).

Assessment

A clinical examination of the infant or child is the best way to establish a diagnosis (Alman & Goldberg, 2006). Joint contractures are present at birth, and the newborn may suffer fractures during the delivery (Hawk & Bailie, 2007). The limbs are striking in appearance and position: they are featureless and tubular, without normal skin creases (Alman & Goldberg, 2006) and with deep dimples over the joints (Hawk & Bailie, 2007). Muscle mass is reduced, although in infancy there is often abundant subcutaneous tissue. Typically the shoulders are adducted and internally rotated, the elbow more often extended than flexed, and the wrist flexed severely, with ulnar deviation. The fingers are flexed, clutching the thumb. In the lower extremities, the hips are flexed, abducted, and externally rotated; the knees are typically in extension, although flexion is possible; clubfeet are the rule. Motion of the joints is restricted. The hips may be dislocated unilaterally or bilaterally (Alman & Goldberg, 2006). One third of patients may have scoliosis (Hawk & Bailie, 2007). As a consequence of the general muscle weakness, there is a 15% incidence of inguinal hernia. The face is not particularly dysmorphic. A few subtle features such as a small jaw, narrowing of the face, and limited upward gaze (secondary to ocular muscle involvement) may be present. A frontal midline hemangioma may help with the diagnosis (Alman & Goldberg, 2006).

An assessment of the infant or child includes the presenting symptoms and a parental report of the onset, progression, and previous treatment of the condition. The family history is usually negative for relatives with arthrogryposis. The developmental history typically reveals normal intelligence, but the child likely will have functional limitations due to limb contractures and/or position. There may be a history of difficult feeding secondary to a stiff jaw or an immobile tongue (Hawk & Bailie, 2007), which leads to respiratory infections and failure to thrive (Alman & Goldberg, 2006).

Radiographs will reveal that the joints are normal, but that changes are adaptive and acquired over time as a consequence of their fixed position. There is also evidence of a loss of subcutaneous fat and tissue. Electromyograms and muscle biopsies are of questionable diagnostic value and have been used to separate patients with primarily neuropathic changes from those with myopathic changes, but the clinical implications of such distinctions are not clear. A diagnosis of arthrogryposis can be suspected when prenatal ultrasound detects an absence of fetal movement, especially if seen in combination with polyhydramnios (Alman & Goldberg, 2006).

Although many patients with AMC have been treated at large medical centers, the natural history and long-term outcomes are not well known. While some contractures seem to worsen with age and the joints become stiffer, no new joints become involved. At least 25% of affected patients are nonambulatory, and many others are limited household walkers. Typically those with arthrogryposis who are very weak as infants stay weak, and those who appear stronger as infants stay strong. The dependency on adults seems to be related to education and coping skills more than to the magnitude of contractures of the joints (Alman & Goldberg, 2006).

Common Therapeutic Modalities

The prognosis of an infant or child with arthrogryposis is better than might be expected, based on the clinical findings at birth. Primary treatment goals include the alignment and stability of the lower extremities to allow weight-bearing and ambulation, and positioning and motion of the upper extremities to allow independent ADLs. Complex problems are best managed by a comprehensive multidisciplinary team that includes a pediatrician, neurologist, orthopaedist, geneticist, nurse, social worker, physical therapist, and occupational therapist (Hawk & Bailie, 2007).

To treat contractures non-surgically, aggressive physical therapy (PT) and occupational therapy (OT) should begin immediately after birth (Hawk & Bailie, 2007) if feasible, and after neonatal fractures are ruled out (Alman & Goldberg, 2006). Frequent passive range of motion (ROM) of the affected extremities should be done, in addition to splinting of the joints in a position of function. Casting should be avoided, but the use of bracing and assistive devices is advocated (Hawk & Bailie, 2007).

Surgical outcomes seem better if surgery on the joints is done when children are younger, usually before adaptive intrarticular changes occur between ages 4 and 6 (Alman & Goldberg, 2006). It is also important to consider how one contracture relates to another when planning surgical intervention (Hawk & Bailie, 2007). Realignment osteotomies are usually performed later in adolescence, closer to the completion of growth. Early motion and avoidance of prolonged casting may increase joint mobilization, thereby improving function (Alman & Goldberg, 2006).

Hip Displasia. Although approximately two thirds of patients have developmental dysplasia of the hip or frank dislocation, there is controversy about the management of the hips in these children. Closed reduction is rarely successful. Operative reduction of a dislocated hip should be performed if it will improve function or reduce pain, although studies to date have not found pain to be a problem with these hips. The ROM of the hips may be important for functioning because hip contractures—especially those that cause flexion deformity—adversely affect the gait pattern. Consequently, operative procedures to locate dislocated hips have the potential to worsen function if they produce significant contractures (Alman & Goldberg, 2006).

Knee Deformities. Knee flexion contractures of more than 30 degrees can be addressed by a posterior capsulotomy before age 2. Supracondylar osteotomies of the femur are recommended toward the end of growth to correct residual deformity (Hawk & Bailie, 2007). A femoral shortening may be included in the osteotomies, especially in cases where the neurovascular structures will be stretched by correcting the deformity. Hyperextension deformities of the knee can be treated without surgery, but quadriceplasty may be needed in cases with residual lack of motion. In children with a persistent hyperextension contracture, late osteoarthritis seems more common (Alman & Goldberg, 2006).

Clubfoot. A severe and resistant clubfoot is characteristic. It is rare for the arthrogrypotic clubfoot to respond to PT and casting, and surgical intervention is usually necessary. Although surgical treatment of clubfeet was previously delayed until after age 1, as other joints were attended to first, combined procedures with minimal immobilization earlier in life are gaining in popularity. Recent reports show good outcomes with a circumferential release if done before age 1. A triple arthrodesis is often done during adolescence to treat a residual clubfoot deformity, with the goal of maintaining the subtalar joints while producing a plantigrade foot (Alman & Goldberg, 2006). Further discussion of clubfoot is found in the section of this chapter devoted to this condition.

Upper Extremities. While most patients do not require upper extremity surgery, if surgical intervention is being considered, a functional assessment should be made before deciding on an operation (Alman & Goldberg, 2006). Two key goals in treatment of the upper extremities are self-help skills, such as feeding and toileting, and mobility skills, such as pushing out of a chair and using crutches. A tendon transfer of the elbow for active flexion may be done if 90 degrees of passive motion is present, and should only be done on one side (Hawk & Bailie, 2007). A distal humeral osteotomy, designed to place the elbow into flexion and to correct some of the shoulder internal rotation deformity, can be performed toward the end of the first decade and is designed to improve hand-to-mouth function (Alman & Goldberg, 2006).

Nursing Considerations

Nursing Diagnoses. Nursing diagnoses for this condition are expanded upon in the Appendix.

- Anxiety.
- Body image, disturbed.
- Growth and development, altered.
- Mobility: physical, impaired.
- Parenting, altered.
- Self care deficit: bathing/hygiene, dressing/grooming, feeding, toileting.
- Social interaction, impaired.

Nursing Interventions. Nursing interventions that focus on anxiety and altered parenting include recognizing that parents have fears and concerns related to the diagnosis, along with guilt, to which counseling and education must be targeted. Provide information about the condition and available resources to help parents adapt to their roles in rearing a child with a neuromuscular disorder and demonstrate methods they can utilize while interacting with their child despite limitations related to treatment. Support parents' role in their decision-making regarding treatment options, and promote family cohesion by enabling privacy, visitation, and caregiving by family members. New parents may be comforted by knowing that contractures are worse at birth and that the infant's condition improves with treatment. Provide ongoing parental support as continuous caregivers because they are an integral part in the success/failure of treatment. Reassure parents that intelligence and life expectancy are usually not altered by AMC, and offer information about support groups such as the National Arthrogryposis Foundation.

Interventions related to altered growth and development, impaired social interaction, disturbed body image, and deficient self-care include promoting the accomplishments of developmental tasks and peer interactions, planning alternative methods of stimulation, establishing developmental tasks to compensate for physical restrictions, encouraging independence in ADLs, praising the accomplishments of age-related tasks, encouraging involvement of age-related activities, encouraging and supporting involvement and interactions with peer groups, and focusing on the positive aspects of the child's appearance, such as their hair, eyes, etc. Positive outcomes for these interventions are the achievement of appropriate developmental tasks, the establishment of positive peer relationships, and the participation in age-related activities (Hawk & Bailie, 2007).

Interventions focused on impaired physical mobility include promoting mobility within limitations, teaching significant others how to hold the child with immobilization devices, planning methods of self-care taking into account limitations of motion, reinforcing prescribed exercise programs—such as gait and balance training or stretching, strengthening, and ROM exercises—and stressing the importance of an aggressive therapy program starting at birth and how this relates to the most optimal outcome for the child (Hawk & Bailie, 2007).

Blount's Disease

Overview

Blount's disease, also known as Blount disease or tibia vara, is a pathologic bowing of the legs (Schoenecker, 2006). It is considered a growth disorder involving the medial portion of the proximal tibia growth plate that produces a localized varus deformity (Staheli, 2008e) and has either an early onset (infantile) or a late onset (juvenile/adolescent) (Hawk & Bailie, 2007). Although the etiology of Blount's disease is unknown, it has been theorized that mechanical stress damages the proximal medial growth plate in susceptible individuals, thus converting physiologic bowlegs into tibia vara

(Staheli, 2008e). There is no known genetic element in tibia vara, but frequently there is a familial tendency for the condition (Hawk & Bailie, 2007). The incidence of Blount's disease is greater if the child is black, obese, and resides in certain geographical locations such as the southeastern part of the United States (Staheli, 2008e). The incidence of adolescent Blount's disease has markedly increased in the past 20 years, corresponding to the development of earlier and more severe adolescent obesity (Schoenecker & Rich, 2006).

Asymmetric local pressure on the posteromedial aspect of the proximal tibial epiphysis and physis (growth plate) is followed by selective growth slowing. This results in an intra-articular deformity in the posteromedial area of the tibial plateau and causes progressive, localized tibial bowing and premature closure of the medial tibial physis (Hawk & Bailie, 2007). Persisting articular deformity often leads to degenerative arthritis in adulthood (Staheli, 2008e).

Physiologic bowing is a normal finding in many infants and toddlers, and usually resolves after the child's second birthday. Early onset or infantile Blount's disease may begin as exaggerated physiologic bowing that progresses to pathologic bowing (Schoenecker & Rich, 2006). Early walking may exacerbate tibial bowing with increasing knee sag, when combined with internal tibial torsion and ligamentous laxity at the knee (Hawk & Bailie, 2007).

Weight-bearing stresses on a bowed leg are sufficient to cause growth disturbance, and obesity increases the potential for a growth plate injury. The proximal medial tibia fails to grow normally, and tibia vara of variable severity develops. This results in extremity shortening and intra-articular depression of the medial condyle. Infantile Blount's is usually bilateral, occurs in children 1-4 years of age, and affects slightly more females than males. Infants with aphysiologic bowing deformity cannot be clearly distinguished from those with infantile Blount's disease. Physiologic bowing and Blount's disease ought to be perceived as two points within the same spectrum, with Blount's disease being the pathologic result of unresolved infantile bowing. Frequently, one extremity will have physiologic bowing, with Blount's disease affecting the contralateral tibia (Schoenecker & Rich, 2006).

Late onset or juvenile/adolescent Blount's disease is typically seen in overweight males. The varus deformity typically involves the proximal medial tibia and the distal femur, in contrast to early-onset or infantile Blount's disease where there is varus of the tibia only (Schoenecker & Rich, 2006). Juvenile Blount's disease occurs between ages 4 and 10, and adolescent Blount's disease occurs after age 11. Juvenile and adolescent Blount's disease tends to be unilateral compared to the typical bilateral involvement seen in infantile Blount's disease.

Assessment

The child's presenting symptoms should be ascertained, including the onset, progression, and prior treatment of the angular deformity. The child may complain of pain/tenderness over the lateral prominence of the proximal tibia, a history of pain with activity that limits physical activity (which can cause further weight gain), and an awkward gait that predisposes the child to sprains and fractures. The developmental history should be obtained, along with the past medical/surgical history and family history. The developmental history may establish that the child ambulated early, and a review of the symptoms may reveal a child who has difficulty walking, especially after longer distances. The radiograph in Figure 11.1 reveals left tibia vara.

Figure 11.1.
Lower Extremities: Left Tibia Vara

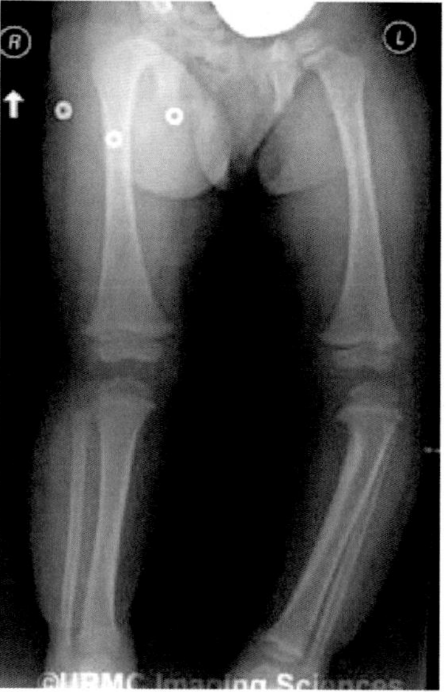

From Musculoskeletal Imaging Case of the Month *by M. Bakman, C. Bang, G. Seo, and J. Monu, 2002, http://urmc.rochester.edu/smd/Rad/MSKcases/MSK02. Reproduced with permission.*

The child's height and weight should be recorded (Hawk & Bailie, 2007). The child should be observed walking toward and away from the examiner, who should note gait mechanics and, specifically, the presence of a limp or lateral thrust to one or both knees (Schoenecker & Rich, 2006). A medial or lateral knee thrust may be present, indicating joint instability or ligamentous laxity. The femoral-tibial angle should be measured with a goniometer. A measurement of more than 20 degrees indicates tibia varus, and a sharp lateral angulation of the proximal tibia may be present, along with a 2-3cm leg length discrepancy. There also may be a palpable bony prominence over the medial aspect of the proximal tibial condyle (Hawk & Bailie, 2007). The older child may have characteristically wide thighs, a proximal tibial procurvatum producing a relative knee flexion deformity,

Table 11.1. Genu Varum versus Blount's Disease		
Physiologic Genu Varum	**Pathologic Genu Varum**	**Blount's Disease**
■ 2.5 cm or greater between medial femoral condyles when medial malleoli are together when child is standing and patellae are facing forward ■ Normal in infants and toddlers ■ Usually bilateral ■ No lateral thrust at knee with ambulation ■ X-rays normal ■ No treatment required	■ Occurs outside of normal developmental sequence ■ Severe malalignment ■ Asymmetry ■ Rapid progression ■ Positive family history ■ Height less than 5th percentile ■ Usually bilateral ■ Lateral thrust at knee evident with ambulation **X-rays** ■ Medial tilting of transverse plane of knee and ankle joints ■ Obvious angulation but epiphysis appears normal Treatment depends on age and severity Surgery	■ A sharp, localized genu varum associated with growth suppression of posteromedial area of proximal tibial physis ■ Asymmetry ■ 50% unilateral ■ Lateral thrust at knee evident with ambulation **X-rays** ■ Changes in medial metaphyseal contour evidenced by "breaking" ■ Medial height of proximal tibial epiphysis is decreased Prominent localized tibial bowing **Always requires treatment** ■ Bracing ■ Surgery

From Core Curriculum for Orthopaedic Nursing (6th ed., p. 280), 2007, National Association of Orthopaedic Nurses, Boston, MA: Pearson. Reproduced with permission.

CHAPTER 11

anterior knee pain secondary to holding the knee in a flexed position, or medial knee pain secondary to medial knee joint stress. The hips should also be examined for evidence of a slipped capital femoral epiphysis (Schoenecker & Rich, 2006).

The irregular metaphyseal ossification changes in Blount's disease are often indistinguishable from physiologic bowing (genu varum) until the child is 2-2 1/2 years old (Schoenecker & Rich, 2006). In a child older than this, standing anteroposterior (AP) and lateral radiographs of the legs should be done, and changes in the medial metaphyseal contours may be seen. There may be a local prominence, or "beaking," and a decrease of the height of the proximal tibial epiphysis. The middle part of the medial half the epiphyseal plate is narrowed, with increased bony density on its other side. The tibiofemoral angle on the radiograph will measure about 25 degrees of varus, and internal tibial torsion will also be visible. If there is a question of a systemic disease such as rickets, laboratory studies should be done (Hawk & Bailie, 2007). See Table 11.1 for a comparison of genu varum and Blount's disease. Genu varum/genu valgum is discussed at length in a dedicated section of this chapter.

Common Therapeutic Modalities

Management of a child with tibia vara is based on the stage of tibia vara and the age of the child (Staheli, 2008e). If observation is being done, follow-up visits with radiographs at 3-month intervals to evaluate a progressive deformity are typical. Bracing is an option to relieve excessive stress on the medial tibial metaphysis, to provide lateral stability to the knee joint, and to externally rotate the leg. For a child up to 24 months old with a progressive deformity, a hip-knee-ankle-foot orthosis (HKAFO) can be worn (Hawk & Bailie, 2007). Others recommend a long-leg brace with a fixed knee (KAFO) that incorporates valgus loading (Staheli, 2008e). The KAFO that prevents knee flexion is worn for 23 hours a day. The locked brace counteracts the pathologic medial compressive forces, allowing resumption of more normal growth and correction of genu varum.

The pathologic radiographic changes at the proximal medial tibial metaphysis, physis, and epiphysis are slow to remodel. In children who are compliant with brace-wearing, the proximal tibia varus should decrease within 12 months. Treatment is continued until the bony changes in the proximal medial tibia resolve, which typically takes about 1 1/2 -2 years.

Surgical interventions are indicated when there is a failure in response to bracing after 6 months of treatment (Hawk & Bailie, 2007) or in a child with Blount's disease older than age 3 who is either noncompliant or not a good candidate for brace treatment because of obesity or bilateral involvement. The radiographic appearance of the medial epiphysis and metaphysis should normalize by age 5. If radiographic improvement is not seen, a varus-correcting osteotomy should be recommended. The osteotomy unloads the medial compartment of the knee and facilitates growth of the proximal medial physis. Restoration of normal growth in the medial tibial physis is less likely to occur if surgery is delayed. Simple osteotomy after age 5 does not assure permanent correction and carries a higher risk of recurrent deformity because of the greater pathologic change and potential for physeal bar formation (Schoenecker & Rich, 2006).

Surgery is also recommended when irreversible changes in the medial tibial physis are seen. The architecture of the proximal tibia is distorted, including the tibial condylar surface. These changes are typically seen in children older than age 10 but may be seen in children as young as age 6. The proximal tibial varus deformity is characterized by severe depression of the medial tibial plateau, often with ligamentous laxity. In severe cases, the tibia will be subluxed medially on the femur. Left untreated, degenerative arthritis is likely to occur early in life. For a lasting satisfactory outcome, the surgical goal is to correct both the abnormal limb alignment and the pathologic depression in the medial tibial plateau, and a combination of a medial tibial plateau elevation and realignment osteotomy of the proximal tibia is done. If significant distal femoral valgus is present, an osteotomy of the distal femur is performed as well. This procedure will produce a marked correction of the varus deformity, but a proximal varus-correcting osteotomy is often needed to restore normal tibial alignment. A distal femoral osteotomy may also be required to correct a valgus deformity. Alternatively, a hemiepiphyseal stapling of the distal lateral femur can be done for gradual correction. After correction of the angular deformity, a significant leg length difference may remain. This can be managed by an epiphysiodesis of the contralateral limb, or a combination of lengthening and shortening may be required to equalize limb lengths.

In patients with adolescent Blount's disease whose growth plates are still open and the varus deformity is not too severe, a hemiepiphysiodesis is indicated. Once this is performed, patients are closely monitored clinically and radiographically. Most patients with moderate to severe adolescent Blount's disease will require an osteotomy of the proximal tibia and sometimes the distal femur, or a combination of hemiepiphysiodesis and osteotomy to achieve a normal mechanical axis and joint orientation (Schoenecker & Rich, 2006).

Nursing Considerations

Nursing Diagnoses. Nursing diagnoses for this condition are expanded upon in the Appendix.

- Anxiety.
- Peripheral neurovascular dysfunction, risk for.
- Self-concept, readiness for enhanced.

Nursing Interventions. Interventions addressing anxiety includes supporting the patient/family during treatment. If surgery is recommended, stress that angular correction is a gradual process that can last up to 6 months. An optimal outcome is a patient/family with knowledge of the condition, treatment, and surgical goal.

Nursing interventions that focus on the risk for peripheral neurovascular dysfunction include frequent assessment of dorsiflexion and plantarflexion of the affected foot and use of a resting splint to prevent a heelcord contracture. An ideal outcome is an intact neurovascular status. See Compartment Syndrome in Chapter 8—Complications.

Interventions focusing on a disturbed self-concept include focusing on the child as a whole, not just on the affected part, accentuating the child's personal strengths and skills, and recognizing that reactions of parents/significant others influences the child's response. The best outcome is a child with a healthy self-concept who is attaining age-appropriate developmental skills (Hawk & Bailie, 2007).

Cerebral Palsy

Overview

Cerebral palsy (CP) is a disorder of movement and posture, causing activity limitation due to a static defect or lesion of the developing brain. Rather than a specific diagnosis, it encompasses a spectrum of neurodevelopmental syndromes characterized by persistent motor delay, abnormal neuromotor examination, and often an extensive range of nonmotor-associated disabilities in cognitive, neurobehavioral, neurosensory, orthopaedic, and other areas. These associated disabilities reflect the fact that motor centers of the brain are rarely affected in isolation.

CP, a clinical diagnosis, may be due to a wide range of genetic and environmental insults to the developing brain. When the clinical diagnosis of CP is established, it is important to investigate the etiology, which may be important to treatment, prognosis, risk of recurrence, and parental understanding. Although the brain lesion is nonprogressive, its motor and nonmotor manifestations can be expected to change with the child's development (Palmer & Hoon, 2011).

CP occurs in about 2-3 per 1,000 live births, with 50% born at term and 50% born preterm (Palmer & Hoon, 2011). CP is more prevalent in black term infants and black males who are more likely to be born prematurely at a lower birth weight (Berry et al., 2010). CP is also more common in twin pregnancies (Hawk & Bailie, 2007). Severity of illness influences CP survival rates; in one study, 80% of children with CP who could feed themselves survived to the age of 16 compared with 20% who were nourished with a feeding tube. Results of some studies have shown that up to 99% of children with mild CP survive to adulthood (Berry et al., 2010).

Despite more than a century of research, specific etiologic factors responsible for the motor impairment remain uncertain in many children with CP, especially in children born at term. Large studies have shown that brain injury occurring at birth is the cause in only 8%-12% of cases. Developmental brain anomalies or prenatal insults are the most common etiologies. In premature children, both prenatal and perinatal factors are believed to play a role. Postnatal etiologies, such as traumatic brain injury and meningitis, account for 10% of CP (Palmer & Hoon, 2011).

Other postnatal causes of CP include hypoxic-ischemic encephalopathy with multi-organ failure, periventricular leukomalacia, intracranial or intraventricular hemorrhage, and hyperbilirubinemia (Hawk & Bailie, 2007). Maternal and/or fetal infection/inflammation has been noted as an important antecedent of CP in both term and preterm infants. Thrombophilia (including the Factor V Leiden mutation), the most common cause of familial thrombosis in neonates, infants, and children, may be an important contributor to intrauterine stroke. Advances in neuroimaging and molecular genetics are greatly improving the understanding of etiology and options for prevention (Palmer & Hoon, 2011).

Clinical classification of CP is based on the nature of the movement disorder, muscle tone, and topography. Classification by type is essential to management and anticipation of associated disabilities and future needs.

Spastic CP. Spastic CP affects 65% of children with cerebral palsy. Most children with CP have spasticity, an upper motor neuron syndrome consisting of persistent velocity-dependent hypertonus (increased muscle tone of clasp-knife character), increased deep tendon reflexes, pathologic reflexes, spastic weakness, and loss of motor control and dexterity. Spastic CP is further classified on the basis of topography. *Hemiplegia*, the diagnosis for 30% of children with CP, is the primary unilateral involvement, often with the arm more affected than the leg. *Quadriplegia*, the diagnosis for 5% of children with CP, is the involvement of four limbs with the legs frequently more involved than the arms, but with functionally limiting arm movement. *Diplegia*, the diagnosis for 30% of children with CP is the involvement of four limbs with the legs much more involved than the arms, which may show only minimal impairment and no functional limitation.

Dyskinetic CP. Dyskinetic CP, which accounts for 19% of children with CP, is the other physiologic category, and is due to prominent involuntary movements, fluctuating muscle tone, or both. *Choreoathetotic* and *dystonic* are the two most common subtypes. Most children with dyskinetic CP have relatively symmetric four-limb involvement.

Ataxic CP. Ataxic CP accounts for up to 10% of children with CP. It often has genetic underpinnings and is associated with significant comorbidities in vision, hearing, cognition, feeding, and epilepsy (Palmer & Hoon, 2011). Affected children have balance disturbances due to a brain lesion located in the cerebellum (Hawk & Bailie, 2007).

Worster-Drought Syndrome. Also known as bulbar CP, this classification should be considered in the child whose motor disability is primarily of a cranial nerve distribution. It may be associated with underlying perisylvian microgyria on neuroimaging and may be familial (Palmer & Hoon, 2011).

CP usually presents with significant motor delay, although the delay may not be recognized in the first months of life. Common presenting concerns include poor head control, hypertonia (especially during activities such as bathing or diapering), generalized hypotonia, early preferential hand use, absent weight-bearing, and feeding problems. Experienced observers may note abnormalities in spontaneous general movements during the first weeks of life (Palmer & Hoon, 2011).

Associated disabilities in children with CP often affect the child's future needs. An intellectual disability, present in 30%-77% of children with CP, is the most important factor influencing habilitation. A language disorder or learning disability, present in about 40% of children with CP, can be due to an oromotor dysfunction, dysphasia, or hearing loss. Neurobehavioral disorders, present in up to 50% of children with CP, cover the spectrum from attention-deficit/hyperactivity disorder to autism, and may be primarily a neurologic symptom or reflect discomfort from an underlying medical problem, such as a hip subluxation, gastroesophageal reflux disease (GERD), or skin breakdown. Visual disorders, present in 50%-90% of children with CP, may have a bearing on education. Hearing disorders, present in 10% of children with CP are easily missed. Somatosensory deficits are present in up to 50% of children with hemiplegic CP, and stereognosis is the most common deficit. Seizures, present in 30%-40% of children with CP, are often associated with spasticity and lower cognition. Growth failure, with undernutrition a frequent problem, is multifactorial in origin. Other health problems include genitourinary issues and drooling, which is a mainly cosmetic problem and may be exacerbated by antispasticity drugs (Palmer & Hoon, 2011).

Although the achievement of normal developmental milestones is delayed or absent in children with CP, early intervention stimulates the cognitive, language, and social development in infants and toddlers. CP is nonprogressive, but the physical deformities and functional impairments may change due to a child's abnormal tone or postural reflexes. Scoliosis and hip dislocations may develop during childhood, and disuse osteopenia may predispose a child with CP to fractures (Hawk & Bailie, 2007).

Assessment

Information about the onset and progression of the presenting symptoms should be obtained, along with a history of the child's general health. Details of the pregnancy and birth history should be elicited. Specific information about the developmental milestones should be obtained, including any delays, failure to follow the normal pattern of gross and fine motor development, and persistence of primitive reflexes. Functional limitations should be noted. Inquire about any history of seizures, nutrition and growth history, bowel/bladder patterns

Table 11.2. Clinical Findings in Cerebral Palsy

	Spastic Diplegia	Hemiplegia	Quadriplegia	Dyskinetic (Dystonic, Athetoid)
	■ LE more affected than UE or face	■ Unilateral spastic motor weakness	■ Involvement of head, neck, and all four limbs	■ Motor restlessness; intermittent movement of head, neck, limbs, hands, and/or feet
Commonly related to	■ Prematurity	■ Congenital or acquired	■ Full-term infant with cortical injury from hypoxemia-ischemia ■ Prematurity	■ Kernicterus ■ Cardiac bypass surgery
Early signs **Later signs**	■ Hypotonia ■ Episodes of increased general tone caused by change in posture ■ Increasing spasticity	■ Rarely suspected in newborn ■ "Hand preference" at 4-5 months ■ Delayed or absent pincer grasp		■ Variable hypotonia or postural instability ■ Insidious development of adventitious movements at 6-12 months
Head/UE involvement	■ Functional use of hands	■ Held in abduction with flexion at wrist and hyperextension of fingers ■ Slower growth of affected side	■ Weakness of facial and pharyngeal musculature: dysphagia, GE reflux ■ Cranial nerve palsies	■ Tongue thrusting ■ Chewing movement ■ Orofacial grimacing ■ Hypotonia of neck and trunk
LE involvement	■ Sitting: flexion of hips and knees ■ Standing: "scissoring" of legs	■ Ambulates within normative time	■ Paucity of lower extremity movement	■ Extensor posturing of foot
Speech/ swallowing	■ Minimally affected	■ Language impairments with injury to either hemisphere	■ Fail to acquire complex speech or language	■ Marked impairment in language
Seizures	■ Uncommon	■ Common	■ Common	
Sensory impairment	■ Visual-spatial deficits ■ Strabismus		■ Cortical blindness ■ Sensorineural hearing loss	■ Hearing loss ■ Visual disturbances
Cognitive development	■ Normal/near normal intelligence	■ Intelligence variable: correlated with severity of seizures	■ Variable: influence by underlying pattern of brain injury ■ Generally some degree of mental retardation exacerbated by seizures ■ Constipation/fecal impaction	■ Receptive language and intelligence near normal
Treatment goals	■ Independent ambulation		■ Maximal functional independence and social adaptation	■ Good posturing to support trunk and head ■ Language and communication

From Core Curriculum for Orthopaedic Nursing *(6th ed., p. 313), 2007, National Association of Orthopaedic Nurses, Boston, MA: Pearson. Reproduced with permission*

including success of toilet training (if appropriate), and social interactions/relationships with peers (Hawk & Bailie, 2007).

There may be a history of difficulty separating the legs when changing diapers, tremors in the arms or legs after a sudden movement or crying, and variations in the quality of muscle tone or stiffness when the child is being handled. Parents or caregivers may report hyperextension of the neck when the head is unsupported, scissoring of the legs when the child is being lifted, tight clenching of the thumb in the palm after the age of 4 months, and kicking of the legs in unison. Continuous tongue movement in and out of the mouth may also be reported, along with excessive sleeping difficulties and overreactions to stimuli. There may be delayed or impaired speech, vision, or hearing (Hawk & Bailie, 2007).

The physical examination of the infant or child starts with accurately weighing and measuring the child (Hawk & Bailie, 2007), including the head circumference. An abnormally increasing frontal-occipital circumference may indicate hydrocephalus, whereas a flat line on the circumference curve may indicate that the brain is not growing adequately; microcephaly in children with CP is associated with mental retardation (Watemberg, Silver, Harel, & Lerman-Sagie, 2002). On neuromotor examination, muscle tone may vary from excessive hypotonia to hypertonia (spastic, dystonic, or mixed in character). Hypotonia in an infant may be manifest as head lag on pull to sit up, slip-through at the shoulders, or an exaggerated curve in ventral suspension. Hypotonia with significant weakness and diminished tendon reflexes is uncommon in CP and suggests a neuromuscular disorder. Early hypotonia may persist, normalize, or evolve into hypertonia (Palmer & Hoon, 2011).

The examination of the infant or child should include an assessment of oromotor and ocular function, focusing on dysmorphic features, neurocutaneous signs, retinal abnormalities, organomeagly, and other findings that could suggest a specific etiology. The presence of orthopaedic abnormalities, including scoliosis, joint contractures (Palmer & Hoon, 2011), angular/rotational deformities, and hip subluxation/dislocation, should also be noted. If the child is able, standing/walking postures should be observed, along with gait and balance. Hip ultrasounds or radiographs are done to evaluate hip subluxation/dislocation, and spine radiographs are done to monitor the presence and progression of scoliosis (Hawk & Bailie, 2007). The child with CP is at risk for hip disorders due to progressive hip adduction and flexion, leading to femoral anteversion, subluxation, deformities of the femoral head, and hip dislocations, which can progress to painful degeneration (Morrell, Pearson, & Sauser, 2002).

Serial examinations are important to monitor progress when there is a suspicion of CP. The diagnosis is often easier if known brain damage is documented by cranial ultrasound, computed tomography (CT), or magnetic resonance imaging (MRI). Generally, the more severely affected child frequently can be diagnosed by 6 months of age, with the more mild cases taking longer (Bennett, 1999).

In children with atypical clinical findings—especially choreoathetosis, which involves irregular, involuntary movements—metabolic disorders should be suspected. Plasma lactate, plasma amino acids, urinary organic acids, and selective use of other tests can be important. A karyotype, chromosomal microassay, or targeted fluorescence in-situ hybridization (FISH) may be revealing in children with apparent prenatal onset of CP and additional, even minor malformations (Palmer & Hoon, 2011). To evaluate the presence of seizures, an electroencephalogram (EEG) is indicated. To assess for GERD, a pH probe or barium swallow is done. Blood tests to evaluate the child's nutritional status may include total serum protein and albumin, iron, iron-binding capacity, transferrin levels, hemoglobin, erythrocyte mean corpuscular volume, and total lymphocyte count. A gait analysis is indicated preoperatively if surgery is being considered in an ambulatory child (Hawk & Bailie, 2007). See Table 11.2 for a discussion of clinical findings.

Common Therapeutic Modalities

The primary goals in the management of a child with CP are to work with the child and family to help the child function as effectively and normally as possible in the home, school, and community; to provide a foundation for the child to function independently as an adult, minimizing the activity limitations imposed by the neurodevelopmental and associated disabilities; to assist the parents in accepting and assuming their roles as primary advocates for their child's needs; to coordinate the recommendations of the many medical and other providers into an integrated health care plan; and, when needed, to assist with adolescents, young adults, and their families to transition care to adult providers in an efficient, effective, and coordinated manner as possible.

The severity of the individual case should help determine the aggressiveness of treatment. Parents should be included in any therapy and should incorporate techniques into their everyday activities with the child. Therapists and intervention programs should be kept informed about the child's health and should keep the clinicians informed of their activities (Palmer & Hoon, 2011).

Thorough academic and psychologic evaluations should be done to develop a comprehensive program for preschool and school-aged children. As the child grows, the family/caregivers may experience difficulty managing daily care. Functional priorities are communication, ADLs, mobility in the environment, and walking. Nonsurgical interventions include positioning to

Table 11.3. Medications Used in Cerebral Palsy				
	Drug	**Medication Classification**	**Side Effects**	**Nursing Implications**
Muscle spasms	■ Diazepam (Valium®) ■ Baclofen (Lioresal®)	■ Skeletal muscle relaxant; anxiety agent ■ Skeletal muscle relaxant; antispasmodic	■ Drowsiness; hypotension; fatigue ■ Drowsiness; dizziness; weakness	■ Used primarily in the postoperative period to reduce muscle spasms and tone. ■ Taper doe when discontinued; withdrawal side effects includes seizures. ■ When teaching patient/family about medication, set realistic expectation of what drug can do: does not cause dramatic reductions in muscle spasms/tone. ■ May be injected intrathecally.
	Local anesthetic		■ Sensory loss along nerve pathway	■ Injected in immediate vicinity of specific nerve as nerve block. ■ Short acting, reversible conduction block.
	Alcohol		■ Local pain at injection site	■ Inject into muscle fibers in region distribution. ■ Inhibits nerve transmission and muscle contractions.
	Phenol		■ Local pain at injection site	■ Permanent nerve effect.
	Botulinum-A toxin	Neurotoxin		■ Injected into sites of nerve branching in muscles. ■ Blocks release of acetylcholine from synapses at myoneuronal junction. ■ Effect begins 12-72 hours, lasts 3-6 months. ■ Contraindicated for fixed joint contractures.
Seizures	Phenytoin (Dilantin®)	Anticonvulsant	■ Slurred speech ■ Confusion ■ Nystagmus ■ Gingival hyperplasia	■ Therapeutic levels should be checked to achieve optimal dosage adjustments. ■ Give drug with or after meals to reduce gastric distress. ■ Instruct patient/family on importance of not missing doses. Instruct patient/family on importance of meticulous oral hygiene.
	Carbamazepine (Tegretol®)	Anticonvulsant	■ Dizziness; drowsiness; hematologic changes; nausea, vomiting	■ Pretreatment blood studies to identify any abnormalities. ■ Periodic evaluations necessary, especially with symptoms of potential hematologic problem. ■ Effective in partial seizures and tonic/clonic seizures.
	Valproic acid (Depakene®)	Anticonvulsant	■ Nausea, vomiting; sedation; hepatotoxicity	■ Liver function tests prior to initiation of therapy and at regular intervals. ■ Take meals to prevent GI distress. ■ Effective in myoclonic seizures and absence (petit mal) seizures.
	Phenobarbital (Luminal®)	Anticonvulsant (barbiturate)	■ Excitement and hyperactivity in children; drowsiness; GI upset	■ Withdraw drugs gradually to prevent convulsions, tremors.
GE reflux	Metoclopramide (Reglan®)	Antiemetic	■ Restlessness; agitation; seizures	■ Contraindication in patients with seizures. ■ Administer 30 minutes before meals.

From Core Curriculum for Orthopaedic Nursing *(6th ed., pp. 315-316), 2007, National Association of Orthopaedic Nurses, Boston, MA: Pearson. Reproduced with permission.*

address tone and movement abnormalities with the purpose of promoting skeletal alignment, compensating for abnormal posture, and preparing the child for independent mobility. Devices that address positioning include side-lyers, prone wedges, standers, and specially designed seating systems.

PT can utilize various modalities to attempt to modify the central nervous system (CNS) by externally applying stimuli and may include neurodevelopmental treatment (Bobath approach), sensory integration therapy, patterning, conductive education, pressure-point stimulation, bracing/stretching, and recreational therapies. A home program with strong parental involvement is extremely important to maintain strength and ROM. Postoperative rehabilitation to maximize the benefits of surgery and to regain preoperative strength is also vital, and assistance using adaptive and therapeutic equipment may be needed for short-term use.

The purpose of bracing and splinting in a child with CP is to prevent deformity, provide support to the joint by substituting for the weakened muscles, and protect the weakened part. Many children with CP wear molded ankle-foot orthoses (AFOs) to prevent plantar flexion of their feetand/or a hand splint to keep the thumb adducted and the wrist in a neutral position. Manipulation and serial casting are done when indicated (Hawk & Bailie, 2007). Medications are used as needed to manage seizures and GERD (see Table 11.3).

Nerve block and motor-point blocks may be done with the goal of weakening the muscle to balance forces across a joint, which may allow an improved stretching/strengthening program. A nerve block is the direct injection into the motor nerve, and a motor-point block is an injection interrupting the nerve supply at the entry site without compromising sensation. The injections may need to be repeated and can be painful. Injections of the potent neurotoxin Botulinum-A directly into spastic muscles may be advocated to reduce spasticity for a short-term, 3-6 month, benefit. A Baclofen pump may be recommended for the severely spastic child. OT and speech therapy, with use of a hearing aid as needed, are utilized by many children with CP for fine motor and speech/oral-motor issues (Hawk & Bailie, 2007).

Surgical interventions may prevent or correct serious structural changes (Hawk & Bailie, 2007) when function is impaired, care is limited, or pain is caused by deformity, contracture, or muscle imbalance. Goals of surgery should be clearly understood by families, and the common parental expectation for unreasonable functional gains should be anticipated (Palmer & Hoon, 2011). Osteotomies can correct fixed bony deformities and stabilize joints. Tendon lengthening (of the heelcords, adductor tenotomies, or myotomies) and hamstring releases/lengthenings are often done to address specific deformities, such as tight heelcords or knee flexion contractures. Tendon transfers are indicated to restore muscle balance. To treat progressive scoliosis, an anterior release and posterior spinal fusion with instrumentation are performed (Hawk & Bailie, 2007).

To address spasticity, intrathecal baclofen (ITB) and selective dorsal rhizotomy (SDR) are employed in many centers for children with spastic diplegia. Both are costly and require surgeons with expertise. When patients are carefully selected and followed in a specialized program, there may be benefits both in ease of care and function. An important difference is that an ITB pump may be removed, whereas SDR is permanent. ITB requires close, ongoing management, and SDR is a single procedure. ITB is an important therapeutic approach for children with refractory spasticity or dystonia, an involuntary muscle contraction causing twisting of the body part. The pump delivers baclofen into the intrathecal space via an implanted, programmable system. ITB allows titratable reductions in spasticity using doses of baclofen in microgram amounts, rather than milligram amounts with oral use and it avoids the adverse effects often associated with higher doses of oral baclofen. Specific goals for functional improvement should be clear before deciding on surgical interventions (Palmer & Hoon, 2011).

Nursing Considerations

Nursing Diagnoses. Nursing diagnoses for this condition are expanded upon in the Appendix.

- Anxiety.
- Aspiration, risk for.
- Grieving.
- Mobility: physical, impaired.
- Nutrition, imbalance: less than body requirements.
- Pain, chronic.

Nursing Interventions. Interventions focused on patient/parental anxiety include developing a plan of care with the child's (if appropriate) and caregivers' input, educating them about the pathology, typical developmental progression, treatment, and available resources. This promotes their active participation and greater understanding of the chronic nature of CP, and allows them to express their fears/concerns related to the diagnosis/treatment. Ideally, the outcome is a family that understands CP and how it changes as the child grows/matures.

Interventions focused on the risk for aspiration include a prior assessment of the child's ability to chew and swallow, positioning the child in an upright or partially upright position, assisting with feeding/drinking as needed, offering foods and fluids of an appropriate consistency, placing food or medication to one side of the mouth or behind the tongue to facilitate swallowing, stroking from the neck to the chin to stimulate swallowing, providing smaller and more frequent meals as needed, allowing rest periods during meals if needed, keeping suction equipment at the bedside, and suctioning secretions prior to when nutrition is offered. An ideal outcome is a child who does not aspirate (Hawk & Bailie, 2007).

Nursing measures that focus on chronic grief include encouraging the verbalization of feelings/fears related to perceived losses. Provide ongoing support to the patient/family through the diagnostic period and assist them in identifying lifestyle modifications, as indicated. Help the family identify sources of support, and refer them to appropriate condition-related support groups (Hawk & Bailie, 2007), such as the United Cerebral Palsy Association, The Council for Disability Rights, and the American Academy for Cerebral Palsy and Developmental Medicine (Palmer & Hoon, 2011). Help family members recognize their child's strengths and skills while acknowledging limitations. The best outcome is a family that is supported through the grieving process.

Measures focusing on imbalanced nutrition include completing a dietary assessment that includes a feeding history and caloric/nutritional intake. Assess for GERD, and identify high-calorie foods that the child can tolerate. If indicated, caregivers should be taught enteric feeding regimens, whether they are nasogastric, gastric, or jejunal feedings. The optimal outcome is a child who receives adequate nutrition as evidenced by a stable growth curve.

Interventions focused on chronic pain include assessing the child for signs of discomfort related to spasticity (in general or post-surgery), and differentiating between soft-tissue/bony pain and muscle spasms. Avoid startling the child, approach slowly and speak softly, and initiate physical contact with firm but gentle pressure. Preoperatively, explain to the child/family the likely occurrence of muscle spasms postoperatively, and assess the degree of muscle spasms before surgery: involved muscles, usual patterns, and usual management. Discuss postoperative spasm management such as comfort measures that may be impeded by immobilization, the use of muscle relaxants (commonly diazepam), and the ineffectiveness of opiates to control spasms. Administer muscle relaxants around the clock for 48-72 hours postoperatively. Signs/symptoms of spasms include alternating crying/calmness, sudden, jerky movements of the limb followed by crying, and waking from sleep. Spasms are often relieved by a change in position, especially to the prone position, and by the administration of muscle relaxants, but not with analgesics alone. An ideal outcome is a child who achieves a maximal level of comfort (Hawk & Bailie, 2007).

Interventions focused on impaired physical mobility are assisting with active/passive ROM of the joints to maintain and promote mobility, lifting the child in a flexed, sitting position, encouraging bilateral hand movement through the use of play when the child is prone, and using an adaptive wheelchair to maintain proper body alignment. An ideal outcome is parental understanding of the exercise/activity program (Hawk & Bailie, 2007).

Clubfoot

Overview

Clubfoot, also referred to as talipes equinovarus, is a congenital foot deformity characterized by equinus of the hindfoot, adduction of the midfoot and forefoot, and varus through the subtalar joint complex. A cavus deformity through the midfoot also accompanies most clubfeet (Kasser, 2006). These characteristics are present in varying degrees and are rigid (Hawk & Bailie, 2007).

The etiology of clubfoot is multifactorial and influenced by genetics and the intrauterine environment. Clubfoot in general is idiopathic, occurring in otherwise healthy children (Kasser, 2006; Staheli, 2008a), but it can also be associated with other congenital abnormalities, such as neural tube defects, anomalies of the urinary or digestive system, and other musculoskeletal irregularities. The clubfoot deformity can have different causes, as evidenced by the variability of expression and response to management (Staheli, 2008a). Prenatal factors, such as intrauterine crowding and oligohydramnios with amniotic band formation, and chemical insults, such as sodium aminopterin ingestion to induce abortion and tubocurarine chloride for treatment of tetaunus during the first trimester of pregnancy, are known causes of clubfoot (Hawk & Bailie, 2007). Maternal smoking has also been identified as a risk factor in clubfoot etiology (Kasser, 2006).

The pathophysiology of clubfoot is typical of a dysplasia. The tarsals are hypoplastic. The talus is most deformed; the size is reduced, with a shortened talar neck that is deviated in a medial and plantar direction. The navicular articulates with the medial aspect of the neck of the talus due to the abnormal talar shape. The relationship of the tarsals is abnormal, with the talus and calcaneus parallel in all three planes. The midfoot becomes medially displaced, and the metatarsals are adducted and plantarflexed. In addition to the cartilage and bony deformities, the ligaments are thickened and the muscles are hypoplastic. This results in a generalized hypoplasia of the limb with a small calf and a small, shortened foot, which is proportional to the severity of the clubfoot. Since the hypoplasia mainly involves the foot, the limb length difference is usually less than one centimeter (Staheli, 2008a).

Clubfoot can be classified into three subgroups:

- Positional clubfoot results from intrauterine position in late gestation and resolves quickly with serial casting;
- Idiopathic clubfoot is multifactorial in etiology and has a moderate degree of stiffness.
- Teratologic clubfoot is associated with neuromuscular disorders and syndromes. This type of clubfoot is very rigid and more difficult to manage.

Classifications are based on the probable cause. The Dimeglio classification is based on stiffness, and points are given for ROM in equinus, adduction, varus, and medial rotation. The sum of these points determines the severity (Staheli, 2008a).

The incidence of clubfoot is about 1 in 1,000 births, is bilateral in half the cases, and affects males more frequently. Complications of an untreated clubfoot produce considerable disability, and the dorsolateral skin becomes the weight-bearing area. Calluses form, and walking becomes limited (Staheli, 2008a). An operatively treated clubfoot is often weak, stiff, and may be in varus. There is potential for a leg length inequality and a rocker-bottom deformity, which is caused by pushing up on the metatarsals while correcting equinus during serial casting. Neurovascular compromise may occur secondary to stress on nerves and blood vessels from overzealous equinus correction or incorrect casting. Postoperative infection and recurrent and/or residual deformity may also occur (Hawk & Bailie, 2007).

Assessment

The assessment of a clubfoot includes obtaining the prenatal, birth, and developmental history, past medical and surgical history of the clubfoot and other diagnosed conditions, and the family history. Parental concerns about the appearance and function of the foot should be elicited also (Hawk & Bailie, 2007).

The diagnosis of clubfoot is not difficult and is seldom confused with other foot deformities. Sometimes severe metatarsus varus is confused with clubfoot, but the equinus component of clubfoot makes the differentiation clear. The presence of clubfoot should prompt a careful search for other musculoskeletal problems. The back should be examined for dysraphism, the hips for dysplasia, and the knees for deformity. Note the size, shape, and flexibility of the feet. Clubfoot is not associated with developmental dysplasia of the hips or spinal deformity, and radiographs of the pelvis or spine should only be done if abnormalities are found.

Note the degree of stiffness of the foot, and compare the size of the foot with the uninvolved foot. Marked differences in foot length suggest that the deformity is severe and foretell the need for operative correction. Document the components of the clubfoot deformity: the equinus, cavus, heel varus, forefoot adductus, and medial rotation. Equinus is due to a combination of a plantar flexed talus, posterior ankle capsular contracture, and shortening of the triceps. Cavus is due to a contracture of the plantar fascia, with plantar flexion of the forefoot on the hindfoot. Varus results from inversion of the subtalar joint. Adductus and medial rotation are due to medial deviation of the neck of the talus, medial displacement of the talonavicular joint, and metatarsus adductus. Tibial rotation is normal (Staheli, 2008a).

The diagnosis of clubfoot can be made prenatally, as it can be seen on fetal ultrasound during the first trimester of pregnancy. Because active treatment usually occurs during early infancy, when ossification is incomplete, the value of radiographic studies is limited. Radiographs become increasingly valuable with increasing age (Staheli, 2008a). To optimize these studies, the foot should be held in the position of best correction: AP and lateral weight-bearing in a child, or a simulated weight-bearing position or forced dorsiflexion in an infant or nonambulatory child. Angles are measured to assess clubfoot severity and treatment response. The use of computed tomography (CT) scan and MRI is not indicated (Hawk & Bailie, 2007).

Common Treatment Modalities

The primary objectives of clubfoot management are to correct the deformity and to retain mobility and strength. The foot should be plantigrade and have a normal load-bearing area. Secondary objectives include the ability to wear normal shoes. Treatment should start as early as possible after birth and includes serial manipulation and casting, which corrects the cavus, rotates the foot from under the talus, and corrects the equinus. Ponseti casting and rotational splinting have been refined over a period of 50 years, have shown excellent long-term results, and are becoming the management standard throughout the world (Staheli, 2008a). A percutaneous tenotomy is often done to facilitate equinus correction during infancy, at age six weeks or later (Hawk & Bailie, 2007). The French taping method emphasizes prolonged intense manipulation and splinting (Staheli, 2008a).

Surgical management is typically planned when non-operative correction has plateaued and may include soft tissue releases. Tendon transfers are commonly done in early childhood to correct the muscle imbalance about the foot, and bony procedures should be performed at the end of growth. More than 90% of children can expect to have an excellent result with a foot that is plantigrade, mobile, and strong. The results are far superior to those achieved by surgery with the traditional posteromedial release procedure. Surgically corrected feet usually become painful during adolescence or early adult life (Staheli, 2008a).

Nursing Considerations

Nursing Diagnoses. Nursing diagnoses for this condition are expanded upon in the Appendix.

- Anxiety.
- Peripheral neurovascular dysfunction, risk for.
- Skin integrity, impaired.

Nursing Interventions. Interventions focused on anxiety include involving the parents/caregivers as much as possible throughout treatment. Encourage parents to express their fears/concerns related to the diagnosis and treatment, include them in the decision-making process, and educate them regarding the pathology, normal progession, treatment, and appropriate community resources, if indicated. The best outcome is a family that is able to express their concerns, understands the child's condition, and fully participates in the treatment plan.

Instruct parents/caregivers how to assess the color, temperature, capillary refill, and motor/sensory function of the affected foot. If capillary refill is slow, the casted foot should be elevated and reassessed after several minutes. If there is no improvement in the function/appearance of the foot, parents should be instructed in advance whom to contact for further instructions (Kunkler, 2007). The best outcome is a foot that is neurovascularly intact.

Since clubfoot treatment typically involves frequent cast applications, interventions should focus on teaching parents cast care and recognizing signs of skin issues. The cast should be kept clean/dry, and the infant/child should be sponge-bathed while casted. Cast removal should be done the evening prior to the next appointment. If there is a plaster cast cast, parents may use a vinegar/water solution (1:10) to soak the cast. Once softened, parents should unwind the cast or use blunt scissors to remove it. If the cast is made of semi-rigid fiberglass, they may unroll it. The infant should be bathed, and the affected leg and foot should be gently washed, with careful attention not to scrub the skin. The skin should be assessed for areas of erythema or breakdown, and parents should notify their health care provider of skin issues. Areas of breakdown and bony prominences should have extra layers of cast padding, and cast edges should be smooth. An ideal outcome is intact skin (Hawk & Bailie, 2007).

Developmental Dysplasia of the Hip

Overview

Developmental dysplasia of the hip (DDH) is a generic term describing a spectrum of anatomic abnormalities of the hip that may be congenital or develop during infancy or early childhood. The spectrum covers mild defects such as a shallow acetabulum to severe defects such as teratologic dislocations (Staheli, 2008c). Previously referred to as congenital dysplasia of the hip (CDH), DDH is a more representative term of the wide range of abnormalities seen in this condition. The term "developmental" is more encompassing and is taken in the literal sense of organ growth and differentiation, including the embryonic, fetal, and infantile periods. This terminology includes all cases that are developmental, incorporating subluxation, dislocation, and dysplasia of the hip (Weinstein, 2006a).

For the hip joint to grow and develop in a normal way, there must be a genetically determined balance of growth of the acetabular and triradiate cartilages, and a well-located and centered femoral head. Acetabular development continues throughout intrauterine life, particularly by means of growth and development of the labrum. In the normal hip at birth, the femoral head is deeply seated in the acetabulum and held within the acetabulum by the surface tension of the synovial fluid. After birth, continued growth of the proximal femur and the acetabular cartilage complex is extremely important to the continuing development of the hip joint. The growth of these two components of the hip joint is interdependent. In the newborn with DDH, the tight fit between the femoral head and acetabulum is lost. The femoral head can be made to glide in and out of the acetabulum, with a palpable sensation or "clunk" known clinically as the Ortolani sign. Another diagnostic test, the Barlow maneuver, is a provocative maneuver in which the hip is flexed and adducted, and the femoral head is palpated to exit the acetabulum partially or completely over a ridge of the acetabulum (Weinstein, 2006a). The acetabulum is most shallow at birth, and the combination of this and the normal joint laxity of the newborn makes the time surrounding delivery high-risk for dislocation (Hawk & Bailie, 2007).

The etiology of DDH is multifactorial, involving genetic and intrauterine factors. It is more commonly seen if a parent or sibling had DDH and in firstborn females. It is thought that the greater susceptibility of girls to the maternal relaxin hormone increases ligamentous laxity. Prenatal conditions leading to decreased fetal movement may be associated with DDH and include oligohydramnios, large birth weight, first pregnancy, and breech position. Unstretched abdominal muscles and the uterus in primagravida women force the fetus against the mother's spine and may result in hip dysplasia (Hawk & Bailie, 2007).

Postnatal environmental factors such as laxity in the hip capsule may influence the development of DDH. Cultural practices such as swaddling, with the hips forced into adduction and extension, increase the likelihood of DDH, possibly as a result of the forceful position of the legs in extension and adduction, counter to normal newborn hip flexion (Weinstein, 2006a).

The incidence of DDH, which is the most common disorder of the hip in children younger than age 3 (Hawk & Bailie, 2007), depends on how much of the spectrum is included. At birth, hip instability is noted in 0.5%-1% of joints, but classic DDH occurs in about 0.1% of infants (Staheli, 2008c). The incidence of mild dysplasia contributing to adult degenerative arthritis is substantial. It is thought that half of the women who develop degenerative arthritis have preexisting acetabular dysplasia (Staheli, 2008c). The left hip is more often affected than the right hip, and DDH can be associated with congenital torticollis, metatarsus adductus, and other lower limb deformities (Hawk & Bailie, 2007).

A dysplastic hip has a shallow acetabulum in which the femoral head does not fit well. A subluxable hip is a femoral head that moves partly out of the acetabulum. A dislocatable hip is a femoral head that moves completely out of the acetabulum. A dislocated but reducible hip is one in which the femoral head is out of the acetabulum but can be reduced. A dislocated and irreducible hip is a femoral head that is out of the acetabulum and cannot be reduced. If the femoral head is not reduced and stabilized, normal growth and development of both the femoral head and the acetabulum are affected. If the hip remains dislocated or subluxated, secondary changes can occur, such as shortening of the adductor longus and iliopsoas, anteromedial constriction of the hip capsule, thickening or elongation of the ligamentous teres, inversion and hypertrophy of the labrum, and development of a false acetabulum.

Some pathologic changes are reversible, particularly when treated early. It is estimated that 95% of newborns are successfully treated with abduction devices, such as a Pavlik harness, but the outcome is more difficult to predict for late-diagnosed cases (Hawk & Bailie, 2007). If the diagnosis of DDH is not made early, secondary adaptive changes develop. The most reliable physical finding in late-diagnosed DDH is limitation of abduction.

Other manifestations of late-diagnosed DDH may include apparent femoral shortening (or Galeazzi sign), asymmetry of the gluteal, thigh, or labial folds, and limb length inequality. In patients with bilateral dislocations, clinical findings include a waddling gait and hyperlordosis of the lumbar spine. If DDH goes undetected, normal hip joint growth and development are impaired. With increasing age at detection and reduction, and in children older than six months, the intra-articular and extra-articular obstacles to concentric reduction become increasingly difficult to overcome by simple treatment methods such as use of the Pavlik harness (Weinstein, 2006a). Sequelae of DDH include residual femoral and acetabular dysplasia, growth disturbance of the proximal femur, failed reduction, avascular necrosis of the femoral head, neurovascular injury related to surgery, degenerative joint disease, an unstable gait, pain with ambulation, functional scoliosis, valgus deformity of the ipsilateral knee, and low back pain (Hawk & Bailie, 2007).

Assessment

Prior to the examination of the infant/child, ask about the presenting symptoms, such as difficult diapering due to one leg not abducting as much as the other, an awkward gait, a leg length discrepancy, or pain with ambulation in an ambulatory child. Obtain information about the onset and progression of symptoms and previous treatment. The perinatal history (including presentation) should be elicited, along with the developmental, medical/surgical, and family history (Hawk & Bailie, 2007). Although the early diagnosis of DDH is critical to a successful outcome (Staheli, 2008c), it is not always easy to identify in early infancy because the physical findings will vary widely, depending on whether the hip is dysplastic, subluxated, or dislocated. Bilateral dislocated hips may be missed because the physical findings are symmetric (Hawk & Bailie, 2007).

Physical findings may include asymmetric skin creases/gluteal folds, persistent limitation of abduction of a flexed thigh, and a dislocated femoral head (Barlow's maneuver), and the femoral head may be able to be reduced (Ortolani maneuver). There may be an apparent limb length discrepancy, as the femur looks shorter on the affected side (Galeazzi sign and Allis sign). An unusual positioning of the lower limb may be noticed in the nonambulatory child. In an ambulatory child, toe walking, limping, pain, or a positive Trendelenburg sign or gait may be present. See Chapter 3—Musculoskeletal Assessment for further discussion of these physical findings.

Diagnostic testing for DDH may include a hip ultrasound, which allows the visualization of the cartilaginous components of the acetabulum and the femoral head. An ultrasound to assess the anatomic characteristics and hip motion is recommended for high-risk infants and infants with an abnormal clinical examination (Hawk & Bailie, 2007). The effectiveness of ultrasound imaging depends upon the skill and experience of the examiner, and in the interpretation of the findings. Imaging is appropriate to evaluate a suspicious finding, when hip-at-risk factors are present, and to monitor the effectiveness of treatment. An AP pelvis radiograph is done after the newborn period, by 2-3 months of age, when radiography is reliable (Staheli, 2008c). Some sources advocate an AP pelvis radiograph after the age of 4 months, as that is when the ossific nuclei begin to develop (Kleposki, Abel, & Sehgal, 2010). An intraoperative arthorogram is done to ouline cartilaginous components of the acetabulum and the femoral head, and CT may be done to verify position of the hips after a closed or open reduction (Hawk & Bailie, 2007).

Common Treatment Modalities

Treatment should begin immediately upon the diagnosis of DDH, as success correlates with the age of the child. Treatment goals include reduction of the femoral head, the maintenance of the reduction to allow normal growth and development, and prevention of a proximal femoral growth disturbance.

Initial treatment in the 0-6 month age range is an abduction device, such as the Pavlik harness (see Figure 11.2). This device maintains flexion and abduction, which leads to reduction and stabilization of the hip. It also prevents hip extension and adduction, which leads to dislocation and avoids forced adduction to protect the blood supply to the femoral head. The Pavlik harness is well-tolerated by the infant, who wears it full-time for 6-12 weeks after achieving hip stability (Hawk & Bailie, 2007). See Figure 11.2.

Figure 11.2. Proper Pavlik Harness Fit

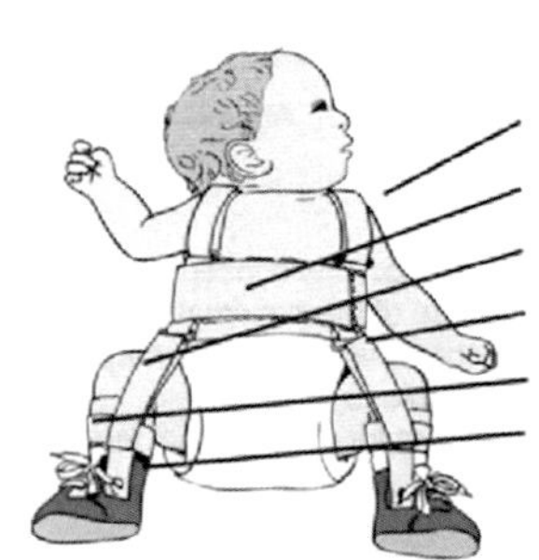

From "Hip and Femur" by L. Staheli, 2008, Fundamentals of Pediatric Orthopedics *(4th ed., p. 211), Philadelphia, PA: Lippincott Williams & Wilkins. Reproduced with permission.*

Possible complications from this treatment include an inferior hip dislocation and a femoral nerve compression from hyper-flexion at the hip, skin breakdown in the groin creases and the popliteal fossa, and damage to the femoral head and the epiphyseal plate. Between the ages of 6 months to 2 years, the Pavlik harness is more difficult to maintain, and a closed reduction and immobilization with a spica cast application may be done, possibly preceded by a period of traction. A spica cast (body cast) immobilizes the pelvis, hips, and legs. Traction stretches the soft tissues until the hip can be reduced without force to prevent avascular necrosis during the reduction.

Modified Bryant's traction (skin traction) with the hips flexed 45-60 degrees, rather than the 90 degrees of true Bryant's traction, can be done at home or in a hospital setting, usually for about 1-3 weeks, although the effectiveness of this has not been documented (Hawk & Bailie, 2007) and the need for traction is controversial (Staheli, 2008c). A closed reduction is tried first. If this is unsuccessful, an open reduction is required. An open reduction also may be necessary to remove tissues blocking the reduction, such as the labrum, ligamentum teres, or the fat pad, or to release soft tissues. This is followed by 12 weeks of immobilization in a spica cast. After the spica cast removal, an abduction brace is worn full-time for several months, then during nap time and during the night until the hip development is normal. In children older than age 2, an open reduction with a pelvic or femoral osteotomy is done to correct the bony deformity, and a femoral shortening may be necessary to prevent excessive pressure on the proximal femur. Both of these procedures are followed by immobilization in a spica cast (see Figure 11.3) (Hawk & Bailie, 2007).

Figure 11.3. Bilateral Long Leg Spica Cast

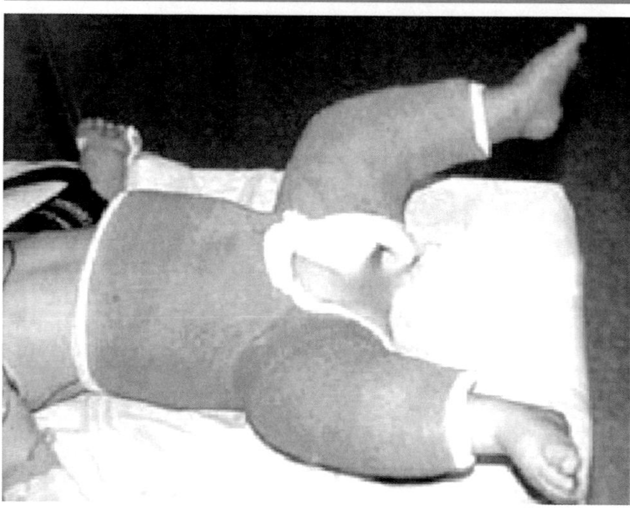

From Massachusetts General Hospital. Reproduced with permission.

Nursing Considerations

Nursing Diagnoses. Nursing diagnoses for this condition are expanded upon in the Appendix.

- Anxiety.
- Compartment syndrome, risk for.
- Mobility: physical, impaired.
- Peripheral neurovascular dysfunction, risk for.

Nursing Interventions. Nursing measures focused on decreasing patient/parental anxiety include developing a plan of care that minimizes undue anxiety, allows the patient/parents to express their fears/concerns related to the diagnosis and treatment plan, and includes the family in the decision-making process as much as feasible. Educate the patient (if appropriate) and parents about the pathology, the normal developmental progression of the diagnosis, the indicated treatment, and appropriate community resources, if applicable. The best outcome is a family that is well-educated about the condition and compliant with the treatment.

Nursing interventions to assess for compartment syndrome include the identification of pain out of proportion to the surgery, pain on passive muscle stretch, pallor of extremity, paresthesia or numbness, and pulselessness. Emergency equipment such as a cast cutter and spreader should be readlily available if needed. The ideal outcome is no evidence of compartment syndrome or, in the event of detection of cast syndrome, the prompt diagnosis and treatment of it (Kunkler, 2007).

Measures focused on the prevention of neurovascular compromise include the frequent assessment of the color, temperature of tissues, edema, pain, capillary refill, motor function, sensory function, and peripheral pulses of the extremity. The extremity should be correctly maintained, positioned, and elevated ("hands above the heart and toes above the nose") as tolerated. The best outcome is an extremity that is neurovascularly intact.

Interventions focusing on impaired physical mobility include promoting mobility within restrictions. Discuss and provide appropriate equipment to assist with mobility, plan alternate methods for patients to achieve developmental tasks to compensate for physical restrictions, teach the family how to hold/cuddle their child, and promote the use of the unaffected extremities. Provide age-appropriate diversional activities to alleviate boredom, stress, and fatigue. An optimal outcome is a content infant/child who is growing/developing despite impaired mobility (Hawk & Bailie, 2007).

Duchenne's Muscular Dystrophy

Overview

Duchenne's muscular dystrophy (DMD) is a hereditary myopathy characterized by progressive weakness in the proximal muscle groups and pseudohypertrophy. The muscular dystrophies are a group of genetic myopathies in which progressive muscle degeneration and weakness prevail. The myopathies primarily involve striate (skeletal) muscle and are not caused by impairment of the central nervous system, anterior horn cells, peripheral nerves, or the neuromuscular junctions. DMD is the most common form of muscular dystrophy (Hawk & Bailie, 2007). It is also referred to as Duchenne syndrome (Staheli, 2008b).

The etiology of DMD is the transmission by an X-linked recessive trait, and the single gene defect is found at the Xp21 region (Hawk & Bailie, 2007) on the short arm of the X-chromosome (Thompson & Berenson, 2006). Females are the carriers of the gene defect (Hawk & Bailie, 2007), and the disease is characterized by its occurrence exclusively in the males, except for rare cases associated with Turner syndrome. In this rare event, the XO karyotype that carries the defective gene may demonstrate the phenotype found in male patients with the disorder. DMD is associated with a high mutation rate, and a positive family history is present in approximately 65% of the cases. DMD occurs in about 1 in 3,500 live male births, with about one third of the children involved having acquired the disease because of a new mutation (Thompson & Berenson, 2006).

Due to the genetic defect, the body does not produce dsytrophin, a component of the surface membrane of a striated muscle cell. Necrosis is caused by the influx of Ca2+ into the muscle fiber through a defective surface membrane, and enzymes are lost from the sarcoplasm of the muscle into the circulation. Eventually there is a decrease in the number of muscle fibers due to the necrosis of fibers and accompanying phagocytosis. The regenerating fibers are structurally abnormal. Hip contractures develop to help maintain a standing posture as weakness in the hip girdle increases, and pseudohypertrophy of the muscles develop, as normal muscle is replaced with adipose and collagen. Cardiac involvement includes tachycardia and right ventricular hypertrophy (Hawk & Bailie, 2007). Life-threatening dysrhythmia or heart failure ultimately develops in approximately 10% of patients (Thompson & Berenson, 2006). Progressive scoliosis develops after ambulation is lost, and obesity may be related to limited physical activity, depression, and boredom. Gastrointestinal tract involvement including megacolon, volvulus, cramping pain, and malabsorption is rare. Patients typically have low-normal intelligence (Hawk & Bailie, 2007), and many also have a static encephalopathy, with mild or moderate mental retardation. Death from pulmonary failure and occasionally from cardiac failure occurs during the second or third decades of life (Thompson & Berenson, 2006).

A first trimester chorionic villous sampling can be done to determine the fetal gender and whether the deletion exists on the X chromosome. Although DMD is clinically evident when the child is between ages 3 and 6, an earlier onset may also occur (Thompson & Berenson, 2006). Most patients with DMD are wheelchair-bound by the end of the first decade, and adolescents are usually able to perform routine daily tasks with their arms, hands, and fingers. Complications of DMD include low back pain with hip flexion contractures, fractures, rapid deterioration of strength after immobilization in bed, pulmonary infections, respiratory insufficiency, sudden cardiac failure, and malignant hyperthermia with anesthesia. Only about 25% of patients survive beyond age 21 (Hawk & Bailie, 2007). See Table 11.4 for a synopsis of clinical features.

Assessment

The assessment of a child with DMD includes a history of the presenting symptoms. There likely will be a history of weakness in the proximal muscles, which descends symmetrically in the lower limbs. The pelvic girdle is

CHAPTER 11

affected first: the gluteus maximus, gluteus medius, and the quadriceps. The tibialis anterior and the abdominal muscles are also affected, with progression to the shoulder girdle and the trapezius, deltoid, and pectoralis major muscles. The lower facial muscles are affected later in the disease process (Hawk & Bailie, 2007). The family may have observed that the child's ability to achieve independent ambulation was delayed or that he has become a toe walker. Children ages 3 and older may demonstrate frequent episodes of tripping and falling, in addition to having difficulty in activities requiring reciprocal motion, such as running or climbing stairs.

Table 11.4. Clinical Features of Major Types of Muscular Dystrophy

	Duchenne's	Becker's	Limb-Girdle	Congenital Muscular Dystrophy	Fascio-Scapulohumeral	Distal
Incidence	Most common type	Less common than Duchenne's	Less common than Duchenne's and Becker's	Rare	Rare	Rare
Age at onset	Generally before age 3	Most between 5-15 years	Usually by second decade	At birth or soon after	Anytime from childhood until adulthood, usually in second decade	20-77 years; mean is 47 years
Sex distribution	Males; rare cases in females with Turner's syndrome	Males	Both sexes	Both sexes	More common in females	Both sexes
Inheritance	Sex-linked recessive gene; 33% due to mutations	Sex-linked recessive gene	Usually autosomal recessive; may occur as autosomal dominant	Not known	Usually autosomal dominant	Autosomal dominant
Pattern of muscle involvement onset	Proximal pelvis muscles; shoulder girdle muscles become involved 3-5 years later	Similar to Duchenne's	Proximal shoulder and pelvic girdle	Generalized muscle weakness, including respiratory and facial muscles	Face, shoulder girdle, upper arm	Distal; intrinsic muscles of hand, anterior tibiali, and calf
Late muscle involvement	All muscles, including facial, oculo-pharyngeal, and respiratory	Face is spared	More distal muscles; brachioradialis, hand, calf		Lower limbs	Proximal
Pseudohypertrophy	Calf muscles	Calf muscles	Occurs in fewer than 1/3 of cases	No	Rare	No
Contractural deformities	Common	Less common	Late, milder than Duchenne's	Severe	Mild, late	Mild, late
Scoliosis/ Kyphoscoliosis	Common late	Not severe	Mild, late	Yes	Mild, late	No
Cardiac involvement	Yes	Yes	Very rare	Not known	Very rare	Very rare
IQ	Decreased	Normal	Normal	Not known	Normal	Normal
Course	Steadily progressive	Slowly progressive	Variable; generally slowly progressive	Variable; rapidly progressive or can stabilize	Insidious with prolonged periods of apparent arrest	Slow progression

From Core Curriculum for Orthopaedic Nursing (6th ed., pp. 319-320), 2007, National Association of Orthopaedic Nurses, Boston, MA: Pearson. Reproduced with permission.

Inability to hop and jump normally is commonly present (Thompson & Berenson, 2006). Obtain information regarding the onset and progression of symptoms, and previous treatment. Ascertain the birth, developmental, and family history, and inquire about the child's current functional status (Hawk & Bailie, 2007).

If the child is ambulatory, observation of their walking will reveal an abnormal gait due to weakness of the hip girdle muscles (Hawk & Bailie, 2007). During gait the cadence is slow, and the child develops compensatory changes in gait and stance as weakness progresses. The child compensates by carrying the head and shoulders behind the pelvis, maintaining the weightline posterior to the hip joint and center of gravity. This produces an anterior pelvic tilt and increases lumbar lordosis (Thompson & Berenson, 2006). The child then develops a waddling (Hawk & Bailie, 2007), wide-based gait with shoulder sway to compensate for gluteus medius weakness (Thompson & Berenson, 2006). To get up from the floor, the child will use a maneuver known as the Gower's sign: the child walks his hands up the thighs to push the trunk into an erect position to compensate for quadriceps and gluteus maximus weakness. It is typically seen by age 5 or 6 (Hawk & Bailie, 2007). Weakness in the shoulder girdle, which occurs 3 to 5 years later, precludes the use of crutches to aid in ambulation. It also makes it difficult to lift the patient from under the arms. This tendency for the child to slip though a truncal grasp has been termed the Meyerson sign. Secondary to the child slipping through a truncal grasp, caregivers and hospital staff should be cognizant about safe lifting and use slings or mechanical devices. Pseudohypertrophy of the calf muscles caused by the accumulation of fat is common, but is not invariably present (Thompson & Berenson, 2006). Pseudohypertrophy can also occur in the vastus lateralis, infraspinous, and deltoid muscles. Deep tendon reflexes will be absent in the upper extremity and knee, but will be present in the ankle until late in the disease (Hawk & Bailie, 2007). Contractures of the iliotibial band and the Achilles tendon are the most consistent deformities noted during an examination of the child (Thompson & Berenson, 2006).

A clinical diagnosis is established by a physical examination, observation of the gait, identification of specific muscle weakness, and notation of the absence of sensory deficits. Myocardial weakness is a constant finding, with electrocardiogram (EKG) changes present in more than 90% of children with DMD (Thompson & Berenson, 2006). Diagnostic tests to confirm a diagnosis include a marked elevation of serum creatine phosphokinase (CPK) of 200-300 times the normal in the early stages of the disease (Hawk & Bailie, 2007). This level decreases as the disease progresses and muscle mass is reduced. There is elevation in other serum enzymes, specifically adolase and serum glutamic oxaloacetic transaminase (SGOT), but the elevations are not unique to striated muscle disease. Although electromyography (EMG) will support the diagnosis of a myopathy, this test is typically not necessary if the clinical findings and CPK are both suggestive of a muscular dystrophy. A muscle biopsy specimen reveals degeneration with subsequent loss of fiber, variation of fiber size, and proliferation of connective tissue and, subsequently, of adipose tissue as well (Thompson & Berenson, 2006). Pulmonary function testing should also be done (Hawk & Bailie, 2007).

Common Therapeutic Modalities

Although there is currently no treatment, surgery, or medication that halts disease progression, treatment with prednisone has been associated with short-term improvement and may prolong ambulation. Orthopaedic-related issues such as the loss of independent ambulation, the development of soft tissue contractures, and spinal deformities can be addressed with orthotics during the early stages of the disease. PT is aimed at prolonging functional muscle strength and preventing contractures, and includes active ROM exercises, gait training, and transfer techniques. Regular daily walking will enhance strength and prevent contractures, and ambulation may be achieved with crutches or walkers. When ambulation is no longer feasible, the child should be fitted with a motorized wheelchair and other appropriate equipment as needed (Hawk & Bailie, 2007).

Tendon releases can be done to address painful contractures or those that interfere with ADLs. These include equinus and equinovarus foot contractures, hip flexion and abduction contractures, and knee flexion contractures. Upper extremity contractures may be common but typically don't require treatment (Hawk & Bailie, 2007). Progressive neuromuscular scoliosis, which is present in 95% of patients with DMD, can be surgically treated with a segmental spinal fusion (Thompson & Berenson, 2006).

Nursing Considerations

Nursing Diagnoses. Nursing diagnoses for this condition are expanded upon in the Appendix.

- Activity intolerance.
- Disuse syndrome.
- Grieving.
- Mobility: physical, impaired.

Nursing Interventions. Interventions focused on activity intolerance include the teaching and promotion of an exercise program to strengthen unaffected muscles and prevent disuse weakness. The use of assistive and ambulatory aids should be encouraged as indicated.

The child's safety related to their ambulatory status and movements during sleep should be assessed, and appropriate aids should be utilized. The patient also should be encouraged to seek assistance as needed for difficult activities. An optimal outcome is a safe physical environment for the child.

Interventions focusing on disuse include maintaining musculoskeletal functioning by providing passive and active ROM to prevent contractures, maintaining functional body alignment, teaching the patient/family to assess body position and promote good positioning, collaborating with PT for exercise guidance and corrective treatment, using braces/splints/assistive devices as needed, and assessing the occurrence of spasms in relation to activity/movement and control them, if possible.

Nursing measures that focus on grieving include the encouragement of the verbalization of feeling/fears associated with perceived losses. Support the patient/family through the diagnostic period, assist them in indentifying lifestyle modifications, help identify sources of support, refer to appropriate disease-related support groups, provide spiritual counseling or psychological support as needed, and help the family recognize the child's strengths and skills while acknowledging limitations. Offer patient/ family information about the national and local chapter of the Muscular Dystrophy Association

Nursing measures that focus on impaired physical mobility include the promotion of mobility within the restrictions due to DMD. Discuss and provide appropriate equipment for mobility, and plan alternate methods for the patient to achieve developmental tasks to compensate for physical restrictions. Promote the use of unaffected extremities, and provide diversional activities to reduce boredom, stress, and fatigue. The best outcome is a content patient who is occupied, engaged in age-appropriate activities, and maintains mobility within the disease limitations (Hawk & Bailie, 2007).

Genu Valgum/Genu Varum

Overview

Genu valgum and genu varum are frontal plane deformities of the knee angle that fall outside the normal range of + or – 2 standard deviations of the mean. Knee angle variations that fall within the normal range are referred to as bowed legs, knock-knees, and physiologic variations (Staheli, 2008d) or physiologic bowing. The normal knee alignment at birth is 10-15 degrees of varus, which remodels to a neutral femoral-tibial angle at about 14 months of age (Schoenecker & Rich, 2006).

Genu varum is characterized by an increased distance (greater than 2.5 centimeters) between the knees when the child stands with the ankles together, and is often accompanied by internal tibial torsion. *Genu valgum* is characterized by in an increased distance (greater than 2.5 centimeters) between the ankles (medial malleoli) when the child stands with the knees together (Hawk & Bailie, 2007). Parents may be concerned with the cosmetic appearance of a bilateral bowing deformity and the associated problem of excessive tripping, but despite their bowlegged, toed-in gait, these young children are typically very agile walkers. Parental concerns regarding knock-knees are less common than those regarding bowed legs (Schoenecker & Rich, 2006).

The natural history of physiologic bowing is spontaneous correction by age 2. Physiologic vaglus develops between ages 3 and 4. Typically, valgus knee position becomes apparent after age 2, reaching a maximum femoral-tibial angle of 8-10 degrees at about age 3-4 and decreasing to an adult level of about 5-7 degrees by age 6-7. Although the conditions may persist into late childhood, this is uncommon.

Children with either physiologic or pathologic bowing are typically early walkers, achieving independent walking before the first year of life, and often there is a family history of bowed legs. *Physiologic bowing* is considered a normal developmental variation, and the entire lower extremity will appear to be bowed. In contrast, *pathologic bowing* has a more focal deformity limited to the proximal tibia, and occurs in infantile tibia vara (Blount's disease), metabolic bone disease (rickets), and skeletal dysplasias such as achondroplasia or pseudoachondroplasia. Pathologic genu valgum may be caused by:

- Rickets;
- Partial epiphyseal arrest on the lateral aspect of the proximal tibial or distal femoral epiphysis caused by a bony bar;
- Trauma;
- Osteomyelitis;
- Overgrowth of the tibia in relation to the fibula due to fracture of the proximal tibial metaphysis;
- Overgrowth due to chronic synovitis of juvenile arthritis; or
- Severely pronated feet (Hawk & Bailie, 2007).

A child with achondroplasia will be short, typically below the fifth percentile. A child with pseudoachondroplasia may present with a varus deformity, although a valgus deformity is sometimes present in association with ligamentous laxity. Metaphyseal chondrodsyplasia (Schmid or McKuscik type) typically presents with persistent bowing and short stature in an otherwise normal-appearing child (Schoenecker & Rich, 2006).

Angular variations are a normal part of growth and development. All infants are born with bowed legs, which typically improve by 18 months to 2 years of age. Knock-knees develop around age 2-3 and increases until age 3-4. It typically improves around age 7-8. The normal alignment in adults is slight varus.

Pathologic genu varum and genu valgum are beyond the normal developmental sequence, and the deformities rapidly progress. Heuter Volkmann's law of epiphyseal growth states that compression inhibits growth and distraction stimulates growth. Compression on one side of the physis will slow growth and lead to continuing deformity as the opposite side grows normally (Hawk & Bailie, 2007).

The clinical and radiographic features associated with metabolic bone disease or skeletal dysplasia readily differentiates these pathologic conditions from physiologic bowing (Schoenecker & Rich, 2006). Physiologic knock-knees are usually symmetric, and the severity of the deformity can be easily assessed and documented. Genu valgum is a persistent knock-knee in a young child, but more often develops during early adolescence. Knee pain is a common feature, along with medial foot pain. The clinical deformity is often more striking than the radiographic appearance, and it may be associated with an out-toeing gait and a flat foot, or pes planus. Pathologic genu valgum arises from asymmetric growth in the distal femur that does not spontaneously resolve. In some cases, the proximal tibia is also abnormal. Skeletal dysplasias most typically associated with genu valgum are chondroectodermal dysplasia (Ellis-van Creveld), mucopolysaccharidosis type IV, and spondyloepiphyseal dysplasia tarda. Benign neoplastic processes such as multiple hereditary exostoses and focal fibrocartilaginous dysplasia may also produce a genu valgum deformity. Many children with genu valgum are above the 90% in height and weight (Schoenecker & Rich, 2006). The incidence of bowed legs or knock-knees is common in some families, and genu varum and genu valgum tend to occur more often in African American and Asian children (Hawk & Bailie, 2007). See Table 11.1 in the section on Blount's disease for a comparison of the conditions.

Assessment

The assessment of a child with physiologic or pathologic alignment issues includes obtaining information about the presenting symptoms, as well as the onset, progression, and prior treatment. Possible symptoms may be pain, difficulty with ambulation, or fatigue associated with walking long distances. The birth, developmental, past medical/surgical history, and family history should be elicited, in addition to parental concerns such as cosmesis or concerns with the child's gait or function (Hawk & Bailie, 2007).

Accurate measurements of the child's height and weight should be recorded. The child should be evaluated, noting rotational abnormalities of the lower limbs and whether they are symmetric or asymmetric. The child should be observed walking and running, with attention to a medial or lateral thrust, which indicates joint instability or ligamentous laxity. Genu varum can be assessed by measuring the distance between the knees when the medial malleoli are touching. Genu valgum can be determined by measuring the distance between the medial malleoli when the medial femoral condyles are touching. An assessment of the child's feet should note the presence or absence of pes planus (Hawk & Bailie, 2007).

If a pathologic deformity is suspected, an AP standing radiograph of the lower extremities with patellae forward is indicated (Hawk & Bailie, 2007), and is best for assessing the mechanical axis and any deviation of joint alignment (Schoenecker & Rich, 2006). A lateral view radiograph should be done if a sagittal deformity is suspected, and a skeletal survey is indicated if skeletal dysplasia is thought to be present. Pathologic genu varum is a femoral-tibial angle of 25 degrees of varus, and pathologic genu valgum is a femoral-tibial angle of 15 degrees of valgus (Hawk & Bailie, 2007). To rule out a physeal bar, an MRI may be indicated (Staheli, 2008d). A metabolic screening panel is indicated if a systemic condition is suspected (Hawk & Bailie, 2007).

Common Therapeutic Modalities

In cases of physiologic bowed legs or knock-knees, no treatment is needed as the leg alignment will correct over time without any interventions. The use of bracing has not been shown to alter the natural history of the condition. If a child has a systemic condition such as rickets, treatment should be guided by a pediatric endocrinologist.

In cases of pathologic malalignment, surgical correction is indicated. To address genu varum, an opening-wedge osteotomy of the proximal tibia is indicated, with application of a long-leg cast for 6-8 weeks. The application of an external fixator, after a proximal tibial osteotomy, may be done to stabilize bone fragments and to lengthen the extremity, if necessary. A tibial osteotomy with a plate and screw fixation can also be utilized to correct the deformity. Genu valgum is addressed by a closing-wedge osteotomy of the distal femur and application of a long-leg cast for 6-8 weeks (Hawk & Bailie, 2007). A hemistapling or a hemiepiphysiodesis can be done to stop the growth on one side of the physis so that growth on the deficient side of the bone can catch up. Hemistapling is done after age 10, while the physis is still open. The use of "8 Plate" fixation can also be used for growth arrest, and the timing of these procedures is critical so that remaining growth can correct the angular deformity (Hawk & Bailie, 2007). When correction is achieved, the staples are removed. The use of bone age radiographs and charts indicating a child's remaining growth until skeletal maturity are used to determine the appropriate timing of surgery (Staheli, 2008d).

Nursing Considerations

Nursing Diagnoses. Nursing diagnoses for this condition are expanded upon in the Appendix.

- Anxiety.
- Peripheral neurovascular dysfunction, risk for.
- Self-concept, readiness for enhanced.

Nursing Interventions. Interventions related to patient/parental anxiety include allowing the family to express their fears/concerns related to the diagnosis and treatment plan. Include the patient/family in the decision-making process, and provide education regarding the underlying pathology, the normal developmental progression, treatment, community resources, and genetic counseling. If a child is symptomatic, as in knee pain associated with the angular deformity, suggest rest, elevation, use of over-the-counter analgesics, and heat or ice. If treatment includes surgery with an external fixator, reinforce the idea of gradual correction of the deformity over 3-6 months and emphasize the need for weekly appointments during the correction phase. The prescribed pin care should be explained and demonstrated, and the signs/symptoms of a pin site infection should be taught. The best outcome is a patient/family able to express their fears and concerns, understand the pathology and developmental progression of the condition, and comply with the recommended treatment plan (Hawk & Bailie, 2007).

Interventions focused on risk for peripheral neurovascular dysfunction include the frequent assessment of the affected extremity and a resting splint to prevent a heelcord contracture. The family should be taught how to assess the extremity and whom to contact if a problem arises. (See Compartment Syndrome in Chapter 8—Complications). The best outcome is a neurovascularly intact extremity (Hawk & Bailie, 2007).

Nursing measures for a disturbed self-concept include the promotion of a positive self-concept by focusing on the whole patient, reinforcing the child's personal strengths and skills, recognizing the reaction of parents/caregivers as influencing the child's response, encouraging the attainment of developmental skills consistent with age, providing consistent feedback, and praising the mastery of each new skill. Allow the child to regain as much control as possible over self-care by allowing choices when possible, such as with the daily routine, food choices, etc. Encourage the child to visually explore and touch the affected part, and slowly help the child to care for the area and become self-sufficient. Teach the child self-help skills, and provide opportunities for the child to demonstrate independence in self-care. An ideal outcome is the identification of strengths and weaknesses and the attainment of developmental skills that are consistent with the child's age (Hawk & Bailie, 2007). If a child has a systemic condition that causes the malalingnment, promote medical follow-up and management (Hawk & Bailie, 2007).

Legg-Calve-Perthes Disease

Overview

Legg-Calve-Perthes Disease, or simply Perthes, is an idiopathic juvenile avascular necrosis of the femoral head (Staheli, 2008c). Also known as coxa plana, it is a self-limiting condition affecting children of both genders, although boys are diagnosed more frequently than girls. Perthes remains one of the most controversial topics in pediatric orthopaedic surgery, and debate about its etiology, pathogenesis, and treatment continues (Weinstein, 2006b).

Although the etiology remains unknown, there are many theories regarding its cause. Affected children are usually small and delayed in maturation, which suggests a constitutional disorder. Vascularity is tenous during early childhood, and developmental variations in vascular pattern are more common in boys, which predisposes some individuals (Staheli, 2008c). Other causal theories include heredity, metabolic, chemical, or mechanical pathology, such as trauma, synovitis with increased fluid pressure within the joint, excessive femoral neck anteversion, endocrine, or metabolic disorders (Hawk & Bailie, 2007). Alterations in blood coaguability (Staheli, 2008c), including protein C and S deficiencies, may also contribute to the development of Perthes (Weinstein, 2006b). There are possibly several factors that combine to cause the condition (Staheli, 2008c).

The pathology of Perthes is consistent with repeated bouts of infarction and subsequent pathologic fractures. Synovitis and effusion, cartilaginous hypertrophy, bony necrosis, and collapse are present (Staheli, 2008c). Cellular changes in the epiphyseal and physeal cartilage occur, and disorganization of the physeal plate, along with minimal trauma, may interrupt blood vessels to the femoral head and cause necrosis (Staheli, 2008c). In the physeal plate, premature closure with resultant deformity, such as central physeal arrest, causes shortening of the neck of the femur and trochanteric overgrowth (Weinstein, 2006b). Widening and flattening of the femoral head follow.

Most deformity occurs in the fragmentation phase. If necrosis is extensive and the support of the lateral pillar is lost, the femoral head collapses, mild subluxation of the hip occurs, and pressure from the lateral acetabular margin creates a depression or "furrow" in the femoral head (Staheli, 2008c).

During the healing phase, the blood supply starts from the periphery and progresses centrally, and irregular areas of bone deposition and resorption occur (Hawk & Bailie, 2007). During this time, the femoral head will deform according to the asymmetric repair process and the applied stresses. The molding action of the acetabulum during new bone formation may also play a role in this process. With deformity of the femoral head, the acetabulum—particularly its lateral aspect—is deformed secondarily. In addition, there is abnormal ossification of the disorganized matrix of the epiphyseal cartilage. Finally, there is periosteal bone growth and reactivation of the physeal plate along the femoral neck, with abnormally long cartilage columns leading to coxa magna and a widened femoral neck (Weinstein, 2006b).Although the blood supply returns, the duration of the disease process is unpredictable. The residual deformity will vary, depending on the effectiveness of treatment (Hawk & Bailie, 2007) and the duration of the disease. This is proportional to the extent of epiphyseal involvement, the age of the patient at disease onset, the remodeling potential of the patient, and the stage of disease when treatment is initiated. Another factor is the type of treatment chosen (Weinstein, 2006b). In young children, the deformity remodels, and the acetabulum becomes congruous. At maturation, the head is reasonably round, and the prognosis is fair to good. If growth arrest occurs, or if the child is older, remodeling is limited, and the capacity of the acetabulum to remodel to congruity is reduced and osteoarthritis is likely in adult life (Staheli, 2008c).

Perthes occurs in about 1:10,000 children and is seen predominantly in males 4:1 (Hawk & Bailie, 2007). It most commonly occurs between ages 4 and 8, but cases have been reported from age 2 into the late teenage years. There is a higher incidence of Perthes in lower socioeconomic groups, and it is more common in certain geographic areas, particularly in urban rather than rural communities. There is also a reported association (33% of patients with the condition) with the psychological profile associated with attention deficit hyperactivity disorder (Weinstein, 2006b). Although bilateral involvement occurs in 10%-15% of cases, (Hawk & Bailie, 2007), with usually more than a year interval between onsets, bilateral symmetrical involvement is very rare (Staheli, 2008c).

The prognosis for Perthes is fair. The most important prognostic factor is the sphericity of the femoral head at skeletal maturation, and this sphericity is related to the age of onset of the condition. The younger the child's age, the more likely the femoral head will be spherical. The longer the period between the completion of healing and skeletal maturity, the longer the period of remodeling. This remodeling cannot occur if a physeal bridge develops. Although physeal bridging occurs more frequently in the older child, it can occur in young patients and accounts for the occasional poor result seen in these young children.

During late childhood and adolescence, children may experience episodes of pain with vigorous activity. These painful episodes are transient, often lasting a day or two (Staheli, 2008c). Most affected children are active and pain-free in adulthood (Hawk & Bailie, 2007), but more persistent disability may develop during late adult life due to osteoarthritis.

In children diagnosed after age 8-9, the need for a total joint replacement will be increased. Complications including hip subluxation, a subchondral fracture, and deformity of the epiphysis may occur, and residual deformities such as coxa magna, premature epiphyseal closure, and an irregular femoral head may result (Staheli, 2008).

Assessment

The child's presenting symptoms may be an antalgic limp or mild pain (Staheli, 2008c), localized to the groin or the medial aspect of the thigh or knee (Hawk & Bailie, 2007). Frequently the child has had pain and a limp for several months being before seen (Staheli, 2008c). The child's history often reveals pain that has been aggravated by physical activity and relieved by rest. The onset and progression of symptoms should be elicited, along with changes in the child's pattern of play or physical activities. The child's height and weight should be recorded to rule out a growth disorder or systemic problem (Hawk & Bailie, 2007). The child will most likely be comfortable, and the examination will be normal except for the involved leg (Staheli, 2008c). The child may position the affected leg in slight flexion and abduction, and may have a hip adduction contracture (Hawk & Bailie, 2007). A Trendelenburg sign may be present, and mild atrophy is often seen. The most prominent finding is stiffness and limited internal rotation of the hip. Abduction is almost always limited, and flexion is the least affected (Staheli, 2008). Pain with abduction and internal rotation is likely to be present, and muscle spasms and a limb length inequality also may be noted (Hawk & Bailie, 2007).

In the majority of cases, only AP and frog-leg lateral view radiographs of the pelvis/hips are necessary to establish the diagnosis of Perthes and provide management (Hawk & Bailie, 2007; Staheli, 2008c), but an arthrogram may be indicated to determine if the femoral head can be contained in the acetabulum (Hawk & Bailie, 2007). Radiographically, Perthes can be classified into four stages: initial, fragmentation, reossification, and healed.

1. In the *initial* radiographic stage, one of the first signs is failure of the femoral ossific nucleus to increase in size because of a lack of blood supply.

The affected femoral head appears smaller than the opposite, unaffected ossific nucleus. Widening of the medial joint space is another early radiographic finding. Some researchers have theorized that widening is caused by synovitis, and other have proposed that this finding is secondary to decreased head volume caused by necrosis and collapse and a secondary increase in blood flow to the soft tissue parts, causing the head to displace laterally.

2. The second radiographic stage is the *fragmentation* phase, when the repair aspects of the condition become more prominent. The bony epiphysis begins to fragment, and there are areas of increased radiolucency and increased radiodensity. (See Figure 11.4)
3. The third radiographic stage is the reparative or *resossification* phase. Radiographically normal bone density returns, with radiodensities appearing in areas that were formerly radiolucent. Alterations in the shape of the head and neck become apparent.
4. The final radiographic stage is the *healed* phase. In this stage, the proximal femur may have residual deformity from the disease and repair process (Weinstein, 2006b).

Numerous other disorders cause clinical and radiographic changes similar to Perthes. Although these are relatively rare, they should at least be considered before the conclusive diagnosis of Perthes is made: multiple epiphyseal dysplasia, spondyloeiphyseal dysplasia, sickle cell disease, lupus erythematosis, hypothyroidism, septic arthritis, femoral neck fractures, toxic synovitis, and lymphoma.

Figure 11.4.
Second Radiographic Stage of Perthes

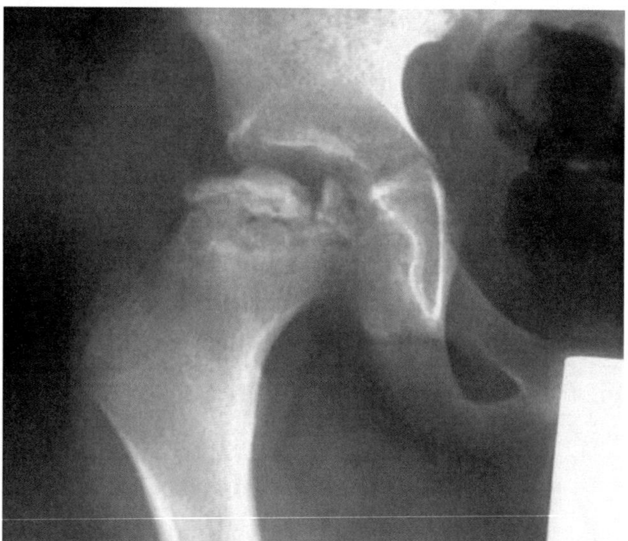

From "Hip and Femur" by L. Staheli, 2008, Fundamentals of Pediatric Orthopedics, *(4th ed., p. 218), Philadelphia, PA: Lippincott Williams & Wilkins. Reproduced with permission.*

Common Therapeutic Modalities

The management objective of Perthes is to preserve the sphericity of the femoral head to reduce the risk of stiffness and degenerative arthritis while preserving the emotional well-being of the child. The management of Perthes is very controversial; in the past, treatment regimens have varied from operating on every case to no treatment at all. Children of any age with minimal involvement do not require treatment. In some cases of Perthes, providing containment of the femoral head to maintain or improve the sphericity of the head requires positioning of the hip in abduction in a brace, or a surgical procedure that increases acetabular coverage of the femoral head. An abduction orthosis, such as a Scottish Rite orthosis, maintains the femoral head in an abducted and internally rotated position, maintains desirable hip ROM, and allows for weight-bearing. This orthosis is not always psychologically acceptable (Hawk & Bailie, 2007) and may be especially difficult for an emotionally dysfunctional child (Staheli, 2008c). Gaining motion by curtailing activity has its limits. What constitutes satisfactory ROM is seldom defined, but a minimum of about 20 degrees of abduction is acceptable. Some experts cite controlling the cost of management and advocate conventional radiographs, rest at home, and the selective use of imaging and procedures, which provides optimum care at the least cost (Staheli, 2008c).

Surgical treatments include a varus osteotomy of the proximal femur, with or without derotation, which positions the femoral head in the acetabulum, and an inominate osteotomy of the pelvis to redirect the acetabulum to provide better anterolateral coverage of the femoral head (Hawk & Bailie, 2007).

Criteria for salvage treatment options include a patient who presents at a later stage of the condition, a hip deformity that cannot be contained using other methods, and a femoral head that has lost containment. In these cases, salvage procedures may include an abduction extension osteotomy, lateral shelf arthroplasty, Chiari ostoetomy, and cheiliectomy (Weinstein, 2006b).

Nursing Considerations

Nursing Diagnoses. Nursing diagnoses for this condition are expanded upon in the Appendix.

- Anxiety.
- Pain, acute.
- Physical activity, impaired.

Nursing Interventions. Interventions focused on anxiety allow the patient/family to express fears/concerns related to the diagnosis/treatment plan and include the family in the decision-making process. Provide education regarding the underlying pathology, the normal developmental progression (with an emphasis on the erratic improvement and possibly uncertain prognosis of Perthes), the treatment, and appropriate community resources, as indicated. The best outcome is an expressive patient/family with an understanding of the pathology, progression, and treatment of Perthes, along with knowledge of community resources.

Interventions related to acute pain include promoting appropriate pharmacologic and nonpharmacologic techniques such as analgesics/NSAIDs, distraction, play activities, heat, and relaxation. Encourage age-appropriate diversional activities and control environmental factors that precipitate or increase the pain in children with Perthes such as vigorous physical activity. The best outcome is a comfortable child.

Interventions focused on impaired physical activity include teaching the family and child (as appropriate) ways to promote mobility within activity restrictions related to the disease process. Discuss and provide equipment to assist with mobility, help plan alternate methods for the child to achieve developmental tasks to compensate for physical restrictions, promote the use of unaffected extremities, and provide diversional activities. Also support the family's efforts to enforce the prescribed activity restrictions. An optimal outcome is a child who maintains mobility within activity restrictions and who is able to complete normal developmental tasks (Hawk & Bailie, 2007).

Leg Length Discrepancies

Overview

Leg length discrepancies, leg length inequality, and leg length differences (LLD) are also known as anisomelia (Staheli, 2008e). LLDs are most commonly due to length differences in the tibia and/or femur (Hawk & Bailie, 2007). LLDs may be functional secondary to a joint contracture, which produces an apparent discrepancy in length, or structural, which may occur in any site of the limb or pelvis. Often, only discrepancies of the tibia or femur are measured. The height of the foot and pelvis also should be included in calculating the total disparity (Staheli, 2008e).

The causes of LLD are numerous (Staheli, 2008e) and may result from the process that changes the length of the leg directly or that alters growth. Direct changes in leg length can result from trauma such as fractures, bone loss, unreduced dislocations, a malunion due to overriding or an angular deformity, a congenital limb shortening or deficiency, or an angular malalignment. A LLD may also occur due to inhibition of growth, as seen in congenital short bones possibly due to faulty genetic programming, injury to the physis from trauma, infection, or tumor, avascular necrosis, or paralysis, in which there is slowing of bone growth due to lack of compression forces across the growth plate. Growth may be stimulated by a tumor, such as vascular malformations, or hemangiomatosis, which produces growth stimulation involving all physes, or certain nonvascular tumors, seen in fibrous dysplasia, neurofibromatosis, or Wilm's tumor. Inflammation and subsequent overgrowth may occur from increased blood flow. Overgrowth after a fracture is thought to result from increased blood flow and may also be a cause of a leg length difference (Hawk & Bailie, 2007). Minor LLDs are seen in clubfeet, hip dysplasia, and Perthes disease, and major discrepancies are seen in tibial, fibular, and femoral agenesis (Staheli, 2008e).

Growth in the leg occurs at four epiphyseal growth plates at the proximal and distal femoral physes and at the proximal and distal tibial physes. Seventy percent of growth occurs at the growth plates around the knee. Inhibition or stimulation of growth at any physis can result in a LLD, and a congenital or acquired loss of bone can change the leg length directly. The difference in leg length will increase proportionately as a child grows. Consequences of a LLD include an abnormal gait, difficult ambulation, contractures in the contralateral leg, and degenerative joint disease (Hawk & Bailie, 2007). A limb length difference in childhood does not lead to an increased risk of structural scoliosis or back pain in adults (Staheli, 2008e).

Assessment

A complete history of the patient, the discrepancy, and its previous treatment should be obtained. The cause of the LLD is important because knowledge of whether length, growth, or both is affected is essential to understanding the growth pattern. Also important is knowledge of the affected physeal plates because this permits an estimation of the future increase in the discrepancy. The history of surgery, including surgery to correct angular deformity, is needed because the numeric data about leg lengths can be misinterpreted if the examiner is unaware of previous surgery that might have affected the leg lengths. The history, which delineates the cause, associated deformity, and neuromuscular deficits, is referred to during selection of the treatment goal. The fact that a patient's discrepancy is of congenital origin suggests increased risk and indicates certain precautionary steps to avoid complications in conjunction with lengthening. Instability of an adjacent joint can preclude lengthening. Weakness of the leg suggests that the weak leg should be left a little short to facilitate floor clearance during swing phase (Moseley, 2006).

The child's presenting symptoms such as a limp or awkward gait, knee or hip pain, unhappiness with the physical appearance of the inequality, or difficulty with physical activities related to the LLD should be elicited, in addition to parental concerns about the gait, function, or cosmesis (Hawk & Bailie, 2007). The physical examination of the child should record accurate height, evaluate the spine to assess for deformity or scoliosis, assess the pelvis for obliquity, and measure the apparent and real leg lengths. The apparent leg length, determined by a tape measure from the umbilicus to the tip of the medial malleolus, is affected by pelvic obliquity, hip position, and contractures of the hip and knee. The real length of each leg is measured from the anterior superior iliac spine to the tip of the medial malleolus. Soft tissue contractures of the knee and hip tend to shorten the leg, and heelcord contractures (equinus) tend to lengthen the leg length (Hawk & Bailie, 2007). A difference between the measured real and apparent discrepancies indicates that pelvic obliquity is present (Moseley, 2006).

Radiologic measurements of the leg lengths are more accurate than clinical methods, but each has its advantages and disadvantages (Moseley, 2006). Generally, a series of radiographs over time are needed to evaluate an altered pattern of growth. Measurements from the radiographs are plotted on the Moseley graph to evaluate the growth pattern, which helps predict future discrepancies and the timing of surgical procedures (Hawk & Bailie, 2007).

A teloradiograph is a single exposure of both legs on a long film, usually with the child standing and with a radiopaque ruler placed on the cassette. Its advantage is showing angular deformities with a single exposure, and its disadvantage is measurements that are subject to magnification because of parallax of the x-ray beam.

The orthoradiograph avoids the magnification factor by taking separate exposures of the hip, knee, and ankle so that the central beam passes through the joints, giving true readings from the scale. This requires multiple exposures and introduces the risk of error if the child moves.

The scanogram also takes separate exposures of the hip, knee, and ankle, and avoids magnification in the same way, but reduces the size of the resulting film by moving the film cassette beneath the patient between exposures.

Digital photography can be used to measure leg length, and CT can be used to measure the distances between points on the radiographic film, reducing errors from angular deformity. If the examination is done specifically for this purpose, the cost is comparable with more traditional techniques, multiple sections are unnecessary, and the radiation exposure is less, especially with microdose techniques. (Moseley, 2006).

A standing AP view of the spine to evaluate scoliosis, standing AP view of the pelvis to evaluate pelvic obliquity, and a bone age x-ray to determine skeletal maturity can also be done to assist with planning appropriate treatment (Hawk & Bailie, 2007). Whatever technique is used to measure leg length, it is important to be consistent and to not mix true and magnified measurements when analyzing data. Because errors are possible with all techniques, the resulting measurements should be compared with, and correspond to, the clinical measurements (Moseley, 2006).

Common Treatment Modalities

The choice of treatment of a LLD depends on the expected size of the discrepancy at skeletal maturity. For differences of 0-2cm, no treatment is necessary. For differences of 2-6cm, a shoe lift, epiphysiodesis, or shortening is typically recommended. For differences of 6-20cm, a lengthening procedure, which may or may not be combined with other procedures, is suggested. A limb lengthening process with external fixation is common. The process involves applying an external fixator with threaded bars that will cause the fixator ends to move apart when the threaded bar or bars are turned, typically a quarter turn every 6 hours. The cortex of the bone is cut circumferentially, and the bone ends are slowly drawn apart by the micro-turns over the course of months. This continued movement of the bone ends, away from each other, prevents the bone from healing and produces new bone, making cells to fill the gap. When the desired bone length is achieved, the turning schedule stops and the bone is allowed to heal. The fixator is dynamized (allowing compression of the bone) and later removed when the new bone is deemed strong enough. This is typically done in adolescence and takes months to a year to complete. The process creates challenges and can be quite painful for the patient. For differences of more than 20cm, fitting with a prosthesis is recommended. There is some flexibility in these guidelines to account for factors such as environment, motivation, intelligence, compliance, emotional stability, patient's and parents' wishes, and associated pathology in the limbs (Moseley, 2006).

Discrepancies of less than 2cm are of no functional consequence and do not require treatment. Lengthening of a limb is not generally done for discrepancies of less than 6cm because of the high morbidity and complication rate of lengthening. In these cases, other alternatives are more favorable, such as an epiphysiodesis or shortening procedure. The site of correction is chosen with the ultimate goal of making the patient's body as symmetrical as possible, with knees being as level as possible (Moseley, 2006).

Nursing Considerations

Nursing Diagnoses. Nursing diagnoses for this condition are expanded upon in the Appendix.

- Infection, risk for.
- Mobility: physical, impaired.
- Pain, acute.

- Pain, chronic.
- Peripheral vascular dysfunction, risk for.
- Self-concept, readiness for enhanced.
- Skin integrity, impaired.

Nursing Interventions. Nursing interventions are based on the amount of leg length inequality and the recommended treatment. Postoperatively, children with external fixators need regular skin assessment. Frequent turning/positioning to keep the skin clean/dry/intact should be done in the hospital setting and at home using pressure-reducing or pressure-relieving devices such as air mattresses or special beds. Parents should be taught how to lengthen the device and develop/post a schedule for turning, assess the skin and its neurovascular status, check for signs/symptoms of compartment syndrome, properly align the affected limb, and avoid thermal injuries from external fixators being exposed to extreme temperatures. The caretakers also need to be taught proper pin care and to be aware of signs/symptoms of an infection, such as erythema, edema, or drainage at the pin sites. If fever and/or malaise are present, caretakers should know whom to contact so that child can be assessed by an appropriate provider and so the appropriate treatment can be started, as indicated. The best outcome is the maintenance of skin integrity (Hawk & Bailie, 2007). See Chapter 6—Effects of Immobility and Chapter 10—Therapeutic Modalities.

Interventions focusing on both acute pain and chronic pain include the frequent assessment of the child's pain using an age-appropriate assessment tool and observing for nonverbal cues, especially in those who cannot communicate effectively. Promote patient comfort by using appropriate pharmacologic and nonpharmalogic techniques such as muscle relaxants, antispasmodics and analgesics, rocking, holding/cuddling, distraction, play activities, moist heat, ice, and relaxation. Handle the child gently, and position the child to prevent problems such as muscle spasms. Encourage diversional activities, and control environmental factors that precipitate or increase the pain experience. Discuss coping methods with the patient/family, and promote family participation in providing comfort. See Chapter 7—Pain. An ideal outcome is a patient who demonstrates a maximal degree of comfort.

Measures focused on preventing and identifying ineffective tissue perfusion include performing frequent bilateral neurovascular assessments. The limbs should be evaluated for color, temperature of the tissues, pain, capillary refill, motor function, sensory function, and peripheral pulses. Symptoms suggestive of compartment syndrome include pain that is out of proportion to the surgery, pain on passive muscle stretch, pallor of extremity, paresthesia or numbness, and pulselessness. Emergency equipment such as a cast cutter and spreader should be readily available if needed. Ice bags can be used to reduce edema for 48 hours, and heat can be used after 48-72 hours. The best outcome is an intact neurovascular status, which includes capillary refill within 1-3 seconds, strong peripheral pulses, and an extremity that is pink in color or normal compared to the unaffected limb (Kunkler, 2007).

Interventions focused on promoting mobility with restrictions include the discussion and provision of equipment to assist with mobility, planning alternate methods for the patient to achieve developmental tasks to compensate for physical restrictions, and promoting the use of unaffected extremities. Age-appropriate diversion should be offered to the child to alleviate boredom, stress, and fatigue. An ideal outcome is a child who maintains mobility within activity restrictions and who participates in diversional activities.

For those children with a major difference, interventions to promote a positive self-concept include focusing on the whole patient, reinforcing personal strengths/skills, encouraging the attainment of developmental skills consistent with the patient's age, providing consistent feedback, and praising the mastery of new skills. When possible, allow the child to make choices and provide opportunities for the child to demonstrate self-care. An optimal outcome is a child whose strengths and skills are identified and who attains appropriate developmental skills (Hawk & Bailie, 2007).

Metatarsus Adductus

Overview

Metatarsus adductus, the most common foot deformity of infants and children, is characterized by a flexible convexity of the lateral aspect of the foot. It is a positional deformity that occurs in late intrauterine life. It is a common, flexible, and benign condition, and 90% of cases resolve spontaneously (Staheli, 2008a).

The varus deviation is located at the tarsometatarsal joints and is most prominent at the first joint. The deviation decreases in severity from the great toe to the small toe, and the hindfoot usually remains in a neutral position. In a severe case, the exaggerated convexity of the lateral foot border may lead to excessive weight-bearing forces on the fifth metatarsal, varying degrees of supination, and improper fitting of shoes. Metatarsus adductus tends to run in families and is seen more often with twin pregnancies. It occurs in 1 in 1,000 births, affecting boys and girls equally. The condition generally improves as a child grows and matures (Hawk & Bailie, 2007).

There are two clinical classifications systems to define this condition. One is known as the heel bisector, in which the heel is placed on a photocopy machine, and the axis of the heel is projected through the forefoot or a similar line is drawn on the plantar surface of the foot. The heel bisector moves laterally across the toes with increasing severity of the condition. The second classification defines metatarsus adductus based on flexibility by holding the heel with a thumb, providing a fulcrum over the fifth metatarsal head, while pressure is applied laterally to the forefoot. The degree to which the lateral border of the foot can be corrected determines the flexibility of the foot (Kasser, 2006).

Assessment

The assessment of the patient includes obtaining the birth and developmental history, past medical and surgical history, and the family history. Parental concerns regarding gait, function, and cosmesis should be ascertained also. The examination of the foot will reveal an adducted forefoot that may be mildly supinated. The great toe will be in varus, with a widened interval between the first and second toes. Ankle and foot dorsiflexion will be normal. The forefoot will be correctable to neutral, but will return to adduction when released (Hawk & Bailie, 2007).

Because metatarsus adductus is associated with hip dysplasia in 2% of cases, a careful hip evaluation is essential (Staheli, 2008a). The use of radiographs is not indicated for diagnosing metatarsus adductus, as the diagnosis is based on clinical findings. When a persistent deformity is present, however, a standing or simulated weight-bearing x-ray of the foot will demonstrate a trapezoidal shape to the medial cuneiform and medial deviation of the metatarsals (Kasser, 2006).

Common Treatment Modalities

The management of metatarsus adductus is based on its flexibility and consideration of the child's age. Manage metatarsus addcutus by serial casting or bracing. Long-leg bracing is useful in the toddler, and serial casting is most effective. The deformity yields much more rapidly when the cast is extended above the flexed knee (Staheli, 2008a), and the infant is less likely to kick off the casts as easily. The long-leg cast allows walking in ambulatory children, effective correction, and controls tibial rotation (Hawk & Bailie, 2007).

Surgical interventions may be required with a severe, residual deformity in the older child (Hawk & Bailie, 2007), although some experts advocate accepting the deformity, as it does not cause disability. In severe cases, opening-wedge cuneiform osteotomies and closing-wedge cuboid osteotomies are recommended (Staheli, 2008a), which can be combined with osteotomies of the second, third, and fourth metatarsals at the bases, to provide better correction (Kasser, 2006).

Nursing Considerations

Nursing Diagnoses. Nursing diagnoses for this condition are expanded upon in the Appendix.

- Anixety.
- Peripheral neurovascular dysfunction, risk for.
- Skin integrity, impaired.

Nursing Interventions. To address parental anxiety, provide reassurance and support to parents about the usual benign nature of metatarsus adductus and its probable spontaneous resolution as the infant grows. Provide education regarding the pathology, normal developmental progression, and treatment of observation over time. The best outcome is a family that understands the probable resolution of the condition and possible future serial casting or surgical intervention if the condition does not resolve (Hawk & Bailie, 2007).

To prevent and/or identify peripheral neurovascular dysfunction and ineffective tissue perfusion, the extremity should be frequently assessed. The color, temperature of tissues, edema, pain, capillary refill, motor function, sensory function and peripheral pulses should be evaluated in the affected extremity, and the unaffected extremity should also be assessed and compared with the affected limb. An ideal outome is an extremity with capillary refill within 1-3 seconds, strong pulses, and normal color as compared to the unaffected limb (Kunkler, 2007).

Myelomeningocele

Overview

Myelomeningocele is a neural tube defect (NTD) involving the spinal cord, the meninges, and the vertebral bodies. The neural tube eventually develops into the brain and spinal cord (Hawk & Bailie, 2007). NTDs are grouped together under the generic terms myelodysplasia, spinal dysraphism, and spina bifida aperta (not to be confused with spina bifida occulta, a term that refers to a laminar or spinous process defect that is commonly seen on plain radiographs).

Myelomeningocele consists of a spinal cord that has failed to fuse, resulting in an open defect with no dura, bone, muscle, or skin covering. It occurs mostly in the low thoracic and lumbosacral regions, and may present rarely in a cervical location. Cervical dysraphia are usually skin-covered and have more normal neurologic function. In thoracic or lumbosacral myelomeningocele, the neural elements are abnormal (Noonan, 2006) and are part of the sac. There is a neurologic deficit at, and caudal to, the level of the lesion, and the affected infant may have central nervous system abnormalities such as an Arnold-Chiari malformation (Hawk & Bailie, 2007) and hydrocephalus (Noonan, 2006). Other NTDs include spina bifida cystica, which is a term applied to all midline fusion defects in the spine in which there is external evidence of herniation of the meninges.

Meningocele is the condition of unfused vertebral arches with a visible meningeal sac along the spinal axis, and it accounts for less than one third of all cases of spina bifida cystica. The sac contains cerebrospinal fluid (CSF) and is composed of dura, or dura and arachnoid but no nerve tissue, and there are usually no neurologic deficits. Lipomeningocele is associated with lobules of fat tissue. The sac contains a lipoma that is intimately involved with the sacral nerves, and the lesions are epithelialized at birth. The infant may not have hydrocephaly or other CNS abnormalities, but neurologic function may become impaired with growth. An encephalocele is a congenital gap in the skull, often with herniation of the brain or the meninges. Anencephaly is the absence of development above the brain stem.

The etiology of myelomeningocele is unclear but thought to be multifactorial (Hawk & Bailie, 2007). Some NTDs are associated with chromosomal abnormalities and others are caused by single-gene mutations. Environmental factors, such as exposure to valproic acid, may cause NTDs independently of any genetic variables. Another important environmental factor is the lack of folate in the diet of expectant mothers who may have an unrecognized disorder of folate metabolism (Noonan, 2006).

Development of the neural tube, which normally occurs during day 21-29 of embryonic life, is disrupted. Two etiologic theories proposed include a partial or complete failure of the neural tube to close, or the rupture of a neural tube that is overdistended with ventricular fluid. There is partial or complete paralysis and sensory loss below the affected neurosegmental area. The lesion can occur at any level of the spine. Most lesions are posterior, with rare instances of anterior or lateral lesions. The cause of the neurologic deficit is unclear, but may be due to the malformed spinal cord, the combination of malformation and the inflammatory effect of the chronic exposure of the open cord to amniotic fluid, or the direct abrasion of the cord against the uterine wall as the fetus grows. Secondary trauma may occur during delivery (Hawk & Bailie, 2007).

Hydrocephalus occurs in almost 90% of patients and results from the obstruction of the flow of CSF at the fourth ventricle or from the obstruction of flow from an Arnold-Chiari malformation, which is displacement of the brain stem through a small foramen magnum. If hydrocephalus is not shunted, the fluid pressure increases in the brain and the spinal cord, causing brain atrophy, hydromyelia, and eventually syringomyelia. Most children (90%) require ventriculoperitoneal (VP) shunting as a means of avoiding further damage to the CNS (Noonan, 2006).

The two types of Arnold-Chiari malformations are Chiari Type II deformity (the most common type), which is displacement of the cerebellum, and Chiari Type III deformity, which is displacement of the entire cerebellum and lower brain stem. Cognitive impairments are associated with diffuse changes in the cerebral cortex. Other consequences of a NTD are abnormal spinal curves, which result from bony malformations of the spinal column and the lack of muscle tone in the trunk. These abnormalities can include hemivertebrae, unsegmented bars, or diastematomyelia. The incidence of scoliosis increases as the level of the spinal defect moves proximally, and lordosis may develop in relation to hip flexion contractures. Lower limb deformities result from abnormal neurologic development and muscle imbalance. The risk of hip dislocation in high lumbar (L1, L2, L3) myelomeningocele is also due to muscle imbalance. Foot deformities are also quite common in children with myelomeningocele (Hawk & Bailie, 2007).

In virtually all cases, some form of bowel and bladder dysfunction is present, due to the bladder, urinary outlet, and rectum being controlled by the nerves that leave the spinal cord in the sacrum. The child may have difficulty storing urine and emptying the bladder. Bowel issues are the result of uncoordinated propulsive action of the intestines, the ineffectual anal sphincter, and the lack of anal sensation (Hawk & Bailie, 2007).

Myelomeningocele remains the most common congenital birth defect (Noonan, 2006), with an incidence of 4.5 per 10,000 births (Hawk & Bailie, 2007). The overall incidence would likely be higher, as it estimated that 23% of pregnancies with myelodysplasia are terminated (Noonan, 2006). After folic acid fortification became standard practice during prenatal care, NTD prevalence decreased from 24.9-37.8 to 20.1-30.5 per 100,000 live births. Mexico-born women in the United States have a two-fold higher risk of neural tube defect-affected pregnancies, possibly because of unfortified diets. In the early 1980s, about 50% of children with myelodysplasia survived to the age of 20, compared with 80%-85% today (Berry et al., 2010). Myelodsyplasia is more common in females than males. Families with one child with a neural tube defect have a 30-fold higher risk of having a second child with a neural tube defect, and adults with spina bifida have a 1:23 risk of bearing a child with a NTD (Hawk & Bailie, 2007).

Prevention programs aimed at reducing the likelihood of spina bifida have increased awareness of the need for folic acid supplementation. When folic acid supplementation is initiated before conception and within the first month of pregnancy, it has been shown to reduce the rate of neural tube defects by 70%; supplementation may not have any effect in women after the first month of pregnancy (Noonan, 2006).

Prenatal screening is performed between 16 and 18 weeks of gestation in all pregnant women, to look for elevated levels of serum alphafetoprotein (AFP); this test can detect 75%-80% of affected pregnancies. If the levels are high, special diagnostic procedures such as a detailed ultrasound, ultra-fast MRI scan, and amniocentesis for AFP and acetylcholinesterase (ACH) are indicated. Ultrasound examination of the fetal spine provides important information about the presence and location of a neural tube defect, and is a sensitive and efficient test in pregnancies at high risk for a neural tube defect. A prenatal diagnosis of myelomeningocele will give the family the option to either terminate or continue the pregnancy. The decision to continue the pregnancy implies that the disorder will be treated in the postnatal period, but the option of antenatal can be considered with fetal surgery to correct the defect (Noonan, 2006). This surgery is done between 22 and 30 weeks of gestation. Early results of fetal surgery have shown less neurologic damage, relative to the level of defect, and a decreased incidence of Arnold-Chiari malformation, but long-term results are unknown. A planned delivery by cesarean section before the onset of labor or the rupture of the fetal membranes is recommended to prevent trauma to the exposed nervous tissue.

Neurologic function in an affected child is not progressive and should remain steady throughout growth. If neurologic function deteriorates, this indicates a complication that requires prompt evaluation and treatment. As the child reaches adolescence, a changing relative strength and shift in the center of gravity may decrease the ability to ambulate (Hawk & Bailie, 2007).

Altered, decreased stature is seen in 50%-60% of individuals with myelomeningocele. Stature and bodily dimensions are altered by skeletal deformities and nutritional factors that may lead to obesity. Growth may be diminished by alterations in the hypothalamic-pituitary axis. These abnormalities result in precocious puberty and growth hormone deficiency (Noonan, 2006). Sexual dysfunction in adolescents and adults is common and although 75% of males with myelomeningocele are capable of erections, this may not be controlled. There is normal fertility in females, but affected women have decreased genital sensation (Hawk & Bailie, 2007).

Consequences of spina bifida include a latex allergy, which is characterized by swelling or itching of the lips after latex exposure, swelling of the skin after contact with rubber products, hand eczema, wheezing, or bronchospasm. High-risk patients report oral itching after eating bananas, chestnuts, or avocados, or report multiple surgical procedures in infancy. A complication in a child with spina bifida with shunted hydrocephalus is a ventriculoperitoneal shunt infection or malfunction. Hydrosyringomyelia may develop from the increased fluid pressure in the spinal canal when the shunt malfunctions. Symptoms include increasing paralysis and/or spasticity of the lower limbs, weakness of the hands and upper limbs, and occasional back pain.

Tethering of the spinal cord is a complication that occurs due to the normal cephalad migration being impeded by the ectodermal attachment of the cord as part of the initial defect, or by adhesions after surgery. Symptoms may include increasing paralysis and/or spasticity in the lower limbs and pain in the lower back and along the sacral nerve roots. Urologic complications include frequent urinary tract infections (UTIs), vesicoureteral reflux, and hydronephrosis. Bowel complications include impaction and rectal prolapse. Patients are prone to

Table 11.5. Functional Level in Myelomeningocele

Spinal Level	Motor Function/Sensation	Orthopaedic Problems	Mobility
Thoracic	■ No motion in legs ■ Extremities lie in abduction, external rotation, and flexion ■ Variable weakness and sensory loss in abdomen and LE	■ Flexion-abduction-external rotation contracture	■ Requires extensive orthotics 1. Parapodium 2. Reciprocal gait orthosis 3. HKAFO
Upper lumbar L1-L2	■ Hip inflexion and adduction ■ Sensation in anterior hip joint and thigh	■ Flexion contracture at hip ■ Hip dislocation	
Mid to lower lumbar L3-L5	■ Hip flexion and adduction ■ Knee extension ■ Weak knee flexion ■ Foot dorsiflexion and eversion ■ Sensation to below the knee	■ Flexion contracture at hip ■ Decreased hip abduction ■ Predisposed to progressive hip subluxation ■ Clubfeet	■ Less extensive orthotics ■ Able to use crutches
Sacral	■ Mild weakness of ankles and toes	■ Cavus foot	■ Minimal or no bracing ■ Ambulates with or without crutches

From Core Curriculum for Orthopaedic Nursing *(6th ed., p. 307), 2007, National Association of Orthopaedic Nurses, Boston, MA: Pearson. Reproduced with permission.*

pressure ulcers and skin breakdown due to insensate areas. Fractures of the tibia and fibula can occur, with the peak at age 3-7, and knee arthropathy occurs in the early 20s due to a valgus-external rotation thrust during ambulation. Charcot arthropathy often occurs and is characterized by a progressive degeneration of the metatarsal-phalangeal joint of the great toe in an insensate foot. Minor trauma causes swelling and redness around the joint, resembling cellulitis, and this progresses as the patient continues to walk on the injured foot (Hawk & Bailie, 2007).

Assessment

An initial assessment of the child starts with the presenting symptoms, including the onset and progression of symptoms and previous treatment. (See Table 11.5.) Any deterioration in neurologic status warrants careful evaluation, and symptoms may include an increased frequency of UTIs and increased shunt malfunctioning. Symptoms of hydrocephalus can include a high-pitched or shrill cry, malaise (vague signs of not feeling well), nausea/vomiting, severe headaches and/or neck pain, decreased upper limb strength, increased paralysis of the lower limbs, a bulging fontanel, and sunset eyes (characterized by a broad forehead and eyes deviated downward) in infants/young toddlers. Symptoms of a shunt malfunction may include the aforementioned signs, along with blurred vision, increased irritability, decreased perceptual motor function, a short attention span, and coma.

Information regarding the pregnancy and birth history should be elicited, in addition to any history of latex allergy or sensitivity. The child's developmental history, neurologic and functional status, bowel/bladder patterns, and social interactions/relationships with peers should be obtained, along with a family history.

The physical examination of the child includes an accurate height, weight, and head circumference. The skin should be assessed for pressure ulcers from orthotics, or from sitting in a wheelchair, and from abrasions on insenate areas. The surgically repaired spine should be assessed for scoliosis, kyphosis, or kyphoscoliosis. The eyes should be examined for nystagmus, involuntary rhythmic movements of the eyes that may be horizontal, vertical, rotary, or mixed. A musculoskeletal examination also includes an assessment of the upper and lower limbs, and observation of any contractures or deformities. Upper limb strength should be assessed, along with the level of motor deficit. If the child is ambulatory, the gait should be observed. A neurologic examination includes the recognition of signs/symptoms of increased intracranial pressure. Signs of an Arnold-Chiari malformation are an abnormal gag reflex, staring spells, nystagmus, apneic spells, a changed level of sensory deficit, and abnormal reflexes of the upper or lower limbs. If a child or parent mentions a change in the urologic status, this should prompt a visit to the pediatric urologist.

Radiographs to evaluate bony abnormalities are done as needed of the spine, hips, knees, or feet. To evaluate VP shunt functioning, shunt series x-rays can be done. MRI or CT of the head, spine, or hips is performed when indicated. To assess for urologic function, an ultrasound of the kidneys, urodynamics, and a voiding cystouretrhogram are done as recommended by the child's urologist (Hawk & Bailie, 2007).

Common Treatment Modalities

Before surgical repair, key objectives are the prevention of infection of the sac, protection of the exposed spinal cord and the nerves from injury, and prevention of skin breakdown while the infant is in a prone position. After surgical repair, treatment objectives are the prevention of complications and maximizing independence in ADLs.

Care of the infant with myelomeningocele requires the coordinated efforts of an interdisciplinary team (Hawk & Bailie, 2007). An ideal interdisciplinary team includes a urologist, an orthopaedist, a neurosurgeon, a social worker, physical and occupational therapists, educators, a pediatrician, and a nurse-specialist. These integrated programs have evolved with time and offer improvements unimagined 30 years ago (Noonan, 2006).

Neurosurgical interventions include the surgical closure of the defect within the first 24-48 hours after birth and placement of a VP shunt to treat hydrocephalus, which drains the fluid into the peritoneal cavity. Potential issues include the shunt becoming blocked, kinked, or infected. If these occur, a shunt revision is needed. Release of a tethered cord may be necessary and is also performed by a neurosurgeon.

Orthopaedic interventions include recommending orthotics to support the trunk in sitting and standing, stabilizing weight-bearing joints, treating hip dysplasia, and maintaining corrected position after surgical procedures. The use of parapodiums, standing tables, and other devices are advocated to maintain the child's upright balance, to teach ambulation, and to place weight through the lower limbs. Serial casting to treat clubfeet can be done in preparation for surgery. Surgery may be advised to release soft tissue contractures and to correct knee, ankle, or foot deformities. To stabilize and prevent the progression of scoliosis or kyphoscoliosis (Hawk & Bailie, 2007), treatment options include observation, bracing, and surgery. Scoliosis tends to be uniformly progressive, worse in younger patients with larger curves. Curve progression in these patients is usually more rapid than in patients with idiopathic scoliosis and tends to worsen with time and age, irrespective of the magnitude of the curve (Noonan, 2006).

Urologic interventions include a timed voiding schedule, with or without pharmacologic adjuncts, or a clean, intermittent catheterization program. To decrease bladder wall contractions, an anticholinergic medication such as oxybutynin chloride (Ditropan®) can be prescribed, and pseudephedrine (Sudafed®) or imipramine chloride (Tofranil) may be prescribed to increase the storage of urine. Urologic surgery consisting of bladder augmentation may be recommended. During this procedure, a piece of the colon or gastric tissue is used to enlarge the bladder. An appendicovesicostomy is a procedure in which the appendix is used as a conduit to catheterization. A procedure to make an artificial urinary sphincter may help to control continence in a very select group of patients. It is vital that hospital staff be cognizant that the child is at high risk for a latex allergy, and strategies should be in place to guarantee latex avoidance during surgical procedures for these children (Hawk & Bailie, 2007).

It is imperative that a child with myelomeningocele receive routine pediatric care. The primary care provider monitors the neurologic status and developmental progress, refers the child to early intervention programs, and oversees developmental and academic needs. There is a high incidence of learning disabilities in this population, as well as visual/spatial and perceptual problems, in addition to attention deficit disorders. The child's weight should be monitored because obesity is a common issue. Early and ongoing education of the child's family regarding nutritional needs, common problems of gagging, and delays in accepting different-textured foods is also important (Hawk & Bailie, 2007).

Nursing Considerations

Nursing Diagnoses. Nursing diagnoses for this condition are expanded upon in the Appendix.

- Mobility: physical, impaired.
- Nutrition, imbalanced: more than body requirements.
- Skin integrity, impaired.
- Tissue perfusion: cerebral, risk for ineffectiveness.
- Urinary elimination, impaired.

Nursing Interventions. Nursing interventions relating to bowel incontinence include inquiring about the patient's bowel movement pattern and teaching the child/family an appropriate bowel regimen. This should be started at age 2-3 and should include a morning and evening routine. The child/family should be taught how to use digital stimulation, a suppository, and an enema, as needed. The importance of an adequate fluid intake and use of oral adjuncts, as needed, should be stressed, along with a diet full of high-bulk foods. Mobility/physical activity should be encouraged as much as feasible. An optimal outcome is regular bowel elimination and social continence (Hawk & Bailie, 2007).

In the hospital setting, the child should be assessed for a latex sensitivity or allergy. The administration of premedications every 6 hours for 3 doses prior to surgery is often ordered and includes a corticosteroid, IV or PO, an H1-Blocker, IV or PO, and an H2-Blocker, IV or PO. A latex allergy alert should be documented, and latex-free products should be used whenever possible. Latex products should not be in contact with the child's skin, powder-free gloves should be used to prevent air-borne particles, and nurses should be alert for new reactions in high-risk patients. The child's normal bowel/bladder regimen should be maintained when possible, and nursing staff should be aware of the increased risk of postoperative infections in this population due to low-grade UTIs and the poor quality of the soft tissues (Hawk & Bailie, 2007).

Interventions regarding imbalanced nutrition (i.e., more than the body requires) consist of monitoring a child's height/weight and ongoing counseling, starting during infancy, explaining that the child is prone to excessive weight gain that may interfere with ambulatory potential/function, self-care, and self-concept. Provide information and support to parents/caregivers regarding possible gagging during eating and when introducing new textures. The best outcome is a child with a healthy body weight evidenced by a weight for height on the pediatric growth chart no higher than the 80th percentile (Hawk & Bailie, 2007).

Interventions focused on impaired physical mobility include encouraging the patient to work toward maximum mobility, stressing the benefits of ambulation, strengthening the upper limbs, protecting against obesity, improving bone density, preventing lower limb contractures, increasing independence, and encouraging a wider range of life experiences. When ambulation is unrealistic, help the family/significant others to secure appropriate mobility devices, such as a wheelchair, cart, or parapodium. Also encourage the child/family to maximize mobility by using prescribed orthotic devices, such as a parapodium during toddlerhood and leg braces when the child grows older. Emphasize how bracing promotes ambulation and normalizes the child's life, and how a program of active/passive ROM prevents contractures and promotes mobility. The best outcome is the achievement of optimal mobility.

Nursing interventions related to impaired skin integrity consist of teaching the child/family the importance of daily hygiene and skin checks for redness, cuts, and sores. The older child should be taught to check the soles of the feet with a hand mirror, and to protect the soles from rough surfaces. The importance of protecting the skin from temperature extremes should be stressed, such as testing bath water to prevent burning of insensate skin, and wearing layers of warm clothing to prevent frostbite. The patient should be taught to gradually wean into new orthotics and shoes to prevent the development of pressure sores. Assess the child's wheelchair needs and provide proper seating. Instruct the wheelchair-bound patient to do "wheelchair push-ups." An ideal outcome is a patient with intact skin evidenced by lack of sores or ulcers (Hawk & Bailie, 2007).

Interventions focusing on altered tissue perfusion include instructing the child/family on signs/symptoms of increased intracranial pressure and shunt malfunction, and stressing the importance of regular neurosurgical follow-up to assess shunt functioning and to monitor the child's status. The child's neurological status should be evaluated at each visit, and the ideal outcome is a child without signs/symptoms of increased intracranial pressure (Hawk & Bailie, 2007).

Interventions regarding altered patterns of urinary elimination include emphasizing the importance of adequate fluid intake and good perineal skin care. Counsel the patient/family on long-term urologic management, and assist/instruct the family in a bladder continence regimen as needed. Provide teaching/demonstration of a clean, intermittent catheterization program, educate the child/family on medications that supplement the program, and facilitate the program by communicating to the school nurse/teacher as needed. Teach the child/family the signs/symptoms of UTIs. Support the child in developing social and age-appropriate developmental skills. A successful outcome is the establishment of bladder training with social continence and infrequent/no UTIs (Hawk & Bailie, 2007).

Neurofibromatosis

Overview

Neurofibromatosis (NF) is a progressive disorder characterized by multiple tumors within the nervous system (central and peripheral) and is associated with variable abnormalities of the skin, skeleton, and soft tissues (Hawk & Bailie, 2007). The most common types are neurofibromatosis Type 1 (NF1) and neurofibromatosis Type 2 (NF2). (See Table 11.6.)

In *NF1, the peripheral form* of the disorder, café-au-lait spots and fibromas are present, and orthpaedic involvement is common. NF1 is also called von Recklinghausen disease. In *NF2, the central form*, bilateral acoustic neuromas are common (Hawk & Bailie, 2007), orthopaedic manifestations are rare (Alman & Goldberg, 2006), and there are a few peripheral findings. Numerous other types of NF have been identified, including familial spinal neurofibromatosis, which is characterized by extensive and multiple spinal neurofibromas. The focus of this section will be on NF1.

NF1 is the most common single-gene disorder in humans, affecting 1 in 3,000 newborns (Alman & Goldberg, 2006). The affected gene has been mapped to the long arm of chromosome 17 (Hawk & Bailie, 2007). There is an autosomal dominant inheritance pattern with 100% penetrance, but half of all cases are sporadic mutations associated with an older-than-average paternal age. A mutation that results in dysregulation of a pathway can cause increased cell proliferation, resulting in overgrowth of a cell type or organ. The type of tissue or organ involved depends on the cell type in which the gene is expressed. In a syndrome such as NF, the tissues of the musculoskeletal system are affected, resulting in obvious bone or soft tissue abnormalities (Alman & Goldberg, 2006).

In NF1, the protein neurofibrinomin, which has a role in tumor suppression, is decreased or absent. This results in uncontrolled cell proliferation and tumor growth. The growth disturbance is apparent in neural crest cell growth and function (Hawk & Bailie, 2007). The cells of the neural crest migrate (Alman & Goldberg, 2006) to become the pigmented cells of the skin, brain, spinal cord, peripheral nerves, and the adrenals (Hawk & Bailie, 2007), which explain the common sites of abnormalities of the disorder (Alman & Goldberg, 2006).

Cutaneous manifestations of the disease include café-au-lait spots, which are discrete spots the color of "coffee with milk." People affected by NF1 have a wide variation in the number, shape, and size of the spots, and they are found in skin areas not typically exposed to sun. They are primarily a cosmetic problem (Hawk & Bailie, 2007) and often appear after 1 year of age. The spots have a smooth edge, often described as similar to the coast of California, as opposed to the ragged edge of spots associated with fibrous dysplasia, which are described as similar to the coast of Maine (Alman & Goldberg, 2006). Freckling in the axillae, groin, and other skin folds is commonly seen in those with NF1 (Hawk & Bailie, 2007) and serve as good diagnostic markers because such freckling is exceptionally rare except in people with NF1 (Alman & Goldberg, 2006).

Cutaneous neurofibromas are composed of benign Schwann cells and fibrous connective tissue, can occur anywhere, and are usually present just under the skin. They are generally evident by age 10, and there is usually no neurologic impact. With puberty there is a rapid increase in their number. When many are grouped together on the skin, it is known as fibroma molluscum (Alman & Goldberg, 2006).

Table 11.6. Clinical Features of Neurofibromatosis Types 1 and 2		
	NF1	NF2
Diagnostic criteria	**Two or more of the following:** ■ At least 6 café-au-lait spots 1. Larger than 5 mm in children 2. Larger than 15 mm in adults ■ Two neurofibromas or single plexiform neurofibroma. ■ Freckling in the axillae or inguinal region. ■ An optical glioma. ■ At least two Lisch nodules (white bumps on the iris). ■ A distinctive osseous lesion, such as vertebral scalloping or cortical thinning. ■ A first-degree relative with NF1.	**Confirmed NF2** ■ Bilateral vestibular schwannomas (VS) or family history of NF2 plus: 1. Unilateral VS 2. Any two of the following: a. Meningioma b. Glioma c. Neurofibroma d. Schwannoma e. Posterior capsular lenticular opacities (SLO) **Presumptive NF2** ■ Unilateral VS diagnosed before age 30 plus any two of the following: 1. Meningioma 2. Glioma 3. Neurofibroma 4. Schwannoma 5. SLO ■ Two or more meningiomas plus: 1. Unilateral VS diagnosed before age 30 2. Any two of the following: a. Glioma b. Neurofibroma c. Schwannoma d. Cataract e. Cerebral calcification
Genetics	■ Autosomal dominant ■ Defect on chromosome 17 (17q11.2) ■ Lack of protein neurofibrinomin	■ Autosomal dominant ■ Defect on long arm of chromosome 22 (22q12.2) ■ Lack of gene product merlin or schwannomin
Incidence	■ 1/3,000	■ 1/40,000

From Core Curriculum for Orthopaedic Nursing *(6th ed., p. 323), 2007, National Association of Orthopaedic Nurses, Boston, MA: Pearson. Reproduced with permission.*

Plexiform neurofibromas are the result of the proliferation of cells in a nerve sheath extending along the length of a nerve. They may be visible, or internal and without external evidence. Soft tissue overgrowth results in hemihypertrophy, which is usually present at birth. They tend to grow in early childhood and during periods of hormonal changes, such as adolescence and pregnancy, and can undergo malignant transformation (Hawk & Bailie, 2007). The overlying skin is often darkly pigmented. They are highly vascular and lead to limb giantism, facial disfigurement, and invasion of the neuroaxis (Alman & Goldberg, 2006).

In both NF1 and NF2, cerebral tumors including gliomas can be seen, particularly an optic pathway glioma, which can block the flow of cerebrospinal fluid. The peak incidence of an optic glioma is age 4-6, and although the majority of gliomas are asymptomatic, they are capable of causing vision loss.

In NF2, medulloblastomas and ependymomas of the brain stem have a more indolent course than other tumors seen in oncology patients, but 50% of people with NF2 show clinical or radiological progression of them. Intraspinal and intermedullary tumors may occur and can become symptomatic, causing pain, loss of sensation, and loss of reflexes at the level of the tumor. These tumors are slow to progress and difficult to treat. Spinal root neurofibromas can occur also (Hawk & Bailie, 2007). Spine involvement in NF1 is common. There may be bony dysplasia associated with scoliosis. If dysplastic features are present, MRI or CT studies should be considered. Because rapid progression may occur with growth, these curves should be followed carefully. Dystrophic scoliosis is often characterized by short, angular, progressive curves for which brace treatment is ineffective. Correction is accomplished by a combined anterior and posterior spinal fusion, with the inclusion of the entire structural levels in both the fusion masses (Staheli, 2008f). Vertebral abnormalities such as scalloping of the posterior body, enlargement of the neural formina, and defective pedicles may occur in NF1. Dural ectasia may erode and thin the posterior vertebral elements.

Dysplasia of the long bones may occur with angular deformities ranging from bowing to pseudoarthrosis. This is seen most commonly in the tibia, but can arise in the ulna, radius, clavicle, or femur. Lytic areas resembling fibrous cortical defects and scalloping of the cortex may also be present (Hawk & Bailie, 2007).

NF cannot be diagnosed in many infants and children using the standard criteria, but health care providers should be alert to consider the diagnosis of NF1 if an unusual scoliosis, overgrowth of a part, or a congenital pseudoarthrosis lesion is seen on a radiograh (Alman & Goldberg, 2006). By age 8-10, numerous clinical manifestations of the condition are present in most affected children, who also may have a learning disability in 30%-60% of cases.

Complications of NF1 include cutaneous or plexiform neurofibromas that may affect the appearance of an individual, depending on their size and location, and fractures characterized by poor healing and progressive pseudoarthrosis. The start of seizures may signal the existence of an unrecognized tumor, hydrocephalus, or cerebrovascular disease. Hydrocephalus may result from aqueductal stenosis, and cerebrovascular disease is related to the intrinsic abnormalities of the intracranial vasculature. Spinal meningoceles can cause headaches, minor neurologic symptoms, and paraparesis, or muscle weakness especially of the legs that limits movement. Neurofibromatosis neuropathy is due to the accumulation of multiple peripheral neurofibromas, and malignant changes in the peripheral cell tumors or plexiform neurofibromas can occur. Hypertension can arise due to renal artery stenosis. There is an increased incidence of childhood leukemia and multiple sclerosis in those with NF1, and a shortened life expectancy is frequently noted (Hawk & Bailie, 2007).

Assessment

The presenting signs of the child should be elicited and may include pain, visual complaints, or neurologic symptoms. There may be a history of progressive neurologic deficits such as changes of bowel or bladder function, weakness, seizures, and headaches. Cutaneous changes may be noted also. Obtain the history of the development of the condition, along with present and past treatments. Ask about family history, specifically if first- and second-degree relatives have had skin lesions or tumors. Also inquire about any musculoskeletal findings, cognitive or psychomotor deficits, and the child's play/physical activities (Hawk & Bailie, 2007).

The physical examination of the child may reveal café-au-lait spots. These should be counted and measured. There may be freckling in the axillae, groin, or other skin folds. Cutanueous neurofibromas, discrete nodules palpable just below the skin and located in any body area, may be seen. These nodules may cause itching, but are rarely painful. A plexiform neurofibroma may be visible or may be internal, and hypopigmented skin may be seen. The area may be tender or painful upon palpation. Hemihypertrophy from overgrowth of the soft tissues may be noticed, and this may affect the cranial nerves.

Lisch nodules of the iris may be evident, which are gelatinous elevations from the iris surface, ranging in color from clear to yellow to brown. To evaluate Lisch nodules, a slit lamp eye exam is necessary (Hawk & Bailie, 2007).

Scoliosis may be present and can occur at an early age. Tibial bowing, with the apex anterolaterally, is often evident by age 2, and pseudoarthrosis of the long bones may be evident on radiographs. Radiographs are done to monitor the child's scoliosis, to evaluate intraspinal or paraspinal neurofibromas, and to evaluate abnormalities of the long bones.

MRI to delineate the extent of plexiform neurofibromas and to evaluate central nervous system tumors can be done. "Unidentified bright spots" are incidental findings on MRI and are areas of spongiform myelinopathy in the basal ganglia, cerebellum, brain stem, and pons. They are common in children and rare in adults, and do not cause overt neurologic symptoms, but they may be related to cognitive impairment.

A prenatal diagnosis of NF1 is possible with chorionic villa sampling, through genetic linkage, or by mutation (if the family mutation is known), but the severity of the clinical manifestations cannot be determined prenatally.

Common Therapeutic Modalities

The treatment of NF1 is based on the symptoms and complications of the condition. Nonsurgical interventions include bracing to protect the long bones when pseudoarthrosis is present. Bracing does not prevent curve progression in dystrophic scoliosis. Idiopathic scoliosis in children with NF1 is managed with a protocol similar to other populations, but dystrophic scoliosis is treated with surgery. Curves between 20-40 degrees are treated with a posterior spinal fusion with instrumentation, and curves greater than 40 degrees are treated with a combined anterior/posterior spinal fusion with instrumentation. Postoperative bracing is recommended. Symptomatic neurofibromas are surgically removed. To address pseudoarthrosis, resection of the dysplastic bone with grafting, transplant of the vascularized fibular, or bone transport with an external fixator may be recommended (Hawk & Bailie, 2007).

Nursing Considerations

Nursing Diagnoses. Nursing diagnoses for this condition are expanded upon in the Appendix.

- Anxiety.
- Pain.
- Self-concept, readiness for enhanced.

Nursing Interventions. Interventions focused on anxiety include the development of a plan of care that minimizes patient/family anxiety, allows the patient/family to express their fears and concerns related to the diagnosis and treatment plan, and includes the patient/family in the decision-making process. Provide education regarding the underlying pathology, normal developmental progression, indicated treatment, community resources, and genetic counseling as indicated. The best outcome is the family unit that expresses their fears/concerns related to the diagnosis/treatment, demonstrates understanding of the pathology, progression, and treatment, and has awareness of community resources/genetic counseling.

Interventions that assist in minimizing back pain include teaching relaxation techniques, teaching appropriate use of analgesics, and teaching and encouraging the use of a back brace. The ideal outcome is decreased or relieved pain.

Interventions focused on a disturbed self-concept should promote a positive self-concept by focusing on the patient as a whole, not just on the affected part or dysfunction. Reinforce personal strengths and skills, recognize that the reaction of parents/significant others influences the child's response, encourage attaining developmental skills consistent with the child's age, provide consistent feedback, and praise the mastery of new skills. The child should be allowed to have control over self-care and to make choices regarding daily routine, food choices, etc. Encourage the child to become more self-sufficient, to learn self-help skills, and to demonstrate independence in self-care. The best outcome is a child in whom strengths and weaknesses are identified and who attains developmental skills consistent with their age. Also offer the family information about the Neurofibromatosis Foundation (Hawk & Bailie, 2007).

Osgood-Schlatter Disease

Overview

Osgood-Schlatter disease (OSD) is a traction apophysitis of the tibial tubercle, which causes painful swelling of the knee (Hawk & Bailie, 2007). The apophysitis is due to repetitive tensile microtrauma and occurs in 10%-20% of children participating in sports (Staheli, 2008d). (Also see Chapter 22—Knee.)

The tibial tubercle develops as an extension of the epiphysis of the proximal tibia, and the ossification center (apophysis) is susceptible to repeated trauma at the patellar tendon insertion. As a result, apophysitis and tendinitis occur and cause pain at the tibial tubercle. Partial or complete separation of the tibial tubercle can occur, interrupting the blood supply resulting in necrosis. At skeletal maturity, the apophysis fuses to the tibia, and the symptoms stop when the apophysis is fully ossified.

Although OSD is usually a self-limiting condition, rare complications can ensue such as the persistent enlargement of the tibial tubercle that causes a bony prominence, fracture of the tibial tubercle, premature closure of the tibial tubercle apophysis causing a recurvatum deformity, and ossicle development in the tendon causing pain and tenderness (Hawk & Bailie, 2007). In about 10% of knees, some residual prominence of the tibial tubercle or persisting pain from an ossicle may cause problems (Staheli, 2008d).

Rapid growth and increased physical activity predisposes the early adolescent to the development of this condition. The immature patellar tendon-tibial tubercle junction is highly susceptible to submaximal, repetitive tensile stress resulting from high-intensity sports activity. The underlying pathology is suggestive of minor avulsions at the site and subsequent inflammatory reaction (Patel, 2009b). It occurs most frequently during the rapid growth before puberty, age 11-14 (Hawk & Bailie, 2007), and is commonly seen during Tanner stage 2 or 3. It is most commonly seen between ages 11 and 13 in girls and 12 and 15 in boys.

There may also be a familial component. In one study, the incidence is higher in athletes compared to non-athletes, 21% compared to 4.5% (Patel, 2009b). In most cases, the condition is unilateral (Staheli, 2008d), but in 20%-30% of cases there is bilateral involvement. The associated pain is aggravated by sports involving jumping, squatting, and kneeling, and is relieved by a period of rest (Patel, 2009b).

Assessment

The child's presenting symptoms should be elicited (Hawk & Bailie, 2007). Patients commonly complain of localized pain and swelling over the tibial tubercle (Patel, 2009b), which increase with activities such as running, bicycle riding, and stair-climbing, and which decrease or are completely relieved with rest. Obtain information regarding the onset, progression, and prior treatment of the symptoms and the child's level of physical activities or limitations. The parent may report a rapid growth spurt prior to the onset of symptoms.

The physical examination of the child typically reveals a tender, bony prominence over the tibial tubercle and localized pain at the anterior aspect of the knee. There may be subcutaneous swelling of the soft tissues over the tibial tubercle. The child may experience pain with forced knee extension against resistance and/or with squatting with full knee flexion.

The diagnosis of OSD is based on the history and clinical examination. AP, lateral, and oblique view x-rays may show irregular areas of bone deposition and resorption of the proximal tibial tubercle (Hawk & Bailie, 2007), or fragmentation of the tibial tubercle, and sometimes an ossicle in the patellar tendon is seen (Patel, 2009b). Diagnostic testing beyond plain x-rays is rarely indicated (Hawk & Bailie, 2007).

Common Therapeutic Modalities

The treatment objective for OSD is to reduce stress on the apophysis (Hawk & Bailie, 2007). Conservative treatment focusing on symptom management, such as decreased activity and promotion of rest, will result in significant improvement of pain. Because it is a self-limiting condition, overtreatment should be avoided.

In some athletes, it is not uncommon for recurrent pain to last up to 2 years before complete resolution. The adolescent should be allowed to participate in all sports as tolerated, but hamstring and quadriceps stretches should be done on a regular basis to improve and maintain flexibility (Patel, 2009b). Application of ice after sports activities is useful, and protective pads or knee sleeves may also benefit the athlete (Hawk & Bailie, 2007). If pain is severe or persistent, the use of a knee immobilizer for 7-10 days to relieve inflammation may be helpful. The use of nonsteroidal anti-inflammatory durgs (NSAIDs) can also be beneficial (Staheli, 2008d). The most common complication is a persistent, localized swelling, which may only be of cosmetic concern. Ossicle formation in the patellar tendon may be a source of chronic pain in some athletes, and removal of an ossicle may be indicated. Presence of OSD does not necessarily predispose the athlete for complete avulsion of the patellar tendon from the tibila tuberosity. This is only a potential concern during the rapid growth phase just prior to fusion of the tubercle to the tibia (Patel, 2009b).

Nursing Considerations

Nursing Diagnoses. Nursing diagnoses for this condition are expanded upon in the Appendix.

- Activity intolerance.
- Anxiety.
- Pain, acute.

Nursing Interventions. Interventions related to alteration in activity include discussing activity limitations, managing symptoms, and supporting the family's efforts to balance symptoms and activity. The best outcome is agreement on restrictions on planned activities related to the condition.

Interventions that focus on anxiety include developing a plan of care in which the patient/family can express their concerns related to the diagnosis and treatment plan. Provide education regarding the underlying pathology, normal developmental progression, and treatment. The best outcome is a patient/family that understands the pathology, developmental progression, and treatment of OSD.

Interventions related to acute pain include promoting patient comfort using pharmacologic and nonpharmocologic techniques, such as ice, diversional activities, and coping methods. Environmental factors that precipitate or increase pain should be identified. The best outcome is a patient who demonstrates a maximal degree of comfort (Hawk & Bailie, 2007). See Chapter 7—Pain.

Osteogenesis Imperfecta

Overview

Osteogenesis impefecta (OI) is an inherited connective tissue disorder that affects bone and soft tissues. It is also referred to as "brittle bone disease" (Hawk & Bailie, 2007) because the hallmark features OI are fragile bones that fracture easily. The clinical features and their severity vary, depending on the type of OI (see Table 11.7). OI affects both bone quality and bone mass, and people with OI have less collagen than normal and a poorer quality than normal. In some people with OI, height, hearing, skin, blood vessels, muscles, tendons, and teeth may be affected also. Children with OI have life-long medical issues, but they often lead healthy, productive lives despite the disorder. It is estimated that OI occurs in every 12,000-15,000 births. It is also estimated that 25,000-50,000 people in the US have OI (Glorieux, 2007).

In most cases, OI is caused by a dominant mutation in the COL1A1 or the COL1A2 genes that encode type I collagen (Glorieux, 2007). The genetic defect is usually transmitted as autosomal dominant (Hawk & Bailie, 2007), and fewer than 10% of OI cases are believed to be caused by recessive mutations in other genes in the collagen pathway. Mutations in the genes for prolyl 3-hydroxylase (LEPRE1) and for cartilage-associated protein (CRTAP) have also been identified. People with OI Types V and VI do not have evidence of mutations in the type I collagen genes. Spontaneous new mutations are common, and they account for most cases of OI in children born to unaffected parents. The mutation will usually be identical within families, but its expression (the degree of severity and the number of fractures, etc.) may differ among family members (Glorieux, 2007).

Table 11.7. Types of Osteogenesis Imperfecta

	Type I	Type II	Type III	Type IV
Inheritance	Autosomal dominant	Autosomal recessive	Autosomal recessive	Autosomal dominant
Incidence	1/15-20,000	1/20-60,000	1/70,000	1/200,000
Onset of fractures	■ Fractures usually begin when child starts to walk ■ Frequency of fracture decreases after puberty ■ Increase in frequency in women after menopause; in men, 60-80 years	Multiple fractures in utero	Fractures at birth or within first year of life	■ Fracture in utero, during labor and delivery, or in newborn period ■ Fracture frequency increased when child starts to walk ■ Fractures decrease after puberty ■ Increase in frequency in postmenopausal women
Physical manifestations	■ Mildest form ■ Mild to moderate bone fragility without deformity ■ Easy bruising ■ Mild joint hypermobility ■ Mild shore stature	■ Most severe form ■ Extreme fragility of connective tissue ■ Intrauterine growth retardation ■ Soft, large cranium ■ Extremities short ■ Legs bowed ■ Small thoracic cavity	■ Severe fragility of bone ■ Fractures heal with deformity and bowing ■ Long-bone deformity noted within first 2 years of life ■ Relative macrocephaly with triangular facies ■ Extreme short stature ■ Severe kyphoscoliosis	■ Skeletal fragility and osteoporosis more severe than Type I ■ Bowing of long bones ■ Moderate joint hypermobility ■ Basilar impression results in brain stem compression ■ Mild to severe scoliosis
Appearance on x-ray	■ Mild osteopenia with recurrent fractures ■ Slender and gracile bones	■ "Crumpled" bones ■ Skull severely osteopenic ■ "Beaded" ribs	■ Progressive bone deformities ■ Undermineralized skull ■ Wormian bones ■ Short, deformed long bones ■ Severe scoliosis	■ Osteopenia with recurrent fractures ■ Bowing of long bones
Color of sclera	Blue	Dark blue	■ Pale blue at birth ■ Fade to white	Grayish to white
Dentinogenesis Imperfecta	■ Type A: No ■ Type B: Yes (Uncommon)	Not known	■ Yes	■ Type A: No ■ Type B: Yes
Other clinical findings	■ Early onset hearing loss ■ Most achieve developmental milestones on time	■ Associated with prematurity and low birth weight ■ Poor feeding	■ Hearing loss common ■ Abdominal pain and chronic constipation or bowel obstruction due to protrusion acetabula ■ Motor development severely delayed ■ Muscle weakness and joint contractures from immobility	Hearing loss in some families
Life expectancy	Normal life expectancy	Lethal in perinatal period – 80% mortality in 1st month ■ Pulmonary insufficiency ■ Congestive heart failure ■ Infection	Shortened life expectancy ■ Cardiac decompensation ■ Pulmonary insufficiency ■ Brain stem compression from basilar impression	Near-normal life expectancy

From Core Curriculum for Orthopaedic Nursing (6th ed., pp. 301-302), 2007, National Association of Orthopaedic Nurses, Boston, MA: Pearson. Reproduced with permission.

The basic defect of OI is in type I collagen synthesis, resulting in a decreased amount or inferior quality. Epiphyseal and articular cartilage is normal, as are amounts of bone minerals. The skin of children with OI is thin, translucent (Hawk & Bailie, 2007), stiffer, and less elastic than normal, and children with OI may be prone to scar from sutures. Increased capillary fragility causes a tendency to bruise easily, and specific mutations in collagen genes may predispose people to aortic aneurysm (Glorieux, 2007), but major aneurysms are rare (Hawk & Bailie, 2007). People with OI have reduced muscle strength. Laxity is common and can lead to frequent sprains and dislocations of the hips, shoulders, and radial heads (Glorieux, 2007).

Skeletal manifestations of OI include generalized osteopenia (Hawk & Bailie, 2007), which is apparent on x-ray or with bone density tests (Glorieux, 2007). Bone trabeculae are thin, frail, and sparsely distributed, and endochondral and intramembranous bone formation can be abnormal. Fractures heal readily, and the callus is plastic and easily deformed (Hawk & Bailie, 2007).

Basilar impression may result from deformation of the soft bones of the skull. Elevation of the floor of the posterior cranial fossa, including the occipital condyles and the foramen magnum, compresses the brain stem. This occurs most frequently in children with OI Type IV, and may be prevented by delaying the upright positioning of an infant (Hawk & Bailie, 2007). The cause of related metabolic abnormalities is unclear, such as sensitivity to heat and cold, excessive diaphoresis, and resting tachycardia and tachypnea (Hawk & Bailie, 2007). Young women with OI may start menstruating later than unaffected women (Glorieux, 2007). The incidence of OI depends on the type (see Table 11.7) (Hawk & Bailie, 2007).

Fracture onset varies with the type of OI (see Table 11.7). In general, the frequency of fractures will decrease after puberty but will increase again in later years. Life expectancy ranges from neonatal death (OI Type II) to normal life expectancy (OI Type I). Early death is related to pulmonary insufficiency, cardiac decompensation, or brain stem compression (Hawk & Bailie, 2007), which is also referred to as basilar invagination. The most severe form, OI Type II, is also the rarest (Glorieux, 2007). Complications of OI may include progressive deformities, severe growth failure, pulmonary insufficiency related to a small thorax and/or kyphoscoliosis, cardiac decompensation related to aortic insufficiency or mitral regurgitation, and brain stem compression from basilar impression (Hawk & Bailie, 2007).

Microscopic studies of OI bone have identified a subset of people who are clinically within the OI Type IV group but have distinctive patterns to their bone. Review of the clinical histories of these people uncovered other common features. As a result of this research, 2 types—Type V and Type VI—have been added to the OI classification. It is important to know that these types do not involve Type I collagen, treatment issues are similar to Type IV, and diagnosis requires specific radiographic and bone studies (Glorieux, 2007).

OI Type V is moderate in severity and is similar to OI Type IV in terms of frequency of fractures and the degree of skeletal deformity. The most conspicuous feature of this type is large, hypertrophic calluses in the largest bones at fracture or surgical procedure sites. OI Type V is dominantly inherited and represents 5% of moderate-to-severe OI cases. OI Type VI is extremely rare. It is moderate in severity and similar in appearance and symptoms to OI Type IV. This type is distinguished by a characteristic mineralization defect seen in biopsied bone. The mode of inheritance is probably recessive, but it has not yet been identified (Glorieux, 2007).

Assessment

The history of an infant or child with OI will vary, depending on the type and severity (Hawk & Bailie, 2007). A person who has OI might exhibit only a few of the common characteristics, and some characteristics are age-dependent, and will not be seen in an infant or young child. Other features are present only in certain types of OI. Additionally, an infant or young child with a mild form of OI might not have bone deformity (Glorieux, 2007).

Elicit the pregnancy and birth history. Typically the child's intellect is normal, but a review of the developmental history may reveal gross motor delay due to fractures and/or hypotonia (Glorieux, 2007). Independent sitting by 10 months is an important indicator for the potential for independent ambulation. Developmental delays can include self-care deficits, delays in ambulation, and difficulty transferring from wheelchairs. Inquire about the child's usual physical activities and play. Ask about the onset and frequency of fractures, and past and current treatments. Also obtain a family history.

The physical examination should include the height, weight, and head circumference (Hawk & Bailie, 2007). The fontanels may close later than usual, and a triangular facial shape is characteristic in the more severe forms (Glorieux, 2007). Short stature may be present, or there may be a history of failure to thrive (Hawk & Bailie, 2007). The head circumference may be greater than average, or the head may appear large relative to the child's small body. Infants may have a low weight for their age, and older children are frequently overweight for their size. The body may be disproportional. The length of the arms and/or legs, or the child's overall height, may be shorter than expected when compared with unaffected children. The child's torso may be short when compared with his or her arms and legs due to vertebral compression. The child may be barrel-chested. The joints may be lax and unstable, which can lead to frequent sprains and dislocations. The feet may be flat. Bone malformations can include abnormal rib shape, pectus carinatum or pectus excavatum, curving of the long bones, scoliosis, mild kyphosis, and an abnormal skull shape.

Wormian bones (small bone islands found at the sutures of the skull) are present in 60% of people with OI. The sclerae might appear darker than normal, with a blue or gray tint. Although tinted sclerae are a frequently mentioned characteristic of OI, they are not necessarily indicative: they are seen in only 50% of OI cases, and pale blue sclera can occur in unaffected children up to 18 months of age. Intense scleral hue and/or its presence past age 2 might warrant further evaluation for OI. In those who have blue sclera, the color intensity will vary, and may fade considerably as the child gets older. Most children with OI have decreased muscle mass and associated muscle weakness. Some children experience multiple fractures of the long bones and vertebrae, and have chronic pain (Glorieux, 2007). There also may be a history of abdominal pain and chronic constipation (Hawk & Bailie, 2007).

Dentinogenesis imperfecta, characterized by transparent, discolored, and fragile teeth that fracture easily, is evident in about 50% of people with OI, particularly in those with severe forms. Dental abnormalities are usually apparent when the first tooth erupts. A child with healthy baby teeth will not develop dentinogenesis imperfecta, and the condition tends to run in families.

OI is a clinical diagnosis. Negative results on molecular or biochemical tests do not exclude the condition because some forms of OI result from mutations in genes other than those tested for. Family members should carry documentation of the OI diagnosis to avoid accusations of child abuse at emergency rooms. Other medical conditions that share some of the same clinical signs as OI include hypophosphatasia, juvenile Paget's disease, rickets, idiopathic juvenile osteoporosis, some inherited defects of vitamin D metabolism, Cushing's disease, and calcium deficiency and malabsorption (Glorieux, 2007).

If signs of basilar impression or basilar invagination are present—including facial spasm, nerve paresis, pyramidal signs, proprioceptive defects, papilledema, extremity weakness, or bladder dysfunction—the child should be taken to an emergency room for further evaluation.

Radiographs of a child with OI are done to evaluate for fractures, bony deformities, and scoliosis (Hawk & Bailie, 2007). Other findings may include osteopenia, subclinical or old/healing fractures, bowing of the long bones, vertebral compressions, and wormian bones in the skull sutures. Laboratory testing is available for the dominant and recessive forms of OI and includes collagen molecular testing, collagen biochemical testing, and separate studies that utilize a skin biopsy and sequencing of the genes for cartilage-associated protein (CRTAP) and prolyl 3-hydroxylase (LEPRE1) to test for the recessive forms of OI. Duel-energy x-ray absorptiometry (DXA) is a bone mineral density test that provides information about bone quantity, not quality. A low reading might be prognostic for a predisposition to fracture, but is not restricted to OI. A bone biopsy can identify all types of OI, but it is invasive and requires general anesthesia. A child must weigh at least 22 pounds (10 kilograms) to be a candidate for the procedure. A bone biopsy also may be obtained during orthopaedic surgery (Glorieux, 2007).

Common Therapeutic Modalities

The medical management of a child with OI needs to be customized to meet the needs of each child. Because there is no cure for OI, treatment focuses on minimizing fractures, surgically correcting deformities, reducing bone fragility by increasing bone density, minimizing pain, and maximizing mobility and independent function (Glorieux, 2007).

Bisphosphanates (specifically Pamidronate®), a class of drugs that are potent inhibitors of bone resorption, have been used to treat patients with OI since the 1990s. They have been used off-label because they have not received approval by the U.S. Food and Drug Administration (FDA) for use in OI. Research on bisphosphonates started in the 1990s and continues today into the use in OI treatment and other bone diseases. Current knowledge about bisphosphonate use indicates fewer fractures, improved bone density, normalization of diaphoresis, and pain reduction. The combination of bisphosphonates and PT has been reported to increase mobility in people with OI. Most severely affected infants and children seem to benefit the most from bisphosphonate treatment, and the maximum benefit of the treatment appears within the first 3-4 years of treatment. The drug effect is growth-dependent: the younger the patient, the more striking the response. Bisphosphonate treatment can begin in early infancy, but severely affected infants may experience respiratory problems during the first infusion. Short-term side effects might include an acute phase reaction with flu-like symptoms after the initial infusion, gastrointestinal upset from oral bisphosphonates, and weight gain. Bisphosphonate treatment is not recommended for women who are pregnant or who plan to become pregnant (Glorieux, 2007).

Coordinated, interdisciplinary care is beneficial for children with OI. Specialists may include geneticists, endocrinologists, neurologists, orthopaedists, rehabilitation experts, and otolaryngologists. Speech therapy, nutrition counseling, and access to adaptive equipment may also be necessary (Glorieux, 2007). PT can strengthen soft tissues and prevent joint contractures, and a program that promotes upright standing may prevent disuse osteopenia and fractures. Developing a child's ambulatory potential using orthotics and assistive devices as necessary is helpful as well (Hawk & Bailie, 2007).

The best management of a child's fractures is with closed reduction, if possible, and fracture alignment should be precise to prevent deformities. In some small children, deformity will be accepted, pending corrective osteotomies when the child is older (Hawk & Bailie, 2007). Plates and screws are not recommended for the surgical repair of fractures in children with OI due to the creation of a short, stiff segment within the bone, which is likely to break above or below the plate. Pins and screws do not anchor well in OI bone, and long-term use can lead to thinning of the bone underneath the plate. Because immobilization reduces bone density and heavy casts can cause new fractures, orthopaedists with experience in OI advocate using the lightest possible casting materials, immobilizing for the shortest time possible, and limiting the use of the spica cast. Bones affected by OI mostly heal at the same rate as healthy bone, but delays in healing and nonunions can occur.

When an open reduction of a fracture is necessary, different types of rods (surgical nails) are available to address issues related to surgery, bone size, and the prospect for growth. The two major categories of rods are telescopic and nontelescopic. Telescopic rods are designed to lengthen during growth and consequently postpone the need for replacement. An example is the Fassier-Duval rod. Nontelescoping rods do not expand and need to be replaced if the child's bone lengthens and begins to bow. This type of rod may be the only option for children with very short, thin bones. Two examples are Rush rods and Kirschner wires (K-wires). The use of bracing to address scoliosis in a child with OI is of limited value, and a rapidly progressing curve may require fusion surgery (Glorieux, 2007).

Nursing Considerations

Nursing Diagnoses. Nursing diagnoses for this condition are expanded upon in the Appendix.

- Injury, risk for.
- Pain, chronic.
- Physical mobility, impaired.

Nursing Interventions. Interventions focused on risk for injury include teaching the child/family how to prevent fractures/recognize injuries; how to handle the child gently by supporting the body when moving, positioning, and lifting; and planning with the child/family methods to achieve developmental tasks that lessen the chance of fractures (Hawk & Bailie, 2007). Obtaining a blood pressure measurement of a child with OI may cause a fracture and an automated blood pressure cuff should not be used. If possible, avoid taking the measurement on an arm that has repeatedly fractured or is bowed. When diapering an infant with OI, slide one hand under the infant's buttocks to lift him or her and use the other to remove and replace the diaper. Lifting of the infant by the ankles should not be done due to the risk of a fracture (Glorieux, 2007). The best outcome is the prevention, recognition, and treatment of fractures. See Chapter 15—Trauma: Fractures.

Interventions focused on chronic pain include promoting patient comfort by handling the child gently and relieving pain with appropriate nonpharmacologic and pharmacologic techniques such as massage, stretching, moist heat, ice, relaxation, and analgesics, as indicated (Hawk & Bailie, 2007). Infants and children with chronic and acute pain, especially from femur fractures, will often require pain medications more powerful than ibuprofen for short periods of time. Titrate medication dosage to a child's weight, not age, even with older children and teens. Some nonsteroidal anti-inflammatory drugs (NSAIDS) have been linked to delayed bone healing after fracture. The use of drugs that contain steroids should be minimized because of their negative effect on bone metabolism (Glorieux, 2007). Position the child to prevent problems such as muscle spasms and encourage diversional activities. Discuss coping methods with the patient/family. An ideal outcome is a patient who achieves a maximal degree of comfort. See Chapter 7—Pain.

Interventions focused on impaired physical mobility include the promotion of mobility. Provide gentle, consistent exercises to the extremities to avoid disuse atrophy, assist with early weight-bearing, possibly using a tilt-table or a standing frame or lightweight orthoses whenever possible. The best outcome is a child who attains independent mobility (Hawk & Bailie, 2007).

Pediatric Fractures

Overview

A fracture is defined as a disruption in the continuity of a bone. It may be an open or closed injury, caused by trauma, sport-related damage, or pathology (Hawk & Bailie, 2007). Fractures in the pediatric population are becoming more common as participation in sports activities increases. Due to a low bone mineral content, children with generalized disorders such as renal diseases, cystic fibrosis, diabetes mellitus, OI, and growth hormone deficiencies are more at risk. Children with CP, spina bifida, and arthrogryposis are fracture-prone because of the combination of poor mineralization and joint stiffness (Staheli, 2008g).

Fractures in children are different from those in adults due to the differences in their musculoskeletal system (Hawk & Bailie, 2007). These differences gradually diminish with age, so that fractures in adolescents are similar to those in adults. The most obvious musculoskeletal difference is that the child has a growth plate. The relative strength of the growth plate, compared to adjacent bone, changes with age. As an example, the physis in infants is stronger than the adjacent bone, so diaphyseal fractures are most common. The growth plates in children usually help in managing fractures, and growth facilitates remodeling that corrects residual angulation. The potential for remodeling depends on the growth rate of the adjacent physis and on the remaining growth of the child. Just as the physis can resolve deformity, asymmetrical physical growth causes deformity (Staheli, 2008g).

A child's bones contain more collagen and are more porous than an adult's bones. They are also more likely to fail in both compression and tension, resulting in buckle fractures (Hawk & Bailie, 2007). The periosteum is thick and more metabolically active in the child than in the adult, which explains the abundant callus seen in the infant and the rapid union and increased potential for remodeling present throughout childhood (Staheli, 2008g). The relatively thicker periosteum and flexibility of the immature bone allows it to bend, and this causes children to sustain more avulsion-type injuries. The younger the child, the greater the ratio of cartilage to bone. This makes x-ray interpretation more difficult (Hawk & Bailie, 2007) but improves resilience in a child (Staheli, 2008g). Compared to adults, children have a greater potential for fracture remodeling, which is the combination of bone being formed on the concave side of the deformity and bone absorption on the convex side. Most remodeling occurs 1-2 years after injury but may continue for 5-6 years. The younger the child, the more remodeling that can occur. The Salter-Harris classification, a system of growth plate fractures, is the most common method used to classify physeal injuries (Hawk & Bailie, 2007). A Type I fracture is separation of the physis; Type II, is a fracture through the physis and adjacent metaphysis; Type III is a fracture through the physis and adjacent epiphysis; Type IV is a fracture through the physis, adjacent metaphysis and epiphysis; Type V is a crush injury of the physis (Patel, 2009a).

Upper Extremities. Common childhood *forearm* fractures include greenstick fractures, distal radius/ distal ulna (or both bone) fractures, midshaft fractures, and Monteggia or Monteggia equivalents. The wrist is the most frequent site of injury (Staheli, 2008g). *Elbow* fractures include supracondylar fractures of the distal humerus, lateral condyle/medial condyle fractures, radial head and neck fractures, olecranon fractures, elbow dislocations, and nursemaid's elbow (see Chapter 19—The Elbow). *Shoulder* fractures include proximal humerus fractures and clavicle fractures. *Hand* fractures include phalanx and tuft fractures (Hawk & Bailie, 2007).

Trunk. *Spine* fractures include SCIWORA: spinal cord injury without radiologic abnormality. *Pelvic* fractures are associated with polytrauma or other injuries.

Lower Extremities. *Femur* fractures may be proximal, midshaft, or distal. Knee fractures include a tibial spine fracture, an osteochondral fracture, and a patellar dislocation or fracture. *Tibia* fractures include a tibial shaft fracture, a proximal tibial metaphyseal fracture, or a toddler's fracture. *Ankle* fractures include physeal fractures, a Tillaux fracture, or a triplane fracture. Fractures of the *foot* include metatarsal fractures, calcaneal fractures, or cuboid fractures.

Other Fractures. Other fractures are *stress fractures* of the upper or lower limbs, ribs, pubic ramus, pelvis, or spine (Cline & Patel, 2009). *Pathologic fractures* are relatively common in children and frequently occur through osteopenic bone in children with neuromuscular disorders, such as CP, spina bifida, OI, and dysplasia. Pathologic fractures also occur through bone weakened by tumors, unicameral bone cysts, or nonossifying fibromas (Staheli, 2008g).

Fractures comprise about 15% of all injuries in children in the United States (Hawk & Bailie, 2007). Fractures are more common in boys than in girls (Hawk & Bailie, 2007), and age affects the pattern of injury (Staheli, 2008g). About 200,000 children with injuries related to playground equipment are treated in hospital emergency departments each year (Horn, 2010), and trauma is the leading cause of death in children (Hawk & Bailie, 2007).

Children usually require a shorter period of immobilization than adults, and intra-articular fractures can result in early osteoarthritis. Some fractures, such as a femoral neck fracture, have a greater incidence of avascular necrosis. Complications of fractures may include loss of reduction, malunion or nonunion, compartment syndrome, cast-related issues in a non-communicative child, internal fixation issues, a misdiagnosis, physeal injuries, and avascular necrosis (Hawk & Bailie, 2007). Supracondylar fractures, the most common pediatric elbow fracture, are at high risk for neurovascular compromise (Patel, 2009a). A pink, pulseless hand in a child who has been casted for a supraconylar fracture may appear to have sufficient circulation, but has inadequate perfusion secondary to insufficient collateral circulation. This can lead to anoxia of the tissues and compartment syndrome, and is the leading cause of litigation after upper extremity casting.

Assessment

The history should include the mechanism of injury and the situation surrounding the injury (Hawk & Bailie, 2007). If the child was involved in a physical activity, key elements of the history include when the injury occurred or when symptoms started, the type of sport/activity, the playing conditions, the position being played, and the level of competition. Other important information to obtain is the immediate presence of pain, swelling, deformity, or loss of movement. Ascertain any immediate intervention such as ice application, any subsequent intervention such as PT, the need for pain medication, and previous injury to the same area (Patel, 2009a).

The thorough physical examination requires the removal of all bandages and splints (Hawk & Bailie, 2007). The child may be uncooperative, but it is important to look at the whole child, along with spontaneous movement. Pseudoparalysis in the infant or child is commonly due to trauma (Staheli, 2008g). Depending on the child's presentation, obvious or subtle deformity or swelling may be present, along with decreased or painful movement. Heat or warmth at the fracture site from the hyperemic response of the fractured bone may be the best clue in children who are unable to communicate. Find the point of maximum tenderness, and evaluate capillary refill and peripheral pulses (Hawk & Bailie, 2007).

Observe the patient's reaction while extending the finger or toes. Pain on passive stretching is an early sign of ischemia. Compartment syndrome may be silent in children (Staheli, 2008g). Observe the patient for pain behaviors. In a polytrauma patient, the orthopaedic injuries may not be a priority, but the secondary survey of the child may indicate fractures (Hawk & Bailie, 2007). In the poly-traumatized child, musculoskeletal injuries seldom cause death but are a common cause of residual disability (Staheli, 2008g).

When a fracture is suspected, radiographs of the joints above and below the fracture site are indicated. An arthrogram may be needed in a young child due to the high ratio of cartilage to bone. A CT scan may be useful in complex or intra-articular fractures, and MRI is useful in knee and spine injuries in children. A bone scan may be used as a screening tool in suspected child abuse cases (Hawk & Bailie, 2007). Depending on the child's age and level of cooperation, sedation may be needed for some diagnostic studies. Ultrasound studies should be utilized when evaluating such conditions such as a possible physeal separation of the distal humeral epiphyseal complex in the newborn (Staheli, 2008g).

Common Therapeutic Modalities

The treatment modalities of children's fractures are dependent upon the type of fracture, the location of the fracture, the child's age, the amount of growth remaining, psychosocial issues, and any pre-existing medical conditions.

Casting of a childhood fracture is the most common method of treatment (Hawk & Bailie, 2007). Children with an underlying condition in which osteopenia is likely (such as CP, spina bifida, or OI) should be treated with a minimum period of immobilization. Cast treatment for conditions such as developmental dyplasia of the hip increases the risk of fracture. The period of greatest vulnerability is shortly after cast removal, as joints are stiff and bone is weakened by immobilization (Staheli, 2008g). Splints, immobilizers, and other orthotics can also be used in some instances. A closed manipulation or reduction may be attempted before casting, and this may require sedation or general anesthesia in the operating room.

Surgical interventions to reduce some fractures are sometimes necessary, with or without internal fixation. Younger children often require minimal fixation. A wide variety of surgical implants can be used, including K-wires, flexible intramedullary nails, plate and screw fixation, external fixation devices, rigid intramedullary fixation, bioabsorbable fixation, and cannulated screws (Hawk & Bailie, 2007).

Nursing Considerations

Nursing Diagnoses. Nursing diagnoses for this condition are expanded upon in the Appendix.

- Mobility: physical, impaired.
- Pain, acute.
- Peripheral neurovascular dysfunction, risk for.

Nursing Interventions. Interventions that focus on acute pain and promote comfort include using ice, elevating the extremity, and utilizing pharmacologic/nonpharmacologic techniques. The ideal outcome is a child who demonstrates a maximal degree of comfort (Hawk & Bailie, 2007).

Measures focusing on the prompt identification of ineffective tissue perfusion include the frequent assessment/comparison of the affected extremity and the unaffected extremity. The color, temperature of the tissues, edema, pain, capillary refill, motor function, sensory function, and peripheral pulses should be evaluated. Proper alignment and positioning of the limb should be maintained ("hands above the heart and toes above the nose") as tolerated. Symptoms suggestive of compartment syndrome such as disproportionate pain in relation to the injury, pain on passive muscle stretch, paresthesia or numbness, and pulselessness warrant prompt attention by an appropriate provider or in an emergency department. The optimal outcome is an intact neurovascular status of the extremity, including capillary refill within 1-3 seconds, strong peripheral pulses, and an extremity that is normal in color compared to the unaffected extremity (Kunkler, 2007).

Teaching caregivers how to perform a neurovascular assessment should be done prior to hospital or clinic discharge. The importance of radiographic follow-up in 7-10 days to assess for loss of reduction and to evaluate for any other issues should also be stressed to the caregivers. Help coordinate special car seats/seat belt restraints and the child's hospital discharge when needed. Home care considerations include encouraging parents to allow the child as much activity as possible within activity restrictions and to maintainany prescribed therapy program. Encourage self-care, educational, and diversional activities. Promote home tutoring or special school arrangements while on bedrest, in braces, or in casts, along with frequent neurovascular assessments of the limb.

Interventions include discussing/providing appropriate equipment to assist the child with mobility, teaching the prescribed exercise program (if applicable), planning activities which accommodate any restrictions, planning methods to allow expression of normal developmental tasks, and providing age-appropriate diversional activities to alleviate boredom, stress and fatigue. The optimal outcome is a patient who maintains restricted mobility (Hawk & Bailie, 2007).

Physical Abuse

Overview

The Federal Child Abuse Prevention and Treatment Act (CAPTA) defines child abuse and neglect as "any recent act or failure to act on the part of a parent or caretaker that results in death, serious physical or emotional harm, sexual abuse or exploitation, or an act or failure to act that prevents an imminent risk of serious harm to a child." Physical abuse is characterized by the infliction of physical injury as a result of punching, beating, kicking, biting, burning, shaking, or otherwise harming a child. CAPTA further states that the parent or caretaker may not have intended to harm the child; rather, the injury may have resulted from overzealous discipline or physical punishment (Hornor, 2005). Another source defines child physical abuse as acts of commission involving physical violence that results in injuries (Barron & Jenny, 2011).

Child abuse is not a diagnosis, but a symptom of severe family dysfunction (Hawk & Bailie, 2007) that crosses all socioeconomic, religious, and educational boundaries. It is generally repetitive and tends to escalate over time (Hornor, 2005). It is the result of an interaction between the child and caregiver, a specific event, and the environment (Hawk & Bailie, 2007).

Although there is no singular cause of child abuse, examining the psychosocial profiles of known abusers can be used to identify potential risk factors (see Table 11.8). Certain characteristics of children predispose them to physical abuse, including young age, prematurity, developmental delay/disability, behavioral problems, and placement in foster care. Precipitating factors such as inconsolable crying in infants or toilet training issues in toddlers predispose these populations to potential physical abuse. Environmental risk factors for child abuse include multiple stressors such as domestic violence, mental illness, and lower employment/educational status of parents (Hornor, 2005). Children who live in homes where domestic violence is present are more likely to be victims of physical abuse (up to 15 times the national

Table 11.8. Factors in Child Abuse

Caregiver Characteristics	Child Characteristics	Environmental Characteristics
■ Past or present victim of abuse ■ Negative relationship with parents ■ Difficulty controlling aggressive impulses ■ Inadequate knowledge of normal child development ■ Expect learning to take place automatically ■ Expect child to have maturity and responsibility of an adult ■ Low self-esteem and distrust of others ■ Often live in social isolation with few support systems ■ May be substance abuser	■ Temperament ■ Position in family ■ Additional physical needs due to illness/disability ■ Activity level ■ Sensitivity to parental needs ■ May be illegitimate or unwanted ■ May have cognitive or physical disabilities ■ History of prematurity ■ Age less than 1 year ■ Stepchild ■ Usually only one child abused	■ Chronic stress in family, including divorce, financial difficulties, unemployment, poor housing ■ Substance abuse in family ■ Inadequate social supports ■ Not related to one educational, social, or economic group ■ Lower socioeconomic group may be predisposed due to stress levels ■ Cases in lower socioeconomic group more likely to be reported ■ Upper classes more likely to conceal abuse/less likely to be reported

From Core Curriculum for Orthopaedic Nursing (6th ed., p. 271), 2007, National Association of Orthopaedic Nurses, Boston, MA: Pearson. Reproduced with permission.

average), and the most frequently reported cause for neglect and abuse of children is parental substance abuse (Barron & Jenny, 2011).

The characteristics and presentation of child abuse (highlighted in Table 11.9.) vary considerably, depending on the child's age. Many children with severe injuries at the time of diagnosis have previously presented with less severe injuries, and physical abuse was overlooked (Hornor, 2005). When the diagnosis of child abuse is missed, recurrent injuries occur in about half and are lethal in 10% of infants and children (Staheli, 2008g). An abused child often has multiple injuries that may include bruising/lacerations/abrasions, burns, fractures/dislocations, abdominal injuries, and head injuries. A history of unexplained and repeated poisonings, drug overdoses, alcohol ingestion, or other unusual circumstances should be regarded as red flags and warrant a thorough investigation of the child's injuries (Hawk & Bailie, 2007).

Statistics from the National Incidence of Harm Standard Maltreatment-4 (NIS-4, 2005-2006) estimate the total number of maltreated children to be 1,256,600, or 17.1:1000. This was a decline in all categories of abuse since the NIS-3 (1993) but the same level as reported in the NIS-2 (1986). The NIS-4 findings cite race differences, with higher maltreatment incidence rates for African-American children, and a strong correlation between socioeconomic status and maltreatment. The NIS-4 states that a large percentage (44%, or an estimated total of 553,000) of maltreated children were abused, while most (61%, or an estimated 771,000) were neglected (Sedlak et al., 2010).

The 2006 Kids' Inpatient Database (KID) focused an analysis of hospitalized children younger than age 3 because most serious injuries attributable to abuse occurred among young children. A relatively high incidence of cases of traumatic brain injuries and/or fractures attributable to abuse was found in the youngest age group, age newborn to 11 months, likely due to their vulnerability to injuries caused by caretakers and the increased challenges of caring for young infants. Among children less than 1 year of age, traumatic brain injuries and/or fractures occurred in 1 in 2,000. For children with fractures, the number of abusive injuries peaked during the first months of life. The proportion of children on Medicaid or without insurance was largest for these injuries, compared to other causes of injury. A hypothesis explaining this difference may be the bias in the diagnosis of abuse, as previous studies demonstrated that physicians are more likely to report abuse to protective services for minority children who are more likely to have Medicaid as their health insurance (Leventhal, Martin, & Asnes, 2010). Although reporting of suspected child abuse is legally mandated, and a concerned adult can contact child protective services without penalty for

Table 11.9. Common Injuries in Child Abuse

Injuries	Description/Location
Bruises, welts, lacerations, abrasions	■ Particularly on the buttocks, perineum, trunk, back of legs, back of head, or neck ■ Found on several body surfaces ■ Bruises on young infant ■ Multiple injuries at different stages of healing ■ Geometric shapes ■ Shapes of object that caused injury; electric cord, belt buckle, hand ■ Bite marks ■ Severe bruising that cannot be explained by history
Burns	■ Circular burns (cigarettes), especially on soles of feet, palms, back, or buttocks ■ Immersion burns ■ Sock- or glove-like ■ Symmetric, regular, "water-mark" edge ■ On perineum, upper thighs, lower torso ■ Splash/spill burns ■ Rope burns on arms, legs, neck, or torso ■ Burn in shape/pattern of object used: iron, radiator, stove burner ■ Infected burn indicating delay in treatment
Fractures, dislocations	■ Metaphyseal "corner" fractures ■ Lower extremity fractures in nonambulatory child ■ Bilateral acute fractures ■ Spine or rib fractures ■ Physeal fractures in young children ■ Multiple fractures in various stages of healing ■ Fractures of hands and feet in infants and young toddlers
Abdominal injuries	■ External bruises ■ Ruptured pancreas ■ Laceration of liver and/or spleen ■ Intramural hematoma of bowel ■ Retroperitoneal hemorrhage ■ Kidney contusion ■ Rupture of ureter or bladder
Head injuries	■ Subdural or subarachnoid hemorrhage ■ Skull fracture ■ Scalp swelling ■ Bald patches on scalp ■ Retinal hemorrhage ■ Black eye(s)

From Core Curriculum for Orthopaedic Nursing *(6th ed., p. 272), 2007, National Association of Orthopaedic Nurses, Boston, MA: Pearson. Reproduced with permission.*

unsubstantiated cases, it is estimated that up to 68% of child abuse cases may not be reported, especially in older children (Hawk & Bailie, 2007).

Assessment

The assessment of child who may have been abused includes obtaining a complete history from the parents or caretakers who accompany the child (Hawk & Bailie, 2007; Hornor, 2005). All caregivers should be interviewed separately (Barron & Jenny, 2011). The date, time, location, and mechanism of injury should be obtained, along with the name and relationship of any witness to the event. Allow the parent/caregiver to lead the interview with a narrative and timeline of the injury, noting any delay in treatment (Hawk & Bailie, 2007; Hornor, 2005). Record the information using exact quotes when possible (Barron & Jenny, 2011). The child's developmental history, past medical and surgical history, and family history should be obtained. Note any history of minor trauma with extensive injuries, history of trauma that is incongruous, inconsistent, or not plausible in relation to physical findings, or history of self-inflicted injury that is incompatible with the child's developmental level (Hawk & Bailie, 2007). A family tree may provide invaluable information regarding the current living situation, number of siblings, and number of partners the mother has had children with. Families should also be screened for psychosocial risk factors. If age and development allow, the child should also be questioned about how the injury occurred (Hornor, 2005). Verbal children should be interviewed separately and should be interviewed at eye level, using age-appropriate language. It is important to ask open-ended questions and to avoid asking direct or leading questions. Record the child's disclosures using exact quotes. Further detailed interviews should be completed by trained professionals in response to a report of suspicious injuries to the child welfare agency (Barron & Jenny, 2011).

The child's height, weight, and head circumference (age 2 or younger) should be noted, along with their general state of health, hygiene, and behavior (Hornor, 2005). To put the child at ease, the physical examination should be completed in a child-friendly examination room with adequate lighting. An entire examination should be completed, not simply an exam focused on areas of obvious injury. All children should be examined in a gown, with inspection of the entire skin surface. Clear documentation of any injuries should be completed using color photography and drawings to describe location, size, and pattern of injuries (Barron & Jenny, 2011). The assessment should include symmetry or asymmetry of injuries, degree of pain or bony tenderness, and evidence of old injuries. The examiner should be cognizant of the caregiver's behavior, especially their awareness or indifference to the child's needs and the seriousness of the injury. Child-caregiver interactions also should be assessed, as the child may not look to the caregiver for emotional support or may behave unusually toward the caregiver. Diagnostic testing should be initiated, depending on the presentation of the child (Hawk & Bailie, 2007). Children younger than age 2 with suspected physical abuse require a complete skeletal survey to identify occult osseous trauma. Children with acute injuries should receive a second skeletal survey 2 weeks after the first (Barron & Jenny, 2011). Be suspicious of any long-bone fractures in an otherwise normal infant in the first year, as many femoral shaft fractures in early infancy are due to abuse. Keep in mind, however, that children with undiagnosed, generalized disorders such as OI, renal disease, cystic fibrosis, diabetes mellitus, and growth hormone deficiencies are at risk for fractures (Staheli, 2008g) and initially may be thought to be abused.

When abusive head injury is suspected, a CT of the head is the most rapid, reliable diagnostic tool. If abdominal trauma is suspected, an abdominal CT, urinalysis, and liver enzymes should be done (Hornor, 2005). Consider a pediatric surgery consult for abdominal distension and/or tenderness (Barron & Jenny, 2011). When bruising is seen, diagnostic tests to rule out a systemic cause such as a coagulopathy include a CBC, PT/PTT, platelet count, and bleeding time. Neurologic, ophthalmologic, or gynecologic examinations should be done as indicated by the injuries (Hawk & Bailie, 2007).

Common Therapeutic Modalities

The primary goal for the clinician addressing possible child abuse is to make the diagnosis, provide needed treatment, report suspicious injuries to the child welfare agencies, and ensure the safety of the patient and other children within the same environment. In all states, clinicians are responsible by law for reporting abuse suspicions to child welfare agencies. Suspected child abuse cases require a multidisciplinary approach from medical personnel, child welfare authorities, and law enforcement officials (Barron & Jenny, 2011).

Physical sequelae of child abuse are often apparent and may include disfigurement, disability, neurologic impairment, blindness, and death (Hawk & Bailie, 2007). Less noticeable effects of physical abuse are the emotional and behavioral changes in a child, including changes in neurodevelopement and motor ability, post-traumatic stress disorder (PTSD), and higher lifetime rates of anxiety disorder, alcohol abuse, and antisocial behavior. In cases of sexual abuse, most children will be moderately to severely symptomatic at some point in their lives. Externalizing behaviors, such as delinquency and heavy drinking, are seen more often in boys. Internalizing behaviors, such as depression and disordered eating, are seen more often in girls. Certain developmental milestones also can trigger emergence or re-emergence of PTSD symptoms, such as the initiation of sexual activity or the birth of a child (Hornor, 2005; Hornor, 2010). See Chapter 15—Trauma.

Nursing Considerations

Nursing Diagnoses. Nursing diagnoses for this condition are expanded upon in the Appendix.

- Injury, risk for.
- Nutrition, imbalanced: less than body requirements.
- Parenting, impaired.
- Social interaction, impaired.

Nursing Interventions. Interventions focused on protecting the child from further injury include monitoring the child/caregiver interactions and visits from family/friends. A therapeutic environment should be provided, with consistency in professional caregivers. Play therapy should be used to relieve tension, investigate relationships, establish normalcy, and provide support during interactions, tests, and treatements. Thorough and objective documentation of the physical findings/behavioral responses should be done, and a referral to a Child Abuse/Protective team or outside agency should be made.

If the child is inadequately nourished, provide information about appropriate food choices for the child, and enlist the assistance of a dietician. Observe child/caregiver interactions during feedings/meals, and assist in developing positive connections during these times.

Interventions focused on the perpetrator includes the promotion of adequacy, inclusion as part of the child's care and recovery, teaching and reinforcing appropriate childcare activities, and the fostering of a healthy parent-child relationship. While teaching parenting skills, promote the parent's development of coping strategies to complement the child's temperament and techniques to manage the child's developmental issues such as toilet training or independence. Endorse age- and developmentally-appropriate discipline techniques. Encourage the use of outside social support agencies, as indicated, along with a person or agency to contact in a crisis. If the child will be cared for at home, teach the management of the child's casts, dressings, or diet, enlisting the assistance of a home health care agency as needed.

To facilitate change in a caregiver's behavior, mutually agreed-upon goals should be established. The caregiver should be encouraged to take personal responsibility and not project blame on others. Assist in the development of insight into the emotional climate of the family by addressing the caregiver's needs first, and help identify contributing factors of the abusive behavior. Appropriate referrals to community agencies such as parenting classes, individual and family counseling, substance abuse treatment programs, financial and food assistance programs, and daycare programs may help increase self-esteem and decrease chronic stress (Hawk & Bailie, 2007).

Interventions focused on impaired social interactions include promoting socialization after assessing for diminished self-esteem, assessing interest and skills as sources of diversional and social activities, providing age-appropriate diversional activities, facilitating participation in activities appropriate to the patient's physical and mental capacities, developing althernate communication techniques as needed, removing physical/structural barriers to participation whenever possible, and investigating community resources that may be of assistance in achieving socialization and diversional activity goals. An ideal outcome is a patient who participates in diversional/social activities (Hawk & Bailie, 2007).

Slipped Capital Femoral Epiphysis

Overview

Slipped capital femoral epiphysis (SCFE) is defined as the displacement of the proximal femoral head relative to the femoral neck and shaft (Kay, 2006). It is characterized by the posterior displacement of the proximal femoral epiphysis on the metaphysis due to disruption of the epiphysis, or growth plate (Hawk & Bailie, 2007). It is the most common adolescent hip disorder (Staheli, 2008c).

SCFE is classified as unstable or stable. An *unstable slip* (previously called an acute slip) occurs suddenly and accounts for 5%-10% of all slips. In an unstable slip, avascular necrosis (AVN) is more likely to occur. In a *stable slip* (previously called a chronic slip), there is gradual displacement of the femoral head (Hawk & Bailie, 2007). A "pre-slip" has been defined as a symptomatic hip with evidence of physiolysis prior to true movement of the femoral neck relative to the femoral head (Kay, 2006).

Although the exact cause of SCFE is unknown, it is believed to be multifactorial (Hawk & Bailie, 2007). In early adolescence, the growth plate is relatively weaker, as evidenced from the incidence of physeal injuries at other sites at this age. The hip is particularly vulnerable because it carries about four times its weight (Staheli, 2008c). Biomechanical factors may help explain the increased incidence in this population, such as the proximal femur being subjected to shear stress as a result of certain body weight and rapid growth, and the predisposition of some children to slippage due to decreased femoral anteversion (Hawk & Bailie, 2007) or relative retroversion in obese adolescents (Kay, 2006).

Retroversion (or a reduced neck shaft angle) may increase the verticality of the growth plate, making it mechanically less stable (Staheli, 2008c). Hormonal or endocrine factors may have a role in the etiology of SCFE (Hawk & Bailie, 2007) and appear to account for 5%-8% of SCFE cases. It is 6 times more common in patients who have an endocrinopathy than in those who do not.

The most common endocrinopathies in children with SCFE are hypothyroidism, panhypopituitarism, growth hormone (GH) abnormalities, and hypogonadism. The increased prevalence of hypothyroidism in children with Down syndrome is a likely explanation for the increased risk of SCFE in these children. The initial diagnosis of hypothyroidism is often made after the diagnosis of SCFE; in most children with SCFE and GH deficiency, the endocrine abnormality is known prior to the diagnosis of SCFE. Other systemic medical conditions (such as renal osteodystrophy) are due to secondary hyperparathyroidism. The complex interplay of hormones during puberty may put the hips at risk for SCFE. Laboratory studies in rats have also shown decreased physeal strength at puberty (Kay, 2006).

Previous radiation to the region of the femoral head also increases the risk of SCFE. Unlike the typical patient with SCFE, children with SCFE following previous radiation therapy have been reported to have a median weight at the 10th percentile (Kay, 2006). Treatment with chemotherapy has also been thought to contribute to SCFE (Staheli, 2008c), and immunosuppressive therapy after organ transplantation, particularly kidney, also may be an etiologic factor (Hawk & Bailie, 2007). Elevated levels of serum immunoglobulins and the C3 component of complement have also been reported in patients with SCFE. Although a genetic basis for SCFE has not been definitively established, incidence of the disease has been reported in a second family member in 3%-7% of the cases in most studies carried out. SCFE has been reported in identical twins and has been found to have an autosomal dominant inheritance with variable penetrance in familial cases. Whether this is due to a tendency toward other risk factors (such as obesity) remains unclear (Kay, 2006).

In SCFE, the femoral head is stabilized in the acetabulum, but the femoral neck and shaft move, relative to the femoral head and acetabulum. In almost all cases of SCFE, the proximal femoral neck and shaft move anteriorly and rotate externally, relative to the femoral head. If progression occurs to the point at which the femoral neck is completely anterior to the femoral head, proximal migration of the femoral neck occurs as well (Kay, 2006). The "slip" occurs through what would normally be the zones of cartilage cell hypertrophy and provisional calcification of the physis. The physeal plate abnormality apparently precedes the slippage. A superimposing acute trauma or the chronic stress of weight-bearing may initiate the displacement.

The proposed sequence of events includes rapid growth, which may cause weakening of the proximal femoral physis, and the shear stress of incumbent body weight, which may cause displacement. Often the force that is required for the slip is minimal. As the slip progresses, bone resorption occurs at the anterior superior border of the femoral neck, and bone deposition occurs in the posterior inferior corner. Once the slippage has begun, it will continue until the growth plate is stabilized by either natural or surgical closure (Hawk & Bailie, 2007). Following slippage, remodeling may reduce the deformity (Staheli, 2008c).

The male population with SCFE outnumbers the female population by 1.4:2.0 in most studies (Kay, 2006). It occurs in about 1 in 50,000 adolescents, most commonly in obese boys. The condition peaks at age 13 for boys and age 11 for girls, with a range from middle childhood to maturity (Staheli, 2008c). In girls, it is rarely seen after menarche (Hawk & Bailie, 2007). SCFE is bilateral in about one fourth of cases, with possibly slight silent slippage in even more (Staheli, 2008c). SCFE is about twice as common in African-American children as in Caucasian children, and those with Pacific Islander heritage have the highest rate of SCFE of any population (Kleposki et al., 2010).

Patients with SCFE have a normal acetabulum, and the articular cartilage is often preserved. Despite the presence of significant deformity, many do well for many decades. Chondrolysis and avascular necrosis cause early degeneration. There is a higher-than-normal risk of developing degenerative arthritis in patients with SCFE, and long-term prognosis is dependent upon the amount of displacement (Staheli, 2008c). Other complications include limitation of motion, shortening of the affected extremity, and malunion of the femoral head on the femoral neck. More severe slips have a greater likelihood of degenerating in later life, and joint arthroplasty, or arthrodesis, may be necessary to improve function or position (Hawk & Bailie, 2007).

Assessment

A history of the presenting symptoms, including the presence, location, duration, and intensity of pain, should be obtained. The pain is often located in the groin and may be referred to the anteromedial aspect of the thigh and knee. Typically the pain is dull and vague, and it may be intermittent or continuous. It is often exacerbated by physical activity, and usually there is no pain at rest. There may be a history of limited motion of the hip (Hawk & Bailie, 2007). Hip or groin pain an obese, prepubertal child is highly suggestive of SCFE. Hip pain is absent in as many as 50% of children with

SCFE, however, including up to 8% with a painless limp. The onset of the symptoms, progression, and prior treatment should be elicited, along with a medical history that may include endocrine issues. There may be a history of an inciting event, such as mild trauma (Kay, 2006). An *unstable SCFE* will reveal a sudden onset of severe pain with an inability to bear weight, whereas a *stable SCFE* typically reveals an insidious onset of symptoms over several months. Long-standing slips will also produce an out-toeing gait, an abductor lurch, and limb atrophy (Staheli, 2008c) of the proximal thigh (Hawk & Bailie, 2007).

The physical examination of the child/adolescent will reveal an antalgic limp (decreased stance phase on the affected limb) (Kay, 2006) in the affected leg in a laterally rotated position. ROM may be limited, depending on the severity of the slip, and internal rotation and abduction are restricted. At rest, the limb usually lies in an externally rotated position. Flexing the involved limb produces concomitant external rotation. Shortening of the affected limb may be present, and often there is a positive Trendelenburg test (see Chapter 3—Musculoskeletal Assessment).

An AP view radiograph of the pelvis and lateral view radiographs of both hips should be obtained to confirm the diagnosis. A frog-leg lateral x-ray may exacerbate instability, and a cross-table, true lateral view should be done if there is a high suspicion of an acute, unstable hip. In an *unstable SCFE*, the contours of the femoral neck and head are sharp and easily defined. In a *stable SCFE*, remodeling has likely occurred, and the outlines may be blunted (Hawk & Bailie, 2007).

The degree of slip is commonly quantified as the amount of femoral head displacement as a percentage of the femoral neck diameter (Kay, 2006), with the following classifications:

- "Pre-slip": Widening and irregularity of the growth plate with no actual displacement of the epiphysis;
- Grade I slip: Displacement of less than one third of the diameter of the femoral neck, termed a minimal slip;
- Grade II slip: Displacement between one third and one half the diameter of the femoral neck, termed a moderate slip; and
- Grade III slip: Displacement of greater than one half is termed a severe slip (Hawk & Bailie, 2007).

Although frequently used, this measurement can be inconsistent because of variations in patient positioning and can change over time because of proximal femoral remodeling. Some experts recommend using this measurement only in the evaluation of SCFE prior to remodeling (Kay, 2006). A CT scan may be done to diagnose an early slip in patients who have symptoms, but normal radiographs (Hawk & Bailie, 2007) and ultrasound imaging will demonstrate "step-off" at the site of displacement. Although seldom necessary, a high-resolution bone scan will show increased uptake and can diagnose a pre-slip, and the MRI shows AVN or an altered femoral head position (Staheli, 2008c). Labwork to rule out hypothyroidism is recommended in patients who are obese, age 10 or younger, and with other clinical signs of hypothyroidism. Screening of all patients with SCFE is not recommended (Hawk & Bailie, 2007).

Common Therapeutic Modalities

Treatment of a SCFE should be initiated immediately after the diagnosis to prevent further slippage and to decrease the possibility of complications. No weight-bearing on the affected side is permitted once the diagnosis has been made, and the child should be put on bedrest at home or in the hospital to prevent further slippage prior to surgery.

The goal of surgical intervention is to cause physeal closure, which is when the cartilage cells convert to bone and when the femoral head will be fused to the neck of the femur. Surgical pinning is the most common procedure and is typically done with in situ fixation with a single cannulated screw, which prevents further slippage and induces physeal closure (Hawk & Bailie, 2007). In the child younger than age 8, a smooth pin is used to allow growth (Staheli, 2008c). Postoperatively, the child or adolescent will remain non-weight-bearing or touchdown weight-bearing with crutches for 6 weeks. Subsequent removal of the screw is typically not done (Hawk & Bailie, 2007). Bilateral slips occur in about 25% of patients, and prophylactic pinning is done on the apparently uninvolved side if an early slip is suspected, or if some underlying metabolic disorder is present. Other factors increasing the risk for the other hip to slip are an age younger than 10 and severe obesity (Staheli, 2008c).

Other surgical procedures include a bone graft epiphysiodesis, when a bone graft is used to bridge the femoral neck and the head of the femur (Hawk & Bailie, 2007) to prevent progression (Kay, 2006). Osteotomies of the femoral neck and intertrochanteric and subtrochanteric regions can be done, and are indicated for some chronic slips to restore more normal anatomy and mechanics. These are considered salvage procedures and have varying complication rates. Reconstruction by arthroplasty and arthrodesis can be done. Prior to the arthroplasty, distraction of the joint using an external fixator may be needed to pull the femur down, stretch the soft tissues, and provide better alignment. Joint replacement in the adolescent age group is not recommended (Hawk & Bailie, 2007).

Nursing Considerations

Nursing Diagnoses. Nursing diagnoses for this condition are expanded upon in the Appendix.

- Anxiety.
- Mobility: physical, impaired.
- Pain, acute.

Nursing Interventions. Interventions related to anxiety include developing a plan of care that minimizes patient/parental anxiety by allowing the expression of fears/concerns related to the diagnosis and treatment plan. Provide education regarding the underlying pathology, normal developmental progression, and treatment. The best outcome is a patient/family with the ability to express their fears/concerns about the diagnosis/treatment and to understand the pathology, progression, and treatment plan (Hawk & Bailie, 2007).

Interventions focused on acute pain include assessing the patient for pain and observing for nonverbal cues, especially in those who cannot communicate effectively. Promote patient comfort with appropriate pharmacologic and nonpharmacologic techniques. Encourage diversional activities, and discuss coping methods with the patient/family. The best outcome is a patient who experiences a maximal degree of comfort. See Chapter 7—Pain.

Interventions that focus on impaired physical mobility include instructing the patient/family on mobility restrictions before and after surgery. The patient will require crutch training (or walker training if this is deemed safer more the child). Help coordinate PT, if needed, to restore mobility. Home care considerations include reinforcing the need for protected ambulation, restricting activity, and explaining the signs/symptoms of a slip of the opposite hip (Hawk & Bailie, 2007).

Torsional Issues

Overview

Torsional issues of in-toeing and out-toeing often concern parents (Staheli, 2008e), although rotational profiles are highly variable, particularly in toddlers who have not mastered the basic skills needed for normal walking. Internal and external rotational variations are differences, not pathologic conditions.

Foot position during walking is described by the direction of the foot relative to the body's line of progression during the gait cycle (internal, external, or neutral). It results from the summation of several factors, including version, capsular pliability, and muscular control. Version is tilt or inclination within a bone, such as the relation of the femoral head/neck to the shaft of the femur. Similarly, capsular laxity may allow a greater-than-normal arc of motion. Arthrosis or incongruity may also restrict motion. The balance between opposing muscle groups is also a determinant of foot position and may introduce a significant, dynamic component to the rotational profile. Age is another important variable because version, soft-tissue pliability, and muscle coordination change as the child matures.

No treatment is necessary in most children. The natural history of rotational variations is gradual normalization, usually accomplished by age 5-6 (Schoenecker & Rich, 2006), although some torsional problems may not improve until age 8-10. Severe torsional problems may persist into adulthood, and early osteoarthritis of the hip may be associated with femoral anteversion. Although clinically the words "torsion," "rotation," and "version" are used interchangeably (Hawk & Bailie, 2007), some references define torsion as variation beyond two standard deviations, either plus or minus (Staheli, 2008e).

Internal tibial torsion, or medial tibial torsion, is quite common (Schoenecker & Rich, 2006) and describes the rotation of the tibia along the long axis. It is defined as the distal tibia rotated medially in relation to the proximal tibia. At birth, internal tibial torsion is between 0-20 degrees, and growth alone produces correction in more than 90% of cases. Internal tibial torsion may aggravate or compensate for rotational variations in the femur. In adulthood, 20 degrees of internal tibial torsion is considered normal. It is often asymmetric, with the left side affected more than the right. Persistent, disabling internal tibial torsion is rare.

External tibial torsion, or lateral tibial torsion, is less common and is defined as the distal tibia rotated laterally in relation to the proximal tibia. External tibial torsion is often unilateral and more common on the right side. Torsional changes in the lower extremities occur as a normal part of in utero development and are influenced by genetic factors and intrauterine positioning. Postnatal influences such as prematurity and prone positioning can result in external tibial torsion (Hawk & Bailie, 2007).

Femoral anteversion, or medial femoral rotation, describes the torsion of the femur along its long axis. It is caused by the anterior rotation of the femoral neck in relation to the femoral shaft and is rare in a pure form. Femoral anteversion is about 30-40 degrees at birth, and nearly all children exhibit some femoral anteversion. It gradually decreases to about 10-15 degrees by skeletal maturity. It is considered excessive when it is greater than 50 degrees or if it creates a functional disability. It is often associated with sitting in a "W" position, which is when a child sits with knees bent and feet outside of the hips (Hawk & Bailie, 2007). Femoral anteversion is often familial, usually bilateral, and affects females more than males (Staheli, 2008e).

Infrequently, pathologic conditions will cause a rotational abnormality. Residual foot deformities, disorders of the hip, and neuromuscular diseases are the most common causes of pathologic in-toeing or out-toeing. *In-toeing* may be caused by residual foot deformity from metatarsus adductus, clubfoot, or skewfoot. In-toeing, which is only apparent during swing phase, may be the result of overpull of the posterior tibial tendon, often seen in spastic hemiplegia. Femoral antetorsion is often seen in spastic diplegia or quadriplegia. This may be a combination of excess femoral anteversion with contracture of the adductor and medial hamstring muscles. Excess valgus and pronation of the foot, which contribute to an out-toed foot progression, may also be seen. For some children with spasticity, extremes in rotational posture are a compensatory mechanism for limited hip, knee, or ankle motion (Schoenecker & Rich, 2006). Pathologic *out-toeing* may result from the severe pes planovalgus often associated with external tibial torsion. This may be secondary to tarsal coalition, but may also be seen in adolescents with rigid flat feet without a coalition. The combination of femoral retrotorsion, external tibial torsion, and pes planovalgus can also be seen, particularly in large adolescents, which produces a striking out-toed gait (Schoenecker & Rich, 2006). Femoral retroversion may increase the risk of SCFE (see separate section in this chapter) and has been associated with degenerative changes of the hip (Staheli, 2008e). SCFE should be considered in a differential diagnosis of out-toeing, particularly when the deviation is asymmetric or of recent onset. Hip dysplasia can alter rotation, but its effect is highly variable (Schoenecker & Rich, 2006).

Most children brought in for concerns of in-toeing or out-toeing are normal. Internal tibial torsion is more common than external tibial torsion in toddlers. It is often associated with physiologic bowing and decreases 1-2 years after resolution of the bowing. Occasionally, it will persist into preadolescence. External tibial torsion is less common but is more likely to persist through adolescence (Schoenecker & Rich, 2006). See Table 11.10 and Table 11.11 for summaries of pediatric rotational problems.

Assessment

The child's presenting symptoms, such as the type of torsional problem, difficutly with ambulation, or knee pain, should be elicited (Hawk & Bailie, 2007). Obtain the birth and developmental history. A delay in walking may suggest a neuromuscular disorder. Elicit a family history. Rotational problems are often inherited, and the status of the parent foretells the child's future (Staheli, 2008e). Also ask about the past medical and surgical history and parental concerns regarding the child's gait, function, and cosmesis (Hawk & Bailie, 2007). The child's spine should be examined, and a brief neurological assessment should be done to rule out a neuromuscular disorder such as CP, and the hips should be examined to rule out DDH.

The child should be observed walking and running, and the foot progression angle (FPA) should be estimated. This is the angular difference between the axis of the foot and the line of progression. A minus value is assigned to an in-toeing gait in the following levels:

- -5 to -10 degrees is mild;
- -10 to -15 degrees is moderate; and
- More than -15 degrees is severe.

A rotational profile of the lower extremities should be done to establish the level and severity of any torsional problem, and the values should be recorded with the child prone, the knees flexed to a right angle, and the pelvis level. Assess both sides at the same time.

Table 11.10. Rotational Problems Related to Pediatric Age Groups

Age	Torsional Problem	
1st year of life	**IN-TOEING**	**OUT-TOEING**
	Metatarsus adductus	Generally normal
Toddler	Internal tibial torsion	Generally continues to be normal
Preschool/early school-age	Femoral anteversion	Begin to see external tibial torsion
Late school-age	Internal tibial torsion and femoral anteversion usually resolve	External tibial torsion may increase
Adolescence	Malalignment syndrome – combination of femoral anteversion and external tibial torsion	Malalignment syndrome – combination of femoral anteversion and external tibial torsion

From Core Curriculum for Orthopaedic Nursing (6th ed., p. 276), 2007, National Association of Orthopaedic Nurses, Boston, MA: Pearson. Reproduced with permission.

Table 11.11. Rotational Problems: Assessment Areas

Tibial Torsion	Femoral Anteversion
In-toeing gait (internal tibial torsion) or out-toeing gait (external tibial torsion)	In-toeing gait Abnormal rotation of hips Ligamentous laxity Internal rotation of entire lower extremity

From Core Curriculum for Orthopaedic Nursing (6th ed., p. 277), 2007, National Association of Orthopaedic Nurses, Boston, MA: Pearson. Reproduced with permission.

Internal rotation is normally less than 60-70 degrees. If hip rotation is asymmetrical, evaluate further with a radiograph. To quantitate tibial version, assess the thigh foot angle (TFA). With the child prone and the knee flexed to a right angle, the TFA is the angular difference between the axis of the foot and the axis of the thigh. The TFA measures the tibial and hindfoot rotational status. Also assess the borders of the foot for forefoot adductus, which is identified by a convexity of the lateral border of the foot (Staheli, 2008e).

In an older child with a gait abnormality or with complaints of pain, a cross-table lateral radiograph is optimal to detect a minimally displaced SCFE (Schoenecker & Rich, 2006). If correction of the torsion is being considered a standing AP view of the lower extremities (hips to ankles) on one cassette is indicated (Staheli, 2008e).

Common Therapeutic Modalities

Observational management is indicated for most children with torsional problems, as 90%-95% of rotational issues remodel with growth (Hawk & Bailie, 2007). Measures such as shoe wedges or inserts and daytime bracing with twister cables are ineffective. Night splints that laterally rotate the feet are better tolerated and do not interfere with the child's play, but probably have no long-term benefit (Staheli, 2008e).

Operative treatment to address significant cosmetic and functional deformities in an older child or adolescent is done only if the severity of the condition justifies the risks of the procedure. In this situation, the best options are a femoral rotational osteotomy performed at the intertrochanteric level or a tibial ostetomy performed at the supramalleolar level. Treatment for rotational, or miserable, malalignment syndrome is a major undertaking, as it usually requires a 4-level procedure (femoral and tibial). The site of the tibial osteotomy may be distal (most safe) or proximal (Staheli, 2008e). In patients with physeal closure and with symptomatic lateral torsion of the tibia which fails to correct with growth, the excessive lateral twist of the tibia results in excessive valgus force at the knee and predisposes the knee to patellar instability, osteochondral defects, and anterior knee pain. Some experts advocate a tibial rotational osteotomy using an intermedullary rod fixation to correct the torsion, and removing the excessive strain on the knee is indicated (Stotts & Stevens, 2009).

Nursing Considerations

Nursing Diagnoses. Nursing diagnoses for this condition are expanded upon in the Appendix.

- Anxiety.
- Self-concept, readiness for enhanced.

Nursing Interventions. Interventions focused on reducing anxiety include developing a plan of care that minimizes the anxiety of the patient/family by allowing them to express fears/concerns. The patient and family members should be included in the decision-making process and should receive education regarding the underlying pathology, normal developmental progression and treatment. An optimal outcome is a patient/family that expresses their fears/concerns related to the diagnosis and treatment and understands the pathology, usual progression, and treatment plan.

Interventions for a disturbed self-concept promote a positive self-concept by focusing on the patient as a whole, not on the affected part, and reinforcing personal strengths and skills. The best outcome is a child in whom strengths and weaknesses are developed and who developments the skills consistent with the child's age (Hawk & Bailie, 2007).

Summary

The diagnosis of a pediatric orthopaedic condition can be life-altering and overwhelming for the child and the family. With guidance from knowledgeable and compassionate nurses, however, parents can evolve from novice bystanders to educated advocates, helping their child live a happy and meaningful life.

References

Alman, B.A. & Goldberg, M.J. (2006). Syndromes of orthopaedic importance. In R.T. Morrissy, *Lovell and Winter's Pediatric Orthopaedics* (6th ed., Vol. I.). Philadelphia, PA: Lippincott Williams & Wilkins.

Barron, C. & Jenny, C. (2011). Child physical abuse. In M.Z. Augustyn, *The Zuckerman Parker Handbook of Developmental and Behavioral Pediatrics for Primary Care* (3rd ed.). Philadelphia, PA: Lippincott Williams & Wilkins.

Bakman, M., Bang, C., Seo, G., & Monu, J. (2002). *Musculoskeletal Imaging Case of the Month*. Retrieved from http://urmc.rochester.edu/smd/Rad/MSKcases/MSK02

Bennett, F. (1999). Diagnosing cerebral palsy—The earlier the better. *Contemporary Pediatrics, 16*, 208-216.

Berry, J., Bloom, S., Foley, S., & Palfrey, J. (2010). Health inequity in children and youth with chronic health conditions. *Pediatrics*, S111-S116.

Cline, S. & Patel, D. (2009). Stress fractures. In D. G. Patel, *Pediatric Practice Sports Medicine*. New York, NY: McGraw Hill.

Glorieux, F. (2007). *Guide to Osteogenesis Imperfecta for Pediatricians and Family Practice Physicians*. Bethesda, MD: National Institutes of Health Osteoporosis and Related Bone Diseases.

Hawk, D. & Bailie, S. (2007). Pediatrics/congenital disorders. In National Association of Orthopaedic Nurses, *Core Curriculum for Orthopaedic Nursing* (6th ed., pp. 259-326). Boston, MA: Pearson Custom Publishing.

Horn, P.B. (2010). A new zip in playground injuries. *Consultant for Pediatricians, 9*(9), 313.

Hornor, G. (2010). Child sexual abuse: Consequences and implications. *Journal of Pediatric Health Care, 24*(6), 358.

Hornor, G. (2005). Physical abuse: Recognition and reporting. *Journal of Pediatric Health, 19*(1), 4-11.

Kasser, J.R. (2006). The foot. In R. T. Morrissey, *Lovell and Winter's Pediatric Orthopedics* (6th ed., Vol. II, pp. 1257-1328). Philadelphia, PA: Lippincott Williams & Wilkins.

Kay, R.M. (2006). Slipped capital femoral epiphysis. In R. T. Morrissy, *Lovell and Winter's Pediatric Orthopaedics* (6th ed., Vol. II, pp. 1085-1124). Philadelphia, PA: Lippincott Williams & Wilkins.

Kleposki, R., Abel, K., & Sehgal, K. (2010). Common pediatric hip diseases in primary care. *The Clinical Advisor 6*, 23.

Kunkler, C.E. (2007). Therapeutic modalities. In National Association of Orthopaedic Nurses, *Core Curriculum for Orthopaedic Nursing* (6th ed., pp. 227-258). Boston: Pearson Custom Publishing.

Leventhal, J.M., Martin, K.D., & Asnes, A.G. (2010). Fractures and traumatic brain injuries: Abuse versus accidents in a US database of hospitalized children. *Pediatrics, 126*(1), 104-115.

Massachusetts General Hospital. (n.d.) *Bilateral Long Leg Spica Cast.* Retrieved from http://massgeneral.org/ortho/assets/images/pediatrics/spica-cast-babyincast1.jpg

Morrell, D., Pearson, J., & Sauser, D., (2002). Progressive bone and joint abnormalities of the spine and lower extremities in cerebral palsy. *Radiographs, 22*, 257-268.

Moseley, C.F. (2006). Leg-length discrepancy. In R.T. Morrissy, *Lovell and Winter's Pediatric Orthopaedics* (6th ed., Vol. II, pp. 1213-1256). Philadelphia, PA: Lippincott Williams & Wilkins.

Noonan, K.J. (2006). Myelomeningocele. In R.T. Morrissy, *Lovell and Winter's Pediatric Orthopaedics* (6th ed., Vol. I, pp. 605-648). Philadelphia, PA: Lippincott Williams & Wilkins.

Palmer, F. & Hoon, A. (2011). Cerebral palsy. In M.Z. Augustyn, *The Zuckerman Parker Handbook of Developmental and Behavioral Pediatrics for Primary Care* (pp. 164-170). Philadelphia, PA: Lippincott Williams & Wilkins.

Patel, D. (2009a). Muscouloskeletal injuries: Basic concepts. In D.R. Patel, *Pediatric Practice Sports Medicine*. New York, NY: McGraw Hill.

Patel, D. (2009b). Overuse injuries of the knee. In D.R. Patel, *Pediatric Practice Sports Medicine*. New York, NY: McGraw Hill Medical.

Sedlak, A.J., Mettenburg, J., Basena, M., Petta, I., McPherson, K., Greene, A., & Li, S. (2010). *Fourth National Incidence Study of Child Abuse and Neglect (NIS-4)*. Report to Congress. Washington, DC: US Department of Health and Human Services, Administration for Children for Children and Families.

Schoenecker, P.L. & Rich, M.M. (2006). The lower extremity. In R.T. Morrissy, *Lovell and Winter's Pediatric Orthopaedics* (6th ed., Vol II, pp. 1157-1212). Philadelphia, PA: Lippincott Williams & Wilkins.

Sponseller, P.D. & Ain, M.C. (2006). The skeletal dysplasias. In R.T. Morrissy, *Lovell and Winter's Pediatric Orthopaedics* (6th ed., Vol. I, pp. 205-250). Philadelphia, PA: Lippincott Williams & Wilkins.

Staheli, L.T. (2008a). Foot. In L.T. Staheli, *Fundamentals of Pediatric Orthopedics* (4th ed., pp. 157-185). Philadelphia, PA: Lippincott Williams & Wilkins.

Staheli, L.T. (2008b). Growth. In L.T. Staheli, *Fundamentals of Pediatric Orthopedics* (4th ed., pp. 1-23). Philadelphia, PA: Lippincott Williams & Wilkins.

Staheli, L.T. (2008c). Hip and femur. In L.T. Staheli, *Fundamentals of Pediatric Orthopedics* (4th ed., pp. 201-230). Philadelphia, PA: Lippincott Williams & Wilkins.

Staheli, L.T. (2008d). Knee and tibia. In L.T. Staheli, *Fundamentals of Pediatric Orthopedics* (4th ed., pp. 186-200). Philadelphia, PA: Lippincott Williams & Wilkins.

Staheli, L.T. (2008e). Lower limb. In L.T. Staheli, *Fundamentals of Pediatric Orthopedics* (4th ed., pp. 135-156). Philadelphia, PA: Lippincott Williams & Wilkins.

Staheli, L.T. (2008f). Spine and pelvis. In L.T. Staheli, *Fundamental of Pediatric Orthopedics* (4th ed., pp. 231-258). Philadelphia, PA: Lippincott Williams & Wilkins.

Staheli, L.T. (2008g). Trauma. In L.T. Staheli, *Fundamentals of Pediatric Orthopedics* (4th ed., pp. 57-76). Philadelphia, PA: Lippincott Williams & Wilkins.

Stotts, A. & Stevens, P. (2009). Tibial rotational osteotomy with intramedullary nail fixation. *Strategies in Trauma and Limb Reconstruction, 4*(3), 129-133.

Thompson, G.H. & Berenson, F.R. (2006). Other neuromuscular disorders. In R.T. Morrissy, *Lovell and Winter's Pediatric Orthopedics* (6th ed., Vol. I, pp. 649-692). Philadelphia, PA: Lippincott Williams & Wilkins.

Watemberg, N., Silver, S., Harel, S., & Lerman-Sagie, T. (2002). Significance of microcephaly among children with developmental disabilities. *Journal of Child Neurology, 17*(2), 117-122.

Weinstein, S.L. (2006a). Developmental hip dysplasia and dislocation. In R.T. Morrissey, *Lovell and Winter's Pediatric Orthopedics* (6th ed., Vol. II, pp. 937-1038). Philadelphia, PA: Lippincott Williams & Wilkins.

Weinstein, S.L. (2006b). Legg-Calve-Perthes Syndrome. In R.T. Morrissy, *Lovell and Winter's Pediatric Orthopaedics* (6th ed., Vol II, pp. 1039-1084). Philadelphia, PA: Lippincott Williams & Wilkins.

CHAPTER 11

Chapter 12
Special Geriatric Considerations

Laura M. Criddle, PhD, RN, ACNS-BC, ONC, FAEN

Objectives

- Predict the impact of the growing older adult population on orthopaedic nursing practice.
- Summarize age-associated changes—physiologic and pathologic—to each body system.
- Explain the impact of aging transformations on the musculoskeletal system.
- Explicate the effects that changes in the cardiovascular, respiratory, neurological, and gastrointestinal systems have on the patient with an orthopaedic disorder.
- Discuss common orthopaedic nursing concerns in the geriatric patient.

Americans are living longer than ever before, and the number of citizens ages 65 and older is expected to increase from a current level of 40 million to 75 million by the year 2030, and to 90 million by 2050 (U.S. Department of Health & Human Services [HHS], 2010). This trend is driven not only by huge reductions in infant and young adult mortality over the past century, but by significant longevity gains as well. For example, in the 2-decade interval between 1983 and 2003, mortality rates for males ages 65-74 dropped by almost 30%; mortality rates in men ages 75-84 decreased by 22% (Gilman, Parker, & Tabloski, 2009). Persons older than age 85 now constitute the fastest growing U.S. demographic. In fact, approximately one third of Americans live beyond 85 years, and at least 10% of persons older than age 90 can expect to still be alive at age 99. Currently, 5.8 million Americans are older than age 85 (the "old old"), but this number is expected to reach a staggering 19 million by 2050 (HHS, 2010). Never before in the history of the planet have we seen such demographics. These population shifts are likely to have a profound impact on the number and types of patients seeking care for orthopaedic disorders.

There is lack of consensus regarding the definition of "elderly," and the lower cut-off point for "geriatric" has been variably defined as anywhere between ages 50 and 75. Nevertheless, 65 years—the current age of Medicare eligibility—is the criterion most commonly selected to define "older" adults in the United States. Because an individual may live for more than 100 years, the "elderly" category encompasses a very large group, many of whom may be much closer to age 100 than they are to 50.

The increase in life expectancy during the 20th century has been a remarkable achievement—not without its own complications, however. Senescence (or growing old) predisposes individuals to many diseases and disorders. Almost no one achieves senior status without a history of various medical events. Some physical changes reflect the inevitable and predictable process of aging (physiological or developmental alterations), while other age-associated changes are the result of pathology or cumulative life stressors. Although older Americans generally enjoy good heath, many older adults experience physical disabilities, and a significant proportion suffer from chronic health conditions (Meiner, 2011b).

Orthopaedic problems are not often directly life-threatening in the elderly, but they are among the most common geriatric conditions and contribute significantly to morbidity and mortality, whether they are the presenting complaint or a comorbidity. Age-associated changes to other body systems directly and indirectly impact (and are impacted by) orthopaedic disorders. Moreover, the orthopaedic changes of aging can profoundly affect

Table 12.1. Age-Associated Changes and Their Implications

Body System	Aging Changes	Orthopaedic Implications
Cardiovascular	Hypertension	Chronic hypertension makes it difficult to detect hypotensive episodes.
	Structural changes	Left ventricular wall thickening, myocardial irritability, and calcification of the great vessel reduce myocardial compliance, decreased stroke volume, and blunt the heart's response to stress.
	Cardiac medications	Common medications, (digoxin and beta-blockers) limit compensatory reactions to shock by inhibiting the normal tachycardic response.
	Dependence on preload	Even mild hypovolemia can significantly compromise cardiac function. Hypovolemia worsens renal and coronary perfusion and impairs tissue oxygen delivery. This leads to myocardial ischemia, gut ischemia, and wound-healing failures.
	Hemorrhage risk	Both liver disease and the routine use of warfarin, aspirin, and other anti-clotting agents increase bleeding risk.
Respiratory	Loss of lung elasticity	Reduced pulmonary compliance leads to small airway collapse, uneven alveolar ventilation, and air trapping.
	Declining PaO2	Age-associated parenchymal changes limit the alveolar surface area available for gas exchange creating a ventilation-perfusion mismatch that in turn causes a decline in arterial oxygen tension (PaO2).
	Thoracic skeletal changes	The spine and thorax undergo progressive osteoporotic changes and vertebral collapse, producing kyphosis and making the thoracic skeleton vulnerable to fractures. Contractures of the intercostal muscles and calcification of the costal cartilage reduce chest wall compliance.
	Thoracic muscular changes	Progressive loss of strength in the respiratory muscles is accompanied by a decline in maximum inspiratory and expiratory force by as much as 50%.

Body System	Aging Changes	Orthopaedic Implications
Neurological	Reduced sensory perception	Sensory perception declines steadily with normal aging placing older adults at increased risk for falls and other injuries and complicates patient communication.
	Neuronal atrophy & loss	A progressive, scattered loss of cerebral cortical neurons affects memory and mental processing. Loss is accelerated by Alzheimer's disease and alcohol abuse. Neuronal atrophy and loss predispose to delirium.
	Slowed impulse conduction	Neuronal loss is associated with slowed impulse conduction through the nerves, which diminishes an elder's ability to deal with multiple stimuli and respond to information in order to prevent injury.
	Cerebral blood flow	As brain weight decreases, cerebral blood flow is reduced, placing older adults at increased risk for ischemic insults.
	Cervical spine fractures	The incidence of spine and spinal cord injuries increases with age. These fractures heal very poorly.
Integument & Immune	Subcutaneous fat loss	Loss is particularly pronounced in the fatty pads that protect bony prominences.
	Dermis and epidermis thin	Aging skin is delicate and more susceptible to tears.
	Interstitial tissue changes	Changes in the skin's interstitium predispose older adults to bruising.
	Slowed wound healing	Wound healing responses are greatly diminished and older adults are more vulnerable to wound infection.
	Nail bed changes	Nail bed changes make it difficult to evaluate distal perfusion.
	Immunosuppression	The older adult's ability to mount an adequate response to infection is limited.
Musculoskeletal	Diminished muscle mass	Muscle mass loss reduces overall strength and contributes to fatigability.
	Reduced myocytes functional capacity	Myocyte loss diminishes the muscle's ability to extract and utilize oxygen.
	Osteoporosis	Osteoporosis results in bone fragility, predisposing the older adult to spontaneous fractures and fractures following even minor trauma.

general physical functioning, patient lifestyle, and activities of daily living (ADLs) (Lach, 2007a).

This chapter will focus on the predictable physiological and common pathologic changes of senescence and briefly discuss their relationship to the geriatric orthopaedic patient. See Table 12.1 for an overview of conditions related to geriatric patients. For detailed information on specific orthopaedic conditions and practices, refer to the relevant chapter.

Factors that Influence Aging

Universal Age-Related Changes

Regardless of chronological age, growing old is a highly individual process; no two people age at the same rate or in the same manner. Some age-related changes are universal, however. Over time, the number of normally functioning cells in the body is reduced, oxygen consumption is decreased, and response to physiologic stressors is blunted (Lach, 2007b; Resnick, 2005). Yet the interaction between the genetic, environmental, physiological, psychological, and social aspects of life each exert their influences on the progression of aging. As the years advance, the incidence of disease increases, and cardiovascular and neoplastic disorders replace traumatic events as the most common causes of death. Although physiological decline and disease processes influence each other, it is important to distinguish age-related changes from those associated with chronic conditions or acute illness in order to avoid prematurely attributing findings to advanced age when they are actually caused by a (potentially treatable) disease state (Criddle, 2009b).

The Geriatric Orthopaedic Patient

Orthopaedic nurses need to be cognizant of the differences in outcomes and complications experienced by older adults. Senescence has a profound impact on individual biological performance. In every body system, the elderly patient's physiological reserves are limited, and function can deteriorate rapidly, even with expert medical and nursing attention. Declining physiological status forces seniors to draw upon reserves just to maintain homeostasis. In the face of increased metabolic demands posed by acute illness or surgical stress, organ systems can quickly fail.

In addition to experiencing high rates of acute and chronic illness, the elderly are over-represented in the number of trauma hospitalizations. Both longevity gains and increasingly active lifestyles have contributed to rising injury rates (Criddle, 2009a). In some regions of the United States, the number of elderly women hospitalized for injury exceeds that of young men. In addition, older adults experience a greater number of post-injury sequelae than do their younger counterparts. The elderly suffer an increased incidence of wound healing problems, sepsis, other infections, and multiple organ failure. Pre-existing medical conditions, particularly cardiovascular disease, have a profound effect on patients' ability to manage and recover from the stresses of injury (Criddle, 2009b).

Falls are the leading injury mechanism among persons older than age 65 (Emergency Nurses Association [ENA], 2007). In the over-75 age group, falls are also the leading cause of death from traumatic events. Many factors associated with aging contribute to the high incidence of falls among seniors. Dementia, decreased visual acuity, obesity, neurological and musculoskeletal impairments, gait and balance disturbances, and medication use are all contributory factors (Criddle, 2009b).

By the year 2020, there will be an estimated 40 million drivers in the U.S. older than age 65 (Plummer, 2009). Seniors have a motor vehicle crash rate second only to that of 16- to 25-year-olds; however, the elderly (particularly those ages 75 and older) suffer a post-collision fatality rate greater than that of any other age group. Senescent declines in cognitive function, decreased auditory acuity, changes in direct and peripheral vision, impaired coordination, and increased reaction time all contribute to crashes by geriatric motorists (Criddle, 2009a).

Automobile-versus-pedestrian incidences are a major source of both musculoskeletal and head injury in seniors and are the third-most common cause of traumatic mortality in those older than age 65. In addition to slowed ambulation, many older adults suffer from kyphosis, which produces a stooped posture, making it difficult to raise the head to see oncoming traffic. Delayed reaction time, vision and hearing losses, limited neck rotation, medication use, substance abuse, and poor judgment also contribute to geriatric pedestrian injuries (Criddle, 2009a).

The Impact of Aging on Body Systems

Cardiovascular Concerns

It is difficult to separate cardiovascular decline from normal age-related alterations in body composition, metabolic rate, and general fitness level, all of which affect cardiac performance (Wallace & Grossman, 2008). In the elderly, exercise capacity is commonly restricted by functions that limit exercise ability such as neurological, pulmonary, or orthopaedic disorders.

Aging is associated with changes in the sympathetic and parasympathetic nervous systems that impair the response to beta-adrenergic stimulation. This is particularly important during periods of exercise or other physiological stressors such as illness or injury. In the geriatric population, the predictable loss of sympathetic sensitivity is further aggravated by widespread use of beta-blocking drugs (e.g., metoprolol), putting older adults at risk for postural hypotension, dizziness, and fainting (ENA, 2007). Cardiac function is also limited by the structural changes of aging. Pump function is decreased by progressive fibrosis of the myocardium, left ventricular wall thickening, and stiffening of the aortic and mitral valves. These changes combine to make it more difficult for the aging heart to maintain adequate contractile strength. Dysrhythmias common to older adults—atrial fibrillation and premature ventricular complexes—also serve to reduce cardiac effectiveness (House-Fancher & Lynch, 2007).

Arteriosclerosis and atherosclerosis cause the arteries to become progressively less distensible. Atherosclerotic disease elevates blood pressure, reduces blood flow to vital organs, and decreases physiological reserves (House-Fancher & Lynch, 2007; Miller, 2009). But the vascular changes of aging are not limited to the small vessels. The progressive aortic calcification associated with aging, along with osteoporosis of the thoracic vertebrae, can result in more calcium visible in the aorta than in the spine on the chest radiographs of some elderly patients. Due to these senescent vascular changes, peripheral pulses—particularly in the feet—may be diminished or absent for decades prior to patient presentation and are therefore not reliable indicators of acute circulatory compromise. Older adults are less likely than their younger counterparts to experience chest pain in the presence of acute myocardial infarction. Subtle indicators of cardiac ischemia include new onset fatigue, nausea, anxiety, and diaphoresis.

Seniors are often unable to raise cardiac output to meet increased oxygen demands. Early transfusion—rather than infusion of large volumes of crystalloids or colloids—is, therefore, the safer course of treatment in the geriatric patient in hypovolemic shock (Plummer, 2009). Administration of packed red blood cells enhances oxygen-carrying capacity without adding to interstitial fluid overload. Whenever possible, warm all blood products prior to transfusion to minimize hypothermia. Many elders are at increased risk for bleeding due to the use of warfarin (Coumadin®), aspirin, clopidogrel (Plavix®), or other antithrombotic agents.

Respiratory Concerns

Elderly post-surgical patients have up to a 40% incidence of respiratory complications, depending on the site of surgery. As the result of both chest wall and pulmonary parenchymal changes, a gradual decline in respiratory function accompanies aging. The normal respiratory rate in older adults is 20-22 breaths per minute. Typically, these adaptations occur progressively as age advances and should be insufficient to affect an elderly person's ability to breathe effortlessly at rest. Nonetheless, factors such as frequent exposure to environmental pollutants (particularly cigarette smoke), old pulmonary disorders (e.g., tuberculosis), and recurrent respiratory infections accelerate age-related changes, making it difficult to distinguish expected alterations in pulmonary function from actual disease states (Miller, 2009). Physiological change in senescent lungs leads to loss of elasticity, reduced pulmonary compliance, small airway collapse, uneven alveolar ventilation, and air trapping.

Age-associated alterations reduce the alveolar surface area available for gas exchange, producing a decline in baseline arterial oxygen tension (PaO2) (Miller, 2009). Age alone does not affect ventilation. The partial pressure of carbon dioxide (PaCO2) in healthy elders remains unchanged; however, because many older patients suffer from pulmonary disorders that reduce CO2 elimination (such as chronic obstructive pulmonary disease [COPD]), elevated PaCO2 levels are not an uncommon finding in the geriatric population (ENA, 2007).

With advancing age, the chest wall and thoracic vertebrae undergo progressive osteoporotic changes and vertebral collapse, producing kyphosis. Contractures of the intercostal muscles and calcification of the costal cartilage result in a decline in rib mobility and reduced chest wall compliance. The functional effect of these transformations is a decrease in thoracic wall excursion. Progressive loss of respiratory muscle strength is accompanied by a decline in maximal inspiratory and expiratory force by as much as 50% (Linton, 2007d).

A number of age-related changes diminish the geriatric patient's respiratory defense mechanisms and increase susceptibility to atelectasis and pulmonary infections. Due to atrophy of the epithelial lining, mucociliary clearance is reduced, making it progressively more difficult to clear bacteria from the bronchi. Impaired mucociliary clearance and thickened secretions promote colonization of the upper airways, predisposing patients to pneumonia. Elderly individuals with impaired cough and swallow mechanisms are at heightened risk for pneumonia secondary to aspiration (Linton, 2007d).

Pneumonia and influenza are the fifth-leading cause of death in the geriatric population. Mortality associated with community-acquired pneumonia is high and increases with age. Almost 11% of seniors admitted to the hospital with a specific condition die of the disease. Mortality following a hospital-acquired infection is even higher. Common age-related changes that contribute to respiratory infections include decreased cough reflex, diminished lung elasticity, impaired swallowing, and loss of respiratory muscle strength. The recovery process may be prolonged, involving extended hospitalization and chest radiographic abnormalities that can persist for months.

Older adults are prone to atypical pneumonia presentations characterized by subacute illness and nonrespiratory symptoms such as headache and diarrhea. Cough is less prominent in the elderly, especially among residents of long-term care facilities and seniors with serious comorbidities. Atypical pneumonia symptoms include falling, failure to thrive, altered functional capacity, and deterioration from existing illnesses. Delirium and acute confusion frequently signal pneumonia in older adults (Linton, 2007d).

Due to progressive osteoporosis and reduced chest wall compliance, elderly trauma patients are more likely to have rib fractures—or even a flail segment—than are young adults. Rib fractures and chest wall contusions are intensely painful and lead to splinting and hypoventilation. This is especially detrimental to the geriatric patient with little respiratory reserve. Incentive spirometry, early mobilization, and elevating the head of the bed at least 30 degrees are all well-established nursing practices for reducing respiratory complications.

Prompt and adequate pain relief is essential for promoting pulmonary health in the aged patient with thoracic compromise from injury or surgery. Inadequate pain control increases the work of breathing, elevates oxygen demand, and can easily progress to respiratory failure in seniors. Epidural catheters—infusing a combination of an opioid and a local anesthetic—can effectively control rib fracture and thoracotomy pain while simultaneously minimizing sedation and decreasing the incidence of pulmonary complications. Unfortunately, due to degenerative changes, the elderly spinal canal may not be easy to cannulate. An alternative approach to the management of thoracic orthopaedic pain is a percutaneously implanted anesthetic delivery system, such as the ON-Q PainBuster and SilverSoaker™.

Neurological Concerns

Age-related physiological changes to the nervous system are complex and far-reaching. Sensory perception declines steadily with normal aging, and the incidence of neurological disorders increases with every decade of life (Millsap, 2007). Neuronal loss is a natural consequence of aging. Brain mass decreases by 5% to 17% in older adults, with the majority of cell loss in the frontal and temporal lobes (Barker, 2008). As brain weight decreases, cerebral blood flow is concomitantly reduced. This normal neuronal decline is accelerated by Alzheimer's disease and alcoholism. Neuronal loss slows impulse conduction, diminishing the body's ability to deal with multiple stimuli, respond to information, and recover from stressors (Miller, 2009).

Approximately 12% of the older adult population experiences depression, and the incidence increases with aging. Depression may manifest as somatic symptoms such as constipation, fatigue, anorexia, and psychomotor retardation, as behavioral symptoms including withdrawing, crying, and anxiety, or as cognitive impairment. This latter finding in particular makes distinguishing between depression, delirium, and dementia difficult. Not only are the findings of late-life depression similar to those of dementia, the conditions frequently coexist. Besides social, psychological, and organic etiologies, a number of medications contribute to depression in older individuals. Implicated agents include analgesics, steroids, digoxin, antiparkinson drugs, antibiotics, and antihypertensives (Kazer, 2011).

Sleep disturbances related to aging include longer time to fall asleep, less time spent in rapid eye movement (REM state) sleep, and alterations in sleep patterns such as daytime sleeping. Additional neurological changes typically associated with senescence include impaired judgment, poor memory, and reduced ability to process new information (Miller, 2009). The development of age-associated atherosclerotic disease is not limited to the heart. Vessels in the brain are similarly affected, and the incidence of stroke jumps markedly with age. In addition to ischemic stroke, seniors are also at increased risk for hemorrhagic stroke. Spontaneous intracranial bleeding is associated with the highest case fatality of any stroke subtype. One month after hemorrhage, 50% of patients will be dead; only 20% will have regained functional independence after 1 year (Nyquist, 2010).

Normal senescence is accompanied by anatomic and functional changes in the auditory and vestibular apparatus that cause decreased sensitivity to sound and alter frequency discrimination. Presbycusis, a sensorineural hearing disorder, is the most common cause of hearing loss in older adults. This condition is characterized by a high-frequency hearing loss that is gradual, progressive, bilateral, symmetrical, and associated with poor speech discrimination. Additionally, cerumen production increases with age, and impaction can produce conductive hearing loss. Evaluate patients for cerumen impaction, and remove as necessary (Wallace & Grossman, 2008).

With aging, many transformations occur in the eye and the central visual pathways. These anatomical changes limit visual acuity, depth perception, peripheral vision, tolerance to glare, and speed of eye movements. Impaired light/dark adaptation and other age-related effects heighten an older person's need for ambient light. Furthermore, the high incidence of macular degeneration, glaucoma, retinal tears, cataracts, and diabetic retinopathy in the elderly all contribute to visual impairment (Wallace & Grossman, 2008). Strategies for patient teaching with visually impaired seniors include using materials with large print, selecting contrasting colors for printed items, ensuring adequate glare–free lighting, and facing the patient directly when speaking (Miller, 2009).

Decreased taste perception is associated with declining food intake in the elderly. The satiety center in the hypothalamus can become hypersensitive, leading to anorexia. Likewise, diminished thirst sensation makes older adults less sensitive to their need for hydration (Friedman, 2011; Miller, 2009). Proprioception, balance, and postural control also decline. Elderly persons experience changes in coordination, an altered "righting" reflex, and difficulty with balance (Haywood & Getchell, 2009). These transformations—in conjunction with distorted depth perception and musculoskeletal deterioration—make the older individual less able to respond to environmental changes and more susceptible to falls, particularly in unfamiliar surroundings such as a hospital.

The sensory changes of aging can reduce an elder's ability to perceive, respond to, or express pain, yet pain is one of the most pervasive and undertreated problems of senescence. Geriatric pain—both acute and chronic—is associated with depression, decreased socialization, poor nutrition, sleep disturbance, impaired mobility, and increased health care costs (Wallace & Grossman, 2008). Pain assessment in seniors can be challenging, particularly in those who are cognitively impaired. Assessment may require modifications to traditional pain evaluation strategies. Look for nonverbal expressions of discomfort such as grimacing, guarding, or restlessness. Atypical pain presentations include changes in behavior and function. Other common geriatric pain manifestations are psychobehavioral such as withdrawal, irritability, anxiety, crying, or fearfulness

The person with dementia has a pre-existing or baseline cognitive impairment such as Alzheimer's disease. Although rarely the admitting diagnosis in the orthopaedic patient, dementia is a common comorbidity, predisposing patients to falls and other injuries and greatly complicating patient assessment and care. Because dementia is part of a patient's baseline status, interventions focus on symptom management and not on cure (Miller, 2009). Nevertheless, dementia patients will have a difficult time following discharge instructions or effectively participating in rehabilitative activities, which can negatively impact outcome following orthopaedic injury or disease.

In contrast, the patient with delirium has a transient organic mental syndrome characterized by a cognition disorder, global attention deficits, reduced level of consciousness, abnormal psychomotor activity patterns, and disturbed sleep-wake cycles. Delirium adversely affects mental processing, perception, thinking, memory, and personality. Despite its behavioral manifestations, the root cause of delirium is organic, not psychiatric. Any condition that affects brain function can potentially lead to delirium (Miller, 2009). Established risk factors for delirium include advanced age, pre-existing cognitive impairment, poor functional status, hemodynamic or respiratory instability, ethanol abuse, sensory overload, metabolic imbalances, pain, anxiety, alterations in the sleep-wake cycle, and malnutrition. Treatment of these patients often includes bladder catheterization, sleep deprivation, polypharmacy, and the use of physical restraints. Delirium may also be the first manifestation of a previously unrecognized disease (Millsap, 2007).

Regrettably, the behavioral disturbances of delirium in the ill or injured elder are all too often dismissed as hospital psychosis, and the patient is treated with sedatives and antipsychotic agents. In older adults, the likelihood that delirium is medication-induced is high. Nevertheless, withholding drugs and under-treating pain can also produce delirium. Appropriate assessment and intervention are essential for positive delirium outcomes (Millsap, 2007). Delirium reduction involves a dual approach: 1) prevent or treat the underlying disorder; and 2) appropriately treat delirium at its earliest manifestation.

If the patient becomes acutely agitated or aggressive (hyperactive delirium), small doses of medications such as haloperidol (Haldol®) can sedate and relax the individual. Slowly titrate antipsychotic drugs to effect. The primary treatment goal, however, involves identifying and reversing the underlying causes of delirium. For mild agitation, interventions include decreasing environmental stimuli (lights and noise) and clustering care activities. Visitors or volunteers can help re-orient, mobilize, and feed the patient. Clocks, calendars, family photos, glasses, and hearing aids also promote orientation (Miller, 2009).

Seniors sustain a variety of spinal cord injuries, but one type of cord trauma is more prevalent in the geriatric age group than in other populations. Central cord syndrome, an incomplete injury, is uncommon in younger individuals and usually occurs in older adults with pre-existing cervical stenosis or spondylosis. Central cord syndrome in the elderly is most often the sequela of a forward fall. This mechanism causes cervical hyperextension. Patients with central cord syndrome generally retain lower extremity motor and sensory function, with deficits noted in the upper extremities (Russo-McCourt, 2009).

Musculoskeletal Concerns

Normal senescence is accompanied by a number of important changes to the musculoskeletal system. An overall decrease in muscle mass, strength, and agility leads to alterations in gait (wide-based, shorter steps) and a forward-flexed stance. These alterations, in combination with loss of bone mass, put older persons (particularly individuals with sedentary lifestyles) at risk for musculoskeletal disorders. As the body ages, there is a concomitant decline in the total amount of body water and an increase in the percentage of body fat. Changes in growth hormone metabolism have been implicated in muscle mass decline, as have alterations in androgen secretion. Not only is muscle mass diminished, but the remaining myocytes lose functional capacity. This loss attenuates the muscle cells' ability to extract and utilize oxygen, increases fatigue, and reduces overall muscle strength (Linton, 2007c).

The prevalence of osteoporosis in the geriatric population leads to a fracture incidence greater than that of any other age group. Osteoporosis occurs as a result of decreased osteoblastic activity, which impairs production of new bone cells (Linton, 2007c). The resultant loss of mass is associated with bone fragility, predisposing older adults to fractures following even minor trauma. Much attention has been given to osteoporosis in women, but seniors of both genders have brittle skeletons. Other risk factors for osteoporosis include smoking, sedentary lifestyle, and the use of certain medications such as steroids. With decreased bone density comes concomitant loss of stature, due in large part to compression of individual vertebral bodies. Other degenerative changes to the spine include narrowing of the cervical canal secondary to osteophyte (bony spur) growth (Linton, 2007c).

Osteoarthritis, also known as degenerative joint disease, is the predominant arthritis subtype. This condition is a common accompaniment of aging and a leading etiology of disability in the United States, particularly among women (Miller, 2009). The risk of developing osteoarthritis increases substantially with age, becoming especially common in individuals older than age 60. In fact, prevalence before age 30 is less than 1% (Linton, 2007c).

Osteoarthritis is a disease of both weight-bearing and non-weight-bearing joints. Damage is caused by mechanical stresses that injure areas of articular cartilage and subchondral bone (Upadhyaya, 2011). Biochemical changes in the joint surface, the synovium, and synovial fluid play a role in osteoarthritis etiology as well (Linton, 2007c). Symptoms include joint pain, morning stiffness lasting less than 30 minutes, and varying degrees of loss of function. The amount of connective tissue and collagen in the body continues to increase with age. This is most prominently manifested by the nose and ears, which continue to grow in size. These transformations are largely cosmetic and have few functional implications. Other changes, such as deterioration and drying of the joints and cartilage (Linton, 2007c), have clinical ramifications of joint pain and stiffness.

Although it is unclear whether the incidence of fractures is a surrogate for pre-existing fragility in the elderly or the actual cause of decline, several studies of isolated fractures in older individuals have documented serious outcomes subsequent to even "minor" injuries. Following isolated hip fractures, there is a 60-day mortality of nearly 10%; one third of hip fracture patients will not survive their first post-injury year. Even an isolated distal radius fracture in a geriatric patient is associated with a significantly decreased life span. The cumulative estimated survival at 7 years in a cohort of 325 elderly radial fracture patients was only 57%, compared to the expected value of 71% for the U.S. population (Criddle, 2009a).

The incidence of hip fractures dramatically increases with advancing years. Falls are the most common hip fracture mechanism in geriatric patients; however, evidence suggests that some individuals have hips so osteoporotic that spontaneous fracture actually precedes the fall. Fractures of the cervical spine in older adults tend to be unstable and involve more than one level, commonly occurring at C1-C2. Falls are also the leading cause of bony pelvic injuries in the elderly. Following pelvic fracture, older patients suffer mortality rates three to five times greater than their under-55-year-old counterparts.

Bone healing time can be significantly prolonged in the geriatric patient (Linton, 2007c). Interventions for seniors with musculoskeletal injury (e.g., physical therapy, range of motion [ROM] exercises, occupational therapy) focus on facilitating mobility and maintaining or restoring function while simultaneously preventing complications of immobility such as thromboembolic disease, deconditioning, and pressure ulcer formation (Gilman et al., 2009; Miller, 2009).

Integumentary Concerns

Assessment of an older adult's skin can provide a large amount of information about the patient's medical history, surgical history, social history, and current health status. Look for the presence of peripheral vascular disease, edema, tattoos, deformities, lesions, discoloration, wounds, scars, bruises, scratches, burns, and medical devices. Aging is associated with decreased effectiveness of several of the skin's protective functions. Subcutaneous fat is lost, particularly the fatty pads that protect bony prominences. Both the dermis and epidermis thin, making delicate, aging skin susceptible to tears (Miller, 2009). Changes also occur in the structure of interstitial tissues, which predispose to soft tissue injury.

Loss of skin moisture, decreased elasticity, diminished tensile strength, and reduced turgor all promote wrinkling and skin laxity. Because of these alterations, skin turgor may correlate poorly with hydration status in the elderly (Gilman et al., 2009; Wallace & Grossman, 2008). Both dryness and pruritus are common dermal complaints in older individuals and may lead to chronic scratching. Nevertheless, the number of nerve cells in the skin declines with advancing age, making seniors less aware of dermal injury or ischemia. These changes are accompanied by a reduction in the number melanocytes, which heightens seniors' need for sun protection (Miller, 2009).

All aspects of wound healing appear to be influenced by senescence. Responses in both the inflammatory and proliferative wound healing phases decrease. Angiogenesis, epithelialization, and wound remodeling are each delayed. Fibroblast proliferation and collagen synthesis also diminish with aging. Furthermore, frequent routine aspirin use in the older population, combined with capillary fragility, contributes to ecchymosis and wound bleeding tendencies. Once the body's protective layers are breached, external barriers to bacterial invasion are removed, promoting soft tissue infection. This is aggravated by immune system alterations that accompany aging, which limit the older adult's ability to mount an adequate response to infection. Nutritional deficits, particularly a lack of vitamins A and C, and trace minerals such as zinc, adversely affect the enzyme systems necessary for wound healing (Criddle, 2009b).

In the geriatric patient, atrophic changes in the skin, reduced sensation, and a limited capacity to heal all contribute to the high incidence of pressure ulcer formation. Skin breakdown in the elderly can be initiated by a variety of factors including sensory or motor loss, bed rest, reduced vasomotor tone, hypovolemia, poor nutrition, and age-related changes in skin composition. Pressure ulcers can develop virtually anywhere but are most common over the bony prominences of the sacrum, heels, ischium, elbows, occiput, and on the pinna (Miller, 2009). Intra-operatively, seniors are at heightened risk for dermal ischemia and must be repositioned regularly.

The elderly require exceptional skin care, and skin integrity must be monitored frequently for signs of impairment. Strategies to prevent skin damage in elderly orthopaedic patients include handling the patient gently; avoiding shearing forces; floating the heels; repositioning the patient frequently; and padding bony prominences, casts, splints, or appliances. Use a nondrying cleanser to keep the skin clean. Apply moisturizers and protective lotions liberally, and minimize bony prominence contact with beds and chairs (Miller, 2009). Consult a wound and ostomy nurse for help with selecting the most appropriate interventions including specialty beds.

Urinary Concerns

With increasing age, a substantial number of anatomic and physiological changes occur that directly impact the urinary system. Additionally, alterations to other body systems—such as a decreased sense of thirst and changes in cardiovascular status—have an indirect effect on renal function. Several normal transformations of aging impact voiding, including reduced bladder muscle tone, diminished bladder capacity, and a heightened sense of urgency. In the aging bladder, increased collagen content limits distensibility and impairs emptying. In females, decreased circulating levels of estrogen and limited tissue estrogen responsiveness cause urethral sphincter changes that predispose to urinary incontinence. In older men, prostate enlargement may impede urinary flow, impairing bladder emptying. Together, these factors lead to urinary incontinence in 15% to 20% of older men, 33% to 38% of older women, 50% of all frail elders, and 60% to 80% of nursing home residents (Miller, 2009). Urinary urgency and incontinence play significant roles in orthopaedic injuries in older adults because many falls occurs when seniors are trying to get to a bathroom.

By the eighth decade of life, the number of functional glomeruli has decreased by 35% (Miller, 2009). Nephron loss is accompanied by a drop in the number of renal tubular cells. By age 65, there is an overall reduction in renal mass of 20% to 40%. With an ever-decreasing number of nephrons left to do the work of the kidneys, glomerular filtration rate declines about 1 mL per minute per year, beginning around the age of 40. This reduces the older adult's capacity to maintain fluid and acid-base balance. As renal tubular function wanes, the kidneys' ability to conserve sodium and excrete hydrogen ions is diminished, and serum creatinine levels rise. Dehydration in elderly individuals can be missed due to their limited ability to concentrate urine. In the aged, urine-specific gravity will remain relatively low despite significant fluid losses, making specific gravity an unreliable indicator of volume status in seniors (Miller, 2009).

Changes in renal function have important implications for the type and dosage of drugs used in the elderly. Two categories of medications commonly consumed by older individuals are nonsteroidal anti-inflammatory agents and angiotensin-converting enzyme (ACE) inhibitors. Both of these drug classes have adverse effects on renal regulatory mechanisms. Nephrotoxic substances frequently prescribed to orthopaedic patients include iodinated contrast media and diuretics. Aminoglycosides, such as vancomycin and gentamicin, require careful monitoring of serum peak levels to avoid toxicity in older adults.

The incidence of chronic renal failure increases with age because of anatomic and physiological changes to the kidneys associated with age and comorbidities. In the ill or injured older adult, diminished baseline renal function, polypharmacy, and an elevated risk for nephrotoxicity all combine to increase the incidence of acute renal failure (ARF). Geriatric patients, however, may exhibit atypical signs of uremia. Look for unexplained exacerbations of heart failure that has been previously well-controlled, unexplained mental status, and personality changes. Acute renal failure in the orthopaedic patient is often associated with rhabdomyolysis or sepsis, both of which are life-threatening conditions that require early detection and immediate management.

The urinary tract is among the most common sites of infection in older adults in the community, in long-term care settings, and in acute care facilities. With advanced age comes an increasing incidence of asymptomatic bacteriuria (i.e., a significant bacterial count in the urine, without other symptoms). In older women, the prevalence of bacteriuria may be as high as 20%, and those living in long-term care facilities have the highest incidence of both asymptomatic bacteriuria and symptomatic urinary tract infections (UTIs) (Linton, 2007b). The presence of an indwelling urinary catheter dramatically increases the incidence of bacteriuria, pyuria, and symptomatic UTIs. Early discontinuation of indwelling catheters is highly recommended in the geriatric population.

Gastrointestinal Concerns

Although gastrointestinal (GI) complaints are very common in old age, GI function is generally well-preserved in older adults. A history of multiple abdominal surgeries (particularly bowel surgery), tumors, or adhesions is not unusual in the elderly, however, and each of these factors serves to increase the incidence of bowel obstruction. Importantly, some age-associated changes that affect gastrointestinal function—such as loss of abdominal muscle strength, reduced appetite, and decreased fluid intake—actually originate in other body systems.

Small-bowel motility, and the absorption of most nutrients, is unchanged with aging. Of importance to the geriatric orthopaedic patient, calcium absorption decreases significantly, largely due to a drop in renal production of 1,25-hydroxycholecalciferol and reduced intestinal calcium binding. Iron and many drugs are absorbed more slowly or less effectively in older adults as a result of atrophy of the mucosal lining. Thinning of the mucosal lining also increases the incidence of GI bleeding, especially in the patient taking nonsteroidal anti-inflammatory agents. Diminished bowel muscle tone delays bowel emptying, putting seniors at risk for constipation, diverticular disease, and bacterial translocation. The etiology of constipation in the elderly is multi-factorial: sedentary lifestyle, poor diet, dehydration, anorectal and colonic pathology, systemic illness, and medications can all play a role in abnormal bowel function (Miller, 2009). Unfortunately, both opioid analgesic use and bedrest in the orthopaedic patient contribute significantly to hypoperistalsis.

There are myriad reasons for malnutrition in the elderly, only some of which involve the gastrointestinal system. A variety of social, cognitive, functional, and physiological issues contribute to poor nutritional status in the geriatric population. Factors include limited financial or physical ability to obtain and prepare food, poor dentition, depression, alcohol abuse, anorexia, drug-nutrient interactions, and the loss of a spouse. Additionally, chronic medical conditions—such as congestive heart failure, diabetes, lung disease, and renal failure—make it difficult to keep ill seniors adequately fed and hydrated. Gastroesophageal reflux disease, chronic diarrhea, and many medications also interfere with appetite or nutrient metabolism in the geriatric population (Linton, 2007a).

Malnutrition places the elderly orthopaedic patient at heightened risk for morbidity and mortality. Protein-energy malnutrition and immobility lead to deconditioning, which involves changes to all major organ systems. The incidence of poor wound healing, non-union, pneumonia, and postoperative complications are all increased in patients with nutritional deficits. It is important to start early enteral supplementation in the undernourished or malnourished geriatric patient. Limited data suggest that enteral protein supplementation initiated preoperatively can reduce negative outcomes in malnourished patients (Linton, 2007a). Other interventions to manage malnutrition or deal with feeding problems in older adults include providing small frequent meals to avoid discomfort and to increase intake, encouraging fluids and fiber to improve bowel function, and obtaining early nutritional consultation.

Circulation to the liver decreases by approximately 1% per year in adulthood, so that hepatic blood flow has dropped by almost half at age 85. The most common hepatobiliary disorder in the elderly population is gallstones and gallstone-related complications. The prevalence of cholelithiasis rises steadily with age; biliary stones have been documented in up to 80% of nursing home residents older than age 90, and biliary tract disease is the most common indication for abdominal surgery in older adults (Criddle, 2009b). Standard liver function test norms remain unchanged in healthy seniors, but metabolism of, and sensitivity to, certain substances is altered. Drugs such as warfarin, which acts directly on the liver cells, will produce therapeutic effects at lower doses in the elderly due to increased hepatocyte sensitivity. Some pharmacologic agents have reduced hepatic clearance in older adults (Linton, 2011).

Metabolic and Endocrine Concerns

The metabolic and endocrine changes associated with senescence are wide-ranging, affecting every system in the body. Metabolic responses, in particular, influence the geriatric patient's ability to cope with the stresses of illness or surgery. Caloric requirements are lower in older adults, predisposing them to all the orthopaedic complications associated with obesity. In the face of illness, injury, infection, or surgery, the older patient's increased requirement for carbohydrates and protein is frequently not matched by an equal rise in energy intake. Endogenous protein stores are depleted, declining hepatic function impairs protein synthesis, and serum albumin is consumed just to meet basic metabolic demands.

Decreased muscle mass causes a reduction in strength, which is particularly detrimental to the respiratory muscles. Cells with high turnover (skin, red and white blood cells, GI organs) fail first, leading to loss of barrier function, delayed wound healing, increased susceptibility to infection, and impaired nutrient absorption. Secretion of many hormones decreases with aging. Elderly individuals experience a drop in the production of growth hormone, thyroid hormone, aldosterone, adrenal androgens, testosterone, and estrogen (Hill, 2011). Careful glucose regulation is particularly important in the elderly patient. Closely monitor blood glucose levels, and administer exogenous insulin according to a protocol designed to maintain blood glucose within a stipulated range.

The hypothalamus is the body's thermoregulatory control center. In older adults, declining hypothalamic function and a decreased basal metabolic rate combine to produce an overall reduction in capacity to maintain thermal balance (Miller, 2009). These physiological changes—in association with cognitive and functional decline, certain medications, social factors, loss of muscle mass, thinning skin, and systemic conditions such as thyroid disease, diabetes, and malnutrition—all reduce tolerance to temperature extremes, making body temperature abnormalities both more common and more prolonged in seniors. Hypothalamic, metabolic, and body fat changes reduce baseline body temperature in older adults. Normal temperature drops to 35.5-36.1 degrees Celcius (Miller, 2009). Axillary temperature measurements tend to be poor indicators of core temperature in the geriatric population because skin temperature may be several degrees cooler than core, due to decreased peripheral circulation.

Aging is also associated with a reduction in the threshold for peripheral vasoconstriction and shivering, limiting the body's ability to generate and conserve heat (Miller, 2009). Elderly individuals may present for care in a hypothermic state, and iatrogenically-induced hypothermia also puts seniors at risk. Postoperative patients are particularly vulnerable to cold stress. In the postoperative period, cardiac dysrhythmias, hypertension, angina, and hypoxemia occur more frequently in mildly hypothermic elderly patients than in normothermic individuals. Because seniors are at increased risk for hypothermia, every effort should be made to prevent heat loss (Miller, 2009). Use forced-air heating blankets, warmed intravenous solutions, and heated ventilator circuits, and keep room temperatures high whenever patients are uncovered.

Conversely, because of sweat gland atrophy, the ability to perspire decreases with aging, which reduces the body's capacity to dissipate excess heat. Additionally, many cognitive, social, and functional changes predispose older adults to heat-related disorders. A wide range of drugs, particularly psychotropic medications and those with anti-cholinergic or narcotic actions, further impair sweating in response to heat. Geriatric patients also experience a blunted febrile reaction to infection as a result of immunosenescence. Older adults generate a febrile response less often than their younger counterparts, and this response is often attenuated. With aging, baseline neutrophil counts remain stable, but the ability of the bone marrow to increase white blood cell production in response to infection is impaired. In conjunction with the stresses of illness, injury, or surgery, these cellular changes make it more likely that the geriatric orthopaedic patient will contract an infectious disease and be less able to eradicate existing infection (Miller, 2009).

Drug Metabolism Concerns

Compared to younger adults, the elderly typically take more medications, have more underlying organ dysfunction, experience more inter-individual variations in drug deposition, are more susceptible to malnutrition, and are more likely to have diminished or exaggerated responses to medications (Burchum, 2011). The majority of older patients enter care already taking a number of pharmaceutical agents. Each drug is associated with an adverse risk profile that only worsens when combined with systemic disease and additional medications. This fact underscores the importance of obtaining a thorough medication and health history from the patient, family, or caregiver.

Several age-associated changes alter drug distribution in the elderly. With senescence, the portion of lean body mass decreases, the percentage of body water drops, and the relative amount of total body fat rises. These alterations result in greater distribution of lipophilic drugs into the adipose tissue, producing a longer half-life for agents such as anesthetics, barbiturates, and benzodiazepines (Burchum, 2011).

Age-related biological responses to pharmacologic agents place the elderly at increased risk for adverse drug reactions. Although the total amount of drug absorbed is basically unchanged, elderly patients experience a decline in the rate of drug absorption. Decreased serum albumin levels alter the availability of substances that are protein-bound, enhancing the quantity of bioactive agents. Both liver and kidney function decline with advancing age, which reduces clearance of many substances. The hepatic and renal impairments that occur with senescence can quickly lead to elevated drug concentrations, even in fully compliant patients on standard therapeutic dosing regimens. Agents with a high potential for adverse reactions in older adults include anticoagulants, aspirin, calcium-channel blockers, digoxin, diuretics, narcotics, and theophylline (Burchum, 2011).

The net effect of these senescent changes is an increase in the incidence of drug toxicity related to metabolite accumulation. The first step in reducing adverse pharmacologic reactions in older adults involves obtaining a complete medication history (drug reconciliation) from each orthopaedic patient at the time of initial contact. This history must include prescription medications, over-the-counter agents, recreational drugs, and nutritional supplements, as well as herbal, homeopathic, naturopathic, and folk nostrums. Other strategies for reducing adverse medication events in seniors include weaning drugs as appropriate, increasing doses cautiously, monitoring closely for untoward effects, administering according to renal function, and consulting with a pharmacist regarding age-appropriate dosages. When it comes to analgesic or sedative medications, the adage "start low and go slow" describes appropriate geriatric therapy.

Psychosocial and Functional Concerns

As part of the normal aging process, the elderly experience a number of changes in social interactions. Friends, siblings, spouses, and other family members are often dead or dying. Many geriatric patients have lost their life partner, either as the result of death or due to severe cognitive impairment. Even while dealing with their own health care needs, older adults frequently serve as caregivers for a spouse, parent, sibling, neighbor, child, or grandchild. Many elderly persons are cared for by friends and family members who are senior citizens themselves The individual caring for a 94-year old patient is likely to be the 92 year-old spouse or a 70-year old child. Despite the decremental losses associated with aging, most elders perceive their lives as satisfying. Older adults exhibit a strong need to remain independent, maintain and develop meaningful relationships, and have a purpose in life (Miller, 2009).

Up to half of all geriatric patients admitted to hospitals experience significant decline in function or some loss of ability to perform ADLs. Orthopaedic patients are at heightened risk for this because their conditions frequently affect limb function and locomotion. Assistive devices easily adopted by younger patients may prove impossible for older adults: crutch walking, over-bed trapezes, and halo vests all require upper body strength and a sense of balance that the geriatric patient may no longer possess. Specific factors associated with loss of function in the elderly include pre-existing chronic illness, delirium, immobility, malnutrition, depression, and uncontrolled pain. Sleep disturbance also accelerates functional decline. Sixteen to 68% of American seniors experience sleep disorders ranging from apnea to difficulty falling asleep (Gilman et al., 2009). These disturbances are only exaggerated by the stresses of hospitalization.

Another condition that can cause severe functional decline in elderly persons is alcoholism. When the geriatric patient experiences hallucinations, tremors, or seizures, the possibility of ethanol withdrawal must be considered. Withdrawal onset usually begins within 48 to 72 hours of the last drink. Patients with a known history of alcohol abuse can be prophylactically treated to prevent or attenuate the effects of delirium tremens. Unrecognized or undertreated, ethanol withdrawal can negatively affect the patient's disease course and produce long-term morbidity.

A tremendous amount of health care resources—and a large percentage of Medicare expenditures—are consumed by geriatric patients in the last months or weeks of life. One of the greatest patient care concerns in the elderly is the decision to withhold or withdraw support. This complex decision involves the personal biases of health care providers, patients, and family members (Miller, 2009). Unfortunately, few patients have an advance directive at the time of hospital admission. When they exist, advance directives are often inadequate, except in cases of the most obvious treatment decisions, because they are too vague. Even if a patient's wishes are clear, many health care providers are wary of ignoring the requests of a living surrogate, especially one who is a spouse or other close family member (Meiner, 2011a; Ward & Levy, 2005) because of the litigious nature of American society.

Injury Prevention and the Geriatric Patient

The high frequency and associated morbidity and mortality of geriatric falls have been well-publicized. By the age of 75, falls have surpassed motor vehicle collisions as the leading mechanism of fatal injury. In 2005, nearly 16,000 seniors died of fall-related injuries and close to half a million required hospitalization (Meiner, 2011c). Strategies designed to mitigate fall damage focus on prevention (environmental, behavioral, and medical management) and on limiting the extent of damage should a fall occur (e.g., hip protectors, ground level beds, carpeted flooring).

Beyond falls, however, motor vehicle crashes rank among the top hazards. Elderly drivers pose a significant risk to themselves, others, and property. Again, the approach to injury control is multi-pronged. Interventions may be educational (driver training specially designed for older drivers), engineering-related (safer vehicle design), environmental (left turn traffic light installation), or proscriptive (license revocation).

Other opportunities for injury reduction exist around suicide prevention, particularly with firearms, the method of choice for most geriatric suicides. Older adults are also at increased risk for motor vehicle-versus-pedestrian injuries, thermal injuries (burn, hyperthermia, hypothermia), and accidental toxicologic events including carbon monoxide poisoning (Meiner, 2011c). Injuries by each of these mechanisms are amenable to reduction by employing some combination of the "4 E's" of trauma prevention: Environmental control, Economic incentive, Education, and Enforcement. Importantly, injury reduction strategies must be tailored to the needs of the older adult; safety interventions designed primarily for children or young adults are often poorly suited to seniors. For example, safer playground surfaces and skateboard helmet laws do little to prevent geriatric fall injuries.

Table 12.2. Suggested Online Resources

Resource	Location
American Geriatrics Society	http://www.americangeriatrics.org/
Hartford Geriatric Nursing Initiative	http://www.hgni.org/
Hartford Institute for Geriatric Nursing	http://consultgerirn.org/
National Institute on Aging	http://www.nia.nih.gov/
Portal of Geriatric Online Education	http://www.pogoe.org/

Summary

Demographic shifts, longevity gains, and advances in health care in the past 50 years have dramatically increased the number of seniors with orthopaedic disorders. The proportion of patients who are elderly is projected to increase well into the middle of the 21st century. Senescence has profound effects on the musculoskeletal system, but age-associated changes affect every system in the body, which in turn impacts the care of all geriatric orthopaedic patients. In older adults, normal age-related transformations can be difficult to distinguish from alterations due to illness, environmental exposure, social situation, functional status, and comorbid conditions-yet these changes interact to threaten seniors' ability to survive and recover from orthopaedic surgery, injury, or disease. Table 12.2 provides additional resources for care of the older adult.

References

Barker, E. (2008). The adult neurologic assessment. In E. Barker (Ed.), *Neuroscience Nursing: A Spectrum of Care* (3rd ed.). St. Louis: Mosby.

Burchum, J. (2011). Pharmacologic management. In S. Meiner (Ed.), *Gerontologic Nursing* (4th ed.).

Criddle, L.M. (2009a). 5 year survival of geriatric patients following trauma center discharge. *Advanced Emergency Nursing Journal, 31*(4), 323-336.

Criddle, L.M. (2009b). Caring for the critically ill elderly patient. In K. Carlson (Ed.), *Advanced Critical Care Nursing* (pp. 1372-1400). St. Louis: Elsevier.

Emergency Nurses Association (ENA). (2007). *Trauma Nursing Core Course Provider Manual* (6th ed.). Des Plaines, IL: Emergency Nurses Association.

Friedman, S. (2011). Sensory function. In S. Meiner (Ed.), *Gerontologic Nursing* (4th ed.). St. Louis: Elsevier.

Gilman, P., Parker P., & Tabloski, P. (2009). *Gerontological Nursing* (2nd ed.). Silver Springs, MD: American Nurses Credentialing Center.

Haywood, K. & Getchell, N. (2009). *Life Span Motor Development*. Champaign, IL: Human Kinetics.

Hill, C. (2011). Endocrine function. In S. Meiner (Ed.), *Gerontologic Nursing* (4th ed.). St. Louis: Elsevier.

House-Fancher, M.A. & Lynch, R.J. (2007). Cardiovascular system. In A. Linton & H. Lach (Eds.), *Matteson & McConnell's Gerontologicial Nursing Concepts and Practice* (3rd. ed.). St. Louis: Saunders.

Kazer, M. (2011). Cognitive and neurologic function. In S. Meiner (Ed.), *Gerontologic Nursing* (4th ed.). St. Louis: Elsevier.

Lach, H.W. (2007a). Gerontological nursing: Issues and trends in practice. In A. Linton & H. Lach (Eds.), *Matteson & McConnell's Gerontological Nursing Concepts and Practice* (3rd. ed.). St. Louis: Saunders.

Lach, H.W. (2007b). Gerontology: The study of aging. In A. Linton & H. Lach (Eds.), *Matteson & McConnell's Gerontological Nursing Concepts and Practice.* St. Louis: Elsevier.

Linton, A.D. (2007a). Gastrointestinal system. In A. Linton & H. Lach (Eds.), *Matteson & McConnell's Gerontological Nursing Concepts and Practice* (3rd ed.). St. Louis: Saunders.

Linton, A.D. (2007b). Genitourinary system. In A. Linton & H. Lach (Eds.), *Matteson & McConnell's Gerontological Nursing Concepts and Practice.* St. Louis: Elsevier.

Linton, A.D. (2007c). Musculoskeletal system. In A. Linton & H. Lach (Eds.), *Matteson & McConnell's Gerontological Nursing Concepts and Practice.* St. Louis: Elsevier.

Linton, A.D. (2007d). Respiratory system. In A. Linton & H. Lach (Eds.), *Matteson & McConnell's Gerontological Nursing Concepts and Practice* (3rd ed.). St Louis: Saunders.

Linton, A.D. (2011). Pharmacological considerations. In A. Linton & H. Lach (Eds.), *Matteson & McConnell's Gerontological Nursing Concepts and Practice.* St. Louis: Elsevier.

Meiner, S.E. (2011a). Legal and ethical issues. In S. Meiner (Ed.), *Gerontologic Nursing* (4th ed.). St. Louis: Elsevier.

Meiner, S.E. (2011b). Overview of gerontological nursing. In S. Meiner (Ed.), *Gerontological Nursing* (4th ed.). St. Louis: Elsevier.

Meiner, S.E. (2011c). Safety. In S. Meiner (Ed.), *Gerontologic Nursing* (4th ed.). St. Louis: Elsevier.

Miller, C.A. (2009). *Nursing for Wellness in Older Adults* (5th ed.). Philadelphia: Wolters Kluwer.

Millsap, P. (2007). Neurological system. In A. Linton & H. Lach (Eds.), *Matteson & McConnell's Gerontological Nursing Concepts and Practice* (3rd ed.). St. Louis: Saunders.

Nyquist, P. (2010). Management of acute intracranial and intraventricular hemorrhage. *Critical Care Medicine*, 38(3), 946-953.

Plummer, E. (2009). Trauma in the elderly. In K. McQuillan, M. Makic, & E. Whalen (Eds.), *Trauma Nursing from Resuscitation Through Rehabilitation* (4th ed.). St. Louis: Saunders.

Resnick, B. (2005). The critically ill older patient. In P. Morton, D. Fontaine, C. Hudak, & B. Gallo (Eds.), *Critical Care Nursing: A Holistic Approach* (8th ed.). Philadelphia: Lippincott Williams & Wilkins.

Russo-McCourt, T.A. (2009). Spinal cord injuries. In K. McQuillan, M. Makic & E. Whalen (Eds.), *Trauma Nursing from Resuscitation Through Rehabilitation* (4th ed.). St. Louis: Saunders.

U.S. Department of Health & Human Services (HHS) Administration on Aging (2010). *A profile of older Americans.* Washingon D.C.: Government Printing Office.

Upadhyaya, R. (2011). Musculoskeletal Function. In S. Meiner (Ed.), *Gerontologic Nursing* (4th ed.). St. Louis: Elsevier.

Wallace, M. & Grossman, M. (2008). *Gerontological Nurse Certification Review*. New York: Springer.

Ward, N. & Levy, M. (2005). End-of-life issues in the intensive care unit. In M. Fink, E. Abraham, J. Vincent, & P. Kochanek (Eds.), *Textbook of Critical Care* (5th ed.). Philadelphia: Elsevier.

Chapter 13

Arthritis & Connective Tissue Disorders

Dottie Roberts, MSN, MACI, RN, CMSRN, OCNS-C, CNE

Objectives

- Differentiate the three types of juvenile idiopathic arthritis.
- Describe clinical presentation and treatment for rheumatoid arthritis and osteoarthritis.
- Discuss typical history, physical findings, and treatment for patients with polymyalgia rheumatica, rheumatic fever, polymyositis, and dermatomyositis.
- Describe diagnostic features of fibromyalgia syndrome.
- Identify causes and appropriate treatments for both acute and chronic gout.
- Describe patient symptoms in each stage of Lyme disease.
- Discuss complications of systemic sclerosis.
- Identify clinical presentation and treatment of the three seronegative spondyloarthropathies.
- Identify possible complications of systemic lupus erythematosus.

More than 100 types of arthritic and connective tissue disorders have been identified, and they can affect all age groups. Arthritic conditions can be disabling and debilitating, with profound effects on patients' quality of life and ability to function independently. Orthopaedic nurses play an important role in helping patients understand and live successfully with these chronic diseases. This chapter discusses the etiology, pathophysiology, and treatment options for common disorders such as osteoarthritis and fibromyalgia, as well as less common conditions such as polymyositis and polymyalgia rheumatica. Appropriate nursing interventions and patient teaching also are identified.

Juvenile Arthritis

Overview

Definition. Juvenile arthritis is a group of diseases marked by pain, swelling, stiffness, and loss of joint motion, with onset before age 16 (Abramson, 2008). Children can develop almost all forms of arthritis that affect adults, but the most common type is *juvenile idiopathic arthritis* (JIA). The term *juvenile rheumatoid arthritis* (JRA) with its three subtypes still may be used to classify childhood arthritis; however, the JIA classification system includes more types of chronic childhood arthritis and provides a more accurate description of the three previously identified JRA subtypes. The seven separate subtypes of JIA have characteristic symptoms described below (National Institute of Arthritis and Musculoskeletal and Skin Diseases [NIAMS], 2008).

With *systemic onset JIA* (formerly known as systemic JRA), the affected child develops arthritis with or preceded by a fever that lasts at least 2 weeks. The fever must be documented as intermittent, spiking for at least 3 days, and accompanied by at least one of the following:

1. Generalized lymph node enlargement;
2. Enlargement of the liver or spleen;
3. Pericarditis or pleuritis; and
4. A characteristic rheumatoid rash, which is flat and pale pink, and generally not itchy. The spots are generally the size of a quarter or smaller. They may be present for minutes to hours, and then disappear without causing skin damage. The rash also may move from one part of the body to another. Arthritis will persist even after fever and other symptoms have resolved.

The child with *oligoarthritis* (previously termed *pauciarticular JRA*) has one to four affected joints during the first 6 months of the disease. The recognized subcategories include *persistent oligoarthritis*, with no more than four joints ever affected during the course of the disease, and *extended oligoarthritis*, with more than four joints involved after the first 6 months of the disease. Girls are more likely to develop oligoarthritis than boys. Older children with this form of JIA may have arthritis that lasts into adulthood. Children who develop oligoarthritis before age 7 are more likely to experience resolution of joint symptoms in time, but they are at increased risk for developing inflammatory eye disorders such as iritis and uveitis (NIAMS, 2008).

With *polyarthritis – rheumatoid factor negative* (formerly known as polyarticular RA – RF negative), the child has five or more affected joints and negative tests for RF. The child with *polyarthritis – rheumatoid factor positive* will have five or more affected joints and at least two positive RF tests at least 3 months apart.

The child with *psoriatic arthritis* has both arthritis and the skin disorder psoriasis, or arthritis and at least two of the following symptoms:

1. Inflammation and swelling of an entire finger or toe (dactylitis);
2. Nail pitting or splitting; and
3. A first-degree relative with psoriasis.

The child with *enthesitis-related arthritis* has both arthritis and inflammation of an enthesis (point of ligament, tendon, or joint capsule attachment to a bone), or either arthritis or enthesitis and at least two of the following symptoms:

1. Inflammation of the sacroiliac (SI) joints, or lumbosacral pain and stiffness;
2. Positive blood test for human leukocyte antigen (HLA) B-27 gene;
3. Onset of arthritis in males after age 6; and
4. A first-degree relative diagnosed with ankylosing spondylitis, enthesitis-related arthritis, SI joint inflammation in association with inflammatory bowel disease (IBD), Reiter's syndrome, or acute inflammation of the eye.

Finally, *undifferentiated arthritis* is identified if arthritis manifestations do not meet criteria for one of the other subtypes, or if they fulfill criteria for more than one category.

Etiology. Many forms of JIA are autoimmune disorders, in which the body mistakenly attacks its own healthy tissues. Inflammation results, marked by redness, heat, pain, and swelling, with accompanying joint damage. Although the reason for the autoimmune response is not understood, scientists suspect it is a two-step process. First, the child's genetic makeup predisposes him or her to develop JIA. Then an environmental factor such as a virus may trigger onset of the disease; however, no specific infectious agent has been identified.

On the other hand, not all cases of JIA have autoimmune origins. Recent research found that some persons, including many with systemic arthritis, have what is termed more accurately an *autoinflammatory condition* (NIAMS, 2008). The healthy immune system creates antibodies in response to bacterial or viral invasion. In an autoimmune reaction, these antibodies attach to healthy tissues by mistake (autoantibodies) and signal the body's defense mechanisms to destroy its own tissues. Autoinflammatory conditions also cause inflammation and immune overactivity. They trigger a more primitive part of the immune system, leading to tissue destruction by white blood cells rather than autoantibodies.

Pathophysiology. Chronic inflammation of synovium and joint effusion characterize the rheumatic process, which is marked by eventual erosion, destruction, and fibrosis of articular cartilage. Joint ankylosis follows due to adhesions between articular surfaces, if the process persists. General manifestations of JIA result from joint erosion and synovial thickening. They include stiffness, especially after inactivity, loss of motion due to muscle spasm and inflammation (early disease), and ankylosis and soft tissue contracture (later disease).

Incidence. About 1 in 1,000 children develops some form of arthritis. Arthritis can affect children at any age, though it rarely occurs in the first 6 months of life. Systemic onset JIA affects about 10% of children with arthritis. Oligoarthritis affects about half of all children with arthritis. Other forms of juvenile arthritis occur less frequently (Abramson, 2008).

Complications. JIA may affect bone development, causing a growth delay, and residual joint destruction may affect function in adulthood (NIAMS, 2008). Visual impairment or blindness and ocular complications, such as cataracts and elevated intraocular pressure, also are possible due to chronic uveitis often associated with JIA (Woreta, Thorne, Jabs, Kedhar, & Dunn, 2007).

Special Considerations. Children with JIA should attend school and participate in activities to the fullest extent possible. In addition, parents should become familiar with Section 504 of the Rehabilitation Act of 1973 (www.dotcr.ost.dot.gov/documents/ycr/REHABACT.HTM); this law requires schools to provide accommodations for children with JIA (U. S. Department of Health & Human Services, 2006). A healthy transition to adulthood can be fostered by allowing adolescents to engage in independent activities, such as working part-time or learning to drive. Long-term prognosis is determined by the severity of the child's arthritis.

Assessment

History. JIA typically is marked by an insidious onset of arthritis symptoms in a child younger than age 16. The child complains of or demonstrates joint stiffness after periods of immobility, especially in the morning (Hoffart & Sherry, 2010).

Physical Exam. Examination reveals warm, swollen, painful joints, with decreased range of motion. The child may limp or obviously favor one of the lower extremities. Because the extra-articular symptoms of systemic onset JIA often precede the onset of arthritis, the child first may be evaluated for intermittent high fevers, malaise, anorexia, and weight loss. A transient rash may occur with the fever. The health care provider should evaluate carefully for abnormal pupils (associated with uveitis), lymphadenopathy, hepatosplenomegaly, and pericardial or pleural rubs (Hoffart & Sherry, 2010).

Misdiagnosis often occurs when one of four key points is missed:

1. Arthritis must be present, defined as swelling, effusion, or the presence of two or more of the following: limitation of motion, tenderness, pain on motion, and joint warmth.
2. Arthritis must be consistently present for at least 6 weeks.
3. More than 100 other causes of chronic arthritis in children must be excluded.
4. No specific laboratory/other test can establish the diagnosis of JIA (NIAMS, 2008).

Diagnostic Tests. While rheumatoid factor (RF) remains a standard for screening adults with suspected inflammatory arthritis, it has limited use in evaluating children with musculoskeletal complaints and possible rheumatic disease. According to Jarvis (2008), most children with JIA do not have positive RF tests. In addition, children with positive RF can be identified easily based on history and physical examination; the test does not impact the diagnosis.

Additional laboratory tests can be used to rule out other conditions (e.g., infection, Lyme disease, or systemic lupus erythematosus), as well as to classify the type of JIA a child has. For example, a low hemoglobin and hematocrit may be related more to anorexia than to arthritis progression. General findings also are likely to include an elevated erythrocyte sedimentation rate (ESR), depending on the degree of inflammation present. Antinuclear antibody (ANA) is found in some patients with juvenile arthritis. Its presence suggests the occurrence of connective tissue disease and can help the health care provider refine the diagnosis; positive ANA in a child with oligoarthritis is related to a marked increase in his or her risk for developing eye disease. In addition, testing may be done for anti-cyclic citrullinated peptide (anti-CCP) antibodies. These antibodies may be detected in healthy individuals before the onset of rheumatoid arthritis (RA) and may predict the ultimate development of undifferentiated arthritis into RA (NIAMS, 2008).

X-rays are needed if the health care provider suspects bone injury or unusual bone development. Although x-rays may show soft tissue changes in early disease, they generally are more useful later to identify effects on bones.

Common Therapeutic Modalities

Nurses and other health care providers should partner with the patient and family to address all facets of life that may be affected by a chronic illness: education, peer relations, self-esteem, social adjustment, family dynamics, vocational planning, and financial concerns. Goals include preservation of joint motion and muscle strength, prevention or minimization of anatomic joint damage, and relief of symptoms without potential iatrogenic harm.

Medications. Pharmacologic treatments are used for the articular and ocular manifestations of juvenile arthritis. Nonsteroidal anti-inflammatory drugs (NSAIDs) are often first-line treatment for JIA and may be the only treatment needed for patients with very mild arthritis. Achieving an anti-inflammatory effect requires up to twice the dose used for analgesia and takes an average of 1 month. Many NSAIDs have been evaluated in patients with JIA; overall efficacy rates are similar, though patient response is idiosyncratic. Liquid NSAIDs are often needed in young patients in forms that require less frequent use, especially in school-aged children (NIAMS, 2008). Although most children tolerate NSAIDs well, abdominal pain and anorexia occur commonly. Because of the risk of gastrointestinal distress, they should be given with food. H2 blockers, misoprostol (Cytotec®), or antacids also can be given to minimize complaints. NSAIDs may adversely affect coagulation and liver or renal function, or cause central nervous system side effects (drowsiness, irritability, headaches, tinnitus). Unique skin toxicity (development of pinhead-size blisters) can occur in children taking naproxen; the lesions are minimally symptomatic, but scars often resolve very slowly.

When one or two NSAIDs are ineffective, disease-modifying anti-rheumatic drugs (DMARDs) may be taken singly or in combination to slow or stop JIA progression. Methotrexate, the most commonly prescribed DMARD for juvenile arthritis, is safe and effective for most children. It often is used in combination with a NSAID. No data currently exist about when to initiate methotrexate therapy in children with JIA, or how long to continue treatment (Niehues & Lankisch, 2006). Dosing generally begins at 10-15 mg/m2 body surface area (BSA) administered once weekly by mouth or injection. The weekly dose of parenteral methotrexate can be increased to 15-20 mg/m2 BSA. Therapeutic effects of methotrexate usually are not evident for at least 3–4 weeks. Common side effects are generally mild and do not require alteration in dosage. They include oral ulcers, nausea, decreased appetite, and abdominal pain. Folic acid (1 mg/day orally) often is given to decrease the severity and/or frequency of these side effects. Most pediatric rheumatologists follow American College of Rheumatology monitoring guidelines for methotrexate toxicity, although guidelines have not been evaluated or validated in patients with JIA (Kremer et al., 1994; Saag et al., 2008). Other DMARDs prescribed for JIA include sulfasalazine and hydrochloriquine (Abramson, 2008).

For children who have experienced little relief from other agents, one of five biologic response modifiers may be beneficial. Etanercept, infliximab, adalimumab, abatacept, and anakinra may be helpful in treatment of systemic onset arthritis, extended oligoarthritis, and polyarthritis (NIAMS, 2008). The first three agents work by blocking tumor necrosis factor (TNF), a naturally occurring compound that helps cause inflammation in the body. Anakinra blocks interleukin-1, another inflammatory protein, and abatacept blocks the activation of inflammatory T cells.

Corticosteroids continue to be used for severe life-threatening complications such as pericarditis (NIAMS, 2008), but the lack of evidence that they alter the natural history of articular manifestations makes their routine systemic use unlikely. Intra-articular corticosteroids may be used to decrease pain and inflammation for patients with limited joint involvement, and topical steroids may be indicated for treatment of inflammatory eye disorders.

Physical Management. Individualized treatment programs are designed for children with JIA to preserve joint function and prevent deformity. Joint protection involves splinting an affected extremity to maintain it in neutral position and minimize pain. The child should rest on a firm mattress with a very low pillow or no pillow at all under affected joints to maintain extension and avoid flexion contractures. Nutritional support will be needed to decrease the likelihood of obesity and also help the child avoid growth retardation.

Physical and occupational therapists may consult with school personnel about physical education and classroom adaptations. Physical therapists may prescribe activities to mobilize restricted joints and help the child avoid or correct deformity. Muscle strengthening also is needed to provide joint support. As part of an exercise program, pool activity may be especially beneficial due to the warmth and mild resistance of the water. Swimming promotes range of motion (ROM), and the water's buoyancy alleviates stress over affected joints. In addition, isometric/tensing exercises should be used during peak periods of inflammation to avoid joint motion that may aggravate pain. After disease remission, ROM exercises should continue. Developing and following up on an individualized exercise program are essential to encourage consistent participation. Occupational therapists should build on the child's natural tendency to be active, with a focus on generalized mobility and performance of activities of daily living (ADLs).

Other modalities that have been proven as effective adjuncts for disease management include warm baths and hot packs to reduce joint stiffness and muscle spasm in the nonacute inflammatory phase of the disease. Cold can be used in periods of acute inflammation. Ultrasound and electrical stimulation may decrease pain and increase joint mobility.

Surgery may be considered for joint contractures or unequal growth of extremities. Possible surgical treatments include soft tissue release (tenotomy) for contractures, leg length correction, and joint arthroplasty.

Complementary and Alternative Therapies. Many adults seek alternative treatments for arthritis, including dietary supplements and acupuncture. Research indicates an increasing number of children seeking such complementary therapies as well (NIAMS, 2008). If the health care provider believes an alternative approach has value and does not cause harm, it can be incorporated into the child's treatment plan; however, the nurse should stress the need to maintain the regular health care regimen and seek medical attention for serious symptoms.

Nursing Considerations

Nursing Diagnoses. Nursing diagnoses for this condition are expanded upon in the Appendix.

- Activity intolerance, risk for.
- Body image, disturbed.
- Caregiver role strain, risk for.
- Development, risk for delayed.
- Family coping, compromised.
- Knowledge deficit.
- Mobility: physical, impaired.
- Pain, acute.
- Pain, chronic.
- Self-care deficit: bathing/hygiene, dressing/grooming, feeding, toileting.
- Self-health management, ineffective.

Interventions. The nurse should discuss strategies for the child's success in school. The teacher should be made aware of the child's condition and its potential impact on school performance; the American Juvenile Arthritis Organization (AJAO) offers materials to assist parents in working with teachers and school administrators. The child should be given a backpack to eliminate strain on small joints by carrying books and papers. If possible, parents should obtain two sets of books so the child does not have to carry them between school and home. High-quality running shoes can decrease ankle pain exacerbated by walking at school. Adequate travel time between classes also should be arranged. In completing schoolwork, the child can prevent pain, stiffness, and fatigue in the hands by using a felt-tip pen or a pen covered with a foam wedge. Other strategies for success include scheduling oral rather than written tests, using the computer for long reports, using a chalk holder for work at the blackboard, and using a flip chart and felt-tip pen instead of a blackboard.

Patient Teaching. Parents and care providers of a child treated with corticosteroids must understand that sudden withdrawal of the medications can be dangerous, and that the health care provider's instructions for tapering the medication must be followed exactly. Parents and others involved should be taught to provide age-appropriate care to meet the child's developmental needs. Play activities for toddlers should encourage development of both small and large muscle groups through use of blocks, puzzles, or art projects. School-aged children should be allowed to participate in less strenuous activities, such as board games or collections, to keep involved with their peer groups while conserving energy and preserving joint and muscle movement.

Practice Setting Considerations. Because the majority of an affected child's care occurs in the home, the nurse in a clinic or hospital must help the parent and child cope with and adapt to the limitations of disease. The nurse should question parents sensitively to determine if they have stopped giving medications due to fears about side effects or doubts concerning their efficacy. Parents need encouragement to avoid overprotecting the child, especially if they hold the misconception that inactivity will spare the child pain. The nurse should encourage parents to contact local chapters of AJAO and the Arthritis Foundation for information and ongoing emotional support. Social workers also can help parents to locate resources to cope with the financial demands of chronic illness. Health care providers and parents alike must facilitate the child's understanding that the disease is not his or her fault, or punishment for something the child has done.

Rheumatoid Arthritis

Overview

Definition. Rheumatoid arthritis (RA) is an autoimmune, systemic inflammatory disease with predominant clinical manifestations in the synovial membranes of diarthrodial joints. RA is characterized by unexplained periods of remission and exacerbation. It has long been feared as one of the most disabling forms of arthritis, but recent treatment advances have improved the prognosis for many newly diagnosed patients (Ruderman & Tambar, 2008).

Etiology. No single cause has been identified, and no known risk factors exist for RA. External events that precipitate disease development have not been identified, though infection is thought to be a possible trigger of the disease. RA is believed to be caused by an aberrant immune response in a genetically predisposed host. Complex genetic factors influence the degree of joint destruction and organ involvement. Because women are more likely to develop the disease than men, a variety of hormonal factors may be involved in RA development (NIAMS, 2009b); however, neither breastfeeding nor irregular menstruation appear to alter risk for RA substantially (Karlson, Mandi, Hankinson, & Grodstein, 2004).

CHAPTER 13

Pathophysiology. In Stage I RA, synovitis (or inflammation of the synovial membrane) is mediated by infiltrating lymphocytes. Joint effusions with a high cell count (5,000-60,000/mm3) are likely. X-rays show soft tissue swelling but no destructive joint changes at this point. During Stage II, the inflamed synovial tissue hypertrophies and begins to grow into the joint cavity across the articular cartilage. The characteristic pannus, a highly vascularized fibrous scar tissue, develops during this stage. In Stage III, the destructive pannus erodes and destroys the articular cartilage. Tumor necrosis factor (TNF) is a mediator of cartilage destruction at the cartilage-pannus junction. Subchondral bone erosions and fissures, bone cysts, and bone spurs occur. The pannus also scars and shortens tendons and ligaments to create laxity, joint subluxation, and contractures. With Stage IV (end-stage) RA, the inflammatory process is subsiding. Fibrous or bony ankylosis occurs, ending the functional life of affected joints. Rheumatoid nodules appear as cutaneous masses or pressure points, and are associated with severe disease (Wheeless, 2010c).

Incidence. About 1.3 million people in the United States have RA; however, the actual number of new cases of the disease may be lower than previously estimated because of changes in classification criteria for RA (Helmick et al., 2008). RA can occur at any age, but peak incidence is fourth and sixth decades. About 2–3 times as many women as men have RA (NIAMS, 2009b; Ruderman & Tambar, 2008). The prevalence of RA worldwide is about 1%-2%; however, 3.5%-5.3% of Native Americans develop the disease, suggesting a higher genetic burden for RA risk (Haque & Bathon, 2007).

Complications. RA is the direct cause of death or severe morbidity more often than has been appreciated due to extra-articular manifestations of the disease. For example, obstructive airway disease can occur in persons with RA in the absence of a significant smoking history. Rheumatoid nodules in the lungs can create cavitation similar to cancer or infection, and careful diagnostic differentiation is needed. Pericarditis is the most common cardiac manifestation of RA; patients present with chest pain, fever, and a pericardial rub that may resolve spontaneously. Rheumatoid cardiovascular disease leads to a shorter life span for persons with RA than their age- and sex-matched peers. In addition, sensory peripheral neuropathy can occur in the extremities of a person with RA. Keratoconjunctivitis or Sjögren's syndrome also occurs as a common ocular manifestation of RA (Haque & Bathon, 2007).

Joint destruction begins early, but almost 90% of joints ultimately affected are involved during the first year of disease. Flexion contractures and hand deformity result in diminished grasp strength. Characteristic deformities include ulnar deviation ("zigzag" deformity) of the wrist, swan-neck deformity (flexion of distal interphalangeal

Figure 13.1.
Advanced Hand Deformities in Rheumatoid Arthritis

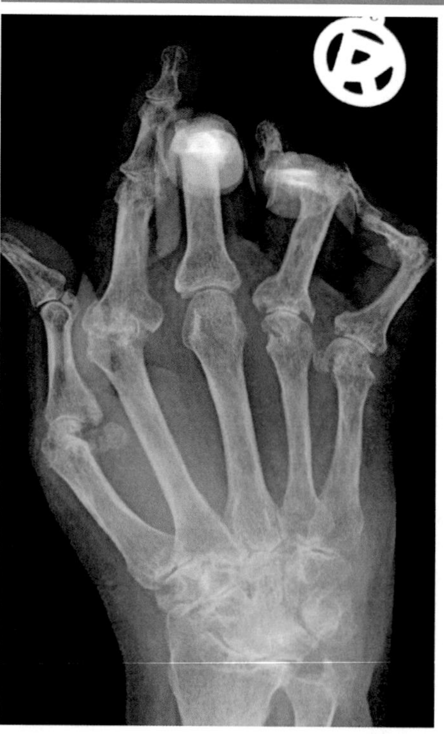

From Rheumatoid Arthritis *by Bernd Brägelmann, http://en.wikipedia.org/wiki/File:RheumatoideArthritisAP.jpg. Reproduced with permission.*

[DIP], metacarpophalangeal [MCP] joints with hyperextension of proximal interphalangeal [PIP] joint), and boutonniere deformity (avulsion of extensors, producing flexion of PIP joint) (Wheeless, 2010b). (See Figure 13.1 for common hand deformities in RA.)

Involvement of the foot and ankle causes greater dysfunction and pain than upper extremity disease. Pronation deformities and eversion of the foot occur due to stretching and erosion of ligaments. Tarsal tunnel entrapment can cause burning paresthesia on the sole of foot, worsened by standing or walking. Metatarsal phalangeal (MTP) arthritis causes deformities of the toes and subluxation of the MTP heads on the sole (Wheeless, 2010a).

Special Considerations. In younger people, RA tends to have a slow, insidious onset. With disease onset after age 60, symptoms tend to be acute, explosive, and widespread, but they have a shorter duration and better prognosis. During pregnancy, genetic differences between mother and fetus may alter disease activity. Most women report marked improvement in joint pain and/or swelling during pregnancy, but low-dose prednisone or NSAIDs may be used if needed in the first and second trimesters without apparent risk to the fetus (Haque & Bathon, 2007). Disease symptoms typically return within about 6 weeks after the baby's birth. Breastfeeding may aggravate the disease (NIAMS, 2009b).

Assessment

History. Early RA can be difficult to diagnose, in large part because symptoms and severity differ from person to person. RA may begin with subtle complaints, such as mildly achy joints or transient morning stiffness. The patient may describe pain in the balls of the feet upon rising from bed. Similar stiffness may occur after long periods of sitting (Haque & Bathon, 2007). The patient also may complain of fatigue, lethargy, and weight loss. He or she may describe increasing difficulty with mobility and performance of self-care activities (NIAMS, 2009b; Ruderman & Tambar, 2008).

Physical Exam. Although not diagnostic for RA, one indicator of joint inflammation is pain on palpation or with passive motion of affected joints. Swelling and warmth may be evident in small joints of the hands and feet, as well as in the elbows, knees, and ankles. Joint range of motion may be limited by edema or structural deformities. Movement may be guarded due to pain, and gait abnormalities may be observed. Spindle-shaped fingers are common in early disease, but permanent joint deformities (claw toes; swan-neck, or boutonniere deformities of the fingers) or frank dislocations are characteristic of later disease (see Figure 13.1 on advanced hand deformities). Intense erythema, common with gout or septic arthritis, is unlikely with RA (Haque & Bathon, 2007).

Diagnostic Tests. Diagnosis of RA is based predominantly on patient history and physical findings, and documentation of inflammatory synovitis is essential. Positive rheumatoid factor (RF) is found in 70%-90% of patients with RA, but titers in early disease may be negative in approximately 25% of patients. High titers do not correlate with disease activity, but patients with high-titer RF are more likely to have severe, unremitting disease marked by erosion, extra-articular manifestations, nodules, and greater functional disability.

Antibodies against citrullinated proteins (anti-CCP) are highly specific for diagnosis of RA. More than 80% of patients with RA have anti-CCP antibodies. When a diagnosis of RA is being considered, both RF and anti-CCP should be ordered because the patient can be negative in one and not the other. A small percentage of patients with RA remain negative for both antibodies throughout the course of their disease.

Antinuclear antibodies are present in some 20%-30% of patients with RA. They are more common in patients with extra-articular manifestations and high-titer RF. The ANA test is not needed unless the diagnosis is in doubt or other systemic symptoms are noted.

Among other diagnostic tests, synovial fluid analysis may be done to distinguish RA from osteoarthritis (OA) (see Table 13.1 for a comparison of RA and OA). In early disease, the fluid is straw-colored and slightly cloudy, with many fibrin flecks and more than 2,000 WBCs/mm3. Synovial biopsy generally is not needed for diagnosis and only performed to rule out infection. Genetic markers also are not necessary as a screening test for RA.

Radiographs generally are not needed to make a diagnosis, but they will show characteristic changes. Loss of articular cartilage leads to narrowed joint space with advanced disease. Joint subluxation and mal-alignment seen on x-ray reflect the destructive changes noted on physical examination. Serial x-rays are likely to monitor erosive changes to joints; however, structural changes can be identified earlier on magnetic resonance imaging (MRI) and ultrasound than on plain films (Haque & Bathon, 2007).

Common Therapeutic Modalities

Goals in the treatment of RA include relieving pain, swelling, and fatigue; slowing or stopping joint damage; preventing disability and disease-related morbidity; and improving the patient's sense of well-being and ability to function.

Medications. Drug therapies remain the most important part of an interdisciplinary care approach. For many years, health care providers prescribed aspirin, NSAIDs, or other analgesics, and only offered more powerful medications if the disease worsened. More recently, providers have recognized that cartilage

Table 13.1. Comparison of Rheumatoid Arthritis and Osteoarthritis		
Characteristic	**RA**	**OA**
Age at onset	2nd - 5th decade	4th - 5th decade
Sex	Females 2 or 3:1 Differences less marked after age 60	Females 2:1 over age 55
Disease course	Exacerbations, remissions	Variable, progressive
Symptomatology	Systemic	Local
Commonly affected joints	Small joints first (PIPs, MCPs, MTPs), wrists, knees	Weight-bearing joints (knees, hips), MCPs, DIPs, PIPs, cervical and lumbar spine
Morning stiffness	1 hour to all day	10-30 minutes after rising
Joint involvement	Symmetric	Asymmetric
Effusions	Common	Uncommon
Synovial fluid	Decreased viscosity; 3000 - 25,000 WBCs	Usually normal viscosity, few cells
Synovium	Thickened, may be severely inflamed	Possible localized synovitis with point tenderness
Nodules	Rheumatic nodules over bony prominences, extensor surfaces, juxtarticular regions	Heberden's nodes (DIPs); Bouchard's nodes (PIPs)
X-rays in advancing disease	Global narrowing of joint space, erosions, subluxations; osteoporosis RT corticosteroid use	Asymmetric narrowing of joint space; osteophytes, subchondral cysts & sclerosis

damage and bony erosions often occur in the first 2 years of the disease (Matsumoto, Bathon, & Bingham, 2010). Use of appropriate medications early in the disease can alter the outcome, severity, disability, and mortality associated with RA. Correct and timely diagnosis is critical to the expedient use of disease-modifying anti-rheumatic drugs (DMARDs) or biologic response modifiers (BRMs) for disease treatment. Their consistent use has been shown to prevent joint erosion and damage, and control the acute synovitis of RA. Persons with long-standing RA do not respond as well to treatment as patients with early disease (NIAMS, 2009b). Choice of drug is based on disease activity and/or progression, the patient's functional status, relevant lifestyle considerations (e.g., affected female of childbearing age), cost, and side effect profile.

Among DMARDs, methotrexate (10-20 mg weekly) is preferred for early treatment of patients with an established diagnosis of RA. Onset of therapeutic effects generally occurs in 6-8 weeks, with minimal side effects and low risk of toxicity. More serious side effects (hepatic cirrhosis, interstitial pneumonitis, severe myelosuppression) occur only rarely, especially with proper monitoring. Complaints of gastrointestinal upset can be reduced when the oral drug is taken at night or can be completely eliminated with subcutaneous administration. Stomatitis, oral ulcers, and mild alopecia (hair loss) are related to folic acid antagonism, and can be improved with administration of folic acid 1 mg daily. Methotrexate not only reduces the signs and symptoms of RA, but also slows or stops radiographic damage (Matsumoto et al., 2010). Additional DMARDs are included in Table 13.2.

Biologic response modifiers are of four types: tumor necrosis factor (TNF) inhibitors, T-cell costimulatory blocking agents, B cell depleting agents, and interleukin-1 (IL-1) receptor antagonists.

TNF is a pro-inflammatory cytokine produced by macrophages and lymphocytes; it mediates joint destruction because of its cellular effects. TNF inhibitors were the first biologics developed for treatment of RA. Three TNF inhibitors are approved for treatment of RA and are similar in their efficacy. They decrease signs and symptoms of the disease, slow or stop radiographic changes, and improve quality of life. Patients receiving a TNF inhibitor are at increased risk for infection due to immunosuppression (Matsumoto et al., 2010).

T-cell costimulatory blockers interfere with the actions between antigen-presenting cells and T lymphocytes, thus lessening the effects in the early stages of RA development. By activating molecules found on the surface of the antigen-presenting cells and the T lymphocytes, these agents decrease the production of T cell-derived cytokines such as TNF (Matsumoto et al., 2010).

B cells, an important inflammatory cell, have multiple functions in human immune response. Depletion of B cells in RA has been shown to reduce signs and symptoms, as well as slow progression of the disease. One B cell depleting agent is currently approved for treatment of RA.

IL-1 is another pro-inflammatory cytokine active in the pathogenesis of RA. IL-1's effects on cartilage lead to damage and inhibited repair. As a potent stimulus to osteoclasts, IL-1 also leads to bone erosion. Only one

Table 13.2. Pharmacologic Treatment Options for RA			
Drug Name	**Dosage**	**Usual Time to Effect**	**Side Effects**
DMARDs			
Methotrexate (Rheumatrex®)	10-20 mg weekly Maximum dose generally 25 mg	As early as 4-6 weeks. Additional 4-6 weeks may be required after a dose increase.	Stomatitis, oral ulcers, alopecia improved with folic acid supplement. GI upset eliminated with subcutaneous administration. Rarely, hepatic cirrhosis, interstitial pneumonitis, severe myelosuppression.
Hydrochloroquine (Plaquenil®)	400 mg daily 600 mg daily sometimes used	2-4 months usual If no response after 5-6 month, drug failure is considered	Eyes: corneal deposits, extraocular muscle weakness, loss of accommodation, retinopathy possibly progressing to vision loss. Baseline opthalmic exam and yearly follow up recommended.
Sulfasalazine (Azulfidine®)	2-3 grams daily in divided doses Often initiated at 1 gram daily and increased to tolerance	6 weeks-3 months	Hypersensitivity, allergic reaction in patients with sulfa allergy. Mild GI complaints common, decreased with use of enteric-coated preparation. Mild cytopenias possible; blood monitoring every 1-3 months based on dose.
Leflunamide (Arava®)	100 mg loading dose daily for 3 days, followed by 20 mg daily Loading period may be shortened, daily dose reduced due to GI effects	4-8 weeks, possibly earlier when loading dose used	Mild diarrhea, GI upset, alopecia. Liver transaminase elevations reversed with drug cessation. Teratogenic effects: women of child-bearing age must be warned of possible fetal risk, cautioned to use adequate contraception.
BRMs – Tumor Necrosis Factor Inhibitors			
Etanercept (Enbrel®)	50 mg weekly by subcutaneous injection Also available as 25 mg dose for twice weekly administration	1-4 weeks Additional improvements seen over 3-6 months	Increased risk for infection. Transient neutropenia, other blood dyscrasias. Mild injection site reactions.
Infliximab (Remicade®)	3 mg/kg by IV infusion, followed by additional dosing at 2 and 6 weeks, then every 8 weeks thereafter Can be increased to 10 mg/kg with infusions every 4-6 weeks Should be given in combination with methotrexate	Days to weeks	Increased risk for infection. Clinical syndrome of fever, chills, body aches, headaches with infusion; can be prevented by slowing infusion rate, administering diphenhydramine (Benadryl®)
Adalimumab (Humira®)	40 mg every other week by subcutaneous injection Frequency can be increased to weekly	1-4 weeks	Increased risk for infection. Mild injection site reactions.
BRMs – T Cell Costimulatory Blocker			
Abatacept (Orencia®)	Dosing on body weight: 500 mg for patients <60 kg, 750 mg for patients 60-100 kg, 1000 mg for patients >100 kg Administered by IV infusion over 30-60 minutes	Within 3 months, with continued improvement over 1 year	Increased risk for infection. Mild infusion reactions.

(continued next page)

Table 13.2. Pharmacologic Treatment Options for RA *(continued)*

Drug Name	Dosage	Usual Time to Effect	Side Effects
BRMs – B Cell Depletion			
Rituximab (Rituxan®)	1000 mg by IV infusion over 3-4 hours Two doses given 2 weeks apart Premedication with acetaminophen (Tylenol®) and diphenhydramine (Benadryl®) Optimal time for readministration not clear	Optimal effects not seen for 3 months after treatment, but may persist for 6 months-2 years	Increased risk for infection. Infusion reactions: hives, itching, swelling, difficulty breathing, fever, chills, BP changes
BRMs – IL-1 Antagonist			
Anakinra (Kineret®)	100 mg daily by subcutaneous injection	2-4 weeks	Modestly increased risk for infection. Injection site reactions: erythema, itching, discomfort generally resolve over 1-2 months Mild-to-moderate neutropenia
Other Immunomodulatory/Cytotoxic Agents			
Azathioprine (Imuran®)	1 mg/kg once or twice daily	8-12 weeks	Cytotoxin typically used for life-threatening effects of extra-articular RA. Bone marrow suppression, cytopenias, nausea, alopecia.
Cyclosporine (Sandimmune®)	2.5 mg/kg daily	1 week-3 months	Increased risk of infection, malignancies. Renal insufficiency. Numerous medication interactions can lead to toxicity.
Cyclophosphamide (Cytoxan®)	1.5-2. 5 mg/kg daily	Weeks-months	Increased risk of infection. Bone marrow suppression, hemorrhagic cystitis, premature ovarian failure, secondary malignancy.
Antibiotic - Tetracycline			
Minocycline (Minocin®)	100 mg twice daily	2-3 months	GI upset, dizziness, skin rash.

Data from Patient Education – Medications *by the American College of Rheumatology, 2009, http://www.rheumatology.org/practice/clinical/patients/medications/; and* Rheumatoid Arthritis Treatment *by A. Matsumoto, J. Bathon, and C. Bingham, III, 2010, http://www.hopkins-arthritis.org/arthritis-info/rheumatoid-arthritis/rheum_treat.html#new#new.*

drug in this class is currently approved for treatment of RA. See Table 13.2 for representative DMARDs, BRMs, and other agents.

NSAIDs are used to improve joint function by decreasing acute inflammation and pain. Importantly, NSAIDs alone do not alter the course of RA or prevent joint damage; they typically are prescribed for use while the patient awaits therapeutic effects of a DMARD or BRM. Aspirin largely has been replaced as the initial choice for inflammation and pain because of its marked gastrointestinal effects and the inconvenience of multiple daily doses. A large number of NSAIDs is available, and most drugs in the class, including both traditional NSAIDs and the single COX-2 inhibitor celecoxib (Celebrex®), are equally effective. Longer-acting drugs that allow daily or twice-daily dosing may improve patient adherence to therapy (Matsumoto et al., 2010).

Corticosteroids can help in symptom relief but are inadequate as a sole therapy for RA. Low-dose prednisone may be used with caution in selected patients to minimize disease activity for a limited time until DMARD effect is seen. Long-term use of oral corticosteroids is associated with development of osteoporosis and avascular necrosis. High doses of systemic corticosteroids are needed only rarely to address life-threatening complications of RA. Direct injection into affected joints can alleviate pain temporarily and address inflammation associated with flare-ups (Matsumoto et al., 2010).

Physical Management. Range of motion (ROM), strengthening, and endurance exercises typically are prescribed for the patient with RA. Passive, active, or assisted ROM exercises can improve joint mobility, while isometric and isotonic exercises build muscles that surround and connect affected joints. Appropriate low-resistance exercises include biking, swimming, golfing, and dancing. Exercise programs should be implemented progressively to achieve optimal long-term benefits. Progressive muscle contraction and relaxation should be used cautiously due to the tendency to exacerbate pain.

Heat and cold applications are important adjuncts to exercise. Superficial heat can be provided with hot packs, hydrotherapy, and paraffin baths; deep heat can be achieved with ultrasound. Cold packs may provide greater relief from pain and stiffness than heat, but they should not be used in patients with Raynaud's phenomenon. Use of splints appears to resolve inflammation more quickly than leaving the joint unsplinted (Krabak & Minkoff, 2010).

Complementary and Alternative Therapies. Some patients with the chronic pain of RA consider complementary and alternative therapies for disease management, in part because of concerns about side effects of conventional medicines. Unfortunately, a great deal of information provided to patients through popular sources is misleading and not based on the quality of evidence required by the U.S. Food and Drug Administration (FDA) for the approval of conventional medicines. Nurses should provide patients with current scientific information regarding any alternative therapies, reinforcing the concerns related to delay in care or exclusion of proven medical treatments for RA (Marcus, 2008).

Acupuncture is more commonly used for treatment of OA than RA, but patients with a variety of arthritic disorders may try acupuncture for pain management. In traditional Chinese medicine, acupuncture is part of a comprehensive treatment plan that also may include herbal therapy, diet, and exercise. In contrast, Western health care providers increasingly use acupuncture as a single therapy. Research findings indicate no significant difference in pain management between sham acupuncture (e.g., insertion of needles at non-acupuncture points) and conventional acupuncture; however, acupuncture has a particularly potent placebo effect that may contribute to pain management and make this therapy an acceptable adjunct to proven medical treatments (Marcus, 2008).

An overall nutritious diet with sufficient calories, protein, and calcium is recommended for patients with RA. In some patients, specific foods have been linked to symptom exacerbation. Unfortunately, elimination of foods has been found to have limited, short-term benefits only; no long-term benefits resulted from this management strategy. Omega-3 fatty acids in some fish or plant seed oils may reduce inflammation, but their use remains controversial. Any benefits are modest and may not appear for several months. In addition, many people are unable to tolerate the large amounts of oil necessary for benefits. Patients who wish to try fish oil should be reminded that some supplements may contain toxic levels of vitamin A or mercury. In addition, fish oil can interfere with blood clotting and increase the risk of strokes (Koch, 2010).

A number of other therapies have only anecdotal support and additional research is needed to demonstrate their efficacy in treatment of RA. These include use of magnets and copper bracelets, t'ai chi and yoga, and homeopathy (Haaz, 2008).

Nursing Considerations

Nursing Diagnoses. Nursing diagnoses for this condition are expanded upon in the Appendix.

- Activity intolerance, risk for.
- Body image, disturbed.
- Coping, ineffective.
- Home maintenance, impaired.
- Mobility: physical, impaired.
- Pain, chronic.
- Powerlessness, risk for.
- Resilience, impaired individual.
- Self-care deficit: bathing/hygiene, dressing/grooming, feeding, toileting.
- Sexuality pattern, ineffective.

Interventions. Use of appropriate and effective coping mechanisms should be reinforced. The nurse should encourage the patient to participate actively in decision-making related to disease treatment and lifestyle changes. The nurse also should discuss the effects of RA on the patient's sexuality and suggest strategies to allow sexual expression. Adaptive strategies for the workplace should be suggested. In addition, the nurse should encourage involvement by the patient and family in support groups through agencies such as the Arthritis Foundation.

In addition, the patient should receive assistance in meeting self-care needs at home. Assistive devices, such as easy-to-grip combs and long-handled brushes, may help with grooming. The use of a long-handled bath brush creates less stress on joints. Clothing can be selected or adapted as necessary to allow self-dressing (e.g., zipper pulls, buttoners, Velcro® closures, pull-on pants). Equipment needs for hygiene care also should be identified (e.g., shower chair, elevated toilet seat). In addition, mobility aids such as a platform cane or walker may be helpful.

Patient Teaching. The patient with RA should receive information about the purpose, dose, frequency, and anticipated side effects of all medications. He or she should know when to report adverse effects to their health care providers, and what to do if a dose of medication is missed. The patient who is taking corticosteroids should be instructed to avoid abrupt cessation of these medications.

The nurse should reinforce the patient's use of a pain management plan. Strategies include analgesics, positioning and joint protection, heat and cold applications, and relaxation techniques (e.g., imagery, rhythmic breathing, music). Energy conservation and joint protection are essential.

Support of family members is critical. They also need instruction on the disease process and planned treatments. They should be encouraged to allow the patient to function independently when able but be available for assistance (e.g., if severe morning stiffness occurs). Family should be encouraged to collaborate with the patient in developing a nutritionally sound diet and in identifying strategies to maximize the patient's sleep and rest.

Osteoarthritis

Overview

Definition. Osteoarthritis (OA) is a slowly progressive, noninflammatory disorder of the cartilage in movable (diarthrodial) joints. It is characterized by gradual loss of articular cartilage combined with thickening of subchondral bone; bony outgrowths (osteophytes) at joint margins; and mild, chronic, nonspecific synovial inflammation.

Etiology. Idiopathic OA is a form of the disease with an obscure or unknown initiating factor. Some health care providers limit use of this identifier to disease of the joints of the hands, while others also include the hips, knees, and spine. The term may become obsolete as research continues into the cause of osteoarthritis. For example, some investigators suggest the cause of idiopathic OA may be unrecognizable or subtle congenital or genetic defects (Stacy & Basu, 2009).

Secondary OA is caused by any condition that damages cartilage directly; subjects joint surfaces/underlying bone to chronic, excessive, or abnormal forces; or causes joint instability. Possible causes of secondary disease include the following:

- Trauma: sprains, strains, dislocations, fractures (possibly leading to avascular necrosis, osteonecrosis);
- Mechanical stress: long-term involvement in repetitive physical tasks or activities, such as athletics or ballet;
- Inflammation in joint structures: inflammatory cells release enzymes that can digest cartilage;
- Joint instability: damage to supporting structures, such as ligaments, tendons, and the joint capsule;
- Neurologic disorders: pain; lost or diminished proprioceptive reflexes leading to increased tendency for abnormal movement, positioning, and weight bearing (diabetic neuropathy, Charcot arthropathy);
- Congenital/acquired skeletal deformities: varus or valgus leg deformity, congenital hip subluxation, slipped capital femoral epiphysis, Legg-Calvé-Perthes disease;
- Hematologic/endocrine disorders: hemophilia with chronic bleeding into joints; hyperparathyroidism with calcium loss from bone; and
- Selected drug use: activity of collagen-digesting enzymes stimulated in synovial membrane (colchicine, indomethacin, steroids) (Altman, 2008a).

OA also is classified based on joint involvement. In localized disease, one or two joints may be affected. Three or more joints are involved in generalized disease.

Pathophysiology. Smooth, glistening, white articular cartilage normally covers synovial joint surfaces. Normal cartilage is characterized by extremely low friction with movement, as well as a shock-absorbing capacity due to its compressibility and elasticity. It is composed of chondrocytes and a matrix made of type II collagen and proteoglycans. Under normal conditions, articular cartilage undergoes a continual remodeling process that involves a balance of degradating and synthesizing enzyme activity. In osteoarthritic cartilage, however, the enzymes responsible for matrix degradation are overexpressed. The balance of activity thus shifts in favor of net degradation, leading to loss of collagen and proteoglycans from the matrix. In response to this loss, chondrocytes proliferate and begin to synthesize increased amounts of proteoglycans and collagen. As the disease progresses, these attempts at repair are exceeded by progressive cartilage destruction. The superficial cartilage layer becomes marked by fibrillation, erosion, and cracking; in time, these changes progress to the deeper layers of cartilage (Ling & Bathon, 2010b).

Fissures cause cartilage fragments to detach into the articular cavity as loose bodies, and subchondral microcysts develop. The fragments cause the mild synovial inflammation of OA, which is typically more focal than the inflammation of RA. Sclerosis of subchondral bone occurs due to apposition of small strips of new bone; osteophytes form around this zone. With disease progression, subchondral sclerosis increases and accelerated turnover causes changes in the architecture of subchondral trabecular bone.

The early pain and stiffness of OA result from inflammatory changes in the synovium and joint capsule. Possible causes include prostaglandin release, microfractures of subchondral trabeculae, joint effusion, irritation of periosteal nerve endings by osteophytes, compromise of circulation to bone, effects on tendons or fascia, and muscle spasm. Because cartilage has no nerve supply, joint surfaces do not become painful until subchondral bone is exposed in the later stages of OA.

Incidence. OA is the most common form of articular disease in the world, and the leading cause of disability and pain among older adults. It affects more than 70% of persons ages 50-78. Women are affected more than men. Hip OA is more common in Western countries, suggesting environment and race may be factors in disease development (Wilke & Carey, 2009). OA demonstrates site specificity: only certain synovial joints show high prevalence. These include the weight-bearing joints (hips, knees); the cervical and lumbar spine; the DIP, PIP, and MCP joints in the hands; and the metatarsophalangeal (MTP) joint in the feet. The knees and hands are affected more often in women, especially after menopause, while the hips are affected more frequently in men.

Risk Factors. OA in younger people often occurs secondary to trauma, joint bleeds, or infection, and may cause lifelong disability. See the discussion of secondary OA above. Some risk factors are based on patient involvement in injury-prone activities and therefore modifiable, while other factors may be related to co-morbid health conditions.

Sex hormones and other hormonal factors also seem to influence disease development and progression. For example, OA occurs more frequently in women over age 50 than in age-matched men; women who take estrogen replacement therapy are less likely to have OA than women not taking estrogen. Excessive parathyroid hormone, which results in hypercalcemia, also can produce skeletal changes. In addition, excessive growth hormone (acromegaly) has adverse effects on bones and joints that can lead to OA. Low intake and low serum levels of vitamin D also appear to be associated with progressive osteoarthritis.

Complications. Resulting limitations in physical activities increase with age. Arthritic involvement of the feet and knees, in particular, may cause an unstable gait and increased risk for falling. Other complications of OA include chronic pain, decreased joint ROM and accompanying loss of function, and decreased independence due to an altered ability to perform ADLs. Emotional and social problems may result from coping with the chronicity, pain, and activity limitations.

Assessment

History. (See Table 13.1 for a comparison of RA and OA.) Joint pain is the dominant symptom and the usual reason for the patient to seek treatment. In addition, a synergistic effect can be medical opinion and a major determinant of disability/functional impairment. Pain typically is localized and asymmetric. The pain generally is described as mechanical in nature ("aching"), with a gradual or insidious onset. The patient may not be able to recall specifically when the pain began. It increases with joint use but is relieved by rest in early disease; night pain and pain at rest are considered features of severe disease. Pain also can be increased with a drop in barometric pressure before inclement weather.

Joint stiffness varies from a simple slowness of movement to pain on initial movement. Early morning stiffness is common, with stiffness also occurring after prolonged periods of inactivity (gel phenomenon). Overuse of an affected joint may cause swelling due to a moderate effusion, with associated stiffness. The joint stiffness of OA usually is short-lived (often less than 30 minutes), compared to the generalized, persistent stiffness of inflammatory arthropathies such as RA.

Functional impairment is likely with OA. For example, knee OA often leads to complaint of joint instability and buckling, especially when the patient is descending stairs or stepping off curbs. Hip OA can cause gait problems, with pain localized to the groin and radiating down the anterior thigh to knee. OA of the hands may cause problems with manual dexterity, especially if the basal joints of the thumbs are involved (Altman, 2008a; Ogiela, 2009).

Physical Exam. Symptoms of OA are localized, not systemic. Bony enlargement of affected joints is common, making them tender to palpation. Point tenderness away from the joint line suggests accompanying periarticular lesions (bursitis) that may be readily amenable to local treatment. Crepitation may be heard or felt during joint movement due to osteophyte formation and irregularity of opposing cartilage surfaces. Reduced ROM is a principal feature of the disease and a contributor to overall disability for the affected patient. Related impact on functional ability is more notable than precise effects on ROM.

Specific joint deformities are unique to OA. Heberden's nodes, which develop on the DIP joints of the hands, indicate osteophyte formation and loss of joint space. They appear most often in women with OA and can occur as early as age 40. Heberden's nodes tend to be seen in families. Bouchard's nodes on the PIP joints indicate similar involvement to Heberden's nodes. Varus or valgus deformities are possible in advanced knee OA. In advanced hip OA, leg length discrepancy may result from loss of joint space. Large effusions are uncommon in OA, but slight to moderate effusion may occur due to mild synovitis. Muscular atrophy may be noted in advanced disease secondary to joint splinting for pain relief. With spine OA, weakness or numbness in the arms or legs may result from nerve root impingement by osteophytes.

Joint warmth can indicate varying degrees of synovitis. It may accompany or precede signs of joint damage. Localized warmth is most evident at the knee or during early development of OA in fingers. Large, warm effusions are uncommon and should suggest alternative pathology (Altman, 2008a; Ogiela, 2009).

Diagnostic Tests. Accurate diagnosis of OA allows prompt initiation of appropriate treatment, as well as prevention of unnecessary suffering, disability, and cost. While radiographs are considered the "gold standard" for diagnosis of OA, changes are evident on plain films only relatively late in the disease. Films may display typical changes: bony proliferation (osteophytes or spurs) at joint margins, asymmetric joint-space narrowing and subchondral bone sclerosis, and bone remodeling with formation of subchondral cysts. Films, however, do not always correlate with the severity of the patient's clinical symptoms. Magnetic resonance imaging (MRI) can allow direct views of the cartilage, but it is rarely needed for diagnosis of OA (Altman, 2008a).

The need exists for a specific biological marker that would allow early diagnosis of the disease. Routine laboratory findings, such as elevated ESR or CRP, are not useful as disease markers, although recent evidence suggests that an elevated CRP is predictive of more rapidly progressing disease. Several isotopes of cartilage components offer some promise as markers of OA. For example, chondroitin sulfate epitope 846 has been identified in OA but not in normal adult cartilage and synovial fluid. Elevated serum hyaluronon also has been correlated with radiographic OA. In addition, elevated cartilage oligomeric protein (COMP) in synovial fluid following trauma may predict the development of OA in the injured joint (Ling & Bathon, 2010a).

Synovial fluid analysis can be performed if necessary to differentiate between OA and other forms of arthritis. Normal synovial fluid is clear to dark yellow in color. In a patient with OA, synovial fluid may be turbid with visible shards of cartilage. Fluid from osteoarthritic joints also may show a mild increase in white blood cells if inflammatory synovitis is present (Altman, 2007).

Common Therapeutic Modalities

Conservative management may be accomplished with physical therapy, drug therapy, and/or self-care modifications. Goals are to manage pain and inflammation, maintain joint function and mobility, prevent or correct deformity, and help the patient achieve maximal role function and independence in self-care. In addition, the nurse should help the patient accept and manage OA as a chronic illness through an individualized therapeutic regiment, using positive coping strategies.

Medications. Because no drug can reverse the structural and biochemical abnormalities of OA, pharmacologic therapy is aimed at pain management. OA frequently occurs in older adults, and treatment may be complicated because they may have other chronic diseases and take multiple medications. Over-the-counter (OTC) medications, for example, may interact adversely with a recommended OA treatment regimen. In addition, older adults often receive health care from multiple providers, possibly leading to drug duplication or polypharmacy. The nurse must be aware of factors that may affect drug therapy in elders, including age-related changes in body composition and the normal functional decline in body systems. Initiation of pharmacologic treatment is based on the need to "start low and go slow."

The simple analgesic acetaminophen (Tylenol®) is recommended as the initial drug of choice for treating osteoarthritis pain, with doses up to 1,000 mg four times daily. The drug should be used cautiously in the patient with existing liver disease or chronic alcohol use. Careful monitoring of the prothrombin time also is needed for the patient who is taking warfarin (Coumadin®) and begins treatment with acetaminophen (ACR Subcommittee on Osteoarthritis Guidelines, 2000).

If acetaminophen proves inadequate for pain management, low-dose OTC NSAIDs or nonacetylated salicylate may be recommended for the patient with normal renal function and no prior history of GI problems. If pain persists, prescription dosages of NSAIDs may be ordered. The analgesic effect of NSAIDs is exerted by inhibition of prostaglandin synthesis via inactivation of cyclooxygenase (COX) enzymes; however, reduction of prostaglandin levels in the stomach and kidneys due to COX-1 inhibition can result in gastric ulceration and renal impairment. Older adults in particular are at higher risk for these side effects due to multiple comorbidities and their diminished physiologic reserve. Less GI and renal toxicity was expected with use of the newer, COX-2 selective NSAID celecoxib (Celebrex®). Unfortunately, this medication and other NSAIDs were identified by the FDA (2005) as contributing to increased risk for adverse cardiovascular events. Careful monitoring of renal function, hemoglobin, and hematocrit always should accompany treatment with NSAIDs. In addition, prophylactic treatment should be considered to reduce the risk of GI ulceration, perforation and bleeding. This generally is recommended in the patient older than age 60 with prior history of peptic ulcer disease, anticipated therapy of more than 3 months, and use of moderate-to-high doses of NSAIDs or concurrent corticosteroids.

Opioid analgesics, such as acetaminophen-hydrocodone (Vicodin®) and oxycodone (Percocet®) combinations, may be used to supplement NSAID therapy for treatment of severe or breakthrough pain, especially if the patient's rest is affected. In addition, clinical trials are underway with an oral salmon calcitonin product for the treatment of OA. It has potential as the first disease-modifying agent for osteoarthritis (Clinical Trials Search, 2010).

Local therapies can be used as adjunctive agents. These include topical creams, such as capsaicin and methylsalicylate. Intra-articular corticosteroid injections may be appropriate for patients with effusions and local inflammation, but four or more injections suggest the need for additional intervention; oral corticosteroids are not appropriate for treatment of OA. Epidural corticosteroids may be considered for the patient with OA of the spine. Periarticular injections also may be effective in treating bursitis and tendonitis that may accompany OA (Altman, 2008a).

Viscosupplementation involves intra-articular injection of hyaluronan, a glycosaminoglycan present in cartilage, or its derivatives (Synvisc®, Orthovisc®, Supartz®). The mechanism of action is unknown. Although anecdotal evidence suggests that therapy may be effective for 1 year following injection, research does not show clear benefits of viscosupplementation. Hyaluronan injections, however, may have more prolonged effects than intra-articular steroids (Bellamy et al., 2006).

Physical Management. Non-pharmacologic management of OA is stressed by the American College of Rheumatology (ACR) guidelines, which cite increasing evidence that people with OA benefit from weight loss, physical therapy, muscle strengthening, and aerobic exercise (ACR Subcommittee on Osteoarthritis Guidelines, 2000). Weight reduction in obese patients reduces biomechanical stress on weight-bearing joints and may relieve pain significantly. Cartilage and subchondral bone are particularly vulnerable to the effects of obesity in middle-aged and older adults. In addition, OA progresses more rapidly in overweight individuals.

ACR guidelines also acknowledge the importance of exercise as an integral part of OA management (ACR Subcommittee on Osteoarthritis Guidelines, 2000). Evidence suggests that joint loading and mobilization are essential for articular integrity. Quadriceps weakness, which develops in early disease, may contribute to progressive articular damage. Exercise prescriptions should focus on cardiovascular conditioning, improvements in strength and flexibility, and increased joint mobility. Aerobic or resistance exercises have led to improvements in physical performance, painful symptoms, and patient reports of disability. Strengthening and weight-bearing ROM exercises have improved gait, strength, and overall function. In addition, low-impact, gravity-limiting activities (bicycle training) increase muscle tone and strength, neuromuscular function, and cardiovascular endurance without excessive force across joints.

The following additional nonpharmacologic therapies may be chosen to relieve pain, improve joint biomechanics, and enhance function:

- Local heat or ice to reduce pain, stiffness.
- Ultrasound to increase collagen elasticity, flexibility.
- Stimulation with electrical devices (TENS) to strengthen muscles.
- Use of orthotic devices, shock-absorbing shoes to reduce discomfort with movement.

Physical therapy also may be ordered to facilitate exercise and help control joint symptoms. The therapist can educate and motivate the patient while monitoring progress toward treatment goals. Therapy should be a transition strategy in almost all cases, with the patient ultimately exercising independently.

Surgery may be considered for patients whose function and mobility remain compromised despite maximal medical therapy. Arthroscopy allows removal of loose bodies or resection of torn tissue when the joint space is sufficiently wide. Tibial osteotomy can be considered for the patient with relatively small varus angulation and stable ligamentous support in the knee. Arthrodesis may be indicated for the patient with widespread joint destruction, as from bleeding into a joint due to hemophilia. Arthroplasty is indicated for the patient with severe varus/valgus deformity (with related ligamentous instability), advanced OA, or ineffective pain relief with other modalities. The procedure could involve total joint replacement or, for the hip, resurfacing of the femoral head. Unicompartmental arthroplasty may be performed for the patient with medical compartment arthritis of the knee. Arthroplasty can be performed on major joints, such as the hip, knee, shoulder, and ankle; disc replacement also is possible in the arthritic spine. In addition, chondrocyte implantation may be considered for the patient with a focal cartilage defect in the knee. (See Figure 13.2.)

Complementary and Alternative Therapies. Non-traditional therapies, including herbal products or supplements, may be used for relief of OA pain. Glucosamine and chondroitin sulfate supplementation

Figure 13.2.
Tibial Osteotomy

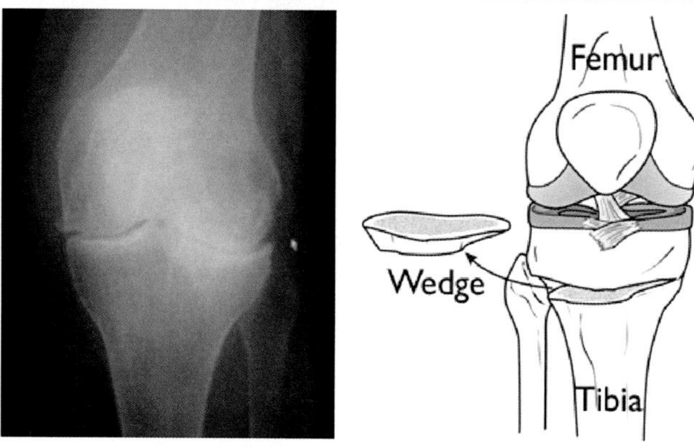

From "Osteotomy of the Knee" by the American Academy of Orthopaedic Surgeons, 2011, OrthoInfo, *http://orthoinfo.aaos.org/topic.cfm?topic=A00591. Reproduced with permission.*

have become popular treatments for OA as the idea of cartilage regeneration has appeared frequently in consumer literature. Chondroitin is part of a protein that gives cartilage its elasticity, while glucosamine is an amino sugar that appears to play a role in the formation and repair of cartilage. Patients with mild to moderate OA may experience pain relief similar to that achieved with NSAIDs, although the supplements may take longer to begin working. Supplements should be taken for 6 weeks and discontinued if no symptom change has occurred by that time. Research on their efficacy is mixed (Altman, 2008a).

Long-term data on use of the dietary supplement S-adenosylmethionine (SAM-e) do not confirm its value in treatment of OA. See the discussion of "Rheumatoid Arthritis" for additional information on complementary and alternative therapies.

Nursing Considerations

Nursing Diagnoses. Nursing diagnoses for this condition are expanded upon in the Appendix.

- Activity intolerance, risk for.
- Body image, disturbed.
- Comfort, impaired.
- Coping, ineffective.
- Mobility: physical, impaired.
- Nutrition: imbalanced, risk for more than body requirements.
- Role performance, ineffective.
- Self-care deficit: bathing/hygiene, dressing/grooming, feeding, toileting.
- Self-health management, ineffective.
- Walking, impaired.

Interventions. Advancing disease may prompt the need for retraining by the patient still in the workforce. OA also can lead to self-care deficits that threaten the patient's independence. The nurse should collaborate with an occupational therapist to obtain assistive devices that facilitate the patient's independence in self-care. The nurse also should discuss the impact on the patient's self-esteem of arthritic deformities and decreased independence. The effects of OA on the patient's sexuality should be considered; the nurse may suggest alternative positions for intercourse, and discuss strategies to relieve pain and stiffness before intercourse (e.g., analgesics, warm bath).

Patient Teaching. Education and counseling are the nurse's primary role in assisting the patient with potentially disabling OA. The nurse can help families become partners with the patient in effective disease management. Educational sessions can be scheduled when key family members can attend with the patient, and content can focus on the concerns of all family members to facilitate care. Education should be provided about the disease process, treatment, and probable impact. In particular, the nurse should discuss the nonsystemic nature and unpredictable course of OA. The importance of exercise and weight management should be stressed, along with use of proper body mechanics and strategies for joint protection. Finally, pharmacologic therapies for OA and other medications taken by the patient should be discussed.

Polymyalgia Rheumatica

Overview

Definition. Polymyalgia rheumatica (PMR) is a clinical syndrome characterized by pain and stiffness in muscles of the shoulder girdle, pelvic girdle, and neck occurring in people over age 50. The stiffness is particularly noticeable in the morning or after a period of inactivity, and it generally lasts longer than 30 minutes. PMR is primarily a pain syndrome rather than one of weakness, swelling, or limitation of motion. Myalgias often are combined with signs of systemic inflammation, such as malaise, weight loss, sweats, or low-grade fever. It was considered previously to be a form of elderly onset RA. The condition rarely occurs in younger persons (ACR, 2009b).

Etiology. The sudden onset of intense inflammation associated with PMR suggests an infectious etiology, but no causative organism has been identified for this condition. In addition, no evidence of disease is present on muscle biopsy. Human leukocyte antigen DR-4 (HLA-DR4) has been found in persons with both PMR and giant cell arteritis (GCA). Occurrence of PMR in siblings also suggests a genetic role in disease development. Some experts hypothesize that an environmental factor, such as a virus, serves as a trigger for monocyte activation in a genetically predisposed person. Systemic activation of monocytes is characteristic of both disorders, but the pattern of T-cell-derived cytokines distinguishes the conditions from each other (Saad, 2010).

Pathophysiology. Infiltrating mononuclear cells lead to mild synovitis. Strong expression of HLA class II antigens appears on synovial and inflammatory cells. Musculoskeletal symptoms may occur before, after, or simultaneously with GCA. About 15% of people with PMR develop GCA, and about 50% of people with GCA have concurrent PMR (Saad, 2010).

Incidence. The incidence of both PMR and GCA peaks between ages 70 and 80. An estimated 700 per 100,000 persons in the United States develop PMR. Caucasian women over age 50 have the highest incidence of PMR (NIAMS, 2010b). Diagnosis of PMR is extremely unlikely in anyone under age 50. Frequency varies by country, with the highest rates occurring in northern Europe (Saad, 2010).

Complications. The condition generally is mild and self-limiting within a few months with treatment unless associated with GCA. Spontaneous disease exacerbations can occur more frequently in the first 2 years, but PMR usually resolves within 1-3 years after onset (Saad, 2010). Myalgias may be reactivated when corticosteroids are tapered; corticosteroid-related side effects also are possible. Patients must be evaluated carefully for associated GCA, which may have severe vascular complications; these include blindness, stroke, and increased risk of aortic aneurysm (Mayo Clinic, 2010).

Assessment

History. Bilateral symmetric proximal myalgia develops typically in the shoulders and hips, with night pain and prominent morning stiffness that can lead to difficulty rising or dressing without assistance. Discomfort may extend to the proximal arms and thighs, as well as the axial muscles. Fever, malaise, anorexia, weight loss, and depression are common. Headache, scalp tenderness, and vision changes may occur with associated GCA. Onset of PMR is often abrupt, sometimes occurring literally overnight (Saad, 2010).

Physical Exam. Pain at rest is noted in affected joints and typically increases with joint movement. Tenderness to palpation is likely. Muscle strength is normal; clinical swelling is not significant. The patient may have transient synovitis of the knee, wrist, or sternoclavicular joints. In later stages of the disorder, the patient may have proximal muscle weakness due to disuse. Contractures of the shoulder capsule may lead to limited passive and active movement (Saad, 2010).

Diagnostic Tests. Diagnosis of PMR is based on clinical presentation rather than laboratory findings. The most typical laboratory findings include elevated ESR and CRP. These results indicate a systemic inflammatory syndrome but are not diagnostic of PMR. Temporal artery biopsy can assist in diagnosis of GCA, but negative biopsy does not exclude vasculitis in large vessels, such as subclavian, axillary arteries, and aorta (NIAMS, 2010b).

Common Therapeutic Modalities

Corticosteroids are the drug of choice for treatment of PMR. In fact, the patient's rapid response to oral corticosteroids generally is taken as confirmation of the diagnosis of PMR. If improvement has not occurred after 2-3 weeks of treatment, the diagnosis of PMR should be questioned (ACR, 2009b). The dose for successful suppression of symptoms and inflammation can vary greatly among patients; however, approximately two thirds of patients respond to initial dose of prednisone 20 mg/day. Some patients require as much as 40 mg/day for complete clinical symptom control; these patients may be at higher risk for progression to GCA. Long-term therapy with low-dose prednisone may be needed to suppress recurrent myalgias and stiffness, but most patients can discontinue treatment after 6 months-2 years. Tapering should occur based on the patient's clinical response (NIAMS, 2010b).

Daily NSAID use also may be prescribed, but most patients do not get relief with NSAIDs alone. Methotrexate, azathioprine, and other immunosuppressant drugs have been used for PMR in an attempt to decrease the need for corticosteroids. No data currently suggest these drugs are superior, however. In addition, they seldom are needed because most patients with PMR respond to low-dose corticosteroids (NIAMS, 2010b; Saad, 2010).

Nursing Considerations

Nursing Diagnoses. Nursing diagnoses for this condition are expanded upon in the Appendix.

- Activity intolerance, risk for.
- Coping, ineffective.
- Infection, risk for.
- Knowledge, deficit.
- Mobility: physical, impaired.
- Pain, acute.
- Powerlessness, risk for.
- Resilience, impaired individual.
- Self-care deficit: bathing/hygiene, dressing/grooming, feeding, toileting.
- Walking, impaired.

Interventions. Corticosteroid use may cause weight gain, and the patient with diabetes may need to increase the insulin dose. In addition, the risk for osteoporosis increases with corticosteroid use. The nurse should encourage the patient to have consistent calcium and vitamin D intake or supplementation. Bone densitometry also should be recommended (NIAMS, 2010b).

Patient Teaching. The nurse should educate the patient on the use and side effects of drug therapy. In particular, both corticosteroids and NSAIDs should be taken with food to decrease negative GI side effects. The patient also should be counseled to avoid abrupt discontinuation of corticosteroids. Because PMR often is associated with GCA, the patient should be told to seek immediate medical attention for headache, changes in vision, or fever (ACR, 2009b). Normal activities, including exercise as tolerated, can be typically resumed once stiffness has subsided.

Rheumatic Fever

Overview

Definition. Rheumatic fever is an acute multisystem inflammatory disease that occurs as a delayed result of pharyngeal infection with streptococcal bacterial. It can affect the heart, joints, skin, and brain. Rheumatic fever is not directly contagious, but the streptococcal infection that triggers rheumatic fever can be highly contagious.

Etiology. Rheumatic fever is caused only by group A (beta-hemolytic) streptococci. It does not follow soft-tissue infection by other strains at other sites. In addition, not all pharyngeal infections lead to rheumatic fever. Experts suspect the disease is due to a hypersensitivity reaction induced by the bacterium. Antibodies to certain strains of streptococci are believed to cross-react with tissue glycoproteins in the heart, joints, and other tissues. Another suggestion is that streptococcal infection evokes an autoimmune response against self-antigens in the affected patient. Although acute rheumatic fever can occur at any age, it is uncommon before age 3 or after age 21. Thus testing for group A streptococcal infection for primary prevention of rheumatic fever is not usually needed in children younger than age 3 with pharyngitis (Pessler & Sherry, 2010).

Pathophysiology. Widely disseminated inflammatory lesions (Aschoff bodies) occur in various sites, most notably the heart. Cardiac damage is cumulative. Diffuse inflammation may affect all three layers of the heart (valves and endocardium, myocardium, pericardium), often leading to valvular thickening, fusion, retraction, or other destruction of leaflets and cups. The mitral valve is the most frequently affected, although any valve can be damaged. In addition to cardiac involvement, migratory polyarthritis generally leaves successive large joints painful and swollen. Joint symptoms often resolve spontaneously and leave no residual damage. In the central nervous system, the occurrence of Sydenham's chorea (a childhood neurological disorder) may be marked by irregular, abrupt, involuntary movements of the face, neck, trunk, and limbs. On the skin, subcutaneous nodules may occur, similar in appearance to those of RA (Pressler & Sherry, 2010).

Recurrent attacks are possible, with the affected person demonstrating increased vulnerability to reactivation of the disease with subsequent pharyngeal infections. Recurrence of fever is relatively common without continued low-dose antibiotics, especially in the first 3-5 years after an initial episode of rheumatic fever. The same manifestations of the disease are likely to reappear, with chorea frequently reactivated and carditis worse with each recurrence. Patients who do not have carditis are less likely to have recurrences and are unlikely to develop carditis if fever does recur (Pressler & Sherry, 2010).

Incidence. International high-risk areas include the tropics, countries with limited resources, and communities with minority indigenous populations. An estimated 95% of cases worldwide develop in these areas (Parrillo, 2010). Rheumatic fever remains the leading cause of heart disease among children and young adults in many developing countries; however, recent local outbreaks in the United States suggest that more rheumatogenic strains of streptococcus are still present in this country (Pressler & Sherry, 2010). Rheumatic fever affects both sexes and all races, although it is most common among American Samoans in Hawaii. No group is known to be free of risk of rheumatic fever if exposed to pharyngeal infection with a causative organism (Parrillo, 2010).

Risk Factors. The incidence of rheumatic fever reflects the worldwide inadequacy of preventive medical care. Under-nutrition, overcrowding, and lower socioeconomic status predispose children to streptococcal infection and subsequent rheumatic fever (Pessler & Sherry, 2010).

Complications. Rheumatic fever is likely to recur, particularly in the first 3-5 years after initial infection. Recurrence is unrelated to intervening streptococcal infection or cessation of antibiotic therapy. Valve replacement may become necessary, particularly with profound mitral regurgitation (Vorvick, 2010).

Inadequately treated infection is most likely the cause of major complications of rheumatic fever. For example, infective endocarditis can lead to the formation of bulky vegetations on heart valves. Valve malformations can increase the risk for embolic events, including cerebral or myocardial infarction. Cardiac hypertrophy and heart failure can result from myocarditis. Atrial fibrillation is possible, especially with mitral stenosis. About 60% of patients with acute rheumatic fever will develop rheumatic heart disease. Age at onset generally determines the order of complications. Young children tend to develop carditis first, while older persons are more likely to develop arthritis first (Parrillo, 2010).

Post-streptococcal reactive arthritis may develop in patients following acute rheumatic fever. It typically involves fewer joints and is less migratory; however, it generally has a more protracted course. It responds less to aspirin but can be treated effectively with NSAIDs (Pessler & Sherry, 2010).

Assessment

History. The patient or family member describes a history of recent group A streptococcal pharyngitis or previous rheumatic fever. Initial symptoms develop 2-4 weeks after infection. Complaints of migratory joint pain, fever, and rash are typical; joint pain in particular occurs early as one of the first manifestations of rheumatic disease. The patient also may exhibit personality changes, emotional lability, or outbursts of inappropriate behavior.

Physical Exam. Arthritis affecting several joints may develop in quick succession, each for only a short time. Joint involvement is more common and more severe in adolescents and young adults than in children. Muscle weakness with jerky, purposeless movements suggests accompanying chorea from central nervous system involvement. These movements usually are more marked on one side of the body, occasionally appearing completely unilateral. Muscle weakness is revealed as the patient attempts to squeeze the provider's hands, with a continuously increasing and decreasing grip (relapsing grip, or "milking sign"). This sign may be overlooked in children, attributed to restlessness or clumsiness if it is the first or only major sign of rheumatic fever.

Subcutaneous nodules and erythema marginatum are characteristic signs of rheumatic fever, but they occur rarely and are overlooked easily. Small, painless nodules appear over bony prominences and in tendon sheaths. The rash is obvious only in fair-skinned patients and generally is hidden by clothing.

The provider may detect a change in heart sounds, marked by a new murmur or a change in a previous murmur; however, murmurs may not be heard at initial examination, and repeated examinations may be needed to determine the presence of carditis. Heart sounds may be weak. A pericardial friction rub, tachycardia, and arrhythmias also may be noted (Parrillo, 2010).

Diagnostic Tests. No specific laboratory test is diagnostic of rheumatic fever. Diagnosis is based on the Modified Jones Criteria (see Table 13.3). Throat cultures are usually negative by the time fever appears, but efforts should be made to isolate the causative organism through antibody testing. Diagnosis may be quite difficult unless clearly indicated by patient presentation. Joint aspiration may be done to rule out other forms of arthritis. In addition, an electrocardiogram is done during initial evaluation, and repeated at time of diagnosis, to identify any abnormalities associated with pericarditis, enlargement of the ventricles or atria, or arrhythmias (Pessler & Sherry, 2010). With diagnosis of rheumatic heart disease in later life, the patient often does not recall a previous attack.

Common Therapeutic Modalities

Detection should lead to prompt treatment to avoid introducing strains of disease-causing bacteria into the community. Whether or not signs of pharyngitis are present at the time of diagnosis, antibiotic therapy should be started with penicillin or erythromycin, maintained for at least 10 days in doses recommended for eradication of streptococcal infection, and then continued after resolution of the acute episode at a prophylactic dose at least until the patient is age 18–21. Salicylates are indicated for routine treatment of inflammation, with dramatic improvement in symptoms usually seen after the start of therapy. Corticosteroids may be indicated for a small minority of patients with severe carditis (indicated by significant cardiomegaly, congestive heart failure, third-degree heart block). Chronic disease management will be based on specific manifestations (Pessler & Sherry, 2010).

Table 13.3. Modified Jones Criteria for a First Episode of Acute Rheumatic Fever
Diagnosis of acute rheumatic fever requires 2 major or 1 major and 2 minor manifestations and evidence of group A streptococcal infection (elevated or rising antistreptococcal antibody titer [eg, antistreptolysin O, anti-DNase B], positive throat culture, or positive rapid antigen test).
Manifestations
Specific Finding
Major
Carditis
Chorea
Erythema marginatum
Polyarthritis
Subcutaneous nodules
Minor
Arthralgia
Elevated ESR or C-reactive protein
Fever
Prolonged PR interval (on ECG)

From "Guidelines for the Diagnosis of Rheumatic Fever. Jones Criteria" by the Special Writing Group of the Committee on Rheumatic Fever, Endocarditis, and Kawasaki Disease of the Council on Cardiovascular Disease in the Young of the American Heart Association, 1992, Journal of the American Medical Association, *268(15):2069–2073.*

Nursing Considerations

Nursing Diagnoses. Nursing diagnoses for this condition are expanded upon in the Appendix.

- Activity intolerance, risk for.
- Comfort, impaired.
- Coping, ineffective.
- Injury, risk for.
- Tissue perfusion: cardiac, risk for decrease.

Interventions. In populations where rheumatic fever remains a problem, causative strains need to be identified and studied. Duration of prophylaxis is risk-dependent; the optimal duration of antibiotic prophylaxis is uncertain (Pessler & Sherry, 2010).

Patient Teaching. Patients should be instructed to complete their prescribed antibiotic regimens even if they feel better. About 6%–29% of treated patients continue to carry group A streptococci after clinical recovery, but the bacteria pose no threat to family and other contacts in populations with a low incidence of rheumatic fever (Pessler & Sherry, 2010).

Gout

Overview

Definition. Gout is a disorder of purine metabolism characterized by monosodium urate crystal deposits in articular, periarticular, and subcutaneous tissues that lead to acute attacks of inflammatory arthritis.

Etiology. Excess production of uric acid, decreased renal excretion of uric acid, or a combination of the two conditions contributes to the development of hyperuricemia in patients with gout. In addition, urate levels can be elevated by increased purine intake; foods high in purine include liver, dried beans and peas, asparagus, mushrooms, and scallops (NIAMS, 2010a). Primary gout (90% of cases) results from an inborn error in either production or excretion of uric acid. Secondary gout (10% of cases) results from drug therapy or another known medical condition (McCarty, 2008; NIAMS, 2010a):

- Various acquired diseases (hematologic conditions, such as hemolytic anemia, lymphoma, leukemia; diseases of cellular proliferation and death, such as psoriasis; renal insufficiency).
- Obesity.
- Lead toxicity.
- Use of certain common drugs (salicylates, thiazide diuretics, niacin, levodopa, alcohol; cyclosporine [Sandimmune®] given to patients following organ transplant).

Pathophysiology. Uric acid is a normal end-product of purine metabolism. It normally is excreted through the kidneys and eliminated in the urine. Humans may accumulate uric acid due to a lack of uricase, the enzyme that breaks down uric acid into more water-soluble products. Hyperuricemia is a risk factor in the development of gout, but gouty arthritis can occur in the presence of normal serum uric acid concentrations. The decreased temperature of peripheral structures (e.g., toes, ears) allows for decreased solubility of monosodium urate, which may explain why crystals typically are deposited in these locations. Urates also become supersaturated in joint fluid, especially in peripheral joints. The tendency for urate crystal deposition in the first MTP joint (great toe) also may be related to repetitive minor trauma.

The first stage of clinical progression for gout is *asymptomatic hyperuricemia* marked by elevated serum uric acid. Treatment generally is not required. Some patients progress to a second stage known as *acute gout* or *acute gouty arthritis*. Hyperuricemia has caused the deposit of uric acid crystals in joint spaces, creating sudden, intense joint pain and swelling. Acute attacks often occur at night, and their pain typically involves only one joint (e.g., the MTP or other joints in the foot and leg). Attacks generally subside in 3-10 days, even without treatment. Another attack may not occur for months or even years, but they do tend to last longer and occur more frequently over time. *Interval* or *intercritical gout* is the period between acute attacks, when patients are free of symptoms. *Chronic tophaceous gout* is the most disabling phase of the disease. It typically develops over a long period of time, marked by permanent damage to affected joints and likely the kidneys as well. Visible deposits of urate crystals, known as tophi, occur during this stage, most commonly on the fingers, hands, feet, ears, elbow, or Achilles tendon. Tophi also can develop in the kidneys. They can become acutely inflamed and painful, often leading to deformities and limited joint motion (McCarty, 2008; NIAMS, 2010a).

Incidence. Gout is predominantly a disease of adult men, with peak incidence in the fifth decade. It rarely occurs in preadolescent men or premenopausal women. Around the world, non-Caucasian populations are more prone to hyperuricemia and gout than are Caucasians (Underwood & Adabajo, 2009). An estimated 3 million people in the United States report having gout at some time in their lives (Schumacher, 2009).

Risk Factors. Dietary trends, including the increased prevalence of obesity and Metabolic Syndrome, appear to be a major contributor to the increasing prevalence of gout in the United States (Schumacher, 2009). Weight management and adherence to a balanced diet will decrease a person's risk of developing gout.

The duration and extent of hyperuricemia directly correlate with the patient's likelihood of developing gouty arthritis, and with age at onset of initial disease manifestations. For example, gout generally is more severe in patients with initial symptoms before age 30 (McCarty, 2008). An initial episode of acute gout usually follows decades of asymptomatic hyperuricemia. A patient with recurrent attacks has longer duration of illness and is more likely to have polyarthritic disease.

Older adults who have diminished renal function or use a diuretic are susceptible to development of polyarticular tophaceous gout. Estrogen promotes renal excretion of uric acid (uricosuric effect) and thus generally protects women against hyperuricemia until menopause (Mahajan, Tandon, Sharma, & Jandial, 2007).

Complications. After an acute attack or following recurrent episodes, a patient is at risk for developing gouty arthritis, tophi, nephrolithiasis, or renal damage. A person with uric acid levels above 9 mg/dL is at risk for the same complications (Watkins, 2010).

Assessment

History. Symptoms of gout often are vague and may mimic other conditions, making diagnosis difficult. Gout is suspected when the patient describes sudden swelling and pain in one or two joints, especially at night and often followed by pain-free episodes (Schumacher, 2009). Family history of gout increases the patient's risk, especially in early-onset disease. Secondary gout may be considered in the differential diagnosis, based on history of specific drug usage or medical conditions described previously (McCarty, 2008; NIAMS, 2010a).

Physical Exam. Swelling, pain, and decreased ROM are noted in affected joints. The MTP joint is classically involved, but symptoms also may be experienced in the fingers, knees, ankles, wrists, and elbows (Schumacher, 2009). (See Figure 13.3.)

Figure 13.3.
Tophi as a Manifestation of Gout

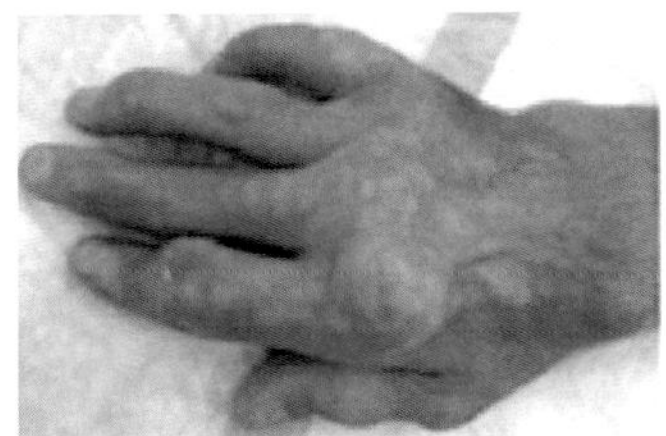

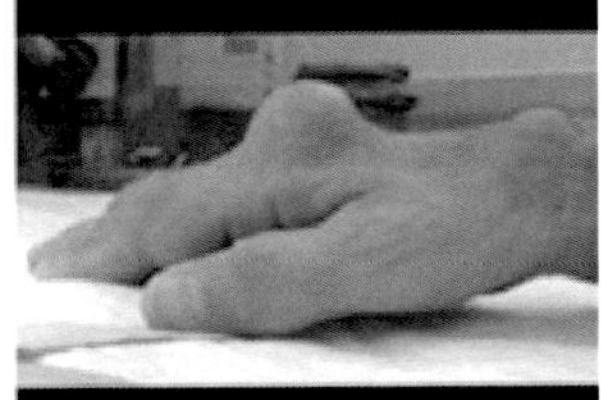

From "Gout Affecting the Hand and Wrist" by B. Fitzgerald, A. Setty, & C. Mudgal, 2007, Journal of the American Academy of Orthopaedic Surgeons, *Volume 15(10), pp 625-635. Reproduced with permission.*

Diagnostic Tests. A health care provider should perform arthrocentesis for synovial fluid analysis on initial presentation of a patient suspected of having acute gouty arthritis. Analysis confirms the diagnosis of gout by identifying needle-shaped urate crystals free in the fluid or surrounded by phagocytes. The fluid during an acute attack also contains white blood cells indicative of inflammation; infectious arthritis can be ruled out by gram stain and culture (McCarty, 2008).

Elevated serum urate level is of limited value in establishing diagnosis because approximately 30% of patients have normal values at the time of an acute gout attack (Schumacher, 2009). Serum urate may be assessed on two or three occasions in the newly diagnosed patient to establish a baseline and then to help the health care provider follow the effects of antihyperuricemic therapy.

X-rays of patients in early stages of gout may reveal intraosseus tophi that are not visible above the skin; however, films generally are not needed if diagnosis has been established by synovial fluid analysis. In chronic gout, x-rays will show "punched out" erosion of bone with overhanging bony margins. These subchondral bone lesions must be at least 5mm in diameter before becoming visible on x-ray. Lesions are not diagnostic of chronic gout, but they almost always precede appearance of tophi (McCarty, 2008).

Evaluation of renal and cardiovascular systems is essential if gout is suspected. In particular, metabolic syndrome and cardiovascular disease increase mortality in persons with gout (McCarty, 2008).

Common Therapeutic Modalities

Treatment goals for the patient with gout include termination of an acute attack, prevention of recurrent attacks, prevention of additional deposition of urate crystals and resolution of existing tophi, and treatment of co-existing conditions (e.g., hypertension, hyperlipidemia, obesity) (McCarty, 2008).

Medications. Symptomatic hyperuricemia requires medication in addition to diet and lifestyle changes. NSAIDs are effective in treating an acute attack, but they do have notable side effects. In particular, older adults are at risk for gastrointestinal upset, hyperkalemia, increased creatinine, and fluid retention when taking NSAIDs. Although indomethacin (Indocin®) often is preferred, almost any NSAID is effective in treating acute gout if prescribed in anti-inflammatory doses. Treatment should be continued for several days after resolution of pain and inflammation in order to avoid a relapse. Attack frequency can be decreased by continuing low-dose NSAID treatment (McCarty, 2008).

Colchicine, a traditional therapy for gout, can be dramatically effective if initiated shortly after onset of symptoms. Joint pain generally decreases after 12-24 hours of treatment and typically ends within a week. Doses of 0.6 mg hourly until symptoms improve are typical but not always well tolerated. Severe diarrhea occurs in up to 80% of patients following this regimen, and dose reductions may be needed. If treatment can be started very early, doses of 0.6-1.2 mg two to three times daily for 1-2 days may be effective and better tolerated. The frequency of acute attacks can be decreased by continuing this regimen, with additional medication taken at the first indication of an attack to abort any flare-up. Intravenous neumonias is much less likely to cause GI symptoms and may be indicated for postoperative patients; however, it should not be given to patients with renal or liver disease, or those already taking oral neumonias, due to risk of bone marrow suppression, shock, and death (McCarty, 2008).

Use of systemic corticosteroids for acute attacks is controversial because inflammation may continue while symptoms are masked by this treatment. They may be a useful therapy for multiple joint involvement, however, especially in the patient who cannot tolerate NSAIDs or colchicines, and should be continued until the attack fully resolves. Intra-articular injection of corticosteroids can be very effective for uncomplicated monoarticular gout (McCarty, 2008).

NSAIDs, colchicines, and corticosteroids do not delay the progressive joint damage associated with gout. Only uricosuric drugs, which decrease serum uric acid by increasing renal excretion, can prevent such damage. These drugs are preferred in persons younger than age 60 with normal renal function, no history of kidney stones, and decreased renal urate excretion. Treatment with probenecid (Benemid®) begins at 250 mg twice daily, increased to a maximum of 1 gram three times daily. Sulfinpyrazone (Anturane®) treatment begins with 50-100 mg twice daily, with increases to 100 mg four times daily. Both drugs are contraindicated in patients with renal insufficiency; their use in older adults frequently is limited due to the physiologic decline in renal function that occurs with aging (McCarty, 2008).

Allopurinol impairs conversion of xanthine to uric acid, thus inhibiting urate synthesis. It is the most commonly prescribed hypouricemic for patients with severe tophaceous deposits, history of impaired renal function, uric acid nephropathy, or nephrolithiasis. Initial treatment of 100 mg daily may be increased to 800 mg to achieve target urate levels, assuming no renal insufficiency. The most common daily dose is 300 mg, however. Prolonged treatment with appropriate doses of allopurinol often leads to resolution of even large, draining tophi, so surgical excision of tophi seldom necessary (McCarty, 2008).

Febuxostat (Uloric®), an alternative to allopurinol, is the first new drug approved for the treatment of gout in 40 years. In three randomized clinical trials, 80 mg of febuxostat was more effective in lowering serum urate to the target level than was allopurinol. The U.S. Food and Drug Administration (2009) has, however, identified a higher number of cardiovascular events in patients taking febuxostat and recommended the collection of additional data by the drug's manufacturer.

Physical Management. Fluid intake of more than 2 liters daily is recommended for all patients with gout, but especially indicated for persons who pass urate gravel or stones. Urine alkalinization with potassium citrate also can be effective for persons with persistent urate stones despite hypouricemic treatment and sufficient hydration. Co-existing hypertension and hyperlipidemia should be controlled. In addition, weight reduction, decreased alcohol ingestion, and decreased consumption of foods with high purine content are recommended (McCarty, 2008). Early research suggests some foods, including low-fat dairy products, may reduce the risk of gout in men by half. In addition, vitamin C may beneficial in the prevention and management of high uric acid (Schumacher, 2009).

Nursing Considerations

Nursing Diagnoses. Nursing diagnoses for this condition are expanded upon in the Appendix.

- Mobility: physical, impaired.
- Pain, acute.
- Skin integrity, risk for impaired.

Interventions. Heat and ice should be used appropriately to alleviate pain in the affected extremity.

Patient Teaching. The patient and family must understand dietary guidelines for appropriate food selections at home and in restaurants if restrictions are recommended. The nurse also should provide information on all gout medications, including their potential interactions with other drugs. The focus of all patient education should be on the prevention and decrease of future attacks through consistent health care.

Lyme Disease

Overview

Definition. Lyme disease (LD) is a tick-borne multisystem inflammatory disease. It often is called the "great imitator" because its symptoms can mimic those of mononucleosis, meningitis, multiple sclerosis, or other diseases.

Etiology. LD is caused by the spirochete *Borrelia burgdorferi* transmitted by a bite from an infected tick, most commonly of the *Ixodes* species (deer tick in United States, sheep tick in Europe). Person-to-person transmission does not occur.

Pathophysiology. The tick's need for a blood meal in order to molt or lay eggs leads to obligatory parasitism on mammals, reptiles, amphibians, and birds in various locales. Humans become suitable alternative hosts when participating in activities in wooded areas where ixodid ticks are prevalent. When a tick in the nymphal stage attaches to a mammalian host, spirochetes (gram-negative, motile, spiral bacteria) begin to migrate to the tick's salivary glands and are regurgitated into the host. This immature tick is more likely to bite people and is harder to notice because of its smaller size. The tick is most likely to transmit infection after feeding 36-48 hours, though the minimum time may be as little as 24 hours (Bratton, Whiteside, Hovan, Engle, & Edwards, 2008). The infective organism may travel rapidly via the blood to any area of body, with special affinity for skin, nerve tissue, synovium, and the heart's conduction system. The disease frequently appears as localized skin lesion but in its disseminated form may affect joints, cardiovascular, and nervous systems.

Early localized disease (stage 1) presents in most cases with the appearance of a typical LD bull's eye rash (*erythema migrans*). The expanding erythematous rash often occurs at the site of a tick bite (axilla, belt line) 2–30 days after exposure (most commonly 7–10 days). Up to 20% of infected patients may not exhibit the characteristic skin manifestations, however. The patient may also describe complaints similar to viral syndrome, including fever, fatigue, malaise, headache, myalgias, and arthralgias; these may precede onset of the rash by several days. Early localized disease usually is cured with 3–4 weeks of antibiotic therapy (Bratton et al., 2008).

Early disseminated disease (stage 2) is associated with hematogenous spread to other body sites within a few days to weeks after the tick bite. During this stage, multiple secondary erythema migrans lesions may occur. In addition, musculoskeletal, neurologic, and cardiac manifestations are likely. Approximately 60% of infected persons experience migratory joint or muscle pain, with or without swelling. Neurologic damage, including lymphocytic meningitis, cranial nerve palsies, and radiculoneuritis, occurs in about 15% of previously untreated persons. Without treatment, about 8% of people develop cardiac manifestations, such as temporary heart block or mild myopericarditis. Complete heart block rarely develops, although temporary pacing may be needed for about 30% of patients with cardiac symptoms (Bratton et al., 2008).

Late disease can occur months to years after initial infection. Approximately 60% of affected persons develop chronic Lyme arthritis if undiagnosed or untreated. Involved joints typically include the knees and hips. In particular, persons with the HLA-DR4 gene have a high risk of developing chronic arthritis. Late neurologic involvement also is possible, including polyneuropathy or encephalopathy. Without treatment, LD may contribute to substantial disability, but it is rarely fatal (Bratton et al., 2008).

Co-infections, which are common with LD, may complicate its diagnosis and treatment. For example, infection with the intracellular protozoan *Babesia microti* also may be transmitted by a tick bite. This infection generally increases the severity of symptoms, including high fever and chills. Babesia infection may be accompanied by mild-to-severe hemolytic anemia and a slightly decreased leukocyte count. It can progress to disseminated intravascular coagulation, heart failure, and acute respiratory distress syndrome. Careful differential diagnosis thus is critical (Meletis, Zabriskie, & Rountree, 2009).

Incidence. The disease was named after Lyme, CT, one of three sites of initial identification in the mid-1970s when groups of children were diagnosed with an unusual rash and arthritis symptoms. LD is reported most commonly in New England, the mid-Atlantic states, the Great Lakes region, and several counties in northwestern California. More than 20,000 cases are reported annually to the Centers for Disease Control (CDC). The age distribution for the disease is bimodal, with children ages 5-14 and adults ages 55-70 most frequently affected (Bratton et al., 2008).

Risk Factors. LD is the most common tick-borne illness in the United States (Kest & Pineda, 2008). Persons who participate in outdoor activities in endemic areas are at risk for tick bites and thus development of LD.

Complications. No accepted definition or diagnostic criteria have been established for the so-called *post-Lyme disease syndrome* or *chronic Lyme disease*. Many health care providers and scientists disagree on its existence as a true medical condition. The term has been applied to patients with continuing or relapsing symptoms, such as fatigue, musculoskeletal complaints, and mood or memory disturbances. These symptoms have been suggested as the result of slowly resolved inflammation in treated patients, rather than a continuing *B burgdorferi* infection, and repeated or intensive antibiotic therapy has done little to address symptoms of pain and altered cognition (Bratton et al., 2008; Walsh et al., 2007).

Preventive Strategies. Because LD is transmitted by tick bite, persons who enjoy outdoor activities should be encouraged to adopt the following preventive strategies:

a. Walk in the center of the path.

b. Tuck long pants into socks.

c. Wear white clothing to make ticks more visible.

d. Check for ticks daily, and remove attached ticks before they are likely to transmit disease.

e. Use a tick repellant (Bratton et al., 2008).

Special Considerations. Because of similarities between Lyme disease and syphilis, initially great concern existed related to possible fetal transmission in pregnancy and teratogenicity. Antepartum LD is uncommon, even in endemic areas, and there appears to be no increased risk to pregnant women who do develop the disease if they receive appropriate antibiotic therapy. In spite of reported transplacental transmission of the spirochete, a fetal immunologic response is lacking. Large-scale studies have concluded that there are no consistent data of adverse fetal effects (Walsh, Mayer, & Baxi, 2007).

Assessment

History. The patient may complain of a localized skin infection. Although he or she may have no memory or awareness of a tick bite, the patient may report activities in areas endemic for LD. The flat rash generally is found on the thorax, in body creases, or in areas where a tick experience an obstacle (hair line, panty line, sock line). The patient also may describe fever, neck stiffness, joint pain, a fluctuating headache, and malaise. Disseminated disease causes systemic complaints 1–4 months after a bite by an infected tick, requiring clinical acumen for accurate diagnosis. Disturbances of memory, mood, and sleep are possible from late neurologic involvement (Bratton et al., 2008).

Physical Exam. Only a minority of patients has the LD-associated bull's eye rash. The rash usually is asymptomatic, although the patient may state it burns, itches, or hurts. The lesion also can present with central necrosis, induration, or vesiculation. The patient who did not get a rash typically presents with symptoms of stage 2 or late disease, including swollen lymph nodes; swollen, stiff, painful joints; facial muscle paralysis (Bell's palsy); and severe headache and neck stiffness from meningitis. An abnormal heart beat also may be noted on examination (Meletis et al., 2009).

Diagnostic Tests. Routine laboratory tests have only a minor role in the diagnosis of this disease; however, history and objective physical findings can be confirmed by serologic testing. The enzyme-linked immunosorbent assay (ELISA) first is used to screen for antibodies to *B burgdorferi.* All positive or equivocal ELISA results are confirmed with a Western immunoblot assay. Sensitivity of the tests is affected by their timing, as antibodies to the spirochete may not be present in early disease and contribute to a false-negative result (Bratton et al., 2008). To optimize the predictive value of a positive finding, serologic testing should be performed only in patients who have clinical features truly suggestive of disseminated disease and are considered to be at risk. The CDC currently does not recommend other studies, including fluorescent antibody tests, high resolution microscopy, and lymphocyte transformation tests (Meletis et al., 2009).

Synovial fluid can be analyzed to exclude other causes of arthritis, and cerebrospinal fluid should be examined in cases of possible neurologic involvement. An electrocardiograph (ECG) is indicated in patients with cardiovascular symptoms.

Common Therapeutic Modalities

Antibiotic treatment is critical, typically with doxycycline hyclate (Vibramycin®) (100 mg orally twice daily) for non-pregnant adults and children older than age 8. Amoxicillin may be prescribed for 2-4 weeks for patients with early stage disease or for younger children. Late or severe disease may require ceftriaxone (Rocephin®) or pencillin G by intravenous administration. Other antibiotics, including erythromycin and tetracycline, also may be used. Pregnant women requiring treatment may receive any customary treatment but tetracycline. Treatment length varies based on the stage and severity of infection. A single dose of doxycycline (200 mg) may be given prophylactically after a tick bite in an endemic area. The drug has good penetration into the central nervous system to address neurological involvement; however, no prophylactic treatments can be recommended for tick bites in children and pregnant women. Patients with symptoms unresponsive to antibiotics may be treated with NSAIDs or corticosteroids (Bratton et al., 2008; Meletis et al., 2009).

Nursing Considerations

Nursing Diagnoses. Nursing diagnoses for this condition are expanded upon in the Appendix.

- Fatigue.
- Infection, risk for.
- Knowledge deficit.
- Pain, acute.

Interventions. Patients with carditis or any symptom more severe than mild PR prolongation should be admitted for cardiac monitoring and possible insertion of≈temporary pacemaker (Bratton et al., 2008).

Patient Teaching. Patient education must focus on disease prevention and prompt evaluation of suspicious symptoms. The nurse should be prepared to counter public sources (Internet, call-in help lines from advocacy groups) that may provide misinformation about Lyme disease. The CDC provides a thorough discussion of LD (http://www.cdc.gov/lyme/) that can be used for this purpose.

Seronegative Spondyloarthropathies

The seronegative spondyloarthropathies are an interrelated group of multi-system inflammatory disorders that affect the axial spine, asymmetric peripheral joints, and peri-articular structures in the absence of serum rheumatoid factor (RF). Inheritance of the HLA-B27 gene is associated strongly with susceptibility to all forms of spondyloarthropathy, but the gene is neither necessary nor sufficient for disease development (Altman, 2008c). Both genetic and environmental factors are likely to play a role in pathogenesis.

According to the European Spondyloarthropathy Study Group criteria (Gomariz et al., 2002), a diagnosis of spondyloarthropathy cannot be made unless the patient demonstrates one of two entry criteria: (a) inflammatory spinal pain; or (b) synovitis that is asymmetric or predominantly in the lower extremities. That will be accompanied by one or more of the following:

- Episodes of alternating buttock pain;
- Radiographic evidence of sacroiliitis;
- Positive family history;
- Psoriasis;
- Inflammatory bowel disease;
- Urethritis, cervicitis, or acute diarrhea occurring within 1 month before onset of arthritis; and
- Enthesopathy (inflammation where tendons, ligaments attach to bones).

The spondyloarthropathies share clinical, laboratory characteristics that make it difficult to distinguish among them in early stages. They include ankylosing spondylitis, reactive arthritis, and psoriatic arthritis.

Ankylosing Spondylitis

Overview

Definition. Ankylosing spondylitis (AS), the first of the seronegative spondyloarthropathies, is a chronic inflammatory disease of the axial skeleton, including sacroiliac joints, intervertebral disc spaces, and costovertebral articulations. It may be associated with extra-spinal lesions. Large peripheral joints and digits also may be affected (Altman, 2008c).

Etiology. The cause of AS is unknown. Genetic predisposition is notable, however. The genetic marker HLA-B27 occurs in 90%-95% of patients diagnosed with AS and 20%-30% of their first-degree relatives; however, it occurs in only 7%-8% of the general population. One theory suggests that HLA-B27 is the receptor for a damaging etiological factor (e.g., bacterium, virus), with the resulting complex producing cytotoxic T-lymphocytes that damage host cells (Ankylosing Spondylitis Center, 2010).

Pathophysiology. A proliferative fibroblastic response leads to the development of dense fibrous scars that tend to calcify/ossify and fuse the articular tissues. Large spurs cause complete ossification between adjacent vertebrae, creating the classic "bamboo spine" appearance on x-ray (Shamji, Bafaguy, & Tsai, 2008). Extra-articular inflammation can affect eyes, lungs, heart, peripheral nervous system, and kidneys.

Incidence. AS is estimated to affect as many as 2.4 million people in the United States, with the male-to-female ratio at 3:1. The disease is 10-20 times more common in people whose parents or siblings have it (Altman, 2008b). The highest prevalence is in some high-risk Native Americans.

AS usually manifests with the onset of chronic low back pain and stiffness during the third decade of life, although onset in adolescence also is relatively common. Disease onset and acute iritis at a younger age generally are linked to the presence of the HLA-B27 gene. It is very unusual for onset of AS to occur after age 45, although the disease may be identified later in life if early symptoms were mild or ignored (Shaikh, 2007).

Complications. Inflammation of the entheses (points of joint capsule, ligament, or tendon attachment) is a classic complication of AS. The sites of inflammation sometimes are called "hot spots," and they often are accompanied by swelling and tenderness. In particular, inflammation of the heel can affect the person's mobility; the Achilles tendon and the plantar fascia are notably involved. The body's attempts to repair the inflamed entheses can lead to scarring, which subsequently causes extra bone formation and ultimate bony fusion. Fusion of the spine can contribute to development of kyphosis, although this is less common with recent advances in AS treatment. Hip involvement can occur in younger patients and is associated with a worse prognosis. Shoulder involvement generally is mild. Patients with AS can have chest pain that mimics angina or pleurisy.

In addition to joint manifestations, inflammation of the eye (iritis) is a common complication of AS that occurs in up to 40% of affected persons. Redness, pain, sensitivity to light, and vision changes are suggestive of iritis, and should be evaluated immediately by a health care provider. Iritis generally is treated with corticosteroid eye drops and mydriatics.

Rarely, people with AS can develop cauda equina syndrome due to scarring of spinal nerves. Long-term treatment with NSAIDs can also contribute to the development of amyloidosis (deposition of amyloid proteins in organs and tissues). A small number of patients will develop chronic inflammation around the aortic valve, leading to valve leakage. They also may experience heart block. Finally, possible effects on the lungs include pulmonary fibrosis that may cause functional impairment (Spondylitis Association of America [SAA], 2009b).

Special Considerations. Variance in prevalence between the sexes occasionally leads to unnecessary delays in diagnosis for women with AS. Some women may have mild disease that is not detected as easily as in men, and the disease may progress more slowly in women than in men. AS can affect different joints in women (e.g., neck, peripheral joints), yet diagnostic criteria are based on men's presentation (e.g., low back, spine). Although there is no tendency, as with RA, for AS to remit during pregnancy, women with the disease have the same rate of miscarriage, stillbirth, and small-for-gestational-age babies as healthy women. Sacroiliac inflammation or ankylosis is not a mechanical hindrance to giving birth. Methotrexate (Rheumatrex®) should not be taken during pregnancy. Although research on effects during human pregnancy is currently reassuring, it is incomplete regarding the tumor necrosis factor (TNF) alpha inhibitors etanercept (Enbrel®), infliximab (Remicade®), and adalimumab (Humira®); therefore, these drugs should not be continued during pregnancy (SAA, 2009e)

Assessment

History. The most common complaint is of a dull ache and stiffness in the neck and back, which varies in intensity from episode to episode and person to person. Pain is often worse at night. Pain may be accompanied by loss of appetite and weight, low-grade fever, fatigue, and anemia. The patient also commonly describes early morning stiffness relieved by activity. In addition, the patient may describe eye inflammation and redness (Altman, 2008d).

Physical Exam. The health care provider will note the patient's restricted back motion with reduced extension, and lateral and forward flexion. Sacroiliac joints are tender to palpation when the patient is in a position of forward flexion. Reduced chest expansion and diaphragmatic breathing are associated with costovertebral involvement in the thoracic spine. The patient may exhibit gait changes due to pain at the plantar fascia and Achilles tendon insertions into the calcaneus (Rizzo & Gunta, 2007).

Diagnostic Tests. Diagnosis of AS is based primarily on physical findings before radiographic changes have occurred. Probable AS is diagnosed based on inflammatory back and buttock pain that is relieved by exercise and NSAIDs. In addition, MRI or CT scan will show early evidence of sacroiliitis. Radiographic appearance of juxtra-articular osteoporosis, irregular bone erosion, and sclerosis may take 7-12 years to become apparent. Later in the disease progression, the "bamboo spine" becomes evident due to calcifications that bridge from one vertebra to the next.

A test for the HLA-B27 gene is not diagnostic of AS but can increase the index of suspicion, especially among Caucasian patients. Only 50% of African-American patients with AS have the gene. Finally, no association exists between AS and rheumatoid factor (associated with RA) or antinuclear antibody (associated with system lupus erythematosus) (SAA, 2009a).

Common Therapeutic Modalities

Treatment goals include mobility maintenance, decreased inflammation, and pain management.

Medications. NSAIDs or salicylates commonly are prescribed to treat the pain and stiffness associated with AS. When NSAIDs are not enough, DMARDs such as sulfasalazine or methotrexate may be added to the treatment regimen. The most recently employed medications are the TNF alpha inhibitors, or biologics. These include etanercept, adalimumab, infliximab, and golimumab (Simponi®). Infliximab is given intravenously, but the other biologics are given by subcutaneous injection weekly, biweekly, or monthly. Patients taking these immunosuppressant drugs should be warned about their increased risk for infection and encouraged to avoid crowds or people with known contagious illness. In addition, corticosteroid eye drops may be indicated for treatment of AS-associated uveitis (SAA, 2009d).

Physical Management. Regular exercise is critical to the patient's ability to maintain normal, upright posture and spinal mobility. Daily stretching and spinal exercise are needed, with active participation in ADL to minimize spinal curvature. Hydrotherapy has been shown to decrease pain and facilitate spinal extension. Light exercise often is more comfortable for the patient than bed rest or a reclining position. Treatment by a physical therapist may be helpful, but a patient-driven treatment is more likely to be maintained. In addition, use of heat can help with stiffness, while ice can alleviate inflammation. In severe cases, surgery in the form of joint arthroplasty may be indicated. Surgical correction of spinal deformities also is possible (SAA, 2009d).

Nursing Considerations

Nursing Diagnoses. Nursing diagnoses for this condition are expanded upon in the Appendix.

- Body image, disturbed.
- Breathing pattern, ineffective.
- Falls, risk for.
- Grieving.
- Pain, chronic.

Interventions. The patient should be encouraged to sleep on the back with a pillow on a firm surface to allow any back or neck fusion to occur in a functional position. The patient also should use office furniture and equipment that reduce spinal flexion, such as a tilting artist's table rather than conventional desk, and maintain correct placement of the computer work station.

Patient Teaching. The patient should be encouraged to continue prescribed exercises at home. Except in severe disease, the patient should be urged to continue normal activities. In particular, the nurse should instruct the patient to seek immediate ophthalmologic examination if painful red eye develops to diagnose/exclude anterior uveitis.

Reactive Arthritis

Overview

Definition. Reactive arthritis (ReA), another seronegative spondyloarthropathy, is a self-limiting form of peripheral arthritis that often appears shortly after certain infections of the genitourinary (GU) or gastrointestinal (GI) tracts. A symptom complex of urethritis or cervicitis, conjunctivitis, and asymmetric arthritis is considered classic, but less than one third of diagnosed cases shows all three clinical signs.

Etiology. Acute inflammation occurs within 1 month after infection of the GI or GU tract in genetically predisposed persons. Presence of the HLA-B27 gene correlates with the severity and chronicity of ReA (Bykirk, 2006).

Pathophysiology. The primary microbial trigger is *Chlamydia trachomatis* GU infection. Other triggers include the enteric pathogens *Salmonella, Yersinia, Shigella,* and *Campylobacter* (Bykirk, 2006). In addition, some evidence suggests respiratory infection with *Chlamydia neumonia* may trigger ReA. It is unclear if the HLA-B27 gene is linked to the pathogenesis of ReA or if it is an immune response-linked gene (NIAMS, 2009a).

Incidence. Men ages 20-40 are most likely to develop ReA. Men are 9 times more likely than women to develop ReA as a result of a sexually acquired infection, but men and women are equally likely to develop the disease as a result of a food-borne GI infection. Almost all cases in elders and children develop after enteric infection. Caucasians are affected more commonly than African Americans and other racial groups with a lower frequency of HLA-B27 (NIAMS, 2009a).

Risk Factors. Unprotected sexual intercourse places the patient at risk for infection that may trigger ReA. Improper food handling, storage, and preparation also place a person at risk for ReA.

Complications. Approximately 20% of ReA patients develop chronic arthritis, though the condition is often mild. A few patients will have severe arthritis that is difficult to control and can cause permanent joint damage. Long-term disability usually is related to chronic foot or heel pain, or vision loss (NIAMS, 2009a). An estimated 15%-50% of patients redevelop symptoms after the initial flare has ended; these relapses may be caused by re-infection. Arthritis and back pain are the most common returning symptoms, but urogenital and eye inflammation also can recur (Mayo Clinic, 2009d).

Preventive Strategies. While food-borne infection may be more difficult to anticipate, risk of transmission can be decreased by carefully washing and thoroughly cooking all foods. Meals away from home should be taken from restaurants with established safety ratings for proper food handling and preparation. In addition, risk of transmission also can be decreased by avoiding unprotected sexual activity.

Assessment

History. With prompting, the patient may describe a history of infection. An episode of dysentery or bacterial gastroenteritis may have been forgotten. A sexually transmitted disease (STD) may not be admitted or discussed readily, but questioning about sexual contacts is essential to appropriate diagnosis. The patient may complain of painful urination, urinary urgency, and possibly blood in the urine. A male may describe penile discharge, edema/erythema at urinary meatus, and painless ulcers on the glans penis. In addition, the patient may describe joint stiffness, muscle aches, and low back pain, as well as chest wall pain from inflamed tendons in the sternum and vertebral attachments. Complaints of eye redness, discomfort, and tearing are not uncommon, and skin lesions similar to those of psoriasis may have appeared (Mayo Clinic, 2009d).

Physical Exam. Examination will reveal asymmetric polyarticular joint involvement with or without edema and effusions. The lower extremities (especially the knees, ankles, and small joints of the feet) are affected more commonly than the upper extremities, with one third of patients having exclusively lower extremity arthritis. Muscle wasting near the affected joints is possible, and gait changes may be noted due to the pain of enthesitis.

Evidence of urethritis includes edema and erythema at the urinary meatus, with muculopurulent drainage likely. Keratoderma blennorhagicum lesions, that present as a scaly rash, may be noted on the soles of the feet and other body surfaces, and may evolve into exfoliative dermatitis. The patient may also have red, irritated eyes (Mayo Clinic, 2009d).

Diagnostic Tests. The greatest problem comes in differentiating ReA from the other two spondyloarthropathies. Diagnosis is based largely on clinical signs and symptoms, and a history of infection. Laboratory testing, especially for *Chlamydia*, can confirm the presence of an STD. Similarly, a stool culture showing the presence of bacteria prior to the development of arthritis can aid in diagnosis. Other laboratory findings are common but not diagnostic. These include anemia and mild thrombocytosis, elevated ESR and CRP, and leukocytosis (during the acute phase of ReA). Urinalysis may reveal pyuria and hematuria. Synovial fluid analysis likely would reveal increased leukocytes and other inflammatory changes, such as turbidity, poor viscosity, and poor mucin clot tests. It is debatable if HLA-B27 screening is worthwhile because it is more likely to be found in patients with chronic or relapsing disease (Bykirk, 2006).

Common Therapeutic Modalities

No treatment regimen has been shown to have a lasting effect on the disease course. Treatment must include patient education and symptom management.

Medications. Although antibiotics are used to treat confirmed infection, they have no effect on arthritis or other symptoms. Joint discomfort initially is treated with NSAIDs, though response is usually incomplete. Local corticosteroid injections may be indicated for severe pain and inflammation in a specific joint. DMARDs (e.g., methotrexate, sulfasalazine) also may be indicated in more severe cases. Topical creams may be prescribed to treat skin lesions, and corticosteroid eye drops or subconjunctival preparations may be needed for eye symptoms (SAA, 2009c).

Physical Management. Splinting is recommended for joint protection. In addition, a managed exercise program is indicated for joint mobility and maintenance of muscle strength. Orthotics may prevent foot contracture and decrease deformity. Knee surgery may be indicated for persistent effusion or popliteal cysts (SAA, 2009c)

Nursing Considerations

Nursing Diagnoses. Nursing diagnoses for this condition are expanded upon in the Appendix.

- Comfort, impaired.
- Health behavior, risk-prone.
- Health maintenance, ineffective.
- Knowledge deficit.

Interventions. Principles of energy conservation and joint protection must be employed, including use of assistive devices as needed. Home exercise also is important for maintenance of joint mobility and muscle strength.

Patient Teaching. The nurse should instruct the patient on the safe use of all medications, including avoidance of alcohol if taking methotrexate. Safe sexual practices also must be discussed. Condom use will help protect the patient from postvenereal exacerbation and re-infection. The patient also should be advised to avoid multiple sexual partners.

Psoriatic Arthritis

Overview

Definition. Psoriatric arthritis (PsA), the third seronegative spondyloarthropathy, is an inflammatory arthritis associated with psoriasis, a common skin disorder.

Etiology. The cause of PsA is unknown, but a combination of immunologic, genetic, and environmental factors is believed to influence disease susceptibility and expression. For example, multiple HLA class I alleles have been related to psoriasis with or without arthritis. A 70% concordance for psoriasis exists in monozygotic twins. In addition, persons with a first-degree relative affected by PsA have a 50-fold increased risk of developing the disease. Environmental factors, such as streptococcal or HIV infection, may be important in disease development. Physical trauma also has been implicated in disease development. The inflammatory and autoimmune nature of PsA is supported by the role of T-cells and various cytokines in its development and perpetuation (Martin, 2010).

Pathophysiology. The scaling of psoriasis occurs when cells in the skin's outer layer reproduce faster than normal, piling up on the skin surface as plaques. Common sites of plaque deposition are the knees, elbows, and trunk. Lesions also may be seen in the scalp or at the hairline, and in the umbilical area. The skin disease precedes joint disease in 85% of patients; however, the extent, pattern, and severity of arthritis generally do not correlate with the extent of skin lesions (National Psoriasis Foundation [NPF], 2010).

Incidence. About 2% of Caucasians in North America have psoriasis. Of those, 5%-7% are affected by some form of arthritis. The incidence is as low as 0.3% in African Americans, Latin American Indians, and persons of Chinese descent. PsA affects men and women equally. Peak incidence is in the fourth through sixth decades (Martin, 2010).

Complications. PsA now is recognized as a progressive and destructive disease, capable of causing significant disability. Considerable social and economic distress is possible due to double disfigurement from psoriasis and arthritis. Factors suggesting a worse prognosis include extensive skin involvement; a strong family history of psoriasis; female sex; disease onset younger than age 20; expression of HLA-B27, -DR3, or -DR4 alleles; and the presence of polyarticular or erosive disease (Martin, 2010).

PsA is accompanied by a high prevalence of joint damage and associated loss of motion. Joint laxity may limit movements needed for the patient's performance of ADL, and ankylosis in the proximal joints (wrists, MCP) can lead to disability. Swollen toes can make it difficult to find shoes that fit properly. Enthesopathy (a disorder of the muscular or tendinous attachment to bone) can cause debilitating foot pain, especially at the Achilles tendon and in the plantar fascia. In addition, spondylitis can occur as a complication of PsA (Mayo Clinic, 2008). Arthritis mutilans, which occurs in 5% of cases, is marked by resorption of the phalangeal bones (Martin, 2010).

Assessment

History. The patient typically has a history of nail changes (pitting, with appearance of fungal infection) and the development of pruritic silver scales on patches of bright red skin. A family history of psoriasis or PsA may be reported. Digits have become swollen and painful, and the patient may describe low-grade back pain with loss of motion and stiffness. The patient also may complain of eye redness and pain (NPF, 2010).

Physical Exam. Asymmetric swelling ("sausage digit") and erythema are noted in small peripheral joints. A tendency exists for "ray" involvement, with inflammation of several joints in one digit. Back pain and loss of motion suggest sacroiliitis. Gait changes also indicate inflammation at areas of tendon or ligament insertion (enthesopathy). The patient is likely to have scaly skin lesions on the knees, elbow, trunk, and scalp, as well as pitted, ridged and partially discolored nails. (NPF, 2010).

Diagnostic Tests. Most rheumatologists agree that diagnosis cannot be made without evidence of skin and nail changes. PsA should be considered in any patient who presents with psoriasis and inflammatory arthritis. Diagnosis is relatively simple if the patient is RF-negative, as is typical. If RF is present as a significant titer, however, it is likely that the patient has coincident psoriasis and RA. Because hyperuricemia may be noted in psoriasis due to rapid cell turnover, gout also must be considered in a differential diagnosis. Laboratory markers of inflammation such as ESR are not diagnostic but may help monitor the disease. On radiograph, PsA shows both bone destruction and proliferation. Erosive arthritis causes the classic "pencil-in-cup" phalangeal deformity with osteolysis and articular ankylosis. Evidence of sacroiliitis also is present with spinal involvement (Martin, 2010).

Common Therapeutic Modalities

Goals of care include symptom relief, disease suppression, and rehabilitation. Treatment remains suppressive rather than curative.

Medications. Treatment generally begins with NSAIDs to address pain and inflammation associated with PsA; however, patients with aggressive or potentially destructive disease need early treatment with DMARDs or biologics. Given its efficacy and tolerability, methotrexate often is the first choice. It is an effective treatment both for the cutaneous and the peripheral articular manifestations of psoriasis. Sulfasalazine may benefit arthritic symptoms but has no effect on cutaneous disease. Cyclosporine is effective for both cutaneous and articular disease, but caution must be used because approximately 20% of treated patients develop hypertension and 17% nephrotoxicity. The biologics etanercept, infliximab, and adalimumab are prescribed often, as they generally are effective and well tolerated in treatment of both psoriasis and PsA. Intra-articular and low-dose oral corticosteroids may be used as a bridging therapy when a DMARD or biologic is instituted, but long-term use is not indicated. Finally, antimalarial drugs, retinoic acid derivatives, or psoralen with UV-A light may provide benefit to varying degrees (Martin, 2010).

Synovectomy and joint arthroplasty may be indicated as in any chronic inflammatory arthritis.

Medical Management. Physical and occupational therapy often are needed to protect involved joints and maintain function. Orthoses may be indicated. Because of the effects of PsA on the small joints of the hands, the patient may need vocational retraining (Martin, 2010).

Nursing Considerations

Nursing Diagnoses. Nursing diagnoses for this condition are expanded upon in the Appendix.

- Pain, chronic.
- Sleep pattern, disturbed.
- Self-care deficit: bathing/hygiene, dressing/grooming, feeding, toileting.
- Infection, risk for.

Interventions. The patient with psoriasis and PsA may experience helplessness and frustration in trying to cope with effects of these diseases. Engaging the patient's partnership is essential to continued participation in therapeutic regimen. Significant image disturbance may result, requiring emotional support from caregivers.

Patient Teaching. A balance of rest and activity is recommended. Education must be provided concerning key treatment strategies for both cutaneous and arthritic manifestations.

Systemic Sclerosis

Overview

Definition. Systemic sclerosis (SS) is a multi-system disease affecting the microvasculature and connective tissue, causing alterations in the skin and in a variety of internal organs. Painful symmetric arthropathy also may develop. SS also is called scleroderma due to the presence of skin induration.

Etiology. The cause of SS is unknown. Both immunologic derangements and vascular abnormalities are believed to play a role in the development of fibrosis. Some cases are linked to chemical exposure, such as silica dust, organic solvents, or urea formaldehyde. SS-like conditions can result from genetic factors (phenylketonuria), metabolic disorders (Hashimoto's thyroiditis), malignancies, post-infection disorders, and neurologic conditions (International Scleroderma Network, 2010).

Pathophysiology. General consensus holds that vasculopathy and fibrosis are secondary to abnormal activation of the immune system. Responding to unknown antigens, activated T cells accumulate in skin and release cytokines, attracting inflammatory cells such as mast cells and macrophages. The accumulated T cells and inflammatory cells release mediators that interact, leading to fibroblast activation and growth, and stimulating the complex development of fibrosis. Vascular mechanisms involved in this process include endothelial cell injury, vasoconstriction, vascular occlusion, and tissue hypoxia. These are potential targets for drug therapy to treat SS (Moore & DeSantis, 2008).

Two major types of SS are described, based on the degree of systemic involvement. The first type, *localized scleroderma*, is the more common form of the disease. Skin changes usually are confined to the face, fingers, and distal extremities without truncal involvement. This form of the disease is not marked by internal organ involvement (Chatterjee, 2009). It often is accompanied by CREST syndrome (Hajj-Ali, 2008b):

- **C**alcinosis: calcium deposits on fingers, forearms, other pressure points; painful ulcers may occur in areas of calcinosis;
- **R**aynaud's phenomenon: intermittent vasospasm of fingertips; often present 1-10 years before other signs of disease become evident;
- **E**sophageal dysmotility;
- **S**clerodactyly: scleroderma of digits; and
- **T**elangiectasias: capillary dilations leading to lesions on face, mucous membranes, hands.

The second type is *diffuse systemic sclerosis*. Inflammatory signs in the early stages of diffuse systemic sclerosis include edematous skin, painful joints/muscles, and occasional tendon friction rubs. Skin changes are rapidly progressive during the first months of the disease. They continue approximately 2-3 years before skin tends to soften, either thinning or returning to normal texture. Severe fibrosis of the skin causes irreversible atrophic changes and tethering to deeper tissues. Diffuse disease also is associated with internal organ involvement (Chatterjee, 2009).

Incidence. SS is a chronic disorder that occurs in only about 20 adults per 1 million in the United States (Chatterjee, 2009). It is rare in children, with peak occurrence in the third to fifth decades of life. Incidence in women is 4 times more common than in men (Hajj-Ali, 2008b). Ethnicity influences survival and disease manifestation: persons who are African American, Native American, and of Japanese descent are at particular risk.

Risk Factors. Because some cases of SS may be caused by chemicals, the person who works with or around possible causative substances, such as silica dust, organic solvents, or urea formaldehyde, should utilize appropriate strategies to minimize exposure (International Scleroderma Network, 2010).

Complications. The 10-year cumulative survival rate is about 80% for patients with disease onset before age 40, and 58% for those who developed SS at age 40 or older (Moore & DeSantis, 2008). Pulmonary fibrosis, pulmonary arterial hypertension, severe gastrointestinal involvement, and scleroderma heart disease are the main causes of death (Chatterjee, 2009). Keeping the disease controlled with pharmacologic treatment helps to decrease the patient's need for hospitalization (Moore & DeSantis, 2008).

Skin fibrosis and flexion contractures can lead to loss of hand grasp ability, contributing to marked functional disability. Trophic ulcers are common, especially at the fingertips and over finger joints. Skin fibrosis also contributes to an inability to open the mouth, creating difficulty with adequate food consumption (Hajj-Ali, 2008b).

Raynaud's phenomenon is a common complication of endothelial damage. It is characterized by temporary vasoconstriction of the small vessels in the fingers, toes, tips of the nose, and earlobes. The resulting temporary ischemia causes pallor or cyanosis, and contributes to numbness and coldness in these peripheral structures. With rewarming, the areas appear red and the patient will note that they are painful and tingling. More than 90% of patients with SS develop Raynaud's phenomenon (Moore & DeSantis, 2008).

Esophageal dysfunction occurs in most patients with SS, generally beginning with dysphagia. Acid reflux can cause esophageal stricture. Bowel hypermotility causes overgrowth of anaerobic bacteria that contributes to malabsorption syndrome. The damaged bowel wall can allow leakage into the abdominal cavity, contributing to development of peritonitis. Air in the damaged bowel wall (pneumotosis intestinalis) often is visible on x-ray. In addition, unique wide-mouthed diverticula may be noted in the colon. Patients with CREST syndrome also may experience biliary cirrhosis (Hajj-Ali, 2008b).

Lung involvement is not rapidly progressive, but it is a common cause of death in patients with SS. Fibrosis caused by SS can impair gas exchange, contributing to exertional dyspnea and restrictive airway disease with eventual respiratory failure. Both pulmonary hypertension and heart failure can develop, and indicate a poor prognosis. In addition, esophageal dysfunction can lead to aspiration pneumonia. Renal involvement often is severe and sudden, typically occurring in the first 4-5 years of diffuse disease progression. It generally is preceded by sudden, severe hypertension. Dialysis and transplantation may become necessary if the patient does not respond to other treatments (Hajj-Ali, 2008b).

Assessment

History. The patient typically describes nonspecific arthralgias and myalgias. He or she may describe a history of esophageal reflux or persistent heartburn, and possible diarrhea or constipation. The patient likely discusses changes in the texture, color, consistency, and moisture of the skin. In addition, the patient notes blanching, cyanosis, and erythema in the fingertips. Fatigue and shortness of breath are not uncommon (Hajj-Ali, 2008b).

Physical Exam. The health care provider notes the patient's edematous hands with thickened or hardened skin, generally accompanied by loss of skin folds or wrinkles (sclerodactyly). In addition, edema and tightening of skin over the forearms, face, legs, and trunk may be apparent. Calcific nodules and dilated capillary loops (telangiectasias) may be observed in the fingers, palms, fingernails, and lips. Complaint of pain and stiffness over the joints generally is out of proportion with objective signs of inflammation. Cardiac assessment may reveal rhythm changes and hypertension, as well as signs of heart failure late in the disease course. The patient displays decreased thoracic excursion. Pulmonary hypertension should be suspected in the patient who is dyspneic at rest (Hajj-Ali, 2008; Siebold & Korn, 2002).

Diagnostic Tests. SS should be considered in patients with Raynaud's syndrome, musculoskeletal or skin manifestations, unexplained dysphagia or malabsorption, pulmonary fibrosis, pulmonary hypertension, or cardiomyopathies. Diagnosis can be obvious in some patients but cannot be made in others based on clinical presentation. In that case, laboratory testing can be performed to increase suspicion of the disease; however, results do not confirm the diagnosis of SS (Hajj-Ali, 2008b). Diagnostic criteria have been proposed by the American College of Rheumatology (see Table 13.4), but limitations in their applicability have led many experts to recommend modifications (Chatterjee, 2009).

Table 13.4. American College of Rheumatology Diagnostic Criteria for Systemic Sclerosis
Major Criterion
■ Sclerdermatous skin changes proximal to MCP joints
Minor Criteria
■ The patient should meet the major criterion OR two or three of the minor criteria:
■ Sclerodactyly
■ Pitting scars to fingertips OR loss of substance of distal finger pads
■ Bibasilar pulmonary fibrosis

From "Preliminary Criteria for the Classification of Systemic Sclerosis (Scleroderma)" by the Subcommittee for Scleroderma Criteria of the American Rheumatism Association Diagnostic and Therapeutic Criteria Committee, 1980, Arthritis & Rheumatism, *23, 581-590.*

All patients suspected of having SS should receive a complete blood count, complete metabolic panel, muscle enzymes, thyroid function test, and urinalysis. A slightly elevated ESR is common, but other results are largely normal. Serologic studies can help predict clinical features and patient survival, but they are not sensitive enough to exclude the disease independently. About 60%-80% of people with localized SS have anticentromere antibodies (associated with CREST syndrome), which occur only rarely in persons with diffuse disease. Antibodies to topoisomerase-1 are present in about 30% of persons with disseminated disease. The presence of either type of antibody is highly specific for diagnosis; it also is highly specific for patients presenting with isolated occurrence of Raynaud's syndrome and thus may be helpful when the syndrome is the initial manifestation of SS (Chatterjee, 2009).

Once the diagnosis is made, the health care provider can identify localized or diffuse disease based on the extent of skin tightening. The modified Rodnan skin score is used widely to assess degree of involvement. A score is derived for each of these skin areas: fingers, hands, forearms, arms, feet, legs, thighs (in pairs), face, chest, and abdomen. The assigned score is 0 for uninvolved skin, 1 for mild thickening, 2 for moderate thickening, and 3 for severe thickening, with a maximum possible score of 51. The score tends to correlate with the extent of dermal fibrosis, which in turn correlates with the extent of organ involvement. With diffuse disease, the score tends to rise rapidly and plateau in the first 3-5 years. The score in localized SS does not progress quickly and is never as high as in diffuse SS (Chatterjee, 2009).

Common Therapeutic Modalities

Medications. No medication substantially alters the course of SS, but pharmacologic treatment can be initiated to address symptoms and dysfunctional organs. NSAIDs can be used to address arthritis symptoms. Corticosteroids may be helpful for overt myositis or mixed connective tissue disease, but their use may predispose the patient to renal crisis. The DMARD D-penicillamine, long used for treatment of skin thickening, has not proven efficacious in recent trials. Immunosuppressants, such as methotrexate, azathioprine, and cyclophosphamide (Cytoxan®), may alleviate pulmonary alveolitis (Hajj-Ali, 2008b). Calcium channel blockers manage pulmonary artery hypertension in 10%-20% of patients; their low cost makes them a logical first-line treatment. Continuous ambulatory intravenous epoprostenol (Flolan®) and treprostenil (Remodulin®), as well as oral bosentan (Tracleer®), also have been approved for treatment of this complication (Seibold & Korn, 2002).

Symptoms of Raynaud's syndrome also may be helped with administration of a calcium channel blocker such as nifedipine (Procardia®) or an angiotensin receptor blocker such as losartan (Cozaar®). In addition to small, frequent feedings, reflux can be addressed with a high-dose proton pump inhibitor. Tetracycline or another broad-spectrum antibiotic can be prescribed for suppressive overgrowth of intestinal flora and alleviate symptoms of malabsorption. For acute renal crisis, prompt treatment with an angiotensin-converting enzyme inhibitor can improve the patient's likelihood of survival (Hajj-Ali, 2008b).

Physical Management. Physical therapy should be initiated early and aggressively in the patient with rapidly progressing diffuse disease and joint contractures. In addition, regular exercise (e.g., mouth excursion) helps improve the patient's overall well-being, as well as keep joints flexible and improve circulation. Rest is appropriate for brief periods of time for the patient with severe myositis or prominent synovitis. Skin protection is critical, especially for symptoms of Raynaud's syndrome and for dry, thick patches of skin from localized SS. The patient should use creams or lotions developed for persons with very dry skin, and should keep the air moist in the home through use of a humidifier. In colder months, the patient should dress appropriately by wearing hat, gloves, and scarf to protect superficial blood vessels. The patient should be encouraged to wear multiple thin layers of clothing, as well as loose-fitting boots or shoes to allow adequate circulation to the feet (Chatterjee, 2009).

Complementary and Alternative Therapies. Because of the difficulty in treating SS, many patients may be tempted to try high-dose supplements or other alternative treatments. Para-aminobenzoic acid, vitamin E, evening primrose oil, an avocado/soybean extract have been evaluated for treatment of SS but have not been demonstrated to be effective. The health care provider should caution the patient with SS about the potential danger of using herbal products and dietary supplements, especially in lieu of allopathic treatments (Simon, 2009). In addition, temperature biofeedback and relaxation remain controversial as potential treatments for Raynaud's syndrome associated with SS (Scleroderma Foundation, n.d.).

Nursing Considerations

Nursing Diagnoses. Nursing diagnoses for this condition are expanded upon in the Appendix.

- Breathing pattern, ineffective.
- Infection, risk for.
- Nutrition: imbalanced, less than body requirements.
- Skin integrity, risk for impaired.
- Swallowing, impaired.

Interventions. Treatment involves shared management of SS as a chronic disease. Ergonomic work interventions may be needed due to the peak incidence of SS during a patient's work life. Nutritional goals should be developed to maintain the patient's weight and minimize elimination problems. Ideal diets include high-calorie, high-fiber, easy-to-swallow foods that do not aggravate existing stomach problems. Eating frequent, small meals may improve digestion and decrease the risk for or symptoms of reflux. For the patient with co-existing Sjögren's syndrome (autoimmune condition marked by dryness of the eyes and mouth), proper dental care is essential because of the risk of dental caries (Chatterjee, 2009).

Patient Teaching. General education is needed regarding the nature, course, and treatment of the disease. In addition to practicing skin protection and exercise, the patient should stop smoking to decrease the risk for vasoconstriction.

Polymyositis and Dermatomyositis

Overview

Definition. Polymyositis (PM) is an inflammatory myopathy of symmetric proximal skeletal muscles. Dermatomyositis (DM) is an inflammatory myopathy of skeletal muscle accompanied by distinctive skin inflammation.

Etiology. The cause of these disorders is unknown, although viruses or autoimmune reactions may play a role. Cancer has been suggested as a possible trigger, with an immune reaction against the cancer cells directed at a substance in the muscle (Hajj-Ali, 2008a).

The response of affected patients to immunosuppressive medications also suggests an autoimmune origin (Diamond, 2008).

Pathophysiology. Pathologic changes in both PM and DM lead to varying degrees of inflammation that cause cellular damage and atrophy. Rhabdomyolysis, the breakdown of muscle fibers resulting in the release of muscle fiber contents (myoglobin) into the bloodstream, is common and can damage kidneys. With DM, immune complexes are deposited in the vessels to generate a complement-mediated vasculopathy (Hajj-Ali, 2008a).

Incidence. PM and DM most often occur in children ages 5-15 and adults ages 40-60. Women are twice as likely as men to develop these conditions. In adults, PM and DM can occur alone or as part of another connective tissue disorder (Hajj-Ali, 2008a). DM is the most common childhood myositis. Figures regarding incidence of the diseases vary widely from study to study because of discrepancies in classification criteria. General estimates are 0.5-8.4 cases per million (Diamond, 2008).

Complications. Up to 50% of persons experience a long remission within 5 years of treatment for PM or DM; however, the disorder may return at any time. Approximately 75% survive at least 5 years after diagnosis (Hajj-Ali, 2008a).

Continued difficulty in swallowing can lead to weight loss and malnutrition, as well as increase the risk for aspiration pneumonia. Weakness of chest wall muscles can contribute to shortness of breath and even respiratory failure. Myocarditis, heart arrhythmias, and heart failure also can occur as a complication of PM and DM. Late in disease progression, calcium deposits can occur in soft tissue (calcinosis) and develop eschar (Mayo Clinic, 2009b).

Pulmonary involvement has been recognized as a major complication of PM and DM, and the cause of increased morbidity and mortality. Aspiration pneumonia, hypoventilation, and interstitial lung disease are frequent complications of myositis. All patients with PM or DM should be evaluated routinely with a chest x-ray, CT scan, and pulmonary function tests (Fathi, Lundberg, & Tornling, 2007).

Special Considerations. Pregnancy can worsen symptoms of active PM or DM. In addition, active PM can increase the risk of premature or stillbirth. Risk is decreased if the disease is in remission (Mayo Clinic, 2009b).

Assessment

History. The patient may describe symptoms of symmetrical muscle weakness, especially in the upper arms, hips, and thighs, often occurring after an infection. Complaints of joint pain are likely, but the patient will not often describe co-existing muscle pain. Increasing fatigue, difficulty swallowing with possible regurgitation of food, and weight loss often occur over several months. A patient suspected of DM will identify all the symptoms of PM, as well as nail or skin changes, including distinctive rashes. Occasionally, the patient describes shortness of breath due to effects on the heart and lungs (Hajj-Ali, 2008a).

Physical Exam. Symptoms of PM are similar in patients of all ages, although they develop much more abruptly in children than in adults. The patient demonstrates difficulty lifting the arms above the shoulders, climbing stairs, or getting out of chairs. If the neck muscles are affected, the patient may have trouble even raising the head from a pillow. No muscle effects typically are noted in the hands, feet, or face. Joint aches and inflammation affect about 30% of patients, but pain and swelling tend to be mild. Poor chest expansion, dyspnea, and crackles on auscultation are likely if pulmonary fibrosis has developed (Hajj-Ali, 2008a).

Characteristic skin changes of DM include a shadowy red or purple rash (heliotrope rash) on the face, with discolored edema around the eyes. An additional scaly, smooth, or raised rash often is found on the knuckles and sides of the hands but may appear elsewhere on the body. Nail beds may be red. When the rashes fade, the skin may show residual brownish discoloration or pale, depigmented patches with scarring or shriveling (Hajj-Ali, 2008a).

Diagnostic Tests. Laboratory tests are helpful but not diagnostic of PM or DM. Increased muscle enzymes, especially creatine kinase, reflect muscle damage. With serial muscle enzyme measurement, levels will fall to normal or near normal with treatment. In addition, abnormalities in muscle electrical activity may be seen on electromyography (Hajj-Ali, 2008a).

Biopsy is the gold standard for diagnosis, which is confirmed after excluding other neuromuscular diseases. Findings in DM classically include endothelial hyperplasia with fibrin thrombi in the intramuscular vessels. In PM, infiltrating CD8 T cells gather with activated macrophages around healthy-appearing muscle fibers (Diamond, 2008). MRI can be used both to identify areas of inflammation and guide the health care provider in biopsy site selection (Hajj-Ali, 2008a).

Common Therapeutic Modalities

Medications. High-dose oral corticosteroids generally are the first line of treatment in a single morning dose of 80-100 mg for 3-4 weeks. Based on the impact of treatment on muscle strength, this will be tapered slowly until the lowest possible dose associated with symptom control is achieved. Most patients respond to corticosteroids. For those who do not, however, a steroid-sparing medication may be indicated. Options include methotrexate, azathioprine, cyclophosphamide, cyclosporine, tacrolimus (Prograf®), or rituximab (Ritusan®) (Gondim, 2010). If medications are ineffective, IV immunoglobulin (IV Ig) may be given (Hajj-Ali, 2008a). Topical immunosuppressants largely have been ineffective in treating the rash of DM (Stringer & Feldman, 2006).

Medical Management. The primary goal of treatment is to improve muscle strength and function in ADL; however, an effective treatment regimen for PM is uncertain due to the lack of large-scale, randomized controlled trials. Modest activity restriction can be beneficial during the initial period of intense inflammation. Muscle strengthening exercises then may be helpful in decreasing serum creatinine kinase (Gondim, 2010).

Nursing Considerations

Nursing Diagnoses. Nursing diagnoses for this condition are expanded upon in the Appendix.

- Family coping, compromised.
- Infection, risk for.
- Injury, risk for.
- Tissue perfusion: cardiac, risk for decreased.
- Swallowing, impaired.

Interventions. The patient will need to return for frequent monitoring of creatine kinase because elevations can indicate poor response to treatment or overuse of muscles. With corticosteroid use, the patient also should be made aware of the increased risk of developing diabetes mellitus, osteoporosis, or avascular necrosis.

Patient Teaching. Patient education should focus on safety, including use of assistive devices and fall prevention strategies. Aspiration precautions also are indicated. The patient should be urged to rest before meals, maintain an upright posture while eating, and select a diet of easily swallowed foods. Education also will be needed regarding corticosteroid or immunosuppressant use. For example, the patient should be urged to report signs of infection, such as low-grade fever, chills, or joint pain, immediately to the health care provider. He or she also should be instructed to never change the cortisteroid dose or discontinue therapy suddenly.

Systemic Lupus Erythematosus

Overview

Definition. Systemic lupus erythematosus (SLE), also known as lupus, is a multi-system inflammatory connective tissue disorder characterized by the production of autoantibodies to the cell nucleus. It occurs in subsets known as discoid lupus erythematosus, subacute cutaneous lupus erythematosus, antiphospholipid syndrome, neonatal lupus syndrome, and drug-induced lupus.

Etiology. Several likely possibilities exist to explain the etiology of SLE. First, lupus is believed to be a disease of immune system dysfunction. Signs and symptoms of the disease can be attributed directly to damage caused by autoantibodies, the deposit of immune complexes, or cell-mediated immune responses. Considerable evidence also suggests that genetics play a role in the development of SLE. For example, occurrence is higher among identical twins than among nonidentical twins or other siblings. Finally, scientists suspect that environmental triggers are implicated in disease development. These include sunlight, stress, exposure to some chemicals and toxins, and infectious organisms such as viruses (NIAMS, 2006).

Pathophysiology. Essentially all persons with SLE have autoantibodies. The antinuclear antibodies (ANA) in particular are present in patients with lupus and target elements in cell nuclei (nucleic acids, proteins, ribonucleoprotein complexes) (NIAMS, 2006). Other antibodies often found in SLE include the anti-Smith (anti-Sm) antibodies, anti-double-stranded DNA (anti-dsDNA) antibodies, and antiphospholipid antibodies. Anti-Ro antibodies will be found in persons with a lupus rash that is very sensitive to the sun (Lupus Foundation, 2010d). Antigen-antibody complexes penetrate the basement membrane of capillaries to affect the kidneys, heart, skin, brain, and joints. These complexes trigger the inflammatory response that leads to tissue destruction.

Studies also suggest that a number of different genes are involved in the development of SLE. These include HLA-DR3, HLA-DR2, and other HLA alleles, as well as genes that control immune complex deposition and programmed cell death (NIAMS, 2006).

Incidence. Approximately 250,000 persons in the United States have lupus (Bartels & Muller, 2010). Certain ethnic groups have a greater risk of developing SLE. These include people of African, Asian, Hispanic, Native American, and Hawaiian/Pacific Island descent. The disease occurs in all age groups but peaks at ages 15-40. Women are affected far more than men (female: male ratio 6-10:1), and the correlation between age and incidence reflects peak years of female sex hormone production (Bartels & Muller, 2010; Centers for Disease Control [CDC], 2010).

Complications. Renal failure is a leading cause of death among patients with SLE. Approximately 75% of persons with lupus develop kidney damage, usually within the first 2 years after diagnosis; however, most lupus-related kidney problems can be treated effectively with medications (Mayo Clinic, 2009a).

Corticosteroids can be prescribed to decrease swelling and inflammation. Other immunosuppresants used for lupus nephritis include cyclophosphamide and retuximab (National Kidney and Urologic Diseases Clearinghouse, 2007).

Myocarditis, endocarditis, pericarditis, and coronary vasculitis are possible expressions of lupus-mediated cardiac damage. Nearly 40% of persons with SLE develop premature atherosclerosis, compared to 15% of same-age peers without the disease. Managing hypertension and hypercholesterolemia are essential for the patient with lupus. Key strategies include smoking cessation and weight management. Lupus also is linked to development of anemia and venous thromboembolism. Vasculitis is responsible for 7% of lupus-related deaths (Mayo Clinic, 2009a).

SLE is linked to increased incidence of pleurisy and pneumonia. In addition, the occurrence of pulmonary hypertension, while occurring less frequently in persons with lupus than in those with systemic sclerosis, is likely to be under-recognized in lupus. Potential causes of death in the patient with lupus include thromboembolic disease, pulmonary vasculitis, and hypoxia and fibrosis from interstitial lung disease. Pulmonary artery hypertension (PAH) has been identified in some studies as a major cause of death in patients with lupus. Standard treatment for PAH can be used along with immunosuppressant medications (Pope, 2008).

Gastrointestinal problems related to SLE range from mild anorexia to life-threatening bowel perforation secondary to mesenteric arteritis. In particular, anorexia, nausea, vomiting, and diarrhea may be related to use of salicylates, NSAIDs, corticosteroids, and immunosuppressant medications. The patient who presents with acute abdominal pain and tenderness needs immediate, comprehensive evaluation to identify possible intra-abdominal crisis. Ascites is found in 10% of persons with SLE, and pancreatitis occurs in about 5% of patients usually secondary to vasculitis. Although abnormal liver enzymes may be noted, they are usually secondary to medication use; active liver disease rarely occurs in SLE (Lupus Foundation of Colorado, n.d.).

Central nervous system effects of SLE may include headaches, dizziness, mood disturbances, hallucinations, and seizures. Approximately 80% of persons with lupus experience cognitive dysfunction, often marked by confusion and memory loss. Many patients have difficulty expressing their thoughts (Mayo Clinic, 2009a).

Having lupus appears to increase a person's risk of developing lung cancer and non-Hodgkin's lymphoma. Immunosuppressant drugs used to treat SLE can increase the risk of cancer. Other than non-Hodgkin's lymphoma, however, people with lupus are less likely to die of cancer than the general population (Mayo Clinic, 2009a).

Special Considerations. Neonatal lupus erythematosus occurs due to passively acquired autoantibodies from a mother with lupus. Skin and liver problems typically resolve by the time the infant is 6 months old; however, the serious manifestation of congenital heart block requires a pacemaker and is linked to approximately 20% infant mortality (CDC, 2010). In older children, lupus once was thought to be more severe than in adults. Although health care providers no longer believe this, children with lupus generally have been ill longer than adults when diagnosis is made and are more likely to have organ involvement than are adults (Lupus Foundation, 2010a).

Adults' adherence to therapy often is a problem, especially in young women of childbearing age using strong immunosuppressant medications (CDC, 2010). In the 1970s, women with lupus were counseled not to become pregnant. A successful pregnancy is possible for most women with lupus, although not without elevated risk. About 10% of pregnancies end in miscarriage, most often after the first trimester, due to antiphospholipid syndrome despite treatment with heparin and aspirin. Premature birth may be due to preeclampsia and premature rupture of membranes. The most important risk, that of a lupus flare, also is the most controversial and not confirmed in all studies. Referral to a high-risk obstetrician always is appropriate (Petri, 2010).

Late-onset lupus is possible in adults over age 55. It affects women 8 times more than men and is found primarily in Caucasians, although any race can be affected. Older adults generally are able to manage the disease with conservative therapy; low-dose corticosteroids may be used. In addition, drug-induced lupus is more likely to occur in older adults because health conditions (e.g., hypertension, heart disease) require treatment that may cause the symptoms of lupus (Lupus Foundation, 2010b).

Assessment

History. Patients being evaluated for SLE almost universally complain of fatigue, even without other manifestations of the disease. About one half of them also often identify weight loss due to decreased appetite and/or gastrointestinal problems. Episodic fever is reported in about 80% of patients, but there is no particular pattern to this occurrence. Many patients complain of chest pain, but evidence of pericardial changes generally is not found on clinical evaluation. Reports of cognitive dysfunction ("lupus fog") and headache also are not uncommon (Lupus Foundation of Colorado, n.d.).

About 95% of patients with SLE complain of arthralgia. In fact, for about half of affected persons, articular pain is identified as the initial symptom. The patient may complain of morning stiffness, as well as joint and muscle aches. Joints may become warm and swollen, but x-rays do not reveal any erosive changes. Also, unlike RA, the arthritis of SLE tends to be transitory (Lupus Foundation of Colorado, n.d.).

About 80% of patients also have a history of skin manifestations, with itching, pain, and disfigurement possible. The classic sign of lupus is the butterfly rash extending over the cheeks (malar area) and bridge of the nose. It can range from a faint blush to a severe eruption with associated scaling, and is very photosensitive. The butterfly rash occurs in 55%-85% of persons at some time during the disease. Other rashes may appear on the face, ears, upper arms and shoulders, chest, and hands. The patient may report that skin changes were associated with exposure to sunlight. Symptoms of Raynaud's syndrome are common. Skin alterations and hair loss can be disfiguring, prompting the patient to limit his or her lifestyle and social involvement out of fear of rejection by others (Lupus Foundation of Colorado, n.d.).

Physical Exam. Use of the 1982 American College of Rheumatology criteria lead to diagnosis of lupus based on both clinical and laboratory findings, and using the acronym SOAPBRAINMD (Bartels & Muller, 2010; Tan et al., 1982):

- **S**erositis – Pleurisy and pericarditis on examination or diagnostic imaging;
- **O**ral ulcers – Oral or pharyngeal ulcers, often appearing on the palate. They generally are painless;
- **A**rthritis – Nonerosive, involving two or more peripheral joints with tenderness or swelling;
- **P**hotosensitivity – Unusual skin reaction when exposed to light;
- **B**lood dyscrasias – Leukopenia, lymphopenia, thrombocytopenia, hemolytic anemia;
- **R**enal involvement – Proteinuria or cellular casts;
- **A**NA – High titers (>1:160) in the absence of medications associated with drug-induced lupus;
- **I**mmunologic phenomena – Anti-Smith antibodies, antiphospholipid antibodies;
- **N**eurologic disorder – Seizure or psychosis without other causes;
- **M**alar rash – Flat or raised fixed erythema over cheeks and nasal bridge; and
- **D**iscoid rash – Erythematous raised-rim lesions with keratotic scaling and follicular plugging, often with scarring.

The presence of 4 of 11 criteria has a sensitivity of 85% and a specificity of 95% for diagnosis of SLE (Bartels & Muller, 2010).

Diagnostic Tests. No specific diagnostic test exists for SLE; however, in patients with high ANA titers (95% sensitivity) or a strong clinical suspicion of the disease, additional testing is indicated. Other antibody testing includes anti-dsDNA, anti-Sm, and anti-phospholipids. Inflammatory markers (ESR, CRP), complement levels (C3 and C4 often depressed), a CBC, and liver function tests also may be ordered (Bartels & Muller, 2010).

Joint x-rays provide little evidence of SLE, although periarticular osteopenia and soft tissue swelling may be evident. Chest x-rays and CT can be used to monitor interstitial lung disease and assess other complications, such as pneumonitis. Magnetic resonance imaging (MRI) or angiography can evaluate central nervous system lupus for white matter changes, vasculitis, or stroke, although these findings are nonspecific. Finally, echocardiography can be used to assess pericardial effusion or pulmonary hypertension (Bartels & Muller, 2010).

Common Therapeutic Modalities

Treatment for active disease depends on the organ systems involved and disease manifestations.

Medications. Medication use is based on the patient's manifestations. NSAIDs are used for relief of arthralgia, fever, and mild serositis. Their use may cause elevated liver function tests in the patient with active SLE. Concomitant use with corticosteroids also may increase the risk of gastrointestinal ulceration. Thus careful patient monitoring is needed during treatment.

Antimalarial agents (e.g., hydroxychloroquine [Plaquenil®]) frequently are used to treat constitutional symptoms, as well as cutaneous and musculoskeletal manifestations of SLE. Combinations of antimalarials commonly are used and are thought to have a synergistic effect. These medications cause immunomodulation without overt immunosuppression. They are useful in preventing and treating skin rashes, constitutional symptoms, arthralgia, and arthritis. They also help to reduce the occurrence of flares, and are associated with reduced morbidity and mortality.

Corticosteroids are used predominantly as anti-inflammatories and immunosuppressants. Methylprednisolone (Solu-Medrol®) may be indicated for acute, organ-threatening exacerbations. Low-dose oral prednisone can be used for milder disease, but more severe disease requires high doses of oral or intravenous agents. The side effects suggest that caution be used in prescribing for long-term use.

Methotrexate addresses inflammation and manages arthritis, serositis, and cutaneous symptoms. Adults would receive 7.5-25 mg weekly; a pediatric dose has not been established. Azothiaprine is indicated in non-renal disease and is a less toxic alternative to cyclophosphamide. Dosing begins at 1 mg/kg/day for 6-8 weeks, followed by 0.5 mg/kg every 4 weeks until response; a pediatric dose has not been established for this drug. Cyclophosphamide is indicated for serious organ involvement, especially CNS symptoms, vasculitis, and nephritis. Both adults and children receive 500-750 mg/m2 by infusion every month. Immune globulin also can be used for serious disease flares. The drug down-regulates pro-inflammatory cytokines, suppresses inducer T and B cells, and augments suppressor T cells. The patient receives 2 mg/kg daily by intravenous infusion. Mycophenolate (Cellcept®) is useful for maintenance in lupus nephritis and other serious manifestations. It inhibits antibody production and is titrated to 1 gram by mouth twice daily. Neither immune globulin nor mycophenolate is indicated for treatment of children with lupus (Bartels & Muller, 2010).

Biologic agents that are popular in the treatment of RA and AS have also been used to treat patients with SLE. The anti-TNF therapies etanercept, adalimumab, and infliximab have been found to cause drug-induced lupus in some people.; however, the condition was reversible when the medication was discontinued (Lupus Foundation, 2010c).

Because hormones are believed to influence the course of lupus and may even play a role in the disease development, many researchers are interested in testing their effects on persons with the disease. Early indications are that hormone preparations once thought to worsen lupus, such as hormone replacement therapy and oral contraceptives, may be appropriate and safe for some women with the disease (NIAMS, 2006). In addition, Prasterone (Prestara™) is being studied as a treatment for corticosteroid-induced osteoporosis in people with SLE (Lupus Foundation, 2010c).

Cutaneous manifestations usually are treated with strict use of sun block, careful use of topical steroids (not all indicated for use on face), and antimalarial therapy. Intralesional injection of triamcinolone acetonide is useful for healing individual lesions. The antileprosy drug dapsone (Avlosulfon®) and retinoids, such as acitretin (Soriatane®) and isotretinoin (Accutane®), may be additional therapeutic options (Callen, 2010).

Physical Management. Regular follow-up and laboratory testing are needed to detect new organ involvement and monitor response to treatment. Urinalysis, CBC with differential, and creatinine should be assessed periodically. Consultation with other specialists may be needed, based on multi-system involvement and patient's complaints of pain (Bartels & Muller, 2010).

Nursing Considerations

Nursing Diagnoses. Nursing diagnoses for this condition are expanded upon in the Appendix.

- Confusion, risk for acute.
- Family processes, interrupted.
- Knowledge deficit.
- Pain, acute.
- Parenting, impaired.

Interventions. The patient with SLE should avoid fatigue by pacing and modifying activities. Stress, including physical illness, may precipitate a disease flare.

Patient Teaching. The nurse should instruct the patient to avoid sun exposure, especially between 11 a.m. and 3 p.m., and wear sunscreen (at least SPF 25) and protective clothing whenever outdoor activities are needed. Drying soaps or powders and harsh household chemicals should be avoided. The patient should maintain a balanced diet; no diet-based treatment of SLE has proven effective. He or she also should be reminded to call the health care provider for temperature over 99.6°, which can indicate possible infection or lupus flare (Bartels & Muller, 2010). A support group may be accessed through the Lupus Foundation of America (www.lupus.org) or the Arthritis Foundation (www.arthritis.org).

Fibromyalgia Syndrome

Overview

Definition. Fibromyalgia syndrome (FS) is a disease of diffuse, nonarticular musculoskeletal pain and tenderness often accompanied by subjective complaints, such as fatigue, memory difficulties ("fibro fog"), and irritable bowel syndrome (IBS). Fibromyalgia is now recognized as one of the central pain syndromes (Buskila, Atzeni, & Sarzi-Puttini, 2008).

Etiology. The multifactorial features of FS contribute to its unknown etiology. The evidence of familial aggregation suggests an autoimmune etiology. Many investigators believe that the cause of fibromyalgia is an aberrant central nervous system function marked by abnormal human stress response or abnormalities in sensory processing. It may coexist with other rheumatic diseases, including RA and SLE. Various triggers, including trauma, stress, and infection, may precipitate the development of FS (Buskila et al., 2008).

Pathophysiology. FS historically was believed to be either an inflammatory or psychiatric condition, but no evidence was found to support either theory. The currently known abnormalities associated with the disease suggest that it may be a condition of central sensitization or abnormal central processing of nociceptive pain input. Biochemical changes in the CNS, low levels of serotonin, four-fold increase in nerve growth factor, and elevated levels of substance P characterize a whole-body hypersensitivity to pain (Gilliland, 2009).

Incidence. Conservative estimates indicate that 2% of the general United States population meets the criteria for FS, making it the second most common disorder encountered by rheumatologists. Approximately 1 in 10 patients evaluated in a medical practice has fibromyalgia, and it costs the American economy over $9 billion annually. The disease is 4 to 7 times more common in women than in men. Although symptoms usually occur in persons ages 20-55, FS can be diagnosed in any age group. It shows no racial predilection (Gilliland, 2009).

Table 13.5. ACR 1990 Criteria for Classification of Fibromyalgia
Patient will be said to have fibromyalgia if both criteria are satisfied. The presence of a different clinical disorder does not exclude the diagnosis of fibromyalgia.
1. History of widespread pain for at least 3 months. **Definition:** pain is considered widespread when all of the following are present: pain in left side of body, pain in right side of body, pain above waist, and pain below waist. In addition, axial skeleton pain (cervical spine, anterior chest, thoracic spine, or low back) must be present. In this definition, shoulder and buttock pain is considered as pain for each involved side. "Low back pain" is considered lower segment pain.
2. Pain in 11 of 18 tender point sites on digital palpation. **Definition:** pain on digital palpation must be present in at least 11 of the following 18 tender point sites: *Occiput:* bilateral, at the suboccipital muscle insertions. *Low cervical:* bilateral, at the anterior aspects of the intertransverse spaces at C5-C7. *Trapezius:* bilateral, at the midpoint of the upper border. *Supraspinatus:* bilateral, at origins, above the scapula spine near the medial border. *Second rib:* bilateral, at the second costochondral junctions, just lateral to the junctions on the upper surfaces. *Lateral epicondyle:* bilateral, 2 cm distal to the epicondyles. *Gluteal:* bilateral, in upper outer quadrants of buttocks in anterior fold of muscle. *Greater trochanter:* bilateral, posterior to the trochanteric prominence. *Knee:* bilateral, at the medial fat pad proximal to the joint line.
Digital palpation should be performed with an approximate force of 4 kg. For a tender point to be considered "positive," the patient must state that the palpation was painful. "Tender" is not to be considered "painful."

From "Criteria for the Classification of Fibromyalgia" by the American College of Rheumatology, 1990, Arthritis and Rheumatism, *33(2), 160-172.*

Complications. The impact of FS is similar to that of RA, with marked social, economic, functional, and emotional impact. About one third of patients with FS report modifying their work to keep their jobs. They may shorten their workday or workweek, or may change to a position that is less physically or mentally demanding. Reports have indicated the inability to achieve career or educational advancement due to the disease, and some patients have cited career loss. Approximately 15% of persons with FS receive disability payments, although estimates go as high as 44% (Gilliland, 2009).

Special Considerations. Before receiving a diagnosis, the average person with FS has seen 15 health care providers and had the condition for 5 years. Misdiagnosis leads to expensive testing and treatments that provide no benefit. Many patients have been told that there is nothing wrong with them and that the condition is imagined. Although they may be relieved when a diagnosis is made, they also may be skeptical that the provider actually knows what is wrong and can offer a treatment plan (Gilliland, 2009).

CHAPTER 13

Assessment

History. A detailed history will save time for both the patient and the health care provider. Because the patient often does not understand that the symptoms are connected, the provider must be prepared to ask questions to develop a full understanding of the patient's condition. The patient with FS does better when an individualized, comprehensive treatment plan is developed, and a thorough history is critical in developing an appropriate regimen. The patient does not look chronically ill but often appears fatigued or agitated. He or she will describe widespread pain on both sides of the body, both above and below the waist, and along the axial skeleton. The pain is described as constant and has lasted more than 3 months. It is described as burning and aching, although the location migrates and the intensity varies. History reveals that the pain is global, not focal, in its distribution. In addition, the patient's partner can be asked about leg movement in bed; about 20% of persons with FS also have restless legs syndrome (RLS). Approximately 40% also describe bloating, cramping, and an increased urge to defecate, most likely related to concomitant IBS. Questioning also may reveal a history of sleep disturbances, with complaints of unrefreshing sleep and morning fatigue (Gilliland, 2009).

Physical Exam. Physical examination should confirm a suspected diagnosis, rule out other systemic diseases, and identify common co-existing disorders. Muscles should be palpated with 4 kg of pressure. To meet diagnostic criteria for FS, the patient should identify pain at 11 of 18 paired tender points. The tender point hurts only when pressure is applied, and the patient has no referred pain. In addition, pain must have been present in all four body quadrants and in the axial skeleton for at least 3 months. (See Table 13.5 for diagnostic criteria.)

Diagnostic Tests. No laboratory tests accurately confirm FS. A new blood test involves antipolymer antibodies, which are present in 50% of persons with fibromyalgia. Routine laboratory and imaging studies are helpful in ruling out other differential diagnosis considered on the basic of the history and physical examination (Gilliland, 2009).

Common Therapeutic Modalities

Medications. Trigger point injection is an important intervention to provide mechanical disruption (myolysis) of the trigger point. This generally is marked by reduced pain, increased ROM, improved exercise tolerance, and better circulation. Most health care providers prefer 1% lidocaine without epinephrine for injections; corticosteroids generally are not indicated. Sterile saline can be used for the patient who is allergic to anesthetics. Contraindications to trigger point injection include local or systemic infection. A patient with a bleeding disorder or one who is receiving anticoagulant therapy should undergo additional evaluation before injection is done (Gilliland, 2009).

Most investigators oppose the use of opioids for FS treatment. In addition, for the patient without concomitant rheumatic illness, corticosteroids generally are not helpful. NSAIDs have not proven beneficial when used alone, but their use with a tricyclic antidepressant may increase efficacy. Muscle relaxants also may be helpful in pain management (e.g., metaxalone [Skelaxin®], baclofen [Lioresal®]). Also prescribed for pain are pregabalin (Lyrica®) 75 mg twice daily, increased to 150 mg, and gabapentin (Neurontin®), 300 mg daily titrated to 300 mg three times daily. In addition, agents that affect serotonin, substance P, norepinephrine, and other neurochemicals may modulate the pain sensation and tolerance. Zolpidem (Ambien®) is an effective medication for sleep onset, and trazodone (Desyrel®) has helped in sleep maintenance.

Physical Management. Because long-term follow-up suggests little symptom improvement over time, a coordinated, multi-disciplinary approach to care is required. Traditional physical therapy may, in fact, worsen the patient's symptoms. Some research indicates that physical therapy-based programs have a positive impact on the patient's well-being but no effect on other disease symptoms. Electrotherapy, cryotherapy, and massage have had positive impact when used to treat pain. When exercising, the patient should begin with gentle, warm-up flexibility exercises and progress to stretching. Low-impact aerobic exercise is encouraged 3 times weekly. The goal is to exercise safely without increasing pain. The patient thus should be encouraged to exercise at the highest level possible without worsening symptoms (Gilliland, 2009).

Complementary and Alternative Therapies. As with many chronic conditions that do not respond well to allopathic treatment, herbal products or supplements may seem promising to the patient with FS who has little hope of symptom management. Black cohosh, which has estrogen-like properties, also has anti-inflammatory and muscle relaxant effects. White willow bark is a source of salicylates that is mild on the stomach. The patient should be cautioned to seek the advice of a trained herbalist and ensure that the allopathic provider is aware of his or her interest in alternative therapies (Dunne, 2007). In addition to herbal products, acupuncture, yoga, and meditation may be helpful for FS management.

Nursing Considerations

Nursing Diagnoses. Nursing diagnoses for this condition are expanded upon in the Appendix.

- Coping, ineffective.
- Fatigue.
- Pain, chronic.
- Powerlessness.
- Self-care deficit: bathing/hygiene, dressing/grooming, feeding, toileting.
- Sleep pattern, disturbed.

Interventions. Vocational training may be indicated if the disease has affected the patient's employability.

Patient Teaching. The nurse should stress the benign, nonprogressive nature of FS, and reinforce the value of aerobic exercise for its analgesic and antidepressant effects. The basics of good sleep practices should be reviewed to maximize sleep behaviors. The patient can be encouraged to try to correlate symptom exacerbation with nutritional triggers and should be urged to consult the health care provider before pursuing an elimination diet.

Summary

The Centers for Disease Control and Prevention (2009) estimate that more than 45 million Americans have doctor-diagnosed arthritis. Nearly two thirds of affected persons are under age 65. By 2030, the number of people with arthritis is expected to reach 40% of the population, or about 67 million. The widespread nature of arthritic conditions supports the need for nurses to understand disease processes and treatments, and to assist patients in their efforts to live with chronic disease.

References

Abramson, L.S. (2008). *Arthritis in Children.* Retrieved from http://rheumatology.org/practice/clinical/patients/diseases_and_conditions/juvenilearthritis.pdf#search=%22JIA%22

Altman, R.D. (2007). Laboratory findings in osteoarthritis. In R.W. Moskowitz, R.D. Altman, M.C. Hochberg, J.A. Buckwalter, & V.M. Goldberg (Eds.) *Osteoarthritis: Diagnosis and Medical/Surgical Management* (4th ed., pp. 201-214). Philadelphia, PA: W.B. Saunders Company.

Altman, R.D. (2008a). *Osteoarthritis.* Retrieved from http://www.merck.com/mmhe/sec05/ch066/ch066a.html

Altman, R.D. (2008b). *Other Types of Inflammatory Arthritis.* Retrieved from http://www.merck.com/mmhe/sec05/ch066/ch066c.html#sec05-ch066-ch066a-439

Altman, R.D. (2008c). *Seronegative Spondyloarthropathies.* Retrieved from http://www.merck.com/mmpe/sec04/ch034/ch034d.html

American Academy of Orthopaedic Surgeons (AAOS). (2011). *Osteotomy of the Knee.* Retrieved from http://orthoinfo.aaos.org/topic.cfm?topic=A00591

American College of Rheumatology (ACR). (2009a). *Patient Education – Medications.* Retrieved from http://www.rheumatology.org/practice/clinical/patients/medications/

American College of Rheumatology (ACR). (2009b). *Patient Education – Polymyalgia Rheumatica.* Retrieved from http://www.rheumatology.org/practice/clinical/patients/diseases_and_conditions/polymyalgiarheumatica.asp

American College of Rheumatology (ACR) Subcommittee on Osteoarthritis Guidelines. (2000). *Recommendations for Medical Management of Osteoarthritis of the Hip and Knee.* Retrieved from http://www.rheumatology.org/practice/clinical/guidelines/oa-mgmt.asp

Ankylosing Spondylitis Center. (2010). *Pathogenesis.* Retrieved from http://www.ankylosingspondylitiscenter.com/pathogenesis.php

Bellamy, N., Campbell, J., Welch, V., Gee, T.L., Bourne, R., & Wells, G.A. (2006). *Viscosupplementation for Treatment of Osteoarthritis of the Knee.* Retrieved from http://www2.cochrane.org/reviews/en/ab005321.html

Brägelmann, B. (2008). *Rheumatoid Arthritis.* Retrieved from http://en.wikipedia.org/wiki/File:RheumatoideArthritisAP.jpg.

Bratton, R.L., Whiteside, J.W., Hovan, M.J., Engle, R.L., & Edwards, F.D. (2008). Diagnosis and treatment of Lyme disease. *Mayo Clinic Proceedings, 83*(5), 566-571.

Bykirk, V. (2006). *Reactive Arthritis.* Retrieved from http://www.rheumatology.org/practice/clinical/patients/diseases_and_conditions/reactivearthritis.asp

Centers for Disease Control and Prevention. (2009). *FAQs: Self-Reported Arthritis Case Definition.* Retrieved from http://www.cdc.gov/arthritis/data_statistics/faqs/case_definition.htm

Chatterjee, S. (2009). *Systemic Sclerosis.* Retrieved from http://www.clevelandclinicmeded.com/medicalpubs/diseasemanagement/rheumatology/systemic-sclerosis/

Clinical Trials Search. (2010). *Efficacy and Safety of Oral Salmon Calcitonin in Patients with Knee Osteoarthritis (OA2 study).* Retrieved from http://www.clinicaltrialssearch.org/efficacy-and-safety-of-oral-salmon-calcitonin-in-patients-with-knee-osteoarthritis-oa-2-study-nct00704847.html

Fitzgerald, B., Setty, A. & Mudgal, C. (2007). Gout affecting the hand and wrist. *Journal of the American Academy of Orthopaedic Surgeons, 15*(10), 625-635.

Gomariz, E.M., del, M., Guijo, V.P., Contreras, A.E., Villanueva, M., & Estévez, E.C. (2002). The potential of ESSG spondyloarthropathy classification criteria as a diagnostic aid in rheumatologic practice. *Journal of Rheumatology, 29*(2), 326-330.

Haaz, S. (2008). *Complementary and Alternative Medicine for Patients with Rheumatoid Arthritis.* Retrieved from http://www.hopkins-arthritis.org/patient-corner/diseasemanagement/cam.html

Hajj-Ali, R.A. (2008). *Systemic Sclerosis.* Retrieved from http://www.merck.com/mmpe/sec04/ch032/ch032h.html

Haque, U.J. & Bathon, J.M. (2007). Rheumatoid arthritis. In N.H. Fiebach, D.E. Kern, P.A. Thomas, & R.C. Ziegelstein (Eds.), *Barker, Burton and Zieve's Principles of Ambulatory Medicine* (7th ed., pp. 1254-1280). Philadelphia, PA: Lippincott Williams & Wilkins.

Helmick, C.G., Felson, D.T., Lawrence, R.C., Gabriel, S., Hirsch, R., Kwoh, C.K.,. . .Stone, J.H., for the National Arthritis Data Workgroup. (2008). Estimates of the prevalence of arthritis and other rheumatic conditions in the United States. Part I. *Arthritis & Rheumatism, 58*(1), 15-25.

Hoffart, C. & Sherry, D.D. (2010). Early identification of juvenile idiopathic arthritis. *The Journal of Musculoskeletal Medicine, 27*(2). Retrieved from http://www.Musculoskeletalnetwork.com/rheumatoid-arthritis/content/article/1145622/1517642

International Scleroderma Network. (2010). *What Is Scleroderma?* Retrieved from http://sclero.org/medical/about-sd/a-to-z.html#causes

Jarvis, J.N. (2008). Commentary: Ordering lab tests for suspected rheumatic disease. *Pediatric Rheumatology, 6,* 19. doi: 10.1186/1546-0096-6-19

Karlson, E.W., Mandi, L.A., Hankinson, S.E., & Grodstein, F. (2004). Do breast-feeding and other reproductive factors influence future risk of rheumatoid arthritis? Results of the Nurses' Health Study. *Arthritis & Rheumatism, 50*(11), 3458-3467.

Kest, H.E. & Pineda, C. (2008). Lyme disease: Prevention, diagnosis, and management. *Contemporary Pediatrics, 25*(6), 57-64.

Koch, C. (2010). *Nutrition & Rheumatoid Arthritis.* Retrieved from http://www.hopkins-arthritis.org/patient-corner/disease-management/nutinra.html

Krabak, B. & Minkoff, E. (2010). *Rehabilitation Management of RA.* Retrieved from http://www.hopkins-arthritis.org/patient-corner/disease-management/ra_rehab.html

Kremer, J.M., Alarcón, G.S., Lightfoot, R.W., Jr., Wilkens, R.F., Furst, D.E., Williams, J.,. . .Weinblatt, M.E. (1994). Methotrexate for rheumatoid arthritis. *Arthritis & Rheumatism, 37*(3), 316-328.

Ling, S.M. & Bathon, J.M. (2010a). *Osteoarthritis – Clinical Presentation.* Retrieved from http://www.hopkins-arthritis.org/arthritis-info/osteoarthritis/clinical-presentation.html#mark

Ling, S.M. & Bathon, J. M. (2010b). *Osteoarthritis – Pathophysiology.* Retrieved from http://www.hopkins-arthritis.org/arthritis-info/osteoarthritis/pathophysiology.html

Mahajan, A., Tandon, V.R., Sharma, S., & Jandial, C. (2007). Gout and menopause. JK Science: *Journal of Medical Education & Research, 9*(1), 50-51.

Marcus, D.M. (2008). *Herbal Remedies, Supplements, and Acupuncture for Arthritis.* Retrieved from http://www.rheumatology.org/practice/clinical/patients/diseases_and_conditions/herbal.asp

Martin, D. (2010). *Psoriatic Arthritis.* Retrieved from http://www.hopkins-arthritis.org/arthritis-info/psoriatic-arthritis/#etiology

Matsumoto, A.K., Bathon, J., & Bingham, C.O., III. (2010). *Rheumatoid Arthritis Treatment.* Retrieved from http://www.hopkins-arthritis.org/arthritis-info/rheumatoid-arthritis/rheum_treat.html#new#new

Mayo Clinic. (2008). *Psoriatic Arthritis: Complications.* Retrieved from http://www.mayoclinic.com/health/psoriatic-arthritis/DS00476/DSECTION=complications

Mayo Clinic. (2009a). *Reactive Arthritis: Complications.* Retrieved from http://www.mayoclinic.com/health/reactive-arthritis/DS00486/DSECTION=complications

Mayo Clinic. (2009b). *Reactive Arthritis: Symptoms.* Retrieved from http://www.mayoclinic.com/health/reactive-arthritis/DS00486/DSECTION=symptoms

Mayo Clinic. (2010). *Giant Cell Arteritis: Complications.* Retrieved from http://www.mayoclinic.com/health/giant-cell-arteritis/DS00440/DSECTION=complications

McCarty, D.J. (2008). *Gout.* Retrieved from http://www.merck.com/mmpe/sec04/ch035/ch035b.html

Meletis, C.D., Zabriskie, N., & Rountree, R. (2009). Identifying and treating Lyme disease. *Alternative and Complementary Therapies, 15*(1), 17-23.

Moore, S.C. & DeSantis, E.R.H. (2008). Treatment of complications associated with systemic sclerosis. *American Journal of Health System Pharmacology, 65*(4), 315-321.

National Institute of Arthritis and Musculoskeletal and Skin Diseases (NIAMS). (2008). *Juvenile Arthritis.* Retrieved from http://www.niams.nih.gov/Health_Info/Juv_Arthritis/default.asp

National Institute of Arthritis and Musculoskeletal and Skin Diseases (NIAMS). (2009a). *Reactive Arthritis.* Retrieved from http://www.niams.nih.gov/Health_Info/Reactive_Arthritis/default.asp

National Institute of Arthritis and Musculoskeletal and Skin Diseases (NIAMS). (2009b). *Rheumatoid arthritis.* Retrieved from http://www.niams.nih.gov/Health_Info/Rheumatic_Disease/default.asp

National Institute of Arthritis and Musculoskeletal and Skin Diseases (NIAMS). (2010a). *Questions and Answers About Gout.* Retrieved from http://www.niams.nih.gov/Health_Info/Gout/default.asp

National Institute of Arthritis and Musculoskeletal and Skin Diseases (NIAMS). (2010b). *Questions and Answers About Polymyalgia Rheumatica and Giant Cell Arteritis.* Retrieved from http://www.niams.nih.gov/Health_Info/Polymyalgia/default.asp

National Psoriasis Foundation. (2010). *Frequently Asked Questions About Psoriatic Arthritis.* Retrieved from http://www.psoriasis.org/netcommunity/sublearn02_psa_faq

Niehues, T. & Lankisch, P. (2006). Recommendations for the use of methotrexate in juvenile idiopathic arthritis. *Paediatric Drugs, 8*(6), 347-356.

Ogiela, D. (2009). *Osteoarthritis.* Retrieved from http://www.nlm.nih.gov/medlineplus/ency/article/000423.htm

Parrillo, S.J. (2010). *Rheumatic Fever.* Retrieved from http://emedicine.medscape.com/article/808945-overview

Pessler, F. & Sherry, D.D. (2010). *Rheumatic Fever.* Retrieved from http://www.merck.com/mmpe/sec19/ch281/ch281a.html

Rizzo, D.B. & Gunta, K.E. (2007). Disorders of the skeletal system: Metabolic and rheumatic disorders. In C.M. Porth (Ed.). *Essentials of Pathophysiology: Concepts of Altered Health States* (2nd ed., pp. 1015-1046). Philadelphia, PA: Lippincott Williams & Wilkins.

Ruderman, E. & Tambar, S. (2008). *Rheumatoid Arthritis.* Retrieved from http://www.rheumatology.org/practice/clinical/patients/diseases_and_conditions/ra.pdf

Saad, E.R. (2010). *Polymyalgia Rheumatica.* Retrieved from http://emedicine.medscape.com/article/330815-overview

Saag, K.G., Teng, G.G., Patkar, N.M., Anuntiyo, J., Finney, C., Curtis, J.R. . . .Furst, D.E. (2008). American College of Rheumatology 2008 recommendations for the use of non-biologic and biologic disease-modifying anti-rheumatic drugs in rheumatoid arthritis. *Arthritis & Rheumatism, 59*(6), 762-784. doi: 10.1002/art.23721

Schumacher, H.R. (2009). *Gout.* Retrieved from http://www.rheumatology.org/practice/clinical/patients/diseases_and_conditions/gout.asp

Scleroderma Foundation. (n.d.). *Raynaud's Phenomenon.* Retrieved from http://www.scleroderma.org/pdf/Medical_Brochures/Raynaud.pdf

Seibold, J.R. & Korn, J.H. (2002). *New Therapies for Pulmonary Hypertension in Systemic Sclerosis.* Retrieved from http://www.rheumatology.org/publications/hotline/0702pahfinal.asp

Shaikh, S.A. (2007). Ankylosing spondylitis: Recent breakthroughs in diagnosis and treatment. *Journal of the Canadian Chiropractic Association, 51*(4), 249-260.

Shamji, M.F., Bafaquh, M., & Tsai, E. (2008). The pathogenesis of ankylosing spondylitis. *Journal of Neurosurgery (JNSPGOnline), 24*(1). doi: 10.3171/FOC/2008/24/1/E3

Simon, H. (2009). *Scleroderma: Other Treatments.* Retrieved from http://www.umm.edu/patiented/articles/what_investigative_alternative_treatments_scleroderma_000088_9.htm

Spondylitis Association of America (SAA). (2009a). *Ankylosing Spondylitis.* Retrieved from http://www.spondylitis.org/about/as_diag.aspx?PgSrch=diagnosis

Spondylitis Association of America (SAA). (2009b). *Complications: How Is a Person Affected?* Retrieved from http://www.spondylitis.org/about/complications.aspx

Spondylitis Association of America (SAA). (2009c). *Reactive Arthritis.* Retrieved from http://www.spondylitis.org/about/reactive_treat.aspx

Spondylitis Association of America (SAA). (2009d). *Treatment of Ankylosing Spondylitis & Related Diseases.* Retrieved from http://www.spondylitis.org/about/treatment.aspx

Spondylitis Association of America (SAA). (2009e). *Women's Health.* Retrieved from http://www.spondylitis.org/patient_resources/women.aspx

Stacy, G.S. & Basu, P.A. (2009). *Osteoarthritis, Primary.* Retrieved from http://emedicine.medscape.com/article/392096-overview

Subcommittee for Scleroderma Criteria of the American Rheumatism Association Diagnostic and Therapeutic Criteria Committee. (1980). Preliminary criteria for the classification of systemic sclerosis (scleroderma). *Arthritis & Rheumatism, 23*(5), 581-590.

Underwood, M. & Adebajo, A. (2009). Gout, hyperuricaemia, and crystal arthritis. In A. Adebajo (Ed.), *ABC of Rheumatology* (4th ed., pp. 59-64). Chichester, West Sussex, England, UK: John Wiley & Sons, Ltd..

U.S. Department of Health & Human Services. (2006). *Your Rights Under Section 504 of the Rehabilitation Act.* Retrieved from http://www.hhs.gov/ocr/civilrights/resources/factsheets/504.pdf

U.S. Food and Drug Administration. (2005). *Information for Healthcare Professionals: Celecoxib (marketed as Celebrex).* Retrieved from http://www.fda.gov/Drugs/DrugSafety/PostmarketDrugSafetyInformationforPatientsandProviders/ucm124655.htm

U.S. Food and Drug Administration. (2009). *FDA Approves Drug for Gout Management.* Retrieved from http://www.fda.gov/NewsEvents/Newsroom/PressAnnouncements/2009/ucm149534.htm

Vorvick, L. (2010). *Rheumatic Fever.* Retrieved from http://www.nlm.nih.gov/medlineplus/ency/article/003940.htm

Walsh, C.A., Mayer, E.W., & Baxi, L.V. (2007). Lyme disease in pregnancy: Case report and review of the literature. *Obstetrical & Gynecological Survey, 62*(1), 41-50.

Watkins, J. (2010). A case of acute gout. *Practice Nursing, 21*(4), 210-211.

Wheeless, C.R. (2010a). Rheumatoid foot. *Wheeless' Textbook of Orthopaedics.* Retrieved from http://www.wheelessonline.com/ortho/rheumatoid_foot

Wheeless, C.R. (2010b). Rheumatoid hand. *Wheeless' Textbook of Orthopaedics.* Retrieved from http://www.wheelessonline.com/ortho/rheumatoid_hand

Wheeless, C. R. (2010c). Stages of rheumatoid arthritis. *Wheeless' Textbook of Orthopaedics.* Retrieved from http://www.wheelessonline.com/ortho/stages_of_rheumatoid_arthritis

Wilke, W.S. & Carey, J. (2009). *Osteoarthritis.* Retrieved from http://www.clevelandclinicmeded.com/medicalpubs/diseasemanagement/rheumatology/osteoarthritis/#cesec2

Woreta, F., Thorne, J.E., Jabs, D.A., Kedhar, S.R., & Dunn, J.P. (2007). Risk factors for ocular complications and poor visual acuity at presentation among patients with uveitis associated with juvenile idiopathic arthritis (JIA). *American Journal of Ophthalmology, 143*(4), 647-655.

Chapter 14
Metabolic Bone Conditions

Lori E. Abel, MEd, RN, ONC

Objectives

- Define the disease process for osteoporosis, osteomalacia, rickets, hyperparathyroidism, hypoparathyroidism, and Paget's disease.
- Describe the pathophysiology, incidence, etiology, and diagnostic findings of common orthopaedic-related metabolic disorders.
- List the treatment modalities, nursing diagnoses, and interventions in the management of common orthopaedic-related metabolic disorders.
- Describe the treatment and care of the patient with hypoparathroidism and include assessment of the clinical signs of hypocalcemia.
- List the treatment criteria for osteoporosis as identified by the World Health Organization that has established guidelines for diagnosing osteoporosis, identifying bone fragility, and highlighting the importance of risk fracture assessments in adults.
- List intrinsic and extrinsic causes of osteomalacia that can be identified as the result of vitamin D deficiency.

Metabolic bone disease results from an inappropriate function of one or several metabolic processes that create physical and chemical changes within the bone. Conditions altering the normal equilibrium that exists in bone remodeling and causing metabolic bone disease include parathyroid malfunction, vitamin, mineral or dietary deficiency, estrogen deficiency, and malabsorption syndrome (Porth, 2007). Metabolic bone disease is caused by defective mineralization of bone. This can occur in both children and adults.

Over the past few decades, a greater focus has been placed on early identification of bone loss and the need for education to prevent these conditions from developing. Identifying strategies for chronic disease prevention, meeting minimum dietary and vitamin/mineral requirements, and getting adequate exercise all promote lifestyle habits that promote healthy bones. Although genetic predisposition to metabolic bone disease has been established, evidence-based prevention strategy principles have been shown to slow the progression of bone loss. Adults and children identified with metabolic bone disease frequently suffer life-altering quality of life issues because of pain, instability, and the effects of chronic disease, which leads to increased risk of injury and falls during basic activities of living.

Recent research is focused on the effects of biochemical parameters that occur in demineralized bone metabolism and the vascular calcifications that occur, especially in adults and children with chronic renal or cardiovascular disease. Metabolic bone disease progression often can be prevented and successfully treated with early identification and education.

Osteoporosis

Overview

Definition. Osteoporosis is a metabolic bone disease caused when the rate of bone resorption is more rapid than the rate of bone formation. This disorder is characterized by porous and fragile bones. A severe reduction in skeletal bone mass predisposes adults with osteoporosis to an increased susceptibility to fractures, commonly referred to as fragility fractures.

During their 2003 summit in Geneva, Switzerland, the World Health Organization (WHO) published their findings that created a standard for evidence-based research that defines bone loss in terms of bone mineral density. Normal bone mass is categorized as a bone density value (T score) between +1 and -1 standard deviations of the mean of bone mineral density of young healthy adults. Osteopenia (low bone mass) is categorized as a T score value for bone density between -1 and -2.5 standard deviations below the mean value for young adults. Osteoporosis is categorized as a statistical value of bone mineral density or content that is 2.5 standard deviations or more below the standardized mean value (T score) of healthy young adults (National Osteoporosis Foundation, n.d.).

Etiology. The causes of osteoporosis are many and include lifestyle factors that can be controlled and changed. Adults reach peak bone mass at the age of 30. Peak bone mass is influenced by genetic factors but also enhanced by exercise, diet, and avoidance of alcohol and tobacco (WHO, 2003). The rate of bone loss is strongly influenced by estrogen and genetics. Risk factors for decreased bone mass include endocrine disorders, chronic diseases, and medications such as corticosteroids, anticonvulsants, and immunosuppressant medications (Prestwood, 2010).

Pathophysiology. Mature bone is composed of connective tissue consisting of cells, fibers, and a gelatinous material containing crystallized minerals, mostly calcium, that makes bones rigid. Bone cells enable bone tissue to grow, repair, and change shape continuously to synthesize new bone tissue to resorb, dissolve, and digest old bone tissue. The fibers in bone are made of collagen that gives bones strength and a ground substance that acts as a medium for the diffusion of nutrients, oxygen, metabolic waste, chemicals, and minerals between bone tissue and blood vessels (Bickley & Szilagyi, 2007).

Bone cells consist of osteoblasts, which are bone-forming cells that lay down new bone. Osteocytes are within the mineralized bone matrix. Osteoclasts resorb or remove and allow for growth and repair of bone cells. The sequencing of bone resorption cycle takes approximately 4 to 5 months.

Compact or cortical bone comprises 85% of the skeleton. Spongy bone or cancellous bone makes up the remaining 15% of the skeleton (Bickley & Szilagyi, 2007). The compact or cortical bone structure is made of the Haversian system, which includes a central canal and concentric layers of bone matrix and osteocytes. Spongy bone is less complex and arranged in plates or bars that create an irregular mesh network. Spongy bone is filled with red bone marrow.

All bones are covered with a double layer of connective tissue called periosteum that consists of blood vessels and nerves that penetrate through the bone channels. The inner layers of periosteum anchor the collagen fibers that penetrate the bone.

The mineral and protein matrix of bone tissue is diminished when disturbances of normal osteoblastic and osteoclastic balance occur. The loss of cortical bone causes a decrease in bone density that creates the susceptibility to fracture (NOF, n.d.).

Incidence and Groups at Risk. In December 2010, the United States Department of Health and Human Services (HHS) launched Healthy People 2020 (www.healthypeople.gov), a detailed agenda for the promotion of health and the prevention of illness and disability for the United States. Osteoporosis education and prevention, including prevention of complications such as fragility fractures, is just one of the initiative's many goals. Specific collaboration among federal agencies monitors the progress of established goals and benchmarks for health-related care, education, and services. The initiative estimates that 5.3 million adults in the United States over the age of 50 have osteoporosis, and an additional 34 million have low bone mass (Healthy People 2020, 2010). Osteoporosis is mostly identified with women who are estrogen-deficient.

Since the advent of noninvasive bone mineral density testing technology, a greater focus has been on the identification of bone loss in all adults and measures to prevent further bone loss and fractures. Women are most at risk, but they are most likely to initiate preventative measures to avoid further bone loss (Richmond, 2007). Hereditary tendencies of women with osteoporosis over the age 60 are 30 to 40%. Men are affected 5% to 10% at this age, with greater prevalence after the age of 70. Adults with small bone structure also are at greater risk. Other risk factors include Caucasian race, tobacco and caffeine use, and regular alcohol consumption. Weight-bearing exercises aid in the prevention of osteoporosis. Adults who are inactive or bedridden due to weight-bearing restrictions on long bones have decreased bone absorption causing osteoporosis. Long-term use of corticosteroids that are commonly used in the treatment of endocrine disorders affects bone health. A lack of estrogen in women or testosterone in men leads to a decrease in the quality of the bone matrix. Eating disorders also affect bone health, and when these conditions are severe in women, they can cause amenorrhea leading to increased bone loss caused by estrogen deficiency (NOF, n.d.).

Complications. A fragility fracture is a pathological fracture resulting from a disease state. This fracture often occurs as the result of a minimal trauma, such as a fall from standing height. A fragility fracture is often the first indication of osteoporosis. Each year, an estimated 1.5 million adults in the United States suffer a fragility fracture related to osteoporosis (WHO, 2003). The most common fragility fractures include vertebral compression fractures leading to thoracic kyphosis, hip fractures, and wrist, forearm, or Colles fractures. Yearly, there are more than 432,000 hospital admissions, 180,000 nursing home admissions, and 2.5 million physician office visits due to fragility fractures caused by osteoporosis. It is anticipated that by the year 2040, the incidence of hip fractures will double or triple in United States (HHS, 2004). This detrimental forecast has intensified the recent focus on early identification of bones loss, prevention, and treatment.

Adults over age 65 are at the greatest risk for a fragility fracture due to osteoporosis that is associated with morbidity and mortality in this population. Hip fracture is the leading incidence of non-fatal injuries and dramatically contributes to the mortality rate in adults after the age of 65. Currently, 20% of patients experiencing a hip fracture will die within 1 year (HHS, 2004).

Preventive Strategies. Bone loss in adults has been identified as a health care concern that is receiving more attention since advancements in health screening and bone mineral density testing guidelines have been established. Prevention strategies begin with identifying the need for education and associated risk factors that predispose adults to metabolic bone disease due to their heredity tendencies. Early identification of these unavoidable risks is important in recognizing bone loss before it has a profound impact on bone health. Since the advent of bone mineral density testing, adults at early risk of bone loss can be identified and educated on the predictability of fracture risk. Regular appointments with health care professionals as part of wellness evaluations are important to identify and educate patients on prevention strategies. Early in any disease process that has an adverse effect on bone health, educating patients on dietary needs and prescribing medication to enhance absorption of calcium and vitamin D are important. Daily amounts of calcium and vitamin D are recommended and are best absorbed as a food source in such food as tuna, salmon, fortified dairy products, and cereals (HHS, 2004) (see Tables 14.4 and 14.5 in the section on osteomalacia for vitamin D intake guidelines and recommended foods containing vitamin D). If supplements are required, recommended dosing has been established based on age and health requirements. Regular weight-bearing exercise to long bones has been identified to assist healthy bone remodeling in adults. Tobacco and alcohol should be avoided, as they impede calcium and vitamin D metabolism (WHO, 2003).

Assessment

History. Because of the hereditary tendency for chronic disease, a thorough family history is indicated to determine early risk of bone loss. Discovery of height and weight loss indicates early compression of the vertebral body of the spine. Onset of menarche and menopause indicates the beginning of the decline of estrogen that preserves bone absorption of calcium. Risk factors for osteoporosis include thin and lean body build; excessive caffeine, tobacco, and/or alcohol intake; sedentary lifestyle; lactose intolerance or avoidance of dairy products; and chronic health conditions, such as renal failure, thyroid disease, and endocrine disorders (WHO, 2003). A thorough history of the medications required to treat these chronic health conditions is needed to determine the extent of their adverse effect on bone health.

Physical Exam. When shortening of height or marked curvature of the thoracic spine (Dowager's Hump) occurs, back pain and the risk of falls leading to a fragility fracture jeopardize the independence in older adults. Deformities of the spine and ribs due to a fragility fracture can cause impaired breathing. Fragility fractures occur through minimal trauma and/or falls. This establishes the severity of injury in osteoporotic bone and the life-changing complications this disease can cause.

Diagnostic Testing. *Laboratory findings:* Laboratory findings indicating osteoporosis include elevated urinary calcium, which may be due to movement of calcium from the bone. Serum calcium, phosphorus, and alkaline levels can still be normal because of the efficient balance of the endocrine system (Guyton, 2011).

Radiographic findings: Osteoporotic changes are not visualized until 30% of bone mass is lost. Diffuse radiolucency of the bone and loss of cortical bone is noted. It is common to note recent and various stages of compression fractures of the vertebral spine due to the advancing bone loss when osteoporosis is initially diagnosed. It is reported that 70% of osteoporotic fractures are identified in patients who are asymptomatic (Richmond, 2007).

Bone Densitometry (BMD) and qualitative ultrasound (QUS) are low-cost screening tools and the only technologies currently available that accurately measure bone mass and predict fragility fracture risk. This is important in identifying the need for implementing disease treatment and prevention strategies. The WHO 2005 guidelines for defining and identifying osteoporosis provide specific parameters for ordering, performing, and interpreting BMD measurement. These guidelines formed the basis of diagnosis in identifying bone mass in adults who have not suffered a fracture based on dual energy x-ray absorptiometry (DEXA) of the spine and femoral neck (WHO, 2005). In general, two sites should be measured: the anteroposterior spine and the anteroposterior hip.

The best alternative to DEXA is quantitative computed tomography (QCT). Although this may offer information not assessed by DEXA, the WHO guidelines do not recommend it for initial diagnostic purposes. Although CT is readily available, it has a higher radiation dose. It is recommended that the same scanner be used after baseline information is obtained in providing comparative results (Richmond, 2007).

Bone biopsy is invasive and reserved for gathering more precise information about metabolic bone activity. This is typically only performed when noninvasive measures have been unreliable or when the patient is not responding to therapy. The iliac crest is the preferred site for bone sampling.

Common Therapeutic Modalities

Once early bone loss can be determined by DEXA scan, prevention and treatment strategies should be started. The use of selective estrogen receptor modulators (SERM) solely for bone loss prevention remains highly controversial (Huether & McCance, 2007). Anti-resorptive bisphosphonate therapy is the most commonly prescribed treatment (Richmond, 2007). (See Table 14.1.)

Table 14.1. Medications for Osteoporosis Treatment

MEDICATION	DOSE
BISPHOSPHONATES	
Aldendronate (Fosmax) ■ Reduces post-menopausal bone loss ■ Increases bone density in spine and hip ■ Reduces risk of spine or hip fractures ■ Impairs function of the osteoclasts **Side Effect:** Esophageal irritation, patient must remain upright 30 minutes after taking medication	**Prevention:** 35mg/week Oral **Treatment:** 70mg/week Oral
Risedronate (Actonel) ■ Used for treatment and prevention of glucocorticoid-induced osteoporosis in men and women on systemic glucocorticoid treatment (7.5mg or more of prednisone or equivalent) for chronic disease ■ Increases bone mass ■ Aids in glucocorticoid-induced bone loss	**Treatment:** 35mg/week Oral
Bisphosphonate A Ibandronate (Boniva) ■ Treatment of osteoporosis	150 mg/month Oral
Zoledronic Acid (Reclast) ■ Postmenopausal Osteoporosis treatment ■ Glucocorticoid osteoporosis treatment ■ Paget's disease treatment	5mg/year Intravenous
HORMONES	
Calcitonin ■ Slows post-menopausal bone loss ■ Increases spinal bone density ■ Reduces risk of spinal fracture ■ Relieves pain associated with bone fracture	Nasal spray most commonly prescribed Parenteral dose 200-400mg 50-100IU/daily or 3x/week Subcutaneous/ Intravenous

HORMONES (continued)	
Forteo ■ Synthetic parathyroid hormone ■ Regulates calcium ■ Reduces risk of spinal fracture **Side Effects:** Orthostatic hypotension and arthralgia Not evaluated beyond 2 years of continuous use. Not recommended for lifetime use. Must be refrigerated at 36-46 degrees at all times.	Injectable subcutaneous administered 20 mcg daily - 28 daily dose multi-dose
SELECTIVE ESTROGEN RECEPTOR MODULATOR (SERM)	
Raloxifene (Evista) ■ Decreases bone loss at the spine and hip ■ May protect against heart disease without increasing the risk of cancer	60mg/day Oral

From Nursing 2011 Drug Handbook *(p. 293), 2010, Philadelphia: Lippincott Williams & Wilkins. Reproduced with permission.*

Complications of Medication. Clinical complications have emerged in the 10 years since the original research that resulted in the 2001 FDA approval of bisphosphonates (Sellemeyer, 2010). Bisphosphonates have shown to reduce vertebral spine and hip fractures in individuals at increased risk of fragility fractures. Cases reported and limited clinical trials have raised concerns in recent years, however, that prolonged bisphosphonate therapy may suppress bone remodeling to the extent that normal bone formation is impaired and fracture risk is increased. Fractures potentially resulting from suppressed bone turnover have been shown to be atypical, affecting sites such as the subtrochanteric femoral area that are infrequently affected by osteoporotic fractures (Sellemyer, 2010). Prior to fracture, thigh pain and no reports of injury or trauma are reported. As a result of these findings, current strategies include extensive fracture risk assessment, targeting bisphosphonate treatment for appropriate individuals at risk, and consideration of a 12-month interruption in therapy after 5 years of bisphosphonate treatment for those patients appropriate for alternative treatment (Sellemyer, 2010).

Osteonecrosis of the jaw (ONJ) is increasing since first identified in patients taking bisphosphonates in 2003 (Sellemeyer, 2010). As such, extensive dental evaluations and treatments are now recommended prior to the initiation of bisphosphonate medications. Those patients reporting severe complications of ONJ were frequently high-risk patients with preexisting dental disease, poor dentition, cancer, Paget's disease, or renal disease (Woo, Hande, & Richardson, 2005). ONJ is often not identified until bone is exposed in the jaw. This quickly presents with pain, soft tissue swelling, and infection following tooth extraction. Prevention measures for patients taking bisphosphonates include dental evaluations prior to the initiation of therapy and yearly dental health assessments to ensure excellent oral hygiene and care (Valverde, 2008).

Exercise. Regular weight-bearing exercises at least 3 times per week for 30 minutes are recommended to promote bone health. High-impact exercises should be avoided and vertebral spine rotation activities discouraged. A focus on balance exercises and core strengthening, to aid in fall prevention, should be incorporated into exercise programs (Carpenito-Moyet, 2009).

Pain Management. To avoid or lessen pain, patients should plan for rest periods between scheduled activities. The alternate application of heat and ice is recommended for comfort. Lumbosacral bracing for vertebral fractures is appropriate for short-term management. Patients may also use medications such as anti-inflammatory, non-narcotic, or narcotic analgesics, as recommended, and should maintain diets high in vitamins, calcium, and protein that promote healing (Carpenito-Moyet, 2009).

Surgical Management/Complication Management. An estimated 1.5 million vertebral compression fractures occur each year in the United States as a result of osteoporosis (HHS, 2004). Vertebral compression fractures cause pain and affect the quality of life due to vertebral deformity that cause height loss, mobility impediments, and balance difficulties, predisposing patients to falls and further injury. Non-surgical management of vertebral compression fracture includes analgesics, bed rest, back bracing, and physiotherapy.

Prior to the 1990s, conventional open surgery for vertebral compression fractures was indicated in patients that had neurological impairment; most were poor surgical risks with less-than-optimal outcomes (Taylor, 2006). During 1990s, vertebroplasty became the treatment of choice for fixation of vertebral compression fractures. Although this surgical option that was minimally invasive, it still proposed some risk. The use of cement injected into the vertebral fracture fixated the spine but did not restore the loss of height or correct the vertebral fracture instability. Complications also include extravasations of the cement into adjacent structures including both the colon and lung (Taylor, 2006).

Balloon kyphoplasty is currently the treatment of choice for vertebral compression fracture. To date, kyphoplasty has been identified as the most effective treatment for vertebral compression fractures (Wardlaw et al., 2009). Kyphoplasty can restore lost height through the balloon inflation technique. The procedure is commonly performed under moderate sedation. The patient may be able to be discharged the same day of surgery, or occasionally an overnight stay is indicated if additional medical concerns need evaluation.

Nursing Considerations

Nursing Diagnoses. Nursing diagnoses for this condition are expanded upon in the Appendix.

- Falls, risk for.
- Injury, risk for.
- Knowledge deficit.
- Nutrition: imbalance, less than body requires.
- Self-health management, ineffective.

Nursing Interventions. Education is focused on prevention strategies through identification and treatment of early bone loss in adults. Minimizing the complications associated with osteoporosis should be a life-long focus that includes healthy diet choices, weight-bearing exercise, and medication supplements as indicated.

Emotional support should be provided to adults diagnosed with metabolic bone disease. Despite a healthy lifestyle, bone loss can occur due to chronic diseases that have a hereditary predisposition, causing life-altering effects. This is due to the risks associated with fragility fractures and immobility.

Patient Teaching. Patient education should focus on nutrition and the importance of food sources high in calcium. Refer to Table 14.2 for recommended daily requirements. Exercises and activity includes weight-bearing exercises on long bones, especially walking exercises. Avoid twisting exercises of vertebral spine and hips. Education focused on medications should cover bisphosphonates and their effect and precautions.

Practice settings should include office and outpatient visits and should focus on early identification and treatment of osteoporosis. This includes post-acute care, especially following fracture follow-up for ongoing treatment and medication compliance. Fracture care follow-up and treatment to promote optimal bone health after hospitalization should also be considered. A focus on the long-term care environment of bed-bound adults is important and should include risk assessment, identification, and treatment, with both diet and medication, as indicated.

Table 14.2. Daily Calcium Requirements

Age	Male	Female	Pregnant	Lactating
Birth – 6 months	210 mg	210 mg		
7 – 12 months	270 mg	270 mg		
1 – 3 years	500 mg	500 mg		
4 – 8 years	800 mg	800 mg		
9 – 13 years	1,300 mg	1,300 mg		
14 – 18 years	1,300 mg	1,300 mg	1,300mg	1,300mg
19 – 50 years	1,000 mg	1,000mg	1,000 mg	1,000 mg
50+	1,200 mg	1,200mg		

From "Dietary Supplements" by the National Institutes of Health, 2009, www.ods.od.nih.gov. Reproduced with permission.

Osteomalacia

Overview

Definition. Osteomalacia is characterized by softening of the bone due to poor mineral content, leading to a marked deformity of weight-bearing bones, distortion of the bone structure, and possible pathologic fractures. Osteomalacia, which is caused by inadequate intake of vitamin D, often is referred to as adult rickets. It is less common than osteoporosis, and unlike osteoporosis, adults report symptoms that include myalgias, fatigue, muscle weakness, and bone pain (see Table 14.3). Osteomalacia is preventable and treatable (Prestwood, 2010).

Table 14.3. Comparison of Osteomalacia and Osteoporosis

Osteomalacia	Osteoporosis
Impaired bone mineralization due to inadequate vitamin D dietary intake and inadequate synthesis of vitamin D in the skin due to lack of exposure to sunlight	Rate of bone reabsorption more rapid than bone formation leading to porous fragile bones
Bone density and bone mass normal	T score representing the bone density in adults falls to - 2.5 standard deviations or below 0. Zero represents T score in healthy adults.
Symptoms include myalgias, fatigue, muscle weakness and bone pain	No pain or symptoms reported
Vitamin D needed for intestinal absorption of calcium	Heredity, decreased levels of estrogen and testosterone, lack of weight-bearing exercises, chronic disease, and side effects of medications can lead to osteoporosis
Less common than osteoporosis	Most common in post-menopause aged women
Treatable and preventable with medications and exposure to sunlight to avoid vitamin D deficiency	Treatment can delay complications With heredity predisposition, symptoms and bone loss can be delayed with healthy diet, exercise and weight bearing exercise and medications.

From Geriatric Review Syllabus: A Core Curriculum in Geriatric Medicine, 7th Ed. *by K. Prestwood, 2010.*

Etiology. Osteomalacia is most commonly attributed to an inadequate intake of vitamin D. Dietary deficiencies can be attributed to abnormal metabolism of vitamin D due to hepatic or renal disease and the side effect of medications used to treat these chronic diseases. Recent research has focused on the long-term effect of inadequate production of vitamin D due to limited sun exposure and metabolic bone disease, especially in adult women (Hathcock, Shao, Vieth, & Heaney, 2007).

Pathophysiology. Calcium is needed for bone formation and resorption in healthy bone. Vitamin D is needed for intestinal absorption of dietary calcium that aids in healthy bone formation, resorption, and remodeling of bone tissue in healthy adults. Osteomalacia is caused by a deficiency in vitamin D, causing difficulty with the protein framework and poor mineralization of bone tissue that leads to symptomatic bone pain. Unlike with osteoporosis, bone density and bone mass is normal but mineralization of bone is lacking. Both vitamin D and absorption of phosphate are needed to treat this mineral deficit. Deformity of weight-bearing bones and distortion of the bone structure leading to pathologic fractures, which are most common in the distal femur, are characterized as symmetric pseudo fractures (Prestwood, 2010).

Incidence and Risk Factors. Osteomalacia is more common in adult women than men. It is more prevalent in women who have not had adequate exposure to sunlight. In the literature, more recent research has focused on elderly women who are residents of institutional long-term care settings. Dark skin does not synthesize vitamin D as easily as fair skin. Those living in high altitudes also do not synthesize vitamin D as readily as those living in lower altitude regions. Vitamin D deficiency often is undiagnosed, and it is estimated that the incidence in acutely ill elderly adults is 3% to 5% (NOF, n.d.). Dietary deficiencies of vitamin D have been identified in strict vegetarians who limit dairy intake, severely malnourished adults, and women who have had multiple frequent pregnancies who breastfeed for extended periods of time between each pregnancy. Severe dietary deficiencies have also been identified in adults who have had partial or total gastrectomy, bypass, or small bowel resections. Those who are overweight and/or obese with poor dietary habits are also at increased risk of osteomalacia. Adults affected by chronic disease of the liver, kidney, and small intestine are affected by the decrease in bone mineralization caused by vitamin D deficiency. Anticonvulsant medications used to treat seizure disorders, phosphate-binding antacids, tranquilizers, sedatives, and muscle relaxants all can have a long-term negative effect on calcium and vitamin D absorption and healthy bone mineralization, increasing the risk of osteomalacia (Guyton, 2011).

Complications. Osteomalacia is characterized by generalized bone pain, myalgias, fatigue, muscle weakness, and distal femur fractures. The fractures are symmetric and often identified as pseudo-fractures that appear as radiolucent bands and occur in poorly mineralized dense bone (Guyton, 2011).

Assessment

History. The clinical manifestations of osteomalacia are subtle. Complaints of bone pain range from mild or aching to extreme tenderness when weight or pressure is applied to long bones. Muscle pain is localized, and strength is weak. The pelvic and dorsolumbar region are also reported as painful to palpation. Pain and weakness are characterized by difficulty ambulating or changing positions, and low back pain. This creates a high risk for falls in adults, especially those with an unsteady gait. A history of multiple fractures may be reported. Additional history may include renal problems, gastrointestinal difficulties, and poor dietary habits related to poor intake and absorption of vitamin D.

Physical Exam. Deformities of the long weight-bearing bones are common in patients with osteomalacia, as is kyphoscoliosis of the spine. Cox vara deformity of the femoral neck is due to the poor mineralization of bone, and pressure on the weight-bearing structure is reported. Poor posture and an unsteady gait increase risk of falls in adults.

Diagnostic Tests. Significant osteomalacia can exist without radiographic identified fracture. Pseudo-fractures are identified when the radiographic changes do occur in poorly mineralized bone. When fractures occur, they are most commonly identified at the distal femur, femoral neck, pubic rami, ribs, and clavicle (Guyton, 2011). Laboratory tests such as serum calcium, phosphate, parathyroid hormone (PTH), and vitamin D levels can identify deficiencies and osteomalacia (Porth, 2007).

These vitamin D levels are most effectively measured from September through March, due to the long-term effect of fat-soluble vitamin D properties of both dietary and vitamin D synthesis in the skin during exposure to sunlight (Moyad, 2009). Normal levels for vitamin D are 30ng/ml or 75 nmol/L. Treatment is focused on increasing the levels to at least 40ng/ml or 100nmol/L. This may take months to correct, with changes in diet, prescription medication, and sun exposure to maintain healthy levels of vitamin D (NOF, n.d.). (Refer to Tables 14.4, 14.5, and 14.6.).

Table 14.4. Adult Recommended Daily Vitamin D Dietary Intake	
Younger than Age 50	400-500 IU Vitamin D Daily
Older than Age 50	800 -1000 IU Vitamin D Daily

From "Dietary Supplements" by the National Institutes of Health, 2009, www.ods.od.nih.gov. Reproduced with permission.

Table 14.5. Foods Containing Vitamin D Essential for Calcium Absorption	
Salmon (sockeye) 3 oz. 794 IU Vitamin D	3 oz. = 50mg calcium
Tuna 3 oz 154 IU Vitamin D	3 oz. = 4 mg calcium
Egg Yolks – 1 25 IU Vitamin D	1 yolk = 21.9 mg calcium
Liver Beef – 3.5oz 46IU Vitamin D	3.5 oz = 5mg calcium
Milk – 1 cup 124 IU Vitamin D	8oz. = 300mg Calcium
Yogurt – 6 oz. 80 IU Vitamin D	6 oz. = 460mg Calcium
Juice Orange 1 cup – 100 IU Vitamin D	1 cup = 300mg Calcium
Breakfast Cereals – 1 cup 40 IU Vitamin D	1 cup = 1104mg Calcium

From "Dietary Supplements" by the National Institutes of Health, 2009, www.ods.od.nih.gov. Reproduced with permission.

Table 14.6. Prescriptive Vitamin D2 Ergocalciferol	
INFANTS	DOSE
0-6 Month	5 mcg/Day or 200 IU
7-12 Months	5 mcg/Day or 200 IU
CHILDREN	DOSE
1-13 Years	5 mcg/Day or 200 IU
TEEN THROUGH MID-ADULT	DOSE
14 – 50 Years	5 mcg/Day or 200 IU
LATE ADULT	DOSE
51 – 70 Years	10 mcg/Day or 400 IU
ELDERLY	DOSE
71 Years +	15 mcg/Day or 600 IU

From "Dietary Supplements" by the National Institutes of Health, 2009, www.ods.od.nih.gov. Reproduced with permission.

Common Therapeutic Modalities

There are two types of vitamin D prescribed. Initial studies showed D3 (cholecalciferol) to be the preferred treatment. Currently, both D2 (ergocalciferol) and D3 are equally effective in vitamin D deficiency prescriptive treatment (NOF, n.d.).

Nursing Considerations

Nursing Diagnoses. Nursing diagnoses for this condition are expanded upon in the Appendix.

- Comfort, impaired.
- Fatigue.
- Knowledge deficit.
- Nutrition: imbalance, less than body requires.
- Pain, acute.
- Pain, chronic.
- Self-health management, ineffective.

Practice Setting Considerations. Education in practice office and outpatient settings should include the importance of follow-up and testing. Within home care, education on dietary requirements with both foods and supplements should be provided to patients both in writing and verbally. Assisting patients in developing a written plan with education, exercise, diet, and medication should be encouraged.

Long-term care should be focused on identification of those patients most at risk for vitamin D deficiency to create a plan with a focus on exercise, healthy diet, and medication to promote health.

The effect of medication on chronic disease and the identification of these needs is an important part of the plan of care. Consideration of sunlight exposure, exercise, dietary intake, and supplements should be evaluated on an individual basis.

Rickets

Overview

Definition. Rickets is a deficiency in the mineralization and formation of the growing skeleton in infants and young children. It is characterized by softened, deformed bones. The organic matrix osteoid growth plate (epiphysis) and newly formed trabecular bone and cortical bone fail to calcify normally. This deficiency is due to inadequate calcium and phosphate deposition in the osteoid-formed growth plate prior to closure. Rickets is rare, and when it does occur, it is most commonly found in infants who have minimal sunlight exposure and are primarily receiving breast milk without supplements (Moyad, 2009). It is important that breast-fed infants receive vitamin D supplements during the first 2 months of life (Neild, Mahajan, Joshi, & Kamat, 2006). Rickets is both treatable and preventable.

Etiology. Rickets was first identified in the literature in 1650. In 1922, medical research identified cod liver oil as both preventative and curative for vitamin D deficiency (Moyad, 2009). Nutritional rickets occurs in infants or young children who fail to ingest recommended daily requirements of vitamin D. This can also occur with insufficient absorption of minerals from gastrointestinal impairment found in children with celiac disease or cystic fibrosis. Vitamin D deficiency is reflected in decreased levels of calcium and phosphorus that affects the organic matrix of bone (Moyad, 2009). (See Tables 14.4, 14.5, and 14.6 in the section on osteomalacia for vitamin D intake recommendations.)

Renal disease in children creates an abnormally high level of excretion of minerals through the kidneys that produces a malfunction of the tubercles and loss of glomerular function. Congenital hypophosphatemia is produced by an inadequate synthesis of calcitriol vitamin D3. Calcification of bone is impaired due to the abnormal absorption of vitamin D and alkaline phosphatase (Moyad, 2009).

Pathophysiology. Both vitamin D and calcium are needed for bone formation and resorption. Growing bones fail to mineralize when inadequate intake of vitamin D and/or calcium occurs. This is due to the nutritional deficit of vitamin D, as well as familial or hereditary hypophosphatemia. The aim is to identify and diagnosis rickets early in life and implement treatment to resolve bone demineralization and prevent complications that lead to deformity or the need for surgical intervention (Nield et al., 2006).

Incidence. The diagnosis of rickets is usually established in infants or young children between 3 months and 3 years of age. Rickets can affect all bones, but the most common deformities are located in the spine and long bones of the lower extremities. Chronic disease and the risk of hereditary tendencies can cause rickets. Children whose parents are vegetarians and children whose parents avoid dairy products, especially breast-fed infants who are not given vitamin Dfortified milk products, are at most risk of rickets. Lack of exposure to sunlight that occurs in winter and non-tropical climates are also established as risk factors for young children (Nield et al. 2006).

Considerations Across the Life Span. Rickets is most identified during infancy and early childhood but rarely detected in adolescents. The most common age group identified is 3 months to 3 years of age (Nield et al., 2006).

Assessment

History. Rickets is usually identified as a nutritional deficiency in breast-fed infants not receiving supplemental vitamin D as part of their routine well baby care. The infant displays increased restlessness at night, profuse diaphoresis, skin pallor, and lack of interest in play for normal development milestones.

Physical Exam. During routine physical examinations or well baby visits, inflammation of the mucous membranes is noted with frequent infections and diarrhea. Recent research identified problems with immune response in relation to vitamin D deficiencies (Nield et al. 2006). If the vitamin deficiency is severe, central nervous system irritability that results in muscle spasm or convulsions can occur. Hypocalcemia can cause tetany. The fontanels of the skull are late in closing, and the cranium is enlarged and square in appearance. A deformity of the chest wall, with enlargement and depression at the sternum, is noted a few inches above the lower costal margin in these infants. This is caused by the pulling of the diaphragm on the softened ribs, while the chest cage is narrowed transversely and elongated anteroposterior. This is commonly referred to as a pigeon breast. Compression fractures of the vertebrae spine can occur, resulting in a twisted spinal column. The abdomen may be enlarged and prominent. The epiphyses (rounded ends of a long bone) delay closure of the growth plate, especially with rapid growth in children found in the knee and wrist during this age. Delayed dentition is noted early on in infancy. Poor muscle tone is common, resulting in the delay of development with walking and crawling. Deformities of the extremities consequent to weight-bearing makes early attempts at ambulation difficult. A short stature is noted, as rickets progresses and bone formation is affected (Weisberg, Scanlon, Li, & Cogswell, 2004).

Diagnostic Tests. *Laboratory findings:* Children affected by nutritional deficiencies have abnormally low levels of calcium and vitamin D. Serum phosphorus is reduced, and alkaline phosphatase is elevated. In patients with renal disease, problems occur with absorption and secretion of these minerals. Serum calcium is decreased, and serum phosphorus is elevated.

Radiographic findings: In the early stages of rickets, the epiphysis of bones is poorly defined and frayed. Cortical bone is reduced, and the bone is coarse and broader. The pelvis is compressed transversely, and the inlet is abnormally narrowed. Long weight-bearing bones are bent, and cortices are thickened on the concave side. Intestinal dilation that affects the absorption of both calcium and vitamin D is noted in children with celiac disease or cystic fibrosis (Benson, Fixsen, & Macnical, 2010).

Common Therapeutic Modalities

The importance of vitamin D nutritional requirements early in life, especially in breast-feeding infants, has been established. Exposure to sunlight for premature infants with feeding difficulties is critical. Supplemental vitamin D is important for children with celiac disease and cystic fibrosis, due to absorption problems of calcium and vitamin D in the intestine. Occasionally, an osteotomy is necessary after growth is complete to correct bone deformities related to the long-term deformity that affects bone structures (Nield et al. 2006).

Nursing Considerations

Nursing Diagnoses. Nursing diagnoses for this condition are expanded upon in the Appendix.

- Injury, risk for.
- Knowledge deficit.
- Nutrition: imbalance, less than body requires.
- Self-health management, ineffective.

Practice Setting Considerations. Education in office and outpatient environments should focus on prevention, diagnosis, and treatment to parents as part of well baby visits. Identify symptoms that require intervention, and consider the need for a home care evaluation. Educate on sunlight exposure and the importance of vitamin D. Teaching needs to include assessment of the home environment, with a focus on safety to avoid injury, fracture, and minor trauma that predisposes to fracture and deformity to weakened bones. Evaluate the need for lifelong dietary alterations and consideration of daily nutritional requirements of vitamin D and supplements.

Figure 14.1.
Endocrine and Mineral Metabolism

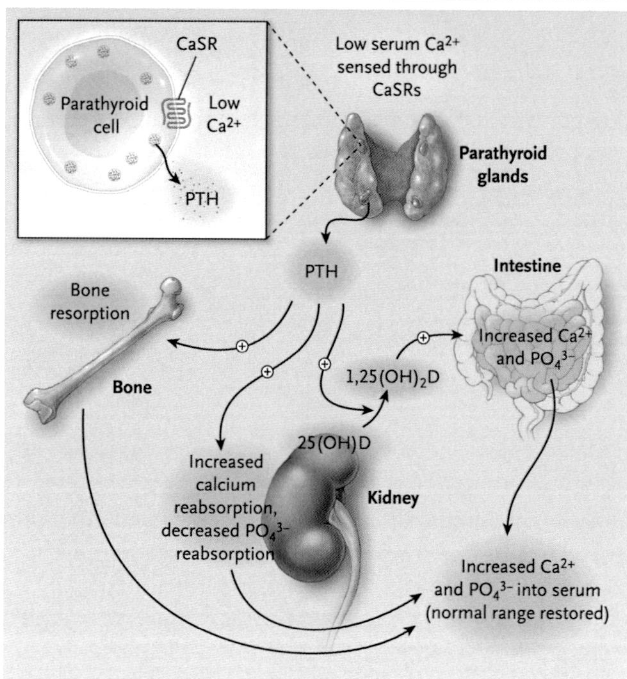

From "Hypoparathryoidism" by D. Shoback, 2008, New England Journal of Medicine, *359:4. pg 393. Reproduced with permission.*

Primary Hyperparathyroidism

Overview

Definition. Hyperparathyroidism occurs when one or more of the four parathyroid glands are enlarged. This results in the excessive secretion of parathyroid hormone (PTH) by the enlarged, overactive gland. This imbalance in PTH interrupts the metabolism of calcium and phosphorus, leading to an elevation in serum calcium (or hypercalcemia).

Etiology. The most common cause of hyperparathryoidism is a benign solitary encapsulated adenoma in a single affected gland. This accounts for 85% to 96% of all primary hyperparathryoidism. Less than 5% of all hyperparathryoidism cases are determined to be malignant. The treatment is often invasive, requiring extensive surgery (Lloyd, 2010).

Pathophysiology. The levels of calcium are controlled by the action of the parathyroid and the secretion of PTH (see Figure 14.1). The extracellular sensing receptors (CaSRs) within the parathyroid gland detect the levels of calcium in the blood. When calcium levels are decreased, increased levels of PTH secretion occurs; when calcium levels are high, PTH secretion is suppressed. PTH stimulates bone resorption that delivers calcium and phosphorus (PO4) into the circulation. When PTH is reduced or absent, homeostasis is impaired, affecting the intestine, kidney, and bone. This may result in hypocalcemia, hyperphosphatemia, and hypercalciuria (Shoback, 2008).

Incidence. Primary hyperparathryoidism occurs in 1 of every 1,000 individuals (Lloyd, 2010). Women are affected twice as frequently as men (Lloyd, 2010). Hyperparathryoidism ranges from asymptomatic to severe. In severe cases, confusion, lethargy, and dehydration may cause rapid deterioration leading to stupor and coma if left untreated. (Refer to Table 14.7.)

Complications. Hyperparathryoidism causes bones to become brittle due to osteoporosis. Renal calculi and nephrolithiasis lead to renal insufficiency, due to the elevation in serum calcium, and can cause chronic renal failure. Peptic ulcer disease can also develop. Central nervous system disorders, ranging from mild personality disorders to severe psychiatric disorders, can occur. Calcium thrombi can develop and migrate to the lungs, heart, or pancreas. Skin necrosis and cataracts can occur (Lloyd, 2010). Hypertension and nephrolithiasis are the most commonly reported complications in most patients. "Kidney stones, painful bones, abdominal groans, lethargic moans, and psychiatric overtones" is a common rhyme frequently associated with complications of hyperparathryoidism in patient assessment findings (Lew & Solorzano, 2009).

Considerations Across the Life Span. Hyperparathryoidism is very rare in children. It is more common in women and seen primarily in patients between the ages of 50 to 70 years of age (Lloyd, 2010).

Assessment

History Physical and Exam. Osteoclastic activity and destruction of the bone may occur, resulting in osteodystrophy and defects in bone development. Bone density is affected, leading to extensive decalcification and the development of punched-out cystic areas of bone that are filled with giant cell tumors (osteitis fibosa cystica). This causes generalized bone weakness. Anemia may result due to the fibrous tissue replacing the bone marrow. Hypercalciuria causes a high calcium level to overwhelm the renal tubular resorptive mechanism. Renal calculi are formed as the excretion of large amounts of phosphates and calcium is present in the urine. Renal calculi and nephrolithiasis result in an obstruction and, if left untreated, can lead to both infection and renal failure. Poliuria will result due to the calcium loss that impairs renal water conservation, interfering with the action of antidiuretic hormone. Hypercalcemia may result in anorexia, nausea, vomiting, and constipation because of the diminished contractility of the muscular walls of the gastrointestinal tract.

The increased secretion of gastrin and pepsin results in a susceptibility to peptic ulcers. There is also an increased incidence of pancreatitis in this population. Cardiac complications are due to an increase in serum calcium, including electrocardiograph changes of shortened QT interval, prolonged PR interval, and dysrhythmias causing heart block and leading to cardiac arrest if left untreated. The central nervous system is depressed, and reflexes become sluggish. Muscles are weak due to the effects of elevated calcium on cell conduction. Renal complications with flank pain can develop, and changes with urinary output may occur. Nephrolithiasis is due to calcium secretion, and clearance within the renal tubule and can develop into problems with renal insufficiency and failure.

Table 14.7. Hyperparathroidism – Incidence and Risk Factors

Primary	Secondary	Tertiary
Benign solitary encapsulated adenoma in parathyroid gland 85-96% of all primary hyperparathyroidism	Hyperplasia excessive parathryroid hormone production Rare underlying disease pathology	Occurs most commonly after renal transplant following end stage renal disease 30% renal transplant patients
1:1000 Adults Women 2x as affected than men 50-70 years of age	Found most common with chronic renal failure 90% cases develop after hemodialysis treatment initiated	All 4 parathyroid glands enlarged. Over secretion of PTH due to enlarged size of gland

From "JAMA Patient Page: Hyperparathyroidism" by J. Troppy, 2005, Journal of the American Medical Association, 293(14), p. 1810. Reproduced with permission.

Diagnostic Tests. Normal serum calcium levels in laboratory studies range from are 8.5mg/dl to 10.4mg/dl in healthy adults. Ninety-five percent of patients with hyperparathyroidism present serum calcium levels greater than 10mg/dl. Serum phosphorus levels fall below 1.8mg/dl due to the inverse relationship with serum calcium elevation. Serum magnesium directly affects PTH secretion. When magnesium levels fall below 1meq/L, PTH secretion is impaired. Serum alkaline phosphatase is increased. This causes acceleration of bone disease, resulting in hypercalcemia that leads to an elevation in serum alkaline phosphatase (Lloyd, 2010). Radiographic studies are helpful in determining the extent of the bone resorption in hyperparathyroidism. Bone density and cyst formation are visible on x- rays showing demineralization and decreased bone density. Bone mineral density (BMD) measurements also report decreased bone density. Localized studies that include parathyroid ultrasound show enlargement of one or more of the parathyroid glands. This may indicate the need for a fine needle biopsy of the thyroid or parathyroid if cancer is suspected.

Common Therapeutic Modalities

Treatment for hypercalcemia with calcium levels over 14mg/dl is indicated. Dialysis may be indicated in patients who have critical calcium levels in emergent situations. Although rare, surgical recommendations may involve removal of the parathyroid gland by subtotal resection. Autotransplantation of the parathyroid remnant to the forearm to prevent subsequent hypoparathryroidism may be the recommended treatment of choice. Autotransplantation of the parathyroid gland is only performed when surgeries require total parathryoidectomy to avoid complications of hypoparathyroidism following surgery. Supplementation of calcium and vitamin D may continue to be indicated (Plitt, Sipple, & Chen, 2009).

Nursing Considerations

Nursing Diagnoses. Nursing diagnoses for this condition are expanded upon in the Appendix.

- Knowledge deficit.
- Nutrition: imbalance, less than body requires.
- Self-health management, ineffective.

It is important to encourage fluid intake up to 3 liters per day to avoid dehydration. Sodium intake should be limited to 8-10grams per day. Phosphorus supplements are important, except for patients with a history of renal calculi. As part of biannual blood work, serum calcium and creatinine clearance tests should be monitored.

Practice Setting Considerations. The importance of providing education regarding diagnosis, treatment, and interventions is indicated. Arrange for outpatient diagnostic care and tests. Provide home care for follow-up teaching and education. Patient teaching should include signs and symptoms of hypercalcemia and hypocalcemia. Long-term care includes life-long monitoring of serum calcium and renal function. BMD evaluation, dietary supplements, and medications for calcium and phosphorus levels should be administered as indicated.

Secondary and Tertiary Hyperparathyroidism

Overview

Definition: Secondary Hyperparathyroidism. Secondary hyperparathyroidism is caused by hyperplasia and excessive parathyroid hormone production. Secondary hyperparathyroidism is a rarity and caused by underlying disease pathology. Although secondary and tertiary hyperparathyroidism are commonly discussed and researched together, they are two distinct and separate disease entities (Soback, 2008). (Refer to Table 14.7 for a comparison of primary, secondary, and tertiary hyperparathyroidism.) Secondary hyperparathyroidism is most commonly due to chronic renal failure. Approximately 90% of all cases develop after hemodialysis treatment is initiated (Shoback, 2008). This is caused by hyperplasia of the parathyroid gland causing difficulty with calcium, vitamin D, and phosphate metabolism.

Definition: Tertiary Hyperparathyroidism. Tertiary hyperparathyroidism occurs primarily in renal transplant patients following renal allograft. With tertiary hyperparathyroidism, all four parathyroid glands are enlarged, and hyperplasia leads to an elevation in PTH levels (Shoback, 2008).

Pathophysiology. Hypocalcemia stimulates the secretion of PTH, which continues to rise along with the serum calcium levels. High PTH levels result in excessive bone resorption. Calcium and phosphorus resorption from the bone matrix cause bone to demineralize and weaken.

Incidence. Primary hyperplasia of the parathyroid gland is most common in patients with end-stage renal disease. It is reported that approximately 30% of all renal transplant patients have persistent hyperplasia of the parathyroid that may initially resolve but reoccur and continue to have an over-secretion of PTH (Shobeck, 2008). The symptoms of this chronic disease state results in hypercalcemia. Management of elevated serum calcium levels is needed, and treatment recommendations are indicated.

Assessment

Same as primary hyperparathyroidism.

Common Therapeutic Modalities

During 2004, the Federal Drug Administration (FDA) approved the calcimimetic medication cinacalcet (Sensipar) that aids in decreasing the amount of serum calcium by signaling the parathyroid to produce less PTH. This is used for patients with chronic kidney disease or parathyroid cancer. The initial dose is 30mg oral administration daily.

Weekly laboratory levels of serum calcium and phosphorus are measured to titrate the medication, as needed, to suppress PTH and lower serum calcium levels. Patients should be instructed on monitoring for signs and symptoms of hypocalcemia. This includes seizures, muscle aches, cramps, and burning or tingling of the lips, tongue, fingers, or feet. These signs and symptoms should be reported to their physician, especially as medication dosing is adjusted. Medical management of patients includes vitamin D therapy, dialysis for patients with end-stage renal disease, and renal transplant if indicated.

Nursing Considerations

Nursing Diagnoses. Nursing diagnoses for this condition are expanded upon in the Appendix.

- Knowledge deficit.
- Nutrition: imbalance, less than body requires.
- Self-health management, ineffective.

Hypoparathyroidism

Overview

Definition. Hypoparathyroidism is a deficiency or absence of PTH due to disease, injury, or congenital malfunction of the parathyroid glands.

Etiology. Hypoparathyroidism can be acute or chronic and is classified as idiopathic, acquired, and/or reversible (see Table 14.8).

Table 14.8. Hypoparathroidism		
Idiopathic	**Acquired**	**Acquired Reversible**
Atrophy of the Parathyroid	Accidental removal or injury during surgery or ischemic infarction	Resulting from any condition that causes hypomagnesemia such alcoholism or malabsortion syndrome that inhibits PTH secretion
DiGeorge syndrome is a childhood disease that results in total absence of the parathyroid gland affects children at birth	Injury to the parathyroid can also be caused by tuberculosis (TB) neoplasms or trauma	Results from any disorder that limits Vitamin D availability such as gastrointestinal surgery, pancreatitis, small intestine malabsorption or hepatic or renal disease.
More common in children	More common in older adults who undergo surgery for hyperparathyroidism	More common in children

Adapted from "Hypoparathryoidism" by D. Shoback, 2008, New England Journal of Medicine, 359*(4) 391-403.*

Pathophysiology. Low PTH levels result in neuromuscular excitability and tetany due to low serum calcium levels as a consequence of low PTH. Decreased renal phosphate excretion and decreased intestinal absorption of calcium create mild metabolic alkalosis. Mental changes and Parkinson-like symptoms are common.

Complications. Tetany, seizures, and laryngospasms can occur due to hypocalcemia. Mental status changes that include psychosis, anxiety, depression, and delirium have been reported. Cardiac dysrhythmias and congestive heart failure are common with decreased serum calcium levels that affect cardiac muscle function. With children, dental abnormalities such as hypoplasia of the enamel and delayed eruption of teeth will occur.

Assessment

History. Chronic diseases may include intestinal absorption difficulties and family history of hypoparathyroidism in both adults and children. Most common is the acquired hypoparathyroidism following recent surgery of the parathyroid due to hyperparathyroidism. During surgery, accidental removal of or injury to the parathyroid gland causes impairment or complete absence of PTH production. Severe metabolic imbalances are reported among adults with long-term alcohol abuse that can lead to hypocalcemia and low PTH levels.

Physical Exam. Neuromuscular irritability and skeletal muscle twitches can lead to tetany as a result of low serum calcium levels. Low serum calcium levels can be indicative of a positive Chvostek sign. To test for Chvostek sign, ipsilateral contraction of the facial nerve is elicited by tapping on the facial nerve just below the zygomatic bone, anterior to the ear. It is reported that 10 to 30% of adults with normal calcium levels can be positive for Chvostek sign (Shoback, 2008). A positive Chvostek sign cannot be used solely as diagnostic unless it was previously assessed as absent. Hyperirritability of the facial nerve can occur in tetany or hypocalcemia.

Cardiovascular changes including electrocardiogram abnormalities with a prolonged QT interval are due to hypocalcemia. Tachycardia and decreased cardiac output with congestive heart failure can occur if left untreated.

Gastrointestinal symptoms include increased gastric motility and hyperactive bowel sounds with abdominal cramping and diarrhea. Skin changes may occur as dry or flaking skin, and nails and hair will be brittle with visible thinning of the eyebrows.

Diagnostic Tests. Laboratory studies commonly report that serum calcium in decreased. Tetany occurs at 6 to 7mg/dl serum calcium levels, and serum phosphorus is increased to greater than 5.4mg/dl. Magnesium, chloride, and uric acid are increased. Vitamin D levels are low. Radiographic studies report that decreased bone density is a late manifestation following chronic hypoparathyroidism. Tooth roots are absent. Calcification of the cerebellum and cerebral basal ganglia causes dementia and delirium in adults.

Common Therapeutic Modalities

Acute hypoparathyroidism is true medical emergency. Emergent care is needed to maintain the airway, prevent laryngeal spasms and seizures, and control tetany. Medical management and treatment can be life-long. Vitamin D supplement with calcium supplement is indicated. Acute life-threatening tetany requires immediate IV administration of calcium gluconate at 10mg to 20mg of 10% solution until tetany can be reversed. Sedatives and anticonvulsants are administered until serum calcium levels are less critical.

Nursing Considerations

Nursing Diagnoses. Nursing diagnoses for this condition are expanded upon in the Appendix.

- Knowledge deficit.
- Nutrition: imbalance, less than body requires.
- Self-health management, ineffective.

Practice Setting Considerations. Education and follow-up, in both the outpatient and office settings, are important. Provide information concerning diagnostic tests and dietary requirements. Instruct the patient to check pulse rates for bradycardia and report if heart rate falls below 60 beats per minute. Instruct on signs and symptoms of hypocalcemia. Provide information to the patient and significant others on seizure precautions, prevention of injury, and contacts for emergency intervention when indicated. Bone density evaluation should be provided initially to establish a baseline, and yearly follow up is indicated.

Paget's Disease (Osteitis Deformans)

Overview

Definition. Paget's disease (osteitis deformans) is a bone loss-associated disease that is marked by rapid bone resorption followed by rapid bone formation. The structure of the bone is disorganized and susceptible to deformity, fracture, and pain. At the sites of affected bone, increased osteoclast activity, with the recruitment of osteoblasts, contributes to excessive new bone formation (Valverde, 2008).

Etiology. The exact cause of Paget's disease is unknown. A genetic predisposition has been reported to be susceptible to a viral response that causes dormant skeletal effects on bone resorption and bone formation, leading to this disease later in life. In the literature, recent research has focused on the exposure to paramyxovirus infection (mumps) as a possible cause (Paget Foundation, 2010). A family history of the disease may be reported in 15% of families with an adult relative diagnosed with this disease (Ralston, Langston, & Reid, 2008).

Pathophysiology. Paget's disease is characterized by focal areas of increased bone turnover. The osteoclastic phase causes excessive bone resorption, followed by an osteoblastic phase that accelerates abnormal bone formation and results in a disorganized weak bone structure. New bone is fragile and susceptible to deformity, fracture, and pain. The bone marrow is frequently replaced by fibrous tissue that has increased vascularity. The abnormal bone is less compact than normal bone. Early stages of Paget's disease are typically asymptomatic; by the time the patient experiences pain, the bone deformity may be extensive (Ralston, Langston, & Reid, 2008).

Incidence. Paget's disease is extremely rare in Asia, the Middle East, Africa, and Scandinavia. In the United States, Paget's disease is second only to osteoporosis in bone loss-associated disease in adults over the age of 50. Approximately 3% of the population in affected (Valverde, 2008). It is slightly more common in males than females.

Complications. Paget's disease is characterized by bone calcification due to disturbed mineral metabolism that contributes to vascular calcifications leading to heart disease and congestive heart failure. As bone deformities of the skull press on cranial nerves, the resulting nerve compression syndrome may cause vertigo, hearing loss, and vision problems. Hypercalcemia and hypercalciuria can cause renal calculi. A waddling gait can be attributed to softening of the pelvic bones and bowing of the femur and tibia. Calcified periarthritis may lead to gout and secondary arthritis. The risk for fractures occurs as bone deformity and weakened bone structure develops.

Assessment

Physical Exam. Patients frequently report persistent and severe bone pain with advancing disease. Pain to the lower extremities increases with weight-bearing activities. The gait may be affected due to impingement on the spinal cord nerves or nerve root. Special consideration to areas of deformity, pain, and neurological deficits identify symptoms that may initially be vague and difficult to distinguish from other diseases. Skull involvement results in an enlarged cranium, with a prominent visible frontal lobe. Kyphosis (with a barrel-shaped chest) affects cardiac and pulmonary function with advancing disease. Bowing and hypertrophy of the femur and tibia may lead to reduced height and problems with ambulation. Gait disturbances put patients at increase risk of falls and fragility fracture. Focal areas are warm and tender to the touch because of increased vascularity at the area of new accelerated bone formation. Fractures at these sites heal slowly, and often non-union of bone is reported (Ralston et al., 2008).

Diagnostic Tests. Often patients are not diagnosed and are asymptomatic early in the disease process. First findings indicate increased levels of serum alkaline phosphatase (ALP), urinary hydroyproline, and serum uric acid due to the rapid abnormal bone metabolism (Ralston et al., 2008). The primary diagnosis of Paget's disease is confirmed with radiological findings. Early phases are characterized by osteolytic lesions, mostly found on the skull and long bones. Adjoining overgrowth of bone appears coarse and irregular in shape. After symptoms are identified, x- rays show characteristic mosaic pattern (Ralston et al., 2008). Radioactive bone scan can assist with diagnosis, showing intense uptake and focal pattern due to abnormal accelerated bone activity. In patients who do not respond to therapy or treatment, a bone biopsy may be indicated.

Common Therapeutic Modalities

Pain management and symptomatic treatment with aspirin, non-steroidal anti-inflammatory medications, or narcotics may be indicated. Calcitonin, commonly prescribed to inhibit bone resorption, acts by lowering serum calcium levels by promoting secretion through the kidneys and decreasing bone lesions. Calcitonin also has an unexplained analgesic effect that aids in decreasing bone pain in most patients. It can be administered subcutaneously or intravenously. Mialcalcin has been most effective by nasal spray administration that avoids gastrointestinal irritation. Bisphosphonates are the treatment of choice, administered to decrease the rate of bone resorption (Ralston et al., 2008).

Medical management is indicated to prevent further bone loss, as is therapeutic diagnostic laboratory monitoring of calcium, phosphorus, and vitamin D. Kidney function, neurological and cardiovascular assessment, and evaluation for advancing disease are important because of the chronic nature of bone vascular calcification and complications.

Surgical evaluation may be indicated due the ongoing risk of pathological fractures caused by poor bone quality, fragility fracture, and deformity. Neurological impairment associated with Paget's disease is due to bone deformity and nerve compression of spinal nerves that contributes to back pain and difficulty with ambulation. Total joint arthroplasty may be indicated as arthritis and bone deformity continues to develop. Medication administered during the perioperative period may increase the risk of bleeding due to excessive hypervascularity of the affected bone.

Nursing Considerations

Nursing Diagnoses. Nursing diagnoses for this condition are expanded upon in the Appendix.

- Comfort, impaired.
- Falls, risk for.
- Health behavior, risk-prone.
- Pain, acute.
- Pain, chronic.
- Self-health management, ineffective.

Practice Setting Considerations. Life-long monitoring of laboratory values that include calcium and serum ALP is needed to monitor ongoing bone remodeling and ongoing assessment of skeletal deformity. Supportive care for progressive complications is needed. Fall risk prevention for fragility fracture includes recommendations for exercises that focus on balance and core strength training. Assessment of the home environment to prevent falls is indicated.

Summary

Metabolic bone diseases and disorders are known to affect skeletal structures caused by defective mineralization of bone. Over the past decade, a greater focus has been placed on early detection and identification of bone loss and the need for education and prevention. The United States Health and Human Services and the Health People 2020 program have established strategies for chronic disease management with prevention, dietary, vitamin and mineral requirements, and exercise have been established to promote life-long habits to preserve and promote bone health. The HealtyPeople.gov initiative focuses on an established agenda and framework to provide prevention and educational strategies for osteoporosis, including fall prevention and risk reduction for fragility fractures in adults. Over the past decade, technology and treatment for metabolic bone disease has advanced in establishing screening and risk stratification for bone density and parameters for evidence-based treatment strategies to avoid bone fragility and the associated risk for fracture and deformity. Chronic hereditary-associated diseases that effect bone health include renal dysfunction, parathyroidism, malabsorption disease of the gastrointestinal system, and Paget's disease. Some metabolic bone diseases are preventable and can be avoided with a healthy diet and exercise plan that focuses on calcium and vitamin D intake. Most important is to identify risk factors related to heredity, to monitor dietary, calcium, and vitamin D intake, and to encourage exercise as part of a focus on bone health.

References

Benson, M., Fixsen, J., & Macnical, M. (2010). *Children's Orthopaedics and Fractures* (3rd ed.). New York, NY: Springer.

Bickley, L.S. & Szilagyi, P.G. (2007). *Bates Guide to Physical Exam and History Taking* (10th ed.). Philadelphia, PA: Lippincott.

Carpenito-Moyet, L.J. (2009). *Nursing Care Plans & Documentation: Nursing Diagnosis & Collaborative Problems.* Philadelphia, PA: Lippincott Williams & Wilkins.

Connor, A. (2009). Newer therapeutic agents and strategies for the management of chronic kidney disease and mineral bone disorder. *Postgraduate Medicine Journal*, 85, 274-279.

Guyton, A.C. (2011). Parathyroid hormone, calcitonin, calcium and phosphate metabolism, vitamin D, bone and teeth. In A.Guyton & J. Hall, *Textbook of Medical Physiology* (12th ed.). Philadelphia, PA: W.B. Saunders.

Hathcock, J., Shao, A., Vieth, R., & Heaney, R., (2007). Risk assessment for vitamin D. *American Journal of Clinical Nutrition.* 85:6-18.

Healthy People 2020. (n.d.). Retrieved 2011 from www. Healthypeople.gov

Huether, S.E. & McCance, K.L. (2007). *Understanding Pathophysiology* (4th ed.). St. Louis, MO: Mosby, Inc.

Lew, J. & Solorzano, C. (2009). Surgical management of primary hyperparathyroidism: State of the art. *Surgical Clinics of North America*, 89, 1205-1225.

Lloyd, R. (2010). *Endocrine Pathology Differential Diagnosis and Molecular Advances* (2nd ed.). Totowa, NJ: Humana Press.

Moyad, M. (2009). Vitamin D: A rapid review. *Dermatology Nursing, 21*(1).

National Institutes of Health. (2009). Dietary supplements. Retrieved January 2011 from www.ods.od.nih.gov

National Osteoporosis Foundation (NOF). (n.d.). Retrieved January 2011 from http://www.nof.org

Nield, L.S., Mahajan, P., Joshi A., & Kamat, D. (2006). Rickets: Not a disease of the past. *American Family Physician, 74*, 619-26.

Nursing 2011 Drug Handbook. (2010). Philadelphia, PA: Lippincott Williams & Wilkins.

Plitt, S., Sippel, R., & Chen, H. (2009). Secondary and tertiary hyperparathryoid: State of the art of surgical management. *Surgical Clinics of North America, 89*, 1227-1239.

Porth, C. (2007). *Essentials of Pathoghysiology: Concepts of Altered Health states* (2nd ed.). Philadelphia, PA: Lippincott Williams & Wilkins.

Prestwood, K. (2010). Osteoporosis and osteomalacia. In *Geriatric Review Syllabus: A Core Curriculum in Geriatric Medicine* (7th ed). New York, NY: American Geriatrics Society.

Raisz, L. G. (2009). Overview of pathogenesis. In *Primer on Metabolic Bone Diseases and Disorders of Mineral Metabolism* (pp. 203-206). Hoboken, NJ: John Wiley & Sons.

Ralston, S., Langston, A., & Reid, I., (2008). Pathogenesis and management of Paget's disease of the bone. *Lancet, 372*, 155-63.

Richmond, B.J., Dalinka, M.K., Daffner, R.H., Bennett, D.L., Jacobson, J.A., Resnick, C.S., …Haralson, R.H. (2007). Expert Panel on Musculoskletal Imaging. *Osteoporosis and bone mineral density*. Reston, VA: American College of Radiology.

Sellmeyer, D. (2010). Atypical fractures as a potential complication of long-term bisphosphonate therapy. *Journal of the American Medical Association, 304*(13),1480-1484.

Shoback, D. (2008). Hypoparathryoidism. *New England Journal of Medicine, 359*(4), 391-403.

Taylor, R.S. (2006). Balloon kyphoplasty and vertebroplasty for vertebral compression fractures: A comparative systematic review of efficacy and safety. *Spine, 31*, 2747-2755.

Torpy, J.M., Cassio, L., & Glass, R. (2005). Hyperparathyroidism. *Journal of the American Medical Association, 293*(14), 1818.

United States Department of Health and Human Services (HHS). (n.d.). Dietary Supplements. Retrieved January 2011 from www.ods.od.nih.gov

Valverde, P. (2008). Pharmacotherapies to manage bone loss associated disease: A quest for the perfect benefit to risk ratio. *Current Medical Chemistry, 15*, 284-304.

Wardlaw, D., ... & Boonen, S. (2009). Efficacy and safety of balloon kyphoplasty compared with non-surgical care for vertebral compression fracture (FREE): A randomized controlled trial. *Lancet, 373*, 1016-24.

Weisberg, P., Scanlon, K., Li, R., and Cogswell, M. (2004). Nutritional rickets among children in the US: Review of cases reported between 1986-2003. *American Journal of Clinical Nutrition* 1697s-7053 80(6suppl).

Woo, S., Hande, K., & Richardson, P. (2005). Osteonecrosis of the jaw and bisphosphonates. *New England Journal of Medicine,* 356(1), 99-102.

World Health Organization, Volume 81, Number 11. November 2003. Retrieved January 2011. WWW.WHO.int/entity/bulletin/volume81/11/en/-26K

World Health Organization. Volume 81, October 7, 2005. Retrieved January 2011. WWW.WHO.int/entity/nutrition/publication/micronutrient/GFF-references-en.pdf

Chapter 15
Orthopaedic Trauma

Kelly A. McDevitt, RN, MS, ONC

Objectives

- Identify mechanisms of injury associated with musculoskeletal trauma.
- Describe common traumatic injuries and their incidence across the life span.
- Summarize nursing assessment for common traumatic injuries.
- Identify therapeutic modalities and interventions typical for common traumatic injuries.
- Evaluate the effectiveness of nursing interventions for common traumatic musculoskeletal injuries.

Trauma antedates recorded history. Anthropological findings have shown that Neanderthal humans sustained a great deal of trauma during their lifetime, as a result of constant exposure to the harsh elements and dangerous encounters with wild animals. Treatment for orthopaedic trauma has been linked to ancient Egypt, where splints have been found on mummies made of bamboo, reeds, and wood, and padded with linens, as well as in ancient Greece, where Hippocrates detailed the care of dislocated shoulders, hips, and knees, as well as treatments for infections.

Many developments in trauma care and orthopaedic treatment have resulted from wartime experiences. A formal systematic trauma system is be credited to Dominique Larrey, a surgeon in Napoleon's French army who introduced the concept of the "flying ambulance" to provide organized rapid transport of the injured away from the battlefield (Trunkey, 2007). During World War I, the use of traction and splinting were more formally developed (Sherk, 2008). World War II saw the German pioneering of intramedulary fixation to speed recovery of soldiers, a system that was quickly adopted by the rest of the world (Sherk, 2008). Currently, traumatic injury is a major public health problem around the world and is predicted to increase worldwide in the 21st century (McQuillan, Makic, & Whalen, 2009).

Trauma refers to any injury that a person sustains as a result of the transfer of energy being absorbed by the body. A traumatic injury can be a major threat to the immediate and often long-term health of individuals. Trauma injuries vary widely in their level of severity. A simple ankle sprain or a laceration from cutting a bagel may seem benign when compared to a skull fracture, gunshot wound, or traumatic amputation; however, they are all types of traumatic injuries. An understanding of orthopaedic trauma can help to minimize the loss of limb function and life. In addition, sound knowledge of orthopaedics is needed during natural disasters or for volunteer work abroad with groups such as Project Cure and Doctors without Borders, as musculoskeletal injuries cross all races, genders, languages, and ages.

Emergency assessment and early intervention lead to the best functional outcomes for traumatic injuries. Generally speaking, prelicensure nursing education does not directly cover trauma or emergency response, and nurses often do not have experience in these areas. Some nurses may seek exposure through professional education such as the Trauma Nursing Core Course (TNCC), or laypersons may attend courses such as a wilderness first aid class, outdoor emergency care through the National Ski Patrol, and American Red Cross emergency first aid courses.

Statistics

Intentional and unintentional injuries sustained by trauma are the fifth leading cause of death for all ages combined in the United States and the leading cause of death for persons ages 1-41 (National Safety Council [NSC], 2007). According to the Centers for Disease Control's (CDC) National Center for Injury Prevention and Control, more than 180,000 lives were lost in 2007 (CDC, 2007) and "the medical and work loss costs for deaths and emergency department-treated non fatal injuries exceeded $90 billion in 2005" (CDC, 2011, p.1). A nurse is likely to encounter orthopaedic trauma (or the result thereof) in many settings and across the patient's life span. Examples of these settings include the acute care hospital, occupational health clinics, primary care clinics, school settings, long-term care facilities, Veteran hospitals, as well as during natural disasters and global relief work.

Incidence

Americans make 30-40 million visits to the emergency department (ED) for unintentional injuries each year (National Safety Council, 2010). In general, most fractures are not life-threatening and are often treated in the field by immobilization until definitive care is determined, starting at the ED. A patient involved in a multitrauma incident is of a higher priority.

In the United States, trauma has a bimodal distribution of incidence: high-energy injuries in the young (ages 16-35) and low-energy injuries in the elderly (ages 70-80+). Motor vehicle crashes (MVC), gun shot wounds, and risky behaviors such as drug and alcohol use account for the majority of trauma injuries of the young (Emergency Nurses Association [ENA], 2007) In the older population, falls and multitrauma in a MVC account for a major cause of death because the elderly are less able to recover from the cumulative effects caused by the initial injury.

According to the CDC, 1 in 3 adults ages 65 and older fall each year, and the total direct costs exceeded $19 billion in 2000 (Stevens, Corso, Finkelstein, & Miller, 2006). Nearly 1 out of 5 elderly hip fracture patients dies within 1 year of their injury (National Institute of Health [NIH], 2010). The patient may not necessarily die from the occult hip fracture but from the adverse effects that may ensue due to immobilization (pneumonia, DVT, and kidney failure). Data related to patterns of injury can be helpful when creating emergency systems, prioritizing specialized rescue equipment, and implementing prevention programs.

Patient Outcomes

Variables that influence survival and patient outcomes related to trauma include age, race, gender, alcohol, drugs, tobacco, and violence (NSC, 2010). In the shipping and farming industries, traumatic injuries can be disfiguring and often fatal. Many traumatic injuries can be prevented by training and common sense. As stated, MVCs account for the majority of trauma injuries. The use of seat belts, advances in car safety such as air bags, proper car seats for children, improvements in road construction, and speed limits have resulted in fewer traumatic injuries over the years. The National Highway Traffic Safety Administration concluded that the use of seatbelts saves more than 13,000 lives per year and that, between 2005 and 2009, motor vehicle crash fatalities decreased by 22% (US Department of Transportation, 2008). Many sports injuries can be prevented with adequate warm-up, proper equipment use, and recognition of warning signs. Guidelines set up by the Occupational Safety & Health Administration (OSHA) are in place to help prevent injuries in the work place.

The underserved suffer a disproportionate amount of trauma deaths and injuries related to MVCs (often as pedestrians), industrial machinery, war and internal conflicts, along with natural disasters (World Health Organization [WHO], n.d.). As we move to a global culture, nurses in the U.S. may care for patients who have sustained these kinds of traumatic injuries in the past or as relief workers when responding to disasters.

Special Patient Populations

Pediatrics

Fractures in the pediatric population differ from those among adults mainly due to physical immaturity. Children, by nature, are physically resilient and can adapt to change; however, trauma is the leading cause of death in children (Oman & Koziol-McLain, 2007). Pediatric bones are more porous and have a higher cartilage-to-bone ratio than adult bones, and children's soft tissues are more flexible than adults' tissue. Children have a greater potential for fracture remolding during the healing process because of these factors. (See Chapter 11—Pediatrics & Congenital Disorders.)

Avulsion fractures are more common in the pediatric population. An example is a bone chip fracture, caused by the tendon being pulled from the bone, as pediatric ligaments may be stronger than bone. In addition, greenstick or buckle fractures are more frequently seen, due to a thick periosteum that limits the fracture line from extending across the entire bone (Oman & Koziol-McLain, 2007).

When treating a pediatric patient with a fracture, consider the location of the fracture in relation to the growth plate. The Salter-Harris Classification (Figure 15.1) is a specific fracture grading system used in the pediatric population to describe fractures related to the epiphyseal (McKeag & Moeller, 2007). Most childhood fractures heal and recover without significant problems; however, fractures that involve the epiphyseal can be problematic due to growth plate involvement. Growth disruption in length, width, or diameter can be affected by a fracture in the pediatric patient. In addition, deformity with resulting dysfunction of a limb or joint can result. Accurate diagnosis at the time of trauma is essential, along with assessing normal bone healing post-treatment.

Figure 15.1. Salter-Harris Classification

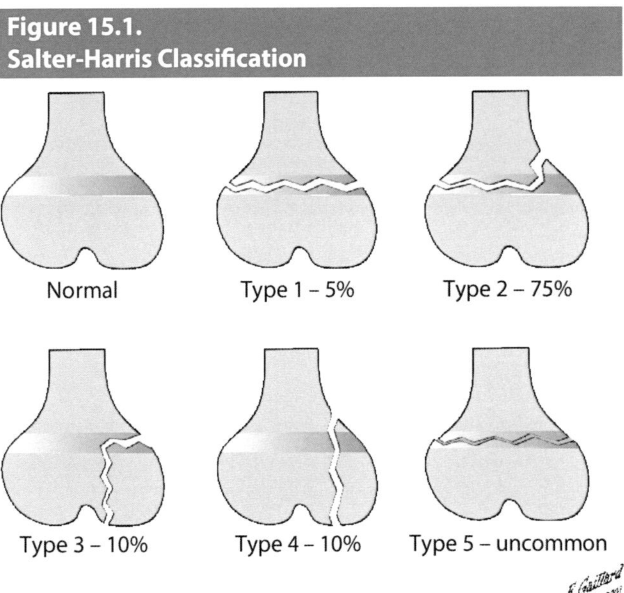

From Salter Harris Fracture Types *by F. Gaillard, 2008, http://en.wikipedia.org/w/index.php?title=File:SalterHarris.svg&page=1. Reproduced with permission.*

CHAPTER 15

Geriatrics

Major trauma is relatively uncommon among the elderly; however; trauma in the geriatric population causes higher mortality and poorer functional outcomes as compared to younger patients. Independent seniors average three chronic medical conditions, and that incidence rises quickly for those in care centers (Ham & Solane, 1997). Assessment of the geriatric patient is more complex, requiring a greater understanding of age-related pathophysiolocial changes and the effects of disease compared to the general public. (See Chapter 12—Special Geriatric Considerations.)

A fall is the most common mechanism of injury for the elder trauma patient. Falls need to be evaluated as to the underlying cause. An unsafe home environment may be corrected, and evaluation for an underlying medical issue such as orthostatic hypotension, arrhythmias, and medication side effects can be treated and prevented. Most seniors are very aware of the potential of losing their independence and the potential for drastic lifestyle changes after injury. Use of their entire health care team—including social work, case management, and rehabilitation specialists—is paramount to keep this special population as independent as possible for the best outcomes.

Psychosocial Impact of Trauma

A traumatic injury often precipitates a crisis for both the patient and the family. The unpredictable nature of the trauma can leave the patient and family feeling vulnerable, overwhelmed, and unprepared to deal with time-sensitive decisions that must be made under pressure. Coping methods people use on a daily basis may not enable them to handle the intense psychological and emotional stress. Psychological consequences of trauma injury can lead to long-term conditions such as social isolation, job loss, economic problems, depression, and post traumatic stress disorder (PTSD).

Emotional responses to crisis include shock, denial, disbelief, anger, guilt, self-blame, sadness or hopelessness, anxiety and fear, withdrawal, and disconnecting. The caregivers' response in this situation is crisis management for the whole family. The focus of crisis intervention is to address the immediate problem, beginning with an assessment of the patient's view of the situation and what resources are available. The three critical factors of crisis intervention are: 1) perception of the event; 2) availability of supports; and 3) effectiveness of the coping mechanisms. A balance of these factors will serve as guardrails for the patient and family (McQuillan et al., 2009).

Nursing interventions for patients and families in crisis include the need for information, the need for compassion, and the need for hope. Providing honest and timely information will prevent inaccurate perceptions and decrease stress. Patients need to feel cared for, and their families need to see that their loved one is cared for with compassion. An adequate amount of time spent at the patient's bedside can be reassuring to both the patient and the family. The caregiver must also display hope, as this may be the only positive emotion that the family feels during the crisis event.

These interventions may take place with the immediate traumatic event and at different times, to different degrees, throughout the inpatient and recovery periods. The use of clinical consults may also prove beneficial, as referrals to clergy, social workers, rehabilitation psychologists, and outside resources such as support groups promote a larger support network for the patient and family.

Injury often comes without warning and can result in either temporary or long-term changes to the patient's life. The patient who experiences a sports injury may not have the associated life threat that a trauma victim might experience; however the situation may be just as traumatic. The high school athlete, for example, may have ambitions for a college scholarship, or a college player may plan for a professional or Olympic career. Even social athletes may define themselves by their sports. These can be sensitive aspects to recovery as the patient, parents, coaches, and therapists may have conflicting goals for recovery and return to play. A team approach with clear goals to guide progressive rehabilitation is the best method for injury recovery.

Energy and Mechanism of Injury

Close attention to the mechanism of injury (MOI) can aid in the identification and treatment of the trauma patient. MOI is the kind of force that acts on the body to cause injury. The fundamental principles of physics can help the caregiver determine injuries at the scene, as well as potential injuries during the assessment phase. Gauging the extent of injury requires basic understanding of physics and the relationship between mass, speed, and energy. Isaac Newton's first law of motion states that "a body in motion will stay in motion unless acted upon by an outside force" and that "an object at rest will stay at rest unless acted upon by an outside force" (Newton's Law, n.d.). A car in motion will remain in motion unless acted upon by an outside force. Similarly, if a car is stopped it will remain stopped unless acted upon. The significance of this is illustrated in the following situation. If Car 1 has stopped at a traffic light and Car 2 hits Car 1, the energy of motion is transferred to Car 1. The passengers in Car 1 potentially would suffer greater injuries than those in Car 2. This is important in predicting injury patterns during the assessment phase.

Several factors play a role in determining the extent of injury from a biomechanical focus, including force, mass, acceleration, potential energy, magnitude, and velocity. The most important aspect of mechanical or kinetic energy is its relationship to speed (ENA, 2007). The importance of speed and mass as related to kinetic energy are depicted in the mathematical equation, or KE = mass X velocity squared / 2, where kinetic energy is equal to half the mass times the velocity squared.

An example of the importance of speed and mass are described in this situation. A truck traveling at 50 mph hits a tree and sustains a certain amount of damage. A smaller car that also travels at 50 mph and hits a tree will sustain more damage. That same car traveling at 100 mph will sustain four times the amount of damage. The larger the mass of the object, the more kinetic energy it may be able to absorb, but as the speed of the object increases, the potential energy increases. A caregiver should expect that deceleration injuries may prove to be more traumatic in severity than a slow action collision.

There are a variety of categories of traumatic injury. Blunt force or compression trauma can be caused by a MVC or collision during a sporting event. Penetrating trauma can include gunshot wounds, stabbings, or blasts such as explosions. The severity of the injury is related to the body's ability to react, resist, and absorb the energy or threat. The body tries to absorb this energy but is often overcome, and thus the energy affects organs, bones, and tissues in a detrimental way. Other forms of energy that can cause injury to the body include thermal, chemical, electrical, and radiant.

Basic knowledge of patterns of injury and an understanding of the MOI will help in the initial assessment of the injury. It will also assist the responder in anticipating the initial course of treatment. Table 15.1 lists the types of energy and the associated mechanism of injury; Tables 15.2, 15.3, and 15.4 list predicted injury related to mechanism and positions types. The caregiver must use this information to develop an index of suspicion to identify both the probability and the likely severity of specific injuries. Knowing these patterns does not, however, substitute for a thorough, systematic, total body assessment.

Table 15.1. Energy Sources and Mechanisms of Injury

Energy Source	Mechanism of Injury
Mechanical or kinetic energy	■ Motor vehicle crash (MVC)/motorcycle crash (MCC) ■ Firearms ■ Falls ■ Assaults
Thermal energy	■ Heat ■ Steam ■ Fire
Chemical energy	■ Plant and animal toxins ■ Chemical substances
Electrical energy	■ Lightening ■ Exposure to wires, sockets, plugs
Radiant energy	■ Rays of light (sun rays) ■ Sound waves (explosions) ■ Electromagnetic waves (x-ray exposure) ■ Radioactive emissions (nuclear leak)
Oxygen deprivation	■ Drowning ■ Asphyxiation from inhalation of toxic substances, carbon monoxide, heat, soot

From Trauma Nursing Core Course *(6th ed., p.11) by Emergency Nurses Association, 2007. Des Plaines, IL: ENA. Reproduced with permission.*

Table 15.2. Patterns of Injury in Unrestrained Occupants of Motor Vehicles

Type of Impact	Predicted Injuries
Frontal impact (down-and-under trajectory)	■ Chest (ribs, heart, aorta most vulnerable) ■ Abdomen (liver, spleen most vulnerable) ■ Posterior dislocation of hip ■ Point of impact (knee, femur, ankle, etc.)
Frontal impact (up-and-over trajectory)	■ Head and neck ■ Chest and upper abdomen
Lateral impact (T-bone impact)	■ Head and face if thrust forward ■ Cervical spine ■ Same side shoulder, clavicle ■ Lateral abdomen (liver of right-side occupant, spleen of left-side occupant
Rear impact	■ Head and neck

From Trauma Nursing Core Course *(6th ed., p.15) by Emergency Nurses Association, 2007. Des Plaines, IL: ENA. Reproduced with permission.*

Table 15.3. Patterns of Injury Related to Pedestrians and Motorcyclists Struck by Motor Vehicles

Mechanism of Injury	Possible Injuries
Adult pedestrian struck by motor vehicle	
When struck	■ Knees ■ Tibia, fibula, femur ■ Pelvis
When thrown on top of vehicle (hood or windshield)	■ Depends on victim's position when struck: □ If struck from the front, truncal injury (ribs, spleen) □ If struck from the back, vertebral column injury
When sliding from vehicle to ground	■ Cranial and spinal injuries
When dragged under vehicle	■ Pelvis
Motorcyclist	
Head-on collision	■ Ejected over bike ■ May strike face and chest on handlebars
Angular collision	■ Lower legs may become trapped
Ejection	■ Cranial and cervical injuries
Lay bike down on side	■ Inside leg fractures, soft tissue injuries

From Trauma Nursing Core Course *(6th ed., p.15) by Emergency Nurses Association, 2007. Des Plaines, IL: ENA. Reproduced with permission.*

CHAPTER 15

Table 15.4. Injury Percent of Unrestrained Occupants and Drivers Injured in Nonfatal MVCs	
Position in Vehicle	**Injuries**
Front-seat passenger (right side of car)	■ Pelvic fractures: 46% ■ Femur fractures: 41% ■ Cranial injuries: 24% ■ Abdominal injuries: 13%
Driver (left side of car)	■ Femur fractures: 65% ■ Pelvic fractures: 46% ■ Chest injuries: 46% ■ Ankle fractures: 39% ■ Facial bone fractures: 37% ■ Cranial injuries: 16%

From Trauma Nursing Core Course *(6th ed., p.15) by Emergency Nurses Association, 2007. Des Plaines, IL: ENA. Reproduced with permission.*

Emergency Response

Assessment of the Environment

To better appreciate the trauma event, one must understand the prehospital sequence of events, as this experience is part of the entire chain of patient care. The first person to render help after a traumatic incident is most often a bystander, spectator, or witness to the injury or accident. The first official responders are usually the police or EMT personnel. There is a systematic approach to trauma assessment that all levels of providers follow. The first assessment is of the environment (the scene size-up). The caregiver simultaneously asks four questions: Is the scene safe to enter? What is the MOI? What is the total number of patients? Are additional resources needed?

Primary Survey

The next step in the care for the trauma patient includes rapid assessment and treatment of life- and limb-threatening problems. The American College of Surgeons (2008) developed Advanced Trauma Life Support guidelines for emergency personnel to follow for a systematic approach to patient assessment. The caregiver at the scene will start with the primary survey known as "the ABCs": **A**irway, **B**reathing, **C**irculation. The prompt initiation of the ABCs and related procedures is especially important during the first 60 minutes of trauma care. Often referred to as the "golden hour," this first hour following injury is a crucial period during which survival rates may be enhanced if critical injuries are identified and properly managed. This concept was first recorded by the French during World War I (trauma.org, n.d.).

The mnemonic ABCDEFGHI is the sequence to be used during the initial assessment, as detailed below. The goal is to ensure that caregivers do not miss important information, which in turn minimizes risk to the patient (ENA, 2007; McQuillan et al., 2009). The first five items (A-E) are considered the primary assessment, and the next four (F-I) are the secondary assessment.

A - Airway

B - Breathing

C - Circulation (pulse and life threatening bleeding)

D - Disability (neurologic)

E - Expose all injuries/environmental, control of the elements: Exposing the injuries will give the caregiver direct visualization of the wound/injury for evaluating treatment in the field. The "E" also reminds the first responder to protect the patient from the environment or elements. Consider a scenario in which a victim fell through the ice in winter. Once removed from the water, keep the patient from sustaining any further exposure to the elements and possibly prevent hypothermia by removing wet clothes and using blankets for warmth. Once the ABCs are established, the neurologic status can be assessed using a quick evaluation of general assessment (AVPU) of the patient's level of responsiveness. (The patient's level of consciousness can be assessed in detail using the Glasgow Coma Scale [see Table 15.5] once there is more time and the patient is out of the initial trauma scene, for example, in the ambulance/helicopter on the way to the ED.)

Table 15.5. Glasgow Coma Scale		
Parameter	**Finding**	**Score**
Eye opening	Spontaneously	4
	To speech	3
	To pain	2
	Do not open	1
Best verbal response	Oriented	5
	Confused	4
	Inappropriate speech	3
	Incomprehensible sounds	2
	No verbalization	1
Best motor response	Obeys command	6
	Localizes pain	5
	Withdraws from pain	4
	Abnormal flexion	3
	Abnormal extension	2
	No motor response	1

From Lippincott Manual of Nursing Practice *(8th ed., p. 475), 2006. Philadelphia, PA: Lippincott, Williams & Wilkins. Reproduced with permission.*

A - Alert

V - Responds to verbal stimulus

P - Responds to painful stimulus

U - Unresponsive

Secondary Survey

The secondary assessment identifies less significant injuries. It includes a full head-to-toe examination of the patient and any medical history or events leading up to the incident that can be obtained.

F - Full set of vital signs/family presence

G - Give comfort measures- including verbal reassurance

H - History and full head-to-toe assessment

I - Inspect the posterior (roll the patient over!) after the

C - spine is stabilized (McQuillan et al., 2009).

The first responder uses yet another mnemonic, SAMPLE, to get a brief history from the patient or bystanders and to gather information surrounding the incident. This information gathered in the field may prove vital, depending on the severity of the trauma and the patient's condition as time ticks on within the golden hour.

S - Signs and symptoms of the injury or the "chief complaint"

A - Allergies

M - Medications and or drugs

P - Past medical history

L - Last meal

E - Events Leading to the injury

Once the victim is stabilized in the field, the patient is transported to the ED, where the same assessment sequence is used but in more depth and with more details. The trauma physician may consult the orthopedic physician at this time for a more detailed assessment and evaluation of the injury and treatment plan related to the musculoskeletal injury.

Bone Structure

The purpose of bones and the entire musculoskeletal system of ligaments and tendons is to give the body support, movement, strength, and protection. Bones themselves are extremely vascular and assist in the production of red blood cells. Specific areas of the bone that may have posttrauma significance include the articular cartilage and the growth plates or epiphyseal plate. Keep these key points in mind when considering traumatic injuries and the potential impact that they have on the particular boney structure. (Details of the anatomy and physiology of bone may be reviewed in Chapter 2—Anatomy & Physiology). Issues to consider include bleeding and shock from hemorrhage, which organs this bone is protecting, range of motion (ROM) of corresponding joints, interruption of future growth due to the location of the fracture, age of the patient as compared to the age of the bone, bone stock and regrowth potential, joint stability, and potential for future osteoarthritis especially if the articular surfaces may be offset post-injury.

Types of Bone Fractures

A fracture is described as a break or disruption in the continuity of the bone. Radiographs (x-rays) are the most frequently used test to diagnose a fracture. Prehospital

Figure 15.2.
Fracture Classification

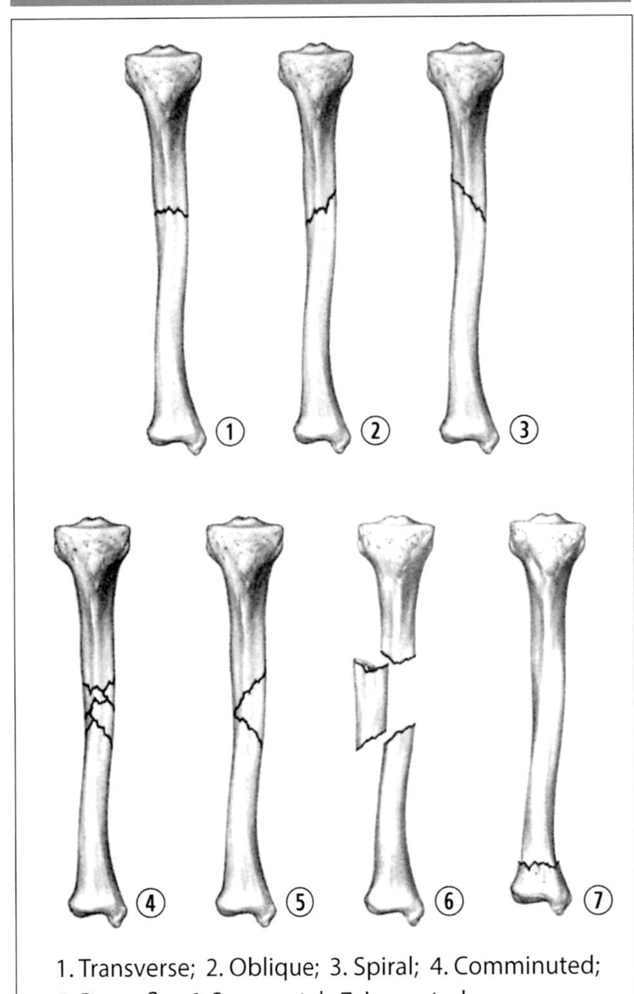

1. Transverse; 2. Oblique; 3. Spiral; 4. Comminuted; 5. Butterfly; 6. Segmental; 7. Impacted.

From Core Curriculum for Orthopaedic Nursing (6th ed, p. 420), by NAON, 2006, Boston, MA: Pearson. Reproduced with permission.

treatment for a suspected fracture is typically with splints and immobility until ruled differently. Fractures are classified (see Figure 15.2) by several different features and descriptors such as:

1. Fracture line: oblique, transverse, spiral, complete, incomplete;
2. Anatomic location: intra-articular, distal, midshaft;
3. Amount of displacement: angulation, impaction, overriding; and
4. Fracture appearance: linear or comminuted.

At the time of injury, long bone fractures are first described as open or closed, which is rather self-explanatory on physical and visual assessment. It is crucial to inspect the integrity of the skin for a possible breach, as a bone end can become recessed at the time of evaluation. If the fracture is open, a grading system (illustrated by Table 15.6) is used to determine the amount of wound contamination. This grade will help to determine treatment course; the greater the contamination, the more challenging the healing of both tissue and bone becomes. (Infections associated with musculoskeletal tissue are described in more detail in Chapter 9—Infections.)

Table 15.6. Wound Contamination Grading System

Grade	Description
Grade I	5. Skin is punctured. 6. Minimal soft tissue injury and contamination. 7. Intact vascular status.
Grade II	1. Accompanied by skin and muscle contusion. 2. Moderate wound contamination. 3. Comminuted bone fragments.
Grade III	1. Extensive soft tissue damage of skin, muscles, blood vessels, and nerves. 2. Usually associated with massive contamination. 3. Highly comminuted or segmental fractures.

From Core Curriculum for Orthopaedic Nursing (6th ed, p. 420), by NAON, 2006, Boston, MA: Pearson. Reproduced with permission.

There are also specific scoring systems related to mangled limbs as a result of trauma to help the physician determine when to attempt limb salvage, opt for reconstruction, or resort to amputation. The Mangled Extremity Severity Score (MESS) is meant to assist the surgeon with the unpleasant and often-devastating process of decision-making when faced with a mangled limb. Several factors require consideration such as the extent of the vascular injury, bone and soft tissue destruction, time of limb ischemia, patient's age and health status, and other traumatic injuries the patient may have suffered. The ultimate goal is to leave the patient with a functional, painless limb.

Anatomic locations are used to describe the fractures in relation to a joint. This is important for the orthopaedic surgeon to prepare tools and proper fixation hardware and for the nurse to predict bone recovery, prevent complications, and prepare for potential needs in the future specifically with patient education. An example is an intra-articular fracture that extends into the joint surface. A distal femur fracture may lead the physician to proceed with standard fixation or possibly a partial/total knee replacement.

Fracture Healing

Healthy bones heal in a predictable manner. Understanding stages of bone healing (Table 15.7) can assist in monitoring bone recovery and aid in identifying interruptions in this normal process.

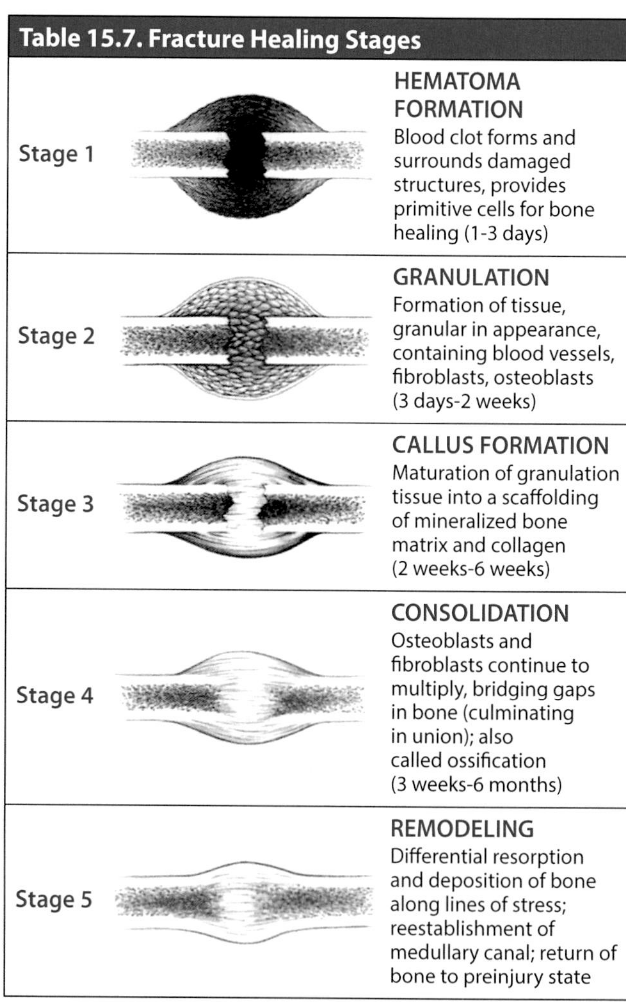

Table 15.7. Fracture Healing Stages

Stage	Description
Stage 1	**HEMATOMA FORMATION** Blood clot forms and surrounds damaged structures, provides primitive cells for bone healing (1-3 days)
Stage 2	**GRANULATION** Formation of tissue, granular in appearance, containing blood vessels, fibroblasts, osteoblasts (3 days-2 weeks)
Stage 3	**CALLUS FORMATION** Maturation of granulation tissue into a scaffolding of mineralized bone matrix and collagen (2 weeks-6 weeks)
Stage 4	**CONSOLIDATION** Osteoblasts and fibroblasts continue to multiply, bridging gaps in bone (culminating in union); also called ossification (3 weeks-6 months)
Stage 5	**REMODELING** Differential resorption and deposition of bone along lines of stress; reestablishment of medullary canal; return of bone to preinjury state

From Core Curriculum for Orthopaedic Nursing (6th ed, p. 423), by NAON, 2006, Boston, MA: Pearson. Reproduced with permission.

Another important concept regarding bone healing is Wolff's Law of Remodeling (Figure 15.3). Julius Wolff developed the theory in the 19th century to explain how healthy bone adapts to loads, or weight (Kushner, 1940). Bone will remodel itself over time to become stronger if loading on a particular bone increases. The outside cortical bone becomes thicker to better withstand a load. The opposite is also true: a bone will become weaker if the loading decreases. This theory has been demonstrated by astronauts who spend significant time in space without gravity and return with "weakened bones." This is the principle behind early initiation of weight-bearing activities during bone healing. If the patient cannot bear weight through the injury, it is important for the limb to be dependent, using gravity to create the load, to help to stimulate bone growth.

Figure 15.3.
Wolff's Law

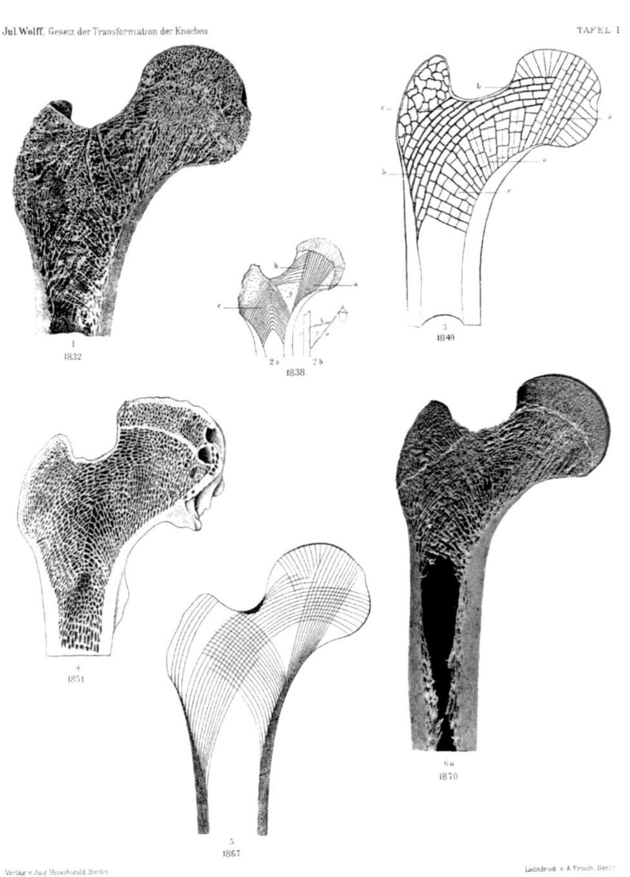

From Das Gesetz der Transformation der Knochen *by Julius Wolff, 1892; reprint 2010. Berlin, Germany: A. Hirschwald. Reprinted with permission.*

In addition to gravity and immobilization, other factors that influence bone healing include trauma severity, bone loss, type of bone, vascular support of the bone, bone health at the time of injury, infection or wound contamination, intra-articular fractures, and fractures involving the growth plates. Comorbidities that may slow the healing process include osteoporosis, peripheral vascular disease, diabetes, age, radiated bone, and smoking (Kunkler, 2006).

OVERVIEW OF ASSESSMENT FOR COMMON ORTHOPAEDIC TRAUMA

The initial on-scene assessment of MOI and evaluation of the chief complaint drives the treatment in the field. Generally the first responder will splint the injury using an array of modalities and then transport the patient to the medical facility. The medical team has, at their disposal, several options for detailed assessment of the injury. The gold standard of orthopaedic evaluation includes history, physical assessment/clinical exam, and radiographs. X-rays are used to identify bone deformity, joint congruity, bone density, and calcification. Computed tomography (CT) uses x-ray beams to take sectional pictures of a particular area to evaluate bone, tumors, nerves, and vessels. Magnetic resonance imaging (MRI) is relied upon to evaluate changes in tissue water content and often used to differentiate tendon, muscle, ligaments, joint structures, and disc disease (Smith, 2002). These diagnostic modalities are discussed in detail in Chapter 4—Diagnostic Studies.

An overview of specific musculoskeletal trauma is reviewed in this chapter as it relates to early accident scene intervention. Specific and ongoing nursing care of pelvic, femur, and hip fractures can be found in those dedicated chapters.

Spine Fractures

Overview

According to the National Center for Injury Prevention and Control, MVCs account for the largest number of spinal cord injuries, about 45% (NCIPC, 2007). A careful assessment at the scene of a MVC is essential. Physical clues that help the rescuer include obvious visualization of the patient's skull and face, a star-patterned crack in a car windshield, use of a helmet or seatbelt, and AVPU assessment of the patient's alertness and orientation (alert, verbal stimuli, painful stimuli, unresponsive).

In the field, a caregiver uses their hands to stabilize the head and neck until a rigid collar can be placed. Because the cervical spine ("c-spine") is difficult to immobilize independently, a backboard and cervical collar are used to prevent movement of the entire spine. The gold standard in the prehospital setting, backboard or spine board use aids in ease of transport while maintaining neutral alignment of the cervical, thoracic, and lumbar spine. The backboard is only used for transport, however; the patient is rolled off immediately upon arrival in the ED.

Research increasingly supports the prompt removal of the patient from the backboard once reaching definitive care. Protocols and guidelines have been established to provide measures to expedite the removal of patients from backboards to prevent skin breakdown, respiratory compromise, false positive pain that distracts from spine examinations, and difficulty with imaging studies. The University of Colorado Hospital Guideline details a timeline of 2 hours for removal after documented physical examination and that specific criteria have been met (Professional Practice Committee, 2010).

Types of vertebral fractures include simple, wedge, burst, and teardrop. A fracture may cause compression of the spinal cord, either at the time of injury or later, as the injury swelling starts to compress on the cord.

Table 15.8. Spinal Fractures

Type of Force	Description of Injury
Flexion	1. Posterior ligaments remain intact and cause wedge compression fractures in minor injuries 2. Severe injuries are associated with posterior ligament injuries and considered unstable 3. Spinous processes are separated and kyphotic angulation is noted 4. Occurs most often in cervical and lumbar spine
Axial loading	1. Burst fractures 2. Spinous process is not separated 3. Anterior and posterior are usually intact 4. If the fracture fragment causes impingement on he spinal canal, it may cause quadriplegia if the fracture is located in the cervical spine or paraplegia if the fracture is located in the lumbar spine 5. If it is comminuted fracture it may be unstable
Flexion/ rotation	1. Fracture dislocation of the spine 2. Posterior ligament is stretched or torn 3. Spinous process separation with paraplegia 4. Unstable when located in the thoracic and lumbar spine
Extension	1. Rare injury 2. Most common in cervical spine 3. Posterior ligaments intact 4. Stable
Distraction	1. Chance fracture result of spine distraction 2. Typically sustained in an automobile crash if only lap belt is used 3. Tear through vertebral body and or ligaments 4. Stable

Data from Core Curriculum for Orthopaedic Nursing *(6th ed.), by NAON, 2006, Boston, MA: Pearson.*

A neurological assessment is, therefore, a"must" for baseline data and continued monitoring. The cervical spine is most vulnerable to hyperextension and hyper flexion injuries, and common types of fractures include Hangman's fracture and Odontiod fracture at C-2. For a more detailed list of spine fractures, refer to Table 15.8.

Assessment

The original assessment of the trauma patient starts with evaluating and stabilizing the ABCs. Once stabilized, the next major concern is the "D" (Disability)—the head, neck, and cervical spine. The purpose of the vertebral column is to protect the spinal cord. Any threat to this bony structure must be stabilized, as it is the safety barrier for the spinal column and brain to control neurological functioning.

If there is any evidence to indicate that the patient lost consciousness or is disoriented, or if the mechanism of injury leads the responder to believe that the patient may have sustained a head injury, the protocol is to immobilize the head and neck immediately. Other confounding variables that can cause patient confusion or disorientation include drugs, alcohol, low blood sugar, and cardiac issues such as a transient ischemic attack (TIA) or a stroke.

Assessment of function is evaluated by using baseline information either gathered at the scene or on admission. For this reason, documentation of circulation, motion, and sensation (CMS) of all extremities is essential to evaluate treatment effectiveness and to monitor for complications.

Common Therapeutic Modalities

Treatment is based on many factors, including location, type of fracture, severity, displacement. Treatment modalities for cervical injuries include skeletal traction, Halo apparatus, and ridged cervical collar. Treatment for a thoracic injury may include bed rest, progressive mobilization, corset, thoracic-lumbar-sacral orthosis (TLSO), and body casting. Surgical procedures for unstable fractures include open reduction, internal fixation (ORIF), spinal instrumentation and decompression fusion. See Table 15.9 for a global listing of types of fractures, MOI, assessment, and treatment.

Prehospital Treatment:

- ABCs;
- Early immobilization to prevent further damage on scene;
- Neurologic assessment documentation is necessary to assist in determining level of injury, gross assessment in the field and further evaluation once the injury is stabilized; and

- Use of log roll techniques in the field—to keep the spine in alignment—1 person stabilizing the head/neck and at least 2 other caregivers to roll in sequence according to the count of the leader at the head of the patient.

ED Treatment Goals:

- ABC's;
- Monitor time patient is on backboard and follow protocols for early removal of immobilization;
- Expedite cervical and other spine films; and
- Monitor ongoing neurological assessment.

Table 15.9. Common Fractures/Dislocations

Fracture/ Dislocation	Mechanism of Injury	Assessment	Treatment	Approximate Healing time
Skull	■ Direct blow, fall, fight, collision	■ Increased intracranial pressure. ■ Observe for lumps, bumps, indentations bleeding	Adult/Child: ■ Conservative: observation and steroids. ■ Surgical: burr holes. ■ Surgical: craniotomy to relieve pressure. ■ Direct pressure to control bleeding.	Adult/Child: 4-6 weeks.
Clavicle	■ Fall on shoulder or outstretched hand	■ Have patient stand or sit upright without back support for observation. ■ Majority: middle third of bone ■ Palpation: tenderness, swelling, deformity, crepitus ■ Inspection: shoulder drops downward, forward, inward. May be tenting around skin	Adult: ■ Conservative: sling, clavicle strap, soft immobilizer □ In cases where no reduction is required, some patients require soft immobilizer while others need only a sling for support. □ Closed reduction followed by immobilization in a soft immobilizer. ■ Surgical: open reduction is generally avoided unless necessary because surgery increases the incidence of nonunion. Surgery is indicated when the bone is considerable fragmented or when underling soft tissues must be repaired or explored for damage. Child: ■ Conservative: sling	Adult/Child: Clavicle fractures heal rapidly but it is difficult to maintain immobility during early stages of healing. 3-6 weeks.
Sternoclavicular joint	■ Fall on shoulder or outstretched hand.	■ Posterior dislocation move clavicle retrosternally ■ Inspection: □ Bleeding in area around neck □ Swelling □ Difficulty □ breathing □ Changes in vital signs	Adult: ■ Conservative: □ Sandbag between scapula will pull medial end out of retrosternal area □ Clavicle strap ■ Surgical: internal fixation	Adult: 6-10 weeks Child: 3 weeks
Shoulder dislocation	■ Fall on outstretched hand ■ Common sport-related injury ■ Loose-jointed children can voluntarily dislocate by suppressing the activity of one muscle group.	■ Most are anterior ■ Inspection □ Position of limb: held in abduction and external rotation □ Selling: bulge over anterior aspect of shoulder ■ Severity of pain and muscle spasm ■ Mobility: unable to touch opposite shoulder, cannot abduct beyond 90 degrees ■ Neurovascular assessment	Adult/Child: ■ Conservative: □ Reduction with analgesia, conscious sedation or muscle relaxant if seen shortly after injury □ Reduction under anesthesia if treatment delayed □ Postreduction: shoulder immobilizer	Adult/Child: At least 2 weeks

Table continued on next page ▶

Table 15.9. Common Fractures/Dislocations (continued)				
Fracture/ Dislocation	**Mechanism of Injury**	**Assessment**	**Treatment**	**Approximate Healing time**
Proximal humeral fracture	■ Fall on outstretched hand or elbow ■ Direct blow	■ Cut away clothing for assessment and treatment: movement may be painful and the motion of bone fragments harmful to soft tissues ■ Inspection: local swelling, tenderness, upper third of arm ■ Mobility: loss of motion of internal rotation and abduction ■ Assess for nerve involvement: axillary, median, redial, ulnar ■ Pain ■ Crepitus ■ Arterial involvement with direct blow ■ Neurovascular assessment	Approximately 85% of proximal humeral fractures are nondisplaced or minimally displaced and are treated conservatively. ■ Conservative treatment in adults: □ Few weeks of rest □ Closed reduction may be needed □ Hanging cast/immobilizer □ Program of exercises post healing ■ Surgical treatment: displaced fracture Open reduction and internal fixation ■ Conservative treatment children: □ Sling □ Splint □ Commercial immobilizer □ Hanging cast should not be used in children under 12 years old	Adult: 4-10 weeks Child: 3-4 weeks
Supracondylar fracture	■ Fall on extended or flexed elbow	■ Injury is obvious, usually displaced ■ Vascular and nerve involvement common at injury site ■ Neurovascular assessment □ Displacement may cause compartment syndrome	Adult: ■ Conservative; closed reduction with casting, posterior splint, and sling ■ Surgical: open reduction or percutaneous pinning if fracture unstable Child: ■ Conservative: closed reduction with casting, posterior splint and sling ■ Surgical: percutaneous pinning if displaced	Adult/Child: 4-8 weeks
Elbow injuries	■ Occur more commonly in elderly or children		Although treatment modalities may vary for differing elbow fractures, the one treatment held in common in all immobilization approaches is prevention of extension contractures by keeping the elbow in at least some degree of flexion during healing. Early motion to prevent contractures.	
Olecranon fracture	■ Direct blow or fall	■ Pain, swelling ■ Inability to extend elbow ■ Neurovascular assessment	Adult: ■ Conservative: aspiration of hemarthrosis, sling, traction (skin or skeletal). ■ Surgical: □ Closed reduction with cast from shoulder to wrist, 45-90 degrees flexion □ Open reduction, screw fixation, wiring Child: ■ Conservative: aspiration of hemarthrosis, sling, traction (skin or skeletal). ■ Surgical: □ Closed reduction with cast □ Closed reduction, percutanesous wire fixation	Adult: 7-12 weeks Child: 4- weeks

Table 15.9. Common Fractures/Dislocations (continued)				
Fracture/ Dislocation	**Mechanism of Injury**	**Assessment**	**Treatment**	**Approximate Healing time**
Elbow dislocation	■ Fall on outstretched hand with elbow extended ■ Children: Pull on arm can dislocate	■ Apparent early deformity ■ Late swelling may mask deformity ■ Neurovascular assessment	Adult: ■ Closed reduction under anesthesia ■ Posterior splint and sling or cast Child: ■ Reduce immediately by supinating and flexing the elbow	Adult: 4-6 weeks Start gentle ROM after 2 weeks Child: Begin motion in couple of days
Radius, ulna fractures	■ Direct trauma ■ Fall on outstretched hand ■ Forearm fracture of ulna alone are rare	■ Localized selling and tenderness ■ In adults, often accompanied by significant swelling ■ Limitation in ROM; painful pronation-supination ■ Neurovascular assessment	■ Nondisplaced: casting, posterior splint for 1-2 weeks followed by a sling and active movement of elbow started ■ Displaced: open reduction and internal fixation	Adult: 12 weeks Child: 6-8 weeks
Colles' fracture	■ Fall on outstretched hand	■ Wrist appears puffy and deformed ■ Hump deformity seen when wrist is viewed from side ■ Neurovascular assessment	■ Nondisplaced: forearm splint or cast, pressure dressing ■ Displaced: manual traction, plaster cast, percutaneous pinning, or external fixation	Adult: 4-8 weeks
Hand fracture	(See Chapter 17, Hand)			
Sternum	■ Direct trauma to chest ■ Usually motor vehicle accident	■ Swelling over sternum ■ Tenderness or pain ■ Sternal and rib fractures may cause flail chest: observe for paradoxical breathing ■ Evaluate for cardiac and lung contusion	■ Conservative: analgesics	Adult: 4-6 week Child: 3-4 weeks
Rib	■ Direct or indirect trauma to chest usually by blows, crushing injuries, or strains caused by coughing or sneezing ■ The fifth to ninth ribs most frequently involved	■ Pain or tenderness to touch ■ Respiratory evaluation for shallow respirations and protective guarding ■ Subcutaneous emphysema/ crepitations	■ Analgesics ■ Pulmonary toileting to prevent respiratory complications ■ Sever: regional nerve block for pain relief	Adult: 6-8 weeks Child: 3-4 weeks

Table continued on next page ▶

Table 15.9. Common Fractures/Dislocations (continued)				
Fracture/ Dislocation	**Mechanism of Injury**	**Assessment**	**Treatment**	**Approximate Healing time**
Pelvis	Severe trauma as with motor vehicle crashes, falls from great heights, and crushing injuries	■ Assess for shock: hemorrhagic ■ Local pain, swelling, tenderness, and crepitus ■ Neurovascular assessment ■ Assess peripheral pulses: absence of peripheral pulses may indicate a tear in the iliac or femoral artery. ■ Sever back pain may indicate retroperitoneal bleed ■ Ongoing assessment for injuries to bladder, rectum, intestines, and intra-abdominal organs. ■ Stable fracture: unilateral fracture of superior and inferior pubic rami, single fracture of iliac ring ■ Unstable fracture; bilateral or unilateral fracture of the superior and inferior pubic rami and the sacroliliac joint or sacrum, or a fracture or dislocation of sacroiliac joint or sacrum and symphysis pubis-hip deformity present.	■ Emergent: external fixation for open book fracture, may be life saving ■ Conservative: bed rest until comfortable ambulation with guarded weight bearing ■ Surgical: open reduction internal fixation; external fixation ■ Stable fracture: bed rest several days then progressive ambulation; analgesics ■ Unstable fracture: external fixation alone or combined with ORIF (anterior and/or posterior).	Adult: 6-12 weeks Child: Assess 6-8 weeks
Hip fracture	Adult: Femoral neck: ■ Trivial or minor injuries ■ Fall: direct blow over greater trochanter ■ Lateral rotation injury—head firmly fixed in acetabulum, neck rotates posteriorly, gets caught in acetabulum, and buckles, ■ Osteoporosis ■ Intertrochanteric: ■ Fall involving direct and indirect forces to greater trochanter ■ Metastatic disease Child: ■ Requires great force as with bumper injuries ■ Severe trauma: falls from heights, motor vehicle injuries, bicycle accidents	■ Neurovascular check distal to injury ■ Femoral neck: impacted □ Slight pain in groin or along medial side of knee □ Antalgic gait □ Discomfort on ROM □ Muscle spasm: extremes of motion □ May have marked valgus ■ Femoral neck: displaced ■ Extreme pain in hip region ■ Leg externally rotated, abducted, and shortened. ■ Patient at risk for disruption of blood supply and avascular necrosis ■ Marked shortening ■ 90 degrees external rotation ■ Selling in hip region, ecchymosis over greater trochanter, rish for great blood loss ■ Movement causes groin pain Child: Femoral neck: ■ Pain in hip ■ Extremity shortened, externally rotated Child: intratochanteric: ■ May only have shortening ■ Pain ■ External rotation	■ Internal fixation with multiple percutaneous pins: followed by early ambulation with weight bearing as tolerated ■ Prosthetic replacement; followed by early ambulation, weight bearing as tolerated ■ Open reduction with internal fixation (nails, plates, screws), ambulation with weight bearing as tolerated ■ Closed reduction, Knowles pins, screws ■ Abduction, hip spica ■ Skeletal traction ■ Cast	Adult: 3-6 months Child: 6-8 weeks

Table 15.9. Common Fractures/Dislocations (continued)				
Fracture/ Dislocation	**Mechanism of Injury**	**Assessment**	**Treatment**	**Approximate Healing time**
Hip dislocation	■ Considerable force needed ■ Anterior: forced abduction and extension ■ Posterior: force applied against flexed knee with hip in flexion ■ Central sever blow to lateral hip while in abduction ■ Child: under age 5 ■ Fall: minimal trauma ■ Acetabulum largely cartilaginous; soft ■ Joint laxity common ■ As age increases, so does degree of force required to dislocate	■ Severe pain, especially with movement ■ Anterior: thigh extended, abducted externally rotated ■ Posterior: thigh flexed, adducted internally rotated, short possible sciatic nerve injury ■ Central: usually with a fracture ■ Neurovascular assessment	Adult/Child: ■ Conservative treatment: □ Closed reduction under analgesia, muscle relaxant followed by: a. Anterior: cast/brace to hold leg adducted, internally rotated b. Posterior: traction, hip spica, or brace Adult/Child: ■ Surgical treatment: □ Open reduction under anesthesia when closed does not work followed by hip spica for child □ Central: skeletal traction, or internal fixation	Adult: 2-6 weeks Child: 6 weeks
Femur, proximal and distal	■ Direct or indirect trauma ■ Falls ■ Motor vehicle crashes	■ Proximal: external rotation, shortened extremity, acute pain, inability to move leg ■ Distal: sever pain, swelling, deformity ■ Possible injury to popliteal nerves and vessels; check neurovascular status ■ Both have extensive soft tissue damage and considerable blood loss—sometimes sever enough to precipitate shock	Proximal: ■ Conservative: skin traction, skeletal traction, cast/cast brace ■ Surgical; reduction internal fixation with intramedullary rod Distal: ■ Conservative: skeletal traction, cast brace, spica cast ■ Surgical: open reduction, internal fixation with intramedullary rod.	Adult: 8-16 weeks Child: 6-12 weeks
Patella fracture	■ Direct blow or fall, torsional injury In older, obese, or poorly conditioned individuals, indirect injury can occur from a bump, descending the stairs, or a forceful squat	■ Pain, swelling, tenderness, effusion ■ Frequently are open fractures ■ Inability to extend knee ■ Audible and painful snap may occur followed by a fall or loss of balance	Adult/Child: ■ Conservative: ice until selling subsides □ Without displaced fragment; aspiration of blood, crutches non-weight-bearing, immobilizer to fully extend knee, cast, if unable to prevent flexion	Adult/Child: 4-6 weeks
Patella dislocation	■ Direct blow to medial side ■ Severe falls, athletic injuries	■ Knee buckling causing a fall ■ Tenderness along medial border ■ Sever pain in anterior knee area ■ Muscle spasm ■ Displaced laterally ■ When knee is extended with hips flexed, patella return to normal position ■ May feel "pop" with dislocation and spontaneous reduction ■ Patellar instability	Adult/Child: ■ Conservative: ice, immobilizer, cast (long-leg), knee immobilized in extension ■ Surgical: if unable to align, repair injured ligaments, knee immobilized in extension	Adult/Child: 6-8 weeks

Table continued on next page ▶

Table 15.9. Common Fractures/Dislocations (continued)				
Fracture/ Dislocation	**Mechanism of Injury**	**Assessment**	**Treatment**	**Approximate Healing time**
Knee dislocation	■ Severe blow with hyperextension of knee ■ Twisting or crushing injury	■ Critical to evaluate and monitor neurovascular status ■ Pain on ROM, evaluate for ligament injury ■ May be displaced anteriorly, posteriorly, laterally, or medially (anterior most common). ■ Swelling, effusion, ecchymosis, tenderness ■ Puffiness, marked fullness popliteal area could mean popliteal artery injury. ■ Observe for sings of vascular insufficiency or severe or increasing pain after reduction which may indicate arterial injury.	Adult/Child: ■ Closed reduction with immobilization by cast, knee immobilizer, or posterior splint ■ Open reduction to repair soft tissue or vascular damage	Adult/Child: 6-8 weeks
Tibia, fibula fractures	■ Direct trauma to shin area, torsional force, stepping into hole ■ Ski boot injury ■ Fibula is non-weight-bearing bone so fractures of fibula alone are rare. ■ Fibula fractures often occur in response to ankle fractures. ■ Open fractures of tibia are more common than any other major bone as much of its surface is just below the skin.	■ Usually occurs in both bones ■ Angulation/deformity ■ Localized pain ■ Neurovascular evaluation with attention to signs of compartment syndrome	Adult: ■ Conservative □ Stable, nondisplaced closed reduction fracture: long-leg cast followed by short-led cast ■ Surgical: □ Comminuted/open: external fixation, open reduction internal fixation Child: ■ Conservative: long-leg cast	Adult: 6-10 weeks
Ankle fracture	■ Inversion/eversion ■ Stepping in a hole, walking on uneven surface, platform shoes, skateboards, steps, curbs, inline skating	■ Pain, swelling, ecchymosis, difficulty bearing weight, pain on flexion, extension, rotation ■ Ligamentous injury produces same symptoms, fracture is usually accompanied by ligamentous injury ■ Neurovascular assessment	Adult: ■ Conservative: closed reduction, short-leg cast, splint ■ Surgical: internal fixation ■ Displaced: external fixation Child: ■ Conservative: long-leg cast ■ Surgical: open reduction internal fixation may be necessary for Salter: Type III and IV fractures	Adult: 8-12 weeks Child: 4-6 weeks
Calcaneus fracture (Don Juan)	■ Fall or jump from high place, landing on heels	■ Evaluate for wrist and spine injuries frequently associated with compression fractures, especially T12, L1, L2 ■ Pain, swelling, ecchymosis ■ Heel is broadened ■ Hollows beneath malleoli are obliterated ■ Movement painful and restricted	Adult: ■ No reduction □ Jones compression dressings ■ Reduction: short-leg cast ■ Non-weight-bearing ■ If displaced: closed or open reduction with a cast or PRAFO Child: ■ Bulky dressing	Adult: 6-8 weeks Child: 4 weeks

CHAPTER 15

Table 15.9. Common Fractures/Dislocations (continued)				
Fracture/ Dislocation	**Mechanism of Injury**	**Assessment**	**Treatment**	**Approximate Healing time**
Metatarsal fractures	■ Direct trauma, crush injury ■ Heavy object falls on foot ■ Jump or fall on ball of foot	■ Pain swelling, ecchymosis ■ Tenderness on palpation	■ Closed reduction and immobilization in walking short-leg cast or hard sole shoe ■ Surgical: percutaneous pinning, open reduction with internal fixation	Adult: 4 weeks
Toe fracture	■ Object falling on toe ■ Stubbing toe	■ Pain, selling, ecchymosis ■ Tenderness on palpation	■ Tape to adjacent toe to stabilize ■ Waling cast or stiff sole shoes may be applied with multiple toe fractures	Adult/Child: 2-4 weeks
Cervical spine fracture	■ Blow to top of head ■ Falls landing on head ■ Hyperextension – striking head on dashboard ■ Hyperflexion – diving in shallow water ■ Hyperextension followed by hyperflexion – rear end collision	■ Associated with skull and facial fractures ■ Neck pain, tenderness over spinous process ■ Neurologic evaluation for paralysis paresthesia ■ Neck pain with motion	■ Immobilize spine, sandbags, or cervical collar ■ Spine board ■ Tongs and traction, halo body jacket ■ Internal fixation/decompression fusion	Adult/Child: 6-8 weeks
Thoracic lumbar spine fracture	■ Acute hyperflexion fall from height, landing on feet or buttocks ■ Deceleration forces – seat belt injury Level of consciousness	■ Back pain, point tenderness ■ Neurologic valuation to determine deficits: most common in T122, L1, L2 ■ Observe: ileus; thromboembolic complications	■ Conservative: spine board, firm mattress, logroll, lumbar, thoracic corsets ■ Surgical: if unstable fusion, spinal instrumentation ■ Decompression	Adult: 12-16 Child: 8-16 weeks

From Core Curriculum for Orthopaedic Nursing (6th ed., p. 404-413) by NAON, 2006, Boston, MA: Pearson. Reproduced with permission.

Postsurgery/Inpatient Unit Treatment:

- Education for patients and family for rational and appropriate use of braces/collars;
- Assess skin at points of pressure with braces/ collars; and
- Activity limits and education regarding return to pre injury activities.

Nursing Considerations

Nursing Diagnoses. Nursing diagnoses for this condition are expanded upon in the Appendix.

- Activity intolerance.
- Coping, ineffective.
- Infection, risk for.
- Knowledge deficit.
- Mobility: physical, impaired
- Pain, acute.
- Peripheral neurovascular dysfunction, risk for.
- Shock, risk for.
- Tissue integrity, impaired.

Interventions. Regarding the patient with a spinal fracture, the nurse should be concerned with self-care deficit concerning bathing/hygiene/grooming, feeding, and toileting. Role performance might also be altered. Nursing interventions are geared toward patient needs. As with all postoperative patients, infection, pain, and other potential complications are also considerations with spine-injured patients.

Pelvic Fractures

Overview

The function of the pelvis is to protect the internal vessels and organs, as well as to provide a weight-bearing structure for the body's torso. The pelvic ring is comprised of the sacrum, ileum, ischum, and pubis bones held together by a complex network of ligaments. The stability of the pelvic ring is dependent on the tension between all these structures. Because of the interdependence for support, once there has been an insult to one area of the pelvic ring, the stability of the entire structure is compromised.

The majority of pelvic ring fractures are stable, but the one third that is unstable is potentially more debilitating and life-threatening. For all ages, pelvic fractures are the most common cause of traumatic death following head injuries, due to the high incidence of hemorrhage (NSC, 2007). Major blood loss can occur secondary to the disruption of the large and numerous arterial and venous plexuses within the pelvis. The amount of energy needed to cause a pelvic fracture is significant and is seen in mechanisms of injury such as MVCs (including motorcycles and all-terrain vehicles [ATVs]), automobile-verses-pedestrian accidents, or falls from a great height (as with construction workers and mountaineering/technical rock or ice climbing).

Assessment

In the prehospital setting, the MOI and patient appearance are noted. One or both of the lower extremities may appear misaligned, at an obscure angle, or shortened in length. Pain is often the chief complaint,

Figure 15.4.
Pelvic Fracture Classifications

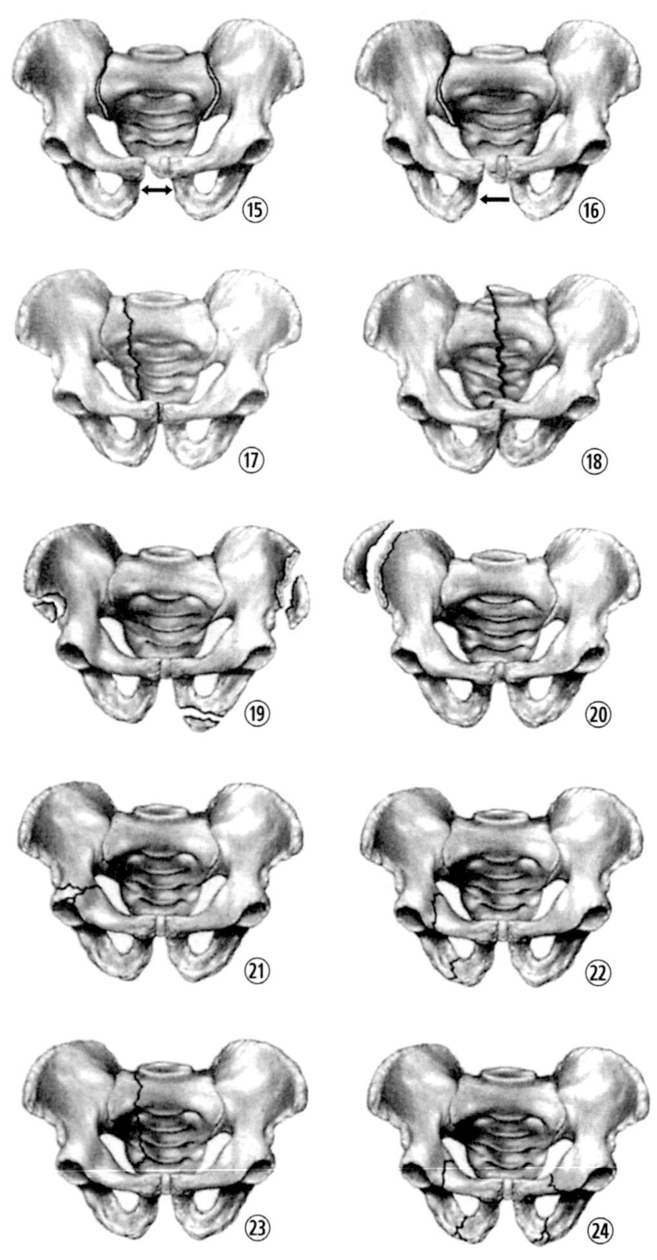

Pelvic Fractures

- Classified according to mechanism of injury and displacement or anatomical location

MECHANISM OF INJURY

- **Open book fracture:** distraction of two sides of the pelvis anteriorly ⑮ ⑯ (at the symphysis pubis)
- **Lateral compression fracture:** two sides of the pelvis are driven into each other, anteriorly (symphysis pubis) and posteriorly (sacrum) ⑰
- Vertical shear fracture: two sides of the pelvis are driven in opposite directions, up/down or forward/backward ⑱

ANATOMICAL LOCATION

- **Avulsion fracture:** ⑱ ⑲
- **Acetabular fracture:** ㉑
- **Stable fracture:** single break in pelvic ring
  - unilateral fracture of ischiopubic rami ㉒
  - fracture of sacrum ㉓
- **Unstable fracture:** double break in pelvic ring
  - **saddle fracture:** bilateral ischial and pubic rami ㉔
  - **Malgaigne fracture:** any combination of one anterior and one posterior fracture or joint disruption ⑮ ⑯ ⑰ ⑱

From Core Curriculum for Orthopaedic Nursing *(6th ed., p. 421) by NAON, 2006, Boston, MA: Pearson. Reproduced with permission.*

as well as inability to move related to the pain. Long board stabilization and emergent transport is the priority. Documentation of CMS is useful at the time of injury for comparison later. Primary diagnosis is determined by physical exam for stability and x-ray for specific location and displacement, which will determine treatment. Pelvic fractures are classified by the type of force that caused the fracture. Detailed illustrations of pelvic fractures are found in Figure 15.4.

Three major categories of pelvic fractures are anteroposterior, lateral, and vertical:

1. *Anteroposterior compression fractures* include classic open-book injury, anterior injury and widening of the symphysis pubis, and posterior disruption of the ileum or sacroiliac joint. An example might be a motorcyclist involved in a crash or an ATV rider who is ejected forward and hits the handlebars at high speed.
2. *Lateral compression fractures* include pubic rami fracture and ileum and sacroiliac joint injury. An example might be a pedestrian hit from the side by a car.
3. *Vertical shear fractures* involve vertical displacement of the hemi pelvis due to fractures at the pubic rami and sacroiliac joints. An example might be a fall from a height as on a construction site or in a mountain climbing incident.

Common Therapeutic Modalities

The immediate treatment in the field is to stabilize the pelvic injury by splinting. Serious complications of pelvic fractures include hemorrhage and hypovolemic shock due to the injury to large blood vessels. The retroperitoneal space can accommodate up to 4 liters of blood before tapenade occurs in the adult. Other complications include neurological injury, colon wounds, and genitourinary damage. The goal of pelvic stabilization is to prevent further displacement and to control bleeding by aligning the fractured bones to create a smaller space for blood to accumulate. Pre-hospital, this can be accomplished with a pelvic sling, a pneumonic air splint, or a criss-crossed bed sheet tied to immobilize the bone fragments. Once the patient is transported to the ED, the goal is more secure fixation of the pelvic ring. Initial stabilization in the ED may include the use of external fixation, like a c-clamp (pelvic stabilizer). This is usually a temporary treatment, and internal fixation is the goal once the patient is hemodynamically stable. This is an example of damage-control orthopaedics, a philosophy that proposes early stabilization of the most traumatic fractures, as well as resuscitation for the polytrauma patient and delayed definitive treatment for those patients most at risk, based on a severity index scale (Carson, 2007).

Treatment of pelvic fractures will vary, according to the severity of the injury. The degree of mobility after a pelvic fracture depends on the type of fracture, the amount of pain associated with the fracture, and the method of treatment. Progressive ambulation without weight-bearing may be allowed per the patient's pain tolerance. In the case of a nondisplaced fracture, the patient may be treated with bed rest and a binder for support and pain control. The use of crutches, walker, and/or wheelchair may be used for protected weight-bearing.

Nursing Considerations

Nursing Diagnoses. Nursing diagnoses for this condition are expanded upon in the Appendix.

- Activity intolerance.
- Body image, disturbed.
- Coping, ineffective.
- Infection, risk for.
- Mobility: physical, impaired.
- Pain, acute.
- Peripheral neurovascular dysfunction, risk for.
- Post-trauma syndrome.
- Self-care deficit: bathing/hygiene, dressing/grooming, feeding, toileting.
- Shock, risk for.
- Skin integrity, impaired.
- Tissue integrity, impaired.

Interventions. The nurse is concerned with treating these aforementioned most common conditions associated with orthopaedic patients. The nurse is also vigilant about potential complications as a result of the acute injury or related to the treatments and inactivity associated with limited mobility such as prevention of pulmonary issues, DVT/PE, fat emboli, infection, and skin breakdown.

Long Bone Trauma: Femur/Hip Fractures

Overview

All bones bleed if fractured. A single fracture may not create shock, but multitrauma may precipitate a hypovolemic situation. The caregivers need to take a proactive approach in the case of the patient with multitrauma. A quick guide accessed from the American Trauma Society (ATS) may be helpful to estimate blood loss per fracture site in anticipating treatment (Table 15.10).

Traumatic femur fractures can also be life-threatening if not recognized in the field and treated expediently,

Table 15.10. Blood Loss by Fracture Site

Site of Fracture	Potential Blood Loss in a Closed Fracture
Pelvis	1,300-1,500ml
Femur	500-1,000ml
Humerus	300-500ml
Tibia/fibula	150-250ml

Data from Trauma Nursing: From Resuscitation Through Rehabilitation *(4th ed., p. 748) by K. McQuillan, M. Makic, and E. Whalen, 2009, St. Louis, MO: Saunders Elsevier.*

due to the potential for significant blood loss. The femur bone is the strongest and longest bone in the body and maintains a large blood supply: 1000mL of blood can be hidden in the soft tissues of the thigh. A considerable amount of force is needed to fracture the femur, which may result in other injuries as well. Femur fracture signs and symptoms may include, pain and inability to bear weight, shortening of the affected leg, internal or external rotation, deformity and swelling of the thigh, and evidence of hypovolemic shock.

Assessment

Early recognition of the injury and treatment are key in the overall outcome for the patient. Splinting of the injury will stabilize the fracture, align the bone in a proper anatomical position, and protect the surrounding tissue from further injury with the use of mechanical aids in the field. Early surgical stabilization of the fracture is key to restoring function (Dobson, 2006).

Common Therapeutic Modalities – Prehospital

- ABC's and full evaluation as described earlier
- Proper splint selection (i.e. traction splint for mid-shaft femur fracture)
- Splint and immobilize the injury
- Immobilize the joints above and below the injury
- Avoid any unnecessary movement to decrease risk for fat emboli
- Ice and elevation
- Document CMS frequently
- Analgesics
- Patient and family education regarding assessment, testing and interventions as related to the initial hospital setting

Nursing Considerations

Nursing Diagnoses. Nursing diagnoses for this condition are expanded upon in the Appendix.

- Coping, ineffective.
- Fluid volume deficit.
- Infection, risk for.
- Injury, risk for.
- Mobility: physical, impaired.
- Pain, acute.
- Pain, chronic.
- Skin integrity, impaired.
- Tissue perfusion: peripheral, ineffective.

Amputations

Overview

Amputations can be complete or partial and usually involve the digits, foot, lower leg, hand, or forearm (McQuillan et al., 2009). This type of injury is often associated with workplace accidents related to machinery in a factory, on a farm, in the fishing industry, when using power tools, and MVCs. Pre-hospital care of the injury involves applying compressive dressings and splinting the wound. A complete amputation will have less active bleeding than a partial amputation because of the retraction of vessels (Oman & Koziol-McLain, 2007). Tourniquets are used in the pre-hospital setting to prevent hemorrhagic shock and in the hospital setting to control bleeding. In all cases, treat for shock and plan for a quick evacuation.

The recommendation for immediate on-scene care of the amputated part is to wrap it in gauze (either dry or moistened with saline) and place in a plastic bag or container. Do not allow the part to freeze. Do not place it directly on ice, and never use dry ice, as it is too cold. The patient and amputated part should be evacuated to the ED immediately for the best chance of surgical reattachment. Research by McQuillan et al. (2009) shows that the best outcome for a viable part is if surgery is performed within 6 hours of warm ischemic time (time of amputation to replantation) and that a properly managed part may be maintained for 6-12 hours before replantation. A guillotine type of amputation has a better chance of successful replantation than the avulsed or tearing types of injuries due to vessel and tissue damage sustained on either end of the wound. Immediate care at the scene should also include splinting the injury to preserve the integrity of the tissue bridge. Constant assessment and documentation of CSM time will be critical when the surgeon makes the final assessment regarding the plan.

Assessment

The amputated part and the amputated site need to be thoroughly assessed to evaluate for replantation success.

With the advances in microsurgery, antibiotic therapies, and the progress in reconstructive surgery, limb salvage has become a viable option. Radiographs of all parts, along with copious irrigation, is necessary to evaluate both bone and tissue status. Areas for consideration for replantation with best outcomes include multiple digits, thumb, wrist, and forearm. The decision to attempt replantation is made by considering technical, aesthetic, medical, and psychological factors (Propehl, 2009). For example, a surgeon in a community hospital without specialized microsurgery equipment may decide not to proceed with this type of surgery.

Common Therapeutic Modalities

Total hemodynamic stabilization of the patient, for blood volume and blood pressure, must take priority as the patient recovers from the traumatic event. If replantation takes place, postoperative care will also include IV antibiotics, strict neurovascular monitoring, assessment and documentation of CSM, limb pulse oximetry, wound care, and pain control. The orthopaedic nurse is also concerned with nutrition and vascular management, as well as limb functioning.

If replantation is not an option, the surgeon will need to consider the extent of wound debridement to formulate a plan to close the tissue preserve function of the remaining stump. Tissue from the amputated part may be used for grafting purposes, so it is prudent to save all amputated parts and transport them with the patient.

Nursing Considerations

Nursing Diagnoses. Nursing diagnoses for this condition are expanded upon in the Appendix.

- Activity intolerance.
- Anxiety.
- Coping, ineffective.
- Infection, risk for.
- Mobility: physical, impaired.
- Pain, acute.
- Shock, risk for.
- Tissue integrity, impaired.

Interventions. Proehl (2009) outlines early treatment of traumatic amputations:

- ABCs;
- Control bleeding;
- Remove jewelry and clothing that may cause constriction;
- Irrigate wounds for debris;
- Splint and immobilize the injury and elevate the stump;
- Assess neurovascular status;
- Keep amputated part (no part is too small) clean and on sterile gauze in an airtight zip-lock baggie;
- Do not freeze the amputated part or use dry ice;
- Radiographs of BOTH the stump and amputated part;
- Culture wounds prior to antibiotic administration;
- Antibiotics and tetanus as indicated;
- Keep patient warm to prevent vasoconstriction;
- Prepare the patient for the operating room by keeping him NPO, OR time secured, consents signed, pre surgery blood work completed;
- Patient and family education—do not give false hope of re-implantation success; and
- Educate the patient post operatively regarding- Do not smoke or ingest caffeine due to the vasoconstriction effects.

Postoperative nursing considerations for the patient with a replanted limb include neurovascular assessment and function. Pain control and phantom pain relief can be challenging for this population. Physical therapy (PT), occupational therapy (OT), and the entire rehabilitation team are vital to evaluate the limb function and the patient's response to trauma.

Considerations for the patient post-amputation include issues surrounding neurovascular status, tissue healing of the stump, and phantom pain. This population also needs to work closely with the rehabilitation team for mobility, balance, training for activities of daily living (ADLs), and prostheses training as appropriate, as well as adaptation to their loss and resulting changes in body image post-amputation.

Special Traumatic Injuries and Wounds

Violence is a public health problem, and orthopaedic nurses are not immune to caring for the results. Injuries from firearms and blast attacks are part of the reality in today's world. Whether intentional or accidental, these types of injuries are intense in their power of tissue destruction. Such trauma can have a widespread and lasting effect on tissue, muscle, and bone. Puncture wounds and crush injuries pose challenges for healing and return to function due to the damage to surrounding tissues. It is important for the nurse to have an understanding of these injuries to be alert to complications and implement early interventions as needed.

Bullet Injuries. Injuries sustained from bullets are directly impacted by the type of firearm, the gauge and velocity of the weapon used, the type of bullet, and the range from which the gun was shot in relation to the tissue injured. Low-velocity bullets, from pistols and revolvers, cause injury by lacerating and crushing tissue as the body absorbs the energy. There will be an entry wound but not necessarily an exit wound. The bullet may be imbedded in the tissue and may need to be retrieved.

Rifles and shotguns are considered to be high-velocity weapons. Injuries sustained from these types of guns often include both entry and exit wounds. Tissue damage is by laceration and crushing forces, along with a high-pressure shock wave that follows the bullet track and cavitation. Cavitation is the formation of a partial vacuum caused by the bullet as it passes through softer tissue. This negative pressure effect draws bacteria and debris into the bullet tract and builds pressure that creates more damage along the way and a larger exit wound (McQuillan et al., 2009). The denser the tissue, the greater the sensitivity to cavitation, resulting in a more extensive wound. The more elastic the tissue, the greater the resistance because bone is dense, inelastic, and highly sensitive to damage (Maher, 2006).

Prior to assessing a patient who has suffered a gunshot wound (GSW) in the prehospital setting, the nurse should be certain to secure the scene before entering. The nurse may feel insulated to these situations; however, violence part of today's landscape. Even in the most benign situation, foremost in the nurse's mind should be personal safety: make sure that the firearm that has been secured before rendering assistance.

CHAPTER 15

First Aid priorities start with the ABCs to assess for any immediate life-threatening injuries such as airway obstruction, chest wounds, and hemorrhage. Initial prehospital treatment to the wound is to control the bleeding, splint the injury, treat for shock, and evacuate. Evaluate for both an entry wound and an exit wound. When the patient is transported to the ED, a similar approach is taken, starting with the ABCs and specific evaluation of the entry/exit wounds.

Blast Injuries. Often associated with the military and terrorism, blast injuries are also found in a variety of domestic settings. Some examples include the mining industry, farming and grain storage, and explosives like fireworks. Blasts are characterized by the release of large quantities of energy in the form of pressure and heat. A blast wave is the result of expanding gases that displace air at a high velocity followed by a wind blast. If the explosive device is filled with objects, the objects will be projected and cause penetrating injury (ATS, n.d.). In the United States, most blast injuries are unintentional and the result of fireworks and occupational hazards. Around the world, undetonated landmines and military explosives are the cause of much civilian and military causality (CDC, 2003).

Factors that contribute to the pattern of injuries include the proximity of the victim to the explosive and whether the explosion occurred inside or outside a building. Explosions that occur in a confined space are worse than those in open areas because the first blast waves continue to reverberate and the toxic gases and smoke are inhaled. Examples of resulting injuries include traumatic amputation, concussion, facial wounds and auditory affects, burns, and grossly contaminated wounds.

Puncture Wounds. All kinds of sharp or dull objects can inflict puncture wounds, including fish hooks, high-pressure spray washers, nail guns, knives, and teeth (animal and human). If the puncture wound is caused by an impaled object like a knife or a tree branch, initial care should never include the removal of the impaled object. This process often results in more tissue damage as the foreign body is retracted. The prehospital goals are to stabilize the object to prevent movement, splint the injury, and evacuate the patient to a higher level of care. In the hospital setting, when and where the removal will take place is determined after thorough evaluation of the organ and tissue involvement, once the potential for hemorrhage is assessed. Impaled objects are evaluated by radiographs and CTs to determine location and potential damage control with removal. Often surgical removal is necessary for complete tissue evaluation and decontamination.

The greatest risk with puncture wounds is the potential for contamination. On examination, the superficial wound may appear benign and the deeper underlying tissue is of concern. The health care provider needs to assess the degree of contamination and evaluate the wound site for any retained parts or foreign material. Deep cleansing of the wound is necessary and may include surgical excision. Drains, frequent irrigation with antibiotic solutions, and leaving the wound open is necessary to prevent bacteria from inoculating itself and sealing over, a potential for sepsis. IV antibiotics and tetanus (if patient is not up-to-date) are given as first line of defense to prevent infection.

Crush Injuries. Crush injuries can result from prolonged entrapment of a limb or digits (such as an arm caught in machinery) or a crushing blow (such as a foot run over by a vehicle). Damage to vessels and nerves are difficult to assess in relation to the different degrees of damage by the compressive forces. Severity of the injury is based on time under compression, and amount and size of the crushed area. Key assessment items are neurovascular status and function of the limb. Crush injuries have a high risk for compartment syndrome (discussed below), infection, and need for amputation. Patients with a crush injury are at risk to develop crush syndrome. Rhabdomyolysis is a result of muscle destruction from the primary injury, which causes a release of myoglobin and potassium. This event can lead to renal dysfunction and failure. Identification of this situation is based on decreased urine output and brown coloring of urine along with serial blood counts. High levels of serum potassium, creatinine, CPK, and urine creatinine, coupled with a history of a crush, would lead to diagnosis. Treatment for this syndrome includes aggressive hydration to prevent kidney damage by flushing myoglobin out of the renal tubules. The effectiveness is evaluated by examining serial blood levels.

Compartment syndrome is a situation in which there is an increase in the compartment pressures of an extremity that leads to circulation and nerve compromise. This can be caused by internal issues such as fractures, dislocations causing vascular compromise, crush injury causing vascular compromise, and burns. Examples of external causes include casts, splints, and dressings that constrict circulation. The most common sites for compartment syndrome are the forearm and the leg (Oman & Koziol-McLain, 2007). Emergent action in this situation is necessary in order to avoid muscle necrosis, loss of nerve function, and loss of limb. A complete treatment of compartment syndrome can be found in Chapter 8—Complications.

Common Sports Injuries: Soft Trauma

Overview

"Sports injuries" are not usually dramatic in nature and fall into the category of soft tissue injuries sometimes referred

Table 15.11. Common Sports Injuries: Fractures, Sprains, Strains, and Dislocations

Anatomic Area	Mechanism of Injury	Common Athletic Assessment	Activities	Acute Management
UPPER EXTREMITY				
Clavicle fracture	■ Fall on shoulder or outstretched arm ■ Direct blow to the clavicle	■ Crepitus ■ Holds arm close to body ■ Unable to raise affected arm above head ■ Can feel movement of both ends of clavicle	■ Contact sports ■ Ice hockey ■ Wrestling ■ Gymnastics	Adult/Child: ■ Sling or shoulder immobilizer ■ Ice NSAIDs
Dislocated shoulder joint	■ Anterior: some combo of hyperextension, external rotation, and abduction ■ Anterior; anterior blow to shoulder ■ Posterior; fall on flexed and adducted arm ■ Posterior; direct axial load to humerus	■ Pain ■ Lack of motion ■ May feel empty socket ■ Uneven posture in compairison to other shoulder ■ Affected arm longer ■ Abduction limited ■ Diagnose with x-ray	■ Rugby ■ Hockey ■ Wrestling ■ Skiing	Adult/Child: ■ Closed reduction ■ Immobilize as directed ■ Pendulum exercises as directed ■ Pendulum exercises as directed
Elbow dislocation	■ Falling on a hand with a flexed elbow ■ Elbow overextended ■ Posterior disclocation is the most common	■ Intense pain ■ Swelling ■ Limited motion ■ Deformity ■ Ecchymosis	■ Football ■ Gymnastics ■ Squash ■ Wrestling ■ Cycling ■ Skiing	■ Immobilization ■ Ice ■ Assess neurovascular status ■ ROM-timing varies
Wrist sprain/ fracture	■ Falling on outstretched are in an attempt to protect yourself	■ Pain, edema ■ Ecchymosis ■ Deformity ■ Limited motion	■ Skating ■ Hockey ■ Wrestling ■ Skiing ■ Soccer ■ Handball ■ Horseback riding	■ Ice ■ Elevation ■ Immobilization ■ Cast, brace, or external fixation ■ Gentle ROM after healing, 4-6 weeks

Table continued on next page ▶

Table 15.11. Common Sports Injuries: Fractures, Sprains, Strains, and Dislocations (continued)				
Anatomic Area	**Mechanism of Injury**	**Common Athletic Assessment**	**Activities**	**Acute Management**
LOWER EXTREMITY				
Knee sprain	Twisting injury that produced incomplete tear of ligaments and capsule around the joint	■ Pain ■ Limited motion ■ Edema ■ Ecchymosis ■ Tenderness over joint ■ Joint appears stable	■ Basketball ■ Football ■ High jump	■ Ice ■ Elevation ■ Compression (ACE) ■ Active ROM ■ Isometric exercises ■ May immobilize
Knee strain	Result of sudden force motion causing muscle to be stretched beyond normal capacity	■ Pain ■ Limited motion ■ Pain aggravated by activity	■ Soccer ■ Swimming ■ Skiing	■ Ice ■ Elevation ■ Rest ■ Gradual return to activities
Meniscal tears of knee	■ Sharp sudden pivot ■ Direct blow to knee ■ Forced internal rotation ■ Wear from repetitive squatting or climbing ■ Torsional weight-bearing force	■ Edema ■ Medial tear: pain in medial knee occurs in hyperflexion hyperextension, and turning in of knee with knee flexed ■ Lateral tear: most common pain in lateral knee on hyperflexion and hyperextension and internal rotation of foot with knee flexed ■ Displaced fragment: inability to extend knee; locked ■ Positive McMurray's sign	■ Hockey ■ Basketball ■ Football	Conservative: ■ PRICE ■ Exercising quadriceps and hamstrings ■ Resistive exercising ■ NSAID's ■ Physical therapy Surgical: arthroscopy
Ankle sprain	■ Foot is twisted, stretching or tearing ligaments ■ ROM has been exceeded	■ Pain ■ Edema ■ Limited motion ■ Ecchymosis ■ Joint laxity in third degree, severe second degree	■ Tennis ■ Basketball ■ Football ■ Skating	■ Ice ■ Elevation ■ Support: ACE wraps, Aircast, short-leg cast
Ankle strain	Sudden forced motion, stretching muscles beyond normal capacity	■ Acute; sever pain ■ Chronic: achy pain	■ Running ■ All ball sports	■ Immobilization in cast, brace ■ Ice ■ Elevation ■ Rest
Ankle fracture	■ Inward turning on sole of foot and front of foot ■ Supination with internal rotation or pronation with external rotation	■ Pain ■ Edema ■ Deformity ■ Inability to bear weight	■ Contact sports ■ Tennis ■ Basketball	■ Ice ■ Elevation ■ Cast 4-6 weeks ■ Surgery if fracture is displaced or unstable
Metatarsal stress fracture	Occurs with repeated loading of bone – often in an unconditioned extremity	■ Forefoot pain that progressively worsens with activity ■ Minimal or no forefoot swelling	■ Running ■ Dance ■ Skating	■ Rest—STOP sport related activity; average of 6 weeks ■ Ice ■ Most are nondisplaced so weight bearing as tolerated

From Core Curriculum for Orthopaedic Nursing (6th ed., p. 398-399) by NAON, 2006, Boston, MA: Pearson. Reproduced with permission.

to as "soft trauma." It is important to note, however, that these types of common soft trauma injuries don't just happen on the ball field but during ADLs as well. Table 15.11 is a more detailed list of common sports injuries, which include fractures, sprains, strains, and dislocations.

Assessment

Assessment of the orthopedic injury is based on the history of the injury, the clinical exam of the injured part, and the diagnostics. X-ray in the case of soft trauma confirms the preliminary diagnosis by ruling out other issues such as an underlying fracture or disease process. CT and MRI may be used for differential diagnosis to identify specific structures involved such as a meniscus tear vs. an anterior cruciate ligament (ACL) tear in a knee injury.

Common Therapeutic Modalities

Immediate treatment involves splinting and supporting the injured body part. After medical evaluation and initiation of rehabilitation of the injury, the goals include tissue healing, reducing pain and swelling, reestablishing nonpainful range of motion (ROM), slowing muscle atrophy, and establishing neuromuscular control of the injury and surrounding joints (McKeag & Moeller, 2007). The standard mnemonic PRICE is used throughout the sports community:

P – Protection: protect through splinting and support

R – Rest: don't use the limb/joint-use crutches or sling

I – Ice: applied for 30 minutes, off and on

C – Compression: wrap to assist in controlling swelling

E – Elevation: just above heart level to help in reducing swelling

Anti-inflammatory medications (NSADS) are used to assist with management of swelling and alleviate pain. Depending on the severity of the injury, mild narcotics may be used to aid in comfort as well.

Nursing Considerations

Nursing Diagnoses. Nursing diagnoses for this condition are expanded upon in the Appendix.

- Anxiety.
- Constipation, risk for.
- Gastrointestinal motility: risk for dysfunctional.
- Infection, risk for.
- Mobility: physical, impaired.
- Nutrition: imbalance, less than body requirements.
- Pain, acute.
- Self-care deficit: bathing/hygiene, dressing/grooming, toileting, feeding.
- Self-concept, readiness for enhancement.
- Skin integrity, impaired.
- Tissue perfusion: peripheral, ineffective.
- Urinary elimination, impaired.

Highlights of nursing considerations include education on injury prevention by warming up prior to activities, using properly fitting equipment (shoes, shin guards), and use of safety gear. Patients and parents (as applicable) need proper education into the rationale of the postinjury treatment plan, as well as their buy-in and motivation for the overall plan of care. Proper documentation and evaluation of return to work/play will be specific to the activity desired. Each injury has specific guidelines for return to play and should be gradual to avoid relapse. The rule of thumb should be pain-free ROM with good strength (McKeag & Moeller, 2007). The nurse is the key player in the recovery phase and may also be the coordinator between the PT and OT departments, as well as with the coach or team trainer.

Common Sports Injuries: Dislocations/Subluxations

Overview

Dislocation is the complete displacement of articulating surfaces within the joint such as when the ball of a joint is forced out of its socket. Subluxation is a partial displacement or brief separation of the articulating surface, which immediately reduces (pops back into place). These injuries are usually caused by a direct or indirect force to the joint; for example, the mechanism for a shoulder dislocation is frequently associated with direct contact while the arm is in abduction and externally rotated, as in arm-tackling in football (Hudson, 2010).

The most significant risk with a dislocation injury is neurovascular dysfunction. If nerves are compressed, stretched, or lacerated, conduction pathways are interrupted (Table 15.12). Blood vessels can also be disturbed, thus compromising blood flow and oxygen to the distal tissues.

Assessment

Dislocations are often recognizable at the time of injury, as the limb looks out of place or unnatural. Comparing one limb to the other may help in this assessment. The limb can also be "stuck" in an awkward position, and ROM is often limited.

Common Therapeutic Modalities

The goal is to restore the limb to its normal anatomical position and early reduction, as soon as possible. Shoulder dislocation is the most common major joint

Table 15.12. Neurovascular Structures at Risk with Joint Dislocation

Joint	Nerve/Vessel
Shoulder	Brachial plexus/axillary artery
Elbow	Ulnar nerve/brachial artery
Wrist	Median nerve
Hip	Sciatic nerve
Knee	Tibial and peroneal nerves/ popliteal artery and vein
Ankle	Tibial artery

Data from Trauma Nursing: From Resuscitation Through Rehabilitation *(4th ed.) by K. McQuillan, M. Makic, and E. Whalen, 2009, St Louis, MO: Saunders Elsevier.*

dislocation. On the field, a sling and swath are applied to stabilize and support the injury. Once the patient arrives at the medical facility, manual force is attempted for reduction; however, conscious sedation may be needed for reduction if muscle spasms prevent relocation. Postreduction x- rays are useful for full evaluation of joint congruity (Hudson, 20010).

Other common upper extremity dislocation sites include the elbow, thumb, and fingers. The elbow is of concern as the ulnar and radial nerves can be compressed and stretched, which may affect the function of the wrist and hand. An elbow dislocation that is not reduced is considered a medical emergency because the potential loss of function in the hand is great. In the pediatric population, nursemaid's elbow is a classic example of a subluxation injury. An example of the MOI in this case is the child at play, being pulled or swinging by one arm (Rodts, 2009). In contrast, a finger dislocation is often reduced by the patient themselves by gently pulling in-line traction and then buddy-taping or splinting the injury. Taping two fingers together can protect the finger enough for the non-athlete to perform ADLs while supporting the injured finger as it heals, and this modality may even create a functional hand where the athlete could continue playing.

Lower extremity dislocations of the knee and hip are medical emergencies. The knee is of concern because of the potential compromise to the peroneal nerve, popliteal artery, and popliteal vein. A delayed reduction of a hip dislocation can lead to permanent disability due to the potential for avascular necrosis of the femoral head because the head of the femur has its own blood supply. These two injuries are often associated with high amounts of force, such as colliding with the dashboard after a MVC.

Gentle support and guidance to return the limb to its normal anatomical position may spontaneously reduce the injury. Force should not be used, and reduction should never be attempted without proper training. Initial care of a dislocation includes splinting the injury and applying ice to reduce swelling and spasms. Documentation of the patient's neurovascular status should be assessed at the time of injury and after any intervention. Medical evaluation should be scheduled following any dislocation or subluxation to determine joint function, to rule out any fractures and assess neurovascular status.

Nursing Considerations

Nursing Diagnoses. Nursing diagnoses for this condition are expanded upon in the Appendix.

- Anxiety.
- Constipation, risk for.
- Gastrointestinal motility, risk for dysfunctional.
- Infection, risk for.
- Mobility: physical, impaired.
- Nutrition: imbalance, less than body requires.
- Pain, acute.
- Self-care deficit; bathing/hygiene, dressing/ grooming, toileting, feeding.
- Self-concept, readiness for enhancement.
- Skin integrity, impaired.
- Tissue perfusion: peripheral, ineffective.
- Urinary elimination, impaired.

Strains

Overview

A strain is defined as a trauma in which the body of the muscle or the attachment of a tendon has been damaged by overstretching, misuse, or overexertion. Strains are caused by sudden muscle overload. This is the most common injury in sports (McKeag & Moeller, 2007). A strain is described as either acute or chronic.

An *acute strain* is further classified according to the degree of the injury:

1. First degree is mild stretching;
2. Second degree is moderate stretching and/or tearing of the muscle or tendon; and
3. Third degree is a severe muscle stretching in which the involved tissue ruptured, tore completely through, or pulled away from the bone, as seen with an Achilles tendon rupture.

A *chronic strain* is a mild-to-moderate overstretching of the muscle or tendon that persists in causing symptomatology for prolonged periods of time. This most often results from improper care of an acute strain or repeated use of muscle beyond normal capacity.

The incidence of a strain can occur in any age group or in any musculotendinous area of the body, and it is often related to particular movements and activity. For example, tendons are more prone to injury in the elderly than in younger people and are more common in middle-aged males than middle-aged women (McKeag & Moeller, 2007) For the athlete, common injuries involve the knee and ankle. If a strain is not properly treated, there is danger of more dramatic injury with the next insult.

Assessment

Assessment of the injured area includes a history from the patient. Inquiring into the MOI usually reveals a history of a recent stress on of the muscles by exercising or a sudden muscle overload by lifting something heavy. In the event of a first degree strain, the patient will complain of a gradual onset of symptoms that did not begin to appear until several hours after the overexertion. Usually the patient describes feelings of stiffness and soreness of the involved areas. A second degree strain history may include overactivity, which results in sudden acute and incapacitating pain that subsides and then leaves the muscle tender. With a third degree strain, the patient complains of a sudden tearing, snapping, or burning sensation in the injured area during the period of overexertion and then a diminished ability to move the injured body part. Physical examination includes a trial of protected ROM, palpation, and visual inspection to determine the degree of strain:

1. First degree: no loss of ROM, tenderness on palpation, and muscle spasm may be noted; edema or ecchymosis may not be seen.
2. Second degree: extreme muscle spasm, passive ROM resulting in increased discomfort, edema will be seen shortly after the injury, and eccymosis will appear after several hours/days.
3. Third degree: severe muscle spasm, point tenderness, edema, inability to contract the muscle/ROM, and may in fact have a muscle bulge above the palpable defect.

The physical exam is often the only tool needed to diagnose a strain. X-rays can rule out avulsion fractures and can be useful to document calcifications in chronic cases. Ultrasound or MRI may show incomplete tears of the tendon and may be used to rule out complete tears if needed to define treatment (McKeag & Moeller, 2007).

Common Treatment Modalities

Acute treatment at the time of injury includes immobilization of the injury, splinting the injury above and below the injured area, and immobilizing the joint above and below the injury to prevent further damage. The standard **PRICE** (**P**rotection, **R**est, **I**ce, **C**ompression, **E**levation) is initiated at the time of injury until further evaluation can be made.

Nursing Considerations

Nursing Diagnoses. Nursing diagnoses for this condition are expanded upon in the Appendix.

- Anxiety.
- Constipation, risk for.
- Infection, risk for.
- Mobility: physical, impaired.
- Nutrition: imbalance, less than body requires.
- Pain, acute.
- Self-care deficit; bathing/hygiene, dressing/grooming, toileting, feeding.
- Self-concept, readiness for enhancement.
- Skin integrity, impaired.
- Tissue perfusion: peripheral, ineffective.
- Urinary elimination, impaired.

Sprains

Overview

A sprain is defined as a traumatic joint injury in which the surrounding ligament fibers have been damaged by overstretching or exertion. This is often caused by a sudden twist or hyperextension of the joint. Sprains are also classified by a grading system:

1. Mild grade/first degree: only a few fibers of the ligament have been torn or separated and hematoma formation is minimal and localized.
2. Moderate grade/second degree: up to half the ligament fibers torn.
3. Severe grade/third degree: the ligament is completely torn through. The torn ends are separated from each other in the belly of the ligament or from the bone at the point of attachment.

The common sprains in the upper extremity are in the wrist, often related to bracing oneself as in a fall on outstretched hand (FOOSH). The most common sprain of the lower extremity occurs in the lateral ligament of the ankle joint (Hupperets et al., 2010). The classic "ankle roll" from missing a step or walking on an uneven surface may result in an inversion of the ankle, stretching the ligaments making the ankle structure weak. Ligaments of the knee are often injured when one is bracing for a direct blow (as in a football tackle) or from a twisting hyperextension (such as "catching an edge" while skiing). The ACL is very vulnerable in these situations. As in the case of strains, sprains can happen to any age group and are more common with the more active population, from professional athletes to "weekend warriors." Another common sprain site is the cervical spine. This injury can happen a result of flexion/extension forces as in a rear-ended MVC.

Assessment

Physical examination of the injury should determine the degree of injury. Diagnosis is dependent on the amount of edema, effusion, ecchymosis, tenderness, and limits in ROM. Mild grade/first degree sprain patients will complain of mild pain, tenderness, and edema. There will be no joint laxity, although edema may decrease ROM. In the case of a moderate grade/second degree sprain, the patient will complain of greater pain and more tenderness and swelling. There may be some joint laxity, and the edema often impairs full ROM. In the case of the patient with severe/third degree sprain, the caregiver will find severe pain, joint laxity, edema, and loss of joint movement/function.

Radiographic findings demonstrate the presence of edema without bone injury or displacement. As with strains, x-rays are useful to rule out any kind of avulsion fractures. MRI or CT are not often used in the initial diagnostic period but may be useful in subsequent surgical planning if needed.

CHAPTER 15

Common Treatment Modalities

Initial treatment of a sprain includes immobilization of the injured area and support of the adjacent joints. For example, in the case of a FOOSH, the chief complaint is an injured wrist. The prehospital caregiver would splint the wrist, using a commercial splint (such as a SAM® splint) or any ridged material. The next step is to limit movement of the joints above and below the injury by using a sling.

After the initial treatment in the field, a physical therapist may compliment therapy with massage, transcutanous electrical nerve stimulation (TENS), acupressure, or acupuncture. The subsequent treatment depends on the severity of the injury:

1. First degree sprain: use of an elastic bandage or soft cervical collar may provide joint protection while healing. Crutches may be used for the lower extremity for supported mobility. Elevation of the extremity and intermittent application of ice are recommended for the first 24-72 hours. Mild analgesics or anti-inflammatory may be prescribed as needed, along with some isometric exercises.
2. Second degree sprain: compression bandage and splinting of the joint will prevent further damage. Protected weight-bearing may be permitted with crutches when the lower extremity is involved. Apply ice intermittently with cryo therapy, ice cups, commercial ice machines that flow cool water to the injury, or cryo cuff.
3. Third degree sprain: a Jones splint (a posterior plaster or fiberglass splint with batting wrapped around the ankle for support and for ease of swelling), a pneumatic fracture boot (a commercial removable splint with an adjustable bladder), or casting may be used (Kunkler, 2006).

Nursing Considerations

Nursing Diagnoses. Nursing diagnoses for this condition are expanded upon in the Appendix.

- Anxiety.
- Constipation, risk for.
- Infection, risk for.
- Mobility: physical, impaired.
- Nutrition: imbalance, less than body requires.
- Pain, acute.
- Self-care deficit; bathing/hygiene, dressing/grooming, toileting, feeding.
- Self-concept, readiness for enhancement.
- Skin integrity, impaired.
- Tissue perfusion: peripheral, ineffective.
- Urinary elimination, impaired.

Summary

Treatment of orthopedic trauma requires a thorough knowledge of not only orthopedics but emergency treatment modalities in general. A nurse with an understanding of orthopedic trauma can help to minimize the loss of life and limb function from assessment to treatment modalities. Emergency assessment and early intervention lead to the best outcomes. Serious trauma injuries often involve many body systems, and a comprehensive "whole-person" approach is best used from initial care through follow-up treatment. A team approach will assure the best treatment outcomes for the patient.

References

American Academy of Orthopaedic Surgeons (AAOS). (n.d.). *Salter-Harris Classification*. Retrieved August 18, 2010, http://orthoinfo.aaos.org/topic.cfm?topic=A00632

American College of Surgeons (ACS). (2008). *ATLS: Advanced Trauma Life Support Program for Doctors* (8th ed.). Chicago: Author.

Carson, J.H. (2007). Damage control orthopaedics: When and why. *The Journal of Lancaster General Hospital, 2*(3), 103-105.

Centers for Disease Control and Prevention (CDC). (n.d.). *Injuries and Violence are Leading Causes of Death: Key Data & Statistics.* Retrieved July 11, 2012 from http://www.cdc.gov/injury/overview/data.html

Centers for Disease Control and Prevention (CDC). (n.d.). *Web-Based Injury Statistics Query and Reporting System (WISQARS).* Retrieved July 11, 2012, from http://www.cdc.gov/ncips/wisquars

Centers for Disease Control and Prevention (CDC). (2003). *Explosions and Blast Injuries: A Primer for Clinicians.* Retrieved September 6, 2010, from http://emergency.cdc.gov/masscasualties/explosions.asp

Centers for Disease Control and Prevention (CDC). (2005). *Acute Injury Care Research Agenda: Guiding Research for the Future.* Retrieved July 6, 2010, from http://www.cdc.gov/injuryresponse/pdf/acragenda-a.pdf

Department of Transportation (USDOT) National Highway Traffic Safety Administration. (n.d.). *Crash Injury Resource and Engineering Network.* Retrieved August 8, 2010, from http://www.nhtsa.gov/Research/Crash+Injury+Research+(CIREN)/CIREN:+Crash+Injury+Research+and+Engineering+Network/

Department of Transportation (USDOT) National Highway Traffic Safety Administration. (n.d.). *Report No. DOT HS 811 346: Analysis of the Significant Decline in Motor Vehicle Traffic Fatalities in 2008.* Retrieved July 18, 2010, from www-nrd.nhtsa.dot.gov/pubs/811346.pdf

Dobson, J. (2006). Bone up on femur traction splinting. *OnScene: The Journal of Outdoor Emergency Care, Summer 2006*, 14-40.

Emergency Nurses Association (ENA). (2007). *Trauma Nursing Core Course* (6th ed.). Des Plaines, IL: ENA.

F. Gaillard (2008). *Salter Harris Fracture Types.* Retrieved from http://en.wikipedia.org/w/index.php?title=File:SalterHarris.svg&page=1.

Ham, R.J. & Sloane, P.D. (1997). *Primary Care Geriatrics: A Case-Based Approach* (3rd ed.). St Louis, MO: Mosby.

Hudson, V.J. (2010). Evaluation, diagnosis, and treatment of shoulder injuries in athletes. *Clinical Sports Medicine, 29*(1), 19-32.

Hupperets, M., Verhagen, E., Heymans, M., Bosmans, J., van Tulder, M., & Mechelen, W. Potential savings of a program to prevent ankle sprain recurrence. *American Journal of Sports Medicine, 38*(11), 2194-2200.

Kunkler, C. (2006). Therapeutic modalities. In National Association of Orthopedic Nurses (NAON), *Core Curriculum for Orthopedic Nursing* (6th ed., 227-258). Boston, MA: Pearson.

Kushner, A. (1940). Evaluation of Wolff's law of bone formation. *The Journal of Bone & Joint Surgery, 22*(3), 589-596.

Lippincott Manual of Nursing Practice (8th ed). (2006). Philadelphia, PA: Lippincott, Williams & Wilkins.

Maher, A. (2006). Trauma. In National Association of Orthopaedic Nurses (NAON), *Core Curriculum for Orthopaedic Nursing* (6th ed., pp. 395-432). Boston, MA: Pearson.

McKeag, D.J. & Moeller, J. (2007). *ACSM's Primary Care Sports Medicine* (2nd ed.). Philadelphia, PA: Lippincott, Williams and Wilkins.

McQuillan, K, Makic, M., & Whalen, E. (2009). *Trauma Nursing: From Resuscitation Through Rehabilitation* (4th ed.). St Louis, MO: Saunders Elsevier.

National Association of Orthopaedic Nurses (NAON). (2006). *Core Curriculum for Orthopedic Nursing* (6th ed). Boston, MA: Pearson.

National Safety Council (NSC). (2010). *Summary of Injury Facts.* Retrieved July 11,2012, from http://www.nsc.org/news_resources/injury_and_death_statistics/Documents/Summary_2010_Ed.pdf

Netter, F. (2006). *Atlas of Human Anatomy* (4th ed.). Philadelphia, PA: Saunders Elsevier.

Oman, K. & Koziol-McLain, J. (2007). *Emergency Nursing Secrets.* St. Louis, MO: Mosby Elsevier.

Physics Classroom. (n.d.). *Newton's First Law of Motion.* Retrieved July 8, 2010, from http://www.physicsclassroom.com/class/newtlaws/u2l1a.cfm

Proehl, J.A. (2009). *Emergency Nursing Procedures.* St. Louis, MO: Saunders Elsevier.

Rodts, M.F. (2009). Nursemaid's elbow: A preventable pediatric injury. *Orthopaedic Nursing, 28*(4), 163-166.

Sherk, H. (2008). *Getting it Straight: A History of American Orthopaedics.* Rosemont, IL: American Academy of Orthopaedic Surgeons.

Smith, J.E. (2002). Diagnostic modalities for orthopaedic disorders. In A. Maher, S. Salmond, & T. Pellino (eds.), *Orthopaedic Nursing* (3rd ed., pp. 211-229). Philadelphia, PA: W.B. Saunders.

Stevens, J.A., Corso, P.S., Finkelstein, E.A., & Miller, T.R. (2006). The costs of fatal and nonfatal falls among older adults. *Injury Prevention, 12*(5), 290-295.

Professional Practice Committee. (2010). *Practice Guidelines: Removal of Backboards From Patients with Suspected or Diagnosed Spinal Injuries.* Aurora, CO: University of Colorado Hospital.

trauma.org. (n.d.). *History of Trauma: Trauma Resuscitation.* Retrieved October 3, 2011, from www.trauma.org/archive/history/resuscitation.html

Trunkey, D. (2007). The emerging crisis in trauma care: A history and definition of the problem. *Clinical Neurosurgery, 54*(32), 200-205.

Wolff, J. (1892; reprint 2010). *Das Gesetz der Transformation der Knochen.* Berlin, Germany: A. Hirschwald.

World Health Organization (WHO). (n.d). *Poverty.* Retrieved February 28, 2011, from http://www.who.int/topics/poverty

Chapter 16

Tumors of the Musculoskeletal System

Colleen R. Walsh, DNP, RN, CS, ONP-C, ACNP-BC

Objectives

- Identify the various types of musculoskeletal tumors that exist, including malignant bone and soft tissue tumors, as well as benign bone and soft tissue tumors.
- Identify surgical options for patients with a malignant bone or soft tissue tumor.
- Describe potential complications that can arise from musculoskeletal tumor surgery, chemotherapy (neoadjuvant and adjuvant), and radiation, which may be used individually or in combination for the treatment of sarcomas or metastatic carcinomas.
- Describe the treatment of multiple myeloma and metastatic carcinoma.
- Discuss nursing care for patients with a diagnosis of sarcoma, metastatic carcinoma, and multiple myeloma.

Tumors of the musculoskeletal system are either benign or malignant. Primary sarcomas are malignant neoplasms that originate in the bone or soft tissue (Virshup, 2010). Benign tumors and tumor-like conditions can also originate in bone and soft tissues. Non-neoplastic bone and soft tissue tumors are called tumor-like conditions. Although these tumor-like conditions do not result in metastasis, the location of these lesions may impinge on surrounding tissues and result in neurovascular compromise (Virshup, 2010).

Sarcomas arise from tissues derived from mesoderm or primitive mesenchyme, such as muscle, bone, fat, fascia, and cartilage. Sarcomas differ from carcinomas by cell origin. Common carcinoma locations include the breast, lung, prostate, thyroid, and kidney and are derived from ectodermal and endodermal tissues. Nerve tumors also arise from ectodermal and endodermal tissues but are characterized as sarcomas because of their behavior (National Cancer Institute, 2007).

Benign Lesions

Bone Cysts

Bone cysts are common benign, fluid-filled lesions usually found in the metaphysis of long bones. The cause is unknown, and they are often incidental findings on a radiograph (Teo & Chew, 2011).

Definitions. *Solitary bone cysts,* either simple (SBC) or unicameral (UBC), are benign, fluid-filled cysts. The fluid is a clear, yellowish, serous fluid unless a pathologic fracture has caused bleeding in the cyst. These cysts are lined with a fibrous membrane usually less than 1mm thick (Schwartz, 2007). They are usually located in the metaphyses of long bones, especially in the proximal humerus and proximal femur. They are asymptomatic, usually found incidentally or when pathologic fractures occur through the weakened bone. Plain radiograph (X-ray) reveals a "fallen leaf sign" where bony fragments fall to the bottom of cyst. Magnetic resonance imaging (MRI) is obtained if the lesion is close to a growth plate (American Academy of Orthopaedic Surgeons [AAOS], 2007). Some 85% of UBCs occur in the first two decades of life with a ratio 2:1 with male predilection. Treatment of small or asymptomatic lesions of upper extremities includes observation with serial plain radiographs. Larger lesions, symptomatic lesions, and lesions in the lower extremities are treated with curettage and bone graft or aspiration and injection of graft. If fracture is noted in upper extremity, treatments include watch as fracture can initiate healing or IM nail. Fractures in the proximal femur should be surgically treated with curettage, graft, and internal fixation with either plate and screws or IM nail (Schwartz, 2007).

An *aneurysmal bone cyst* (ABC) is an expanding osteolytic lesion consisting of blood-filled spaces separated by connective tissue. This usually occurs in the metaphysic or metadiaphysis of long bones, most often the proximal humerus, distal femur, proximal tibia, and ileum. Only 15-20% occur in the lumbar vertebral bodies. These lesions can arise de novo; however, some may be associated with other tumors. Although unproven, it is generally agreed that ABC results from local circulatory disturbance that leads to increased venous pressure and production of local hemorrhage (Schwartz, 2007). About 50%-70% of ABCs occur in the second decade of life; 70%-86% occur in patients younger than age 20, with females having a slightly higher incidence (Eastwood, 2010). Patients usually present with pain, a mass, swelling, a pathologic fracture, or a combination of these symptoms in the affected area. The symptoms are usually present for several weeks to months before the diagnosis is made, and the patient may also have a history of a rapidly enlarging mass. There are several treatment modalities available, and their use depends on the size of the lesion and its proximity to the physis. Selective arterial embolization has promise in small studies, but because the lesion is relatively rare, there are few randomized control studies. With the use of angiography, an embolic agent is placed at a feeding artery to the ABC, cutting off the nutrient supply and altering the hemodynamics of the lesion. Other treatment modalities include intralesional excision and curettage with bone graft or struts to provide strength during healing. Adjunctive therapies are sometimes used to treat areas of the bone not easily accessible, and liquid nitrogen is most commonly used (Eastwood, 2010).

A *juxtaarticular bone cyst,* or intraosseous ganglion, is a benign cystic and multiloculated lesion made of fibrous tissue with mucuoid changes. It is most commonly found in the subchondral bone of long tubular bones and is often an incidental finding on x-ray. The average age range is 20 to 59 years. Many of these do not require treatment, but larger lesions may require curettage and bone grafting (Limb & Agrawal, 2006).

A *metaphyseal fibrous cortical defect* , or nonossifying fibroma, is a bone lesion with the same histological features of benign fibrous histiocytoma. This is usually located in the cortexes of the distal femur and proximal tibia. This is the most common benign bone tumor, found in approximately 50% of children. It can occur in children ages 0-20 years, often self-healing and filling in with mature bone without intervention (Smith, 2009).

An *eosinophilic granuloma* (EG) is characterized by proliferation of reticulohistiocytic elements with leukocytes, lymphocytes, plasma cells, and giant cells. EG is characterized by single or multiple skeletal lesions, and it predominantly affects children, adolescents, and young adults. Solitary lesions are more common than multiple lesions. When multiple lesions occur, the new osseous lesions appear within 1-2 years. Any bone can be involved, with the more common sites including the skull, mandible, spine, ribs, and long bones. Sixty-one percent of patients are younger than age 21, with males having a higher incidence than females. The lesions usually cause local pain, swelling, tenderness, and the erythrocyte sedimentation rate, or "sed rate," (ESR) may be elevated. Bone lesions often resolve spontaneously and do not require treatment unless they cause symptoms, which occurs in less than 10% of cases (Schwartz, 2007). Curettage provides diagnostic biopsy material and is curative. Large lesions may require bone grafts. Injection of high-dose steroids is another option and tends to result in rapid resolution of the lesion, often within 2 weeks (Khan, 2008).

Fibrous dysplasia is a fibro-osseous proliferation of bone, which may be monostotic or polyostotic. It is developmental in nature and consists of fibrous connective tissue that weakens the bone. The medullary bone is replaced by fibrous tissue, which appears radiolucent on radiographs, with the classically described ground-glass appearance (Anand, 2009). It is most commonly found in the proximal femur, tibia, humerus, ribs, and craniofacial bones, and it usually occurs before age 10, with 75% of lesions discovered before age 30. Treatment usually consists of curettage with bone grafts and empiric treatment with bisphosphonate medicines to help prevent fracture (Schwartz, 2007).

Myositis ossificans, or heterotopic ossification (HO), is a locally self-limiting ossifying process that occurs in the muscle and is generally solitary and well-circumscribed. The lesions are thought to be caused by trauma, and the more common sites of ossification include the arm around the elbow, thigh, and buttocks. Patients with spinal cord injuries are more prone to developing HO. The usual age range is 13-30 years, with males having a greater incidence (Banovac & Speed, 2008). Surgery is usually not indicated unless there is significant limitation in the range of motion (ROM) of a joint. Indomethacin is often used to limit the development of HO (McLean, Hargrove, & Woods, 2009).

An *osteoid osteoma* is a small osteoblastic, intracortical lesion that usually measures less than 1cm, and has demarcated outlines with reactive bone formation. This usually occurs in the femur, tibia, and posterior elements of the vertebrae. Eighty percent of lesions occur in patients ages 5-24, with male predominance of 2.5:1 ratio. The classic symptom is pain at night, not related to activity. Pain progresses with time and is often relieved by aspirin or non-steroidal anti-inflammatory drugs (NSAIDs). It is diagnosed by x-rays, bone scans, and computerized tomography (CT) scans (Khan, 2009). The most common treatments include CT-guided percutaneous radiofrequency ablation (RFA) and surgical excision (Schwartz, 2007).

An *osteoblastoma* is histologically similar to an osteoid osteoma but is larger (more than 2cm). There is immature osteoid osteoma production. Approximately 40% of the lesions are located in the posterior elements of the spine, and these lesions are painful and can lead to scoliosis. They can also occur in the skull, long bones, and hands. Patients with osteoblastomas usually present with pain of several months' duration. In contrast to the pain that is associated with osteoid osteoma, the pain of an osteoblastoma is usually less intense, not worse at night, and not relieved readily with NSAIDS. More than 90% of these lesions occur in patients ages 10-25, with male predominance 3:1 (Schwartz, 2007). These lesions usually continue to grow if not treated, and the usual treatment is curettage and bone grafting (O'Connor & Stacy, 2008).

An *osteoma* is a benign bony overgrowth, where new bone grows on older bone. It is well-circumscribed and usually located in the skull or facial bones. The average age is 16-74 years, and females have a greater than 3:1 incidence than males. Often, no treatment is needed, and many of the lesions are asymptomatic (Khan, 2009).

An *osteochondroma* is a cartilage-capped bony projection on external surfaces of bone. It is the most frequent bone tumor encountered, and it does have the rare possibility of malignant transformation (1%) into a low-grade chondrosarcoma. It is usually located in the metaphyses of long bones, especially the proximal tibia and distal femur. The average age range is 0-30 years. It rarely causes symptoms and is often an incidental finding on x-ray (Dickey, 2009). It can, however, present with pain due to mechanical irritation or a painless mass. Sometimes a fracture can occur through the stalk of the lesion, which also causes pain. Watchful waiting is the most common treatment, and occasionally wide excision at the base of the osteochondroma is needed (Schwartz, 2007).

An *enchondroma* is a benign lesion with formation of mature cartilage, but it lacks the histologic characteristic of chondrosarcoma. They are the most common tumor of the hand but can also occur in the feet, humerus, ribs, and femur. The average age range is 20-50 years. The primary significant factors of enchondromas are related to their complications, most notably pathologic fracture, and a small incidence of malignant transformation. Asymptomatic solitary enchondromas should be followed with serial radiographs, but most will not need surgical intervention unless growth is noted (Schwartz, 2007). In the case of large lesions, or lesions that have undergone malignant transformation, excision with bone grafting is the treatment of choice (Chew & Maldjian, 2009).

A *chondroma*, or cartilage tumor, is a benign cartilage growth that form between the cortex and periosteum. More than 50% of these tumors are found in lateral cortex of proximal humerus just proximal to insertion of deltoid muscle. Other lesions are evenly dispersed throughout the long bones. They usually occur after adolescence, and the treatment consists of en-block excision (Wheeless, n.d.).

A *chondroblastoma* is a rare lesion characterized by highly cellular but undifferentiated chondroblast-like cells. Chondroblastomas typically occur in the epiphyses or apophysis of tubular long bones. The distal femoral and proximal tibial epiphyses are most frequently involved, followed by the proximal humerus. Approximately 92% of patients presenting with chondroblastoma are younger than age 30, with male predominance. Presenting symptoms include pain and swelling around joints. The most common treatment is curettage and bone grafting (Morgan & Damron, 2009).

A *chondromyxoid fibroma* is a rare tumor containing chondroid, fibrous, and myxoid tissue growing in a lobular pattern. More than 75% occur in the pelvis and lower extremity, with approximately one third in the knee region (Schwartz, 2007). They primarily affect young adults in their second and third decades of life: 80% of patients are younger than age 36. Patients usually present with pain and occasionally swelling in joints. They are treated with intralesional curettage or en bloc excision (Morgan & Damron, 2008).

A *desmoplastic fibroma* is a locally aggressive tumor characterized by abundant collagen fibers. More than 50% occur in the femur, tibia, humerus, and radius, and 26% in the mandible. They usually occur in first three decades of life, with 90% of patients 15-40 years old. Treatment consists of aggressive curettage and bone graft or wide surgical excision (Schwartz, 2007).

A *giant cell tumor* (GCT), or osteoclastoma, is a benign but aggressive bone tumor with richly vascularized tissue consisting of plump spindle-shaped cells and numerous giant cells. The severity of GCTs varies widely and can range from local bony destruction to local metastasis, metastasis to the lung, metastasis to lymph nodes, or (rarely) malignant transformation. Approximately 50% of GCTs are located around the knee. The most common locations are the distal femur, the proximal tibia, the proximal humerus, and distal radius. The age range is 20-40 years, with more females than males affected. The work-up for GCTs must include testing for pulmonary metastases, as even the benign GCTs can metastasize. Most lesions are treated with "extended" curettage and bone grafting that is often augmented with adjunctive phenol or liquid nitrogen (Lewis & Peabody, 2009). Depending on the amount of bone destruction, resection might be indicated (Schwartz, 2007).

Soft Tissue Lesions

Soft tissue lesions develop in connective tissue other than bone, such as skeletal muscle, fat, tendon, fibrous tissue, nerve, and blood vessels. In general, benign soft tissue tumors occur at least 10 times more frequently than malignant ones, although the true incidence of soft tissue tumors is not well-documented (Shidam, Acker, & Vesole, 2009).

Definitions. *Hemangiomas*, one of the most common soft tissue tumors, comprise of 7% of all benign tumors and are the most common tumor during infancy and childhood (Weiss & Goldblum, 2008). They are lesions of soft tissue or bone that consists of newly formed blood vessels, and can be either capillary, cavernous, or venous types. The head and neck are the most common sites, but they can also be intramuscular or intraosseous. The spine is the most common for intraosseous lesions. Intramuscular hemangiomas may cause pain and swelling, for which patients seek treatment. Hemangioma of bone may be symptomatic or may be purely an incidental finding. Most commonly, hemangiomas are localized to a single area, but multiple hemangiomas may occur in a single individual in a process known as hemangiomatosis. All ages can be affected but are most common in the first three decades of life, with women being affected 3:1 (Kransdorf & Murphey, 2006). Surgery is indicated for symptomatic lesions. Often, soft tissue hemangiomas are treated with embolization to shrink the lesion, which allows for easier resection with less blood loss. Osseous lesions usually require no treatment at all (Katz & Damron, 2008).

Benign fibrous histiocytomas, or dermatofibromas, are characterized by spindle cell fibrous tissue with a storiform pattern and giant cells. They present with a hemosiderin pigment that contains lipid-bearing histiocytes. They are located on the skin, commonly found on the extremities. All age ranges are affected, but they usually develop in young adulthood. Approximately 20% of the lesions occur before age 17. Females are four times more likely to develop these lesions. No treatment is usually needed except for large lesions that are cosmetically unacceptable to the patient (Pierrson & Tam, 2010).

Ganglion cysts are the most common soft-tissue tumors of the hand and wrist, typically in the synovial membrane or tendon sheath. Although anyone can be affected by ganglion cysts, they occur 3 times as often in women as they do in men. The dorsal wrist is generally the most common site. Mucous cysts are found in the distal interphalangeal (DIP) joint and generally present with osteoarthritis and, therefore, are most commonly seen in older patients. Ganglion cysts are predominantly seen in young adults 25-45 years of age and are rare in children. Open removal has been the surgical treatment of choice for ganglion cyst removal, with arthroscopy offering some benefits, including a reduction in intra-operative risks and postoperative complications (Genova & Walsh, 2009). Most cysts can be treated nonoperatively, but a select group is excised, with a very low rate of recurrence (Weiss & Goldblum, 2008).

Lipomas are the most common soft-tissue tumor. These slow-growing, benign fatty tumors form soft, lobulated masses enclosed by a thin, fibrous capsule. They are usually located in the upper back, neck, shoulders, and abdomen. They are also found in the proximal extremities and buttocks. The average age range is 40-60 years, and gender incidence varies, but most report higher incidence in men (Weiss & Goldblum, 2008). Treatment is usually not indicated unless the lesion is cosmetically unacceptable to the patient, or if the lesion causes symptoms (Nickloes, Sutphin, & Radebold, 2010).

Leiomyomas are tumors that arise from smooth muscle. The genitourinary tract and the gastrointestinal track are the most common sites of the lesions, and it is rare for these to develop on the skin and in the deep soft tissue. These can affect all ages, and cutaneous leiomyomas are more likely to occur in adults than in children. Surgical excision is recommended for solitary lesions (Horner, Raugi, & Miethke, 2009).

Rhabdomyomas are rare tumors arising from striated muscle and are far less common than their malignant counterpart, rhabdomyosarcomas. Rhabdomyomas are classified into cardiac and extracardiac. The extracardiac rhabdomyoma is subclassified into adult and fetal. Adult rhabdomyomas are more common in the head and neck (90%), although it may occur at any age. Middle-aged men, with mean age in the sixth decade, are more commonly affected. The male predominance is strong at 2-5:1 (Kransdorf & Murphy, 2006). Patients with adult rhabdomyoma should have surgical resection of head and neck lesions, especially those lesions that compress or displace the tongue and those that may protrude and partially obstruct the pharynx or larynx. Fetal rhabdomyomas are less common than the adult form, with the median age of 4 at presentation, with boys affected much more than girls (2.4:1 ratio). These are usually treated with surgical excision, and local recurrence is uncommon (Kransdorf & Murphey, 2006). They are located in the subcutaneous tissues of the head and neck. In most instances, they can be excised from various parts of the body without much difficulty. Genital rhabdomyomas are very rare, and local excision is the treatment of choice. Open heart surgery may be necessary for the treatment of cardiac rhabdomyomas (D'Silva, Karina, Worrell, & Arora, 2008).

Intramuscular myxomas are painless, palpable masses, histologically appearing very mucoid with loose network of reticular fiber. These are usually located in the large muscles of the thigh, shoulder, buttocks, and upper arm. Peak presentation is between the fifth and seventh decades, with women affected 2:1 ratio over men (Kransdorf & Murphey, 2006). Excision of the lesion is usually curative (Veillette, 2010).

Schwannomas, also called neurilemmomas or neurinomas, are benign, encapsulated tumors of the nerve sheath. Their cells of origin are thought to be Schwann cells derived from the neural crest. These masses usually arise from the side of a nerve and are well-encapsulated. Neurilemmomas can be associated with von Recklinghausen disease. When this is the case, multiple tumors often are present. Neurilemmomas affect persons ages 20-50 years. Common locations for the tumors are the head and flexor surfaces of the upper and lower extremities and the trunk. Surgical excision is the usual treatment, and the nerve is typically able to be separated from the mass to allow native nerve function. If partial resection of mass is necessary to preserve the nerve function, recurrence is still unusual (Kransdorf & Murphey, 2006).

Neurofibromas are the most common benign tumor of type 1 neurofibromatosis. These tumors are composed of Schwann cells, fibroblasts, mast cells, and vascular components. They can develop at any point along a nerve. The nodules can be solitary or multiple as in cases of von Recklinghausen's disease. They are located on the extremities or centrally located on the body. Young adults usually have solitary lesions, while children with von Recklinghausen's disease often have multiple lesions. The average risk of malignant transformation to a neruofibrosarcoma is approximately 5%. When neurofibromas increase in size or cause pain, malignant transformation should be suspected, and excision or biopsy should be performed (Kam & Helm, 2009).

Fibromas are called desmoid tumors. They are benign, fibroblastic lesions that form from fibroblastic stromal elements. They can be located on the torso, shoulder, hip, and buttocks. They are most common in patients between puberty and 40 years of age, with peak incidence between ages 25-35. Women are affected more commonly than men. Complete surgical excision of desmoid tumors with a wide margin is the most effective method of cure. Radical surgery like amputation should be done for palliative purposes only with repeated tumor recurrence or if tumor did response to adjuvant therapy (Weiss & Goldblum, 2008). Extensive cases may require excision plus adjuvant treatment including chemotherapy, radiation, and repeat surgery (Schwartz & Trovato, 2010).

Pigmented villonodular synovitis (PVNS) is a benign proliferative disorder of uncertain etiology that affects synovial lined joints, bursae, and tendon sheaths. Most commonly affected are the large joints, with 75%-80%

occurring in the knee. The disorder results in various degrees of villous and/or nodular changes in the affected structures. They typically invade local tissues. The invasion of the subchondral bone, with resultant cyst formation, is a characteristic finding. It occurs more often in third and fourth decades, affecting men and women equally (Kransdorf & Murphey, 2006). Synovectomy of the affected area is the treatment of choice, and in large lesions that invade bony structures, curettage and bone grafting is the preferred treatment (Monu, 2010).

Nursing Considerations

Nursing Diagnoses. Nursing diagnoses for these conditions are expanded upon in the Appendix.

- Activity intolerance, risk for.
- Anxiety.
- Coping, ineffective.
- Injury, risk for.
- Knowledge deficit.
- Pain, acute.
- Pain, chronic.
- Skin integrity, impaired.
- Tissue integrity, impaired.

Primary Malignant Tumors

Soft Tissue Tumors

Primary malignant soft tissue tumors represent a histologically heterogeneous group. Although most soft tissue tumors of various histogenetic types are classified as either benign or malignant, many are of an intermediate nature, which typically implies aggressive local behavior with a low to moderate propensity to metastasize. Most soft tissue sarcomas develop in extremities (60%) and trunk (30%), and only 9% occur in the head and neck (Shidham et al., 2009). Treatment options for the various conditions will be discussed later in this chapter.

Definitions. *Malignant fibrous histiocytomas* (MFH) are the most common soft tissue tumor in late adult life. MFH occurs most commonly in the extremities (70%-75%, with lower extremities accounting for 59% of cases), followed by the retroperitoneum. Tumors typically arise in deep fascia or skeletal muscle. The tumor occurs with a peak incidence in the fifth and sixth decades, but an age range of 10-90 years has been reported and men account for 70% of lesions (Kransdorf & Murphey, 2006). Although the tumor is rare in children, the angiomatoid subtype is the most frequently occurring variety in patients younger than 20 years. The male to female ratio is about 2:1 (Stacey, 2009). Further MFH discussion is found in the Primary Sarcoma section of this chapter.

Liposarcomas are the second most common soft tissue tumor and are characterized by lipoblastic differentiation. They are found in the deep soft tissues, especially the thigh and retroperitoneum. Metastases are most common to the lungs. The average age range is 40 to 60 years, and males have a slightly higher incidence than females (Shidam et al., 2009). Liposarcomas are exceedingly rare in infants and children (Kransdorf & Murphey, 2006).

Synovial sarcomas are most common in the foot, ankle, and lower extremity. The histologic appearance is biphasic, composed of epithelial and spindle cell components. Intra-articular lesions are very rare, comprising fewer than 10% of cases. It is most prevalent between ages 15 and 35, with males and females affected equally. Local or metastatic disease is noted in approximately 80% of patients, with 16%-25% metastases present at time of diagnosis. The most common location for metastatic disease is the lungs (59%-94%) followed by lymph nodes and bone (Kransdorf & Murphey, 2006).

Epithelioid sarcomas are slow-growing, firm tumors arising from fascia or tendons. These are usually seen in patients between 10 and 39 years old (75%), with men being more affected than women (1.5-2.6:1). They are most common in the distal upper extremity, with approximately 60% occurring in the flexor surfaces of the fingers, hand, wrist. or forearm. The lesion contains a mixture of epithelioid and spindle-shaped cells with deeply eosinophilic cytoplasm, ovioid and indented nuclei, with small amount of chromatin. Local recurrence is noted at 77%. Most common metastatic sites are lymph nodes, lungs, scalp, bone, brain, liver, and pleura (Weiss & Goldblum, 2008).

Rhabdomyosarcomas are the most common soft tissue sarcoma in children. This is a primary mesenchymal tumor in which rhabdomyoblastic differentiation has occurred (Weiss & Goldblum, 2008). It is considered a high-grade tumor, most commonly located in the head and neck, extremities, and trunk. Due to the location, lymph node involvement and metastasis is common. Approximately two thirds of cases develop in children younger than age 10, with a slight male predominance (1.67:1). Caucasians are affected 3 times as frequently as patients of African descent. Approximately 15%-20% of patients present with clinically detectable metastases at diagnosis. Prognosis for this disease has improved, with an increase in survival rate to 75% over the last 20 years. Rhabdomyosarcoma rarely affects adults (Cripe, 2008). Prognosis in adults is far worse than in children, with a 2-year survival of 50% in fifth decade and 20% in seventh decade (Weiss & Goldblum, 2008).

Fibrosarcomas are a fibroblastic malignancy that produces variable amounts of collagen. It typically involves the deep soft tissues of the extremities and trunk. Symptoms are nonspecific, nonpainful enlarging soft tissue mass, dull ache, or tenderness. Fibrosarcoma represents only about 5% of soft tissue sarcomas. They occur primarily in adults, with 60% of patients ages 40-70, with mild male predilection (61%) (Kransdorf & Murphey, 2006). Further discussion of fibrosarcoma is found in the Primary Sarcoma section of this chapter.

Dermatofibrosarcoma protuberans (DFSP) are nodular cutaneous tumors histologically characterized by uniform population of fibroblast, arranged in a distinct storiform pattern. Although rare, it is an intermediate- to low-grade malignancy. Although metastasis rarely occurs, DFSP is a locally aggressive tumor with a high recurrence rate (20%-55%) (Kransdorf & Murphey, 2006). It is most frequently found in the trunk and proximal extremities. DFSP usually occurs in adults ages 20-50 years. Men are more frequently affected than women. Rarely, DFSP has been reported in newborns and elderly individuals (Chen & Siegel, 2009).

Leiomyosarcomas (LMS) are tumors of small muscle origin. Retroperitoneal/abdominal leiomyosarcomas are twice as common (20-675) as those in the somatic soft tissues (12%-41%). Prognosis is guarded, with the overall median 5-year survival rate of 35% (Kransdorf & Murphey, 2006). Rarely, LMS may present as a primary tumor of bone, where it is hypothesized to arise from intraosseous blood vessels, pluripotent mesenchymal stem cells, or intermediate cellular forms such as myofibroblasts. It usually occurs in the fifth to six decade, with women having a reported ratio ranging 2:1-7:1 for retroperitoneal tumors, while peripheral soft tissue masses are more common among men (Kransdorf & Murphey, 2006).

Malignant peripheral nerve sheath tumors are rare aggressive spindle cell sarcomas arising from nerves or neurofibromas. Most cases are associated with neurofibromatosis type 1 (NF1) and occur in adult life, with ages 20 to 50 being the most common age at diagnosis. It can also metastasize to the lungs and cardiac structures (Kitamura et al., 2010).

Angiosarcomas are malignant vascular neoplasms characterized by the formation of rapidly dividing infiltrating anaplastic cells derived from blood vessels and lining irregular blood-filled spaces. They can occur in areas of chronic lymphedema or post-radiation fields. Angiosarcomas have a poor prognosis, despite aggressive wide surgical resection, adjuvant radiation therapy, and chemotherapy. Angiosarcomas are aggressive and tend to recur locally, with early metastases to lung, bone, and lymph nodes. They are usually located in the skin, deep soft tissues, organs, and bone. All age ranges can be affected but most likely present in the elderly, with men twice as likely as women, excluding those associated with lymphedema (Weiss & Goldblum, 2008).

Lymphangiosarcomas are cutaneous angiosarcomas associated with lymphedema. They are most commonly seen after mastectomies or other secondary causes of lymphedema. They are usually located in the extremities and near areas of lymph node dissections. The usual age of onset is in adults (Schwartz & Fernandez, 2009).

Epitheloid hemangioendotheliomas, rare vascular neoplasms that develop either superficially or in the deep soft tissues of the extremities, are characterized by nodules of deeply eosinophilic, cytokeratin-positive cells reminiscent of epitheloid sarcoma (Weiss & Goldblum, 2008). They have an unpredictable clinical behavior and borderline malignant potential. It can metastasize to the lungs, liver, regional lymph nodes, and bone. It can present at any age but rarely occurs in childhood (Gupta, Kolla, Panda, & Sharma, 2008)

Hemangiopericytomas are vascular neoplasms of intermediate aggressiveness of the pericytes, a modified dendritic-like smooth muscle cell encircling blood vessels. The majority are benign, but there are small percentages that are malignant. They are located in the lower extremity, retroperitoneum, head/neck, trunk, and upper extremity. This disease most frequently affects adults in fifth decade, with 80% ages 25-65 years old, except the rare infantile type. Males and females are equally affected (Kransdorf & Murphey, 2006).

Kaposi's sarcomas are endothelial tumors, usually multicentric, that involve the skin and visceral organs. They are usually located on the skin or in lymph nodes. It may be caused by an enteric sexually transmitted agent and is viral-associated or viral-induced. It is associated with immunosuppression (acquired immune deficiency syndrome [AIDS]) and organ transplantation. The usual age of onset is 50-70 years, but that varies widely depending on the age when either viral exposure or organ transplantation occurs (Moses, 2008).

Paget's sarcomas are high-grade malignancies that form in the area of Paget's disease. It occurs as a malignant transformation of Paget's disease into sarcoma of the bone. There is increased bone turnover, increased osteoplastic bone resorption, and irregular bone formation, leading to focally deficient bone. There is increased pain and an enlarging mass at the "pagetic site." It is usually found in the femur and humerus, and it can also occur in healed fracture sites. It is most common in the seventh and eighth decades of life, and males are more likely to develop Paget's sarcoma (Wheeless, 2010a).

Other Malignant Tumors

As with the more common malignant bone tumors, it is important to correctly diagnose these other malignant tumors. The age of the patient, location of a suspected lesion, the amount of periosteal reaction, and the extent of cortical destruction can assist with the differential diagnosis of tumors. The diagnosis of these tumors depends on plain radiographs, CT or MRI scans, and biopsies. Treatment of these tumors is determined by the biopsy results (van der Woude & Smithuis, 2010).

Definitions. *Chordomas* are malignant tumors characterized by a lobular arrangement of tissue made up of cords and sheets of highly vacuolated cells and mucoid intracellular material. Chordomas are thought to arise from primitive notochordal remnants along the axial skeleton. They are usually located on the proximal and distal ends of the vertebral body. The usual age range is 30-50 years (Palmer & Harrison, 2008).

Mesenchymomas are rare tumors that do not fit into any one histological category. They are characterized by two or more unrelated nonepithelial tissue components within the same neoplasm. It is usually located in the retroperitoneum and lower extremities. The majority of cases occur in adults older than age 60, but it has also been reported in children and young adults (Padua, Bhandari, & Pingle, 2009).

Alveolar soft tissue or *alveolar soft part sarcomas* (ASPS) are rare, slow-growing, painless masses. Common locations for metastatic disease are lung, brain, and bone. They are usually present before diagnosis, as they are symptomatic before the slow-growing tumor. It is usually located in the thigh of adults, and in the head and neck in infants and children. The usual age at diagnosis is 15-35, with females having a higher incidence younger than age 30 and males older than age 30 (Weiss & Goldblum, 2008).

Clear cell sarcomas or *malignant melanomas of soft parts* are located deep and near tendons and aponeuroses. They lack epidermal involvement and are considered one of the rarest types of tumors. They are located in the extremities, especially the foot and ankle. The usual age of onset is age 20-40, with females having a higher incidence than males. Recent studies have demonstrated small histologic differences between malignant melanomas and clear cell sarcomas (Handshake, 2010).

Extraskeletal osteosarcomas (ESOS) are rare soft tissue sarcomas, typically characterized by high-grade histological features and a grave prognosis. Tumors present as enlarging soft tissue masses, and they are usually located in the thigh and retroperitoneum. People older than age 40 are usually more affected (Abramovici, 2005).

Extraskeletal chondrosarcomas occur primarily in deep tissue as slow-growing tumors. They are located in the extremities, most common in persons over the age of 35, but they have been reported in children. Males have twice the number of reported cases (Drilon et al., 2008).

Carcinomas are cancers that arise from epithelial tissues and tend to metastasize. The five most common primary sites of metastatic cancer are: breast, lung, prostate, kidney, and thyroid. The most common locations of the metastatic lesions are the vertebrae, rib, pelvis, and proximal long bones. They tend to occur in persons over age 40, but they can occur at any age (Lewis, 2009). See Bone Metastasis in this chapter.

Nursing Considerations

Nursing Diagnoses. Nursing diagnoses for this condition are expanded upon in the Appendix.

- Activity intolerance, risk for.
- Anxiety.
- Coping, ineffective.
- Injury, risk for.
- Knowledge deficit.
- Pain, acute.
- Pain, chronic.
- Skin integrity, impaired.
- Tissue integrity, impaired.

Primary Sarcomas

Overview

Bone sarcomas are classified according to tissue origin as follows: Bone forming, cartilage forming, giant cell tumors, mesenchymal tumors, or vascular lesions. Most common primary bone tumors include osteosarcoma, chondrosarcoma, malignant fibrous histiocytoma of bone, and Ewing's sarcoma (Rosenthal & Hornicek, 2010). Treatment options for the various classifications are discussed later in this chapter.

Definitions. *Osteosarcomas* have many different histologic subtypes, which can range from low-grade to high-grade. The hallmark of osteosarcoma is proliferation of malignant mesenchymal cells associated with production of extracellular matrix osteiod, which may be ossified (Pappo, 2006). They are the most common primary malignant bone tumor in children, with boys having a slightly higher incidence rate. They are can occur in any bone, usually in the extremities of long bones near metaphyseal growth plates (see Figure 16.1). They involve either the intramedullary region or surface of bone. The most common sites are the femur (42%,

75% of which are in the distal femur), tibia (19%, 80% of which are in the proximal tibia), and humerus (10%, 90% of which are in the proximal humerus). Other significant locations are the skull and jaw (8%) and pelvis (8%). Osteosarcoma is very rare in young children. The incidence increases steadily with age, increasing more dramatically in adolescence, corresponding with the adolescent growth spurt (Mehlman & Cripe, 2008).

Figure 16.1. Osteosarcoma—Distal Femur

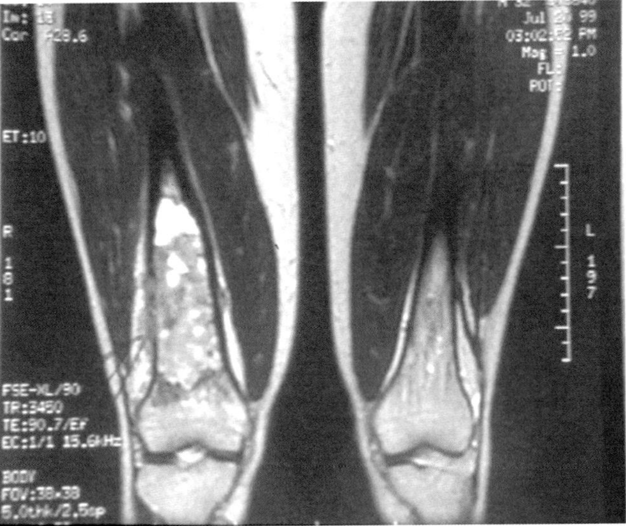

From NAON Orthopaedic Certification Review Course, *2008. Reproduced with permission.*

Surface osteosarcomas are tumors that arise on the cortex, or surface, of bone. They usually occur in metaphyses, especially distal femur. There are three categories of surface osteosarcomas:

1. Parosteal: The most common of the three and occur in the posterior aspect of the distal femur. Ninety-five percent of cases occur in persons ages 15-40, with peak incidence in persons in the second and third decades of life.
2. Periosteal: Most frequently seen on the surface of the proximal tibia, and the age range is similar to parosteal sarcomas.
3. High-grade: The least common of the surface osteosarcomas, and also affects the same age groups. There is a slightly higher incidence in males (Templeton, 2008).

Primary chondrosarcomas are characterized by cartilage forming malignant cells without evidence of direct osteoid formation. It has a higher cellularity and greater pleomorphism than a chondroma. Chondrosarcoma variants are rare and include five types: central, periosteal, mesenchymal, dedifferentiated, and clear cell. The tumor tends to destroy bone and extend into the surrounding soft tissues. The pelvis, proximal femur, and shoulder girdle are the most common sites of the tumor, and the average age range is 30-60 years, with a median age of 45 years. Presenting symptoms include a dull, deep pain in the affected areas that is not associated with activity (Wheeless, 2008).

Secondary chondrosarcomas are benign lesions such as osteochondromas or multiple enchodromatoses that undergo malignant transformation within the cartilage cap of the benign lesion. The most common presenting symptoms may include pain, an irregular border, and an increase in the cartilage cap size after skeletal growth is complete. The lesions are found in the pelvis, proximal femur, and proximal humerus, and average age is 20-60 years (Gelderblom et al., 2008).

Mesenchymal chondrosarcomas are high-grade malignancies that originate in bone (80%) and soft tissue (20%). The lesions contain well-differentiated round or spindle cells with areas of hyaline cartilage. They are found in the maxilla and mandible, pelvis, femur, shoulder, ribs, and sternum. The average age at diagnosis is 30-60 years, but patients of all ages may develop this lesion (Riedel et al., 2009).

Ewing's sarcoma is a tumor composed of densely packed small cells with rounded nuclei. It is considered to be neuroectodermal in origin. It is located on the diaphyseal regions of long bones, especially the femur, as well as the pelvis and axial skeleton. This condition is most common in the second decade of life, with 80% patients less than 18 years old and a median age of 14. Males are more commonly affected than females. This disease is very rare in African-Americans (Pappo, 2006). It is often confused with osteomyelitis, as it presents with fever, anemia, leukocytosis, and an increased sedimentation rate. It is the second most common bone malignancy in children after osteosarcoma (Pappo, 2006). It can be diagnosed by bone marrow biopsy or direct tissue biopsy. Radiographs reveal a classic "onion skin" appearance (Strauss, 2009).

Primitive neuroectodermal tumor of bone resembles peripheral neuroepithelioma of soft tissues. It is histologically different from Ewing's sarcoma due to the neural differentiation, but due to the fact that both tumors were found to contain the same reciprocal translocation between chromosomes 11 and 22, they are considered to fall within the Ewing's sarcoma family of tumors. The age and location of these tumors is similar to Ewing's sarcoma (Toretsky, 2008).

Fibrosarcomas are malignant tumors of fibroblasts, characterized by the formation of spindle-shaped tumor cells of interlacing bundles of collagen fibers, with variable anaplasia and lacking further histologic differentiation. They are usually located in the femur and tibia, and has a wide age range of 5-80 years (Dickey

& Floyd, 2010b). The 2 main types of fibrosarcoma of bone are:

1. Primary fibrosarcoma: a fibroblastic malignancy that produces variable amounts of collagen. It is either central (arising within the medullary canal) or peripheral (arising from the periosteum).
2. Secondary fibrosarcoma: arises from a pre-existing lesion or after radiotherapy to an area of bone or soft tissue. This is a more aggressive tumor and has a poorer prognosis.

Malignant fibrous histiocytomas (MFH), high-grade neoplasms of bone, are composed of fibroblastic and myofibroblastic spindles and pleomorphic cells arranged in characteristic storiform pattern. A significant number of these tumors arise from an underlying condition such as Paget's disease, bone infarctions, or bones that have had prior radiation therapy. Close to 75% of MFH lesions occur at the ends of long bones. Fifty percent of the lesions arise about the knee joint, favoring metaphyseal bone. The lesion can extend into the epiphysis or diaphysis. Rarely is there isolated diaphyseal involvement. MFH is most commonly found in the femur, tibia, pelvis, and humerus. Less common areas include the skull, facial bones, ribs, fibular, spine, scapula and clavicle (Wittig & Villalobes, 2007). These lesions are rarely found in the hands and feet. More than 50% of patients are over the age of 50 at diagnosis; however, it can affect any age group (Schwartz, 2007).

Adamantinomas are rare malignant tumors with the presence of circumscribed masses of epithelial cells surrounded by spindle-cell fibrous tissue. The tumor occurs almost exclusively in the long bones; tumors in the tibia account for more than 80% of cases. The diaphyseal region is the area most commonly affected. Adamantinomas are classified into 2 distinct types: classic and differentiated. Classic adamantinomas usually occur in patients older than 20 years, whereas differentiated adamantinomas occur almost exclusively in patients younger than 20 years. In addition, the 2 classifications of adamantinomas have distinct radiographic and histologic differences (Smelser, Stoffey, Mahaney, Keenan, & Simmons, 2008).

Malignant lymphomas of bone (B-Cell type is most common) are rare tumors where cells are rounded, pleomorphic, and with many indented nuclei. It can occur in any bone, but the most common sites are in short bones such as the ileum and vertebrae, as well as long tubular bones such as the femur and tibia. Primary lymphoma of the bone is rare, but it may present as a symptom of systemic disease, and is classified as a Stage IV lesion. At that stage, regional lymphadenopathy will be present. The age range is 10 to 60 years (Mathur & Damron, 2010).

Multiple myeloma (MM), the most common primary malignant tumor of bone in adults, is a disease where multiple bone involvement is characterized by neoplastic plasma cells with varying degrees of immaturity. There is uncontrolled proliferation of plasma cells, which are highly differentiated B-lymphocytes. MM is associated with abnormal proteins in the blood and urine, as well as anemia and increased sedimentation rate. X-ray reveals "punched out" lesions. This is referred to as the "mosaic pattern." The usual locations of osseous lesions are bones that contain abundant bone marrow, including vertebrae, ribs, skull, pelvis, long bones, and sternum. The median age of patients with MM is 68 years for men and 70 years for women (Grethelin & Thomas, 2010). MM is explained more in-depth in its own section in this chapter.

Incidence. The incidence of primary sarcomas is low. The American Cancer Society (ACS) estimated that, in 2009, 2,507 new cases of bone and joint cancer would be diagnosed, and there would be 1,470 deaths. The number of new soft tissue tumors was expected to exceed 10,660 with 3,820 deaths (ACS, 2009; McCance, 2010).

Etiology. Most etiologies of sarcomas are unknown. While there is no clear-cut correlation between congenital factors and the development of cancer in children, some sarcomas do arise more frequently in children with certain hereditary syndromes such as Beckwith-Wiedemann, neurofibromatosis type I, and Li-Fraumeni (Kline, 2010). Radiation-induced sarcomas have been identified, and these lesions are histologically different than the lesion for which the radiation was given (Rao & Hackbarth, 2009). Trauma draws attention to lesions already present but has no causal relationship with the development of the lesions (Mehlman & Cripe, 2008).

Cancer is caused by alterations in oncogenes, tumor-suppressor genes, and microRNA genes, and it appears that multiple sequential steps are involved in the development of cancer cells (Croce, 2008). Environmental issues such as pollution, exposure to chemicals, and asbestos can accelerate the cellular changes that can lead to the development of sarcomas (Lahat, Lazar, & Lev, 2008). Pelvic and axillary lesions have lower survival rate than extremity lesions (Roque, Mankin, Hornicek, & Nyame, 2007).

Considerations Across the Life Span. Once, cancer was considered a terminal illness. Now, many cancers are considered chronic diseases. The National Cancer Institute reported that nearly 10 million people in the United States have been diagnosed with cancer, and nearly two thirds of those have survived for more than 5 years (Bhatia & Robinson, 2008). There is a need for periodic follow-up for the rest of the patient's life, especially children who have survived because late-onset complications such as cardiomyopathy, pulmonary insufficiency, renal failure, and other malignancies often take years to develop (Geenen et al., 2007). Life-threatening illnesses in childhood that are treated with chemotherapy can affect developmental goals in each stage of growth and development (Kakaki & Theleritis, 2007).

Children with cancer often have impaired socialization, and this is especially true for the school-aged child. These children often require long periods of physical isolation due to the severe immune suppression from chemotherapy, and they often are unable to attend school for long periods of time (Geenen et al., 2007). The children may experience temporary or permanent developmental delays or regression.

Adolescents are significantly impacted by the diagnosis of cancer. Teenagers tend not to ask adults for help or confide about embarrassing physical changes, and that results in receiving their diagnoses much later in the course of their illness than younger children. That usually means that they will require more aggressive and protracted treatments that can lead to lifelong side effects (Rabin, 2010). Issues of autonomy verses dependency, increased reliance on parents, surrender of control, changes in body image, and alterations in sexual development are all issues that adolescents face. Prolonged hospitalizations can alter peer relationships, resulting in a further sense of isolation (Rabin, 2010).

One in 168 Americans develops invasive cancer between ages 15 and 30. Young adults have the lowest rate of health insurance coverage, frequent delays in diagnosis, and the lowest enrollment in clinical trials (Bleyer, 2007). The young adult faces issues of infertility/sterility from chemotherapy, and marriage and family goals may need to be postponed. If the cancer is of genetic origin, the young adult with cancer must decide whether or not to undergo voluntary sterilization (Bleyer, 2007). Finding insurance may be especially difficult if the young adult is unable to find work due to their illness. New health care laws may help mitigate that, as the young adult may be eligible to remain on their parent's health insurance (Bleyer, 2007).

Middle-aged adults with cancer have different challenges. Adults must deal with the cancer's effect on productivity and work ability, which in turn is important to their financial situation, life satisfaction, and social relationships. Career changes may be necessary in order to accommodate the patient's reduced strength and physical endurance, secondary to the effects of the treatments (Tretli & Kravdal, 2008).

Geriatric patients with cancer have unique needs. The majority of cancer incidence and mortality occurs in individuals older than age 65, and the number of older adults with cancer is projected to significantly increase, secondary to the aging of the US population (Pal, Katheria, & Hurria, 2010). Several unique concerns arise in the older adult with cancer. With increasing age, physiologic reserve decreases; however, the pace of this decline varies with each individual. Similarly, variations in functional status, cognition, and comorbidity accompany increased age, likely affecting life expectancy, risk of subsequent functional decline, hospitalization, and other morbidity. These age-related changes can influence tolerance to cancer therapy, as well as the overall risk-benefit ratio of cancer treatment (Pal et al., 2010). The rate of these changes also varies between individuals. Cancer is often viewed as a premature end to productivity.

There is overlap in developmental issues for all age groups. Cancer stigmatizes people, affecting families, friendships, neighborhoods, workplaces, and schools. This is especially true for patients whose cancers may have resulted from personal lifestyle behaviors (Lebel & Devins, 2008).

Complications of Treatment. While cancer treatments have improved and more people are living longer, the treatment regimens often produce serious side effects. Many orthopaedic oncology patients with tumors receive chemotherapy and/or radiation treatments prior to surgical resection, which leaves them immunocompromised (Lewis, 2009). Infection in surgical incisions can occur either early or late in the course of treatment, and this can lead to failure of metal implants or allografts and, subsequently, loss of limb (Lewis, 2009). Many chemotherapeutic agents can cause permanent toxicity, and the cardiovascular complications including heart failure, myocardial ischemia/infarction, hypertension, thromboembolism, and arrhythmias are the most common and potentially lethal (Yeh & Bickford, 2009). Local recurrence of tumors or metastasis of the primary tumor usually results in loss of limb and life (Lewis, 2009).

Assessment

The aims of surgical staging are to determine the surgical margins of resection and to facilitate inter-institutional and interdisciplinary communication regarding treatment data and results. The Enneking system for the surgical staging of bone and soft-tissue tumors is based on grade (G), site (T), and metastasis (M) and uses histologic, radiologic, and clinical criteria. It is the most widely used staging system and has been adopted by the Musculoskeletal Tumor Society (Teo & Peh, 2010)

This information obtained from the G-T-M staging system in turn gives the orthopaedic oncology team and patient information regarding appropriate planning for possible neoadjuvant chemotherapy or radiation treatments, allowing the orthopaedic surgeon to begin planning for possible limb salvage surgery. Additionally, neoadjuvant chemotherapy and radiation therapy may reduce the size of the tumor, thereby possibly making a previously non-operative tumor amenable to surgery. It should be noted that there are other staging systems developed for musculoskeletal tumors, such as the one created by the American Joint Committee on Cancer (Stacey, Mahal, & Peabody, 2006).

History and Physical Exam. When assessing a patient with a suspected musculoskeletal tumor, it is critical to gather information that may assist in diagnosing these tumors. Assessment should include answers to the following questions:

- What is the duration and onset of symptoms?
- Is the pain usually severe, and often occurring at night?
- Is there a palpable mass? If so, note size, tenderness/swelling.
- Is there any family history of malignancies?
- Is there impaired activity or mobility due to pain or mass?
- Are the lymph nodes enlarged?
- Is the liver or spleen enlarged?

This data can help the orthopaedic team develop differential diagnoses that can guide the team in deciding what diagnostic tests need to be obtained. The importance of a thorough and detailed history and physical exam cannot be over-emphasized.

Diagnostic Tests. The orthopaedic team has a variety of diagnostic tests that assist with an accurate diagnosis of musculoskeletal tumors. The team may elect to obtain some or all of the following tests in order to reach a definitive diagnosis:

- High-quality, anteroposterior, and lateral x-ray of involved area;
- CT and/or MRI to detect soft tissue involvement and location of tumor and neurovascular structures in transverse or sagittal planes;
- CT of chest to rule out pulmonary metastases;
- Ultrasound to rule out cystic tumor;
- Arteriogram to identify vessel involvement;
- Complete blood count (CBC) with differential to rule out infection;
- Sedimentation rate;
- Liver function tests (LFTs), serum electrolytes, including calcium, phosphorus, and alkaline phosphate;
- Bence-Jones protein in urine to rule out multiple myeloma;
- Biopsy (see Common Therapeutic Modalities below);
- Bone scan to assess for metastatic disease; and
- Consideration of positron emission tomography (PET) scanning that assists with tumor staging and grading, evaluating treatment, and detecting recurrences (Cripe, 2008; Carsi & Sim, 2009; Lewis, 2009).

Common Therapeutic Modalities

Surgical treatment for sarcoma may be combined with pre- and/or postoperative chemotherapy and/or radiation therapy (Victorian, 2009). In some cases, patients receive intra-arterial chemotherapy aimed at directly delivering chemotherapy into the tumor (Figure 16.2). Bony defects resulting from surgery are replaced with 1) metal implants; 2) allografts with internal fixation; 3) allografts with metal implant combination alloprosthesis; or 4) autografts, such as vascularized or nonvascularized fibular grafts (Beebe et al., 2009; Victorian, 2009). Infection is a serious complication following limb-salvage procedures, but removal of the infected endoprosthesis, the use of antibiotic impregnated spacers, and vascularized free flaps have improved the success rate in treating these devastating infections (Manoso, Boland, Healey, & Cordeiro, 2006). After excision of malignant tumors, some patients receive radiation and chemotherapy, which impairs wound healing. This requires continual surveillance because infection or open wounds can happen early or as many as 1-3 years after surgery. Other factors that negatively affect wound healing include a history of smoking prior to surgery, long-term steroid treatment, diabetes mellitus, hypoproteinemia, and hypothyroidism (Bernard, 2009).

Figure 16.2.
Arteriogram with Intra-arterial Catheter for Chemotherapy

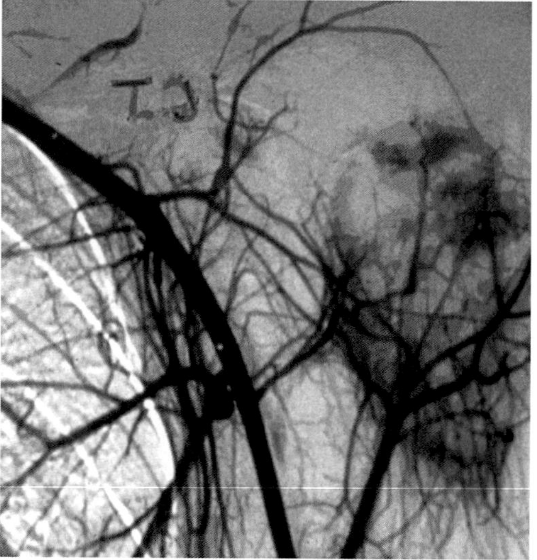

From NAON Orthopaedic Certification Review Course, *2008. Reproduced with permission.*

Skin or muscle deficits may be covered with either split thickness skin grafts or vascularized or nonvascularized myocutaneous flaps. Either local or free flaps can be used, and the size of the resultant defect after wound debridement or tumor resection affects the decision for reconstruction. Typically, muscle flaps are preferred to skin-muscle (myocutaneous) flaps because they conform to the defect better (Bernard, 2009). The types of muscle and myocutaneous flaps available for reconstruction include gastrocnemius, vastus medialis, vastus lateralis, and sartorius flaps (Bernard, 2009).

As discussed previously, there are a variety of treatments for some benign bone lesions. Some of the options available include:

- Curetted and frozen with liquid nitrogen (known as cryotherapy).
- Painted in the cavity with phenol after the lesion has been removed.
- Both phenol and cryotherapy induce further bone tissue necrosis, decreasing the chance of local recurrence.
- Permanently filled with bone graft (synthetic or autograft).
- Occasionally bone cement (methylmethacrylate) is used to fill the defect; however, detection of recurrence is more difficult when bone cement is used (O'Connor & Stacy, 2008).

Indications for these treatment options depend on the tumor, location, whether or not the tumor can be totally removed with tumor-free margins, whether the neurovascular bundle is involved within the tumor, and the skeletal development. Development should be nearly complete in order to minimize leg length discrepancy (Mehlman, 2008).

Biopsy. Biopsies of suspected musculoskeletal lesions continue to be the gold standard for managing patients with suspected musculoskeletal lesions. A biopsy is defined based on what technique is used to obtain the sample. Indications for biopsies include diagnosing a benign versus a malignant mass and obtaining histologic staging, and determining the tissue type to assist with the development of the treatment plan. The most commonly used biopsy techniques are needle, open/incisional, and excisional.

Needle biopsy is used in institutions with pathologists well versed in diagnosing sarcomas. The biopsy is essential for histologic staging of tumors. It is performed in the operating room or under CT guidance, usually by an interventional radiologist. Tissue sample is small; therefore, open biopsy may be warranted if a diagnostic tissue sample is not received. There are two main categories of needle biopsies: 1.) fine needle, used to decrease the amount of disruption to surrounding tissue; and 2.) core needle, used when a larger sample is needed to make a diagnosis and it has a higher accuracy rate than fine needle biopsies.

Open/incisional biopsy is a surgical procedure done in the operating room. It is a procedure in which a small piece of tissue is excised for microscopic examination to determine the type and behavior of the tumor.

Excisional biopsy is a surgical procedure in which a mass, usually benign, is marginally excised. Both incisional and excisional biopsies are used for definitive treatment and microscopic tissue examination to determine the type of tumor (Wheeless, 2010b).

Common anatomic areas that are biopsied include any soft tissue mass, bony mass, or lesion. While these biopsies are very helpful, there are potential problems or complications that occur. There may be inadequate tissue to diagnosis, which is more likely with the needle aspiration or core needle biopsy. Patients may experience delayed wound healing due to infection, and there is the risk of microexpansion of the tumor due to tissue contamination. This may cause distant metastasis (Wheeless, 2010b). There is also a risk of fracture of a biopsied bone due to the presence of a stress riser.

Limb Salvage. Since the early 1970s, limb-salvage or limb-sparing procedures have been the most common method used to treat patients with musculoskeletal sarcomas. It is considered a curative procedure that is performed as an alternative to amputation for the management of sarcomas (Victorian, 2009). The surgical treatment includes removal of the lesion, either bone or soft tissue, with a zone of normal surrounding tissue. Several types of limb-salvage procedures are currently being utilized for bone and soft tissue sarcomas.

Intracapsular or intralesional excision is a procedure done within the pseudocapsule of the lesion (rarely done and done for palliation only). *Marginal excision* is done en bloc extracapsularly within the reactive zone. *Wide excision* is done en bloc through normal tissue beyond the reactive zone but within the compartment of origin, leaving in situ some portion of the compartment.

Radical resection is done en bloc of the lesion and entire compartment of origin, leaving no remnant of the compartment of origin. If performed on a bone lesion, metal implants are placed after the excision to reconstruct the bone (i.e. epiphysis, distal femur replacement prosthesis, or proximal femur).

Rotationplasty is a modified amputation done usually on a skeletally immature child with a malignant tumor near the knee (distal femur or proximal tibia). This procedure is selected due to the tumor's proximity to the growth plate. The procedure involves removing the knee joint and tumor, turning the distal portion of the lower leg 180 degrees and attaching the remaining tibia and foot

Table 16.1. Sarcoma Resections by Site	
Upper Arm: wide excision or radical resection of tumor within the biceps brachialis, coracobrachialis (anterior), or triceps (posterior).	**Groin (Soft Tissue):** wide excision of femoral triangle with sacrifice of nerve, artery, vein, and inguinal lymph nodes; with possible reconstruction by arterial graft and hamstring transfer.
Proximal Humerus: wide excision of tumor within humerus with total shoulder replacement or proximal humeral replacement, proximal allograft, or alloprosthesis.	**Proximal Femur**: wide excision or radical resection of proximal femur, reconstruction using proximal femoral replacement prosthesis, total or hemi-joint replacement, or alloprosthesis.
Proximal Humerus, Glenoid (Shoulder Joint), Distal Clavicle: 1. Modified Tikhoff-Lindberg (resection of humeral head): wide excision or radical resection of scapula, proximal humerus, distal clavicle, acromion, glenoid cavity, deltoid muscle; attach remaining humerus to clavicle with metal rod and/or Dacron® graft and/or allograft bone. 2. Flail shoulder results, and radial nerve palsy (nerve sacrificed) usually occur. 3. Hand and elbow are usually functional.	**Midshaft Femur:** wide resection with allograft, metal intercalary replacement, or total metal femur replacement.
Midshaft Humerus: wide excision of tumor within humerus with allograft or autograft using vascularized or nonvascularized fibula.	**Distal Femur:** 1. Wide excision with long stem distal femoral replacement prosthesis, with or without proximal tibial prosthetic component, allograft or combination, or alloprosthesis. 2. Peroneal nerve may be sacrificed if the popliteal space is involved; therefore, an ankle/foot orthosis will be needed. Some surgeons prefer to perform knee joint arthrodesis using allograft; however, patient satisfaction long-term is low due to the inability to bend the knee.
Scapula: marginal or wide excision of scapula, or modified Tikhoff-Lindberg procedure or custom total scapular replacement.	
Ilium, with or Without Soft Tissue Component: marginal or wide excision of ilium with or without surrounding soft tissue. In certain cases, femoral head will create a pseudoarthrosis.	**Lower Leg/Calf (Soft Tissue):** wide excision or radical resection of lateral or medial gastrocnemius.
Acetabulum and Medial Wall of Pelvis, or Wide Excision of Acetabulum, Medial Wall Pelvis, Femur: surrounding tissues fuse femur to ilium or ischium using internal fixation. A custom-fit pelvic allograft or prosthesis using internal fixation can be inserted (not common due to high risk of failure due to infection).	**Proximal Tibia:** 1. Wide excision with proximal tibial/ knee replacement, allograft, or combination of both. 2. Peroneal nerve may be sacrificed if popliteal space is involved and an ankle/foot orthosis is needed. 3. Some surgeons prefer to perform knee joint arthrodesis with allograft (see "Distal Femur" above).
Pubis, Ischium, and Ischial Tuberosity: wide excision of pubis, ischium, and ischial tuberosity.	**Midshaft Tibia:** wide excision with fibular autograft or allograft (vascularized or nonvascularized).
Upper Leg/Thigh (Soft Tissue): wide excision of radical resection of quadriceps (with or without femoral nerve) anteriorly, hamstrings (with or without sciatic nerve) posteriorly; adductor compartment medially.	**Spine:** laminectomy with or without internal fixation, rods and/or bone graft (with allograft or autograft).

From Musculoskeletal Cancer Surgery: Treatment of Sarcomas and Allied Diseases *by M. Malawer and P. Sugarbaker, 2001, Norwell, MA: Kluwer Academic Publishers. Reproduced with permission.*

to the distal portion of the remaining femur. The ankle joint becomes the new knee joint, and the patient will function as a below-the-knee amputee with a special prosthesis. Before this technique was developed, a child's only option for treatment for a tumor around the knee was an above-the-knee amputation.

Reconstruction. There are a variety of materials that can be used for reconstructions of both benign and malignant boney lesions. *Allografts* are cadaveric human bone that is transplanted to surgically resected bone. The donor must have no history of infection, cancer, hepatitis, HIV, active or chronic systemic viral illnesses, tuberculosis, or chronic intravenous drug use (Meermans, Roos, Hofkens, & Cheyns, 2007). Allografts are stored in -80 degree Celsius deep freezer and can be used only if they have negative 10-day post harvesting cultures. Freezing minimizes immunogenicity so tissue typing or immunosuppressive drugs are not needed (Meermans et al., 2007). Rigid internal fixation is needed, and patients are usually non-weight-bearing for 6–12 weeks. Healing by creeping substitution is a slow process whereby cadaver bone is replaced by the patient's own bone, at least at the junction between the patient's bone and the allograft. The allograft can be ordered with or without soft tissue attachments (tendons and ligaments). It is called an osteoarticular (OA) graft if ordered with the soft tissue attachments (Kayurapan, Makadelok, & Waikiki, 2010). Irradiated freeze-dried tissue (allograft) is also available to fill cavities left by small lesions that are usually benign.

Autografts replace surgically resected bone with the patient's own bone from sites such as the iliac crest, fibula, or rib. They may be vascularized or nonvascularized fibular grafts. While autografts have traditionally been used in bone grafting, advances in screening and retrieval of cadaver bone, as well as the development of demineralized bone matrix (DBM) and recombinant human bone morphogenetic proteins (rh-BMPs), have made autografts far less commonl. Autografts require another surgical incision, and the donor site is usually very painful and not without its own set of complications (Albert, Leemrijse, Druez, Delloye, & Cornu, 2006).

Metallic prosthesis may replace the joint and a large part of the shaft of the bone, or replace the entire bone as is the case with a total femoral replacement. These prostheses can be off-the-shelf or custom made (Holt, Christie, & Schwartz, 2009). Children who have not yet reached skeletal maturity may be treated with expanding endoprostheses that expand as the child achieves longitudinal bone growth. An alloprosthesis is a combination of a metal prosthesis and cadaveric allograft.

Resection. The type and extent of musculoskeletal resections vary by site and tumor type. See Table 16.1 for a list of surgical sites and structures removed.

Amputation. Amputations are defined as the removal of a part of or an entire limb above, below, or through a joint. Although limb salvage is the usual treatment of choice for sarcomas, amputations are used in the treatment of sarcomas when limb-sparing surgery cannot be used. Indications for amputation include the inability to attain tumor-free margins needed for a limb-sparing surgery, extreme neurovascular bundle involvement by tumor, and young children with tumors who would experience significant limb-length discrepancies because of the limb-salvage procedure (Lietman & Joyce, 2010). See Table 16.2 for the different levels for amputations.

Table 16.2. Amputation Levels
1. Symes (just proximal to the ankle)
2. Below the knee (BK).
3. Knee disarticulation (KD).
4. Above knee (AKA).
5. Hip disarticulation (HD).
6. Hemipelvectomy (HP).
7. Hemicorporectomy.
8. Below elbow (BE).
9. Above elbow (AE).
10. Shoulder disarticulation (SD).
11. Forequarter amputation.
12. Rotationplasty (see Rotationplasty under Limb Sparing).

Potential problems abound, and complications are not uncommon following amputations. Proper hemostasis at the time of surgery and proper reattachment of retained muscles over the bone end can help to alleviate some of these complications (Lietman & Joyce, 2010). Common complications include flexion contractures, pressure sores on the distal stump from the prosthesis, development of a neuroma at the site of an amputated nerve, wound dehiscence or infection, excessive swelling at the stump due to improper stump wrapping or not wearing a stump sock, bone overgrowth, especially in children, and phantom sensation and/or pain (Daigeler et al., 2009).

Radiation. Radiotherapy or *radiation therapy* (RT), also called *external beam irradiation* (EBRT), has been shown to decrease the chance of local recurrence in some sarcomas that are radioreceptive. Radiation may interfere with tissue healing, cause joint fibrosis, edema, cessation of growth of extremity due to injury to physis, and permanent bone healing problems. Secondary cancers may occur years later as a result of DNA changes caused by the radiation. These risks are reduced with appropriate planning, although the risk/benefit ratio needs to be evaluated prior to the start of such therapies (Rao & Hackbarth, 2009).

The use of radiation has not shown significantly to increase overall survival; however, retrospective studies show an improved overall survival rate with local control of the sarcoma. The role of RT in the management of bone osteosarcomas or chondrosarcoms is limited. Its primary application appears to be in Ewing sarcoma, for which curative treatment requires combined local and systemic therapy (Sheplan & Juliano, 2010).

The use of RT for palliative pain relief and improved quality of life patients with metastatic bone disease is common. The pathologic fractures are irradiated after internal fixation to destroy tumor growth and improve pain control, thereby increasing mobility and function for the patient (Lewis, 2009). Women older than age 50 are more prone to pathologic fractures after radiation, but that appears to be dose- (rads-) dependent and may be related to the natural course of menopausal osteoporosis (Gridelli, 2007).

Radiation is often used as an adjuvant therapy for soft tissue tumors. It can be administered pre- and/or postoperatively, depending on the size of the tumor or how close the margin area is when the tumor is removed. It can also be used intraoperatively to minimize injury to tissues and structures, such as the bowel or joints that are in close proximity to the excision area. The addition of *intraoperative radiation therapy* (IORT) to conventional treatment methods has improved local control and survival rates in many disease sites in both the primary and locally recurrent disease settings (Willett, Czito, & Tyler, 2007).

Brachytherapy is another option available for the treatment of soft tissue sarcomas. It consists of interstitial radiation therapy that is delivered via iridium. The catheters are implanted at the time of surgery if the margins are not expected to be tumor-free. It is also used to decrease the chance of local recurrence. These catheters are loaded with the iridium approximately 3-5 days after surgery, and the treatment continues for 3-5 days while the patient is kept in a lead-lined room with minimal exposure to staff and family. The implants and catheters are removed after the specific dose of radiation has been administered (Rudert et al., 2010)

Intensity-modulated *photon radiation therapy* is used when there is a need for improved coverage of the tumor volume without increasing the radiation exposure. *Neutron beam therapy* is radiation produced by heavy particle accelerators and is usually used in non-resectable tumors such as the sacrum or vertebrae (Patel & DeLaney, 2008).

Radiation therapy is not without complications. Localized skin redness and irritation, hair loss, nausea, and fatigue are often seen (National Cancer Institute, 2010). Urinary and bowel problems can arise if areas around the pelvis receive large doses (Willett et al., 2007).

CyberKnife® is a newer form of radiation that is a non-invasive alternative to surgery for the treatment of both cancerous and non-cancerous tumors anywhere in the body. CyberKnife® System is the world's first and only robotic radiosurgery system designed to treat tumors throughout the body non-invasively. It provides a pain-free, non-surgical option for patients who have inoperable or surgically complex tumors, or who may be looking for an alternative to surgery (Accuray, 2011).

Chemotherapy. Chemotherapy is another therapeutic option for the treatment of soft tissue sarcomas. The rationale for combination chemotherapy is that many cytotoxic drugs have synergistic effects when administered together. A combination of cell-cycle specific and nonspecific drugs has been demonstrated to have the greatest antineoplastic effect (Jain, Sajeevan, Babu, & Lakshmaiah, 2009).

Preoperative chemotherapy (neoadjuvant) has been used for more than 30 years in the treatment of sarcomas. Its primary purpose is to shrink the primary tumor, making it easier in facilitating en bloc resection of the tumor. It is also used to destroy pulmonary micrometastases or shrink pulmonary macrometastases. It is also used to evaluate the efficacy of the cytotoxic drugs given in the preoperative period (Rosen, 2008).

Postoperative chemotherapy is used in the absence of documented metastatic disease (known as prophylactic or adjuvant chemotherapy). Theoretically, malignant cells have entered the bloodstream either before or during surgery and have traveled to other areas of the body. Metastatic disease would then appear at a later date. The effectiveness of such therapies has been mixed and is dependent on tumor type and grade (Skubitz & D'Adamo, 2007).

Chemotherapy for sarcomas is continually being evaluated by standardized protocols in the attempt to find the best combination of drugs. Chemotherapy regimens for bone sarcomas such as osteosarcoma, Ewing's sarcoma, and malignant fibrous histiocytoma have shown to be effective. For high-grade soft tissue sarcomas in young adults and children (rhabdomyosarcoma, extraosseous Ewing's sarcoma), chemotherapy plays a major role in cures (Skubitz & D'Adamo, 2007). In the majority of adult soft tissue sarcomas, however, chemotherapy has shown no increase in the cure rate (Jain et al., 2009).

Chemotherapy protocols will vary in length of treatment depending on diagnosis. There are multiple drugs that can be used for the treatment of osteosarcoma. The most common drugs used in combination for various osteosarcomas are found in Table 16.3. Several common chemotherapeutic agents, particularly Doxorubicin, are light-sensitive and must be covered with a dark bag to prevent degradation of the drug ("Adriamycin," 2011).

Table 16.3. Commonly Used Chemotherapeutic Drugs
Cisplatin
Cyclophosphamide (Cytoxin™)*
Dacarbazine (DTIC)
Dactinomycin
Doxorubicin (Adriamycin™)*
Etoposide (VP-16)*
Ifosfamide*
Leucovorin
Mesna
Methotrexate
Mitomycin C
Vinblastine
Vincristine*

* This five-drug combination is now the accepted standard of care for the chemotherapeutic management of Ewing's Sarcoma. *From "Sarcoma" by K. M. Skubitz & D. R. D'Adamo, 2007, Mayo Clinic Proceedings, 82(11), 1409-1432. Reproduced with permission.*

Interferons, cytokines that have direct antitumor and immune-stimulating properties, have shown significant activity against osteosarcoma in vitro and on xenograft models, but current studies are underway to if this effect can be reproduced in humans (Whelan et al., 2010).

There are various routes of administration for chemotherapeutic drugs. Oral, intravenous bolus, and intravenous drip routes are most commonly seen in clinical practice. There are several venous access devices that are available to prevent loss of veins from irritating chemotherapy and allow prolonged administration of vesicant drugs. Either external venous catheters or implanted subcutaneous ports can be used. Multi-day infusions of some drugs can be administered via an external pump on an outpatient basis. Arterial infusions of chemotherapy, while not common, are facilitated by placement of arterial ports (Polovich, White, & Olsen, 2009). Patients who are receiving intra-arterial chemotherapy while in the hospital need to be closely monitored for signs of extravasation. Patients must be strictly immobilized to prevent the catheter from being dislodged, which can lead to life-threatening exsanguination. The affected extremity should be immobilized with sandbags or other immobilization devices.

Many of the side effects of chemotherapy can be controlled by good assessment skills and preplanning by the nurses. Common side effects such as nausea and vomiting have decreased, especially with the expanded use of newer antiemetics such as Zofran® (ondansetron). Patients may also be premedicated with dexamethasone, lorazepam, diphenhydramine, metoclopramide, and haloperidol, but they must be monitored closely for sedation, extrapyramidal reactions, anxiety, and diarrhea (Polovich et al., 2009).

Chemotherapy has many side effects, and some of them can be life-threatening (Polovich et al., 2009). Neutropenia, leukopenia, and thrombocytopenia can lead to bleeding, overwhelming infection, and death (Goodwin & Braden, 2009). While bleeding is common in patients with cancer, thrombosis is another complication of cancer and cancer therapies. Due to the release of inflammatory cytokines in patients with cancer, patients are at higher risk for the development of venous thrombosis (Kwaan & Viciuna, 2007).

Table 16.4. Common Chemotherapy Side Effects
Aches and pains
Alopecia and skin changes
Anorexia
Constipation and/or diarrhea
Cystitis
Depression
Depression
Fatigue
Hematopoietic changes (neutropenia, leukopenia, thrombocytopenia)
Metabolic alterations
Reproductive system dysfunction
Stomatitis
Toxicities (cardiac, renal, hepatic, ototoxicity, neuro, and pulmonary)

Patients often complain of fatigue, which is a common side effect of chemotherapy, but fatigue could also indicate cardiorespiratory toxicity. Doxorubicin has long been known to be a factor in the development of cardiomyopathy at high doses, but its effects are exaggerated by the addition of cyclophosphamide even when used at lower doses (Khattry, Malhotra, Grover, Sharma, & Varma, 2009). In order to minimize chemotherapy side effects, many patients try complementary and alternative medicine (CAM) therapies, but there is little evidence that these work. There are too few randomized control trials (RCTs) that support the use of these therapies (Lotfi-Jam et al., 2008). More common side effects can be found in Table 16.4.

Nursing Considerations

The diagnosis of cancer is devastating, and even when child cancer patients are cured, there are many emotional and physical effects that linger into adulthood (Zeltzer et al., 2008). The nurse is in a unique position to assist patients and their families manage the multiple issues related to the diagnosis and treatment of musculoskeletal tumors.

Nursing Diagnoses. Nursing diagnoses for this condition are expanded upon in the Appendix.

- Caregiver role strain
- Coping, ineffective.
- Grieving, complicated, risk for.
- Knowledge deficit.
- Pain, acute.
- Pain, chronic.
- Powerlessness
- Skin integrity, impaired.
- Spiritual distress
- Tissue integrity, impaired.
- Tissue perfusion: cardiac, risk for decrease.

Bone Metastasis

Overview

Definition. Bone metastasis represents one of the most frequent and most debilitating sequelae of malignancy and occurs as a result of the spread of malignant cells beyond their primary site of origin. Sarcomas primarily spread to the lungs (rarely to another bone or soft tissue site), while carcinomas frequently spread to the bone (Peh & Muttrak, 2008). The most common sites and tumor types are presented in Table 16.5.

Table 16.5. Sites of Occurrence of Metastatic Lesions
Thorax and vertebra 50%
Extremities 34%
Skull 22%
Most Common Primary Tumors
Breast
Prostate
Lung
Kidney
Thyroid
Bladder

Etiology. Bone metastasis occurs by three routes:

1. Direct extension: involves spread from a local tumor, such as with multiple myeloma, which arises in the marrow cavity and invades the outer bone;
2. Hematogenous extension: the most common route of spread and results from seeding of micrometastases through the bloodstream and
3. Lymphatic dissemination: usually seen in breast carcinoma (Peh & Muttrak, 2008).

Bone metastases may be osteolytic, sclerotic, or mixed on radiographs. Lesions usually appear in the medullary cavity, spread to destroy the medullary bone, and then involve the cortex. Osteolytic metastases are encountered most frequently, especially in breast and lung carcinomas. Osteolytic lesions occur as a result of increased osteoclastic activity and bone resorption or lysis incited by tumor cells. The specific appearance of bone metastases is often useful in suggesting the nature of the underlying primary malignancy.

Malignancies associated with sclerotic or blastic metastases include prostate cancer, colonic carcinoma, melanoma, bladder carcinoma, and soft-tissue sarcoma (Terris & Rhee, 2010). Blastic lesions are a result of a process similar to callus formation after a fracture in normal bone. The findings of sclerotic metastases virtually exclude an untreated renal tumor or hepatocellular carcinoma (Peh & Muttrak, 2008). Tumor activity evokes a protective response by increased blastic activity in which there is "reactive" bone formation (Chansky & Eady, 2008). Spontaneous or pathologic fracture is less likely to occur than with lytic lesions in which minor stresses can result in fracture (as in prostate carcinoma).

Metastatic bone lesions usually indicate advanced disease. Patients with prostate cancer who have evidence of metastatic lesions have an overall 5-year survival rate of only 29% (Chansky & Eady, 2008). Complications of metastatic bone lesions include impending pathologic fractures, which are defined as the presence of a bony defect that has destroyed at least 50% of the bone over 2.5 cm in diameter and would likely result in a pathologic fracture with physiologic loading (ie, activities of daily living [ADLs]). Prophylactic internal fixation of pathologic or impending pathologic fractures, usually with intra-medullary rods, is generally recommended to facilitate mobility and relieve pain. Because the life span of these patients is limited, the goal of management needs to be centered on returning as much function as possible as rapidly as possible (Chansky & Eady, 2008).

Tumor lysis syndrome is a constellation of metabolic disturbances that may be seen after initiation of cancer treatment. This syndrome usually occurs in patients with bulky, rapidly proliferating, and treatment-responsive tumors. This potentially lethal complication of anticancer treatment occurs when large numbers of neoplastic cells are killed rapidly, leading to release of intra-cellular ions and metabolic byproducts into the systemic circulation. Clinically, the syndrome is characterized by rapid development of hyperuricemia, hyperkalemia, hyperphosphatemia, hypocalcemia, and acute renal failure (ARF) (Krishan & Hammad, 2009). Volume depletion is a major risk factor for tumor lysis syndrome and must be corrected vigorously. Aggressive intravenous hydration not only helps correct electrolyte disturbances by diluting extracellular fluid, but it also increases intravascular volume. Increased volume enhances renal blood flow, glomerular filtration rate, and urine volume to decrease the concentration of solutes in the distal nephron and medullary microcirculation. Ideally, intravenous hydration in high-risk patients should begin 24-48 hours prior to initiation of cancer therapy and continue for 48-72 hours after completion of chemotherapy. Treatment of hyperuricemia should be instituted using allopurinal (Krishan & Hammad, 2009).

Assessment

History and Physical Exam. Patients with cancer need to be monitored frequently during the course of their treatment. If a patient complains of bone pain, it may be suggestive if the patient has a history of a bone-seeking tumor, such as breast or prostate. Localized pain, hyperreflexia, gait abnormality, and loss of bowel/bladder control are often found with metastatic lesions around the spinal cord. Patients will also complain of radicular pain and paresthesias, and these symptoms often are indicative of vertebral collapse and/or tumor pressure on the spinal cord (Terris & Rhee, 2010). The signs and symptoms of vertebral or extremity fractures are discussed in Chapter 15—Trauma: Fractures.

Diagnostic Tests. Frequent diagnostic tests are necessary to monitor for, and detect, bony metastases. Metabolic disturbances, such as hypercalcemia, may be the presenting symptom. Patients may present with nausea, vomiting, alterations of mental status, abdominal or flank pain, constipation, lethargy, depression, weakness and vague muscle/joint aches, polyuria, polydipsia, nocturia, headache, and confusion (Hemphill, 2009). Plain radiographs (x-rays) can detect bony lesions, and bone scans demonstrate increased intake in areas of reactive bone. Alkaline phosphatase is elevated when there is an increase in osteoblastic activity, and other markers may be used depending on the type of primary tumor (Harper, 2007). Bone biopsies may be performed to verify the diagnosis.

Table 16.6. Surgical Treatment of Metastatic Bone Lesions

1. Prophylactic fixation to prevent pathologic fracture, especially of weight-bearing areas, such as femur or tibia.
2. Fracture treatment may involve use of intramedullary rods, pins, and plates, as well as the use of methylmethacrylate to replace larger segments of diseased bone.
3. Spine-preoperative management a. Determine presence or absence of cord compression and stable or unstable spine. b. High-dose steroid therapy for acute edema. c. Treatment options. (1) Asymptomatic: systemic chemotherapy or hormonal therapy. (2) Compression fractures or painful lesion: steroid therapy, radiation therapy and brace if minimal subluxation. (3) Traction (halo apparatus) may be needed with marked subluxation. (4) Lower thoracic and upper lumbar fracture/dislocation. (a) Operative stabilization with metal. (b) Methylmethacrylate. (c) Autogenous bone. (d) Allograft. (5) Cord compression. (a) Radiotherapy. (b) Surgical decompression with stabilization. (c) Anterior and/or posterior approach depending upon the site of the tumor fixation with metal. (d) Methylmethacrylate. (e) Fibular strut autologous bone. (f) Allograft.
4. Solitary metastasis treatment options a. Excise lesion. b. Internal fixation with intramedullary rods or internal fixation and/or methylmethacrylate. c. Endoprosthesis for head, neck, or intertrochanteric fractures of the femoral or humeral head. d. Total hip, shoulder, or knee replacement.

From "Surgical Management of Bone Metastases" by M. Nousiainen, C. Whyne, A. Yee, J. Finkelstein, and M. Ford, 2009, Bone Metastases, Cancer Metastases: Biology and Treatment 12, *New York, NY: Springer Science + Business Media. Reproduced with permission.*

Common Therapeutic Modalities

Management of bony metastasis requires a multidisciplinary team approach. Overall treatment goals include halting the disease progression, relieving pain, preventing or treating pathologic fractures, and preventing metabolic or hematologic complications (Janjan et al., 2009).

Chemotherapy remains the backbone of treatment, and the appropriate cytotoxic agents for the primary tumor type should continue to be administered per the medical oncologist. Radiotherapy promotes rapid destruction of tumor cells, followed by bone healing and recalcification in 3–4 months, and provides relief of pain. Surgery is a major piece in the management of bony metastatic lesions, with a variety of surgical options available (see Table 16.6).

The use of bisphosphonates to help reduce the potential for pathologic fractures from developing, except in spinal cord compression, is now recommended. Starting therapy once the bone metastasis diagnosis is made is preferred to delaying therapy (Costa & Major, 2009). Intravenous bisphosphonates such as zoledronic acid (Reclast®) have been shown to significantly decrease osteoclastic activity and help relieve the pain of bone metastases (Montella et al., 2009). Pain control is a necessary part of the management of bone metastases. See Chapter 7—Pain.

Nursing Considerations

Nursing Diagnoses. Nursing diagnoses for this condition are expanded upon in the Appendix.

- Caregiver role strain.
- Coping, ineffective.
- Grieving, complicated, risk for.
- Injury, risk for.
- Knowledge deficit.
- Pain, acute.
- Pain, chronic.
- Powerlessness
- Skin integrity, impaired.
- Spiritual distress
- Tissue integrity, impaired.
- Tissue perfusion: cardiac, risk for decrease.

Multiple Myeloma

Overview

Definition. Multiple myeloma (MM) is an incurable malignancy of terminally differentiated plasma cells.

B cells proliferate and infiltrate the bone marrow, cause bone destruction, and suppress normal hematopoeisis. These B cells produce high amounts of monoclonal "M" bands of immunoglobulins. The myeloma cells are ineffective in their immune function. They also have an osteoclastic effect that may result in pathologic fractures and hypercalcemia from increased bone destruction (Grethelin & Thomas, 2010).

MM accounts for 1.1% of the malignancies in white United States residents and 2.1% of the malignancies in black residents. The male-to-female ratio of multiple myeloma is 3:2. The median age of patients with multiple myeloma is 68 years for men and 70 years for women (Grethelin & Thomas, 2010).

Etiology. The cause of MM is not understood. Genetic causes appear to play a role, and there is ongoing research investigating whether human leukocyte antigen (HLA)-Cw5 or HLA-Cw2 may play a role in the pathogenesis of MM. Environmental or occupational causes, in case-controlled studies, appear to suggest a significant risk of developing MM in individuals with significant exposures in the agriculture, food, and petrochemical industries. Long-term (>20 years) exposure to hair dyes has been tied to an excessive risk of developing MM. Approximately 19% of patients with monoclonal gammopathy of undetermined significance (MGUS) develop MM within 2-19 years. Radiation has also been linked to MM development (Grethelin & Thomas, 2010).

MM is a disease of the late middle-aged and the elderly. It can be treated and controlled but not cured. Patients may live several months to several years after diagnosis, but essentially all patients with MM will develop some, if not all, of the complications particular to the disease. See Table 16.7 for a list of complications of MM.

Table 16.7. Complications of Multiple Myeloma

1. Pain
2. Pathologic fractures
3. Anemia
4. Dehydration
5. Hypercalcemia
6. Fatigue
7. Renal insufficiency
8. Side effects from chemotherapy

Assessment

History and Physical Exam. The history and physical examination is similar to the one performed for bone metastasis (see Bone Metastasis in this chapter). Patients may experience bone pain with or without fracture, and patients often suffer long bone fractures (Grethelin & Thomas, 2010).

Diagnostic Tests. Diagnostic tests that are used for MM include:

- CBC-Anemia, weakness, infection, weight loss, mental status changes;
- Bone marrow studies: plasma cell infiltration less than 10%;
- Serum and urine electrophoresis: monoclonal spikes;
- Bence-Jones protein in urine is positive;
- Proteinuria, hypercalcuria with spinal cord compression or renal failure;
- X-ray: multiple, lytic lesions, plasmacytomas;
- MRI: used on select patients for more complete skeletal information; and
- Serum B2 macroglobulin is an important prognostic factor (Grethelin & Thomas, 2010).

Common Therapeutic Modalities

If the patient is asymptomatic, frequent monitoring alone may be the initial treatment. Monitoring consists of lab work and radiographs (x-ray). If progression of disease is noted, then there is further treatment with chemotherapy, radiation, and possibly surgery if an impending or pathologic fracture is evident. Common chemotherapeutic drugs used include melphalan, prednisone, VAD (vincristine, doxorubicin, dexamethasone and interferon-alpha.) Radiotherapy and surgery are also often used in the treatment of MM (Grethelin & Thomas, 2010). See Bone Metastasis section in this chapter.

Nursing Considerations

Nursing Diagnoses. Nursing diagnoses for this condition are expanded upon in the Appendix.

- Caregiver role strain.
- Coping, ineffective.
- Grieving, complicated, risk for.
- Infection, risk for.
- Knowledge deficit.
- Pain, acute.
- Pain, chronic.
- Powerlessness
- Skin integrity, impaired.
- Spiritual distress.
- Tissue integrity, impaired.
- Tissue perfusion: cardiac, risk for decrease.
- Urinary elimination, impaired.

Summary

Patients with musculoskeletal tumors, while a small percent of the total cancer diagnoses each year, require care delivered by skilled nurses. The different types of tumors, the age ranges for development of the tumors, and the treatment options for these different types of tumors make it imperative that nurses caring for these patients have the most current knowledge needed to manage the care of these patients.

The complex biopsychosocial implications of musculoskeletal tumors impact not only patients, but also their families and their communities at large. Developmental, physical, psychological, vocational, and alterations in role issues are challenges that patients with musculoskeletal tumors must confront. Nurses are in a unique position to assist patients and families navigate through the process of healing or grieving.

References

Abramovici, L., Hytiroglou, P., Klein, R., Karkavelas, G. Drevelegas, A., Panousi, E., & Steiner, G. (2005). Well-differentiated extraskeletal osteosarcoma: Report of 2 cases, 1 with dedifferentiation. *Human Pathology, 36*(4), 439-443.

Accuray. (2011). CyberKnife® Robotic Radiosurgery system. Retrieved from http://www.cyberknife.com/cyberknife-overview/what-cyberknife.aspx

Adriamycin. (2011). Retrieved from http://www.drugs.com/pro/adriamycin.html

Albert, A., Leemrijse, T., Druez, V., Delloye, C., & Cornu, O. (2006). Are bone autografts still necessary in 2006 ? A three-year retrospective study of bone grafting. *Acta Orthopædica Belgica, 72*(6), 734-740.

American Academy of Orthopaedic Surgeons (AAOS). (2007). Unicameral (simple) bone cyst. Retrieved from http://orthoinfo.aaos.org/topic.cfm?topic=A00081

American Cancer Society. (2008). *Cancer Facts and Figures 2008*. Atlanta, GA: American Cancer Society. Retrieved from http://www.cancer.org/downloads/STT/2008CAFFfinalsecured.pdf.

Anand, M.K. (2009). Fibrous dysplasia. *eMedicine: Radiology*. Retrieved from http://emedicine.medscape.com/article/389714-overview

Banovac, K. & Speed, J. (2008). Heterotopic ossification. *eMedicine: Physical Medicine and Rehabilitation*. Retrieved from http://emedicine.medscape.com/article/327648-overview

Beebe, K., Song, K.J., Ross, E., Tuy, B., Patterson, F., & Benevenia, J. (2009). Functional outcomes after limb-salvage surgery and endoprosthetic reconstruction with an expandable prosthesis: A report of 4 cases. *Archives of Physical Medicine and Rehabilitation, 90*(6), 1039-1047

Bernard, S.L. (2009). Lower extremity reconstruction: Knee. *eMedicine: Plastic Surgery*. Retrieved from http://emedicine.medscape.com/article/1291548-overview

Bhatia, S. & Robinson, L. (2008). Cancer survivorship research: Opportunities and future needs for expanding the research base. *Cancer Epidemiology, Biomarkers, and Prevention*, 17, 1551.

Bleyer, A. (2007). Young adult oncology: The patients and their survival challenges. *CA: Cancer Journal for Clinicians*, 57, 242-255. doi:10.3322/canjclin.57.4.242

Carsi, B. & Sim, F. (2009). *Angiosarcoma. eMedicine: Oncology*. Retrieved from http://emedicine.medscape.com/article/276512-overview

Chansky, H.A. & Eady, J. (2008). Metastatic carcinoma. *eMedicine: Orthopaedic Surgery*. Retrieved from http://emedicine.medscape.com/article/1253331-overview

Chen, C.J. & Siegel, D.M. (2009). Dermatofibrosarcoma protuberans. *eMedicine: Dermatology*. Retrieved from http://emedicine.medscape.com/article/1100203-overview

Chew, F.S. & Maldjian, C.T. (2009). Enchondroma and enchondromatosis. *eMedicine: Radiology*. Retrieved from http://emedicine.medscape.com/article/389224-overview

Costa, L. & Major, P.P. (2009). Effect of bisphosphonates on pain and quality of life in patients with bone metastases. *National Clinical Practice of Oncology, 6*(3), 164-174.

Cripe, T.P. (2008). Rhabdomyosarcoma. *eMedicine: Pediatrics*. Retrieved from http://emedicine.medscape.com/article/988803-overview

Croce, C.M. (2008). Oncogenes and cancer. *The New England Journal of Medicine, 358*(5), 502-511.

Daigeler, A., Lehnhardt, M., Khadra, A., Hauser, J., Steinstraesser, L., Langer, S.,...Steinau, H. (2009). Proximal major limb amputations – a retrospective analysis of 45 oncological cases. *World Journal of Surgical Oncology*, 7, 15. doi: 10.1186/1477-7819-7-15

Dickey, I.D. (2009). Solitary osteochondroma. *eMedicine: Orthopedic Surgery*. Retrieved from http://emedicine.medscape.com/article/1256477-overview

Doenges & Moorhouse Diagnostic Divisions. (2009). *2009-2011 NANDA Diagnoses*. Retrieved from http://www.fadavis.com/related_resources/75_2632_1703.pdf

Drilon, A., Popat, S., Bhuchar, G., D'Adamo, D., Keohan, M., Fisher, C.,...Maki, R. (2008). Extraskeletal myxoid chondrosarcoma. *Cancer, 113*(12), 3364-3371.

D'Silva, K.J., Karina, V.R., Worrell, R.V., & Arora, M. L. (2008). Rhabdomyomas: Treatment & medication. *eMedicine: Pediatric Surgery*. Retrieved from http://emedicine.medscape.com/article/281592-treatment

Eastwood, B. (2010). Aneurysmal bone cyst. *eMedicine: Orthopaedic Surgery*. Retrieved from http://emedicine.medscape.com/article/1254784-treatment

Gelderblom, H., Hogendoorn, P., Dijkstra, S., van Rijswijk, C., Krol, A., Taminiau, A., & Bovée, J. (2008). The clinical approach to chondrosarcoma. *The Oncologist, 13*(3), 320-329. doi:10.1634/theoncologist.2007-0237

Geenen, M., Cardous-Ubbink, M., Kremer, L., van den Bos, C., van der Pal, H., Heinen, R.,...Flora E. van Leeuwen, F. (2007). Medical assessment of adverse health outcomes in long-term survivors of childhood cancers. *Journal of the American Medical Association*, 297, 2705-2715.

Genova, R. & Walsh, J. J. (2009). Ganglion cyst. *eMedicine; Orthopaedic Surgery.* Retrieved from http://emedicine.medscape.com/article/1243454-overview

Gridelli, C. (2007). The use of bisphosphonates in elderly cancer patients. *The Oncologist, 12*(1), 62-71. doi:10.1634/theoncologist.12-1-62

Grethelin, S.J. & Thomas, L.M. (2010). Multiple myeloma. *eMedicine: Hematology.* Retrieved from http://emedicine.medscape.com/article/204369-overview

Goodwin, J.E. & Braden, C.D. (2009). Neutropenia. *eMedicine: Hematology.* Retrieved from http://emedicine.medscape.com/article/204821-overview

Gupta, N.P., Kolla, S.B., Panda, S., & Sharma, M.C. (2008). Epitheloid hemangioendothelioma of urinary bladder. *Indian Journal of Urology, 24*, 253-255.

Handshake, M., Mentzel, T., …Kutzner, H. (2010).Cutaneous clear cell sarcoma. A clinicopathologic, immunohistochemical, and molecular analysis of 12 cases emphasizing its distinction from dermal melanoma. *American Journal of Surgical Pathology, 34*(2), 216-22.

Harper, P. (2007). Update on bone metastases and biomarkers in non-small cell lung cancer: E06-02. *Journal of Thoracic Oncology, 2*(8), S232-S233.

Hemphill, R.R. (2009). Hypercalcemia. *eMedicine: Emergency Medicine.* Retrieved from http://emedicine.medscape.com/article/766373-overview

Holt, G.E., Christie, M.J., & Schwartz, H.S. (2009). Trabecular metal endoprosthetic limb salvage reconstruction of the lower limb. *Journal of Arthoplasty, 24*(7), 1079-1085.

Horner, K.L., Raugi, G.J., & Miethke, M. C. (2009). Leiomyoma. *eMedicine: Dermatology.* Retrieved from http://emedicine.medscape.com/article/1057733-overview

Janjan, N., Lutz, S., Bedwinek, J., Hartsell, W., Ng, A., Pieters, R., Ratanatharathorn, V.,...Rettenmaier, A. (2009). Therapeutic guidelines for the treatment of bone metastasis: A report from the American College of Radiology Appropriateness Criteria Expert Panel on Radiation Oncology. *Journal of Palliative Medicine, 12*(5), 417-426. doi:10.1089/jpm.2009.9633

Kam, J.R. & Helm, T.N. (2009). Neurofibromatosis. *eMedicine: Dermatology.* Retrieved from http://emedicine.medscape.com/article/1112001-overview

Kakaki, M. & Theleritis, C. (2007). Health outcomes in long term survivors of childhood cancer. *Journal of the American Medical Association, 298*(14), 1635-1637.

Katz, D.A., & Damron, T.A. (2008). Hemangiomas. *eMedicine: Orthopaedic Surgery.* Retrieved from http://emedicine.medscape.com/article/1255694-overview

Kayurapan, A., Makadelok, S., & Waikiki, S. (2010). Effect of gamma sterilisation and deep-freezing on length and strength of fascia latae. *Journal of Orthopaedic Surgery, 18*(1), 68-70.

Khan, A.N. (2008). Eosinophilic granuloma, skeletal. *eMedicine: Radiology.* Retrieved from http://emedicine.medscape.com/article/389350-overview

Khan, A.N. (2009). Osteoid osteoma. *eMedicine: Radiology.* Retrieved from http://emedicine.medscape.com/article/392850-overview

Khattry, N., Malhotra, P., Grover, A., Sharma, S.C., & Varma, S. (2009). Doxorubicin-induced cardiotoxicity in adult Indian patients on chemotherapy. *Indian Journal of Medical and Paediatric Oncology, 9*(30), 9-13

Kitamura, M., Wada, N., Nagata, S., Iizuka, N., Jin, Y., Tomoeda, M.,...Tomita, Y. (2010). Malignant peripheral nerve sheath tumor associated with neurofibromatosis type 1, with metastasis to the heart: a case report. *Diagnostic Pathology 2010, 5*, 2. doi:10.1186/1746-1596-5-2

Kline, N.E. (2010). Cancer in children. In K.L. McCance. S.E. Huether, V.L. Brashers, & N.S. Rote (Eds), *Pathophysiology: the biological basis for disease in adults and children* (6th ed., pp. 436-441). St. Louis, MO: Elsevier Mosby.

Kransdorf, M.J. & Murphey, M.D. (2006). *Imaging of soft tissue tumors.* (2nd ed.). Philadelphia, PA: Saunders

Krishan, K. & Hammad, H. (2009). Tumor lysis syndrome. *eMedicine: Oncology.* Retrieved from http://emedicine.medscape.com/article/282171-overview

Kwaan, H.C. & Viciuna, B. (2007). Thrombosis and bleeding in cancer patients. *Oncology Reviews, 1*(1), 14-27.

Lahat, G., Lazar, A., & Lev, D. (2008). Sarcoma epidemiology and etiology: Potential environmental and genetic factors. *Surgical Clinics of North America, 88*(3), 451-481.

Lebel, S. & Devins, G.M. (2008). Stigma in cancer patients whose behavior may have contributed to their disease. *Future Oncology, 4*(5), 717-33.

Lewis, V.O. (2009). What's new in musculoskeletal oncology? *The Journal of Bone and Joint Surgery* (American), *91*, 1546-1556. doi:10.2106/JBJS.I.00375

Lewis, V.O. & Peabody, T. (2009). Giant cell tumor. *eMedicine: Orthopaedics.* Retrieved from http://emedicine.medscape.com/article/1255364-overview

Lietman, S.A. & Joyce, M.J. (2010). Bone sarcomas: Overview of management, with a focus on surgical treatment considerations. *Cleveland Clinic Journal of Medicine, 77*(Suppl 1), S8-S11. doi:10.3949/ccjm.77.s1.02

Limb, D. & Agrawal, Y. (2006). The distribution of bone islands and juxta-articular bone cysts in the growing hand. *Journal of Hand Surgery, 31*(4), 441-444. doi: 10.1016/J.JHSB.2006.03.158

Lotfi-Jam, L., Carey, M., Jefford, M., Schofield, P., Charleson, C., & Aranda, S. (2008). Nonpharmacologic strategies for managing common chemotherapy adverse effects: A systematic review. *Journal of Clinical Oncology, 26*(34), 5618-5629.

Manoso, M.W., Boland, P.J., Healey, J.H., & Cordeiro, P.G. (2006). Limb salvage of infected knee reconstructions for cancer with staged revision and free tissue transfer. *Annals of Plastic Surgery, 56*(5), 532-535. doi: 10.1097/01.sap.0000203990.08414.ad

McCance, K.L. (2010). Cancer epidemiology. In K.L. McCance. S.E. Huether, V.L. Brashers, & N.S. Rote (Eds), *Pathophysiology: The biological basis for disease in adults and children* (6th ed., pp. 398-435). St. Louis, MO: Elsevier Mosby.

McLean, C., Hargrove, R., & Woods, J. (2009). Traumatic heterotopic ossification: Treatment. *eMedicine: Orthopaedic Surgery: Neoplasms.* Retrieved from http://emedicine.medscape.com/article/1254416-treatment

Meermans, G., Roos, J., Hofkens, L., & Cheyns, P. (2007). Bone banking in a community hospital. *Acta Orthopædica Belgica, 73*, 754-759.

Mehlman, C.T. (2008). Unicameral bone cysts. *eMedicine: Orthopaedic Surgery.* Retrieved from http://emedicine.medscape.com/article/1257331-overview

Morgan, H.D. & Damron, T.A. (2008). Chondromyxoid fibroma. *eMedicine: Orthopaedics.* Retrieved from http://emedicine.medscape.com/article/1255062-overview

Morgan, H.D. & Damron, T.A. (2009). Chondroblastoma. *eMedicine: Orthopaedics.* Retrieved from http://emedicine.medscape.com/article/1254949-overview

National Association of Orthopaedic Nurses (NAON). (2008). *NAON Orthopaedic Certification Review Course*. Chicago, IL: NAON.

National Cancer Institute. (2007). Soft tissue sarcomas: Questions and answers. Retrieved from http://www.cancer.gov/cancertopics/factsheet/Sites-Types/soft-tissue-sarcoma

National Cancer Institute. (2010). Radiation therapy for cancer. Retrieved from http://www.cancer.gov/cancertopics/factsheet/Therapy/radiation

Nickloes, T.A., Sutphin, D.D., & Radebold, K. (2010). Lipomas. *eMedicine: General Surgery.* Retrieved from http://emedicine.medscape.com/article/191233-overview

Malawer, M.M. & Sugarbaker, P.H. (2001). *Musculoskeletal Cancer Surgery: Treatment of Sarcomas and Allied Diseases.* Norwell, MA: Kluwer Academic Publishers.

Mathur, S. & Damron, T.A. (2010). Malignant lymphoma. *eMedicine: Orthopaedic Surgery.* Retrieved from http://emedicine.medscape.com/article/1256034-overview

Mehlman, C.T. & Cripe, T.P. (2008). Osteosarcoma. *eMedicine: Orthopaedic Surgery.* Retrieved from http://emedicine.medscape.com/article/1256857-overview

Montella, L., Addeo, R., Faiola, V., Cennamo, G. Guarrasi, R., Capasso, E.,...Del Prete, S. (2009). Zoledronic acid in metastatic chondrosarcoma and advanced sacrum chordoma: two case reports. *Journal of Experimental & Clinical Cancer Research, 28*(7). doi:10.1186/1756-9966-28-7

Monu, J.U. (2010). Pigmented villonodular synovitis. *eMedicine: Radiology.* Retrieved from http://emedicine.medscape.com/article/394649-overview

Moses, S. (2008). Kaposi's sarcoma. *Family Practice Notebook.* Retrieved from http://www.fpnotebook.com/Hemeonc/HIV/KpsSrcm.htm

Nousiainen, M., Whyne, C.M., Yee, A.J.M., Finkelstein, J., & Ford, M. (2009). Surgical management of bone metastases. In D. Kardamakis, V. Vassiliou, & E. Chow (Eds.). *Bone metastases: A translational and clinical approach.* New York, NY: Springer Science + Business Media.

O'Connor, E. & Stacy, G.S. (2008). Osteoblastoma. *eMedicine: Radiology.* Retrieved from http://emedicine.medscape.com/article/392248-overview

Padua, M.D., Bhandari, T., & Pingle, J. (2009). Primary osteoliposarcoma of the bone. *Indian Journal of Pathology and Microbiology*, 52, 80-82.

Pal, S.M., Katheria, V., & Hurria, A. (2010). Evaluating the older patient with cancer: Understanding frailty and the geriatric assessment. *CA: Cancer Journal for Clinicians, 60*, 120-132. doi: 10.3322/caac.20059

Palmer, C.A. & Harrison, D.K. (2008). Chordoma. *eMedicine: Neurosurgery.* Retrieved from http://emedicine.medscape.com/article/250902-overview

Pappo, A. (2006). *Pediatric bone and soft tissue sarcomas.* Toronto, ON, Canada: Springer.

Peh, W.C.G. & Muttrak, M. (2008). Bone metastasis. *eMedicine: Radiology.* Retrieved from http://emedicine.medscape.com/article/387840-overview

Pierson, J.C. & Tam, C.C. (2010). Dermatofibroma. *eMedicine: Dermatology.* Retrieved from http://emedicine.medscape.com/article/1056742-overview

Polovich, White, & Olsen, M., (2009). *Chemotherapy and biotherapy guidelines and recommendations for practice* (3rd ed). Pittsburgh, PA: Oncology Nursing Society.

Rabin, R.C. (2010, March 15). Gaps in dealing with cancer in teenagers. *New York Times.* Retrieved from http://www.nytimes.com/2010/03/16/health/16canc.html

Rao, N. & Hackbarth, D.A. (2009). Post-radiation sarcomas. *eMedicine: Orthopaedic Surgery.* Retrieved from http://emedicine.medscape.com/article/1253714-overview

Riedel, R.F., Larrier, N., Dodd, L, Kirsch, D., Martinez, S., Brigman, B(2009). The clinical management of chondrosarcoma. *Current Treatment Options in Oncology, 10*(1-2), 94-106.

Roque, P., Mankin, H.J., Hornicek, F.J., & Nyame, T. (2007). *Extremity liposarcoma: Prognostic indicators. Therapy, 4*(3), 299-305.

Rosenthal, D. & Hornicek, F.J. (2010). Bone tumors: Diagnosis and biopsy techniques. *UpToDate.* Retrieved from http://www.uptodate.com/patients/content/topic.do?topicKey=~yxxAsidTuaIucr

Rudert, M., Winkler, C.; Holzapfel, B.; Rechl, H.; Kneschaurek, P.; Gradinger, R.,... Röper, B. (2010). A new modification of combining vacuum therapy and brachytherapy in large subfascial soft tissue sarcomas of the extremities. *Journal of Radiotherapy and Oncology, 86*(4), 224-228. doi:10.1007/s00066-010-2046-0

Schwartz, H.S. (Ed.). (2007). *Orthopaedic knowledge update: Musculoskeletal tumors 2.* Rosemont, IL: Musculoskeletal Tumor Society.

Schwartz, R.A. & Fernandez, G. (2009). Stewart-Treves Syndrome. *eMedicine: Dermatology.* Retrieved from http://emedicine.medscape.com/article/1102114-overview

Schwartz, R.A. & Trovato, M.J. (2010). Desmoid tumors: Treatment & medications. *eMedicine: Dermatology.* Retrieved from http://emedicine.medscape.com/article/1060887-treatment

Sheplan, L.J. & Juliano, J.J. (2010). Use of radiation therapy for patients with soft-tissue and bone sarcomas. *Cleveland Clinic Journal of Medicine, 77*(Supp l 1), S27-S29. doi: 10.3949/ccjm.77.s1.06

Shidam, V.B., Acker, S.M., & Vesole, D.H. (2009). Benign and malignant soft tissue tumors. *eMedicine: Orthopaedic Surgery.* Retrieved from http://emedicine.medscape.com/article/1253816-overview

Skubitz, K.M. & D'Adamo, D.R. (2007). Sarcoma. *Mayo Clinic Proceedings, 82*(11), 1409-1432.

Smelser, C.D., Stoffey, R.D., Mahaney, W., Keenan, S.C., & Simmons, G.E. (2008). Adamantinoma. *eMedicine: Radiology.* Retrieved from http://emedicine.medscape.com/article/385977-overview

Smith, S.E. (2009). Fibrous cortical defect and nonossifying fibroma. *eMedicine: Radiology.* Retrieved from http://emedicine.medscape.com/article/389590-overview

Stacey, G.S., Mahal, R.S., & Peabody, T.D. (2006). Staging of bone tumors: A review with illustrative examples. *American Journal of Roentgenology, 186,* 967-976. doi:10.2214/AJR.05.0654

Stacey, G.S. (2009). Malignant fibrous histiocytoma, soft tissue. *eMedicine: Radiology.* Retrieved from http://emedicine.medscape.com/article/391453-overview

Strauss, L.G. (2009). Ewing's sarcoma. *eMedicine: Radiology.* Retrieved from http://emedicine.medscape.com/article/389464-overview

Templeton, K.J. (2008). Juxtacortical tumors. *eMedicine: Orthopaedic Surgery.* Retrieved from http://emedicine.medscape.com/article/1257617-overview

Teo, E.H. & Peh, W.C.G. (2010). Musculoskeletal tumors, staging and treatment planning. *eMedicine: Radiology.* Retrieved from http://emedicine.medscape.com/article/399175-overview

Teo, E. H. & Chew, F. S. (2011). Simple bone cyst imaging. *eMedicine: Radiology.* Retrieved from http://emedicine.medscape.com/article/395783-overview

Terris, M.K. & Rhee, A. (2010). Prostate cancer: Metastatic and advanced disease. *eMedicine: Urology.* Retrieved from http://emedicine.medscape.com/article/454114-overview

Toretsky, J.A. (2008). Ewing sarcoma and primitive neuroectodermal tumors. *eMedicine: Pediatrics.* Retrieved from http://emedicine.medscape.com/article/990378-overview

Tretli, S.A. & Kravdal, S.Ø. (2008). Cancer's impact on employment and earnings: A population-based study from Norway. *Journal of Cancer Survivors, 2*(3), 149-58

Van der Woude, H. J. & Smithuis, R. (2010). Bone tumors: Differential diagnosis. *Radiology Assistant.* Retrieved from http://www.radiologyassistant.nl/en/494e15cbf0d8d

Veillette, C. (2010). Myoma. *Orthopaedia.* Retrieved from http://www.orthopaedia.com:8080/display/PORT/Myxoma

Victorian, B. (2009). Increased sarcoma awareness key in limb-sparing surgery. *Oncology Times, 31*(2), 25, 27-28. doi: 10.1097/01.COT.0000345490.19666.91

Virshup, D.M. (2010). Biology, clinical manifestations, and treatment of cancer. In K.L. McCance, S.E. Huether, V.L. Brashers, & N.S. Rote (Eds) *Pathophysiology: The biological basis for disease in adults and children* (6th ed., pp. 360-395). St. Louis, MO: Elsevier Mosby.

Weiss, S.W. & Goldblum, J.R. (2008). Enzinger & Weiss's soft tissue tumors. (5th ed.). St. Louis, MO: Mosby

Wheeless, C.R. (2008). Chondrosarcoma. *Wheeless Textbook of Orthopaedics.* Retrieved from http://www.wheelessonline.com/ortho/chondrosarcoma

Wheeless, C.R. (n.d.). Periosteal chondroma: (Juxta Cortical Chondroma). *Wheeless Textbook of Orthopaedics.* Retrieved from http://www.wheelessonline.com/ortho/periosteal_chondroma_juxta_cortical_chondroma

Wheeless, C.R. (2010a). Pagets sarcoma. *Wheeless Textbook of Orthopaedics.* Retrieved from http://www.wheelessonline.com/ortho/pagets_disease

Wheeless, C.R. (2010b). Biopsy of musculoskeletal tumors. *Wheeless Textbook of Orthopaedics.* Retrieved from http://www.wheelessonline.com/ortho/biopsy_of_msk_tumors

Willett, C.G., Czito, B.G., & Tyler, D.S. (2007). Intraoperative radiation therapy. *Journal of Clinical Oncology, 25*(8), 971-7.

Wittig, J.C. & Villalobos, C.E. (2007). Other skeletal sarcomas. In H. S. Schwartz (Ed.), *Orthopaedic knowledge update: Musculoskeletal tumors 2* (pp. 197-198). Rosemont, IL: American Academy of Orthopedic Surgeons.

Yeh, E.T.H. & Bickford, C.L. (2009). Cardiovascular complications of cancer therapy. Incidence, pathogenesis, diagnosis, and management. *Journal of the American College of Cardiology,* 53, 2231-2247. doi:10.1016/j.jacc.2009.02.050

Zeltzer, L., Lu, Q., Leisenring, W., Tsao, J., Recklitis, C., Armstrong, G.,...Ness, K. (2008). Psychosocial outcomes and health-related quality of life in adult childhood cancer survivors: A report from the Childhood Cancer Survivor Study. *Cancer Epidemiology, Biomarkers & Prevention, 17,* 435-446. doi: 10.1158/1055-9965.EPI-07-2541

Chapter 17
The Spine

Angela N. Pearce, MS, RN, FNP-C, ONP-C

Objectives

- Identify the most significant spinal pathology, presentation, evaluation, and management for common spinal conditions.
- Describe the common diagnostic testing routinely performed for spine injuries.
- Discuss common conservative nonsurgical treatments.
- List the common surgical procedures utilized in treating spinal conditions after conservative treatment has been exhausted.
- Apply preoperative, intraoperative, and postoperative nursing strategies for patient management.
- Develop home care teaching considerations following spinal surgery.
- Review alternative therapies for patients with spinal disorders.

The spine provides protection to the spinal cord, structure to allow the human body its full range of motion (ROM) from standing erect to curling up like a baby, and stability to the neural elements. The vertebral column consists of 33 vertebrae: 7 cervical, 12 thoracic, 5 lumbar, 5 sacral, and 4 coccygeal. There are four distinct natural curves: cervical lordosis, lumbar lordosis, thoracic kyphosis, and sacral kyphosis. The curves form during the fetal period, with primary curves in the thoracic and sacral areas and secondary curves after weight-bearing of the body and head. Mechanical loading of the spine is important when discussing the etiology of spinal disorders, with compressive loads on the spine being largest during activities of daily living (ADLs). The functional spinal unit consists of two vertebral bodies connected by an intervertebral disc, facet joints, and ligaments (except at C1-2, where there is no intervertebral disc). Damage to the unit often develops into spinal pathology, requiring treatment (Spivak & Connolly, 2006).

Approximately 3% of patients in a trauma registry with blunt trauma sustain a spinal column injury such as spinal fracture or dislocation, and 1% sustain a spinal cord injury. These statistics can be incomplete depending on the inclusion criteria or may be overestimated by including fatal injuries and patients whose neurological deficits rapidly improve, which are often not included. Motor vehicle-related accidents account for almost half of all spinal injuries, with speeding, intoxication, and failure to use restraints being the major risk factors. Other common causes include sporting activities, acts of violence such as gunshot wounds, and falls (Kaji & Hockberger, 2008). Approximately 300,000 anterior cervical surgeries for disc disease are performed each year in the United States. At least 30% of 210,000 patients will involve some kind of arthroplasty (Spivak & Connolly, 2006).

A detailed medical history and physical to establish neurological and musculoskeletal assessment with baseline data are paramount when providing spinal treatment. Patients often have difficulty focusing on their chief complaint and may require guidance in the breakdown of their problems. Mechanical (axial) complaints of pain need to be differentiated from radicular (extremity-involved) complaints. In order to establish an accurate baseline for treatment, the evaluation of motor and sensory testing of the muscles require consistency in their evaluation. Pain management should include a comprehensive assessment of pain with the patient and caregivers, including education on pharmacologic and nonpharmacologic interventions. Conservative treatment of the spine is always the first-line treatment unless there is cauda equina syndrome or progressive neurological decline, which requires urgent evaluation and surgical intervention.

Common Spinal Diagnostic Studies

There are several different studies to assist with the diagnosis of spinal disorders, but most important to remember is a thorough health history and physical examination. Typically the least invasive study is performed first (Wood, Mahoney, & Cooper, 2009).

Plain x-rays, including anteroposterior (AP), lateral, oblique, and flexion/extension views, assess for fracture, instability, lesions and degenerative changes.

Magnetic resonance imaging (MRI) provides visualization of the soft-tissues, bones, discs, and nerves. Its mechanism of use is by a magnetic field and radiofrequency impulses that produce a signal that is processed into a computer, producing sagittal and axial images of the spine. Intravenous injection of gadolinium (contrast) enhancement is useful to differentiate scar tissue from a new problem if surgery has been performed, and to diagnose some tumors.

Computerized tomography (CT scan) produces an image of a cross-sectional plane through an area of the body. It is often used in conjunction with myelograms and discograms as the gold standard of neural compression in spinal stenosis.

Discography is used to reproduce a patient's pain by injecting saline and contrast dye into the disc and to identify concordant pain. It is rarely used but has some merit when identifying a specific level of disease.

Nuclear medicine bone scans, also called bone scintigraphy, are helpful in determining metabolic bone activity by osteoblastic cells. They can be useful in evaluating stress fractures and tumors, or if a fracture causing consistent pain cannot be seen on plain films. Single photon emission computerized tomography (SPECT) studies evaluate the spine in greater detail to assist with the treatment plan.

Electromyography/ nerve conduction velocity (EMG/NCV) is used to identify motor and sensory deficits with nerve root compromise and to identify central versus peripheral causes of neuropathy.

Scoliosis

Overview

Scoliosis is a three-dimensional deformity of the spine. All three planes—sagittal, coronal, and axial—must be considered to maximize patient outcomes. This includes an abnormal lateral and rotational curvature of the vertebral column. Curves may be present in any area of the spine: cervical, thoracic, thoracolumbar, and lumbar. The most common curve is a right-sided thoracic, which can produce a rib prominence or hump. As the curve progresses, the vertebral column rotates around the long axis and causes the ribs to take on a convex pattern in the thoracic region. A thoracic hypokyphosis may be present and, if severe, it decreases the space between the spine and sternum, thus compromising cardiac and pulmonary function. A lumbar curve is usually left-sided and produces an asymmetric waistline and is compensatory to the right thoracic curve. Untreated progressive scoliosis can result in significant deformity and cardiopulmonary compromise in a curve greater than 65 degrees. Pelvic obliquity often causes a leg length discrepancy and altered gait pattern with associated trochanteric bursitis. Debilitating back pain with loss of motor function is seen in the lumbar spine with degenerative scoliosis. There are several types of scoliosis, including idiopathic, adult degenerative, congenital, neuromuscular, posttraumatic, and postinfectious (Spivak & Connolly, 2006).

Scoliosis affects all ages and involves the whole body and its functions. In addition to the pain and functional restrictions, ego integrity and body image can also be negatively impacted. The patient may limit or avoid social interaction. It may be difficult for patients to get well-fitting clothes due to uneven hem lines and different pant leg lengths.

Idiopathic. In 80% of patients with scoliosis, there is no known cause (Larson, 2011). Several theories have been postulated, but no consensus has been reached. These include a genetic predisposition, vestibular dysfunction, muscular weakness, an alteration in collagen metabolism, and the role of melatonin in the pineal gland. The remaining 20% of cases can be divided into two types, based on cause:

1. Structural (functional) causes include congenital deformities of the spinal column, neuromuscular disorders, and syndromic (part of a syndrome).
2. Nonstructural (postural) causes may be posture-related such as leg length discrepancy, pelvic tilt, or hip/knee flexion deformities. Other causes may include spondylolisthesis, tumors, and disc herniations.

Infantile idiopathic scoliosis is more common in males, most common in children of European origin, and usually observed before 6 months of age with many of these curves resolving by age 3. A small number, 0.5% of all cases of idiopathic scoliosis, fall into this category (Wick, Konze, Alexander, & Sweeney, 2009). Most curves are thoracic to the left and may be associated with other congenital anomalies. Progressive curves will be treated with bracing initially, or serial casting may be required. Surgical intervention may be needed if the curve does not respond to bracing.

Juvenile idiopathic scoliosis accounts for 10-15% of all cases in children between the ages of 4 and 9. Females are more common than males after age 6; from ages 3-6, the male-female rate is equal, and the curve is usually left-sided (Wick et al., 2009). This often corresponds with a period of growth deceleration, as opposed to infantile and adolescent scoliosis seen during growth acceleration. Children in this age group are more likely to need surgery and less responsive to bracing.

Adolescent idiopathic scoliosis is diagnosed after age 10, occurs equally in males and females, and is often associated with peak height velocity and/or onset of menarche. The natural history of adolescent idiopathic scoliosis depends on several factors, including the degree of skeletal maturity, curve magnitude, location, and pattern. The determination of cessation of spinal growth is less predictable in males than females. Females tend to have curves that are more progressive, more frequent, and more severe requiring treatment more often (Wick et al., 2009).

Young adults, ages 20-40, may have curves under 40 degrees that remain stable and often are asymptomatic, requiring a watch-and-wait pattern where no treatment is given other than yearly monitoring on radiographs. If the curve progresses and the patient is compromised by pain and a decrease in function, surgery may be required to arrest the curve.

Adult Degenerative. Adult degenerative scoliosis is identified in patients older than age 40. Curves less than 40 degrees are often observed yearly with radiographs and if asymptomatic do not warrant treatment. In severe thoracic scoliosis, progressive curves greater than 65 degrees may cause fatigue, shortness of breath, and cor pulmonale often requiring surgery. In the lumbar spine, degenerative curves are associated with low back pain, fatigue, spinal stenosis, and lumbar radiculopathy, which may require surgery. Osteoporosis and vertebral compression fractures often play a role in this type of scoliosis (Birknes, White, Albert, Shaffrey, & Harrop, 2008).

Congenital. Congenital scoliosis, present at birth, is a fixed spinal deformity caused by an anomaly in the bony structure of one or more vertebral bodies, resulting in longitudinal spinal growth imbalance. This is classified by three types: failure of formation, failure of segmentation, or failure of both. (See Table 17.1.) Girls are affected more often than boys at a rate of 60%:40% (Wick et al, 2009). Location of the abnormality and the potential for growth interference determine the type of deformity: scoliosis, lordosis, kyphosis, or a combination.

Neuromuscular. This includes both neuropathic (nerve-related) and myopathic (muscle-related) categories of scoliosis. Many conditions are included in this category such as muscular dystrophy, cerebral palsy, polio, spina bifida, spinal muscular atrophy, and paralysis from spinal cord injury where the curve is due to muscle imbalance.

Table 17.1. Types of Deformities in Congenital Scoliosis
Failure of Formation Defects (Type I)
Partial (i.e., wedged vertebra): A solid body having the shape of an acute-angled triangular prism.
Complete (i.e., hemi vertebra): A congenital defect of the vertebral column in which one side of a vertebra fails to develop completely (page 2149).
Failure of Segmentation Defects (Type II)
Partial (i.e., bar vertebra): A segment of tissue or bone (i.e., anterior, posterior, lateral, mixed) that unites two or more similar structures (page 867).
Complete (i.e., block vertebra): Congenitally fused hypoplastic vertebral bodies which, on radiographs, give the appearance of a more or less solid bony mass (page 231).
Mixed Defects (Type III)
Formation: The act of giving from and shape (page 761).
Segmentation: The act of dividing into segments (page 1742).

From Stedman's Medical Dictionary *(28th ed.). Philadelphia, PA: Lippincott Williams & Wilkins (2006). Reproduced with permission.*

Children with neuromuscular scoliosis have one of two types: flaccid (floppy and weak muscle control) or spastic (tight and rigid posture). The age of onset and severity are strongly related to the degree of neuromuscular involvement. These patients' neuromuscular disorders should be assessed annually for spinal deformities, in which scoliosis is only one part of this complex condition. Neurofibromatosis can be seen with a sharply angulated curve, scalloping of the vertebra, and unusually thin ribs. In most cases of neuromuscular scoliosis, café au lait spots, cutaneous neurofibromas, and acoustic neuromas are present.

Posttraumatic. Traumatic injuries to the spinal column and iatrogenic injuries to the growth plates by radiation exposure can result in spinal curvature. This includes herniated nucleus pulposus (see separate section in this chapter) and tumors causing a significant trunk shift (list) due to sciatic nerve irritation. Functional or spastic posture shift secondary to primary spondylolisthesis with a spondylolytic defect and hysterical causes, due to emotional crises with a nonstructural scoliosis, is rarely seen.

Postinfectious. Certain infections of the spine, particularly tuberculosis, can cause a postinfectious spinal curvature. These spinal infections are typically found in the thoracic and lumbar areas, although on rare occasions they occur in the cervical spine. They are often observed and treated with antibiotics or antifungal medicines. If the curve progresses, surgical decompression and treatment with pedicle screws may be considered (Chunguang et al., 2010).

Assessment

History. Time must be spent evaluating any patient with scoliosis. Most often there is a familial history, but this is not always present. There is usually a progression of the deformity that is noted. Pain, paresthesias, or weakness may be present and will require further evaluation.

Children are able to relate part of the findings but need their parents to fill in other details, such as gestation, and exposure to teratogens in utero, and family history. Most scoliosis is not identified until school screening exams in seventh grade, regularly scheduled physicals, or while trying on clothing. Most children are asymptomatic; however, as the thoracic scoliosis increases, pulmonary function may be compromised, with shortness of breath and fatigue noted. Restrictive lung disease is secondary to scoliosis. Adults may experience back pain, fatigue, and respiratory compromise, depending on the location of the curve. Menstrual history and obstetric history should be documented, as appropriate.

Physical Exam. The patient is asked to change clothes into a bathing suit of neutral colors. Visualizing the spine is an important part of the physical. The development of a prominent scapula or hip is recorded. Any asymmetry of the shoulders and pelvis is noted. Prominent breasts or rib cages anteriorly are checked for. A plumb line from C7 is observed to see if it passes through the gluteal crease. Adam's Forward Bending Test (Figure 17.1) is performed to assess for spinal movement, as well as rotational

Figure 17.1.
Adam's Forward Bending Test

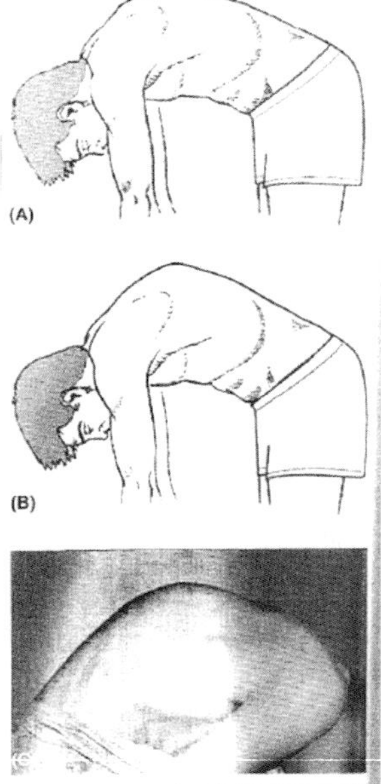

(A) demonstrates a normal spine; (B) and (C) demonstrate rigid hyperkyphosis of the thoracic spine.

From "Scheuermann's thoracic kyphosis in the adolescent patient" by E. Hart, G. Merlin, J. Harisiades, and B. Grottkau, 2010, Orthopaedic Nursing, *29(6), p. 366. Reproduced with permission.*

CHAPTER 17

prominences in the rib area (due to a thoracic curve) and in the paravertebral musculature (due to a lumbar curve). Leg length discrepancies can cause a functional scoliosis. A neurological exam, as well as a cutaneous exam for hairy tufts and café au lait spots, is always performed to rule out underlying neurological conditions.

Diagnostic Tests. Observation and school screening protocols inspect the spine in an upright and forward flexed position from behind the patient, in front of the patient, and to the side of the patient. A scoliometer may be used to quantify a prominence, with readings greater than 10 degrees requiring physician referral.

Standard radiological tests performed for diagnosing scoliosis are standing 36-inch PA and lateral radiographs of the spine. The films are taken posterior to anterior to reduce exposure to the thyroid, breast tissue, and reproductive organs. Shields are used to protect the breast and reproductive organs. Initial radiographs should be obtained after a positive screening and follow-up radiographs after examination and progression is suspected. Side flexion and extension views should be taken for preoperative surgical planning.

The Cobb Method (Figure 17. 2), a universally agreed upon measurement, has been in use since 1948 to measure the magnitude of spinal curves (Wick et al., 2009). The radiologist draws lines parallel to the end plates of the vertebral bodies at the two end vertebrae of the curve to be measured. A second line is drawn perpendicular to each of the lines. The angle formed by the intersection is the Cobb angle. There is a standard measurement error of 3-5 degrees based on the way the film was taken, the position of the patient, and the way the lines are drawn. Documentation of the levels of the curve is important. The Cobb angle is useful as a monitoring tool for curve progression or correction. Rotation is assessed by looking at other indicators such as vertebral pedicle alignment to the midline.

Figure 17.2.
Diagram of the Cobb Method

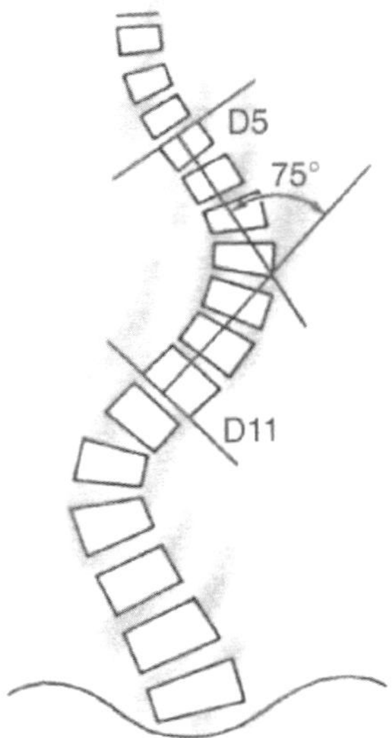

From "Fractures, dislocations, and fracture-dislocations of the spine" by W. Campbell, S. Canale, and J. Beaty, 2008, Campbell's Operative Orthopaedics *(11th ed. Vol. 2, p.1934). Philadelphia, PA: Mosby/Elsevier. Reproduced with permission.*

Somatic sensory evoked potentials (SSEPs) and motor evoked potentials (MEPs) are obtained preoperatively to assess the spinal cord function preoperatively and intraoperatively. Surgery may be stopped and a reassessment of the patient is evaluated before continuation with the procedure if anomalies are detected.

Pulmonary function tests (PFTs) are assessed for curves greater than 65 degrees and for neuromuscular scoliosis. This group of tests measure lung function for both inhalation and exhalation of room air that can be compromised in patients with scoliosis. Normal values are based on age, sex, height, and ethnicity. Pathological conditions associated with scoliosis are discussed in Table 17.2.

Common Therapeutic Modalities

Conservative. Most curves less than 15-20 degrees are observed for progression at 6-month intervals during peak growth and annually otherwise because it is unlikely that they will progress further (Spivak & Connolly, 2006). Postural exercises with an active exercise program are thought to be helpful, although there are no studies to support the theory that exercise can prevent or correct structural scoliosis.

Curves of 20-40 degrees require bracing in a growing child to prevent further progression of the curvature. A brace rarely corrects scoliosis permanently. As the child grows, a new brace needs to be fabricated every 12-18 months. A brace is ineffective in the skeletally mature patient. One treatment option is nighttime bracing for 10-12 hours, and there are several different types of braces available for use. On occasion, serial casting will be prescribed. Skin assessment is vital when using either casts or braces to prevent skin breakdown and pressure ulcers. Maintenance of the curvature at pre-brace degree level is considered successful treatment. Contraindications for bracing include cervico-thoracic and high thoracic curves, thoracic hypokyphosis, curves more than 40 degrees, and emotional intolerance.

Surgical. A patient with a severe, inflexible curve may need more extensive treatment prior to surgery to improve spinal alignment. This may include halo traction, which uses the patient's own body weight to achieve some correction of rigid curves. Counterweights are added to the halo to provide additional traction force. Skin care and pin site care are important nursing interventions. The patient may sleep in a circle electric bed, and additional devices may be modified such as a wheelchair, walker, and tricycle with suspension frames for shower stalls (Wick et al., 2009).

Surgical intervention includes posterior spinal fusion, with instrumentation such as pedicle screws and growing rods, and anterior spinal fusion with instrumentation, which may be in combination with posterior fusion and may be a staged procedure. Growing rods are used to allow for continued controlled growth of the spine. One commonality of these operative systems is the use of pediatric pedicle screws and hooks. In certain situations (such as a child being unable to tolerate bracing), anterior release of the curve is undertaken including intravertebral stapling, in which staples are placed upon the outer (convex) curve of the spine to prevent further progression of the curve and help stabilization. The inner (concave) growth plates will continue to develop and may allow for slight correction of the deformity as growth occurs (Thompson, Lenke, Akbarnia, McCarthy, & Campbell 2007).

In patients with thoracic insufficiency syndrome, surgical placement of vertical expandable prosthetic titanium rods (VEPTR implants) is approved by the United Stated Federal Drug Administration to mechanically stabilize and expand the thorax in skeletally immature patients. The VEPTR device may prevent collapse of the thorax if the spinal curve increases and breathing is compromised. The device is contra-indicated in patients who are either younger than 6 months of age or beyond the age of skeletal maturity, have inadequate bone strength of the ribs to support the implant, do not have proximal and distal ribs to attach the device, lack inadequate soft tissue coverage for the device, have an infection at the surgical site, or have a known allergy to the device. This is inserted using a thoracotomy incision with postoperative chest tube insertion. Variations of surgical plans may be recommended for complex cases (Vaccaro & Baron, 2008).

The use of a thoraco-lumbosacral orthosis (TLSO) may be required postoperatively. This can be removed for bathing and provides reassurance for large surgical

Table 17.2. Pathological Conditions Associated with Scoliosis

Condition	Description
Arachnoid Cyst	A fluid-filled cyst with arachnoid membrane frequently situated near the lateral aspect of the lateral sulcus of the cerebral hemisphere, usually congenital (p.127).
Arnold Chiari Malformation	Malformed posterior fossa structures associated with caudad traction and displacement of the rhombencephalon (i.e., hindbrain, include pons, cerebellum, and medulla oblongata) caused by tethering of the spinal cord; maybe accompanied in some cases by spina bifida and associated anomalies such as meningomyelocele (p.1147).
Cerebral Palsy	A generic term for various types of motor function anomalies present at birth or beginning in early childhood. Causes are both heredity and acquired, and are classified as intrauterine, natal, and early postnatal. Motor disturbances include diplegia, hemiplegia, quadriplegia, choreoathetosis, and ataxia (p.1408).
Congenital Diaphragmatic Hernia	Failure of the left pleuroperitoneal membrane to fuse with the posterior margin of the diaphragm; most commonly occurs on the left side (p.879).
Dextro (scoliosis)	Spinal convexity to the right (p.527).
Diastematomyelia	Complete or incomplete sagittal division of the spinal cord by an osseous or fibrocartilaginous septum (p.534).
Hypotonia	Diminution or loss of muscular tonicity (p.939).
Levo (scoliosis)	Spinal convexity to the left (p.1078).
Lipoma	A benign neoplasm of adipose tissue consisting of mature fat cells (p.1107).
Meningocele	Protrusion of the membranes of the brain or spinal cord through a defect in the cranium or spinal column (p.1183).
Myelodysplasia	An abnormality in development of the spinal cord, especially the lower part; term is sometimes inappropriately used for spina bifida occulata (p.1269).
Syringomyelia	Longitudinal cavities lined by dense gliogenous tissue in the spinal cord, which is not caused by vascular insufficiency; associated with scoliosis of the lumbar spine, although some cases are associated with low-grade gliomas or vascular malformations of the spinal cord (p.1922).
Syrinx Spinal Cord	A pathologic tubular cavity in the brain or spinal cord with a gliotic lining; rarely used synonym for fistula (p.1923).
Tethered Cord Syndrome	Abnormal low positioning of the distal spinal cord by the filum terminale (e.g., below L2 vertebra); associated with incontinence, progressive motor and sensory impairment in the legs, pain, and scoliosis (p.1916).

From Stedman's Medical Dictionary (28th ed.) by T. Stedman, 2006, Philadelphia, PA: Lippincott Williams & Wilkins. Reproduced with permission.

constructs. A custom-made TLSO is typically a plastic molded shell in two pieces (front and back) attached by hook-and-loop (Velcro®) straps protecting the thoraco-lumbosacral area. An off-the-shelf TLSO is constructed of fabric and plastic stays attached with hook-and-loop straps to allow for ease with application.

Nursing Considerations

Nursing Diagnoses. Nursing diagnoses for this condition are expanded upon in the Appendix.

- Activity intolerance; activity intolerance, risk for.
- Anxiety.
- Body image, disturbed.
- Coping, ineffective.
- Development, risk for delayed.
- Disuse syndrome, risk for.
- Family coping, compromised.
- Family processes, interrupted.
- Grieving; grieving, complicated; grieving, complicated, risk for.
- Knowledge deficit.
- Noncompliance.
- Pain, chronic.
- Powerlessness; powerlessness, risk for.
- Self-care deficit: bathing/hygiene, dressing/grooming, feeding, toileting.
- Self-concept, readiness for enhanced.
- Self-esteem, risk for situational low.
- Self-esteem, risk for chronic low.
- Skin integrity, impaired; skin integrity, risk for impairment.

Kyphosis

Overview

Kyphosis is a thoracic convexity of the spine. A natural kyphosis often exists without any complications, but when the convexity is greater than 45 degrees, it becomes abnormal. Severe thoracic kyphosis may cause cardiopulmonary compromise and significant pain.

Congenital kyphosis develops in the embryonic stage of development around 6-8 weeks of gestation. An anomaly in the vertebral structural development occurs, creating a malformation of the bony architecture of the spine.

Postural kyphosis is when a person is able to correct the kyphosis with an alteration of posture in an erect stance with the shoulders pulled backwards. This typically overcorrects on hyperextension of the spine.

Scheuermann's thoracic kyphosis is more prevalent in males. It occurs when there is wedging of three adjacent vertebral bodies greater than 5 degrees with kyphosis greater than 45 degrees between T5 and T12 (Hart, Merlin, Harisiades, & Grottkau, 2010). There is a narrowing of the intervertebral disc spaces and weakened irregular end plates. Hyperextension of the spine does not correct these curves. It is more common in the thoracic spine but can be present in the lumbar spine. Presentation is often with associated back pain, but patients may be asymptomatic. Parental concerns range from cosmesis to the progression of the deformity. The difference between Scheuermann's kyphosis and postural kyphosis on physical exam is the rigidity of the spine. The Adam's forward bend test (see Figure 17. 1) will show a posterior angulation or gibbus deformity of the thoracic spine when viewed from the side. A recent study reviewed 35,000 twins to establish a cohort of symptomatic twins with Scheuermann kyphosis recorded in the Danish twin registry between 1931 and 1982. They found an overall prevalence of Scheuermann kyphosis to be 2.8%, with a prevalence of 2.1% among women and 3.6% among men (Lowe & Line, 2007).

Paralytic kyphosis is secondary to polio and associated with other neuromuscular disorders such as muscular dystrophy, cerebral palsy, spina bifida, and other myopathies characterized with muscle weakness. Traumatic burst fractures or radiation-induced injuries to the spine may cause a significant kyphosis to the bony column.

Postlaminectomy kyphosis can occur following laminectomy for spinal tumors, syringomyelia, or spinal cysts, with vertebral collapse due to loss of bony structures by surgical resection. Allograft strut grafts, and corpectomy, and fusion help prevent this development. Patients with ankylosing spondylitis may develop a significant kyphosis that may need to be treated surgically.

Osteoporosis and vertebral compression fractures are common manifestations of *true senile kyphosis*. Development of this type of kyphosis is most common in postmenopausal women, usually in the high thoracic area (known as a Dowager's hump).

Assessment

History. Refer to the scoliosis assessment earlier in this chapter. In addition, remember that clothing must be removed to adequately assess the spine and its function. The typical presentation includes pain and fatigue, with shortness of breath in some cases. Observe for increased thoracic rounding, asymmetry of the shoulders, and abdominal creases, with tight hamstrings in forward flexion and an inability to toe touch. A neurological exam must be performed to rule out any underlying problems such as tumors. Dermatomal tests must be performed to identify a sensory loss. This is performed anteriorly and posteriorly in the thoracic spine. Abnormal reflexes may be present, with a difference between the upper and lower extremity reflexes. Long tract signs should be tested, as well as pulses to identify vascular anomalies.

Diagnostic Testing. Diagnostics for kyphosis are similar to those found in the scoliosis section. Often patients are identified at the middle school screening protocol or at a routine physical exam.

Common Therapeutic Modalities

Conservative. First-line therapy is observation for progression of the kyphosis. A thoracic curve greater than 45 degrees in adolescents undergoing rapid growth will be evaluated every 6 months with radiographs and clinical exams. Postural exercises may be prescribed to prevent further kyphosis (Hart et al., 2010). Bracing may be helpful for curves greater than 45 degrees to prevent curve progression, often using a Milwaukee brace. Trunk stabilization exercises and hamstring stretching are often prescribed with bracing. Curvature can be corrected with bracing, unlike scoliosis, but the treatment is not indicated until the end of growth. Bracing is ineffective for the skeletally mature patient.

Surgical. Surgery for curves greater than 70 degrees may include anterior and posterior spinal fusions with instrumentation by video assisted thoracoscopic surgery (VATS) or thoracotomy (Vaccaro & Baron, 2008). Paralytic curvatures may require sub-laminar wiring and rods. Often a combination anterior and posterior approach is required for complex cases with allograft strut grafts from the rib or fibula, and a corpectomy may be performed for correction of the curve with osteotomies and pedicle screws. Demineralized bone matrix may be helpful in obtaining solid fusion. Junctional kyphosis can occur if the instrumentation is ended proximal or distal to the Cobb angle (see Figure 17.2). Postoperative bracing often uses a TLSO with an attached neck ring (Minerva brace) or a Milwaukee brace. This helps prevent excessive rotation of the spine and provides reassurance to the patient.

Nursing Considerations

Nursing Diagnoses. Nursing diagnoses for kyphosis are similar to scoliosis. They are expanded upon in the Appendix.

Nursing Interventions. The anterior and posterior surgeries are typically performed approximately 1 week apart, providing there are no serious complications. The risk for superior mesenteric artery syndrome (a medical condition characterized by compression of the transverse process of the duodenum between the aorta and the superior mesenteric artery, causing various degrees of duodenal obstruction) is not insignificant, and patients should remain without food but maintain adequate hydration until the syndrome resolves. Follow-up is surgeon-specific, as with postoperative bracing. Patients receive pain medications and muscle relaxants, and are encouraged to be ambulatory. Follow-up serial radiographs are taken to assess the construct for a solid fusion. Patients are typically followed for up to a year after the surgery. Most activities and physical therapy (PT) are resumed around 12 weeks following surgery.

Herniated Nucleus Pulposus

Overview

Herniated nucleus pulposus is a protrusion of the central portion of the intervertebral disc (nucleus pulposus) through a crack in the outer cartilaginous ring (annulus fibrosis). Spinal disc herniations may occur as a result of trauma to the discs by high-velocity impact such as falls or motor vehicle accidents. More often, however, repetitive stress to the discs though vibration activities such as heavy lifting may cause cracking or fissures in the annulus fibrosis, promoting disc protrusion and herniation. Disc degeneration occurs as a person ages, also causing fissuring and cracks that may develop into disc herniations. See Table 17.3 for the terminology used in discussing disc herniation.

Table 17.3. Terminology of Disc Herniation Progression	
Bulge	An out-pouching of the disc. This is not considered to be a disc herniation but rather a normal part of the aging process.
Protrusion	A herniation of the disc that does not protrude past the posterior longitudinal ligament.
Extrusion	A disc herniation through the posterior longitudinal ligament.
Sequestration	A disc herniation in which a free fragment of disc is no longer attached to the annulus.
The terminology regarding disc herniation can be confusing after MRI is performed.	

The intervertebral disc is one of the primary motion segments of the spine. It is comprised of an outer annulus fibrosis made up of cartilaginous/collagen fibers and an inner nucleus pulposus made up of water-based gelatinous proteoglycans. The disc functions as a "shock absorber" between the two vertebrae and distributes the "load" throughout the spine. The nucleus is stressed by compressive forces such as running or jumping, while the annulus is stressed by rotational forces such as bending and twisting. The disc aids in the flexibility of the spine.

When the nucleus herniates through a crack in the annulus, it may cause pressure and inflammation on the nerve roots creating a radiculitis (extremity pain) to the exiting or traversing nerve roots. Interestingly, most disc herniations occur in the morning soon after the person arises from a supine position. It is hypothesized that the disc rehydrates during sleeping, thereby making it more prone to herniation (Spivak & Connolly, 2006).

Disc herniations, typically seen in the fourth to fifth decade of life, are relatively uncommon in childhood and adolescence. Approximately 2% of the US population is affected by lumbar disc herniations, with 10% (or roughly 600,000 patients) still symptomatic after 3 months (Sarwark, 2010). Males are up to three times more likely to have symptomatic disc herniations, possibly related to occupational influences and recreational activities. The most common sites are L4-5 and L5-1 for lumbar disc herniations and C5-6 and C6-7 for cervical disc herniations, although all discs may be affected. Lumbar disc herniated free fragments may resorb over time and reduce in size.

The most acute potential complication is cauda equina syndrome. This is a medical emergency requiring surgery and should be treated as such. It is characterized with progressive neurological weakness, increase in pain, incontinence of bowel and bladder, perineal and perianal numbness, and loss of rectal sphincter tone. The patient must be evaluated within 2-4 hours at the clinic or emergency room (ER) to prevent permanent nerve damage.

Although disc herniations are not life-threatening, they may be life-altering. Patients may experience financial strain due to lost time at work, and a change in occupation may be necessary if the job requires heavy lifting. Chronic depression and opioid dependence may be seen as a result of diagnosis, as well as chronic pain symptoms (D'Arcy, 2009).

Assessment

History. A thorough assessment of the presenting symptoms is important to ascertain the location of the pain. Is it low back or leg pain? Is it arm or neck pain? Document the patient's history of present illness by asking the following questions:

- Has there been a particular event or injury to cause the pain, or has it been an insidious onset?
- Are there associated pieces of history such as management at the time of injury?
- What is the mechanism of injury? Describe the incident. If the mechanism was a motor vehicle accident, did you lose consciousness? Were you wearing a seat belt? Were the airbags deployed? Did you total your vehicle? Were you the driver or passenger?
- How long have you been experiencing this pain?
- Is there a previous history of pain or past surgery in this body part?
- What are the aggravating or alleviating factors? Describe the characteristics of the extremity pain.
- What past medical history and comorbidities do you have? Is there a family history of back or neck surgery?
- What is your occupational history or disability?
- What is your hand dominance?
- How old are you?
- Are there any constitutional symptoms such as weight loss, fever, or night sweats?
- What is your lifestyle and ADLs? What recreational activities do you participate in, and what is your workout level of activity?
- What is your social history (smoking, alcohol use, and living conditions)?

Subjective complaints are influenced by the mechanism of injury, as well as the level and area of the disc herniation. The duration of the pain is important and may be described as sudden onset or progressively worsening. Radicular pain will typically follow dermatomal patterns, while central disc herniations may not follow radicular patterns. Cervical pain is usually aggravated by cervical flexion and/or extension, lateral rotation and bending, and axial loading in extension. The pain is often relieved by rest. Lumbar disc herniations are usually aggravated by standing, walking, flexion, coughing, or sneezing, and may be relieved by lying supine with knees flexed to reduce nerve root irritation (Sarwark, 2010).

Physical Exam. The cervical spine is assessed for signs of myelopathy. The gait is observed, both with the patient's eyes open and closed while walking, to look for ataxia. L'hermitte's test and Spurling's test assess for nerve root irritation, as well as cervical ROM in flexion, extension, lateral rotation, and bending to assess for pathology. Vascular testing is included of pulses graded 0 - 2+. Conditions with similar symptoms but not of cervical etiology (such as carpal tunnel syndrome and shoulder pathology) should by assessed (Mostofi, 2009). Manual muscle testing and strength are evaluated with reflexes and long tract signs, including the following:

- Hoffmann's Test: with the patient's hand in a relaxed position, flick the first phalanx of the long finger. Look for index finger or thumb flexion as a sign of spinal cord irritation in the neck.
- Babinski Sign: stroke lightly upward on the plantar aspect of the foot, and look for great toe extension and a fanning of the lesser toes as a sign of spinal cord irritation.
- Clonus Test: with the patient in a relaxed position (sitting or supine), grasp the patient's calf with one hand and the foot with the other. Jerk the foot two or three times. If the foot continues to jerk spontaneously, this may be a sign of spinal cord irritation.

The thoracic spine evaluation includes gait, ROM, manual muscle testing, sensation anteriorly and posteriorly to assess dermatomes, reflexes, and long tract signs. The lumbar spine evaluation includes testing the patient's ability to walk on tiptoes, heels, and perform knee squats to assess L4, L5, and S1 nerve roots. Spinal ROM including flexion, extension, lateral bending, and extension rotation identifies painful areas of the spine. Flexion usually indicates discogenic involvement, whereas extension usually indicates spinal stenosis or facet disease. Flattening of the lumbar spine or a trunk shift may indicate muscle spasm. Reflexes are part of the neurological assessment, as well as muscle strength and sensation to assess for muscle weakness and nerve root irritation. Nerve root tension signs may be present when positive straight leg raising is seen, with radiation of pain to the leg in a dermatomal pattern while sitting or supine, or contralaterally. Hip ROM should be assessed for completion of the exam.

Cervical disc herniations may present in the following common dermatomal patterns:

- The **C5** nerve root compression causes a sensory deficit in the biceps and upper lateral arm, a decreased biceps reflex and motor strength decrease in the biceps muscle. After surgery, the C5 nerve root is slow to recover, and it may take up to a year to get full return of strength.
- The **C6** nerve root compression causes a sensory deficit in the thumb, index fingers, and forearm; a decreased brachioradialis reflex; and motor strength decrease in wrist extension.
- The **C7** nerve root compression causes a sensory deficit in the middle finger and medial forearm, a decreased triceps reflex; and motor strength decrease in the triceps muscle and wrist flexion.
- The **C8** nerve root compression causes sensory loss in the medial upper arm, no reflex is tested, and motor strength deficits in finger flexion and hand intrinsics.

Lumbar disc herniations may present in the following common dermatomal patterns:

- The **L1** and **L2** dematomes are associated with lower abdominal and groin involvement. The hip needs to be evaluated for hip pathology, inguinal, and sports hernia.
- The **L3** nerve root compression affects sensory loss in the medial thigh and does not go below the knee. No reflex is tested, and quadriceps strength deficit is often present.
- The **L4** nerve root compression affects sensory loss in the anterior thigh and medial aspect of the calf/shin, diminished or absent patellar reflex, and motor strength deficits with hip flexors, quadriceps supine and sitting, and dorsiflexor strength.
- The **L5** nerve root compression affects sensory loss in the lateral aspect of the thigh, calf, and great toe with no specific reflex and motor strength deficit in extensor hallucis longus (great toe extension). There may be difficulty heel-walking with dorsiflexion weakness.
- The **S1** nerve root compression affects sensory loss in the lateral aspect of the foot, a diminished or absent Achilles reflex, and motor strength deficit with ankle eversion, repetitive plantar flexion, and difficulty toe walking.

Diagnostic Testing. Spine plain radiographs rule out other causes of concomitant pain and include AP, lateral, and flexion and extension films. MRI shows nerve root compromise or impingement from a disc herniation or other problem.

CT shows the bony structures well and nerve root compromise when caused by disc herniations. A myelogram, done in conjunction with a CT scan, is an invasive test whereby a water-soluble contrast dye is injected into the spinal canal and the patient is tilted from a supine position to an upright position to simulate weight-bearing with walking and standing. The nerve roots are often compromised by a disc herniation and stenosis. A myelogram is usually for surgical planning if an MRI cannot be used or if multiple levels are involved.

EMG/NCV is used to identify motor and sensory deficits with nerve root compromise, as well as central versus peripheral causes of neuropathy. Discography is used to reproduce a patient's pain by injecting saline and contrast dye into the disc and identify concordant pain. It is rarely used but has some merit when identifying a specific level of disease.

Common Therapeutic Modalities

Conservative. For 90% of patients with lumbar disk herniation, acute leg symptoms start to improve within 6 weeks and resolve by 12 weeks with conservative care (Gregory, Sego, Wortley, & Shugart, 2008). The natural resolution of disc herniations is typically favorable with nonoperative treatment in the absence of cauda equina symptoms (Sarwark, 2010). This typically includes a period of bedrest (usually 2 days) with medication therapy and easing back into activities as tolerated. Treatment is usually for 4-6 weeks with PT to stretch and strengthen the lumbar musculature. Traction is used in patients with cervical conditions and occasionally in patients with lumbar conditions. Alternating heat and ice modalities is dependent on patient comfort and physician preference. Smoking cessation is emphasized because of the correlation between smoking and healing of bony fusion: patients who smoke tend to have more back and neck pain. Other PT protocols may include massage, and transcutaneous electrical nerve stimulation (TENS) units to provide electrical stimulation of muscles.

Cervical collars relieve stress and tension in the cervical spine. Braces/corsets are typically not recommended because their use can weaken abdominal and lumbar muscles, but they may be helpful on a short-term basis and with elderly patients.

Pharmacologic therapy includes short-term use of analgesics for acute pain. Muscle relaxants can be prescribed if spasm is present. Nonsteroidal anti-inflammatory drugs (NSAIDs) or COX 2 inhibitors can reduce inflammation on the nerve root. A short tapered dose of steroid such as prednisone or a Medroldosepak may be used to decrease inflammation. Cortisone injections using short-and long-acting local anesthetics and an injectable steroid in epidural or selective nerve root injections are useful in reducing inflammation at the site of the disc herniation, sometimes with facet blocks.

Surgical. When conservative treatment has failed, surgical intervention may be instituted. In the cervical spine, the location of the disc herniation determines whether a posterior or anterior approach should be used to shave off the protruding part of the disc. Typically with an anterior discectomy, a fusion is performed either with an intervertebral graft of the patient's iliac crest or an allograft with instrumentation.

In the lumbar spine, several procedures may be performed such as an open microscopic lumbar discectomy, a minimally invasive microscopic discectomy through an endoscope, a laminectomy and discectomy, or a lumbar fusion and discectomy. The fusion is usually performed after all other forms of treatment have been exhausted and when pain is persistent. The decision is physician-determined, based upon clinical examination and available diagnostic studies. See Table 17.4 for a discussion of common surgical procedures, indications, and risks.

Nursing Considerations

Nursing Diagnoses. Nursing diagnoses for this condition are expanded upon in the Appendix.

- Activity intolerance; activity intolerance, risk for.
- Cardiac perfusion, risk for decrease.
- Constipation, risk for.
- Falls, risk for.
- Gastrointestinal motility, dysfunctional; gastrointestinal motility, risk for dysfunction.
- Knowledge deficit.
- Nutrition imbalance, less than body requirements.
- Nutrition imbalance, risk for more than body requirements.
- Pain, acute.
- Pain, chronic.
- Peripheral neurovascular dysfunction, risk for.
- Self-care deficit: bathing/hygiene, dressing/grooming, feeding, toileting.
- Sensory perception: tactile, disturbed.
- Skin integrity, impaired; skin integrity, risk for impairment.
- Social interaction, impaired.
- Tissue perfusion: cardiac, risk for decrease.
- Tissue perfusion: cerebral, risk for decrease.

Nursing Interventions. Pain control is individualized (also see Chapter 7—Pain). Most pain is relieved after the pressure is removed from the nerve root. Comfort measures such as ice topically are provided to the patient postoperatively to provide nonpharmacologic pain relief. The patient is positioned with the knees flexed to relieve nerve root tension. Walking and standing are encouraged once the patient awakens and can tolerate these activities. Sitting for a prolonged period of time increases discomfort in the lumbar spine. The nurse and/or physical therapist will teach the log-rolling technique to get out of bed without excessive twisting of the spine.

After anterior cervical discectomy and fusion, the nurse needs to provide care that is based on hospital protocols and physician preference. Assess the respiratory status for wheezing, distress, or stridor, which may be due to edema or increased bleeding. In the event of respiratory distress, an endotracheal tube and tracheostomy tray must be available on the "crash cart." Provide humidity to prevent drying of secretions. Assess the patient's ability to swallow, and note any voice changes indicative of swelling in the neck area. Assess the wound for excessive bruising or bleeding, and change dressings a needed. The patient will be wearing a hard or soft cervical collar, depending on the number of discs involved in the operation.

Perform neurovascular checks of the upper and lower extremities per unit protocol, assessing for changes, and notify the physician immediately if found. The provision of a soft or hard collar for a period of time, which often may be removed for bathing, is helpful to the patient and relieves tension in the paraspinal muscles. Assess bowel and bladder function for incontinence, and/or constipation, and provide laxatives as needed.

Cervical and lumbar surgery may be complicated by a dural leak of cerebrospinal fluid, which requires the patient to stay flat for a period of time while the leak heals and a spinal headache is averted. This is generally for 24 hours or overnight. Sometimes a spinal drain may need to be placed above the site of the dural leak in order to allow it to heal. Careful monitoring and an aseptic closed drainage system are required to prevent a meningeal infection.

Table 17.4. Common Surgical Procedures for Disc Herniation			
Procedure Type	**Indications**	**Procedure**	**Procedure-Specific Risks**
Percutaneous discectomy	Bulging or herniated lumbar disc	A probe is placed into the center of the disc under fluoroscopic guidance through a small incision. The herniated disc is removed using a cutting cannula at the end of the probe, and removing a portion of the center of the disc so that the bulging or herniated disc retracts back, taking pressure off the nerve.	Nerve root injury, infection, hermatoma, no improvement of symptoms
Microdiscectomy/ limited approach discectomy/ laminotomy and discectomy	Herniated lumbar disc	A small incision is made; a hole is made in the lamina (laminotomy); and with the assistance of magnifying glasses or microscope, the herniated portion of the disc is removed.	Nerve root injury, infection, dural tear, hermatoma, no improvement in symptoms.
Intradiscal electrothermal therapy (IDET)	Degenerated or bulging disc causing discogenic low back pain	The symptomatic disc level is confirmed by discography prior to proceeding. A needle is placed into the disc under fluoroscopic guidance and a catheter is then threaded through and coiled around the center of the disc. The catheter heats the center of the disc in an effort to thicken and contract the disc wall to eliminate it from being a pain generator.	Nerve root injury, infections, no improvement of symptoms.
Laminectomy	Central herniated disc or spinal stenosis	The lamina is removed to either access the area of a centrally herniated disc so that the disc herniation can be removed OR to relieve pressure on the nerve roots caused by spinal stenosis.	Nerve root injury, infections, hematoma, dural tear, no improvement of symptoms.
Posterior spinal fusion Lumbar or cervical	Instability which can be attributed to a variety of causes, such as degenerated or multiple herniated discs, spinal stenosis which requires extensive decompression, spondylolisthesis, or fractures	Bone graft material is placed laterally between the transverse processes and over a period of time heals or "fuses" together creating a bony fusion mass which provides stability to the area.	Nerve root injury, infection, hematoma, dural tear, no improvement of symptoms, failure of the fusion to heal (nonunion), or transitional instability at adjacent segments.
Posterior lumbar fusion with instrumentation and interbody cage (PLIF)	Instability which can be attributed to a variety of causes, such as degenerated or multiple herniated discs, spinal stenosis which requires extensive decompression, spondylolisthesis, or fractures	As above, with the addition of spinal instrumentation (pedicle screws) and interbody cage being placed in an effort to immobilize the fused level and provide a spacer to allow reduction of pressure on the nerve root and aid in the healing of the fusion mass.	As above with the addition of nerve root injury at the time of instrumentation placement; breakage of the instrumentation system; or need for removal of the system in the future.
Anterior lumbar spinal fusion and interbody cage (ALIF)	Instability attributable to a variety of reasons creates anterior instability	An abdominal approach is used to expose the lumbar spine to release discs and a fusion is created using bone graft material or a cage filled with bone material.	Nerve root injury, retroperitoneal hemorrhage, failure of the bowels to regain normal function, sterility in men, failure of the fusion to heal. If cages are used, dislodgement of the cage resulting in injury to the nerves or the aorta, as well as the need for additional surgery, Pneumothorax, hemothorax, pneumonia.

Table 17.4. Common Surgical Procedures for Disc Herniation (continued)			
Procedure Type	**Indications**	**Procedure**	**Procedure-Specific Risks**
Transforaminal lumbar interbody fusion with pedicle screw instrumentation (TLIF)	Instability which can be attributed to a variety of causes, such as degenerated or multiple herniated discs, spinal stenosis which requires extensive decompression, spondylolisthesis, or fractures	Similar to posterior lumbar fusion with or without interbody cage placement and addition of spinal instrumentation (pedicle screws) The cage is placed transforaminally in an effort to immobilize the fused level and provide a spacer to allow reduction of pressure on the nerve root and aid in the healing of the fusion mass.	Nerve root injury at the time of instrumentation placement; breakage of the instrumentation system; or need for removal of the system in the future.
Extreme lateral interbody fusion (XLIF)	Instability which can be attributed to a variety of causes, such as degenerated or multiple herniated discs, spinal stenosis which requires extensive decompression, spondylolisthesis, or fractures	Similar to posterior lumbar fusion with or without interbody cage placement and addition of spinal instrumentation (pedicle screws) The cage is placed extremely laterally in an effort to immobilize the fused level and provide a spacer to allow reduction of pressure on the nerve root and aid in the healing of the fusion mass.	Nerve root injury at the time of instrumentation placement; breakage of the instrumentation system; or need for removal of the system in the future.
Direct lateral interbody fusion (DLIF)	Instability which can be attributed to a variety of causes, such as degenerated or multiple herniated discs, spinal stenosis which requires extensive decompression, spondylolisthesis, or fractures	Similar to posterior lumbar fusion with or without interbody cage placement and addition of spinal instrumentation (pedicle screws) The cage is placed direct laterally in an effort to immobilize the fused level and provide a spacer to allow reduction of pressure on the nerve root and aid in the healing of the fusion mass	Nerve root injury at the time of instrumentation placement; breakage of the instrumentation system; or need for removal of the system in the future. Disruption to the psoas muscle requiring Continuous Passive Motion usage for 24 -48 hours to help with hip ROM
Anterior cervical discectomy and fusion (ACDF)	Cervical herniated disc, stenosis, instability or myelopathy	An incision is made in the front of the neck and the cervical disc is removed. Bone graft autograft from the iliac crest or allograft, is then placed between the vertebrae to create a fusion. This may be done with or without instrumentation.	Nerve root injury, respiratory distress, hematoma, failure of the fusion to heal, difficulty swallowing, iliac crest pain with rare fracture of pelvis, no improvement of symptoms.
Posterior cervical discectomy	Cervical herniated disc	An incision is made posteriorly and the piece of disc is improved	Nerve root injury , hematoma, dural tear, no improvement in symptoms
Cervical laminoplasty	Cervical spinal stenosis with myelopathic features	A motion preserving procedure (nonfusion) used to treat cord compression at multiple levels	Nerve root injury and palsy especially with C5 nerve root with deltoid and biceps weakness, dural leak, continued axial neck pain.
Artificial disc replacement	Degenerative disc disease	The degenerated disc is removed and replaced with a device composed of two metallic endplates and a flexible core that moves between the endplates.	Nerve root injury, breakage of the disc, dislocation of the disc, infection.

Data from "Direct lateral lumbar interbody fusion for degenerative conditions: Early complication profile" by R. Knight, P. Schwaegler, D. Hanscom, and J. Roh, 2009, Journal of Spinal Disorders & Techniques, *22, 34-37; "Spine" by M. Rodts and M. Hickey, 2007,* Core Curriculum for Orthopaedic Nursing *(6th Ed.), Boston, MA: Pearson; "Description of XLIF Surgery" by V. Deviren, 2009, http://www.spine-health.com/treatment/spinal-fusion/description-xlif-surgery; and "Anterior cervical disk arthroplasty, spondyloysis repair, anterior lumbar interbody fusion, transforaminal lumbar interbody fusion, kyphoplasty, veptr opening wedge thoracostomy for congenital spinal deformities" by A. Vaccaro and E. Baron, 2008,* Spine Surgery, *Philadelphia, PA: Saunders/Elsevier.*

Assess the wound for excessive bleeding or bruising, and monitor drainage output. Provide deep vein thrombosis prophylaxis with thromboembolic stockings, early ambulation, and assessment. Log-rolling and the "B,L,T,S,PP" restrictions are taught frequently: limiting **B**ending, **L**ifting no more than 5-10 pounds, **T**wisting and **S**itting no more than 30 minutes, and avoidance of **P**ushing and **P**ulling. Continue to provide education on nutrition, weight loss, and smoking cessation. Monitor activity levels, and encourage continuation of PT, including trunk stabilization, in an attempt to prevent disc herniation recurrence. Assist the patient in finding exercise programs close to home to recondition, maintain muscle tone, and regain flexibility.

Degenerative Disc Disease

Overview

Degenerative disc disease involves increased wear and tear on the intervertebral discs over time. Degeneration is a normal aging process unless accompanied by pain (Madigan, Vaccaro, Spector, & Milan, 2009). A drying up of the water-filled proteoglycans in the nucleus pulposus causes the disc to shrink in size, and the ability to act as a cushion "shock absorber" is decreased. This can cause pressure on the nerve roots with leg pain or acute back pain. It may cause spinal instability and stenosis.

The incidence increases with age, usually starting in the third decade, and progresses at different rates in each individual. This is often not diagnosed until another event causes the patient to seek treatment. Degenerative disc disease may affect cervical, thoracic, and lumbar discs: if it is present in one area of the spine, it is likely to be present in other areas as well. Approximately 95% of the U.S. population appears to have some form of degenerative changes to the spine by age 50 (D'Arcy, 2008). Patients usually experience flare-ups and periods of remission until aggravated by some type of mechanical trauma.

There is often controversy when the diagnosis is made after a motor vehicle accident or work-related accident. In these cases, it is often stated that the pain and other symptoms are identified as an aggravation of a preexisting degenerative disc disease.

This is not a life-threatening disease but a life-modifying condition in which certain activities need to be modified to relieve painful exacerbations and maintain a productive quality of life. Concomitant radicular symptoms must be ruled out by a neurological examination.

Assessment

History. The most common symptom is discogenic back pain with a gradual increase in severity over time. There may or may not be associated radiculopathy. The patient may have a painful ROM in flexion and extension, and may complain of aggravated pain with coughing and sneezing or prolonged activities. A thorough assessment of the presenting symptoms to ascertain the location of the pain. Is it low back or leg pain? Is it arm or neck pain? Document the patient's history of present illness by asking the following questions:

- Has there been a particular event or injury to cause the pain, or has it been an insidious onset?
- Are there associated pieces of history such as management at the time of injury?
- What is the mechanism of injury? Describe the incident. If the mechanism was a motor vehicle accident, did you lose consciousness? Were you wearing a seat belt? Were the airbags deployed? Did you total your vehicle? Were you the driver or passenger?
- How long have you been experiencing this pain?
- Is there a previous history of pain or past surgery in this body part?
- What are the aggravating or alleviating factors? Describe the characteristics of the extremity pain.
- What past medical history and comorbidities do you have? Is there a family history of back or neck surgery?
- What is your occupational history or disability?
- What is your hand dominance?
- How old are you?
- Are there any constitutional symptoms such as weight loss, fever, or night sweats?
- What is your lifestyle and ADLs? What recreational activities do you participate in, and what is your workout level of activity?
- What is your social history (smoking, alcohol use, and living conditions)?

Subjective complaints are influenced by the mechanism of injury, as well as the level and area of the disc degeneration. The duration of the pain is important and may be described as sudden onset or progressively worsening. Radicular pain will typically follow dermatomal patterns.

Physical Exam. The cervical spine is assessed to look for signs of myelopathy. The gait is observed, with the patient's eyes open and closed while walking, to look for ataxia. L'hermitte's Test and Spurling's Test are assessed for nerve root irritation, as well as cervical ROM in flexion, extension, lateral rotation, and bending to assess for pathology. Manual muscle testing and strength are next evaluated with reflexes, as well as long tract signs including Hoffmann's, Babinski's, and Clonus (see the physical exam under "Herniated Nucleus Pulposus").

Vascular testing is included of pulses graded 0-2+. Conditions with similar symptoms but not of cervical etiology (such as carpal tunnel syndrome and shoulder pathology) should be assessed.

The thoracic spine evaluation includes gait, ROM, manual muscle testing, sensation anteriorly and posteriorly to assess dermatomes, reflexes, and long tract signs. The lumbar spine evaluation tests the patient's ability to walk on tiptoes, heels, and perform knee squats to assess L4, L5, and S1 nerve roots. Spinal ROM including flexion, extension, lateral bending, and extension rotation identify painful areas of the spine. Flexion pain usually indicates discogenic involvement, whereas extension pain usually indicates spinal stenosis or facet disease. Reflexes are part of the neurological assessment, as well as muscle strength and sensation to assess for muscle weakness and nerve root irritation. Nerve root tension signs may be present with resisted sitting and supine straight leg raising, and there may be some flattening of the lumbar spine secondary to muscle spasms. Hip ROM should be assessed.

Diagnostic Tests. Plain spine radiographs, including AP, lateral, and flexion/extension films, are taken to assess disc height and instability involvement. If multiple levels are involved, discogram/CT scan may be used to identify the symptomatic level.

Common Therapeutic Modalities

Conservative. Patients are encouraged to modify their activities within comfort levels to avoid acute exacerbations and to allow the acute symptoms to resolve. PT provides stretching and strengthening activities to the affected body parts and increases core strength and flexibility. Heat and ice modalities may be used as comfort measures. Anti-inflammatory medications or a steroid taper may be used in the short term to reduce the pain from inflammation. Epidural steroid injections have been shown to be of some benefit if there is an associated radiculopathy, but this is often temporary. Accupuncture, massage, prolotherapy (a proliferation of the ligament or tendon tissue by injecting the tissue with a sugar-water solution to cause a localized inflammation, increasing the blood supply to the tissue and promoting healing), rolfing (a holistic system of soft tissue manipulation under gravity with movement education for structural integration), yoga, and spinal decompression with chiropractic care are all alternative forms of treatment.

An intermediary procedure known as intradiscal electrothermal annuloplasty (IDET) may be performed when an electrode is placed inside the disc and an electric current is passed through the disc. The heat seems to reduce the pain and seal off the annulus, and the procedure is minimally invasive. Studies and procedures may be performed by pain management specialists who are typically anesthesiologists (Kloth, Fenton, Andersson, & Block, 2008).

Surgical. When conservative treatment has been exhausted and the patient continues to complain of significant pain, surgical intervention will be discussed. This usually involves a fusion (with or without instrumentation) that can be performed anteriorly, posteriorly, direct laterally, far laterally, or transforaminally, depending on the disease and surgeon preference. This is abbreviated with a lexicon of procedures, mostly involving interbody cages and pedicle screw fixation. See common surgical procedures ALIF, PLIF, DLIF, XLIF, and TLIF in Table 17.4.

Nursing Considerations

Nursing Diagnoses. Nursing diagnoses for this condition are expanded upon in the Appendix.

- Activity intolerance; activity intolerance, risk for.
- Cardiac perfusion, risk for decrease.
- Constipation, risk for.
- Falls, risk for.
- Gastrointestinal motility, dysfunctional; gastrointestinal motility, risk for dysfunction.
- Knowledge deficit.
- Nutrition imbalance, less than body requirements.
- Nutrition imbalance, risk for more than body requirements.
- Pain, acute.
- Pain, chronic.
- Peripheral neurovascular dysfunction, risk for.
- Self-care deficit: bathing/hygiene, dressing/grooming, feeding, toileting.
- Sensory perception: tactile, disturbed.
- Skin integrity, impaired; skin integrity, risk for impairment.
- Social interaction, impaired.
- Tissue perfusion: cardiac, risk for decrease.
- Tissue perfusion: cerebral, risk for decrease.

Spinal Stenosis

Overview

Spinal stenosis includes any type of narrowing of the spinal canal or intervertebral foramina by either osseous or soft-tissue structures. Stenosis is most often seen in the cervical and lumbar spine. A spondylolisthesis (see separate section in this chapter), as well as posttraumatic and iatrogenic postoperative conditions, may cause stenosis. Metabolic disorders such as Paget's disease or Cushing's disease are also known causative factors. There are three different types of stenosis: congenital, acquired, and mixed congenital and acquired (Katz & Harris, 2008).

Congenital stenosis may be hereditary, resulting from congenitally short pedicles. Patients tend to become symptomatic in the third, fourth, and fifth decade of life when normal degenerative changes become able to cause symptoms. Athletes in collision injury sports such as football, hockey, wrestling, and rodeo may be found to have congenital cervical stenosis after an injury, which may preclude them from continuation in that particular sport.

Congenital stenosis is usually of the entire canal, whereas *acquired stenosis* is usually limited to one or several segments. Acquired stenosis is always due to degenerative, traumatic, or metabolic changes in the spinal column, causing narrowing and nerve root compromise. This may be due to degeneration of the facet joints, intravertebral discs, and thickening of the ligamentum flavum.

Cauda equina syndrome caused by stenosis is a surgical emergency and needs to be ruled out clinically (see "Herniated Nucleus Pulposus" for additional information regarding this condition). Vascular disease, trochanteric bursitis, osteoarthrosis of the hips, and peripheral neuropathy may mimic some of the stenotic symptoms and need to be ruled out.

Assessment

History. A comprehensive history for all spinal patients is important. (See the history for "Degenerative Disc Disease.") There is often a gradual onset of stenosis over years, most commonly seen when patients have difficulty walking and standing (neurogenic claudication) and when pain is relieved by sitting or bending forward. It is most often seen in the elderly older than age 65. The patient typically is flexed forward, looking for somewhere to sit or lean because this helps open the spinal canal and alleviates nerve compromise.

Physical Exam. A comprehensive physical examination is important. (See the physical exam for "Lumbar Disc Herniation.") Pain may radiate down one or both legs, or may follow a dermatomal pattern. Lumbar extension usually exacerbates the symptoms. Motor strength and falls risk assessment must be completed because this may require more urgent intervention. Bowel and bladder symptoms may be present. A vascular examination may be warranted to assess distal pulses, and a referral to a vascular surgeon is necessitated if abnormalities are found on clinical exam.

Diagnostic Studies. Plain radiographs, including AP and lateral views with flexion/extension films, assess for instability. Myelogram/CT scans identify the area of stenosis and the severity; however, this is invasive, and MRI may be ordered if conservative management is recommended. Occasionally EMG/NCV studies identify other issues such as carpal tunnel syndrome, polysensory neuropathy versus radicular pain.

Common Therapeutic Modalities

Conservative. The goal is to maximize function, maintain independence, and relieve pain. The modification of activities includes the opportunity to sit and rest when necessary and then resume the activity. It may be helpful to suggest that the patient sit on a stool when cooking and avoid extension activities. Treatment with anti-inflammatory medication for a short period may be helpful, but in the older age group, it is necessary to remember to protect the stomach lining with medication to prevent a gastrointestinal bleed. Epidural steroid injections are indicated for acute pain episodes. Sometimes a corset/brace is recommended for acute pain episodes, but long-term this tends to weaken the abdominal and lumbar musculature. PT and aquatic therapy may help to strengthen spinal musculature, maximize function, and relieve pain.

Surgical. (See Table 17.4.) Surgical intervention is the last resort in the absence of cauda equina syndrome, and patients must be medically cleared to undertake surgery because of common pre-existing comorbidities. Quality of life, activity requirements, and a discussion with the surgeon regarding realistic expectations must be addressed preoperatively. Typically a decompressive laminectomy is performed to relieve the stenosis. A fusion is suggested when there is associated instability or if surgery creates instability. The recovery from a fusion is generally twice as long as a decompressive laminectomy and may include postoperative bracing. The length of postoperative hospital stay is approximately 3 days, providing there are no serious complications.

Nursing Considerations

Nursing Diagnoses. Nursing diagnoses for this condition are expanded upon in the Appendix.

- Activity intolerance; activity intolerance, risk for.
- Cardiac perfusion, risk for decrease.
- Cardiac tissue perfusion, risk for decrease.
- Cerebral tissue perfusion, risk for.
- Falls, risk for.
- Gastrointestinal motility, dysfunctional; gastrointestinal motility, risk for dysfunctional.
- Knowledge deficit.
- Nutrition imbalance, less than body requirements.
- Nutrition imbalance, risk for more than body requirements.
- Pain, acute.
- Pain, chronic.
- Peripheral neurovascular dysfunction, risk for.
- Self-care deficit: bathing/hygiene, dressing/grooming, feeding, toileting.

- Sensory perception: tactile, disturbed.
- Skin integrity, impaired; skin integrity, risk for impairment.
- Social interaction, impaired.

Nursing Interventions. Pain control is individualized (also see Chapter 7—Pain). Most pain is relieved after the pressure is removed from the nerve root. Comfort measures are provided to the patient, including ice topically postoperatively to provide nonpharmacologic pain relief. The patient is positioned with the knees flexed to relieve nerve root tension. Walking and standing is encouraged once the patient awakens and can tolerate these activities. Sitting for a prolonged period of time increases discomfort in the lumbar spine. The nurse and/or physical therapist will teach the patient the log-rolling technique to get out of bed without excessive twisting of the spine.

After anterior cervical discectomy and fusion, the nurse needs to provide care that is based on hospital protocols and physician preference. Assess the respiratory status for wheezing, distress, or stridor, which may be due to edema or increased bleeding. A "crash cart" with an endotracheal tube and tracheostomy tray should be available in case of respiratory distress. Provide humidity to prevent drying of secretions. Assess the patient's ability to swallow, and note any voice changes indicative of swelling in the neck area. Assess the wound for excessive bruising or bleeding, and change dressings as needed. The patient will be wearing a hard or soft cervical collar, depending on the number of discs involved. Sometimes patients remain intubated overnight if a staged procedure, anteriorly and posteriorly, is performed.

Perform neurovascular checks of the upper and lower extremities per unit protocol, assessing for changes, and notify the physician if found. The provision of a soft or hard collar (often removable for bathing) for a period of time is helpful to the patient and relieves tension in the paraspinal muscles. Assess bowel and bladder function for incontinence, and/or constipation, and provide laxatives as needed.

Cervical and lumbar surgery may be complicated by a dural leak of cerebrospinal fluid, which requires the patient to stay flat for a period of time while the leak heals and a spinal headache is averted. This is generally for 24 hours or overnight. Sometimes a spinal drain may be needed above the level of the dural leak in order to allow it to heal. Careful monitoring and an aseptic closed drainage system are required to prevent a meningeal infection.

Assess the wound for excessive bleeding or bruising, and monitor drainage output. Provide deep vein thrombosis prophylaxis with thromboembolic stockings, early ambulation, and assessment. Log-rolling and restrictions of "B,L,T,S,PP" (as mentioned earlier in the care of lumbar disc herniations) are taught frequently. Patient education with regards to nutrition, weight loss, smoking cessation, activity levels, and PT (including trunk stabilization) is key to recovery. Assist the patient in finding exercise programs close to home to recondition, maintain muscle tone, and regain flexibility.

Spondylolysis and Spondylolisthesis

Overview

Spondylolysis is a unilateral or bilateral defect of the pars interarticularis. It is the antecedent to forward slippage of the vertebra causing a spondylolisthesis. Spondylolysis may be traumatic in origin or a result of repetitive mechanical stress. Children and adolescents involved in certain sports such as gymnastics, wrestling, tennis, golf, and soccer have a higher incidence related to repeated or exaggerated hyperextension stress on the back at the pars interarticularis (Spivak & Connolly, 2006).

Spondylolysis most often occurs at L4-5 and L5-1 vertebra. It may or may not be associated with spondylolisthesis. This condition has an equal rate in boys and girls in approximately 5% of the US population. It occurs in the lumbar spine most frequently between the ages of 6 and 10, but patients often do not become symptomatic until a traumatic event causes back pain. Spondylolytic defects are typically diagnosed in the early teen years when increased activities put extra demands on the patient, with the defect seen on oblique radiographs and the neck of the "Scottie dog" broken (Hu, Tribus, Diab, & Ghaanayem, 2008; Sarwark, 2010).

Spondylolysis is not a life-threatening condition, but modification of activities with a change in lifestyle may be necessary in order to reduce the painful back condition. Many young athletes are driven to succeed by their parents, and family counseling with both parents (if possible), the child, and the physician is often necessary to make an informed decision for modification of activities. Reasonable alternative noncontact sports should be addressed such as swimming and cycling.

Spondylolisthesis may occur at any level of the spine but is most often seen at L4-5 and L5-1. The condition is commonly diagnosed between ages 7 and 18. The average age of onset for girls is 14 years and 16 years for boys, after peak height velocity and final growth spurt. This is often associated with increased athletic physical activities. This condition may go undiagnosed until it is found at a pre-employment physical examination or after an episode of back pain.

Spondylolisthesis may cause severe pain with radiculitis in an acute or higher grade of defect; however, if the patient is asymptomatic, the spondylolisthesis does not require intervention. The patient may complain of alternating leg pain and/or back pain (Majid & Fischgrund, 2008).

Spondylolisthesis may have a hereditary disposition. The severity is dependent on the type: dysplastic, isthmic, degenerative, traumatic, and pathologic.

1. Dysplastic spondylolisthesis is a congenital defect with an elongation of the pars with or without lysis.
2. Isthmic spondylolisthesis involves lysis of a previously normal pars. This is often seen in young athletes who perform repeated hyperextension activities such as gymnastics, wrestling, and soccer. This type of spondylolisthesis occurs in males 5%-6% of the time and in females 2%-3% of the time. Most patients do not become symptomatic until late childhood or early adolescence.
3. Degenerative spondylolisthesis involve changes in the vertebrae, facet joints, ligamentous structures, and intervertebral discs. This is often associated with general joint laxity and increased mechanical stressors, and causes the vertebra to slip forward. It may be at multiple levels of the spine, most often occurring in the lumbar spine and cervical spine. This type of spondylolisthesis, four times more common in females than males, is often associated with spinal stenosis and typically presents later in life around age 50.
4. Traumatic spondylolisthesis is related to an injury to the area and may occur at any age.
5. Pathologic spondylolisthesis results from a pathologic process such as an infection or tumor. This must be ruled out by further diagnostic testing such as an MRI.

Grades of spondylolisthesis are based upon the amount of vertebral translation (typically anteriorly) when measured on radiographs. They vary from I-V:

Grade I - up to 25% translation
Grade II - up to 50% translation
Grade III - up to 75% translation
Grade IV - up to 100% translation
Grade V - 100% spondyloptosis

Assessment

History. (See the history for "Herniated Nucleus Pulposus.") Cervical pain, radiculopathy, or myelopathy may be noted in the cervical spine; however, low back pain is most often the reason for the clinic visit. It may be acute or chronic in nature, which has worsened, and may involve radiation to one or both legs. It typically presents with exacerbations from an event or insidiously. A comprehensive history avoids missing potential cauda equina syndrome, which may require emergency intervention. This may be due to associated bowel and bladder dysfunction, secondary to nerve compression with severe spondylolisthesis. The onset of pain and the description of the type of pain helps differentiate between mechanical, axial pain and radicular, extremity pain. Presence of paresthesias and a dermatomal pattern are helpful descriptive symptoms. Other helpful details include the number of other physicians the patient has seen, prior back surgeries, and aggravating and alleviating factors. The presence of possible constitutional disease must be addressed to rule out pathological or infectious reasons for pain. Significant family history for hereditary disposition is discussed.

Physical Exam. (See the physical exam from "Herniated Nucleus Pulposus.") The patient must be undressed in a gown and shorts. The gait may be slow or waddling, and there may be an increased lumbar lordosis and protuberance of the abdomen with high grade slips. Single-leg stance and hyperextension may reveal pain either unilaterally or bilaterally. A palpable step-off on the spinous processes may be palpated in patients with a severe slippage of the vertebra and higher grade of spondylolisthesis. There may be muscle spasm present in the paraspinal musculature of the low back. Forward flexion may be limited, and there may be hamstring tightness that produces a false positive on straight leg raise examination. A neurological exam must be given to assess for muscle weakness, paresthesias, reflexes and long tract signs caused by traction of the nerve due to the slippage of the vertebra. Sitting and supine straight leg-raising is performed to assess for a radicular component or hip involvement. A hip examination is performed because lateral hip pain could be from the back or the hip.

Diagnostic Tests. Spine plain radiographs include AP and lateral films to determine the grade of slippage. Flexion/extension views determine any instability or motion at that level. Oblique views enable visualization of the pars defect as represented by the broken collar on the "Scotty dog." This is called a spondylolytic spondylolisthesis.

Lumbar MRI evaluates for the presence of lumbar disc herniations or soft tissue injuries. Myelogram/CT scan evaluates the neural structures in two different positions, (supine and upright), identifies spinal stenosis, and is most often used prior to surgical intervention. EMG/NCV may be used to determine associated nerve root impingement either centrally or peripherally.

Common Therapeutic Modalities

Conservative. Generally, activity is modified until the acute pain resolves. This does not usually require a period of bedrest, but if it does, 2 days' rest is typically sufficient to alleviate symptoms. Patients are urged to avoid lifting heavy objects, or repetitive flexion and extension with twisting. Immobilization for spondylolytic defects above L3 is recommended for 12 weeks. This is done with a TLSO. Analgesics are used for short episodes of pain, but anti-inflammatory medication is not recommended due to interference with bone healing in spondylolytic defects. The use of a bone stimulator has been shown to be beneficial in studies and can be incorporated into the treatment plan. Epidural steroid injections or pars injections may be helpful for temporary relief. PT is helpful after the healing process has begun to provide core strengthening for the abdominal and lumbar musculature (Peer & Fascione, 2007).

Surgical. (See Table 17.4.). Surgical intervention may be recommended with pinning of the pars defects or spinal fusion with instrumentation. This is only considered after conservative treatment has been exhausted and pain persists. The surgical approach is dependent upon the type and degree of slip, as well as surgeon training, philosophy, skill, and preference. For higher grades of slippage, the level of vertebra above the site of slippage may need to be incorporated into the fusion to provide a solid construct, prevent further slippage of the vertebra, and prevent loosening of the hardware.

Nursing Considerations

Nursing Diagnoses. Nursing diagnoses for this condition are expanded upon in the Appendix.

- Activity intolerance; activity intolerance, risk for.
- Body image, disturbed.
- Cardiac perfusion, risk for decrease.
- Constipation, risk for.
- Coping, ineffective.
- Falls, risk for.
- Gastrointestinal motility, dysfunctional; gastrointestinal motility, risk for dysfunction.
- Knowledge deficit.
- Nutrition imbalance, less than body requirements.
- Nutrition imbalance, risk for more than body requirements.
- Pain, acute.
- Pain, chronic.
- Peripheral neurovascular dysfunction, risk for.
- Self-care deficit: bathing/hygiene, dressing/ grooming, feeding , toileting.
- Self-concept, readiness for enhanced.
- Self-esteem, risk for chronic low.
- Self-esteem, risk for situational low.
- Sensory perception: tactile, disturbed.
- Skin integrity, impaired; skin integrity, risk for impairment.
- Social interaction, impaired.
- Tissue perfusion: cardiac, risk for decrease.
- Tissue perfusion: cerebral, risk for decrease.

Home Care Considerations. School-age patients may require a set of books at home and a set at school to avoid the need to carry heavy backpacks. For females, a rolling backpack is helpful. Walking is the therapy of choice for 12 weeks; thereafter, evaluation with x-rays, and PT is recommended for a core stabilization program. Most patients are reminded to avoid smoking, maintain exercises with walking, and avoid gaining weight. The "B,L,T,S,PP" program as mentioned earlier in the care of lumbar disc herniation is stressed. Oral analgesics and muscle relaxants can be taken as needed.

Failed Back Surgery Syndrome

Overview

A definition of failed back surgery syndrome (FBSS) is pain with or without associated leg pain of a chronic, nonmalignant nature that persists after one or more spinal surgical procedures when the outcome of surgery does not meet the established expectations of the surgeon and the patient. The etiology is difficult to determine but includes improper patient selection, incorrect diagnosis of the spinal disorder, incorrect surgical treatment, failure of the patient to respond to a given surgical treatment with failure of the instrumentation, failure of fusion, and reherniation of the vertebral disc. This condition mostly affects adults, and occasionally there is no known cause. There is typically formation of excessive scar tissue from previous surgery, which may compress the nerve roots and cause pain, known as epidural fibrosis. There is also breakdown of the discs at adjacent levels to the surgical site with continued pain. There may also be a psychological overlay.

FBSS affects a relatively small number of patients, considering the high incidence of low back surgery. The incidence has improved due to newer techniques, including minimally invasive procedures, better patient selection, and better explanation of realistic expectations.

Complications include the presence of chronic persistent pain, requiring opioid use that can lead to narcotic addiction and dependency. Illicit drug use, depression, and social isolation are frequent factors that cause patients difficulty in developing interpersonal relationships. Employment changes and the associated financial strain can be present in certain situations. Most FBSS patients are referred to a pain management specialist who generally provides a pain medicine contract with pain medicine refills at precise times, often with an appointment because many drugs may require triplicate prescriptions. After reevaluation, many patients are referred back to the surgeon if there is an identifiable diagnosis. When all spinal surgeries have been exhausted, a trial of a spinal cord stimulator may be suggested. This is a surgical procedure in which implantable electrodes are placed in the spinal column with an implanted pump that provides an electric current to override the pain. If effective, it can reduce the amount of medication taken by the patient and also provide a higher quality of life and functionality (Frey et al., 2009).

Assessment

History. A comprehensive history is more cost-effective than any diagnostic procedure. The patient may bring large amounts of prior history, and the specifics of surgeries, prior testing, and results need to be reviewed. It should be remembered that the patient may have waited a long time for this appointment. The most important details are the specifics related to the surgery and the onset or recurrence of pain. Define the signs and symptoms of pain with the patient. The following questions are important to consider:

- Was the pain ever relieved postoperatively?
- Has there been a reinjury or new injury?
- Was this an insidious progression or a sudden onset of worsening symptoms?
- What is the time period since surgery?
- Is this the same pain as prior to surgery?
- Are there any aggravating or alleviating factors?
- What are the characteristics of the pain?
- Describe all the prior spinal surgeries you have undergone with dates, locations and surgeons.
- What is your quality of life, and recreational activities? Can you cope with activities of daily living?
- Are you able to maintain employment, or are you on disability?
- Who is at home to help you?
- Describe any smoking, alcohol, or illicit drug use?
- Have you tried complimentary medicines or over-the-counter treatments?
- Is there any pertinent family history of prior surgeries?
- Are there comorbidities in the past medical history?
- Have you been referred to pain management? If so, are they required to sign a contract for opioid usage?

Physical Exam. (See the physical exam for "Herniated Nucleus Pulposus.") A physical examination should be performed with the patient dressed in gown and shorts to allow for a thorough exam. Assess whether the patient can ambulate without assistive devices. Ask the patient to walk on toes and heels, and assist them for balance with a gentle squat. An assessment of spinal ROM provides information as to effort of the patient and location of the pain generator. Observe for the presence of spasm, and evaluate for palpable tenderness on the spine or sciatic notch. Manual muscle testing with resistance and sensory testing with light touch and pin prick further elucidate signs of pathology. Assess the reflexes, and monitor for long tract signs. Note the presence of guarding and a positive straight-leg raise. Remember to evaluate the hip, neck, and shoulder if myelopathy is suspected.

Diagnostic Testing. Individualized for every patient, diagnostics may include plain radiographs of AP, lateral, and flexion/extension views for a general overview. The patient may bring numerous prior studies from many years past to be evaluated, and it is important to take the time to do so. A psychological evaluation may be needed and requested.

Common Therapeutic Modalities

Conservative. Nonsurgical treatment is recommended with comfort measures. Validate the patient's symptoms, and provide sufficient time for the patient to thoroughly understand their radiographs. Suggest PT, acupuncture, massage, and local topical heat and ice applications. Consider a brace or corset, and review appropriate use of the medications. Discuss long-term pain management options with intrathecal opioid pumps and spinal cord stimulation. Make a referral to a comprehensive pain clinic for "back school."

Surgical. Surgical intervention should depend on the diagnosis. Achievable goals and realistic expectations should be explained. Documentation in the patient's medical chart should reflect this important surgeon and patient discussion.

Nursing Considerations

Nursing Diagnoses. Nursing diagnoses for this condition are expanded upon in the Appendix.

- Activity intolerance; activity intolerance, risk for.
- Body image, disturbed.
- Cardiac perfusion, risk for decrease.
- Constipation, risk for.
- Coping, ineffective.
- Falls, risk for.
- Gastrointestinal motility, dysfunctional; gastrointestinal motility, risk for dysfunction.

- Knowledge deficit.
- Nutrition imbalance, less than body requirements.
- Nutrition imbalance, risk for more than body requirements.
- Pain, acute.
- Pain, chronic.
- Peripheral neurovascular dysfunction, risk for.
- Self-care deficit: bathing/hygiene, dressing/ grooming, feeding, toileting.
- Self-concept, readiness for enhanced.
- Self-esteem, risk for chronic low.
- Self-esteem, risk for situational low.
- Sensory perception: tactile, disturbed.
- Skin integrity, impaired; skin integrity, risk for impairment.
- Social interaction, impaired.
- Tissue perfusion: cardiac, risk for decreased.
- Tissue perfusion: cerebral, risk for decreased.

Nursing Interventions. The patient often will require a comprehensive pain management program including PT, occupational therapy, biofeedback, social work for financial difficulty, and vocational rehabilitation counseling. Family counseling is often recommended. Encourage the patient to make realistic goals in rehabilitation and to get adequate rest. Provide alternative nonpharmacologic methods of pain control, such as a new mattress, TENS units, or heat and cold modalities.

Spinal Fractures

Overview

Most spinal fractures and ligamentous injuries occur as a result of a high-velocity injury such as a motor vehicle crash, falls, diving, or blunt trauma. The prevalence of each type of spinal fractures depends upon the demographics of the population served by a trauma center. In general, 2%-6% of cervical trauma patients sustain a cervical spine fracture, while thoracic and lumbar spinal fractures account for 30%-50% of all spinal injuries in trauma patients (Spivak & Connolly, 2006). Most thoracic and lumbar spine fractures are related to osteoporosis and involve minimal or no trauma. Neurological injury must be assessed initially in the evaluation of spinal cord injuries, and treatment starts immediately in the ER. (See Chapter 15—Trauma.) Table 17.5 addresses types of spinal fractures

Fractures of the Cervical Spine (Neck). Spinal injury dynamics are complex and incompletely understood. Most patients will present to the health care provider after an acute injury, wearing a hard or soft collar. All patients complaining of neck pain with associated injuries must be evaluated and cleared for fracture before removing a cervical collar. Most missed spinal injuries occur in patients who are obtunded from a closed head injury, unconscious, and/or intoxicated.

The patient with a cervical spine fracture typically presents with severe neck pain, paraspinous spasm, and /or point tenderness to the spine. Pain that radiates to the extremities is indicative of nerve root impingement either centrally or peripherally. Global sensory or motor deficits are suggestive of spinal cord injury. In cases of multiple trauma injuries, the patient may not complain of spine pain until later. The mechanism of injury is always helpful in determining the amount of force incurred to the spine. If the patient can provide a history, this is always helpful but not always given.

General observation of the patient's gait and inspection for swelling, contusions, and bleeding from orifices is important. Palpation for tenderness and spasm may indicate a fracture. A gap or step-off between spinous processes usually is indicative of ligamentous injury in the posterior complex and is often unstable. ROM should be limited to prevent further damage. Motor and sensory function in the upper and lower extremities, as well as anteriorly posteriorly in the thoracic dermatomes, are important to assess. Nerve root impingement signs with reflexes should be assessed, as well as vascular distal pulses. A rectal examination should be performed if spinal cord injury is suspected.

Figure 17.3.
Halo Vest

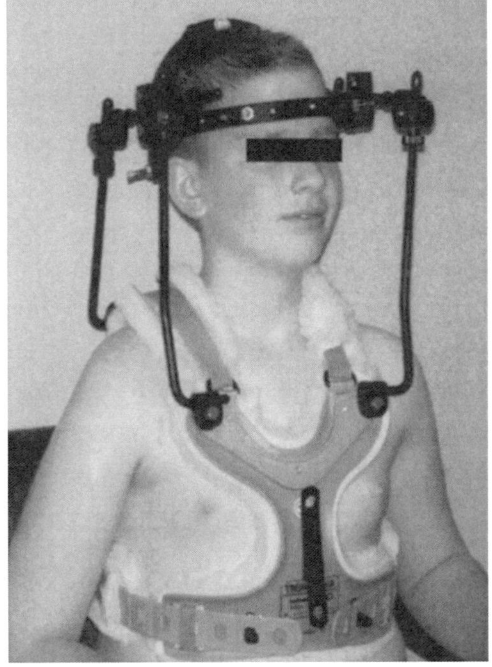

From Orthopaedic Nursing (1st ed., p.288) by A. Maher, S. Salmond, and T. Pellino, 2002, Philadelphia, PA: Saunders. Reproduced with permission.

Table 17.5. Classic Names and Descriptions by Anatomic Location

Name	Description	Common Treatment	Illustration
Chance	Horizontal splitting of spinous process and arch with minimal extension into vertebral body	Stable, heals rapidly with bed rest, logrolling, and corset or brace is desired	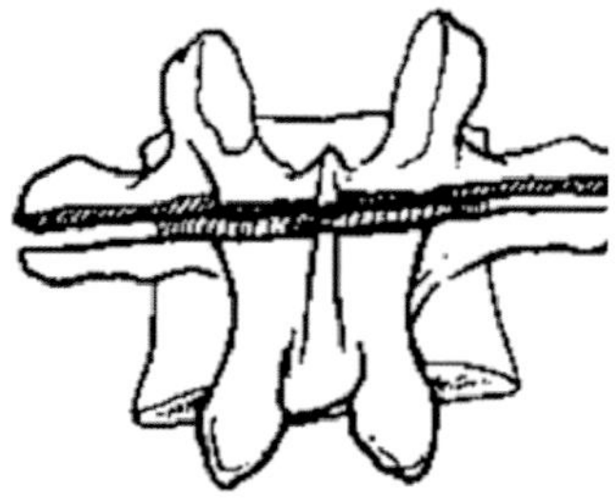
Clay shoveler's	Fracture spinous process(es) C-6, C-7, T-1, T-2, T-3	Stable with no associated neurological damage – no treatment required	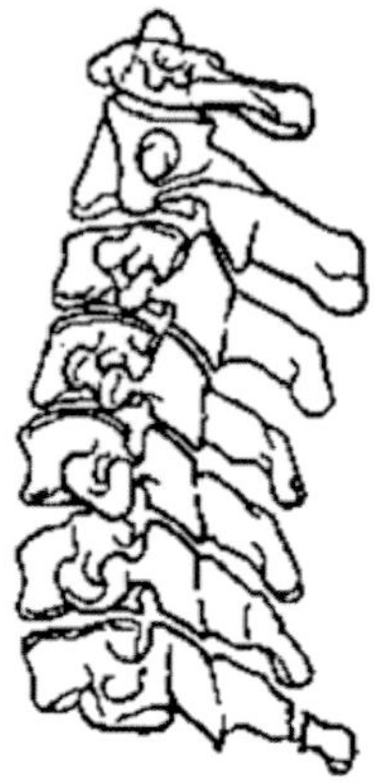
Hangman's (C-2)	Bilateral posterior pedicle fracture of axis (C-2) with subluxation of C-2 on C-3	Avoid hyperextension, keep neck straight to achieve postural reduction, immobilization with halo	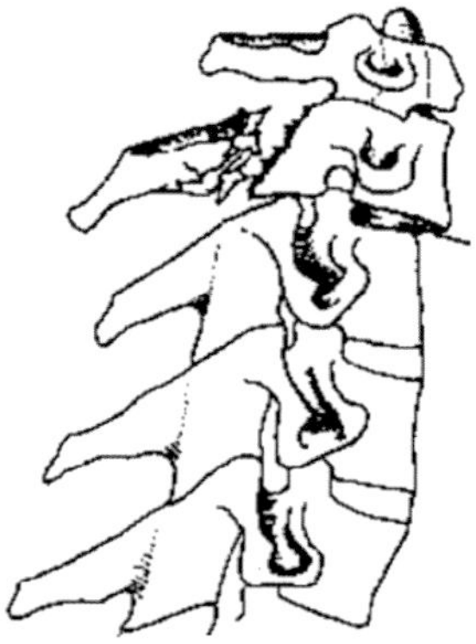
Jefferson (C-1)	Burst fracture disrupting the ring of the atlas (C-1), spinal canal is widened, causes no neurologic deficit	Skull traction or halo (support under neck during halo application permits postural reduction)	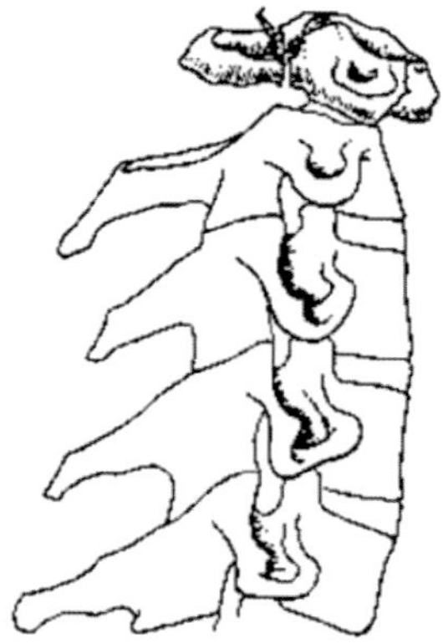
Odontoid process	Fracture at base of odontoid process, which allows the skull, C-1 vertebra, and the odontoid process of C-2 to move relatively independently of the body of C-2 vertebra	Reduction of displacement with skull traction and immobilization without distraction in halo or cervical brace Undisplaced – halo	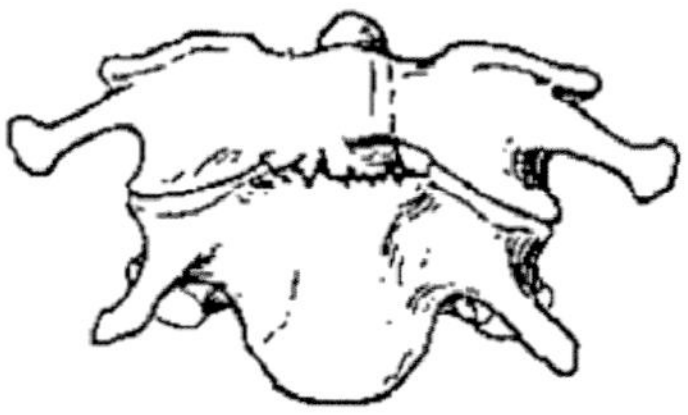

Table 17.5. Classic Names and Descriptions by Anatomic Location (continued)			
Name	**Description**	**Common Treatment**	**Illustration**
Posterior element	Fracture of any spinous process, lamina, facet, pars interarticularis or pedicle	Determined by location and severity Cervical/thoracic – collar 3-4 weeks with head in neutral position Lumbar – bed rest 7-10 days then brace/corset and ambulatory Excision of fragment, cervical – collar Lumbar – corset/brace	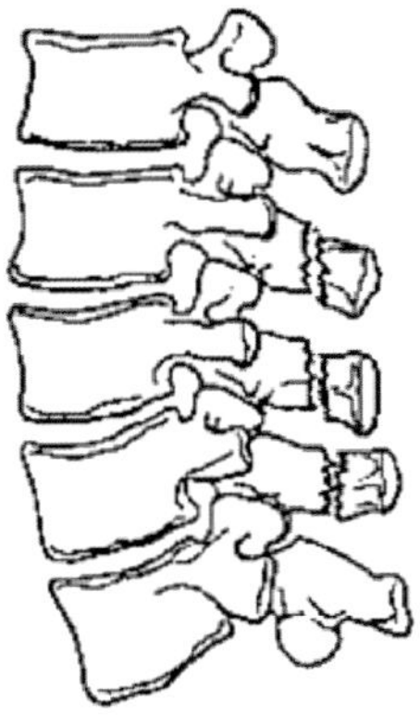
Teardrop	Teardrop-shaped avulsion fracture of anterior lip of cervical vertebral body (comminuted body fracture) fragment displaced in spinal cord	Reduction with increasing weights on skull traction, then anterior stabilization with decompression, fusion, and halo	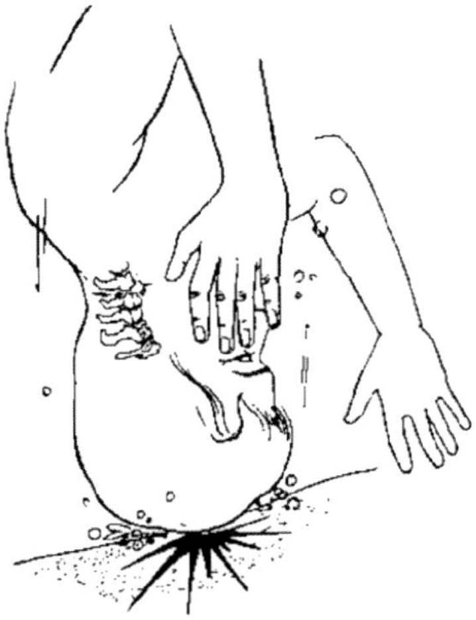
Vertebra plana	Wafer-thin compression fracture of vertebral body from intrinsic cause	Stable – treatment same as wedge fracture	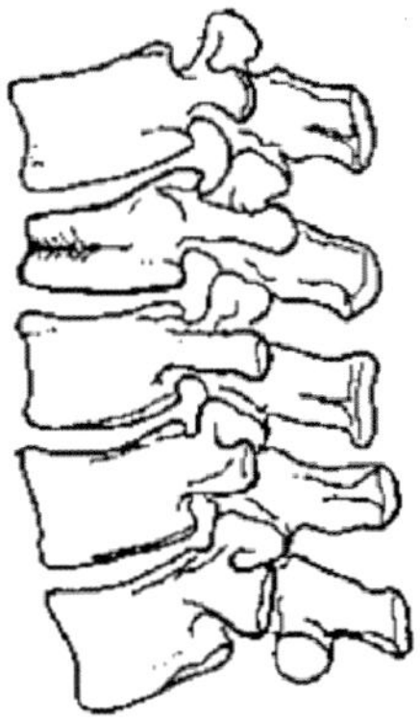
Wedge	Anterior compression fracture of vertebra, most common in thoracic spine	Stable – no reduction or immobilization, bed rest with head of bed <30 degrees, logrolling Unstable – surgical stabilization with spinal instrumentation	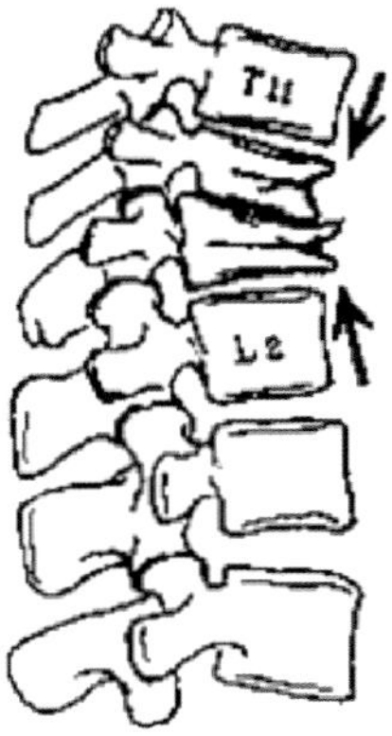 T11 L2

From Orthopaedic Nursing *(1st ed., p.717-719) by A. Maher, S. Salmond, and T. Pellino, 2002, Philadelphia, PA: Saunders. Reproduced with permission.*

Treatment is dependent on the level of stability of the fracture and includes both surgical fixation and/or treatment with immobilization in a hard collar or halo vest. Appropriate imaging must be performed, including CT scans in the ER. Serial x-rays should be assessed weekly for the first 3 weeks to assess for fracture healing and then at 6 weeks, 3 months, 6 months, and 1 year.

A halo vest (see Figure 17.3) may be applied in the ER setting or in the patient's hospital room. Place the patient supine, with the head supported just over the end of the bed by an assistant. Prepare the skin and scalp by washing the hair with a surgical cleansing preparation. Insert a local anesthetic into the pin site areas, usually two anteriorly close to the hairline (avoiding the supraorbital nerves) and two posteriorly in the central channels. Introduce the pins and tighten diagonally. Be certain that the patient closes the eyes during insertion of the anterolateral pins to ensure that traction on the skin does not prevent full closure of the eyes. Continue to tighten with a torque screwdriver to engage all four pins in the skull to prevent migration of the pins. Secure the pins to the halo with appropriate lock nuts and screws. Attach the halo ring to the vest through the anterior and posterior uprights. Tighten the vest with hook-and-loop (Velcro®) attachments. AP and lateral radiographs should be taken to check for alignment. Halo vest care must be taught to the patient and family with regards to pin site care, and skin care, and PT is helpful with early mobilization due to the weight of the halo vest and altered loss of motion in the cervical spine requiring care when ambulating.

Figure 17.4.
Three-Column Classification of Spinal Instability

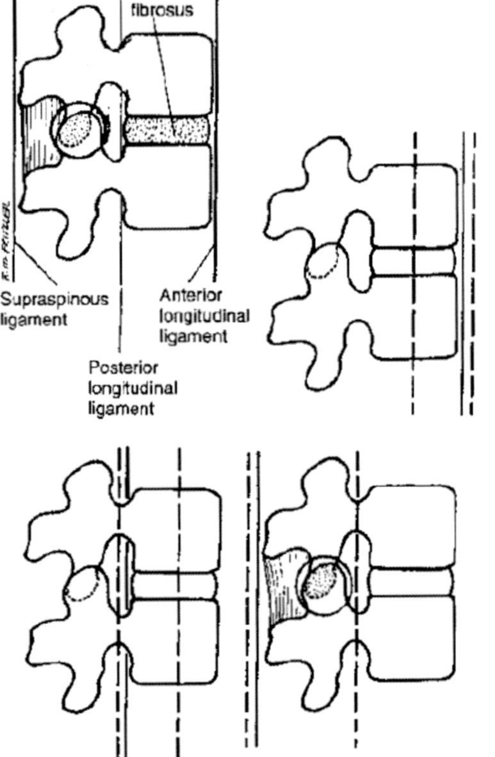

From "Fractures, Dislocations, and Fracture-Dislocations of the Spine" by W. Campbell, S. Canale, and J. Beaty, 2008, Campbell's Operative Orthopaedics *(11th ed. Vol. 2., p.1812), Philadelphia, PA: Mosby/Elsevier. Reproduced with permission.*

Fractures of the Thoracic or Lumbar Spine. Most of these types of spinal fractures occur as a result of a high-energy trauma such as motor vehicle accidents or falls from a height. They may also occur as a result of tumors, infection, osteoporosis, or long-term steroid use. The fracture pattern usually determines the stability of the fracture. Simple compression fractures of the vertebral body are relatively stable; however, flexion-distraction injuries that disrupt the posterior ligamentous complex are highly unstable. Abdominal and bowel injuries accompany these kinds of fractures. Neurological compromise or decline may be indicative of a spinal cord injury. Figure 17.4 describes the three-column classification involving the anterior, middle, and posterior columns of the spine, but other systems of classification are being developed.

In the three-column classification using a series of more than 400 CT scans of thoracolumbar injuries, the anterior column contains the anterior longitudinal ligament, the anterior half of the vertebral body, and the anterior portion of the annulus fibrosus. The middle column consists of the posterior longitudinal ligament, the posterior half of the vertebral body and the posterior aspect of the annulus fibrosus. The posterior column includes the neural arch, the ligamentum flavum, the facet capsules, and the interspinous ligaments. Campbell, Canale, and Beaty (2008) stated that a simple classification of fractures in the thoracolumbar spine would include:

1. Wedge compression fractures after forward flexion and isolated to the anterior column. May be at multiple levels and often associated with osteoporosis;
2. Stable burst fractures due to a compressive load in which the anterior and middle columns fail with no loss of integrity to the posterior column;
3. Unstable burst fractures occurring in compression with failure of all three columns, leading to instability and potential for spinal cord injury;
4. Chance fractures due to horizontal avulsion injuries of the vertebral bodies caused by flexion around the axis anterior longitudinal ligament. The entire vertebra is pulled apart by a strong tensile force;
5. Flexion distraction injuries that are unstable because of complete disruption of the posterior ligamentous complex; and

6. Translational injuries characterized by malalignment of the neural canal. Usually all three columns have been sheared and disrupted, and often occur with a spinal cord injury (page 1812).

With unstable fractures and spinal cord injury, the timing of surgery for decompression and fusion is controversial, based on the spinal cord treatment with steroid protocols and the other associated comorbidities.

Vertebral compression fractures may be treated with a vertebroplasty or kyphoplasty in certain situations, which have been particularly effective for pain control. Complications of further vertebral fractures or extravasation of the cement into and around the spinal cord, however, have been reported in connection with these treatments.

Sacral fractures and lumbosacral dislocation constitute 1% of all spinal fractures (Spivak & Connolly, 2006). They are often associated with pelvic fractures, most commonly from falls or motor vehicle accidents. Any patient with multiple trauma must be examined carefully for sacral root dysfunction. Decreased ankle jerk reflexes and absent bulbocavernosus reflex may suggest root injury. These fractures can be a result of direct or indirect trauma, with most injuries being from the latter. Sacral insufficiency fractures are most often associated with osteoporosis. Typically these fractures elicit pain but few neurological changes.

Assessment

History. A comprehensive history, including the mechanism of injury, is helpful in determining whether a fracture is present. Always remember, that if another fracture is present such as a calcaneous fracture from a fall, the patient should be assessed for another fracture at the thoracolumbar junction. Inquire about constitutional symptoms to rule out pathological causes if no trauma is present. Most fractures present with pain in a localized area, the point of maximum pain. After bad falls, rodeo riders can incur spinal fractures to any part of the spine, and the most important historical questions are associated with their disposition after the fall. (Were you able to walk out of the arena unassisted? Were there any quadraparetic events? How long did the symptoms last?)

Assessment of bowel and bladder habits must be evaluated because thoracolumbar junction compression fractures can cause a paralytic ileus. The duration of the pain is important and may be described as sudden onset or progressively worsening. Radicular pain will typically follow dermatomal patterns. Document the patient's history of present illness by asking the following:

- Has there been a particular event or injury to cause the pain, or has it been an insidious onset?
- Are there associated pieces of history such as management at the time of injury?
- What is the mechanism of injury? Describe the incident. If the mechanism was a motor vehicle accident, did you lose consciousness? Were you wearing a seat belt? Were the airbags deployed? Did you total your vehicle? Were you the driver or passenger?
- How long have you been experiencing this pain?
- Is there a previous history of pain or past surgery in this body part?
- What are the aggravating or alleviating factors? Describe the characteristics of the extremity pain.
- What past medical history and comorbidities do you have? Is there a family history of back or neck surgery?
- What is your occupational history or disability?
- What is your hand dominance?
- How old are you?
- Are there any constitutional symptoms such as weight loss, fever, or night sweats?
- What is your lifestyle and ADLs? What recreational activities do you participate in, and what is your workout level of activity?
- What is your social history (smoking, alcohol use, and living conditions)?

Physical Exam. The age of the patient usually dictates the mechanism of injury causing the fracture; the younger the patient, typically more forces are involved and the more extensive the fracture. An overall assessment of the patient for lacerations, bruising, or spasm is necessary. If the patient is ambulatory, the gait should be observed with toe- and heel-walking. Spinal ROM is noted and will be worse with extension in a patient with a compression fracture. Manual muscle testing, sensory testing, reflex testing, and long tract signs are evaluated for neurological deficits. Generally the joint closest to the affected area is assessed for injury such as the hip and knee with low back pain.

Diagnostic Testing. When assessing spinal fractures with instability, prevention of damage to the spinal cord is the most important factor. Plain radiographs (AP and lateral) and open-mouth odontoid views are taken. Lateral radiographs must include the occiput superiorly and T1 inferiorly. Only obtain flexion and extension views if a spine consultant is present and can read the x-rays to clear the patient for lack of instability and vertebral translation on the lateral views. Widening of the spinous processes may indicate ligamentous injury.

CT scans evaluate the bony structures and evaluate each vertebral level. This best assesses for fractures that may not be seen on plain radiographs. MRI scans evaluate for soft tissue swelling, facet injuries, disc herniations, edema in the spinal cord, and fractures with edema present in the vertebral bodies.

Nuclear medicine bone scans are helpful in determining metabolic bone activity by osteoblastic cells. They can be useful in evaluation of stress fractures and if a fracture cannot be seen on plain films with pain persistence. SPECT studies evaluate the spine in greater detail to help with the treatment plan.

Common Therapeutic Modalities

Preventing neurological injury, restoring stability, and recovering function are the goals of treatment. Isolated transverse process fractures do not affect stability of the spine but do indicate soft tissue muscular injury and possible kidney injury (Sarwark, 2010). Medications for pain, anti-inflammatory agents including steroids in certain situations, and muscle relaxants are helpful in treating spinal fractures. Topical analgesic patches are sometimes useful, depending on the patient. Bracing with collars or TLSO is required for fracture immobilization. Osteoporotic lumbar spine fractures may be treated with a lumbar corset or hyperextension brace for pain relief. Topical ice and heat modalities, as well as modification of activities, may provide some nonpharmacologic pain relief. Occasionally balloon kyphoplasty or vertebroplasty may be suggested for pain control, but recent outcome studies do not advocate this statement (Kallmes et al., 2009).

Nursing Considerations

Nursing Diagnoses. Nursing diagnoses for this condition are expanded upon in the Appendix.

- Activity intolerance; activity intolerance, risk for.
- Body image, disturbed.
- Cardiac perfusion, risk for decrease.
- Constipation, risk for.
- Coping, ineffective.
- Falls, risk for.
- Gastrointestinal motility, dysfunctional; gastrointestinal motility, risk for dysfunction.
- Knowledge deficit.
- Nutrition imbalance, less than body requirements.
- Nutrition imbalance, risk for more than body requirements.
- Pain, acute.
- Pain, chronic.
- Peripheral neurovascular dysfunction, risk for.
- Self-care deficit: bathing/hygiene, dressing/grooming, feeding, toileting.
- Self-concept, readiness for enhanced.
- Self-esteem, risk for chronic low.
- Self-esteem, risk for situational low.
- Sensory perception: tactile, disturbed.
- Skin integrity, impaired; skin integrity, risk for impairment.
- Social interaction, impaired.
- Tissue perfusion: cardiac, risk for decrease.
- Tissue perfusion: cerebral, risk for decrease.

Summary

The spine is a complex collection of bones, providing the main structure for humans to walk on two feet. The functional spinal unit is made up of the columns of the vertebral body, facet joints, and intervertebral discs to provide protection to the spinal cord. Spinal fractures can potentially have life-threatening ramifications and need to be assessed and managed in a timely, competent manner. Assessment for instability and protection of the spinal cord is paramount to good outcomes and functional recovery.

Treatment options will be evaluated on an individual patient basis. Conservative management of spinal conditions is always the first-line treatment unless neurological deficits are present. Spinal surgery is performed with realistic expectations from both the patient and the surgeon as to the surgical outcomes, including possible complications. This requires a detailed discussion prior to surgery, which is usually documented in the patient's medical record, to ensure that everyone involved understands the ramifications of surgery.

References

Birknes, J., White, A., Albert, T., Shaffrey, C., & Harrop, J. (2008). Adult degenerative scoliosis: A review. *Journal of Neurosurgery, 163*(3), 94-103.

Campbell, W.C., Canale, S.T., & Beaty, J.H. (2008). Fractures, dislocations, and fracture-dislocations of the spine. In *Campbell's Operative Orthopaedics* (11th ed., Vol. 2, pp. 1761-850). Philadelphia, PA: Mosby/Elsevier.

Chunguang, Z., Limin, L., Rigao, C., Yueming, S., Hao, L., Qingquan, K,...Jiancheng, Z. (2010). Surgical treatment of kyphosis in children in healed stages of spinal tuberculosis. *Journal of Pediatric Orthopedics, 30*(3), 271-6.

D'Arcy, Y. (2009). Is low back pain getting on your nerves? *The Nurse Practitioner, 34*(5), 10-17.

Frey, M.E., Manchikanti, L., Benyamin, R.M., Schultz, D.M., Smith, H.S., & Cohen, S.P. (2009). Spinal cord stimulation for patients with failed back surgery syndrome: A systematic review. *Pain Physician, 12*, 379-397.

Hart, E., Merlin, G., Harisiades, J., & Grottkau, B. (2010). Scheuermann's Thoracic Kyphosis in the adolescent patient. *Orthopaedic Nursing, 29*(6), 365-71.

Deviren, V. (2009). *Description of XLIF Surgery*. Retrieved from http://www.spine-health.com/treatment/spinal-fusion/description-xlif-surgery

Gregory, D., Seto, C., Wortley, G., & Shugart, C. (2008). Acute lumbar disk pain: Navigating evaluation and treatment choices. *American Family Physician, 78*(7), 835–842.

Hu, S., Tribus, C., Diab, M., & Ghaanayem, A. (2008). Spondylolisthesis and Spondylolysis. *Journal of American Bone and Joint Surgery, 90*(3), 656-71.

Kallmes, D.F., Comstock, B.A., Heagerty, P.J., Turner, J.A., Wilson, D.A., Diamond, T.H.,… Jarvik, J.G. (2009). A randomized trial of vertebroplasty for osteoporotic spinal fractures. *New England Journal of Medicine, 361*(6), 569-579.

Kaji, A. & Hockberger, R. (2008). *Spinal Column Injuries in Adults: Definitions and Mechanisms*. Retrieved from http://www.uptodate.com/patients/content/topic.do?topicKey=~tzBzvl0/kq93/h

Katz, J.N. & Harris, M.B. (2008). Lumbar spinal stenosis. *New England Journal of Medicine, 358*(8), 818-825.

Knight, R., Schwaegler, P., Hanscom, D., & Roh, J. (2009). Direct lateral lumbar interbody fusion for degenerative conditions: Early complication profile. *Journal of Spinal Disorders & Techniques, 22*, 34-37.

Kloth, D.S., Fenton, D.S., Andersson, G.B., & Block, J.E. (2008). Intradiscal electrothermal therapy (IDET) for the treatment of discogenic low back pain: Patient selection and indications for use. *Pain Physician, 160*(5), 280-285.

Larson, N. (2011). Early onset scoliosis: What the primary care provider needs to know and implications for practice. *Journal of the American Academy of Nurse Practitioners, 23*, 392-403.

Lowe, T. & Line, B. (2007). Evidence based medicine. Analysis of Scheuremann's kyphosis. *Spine, 32*(195), 115-119.

Madigan, L., Vaccaro, A.R., Spector, L.R., & Milan, B.A. (2009). Management of symptomatic lumbar degenerative disc disease. *Journal of AAOS, 19*, 102-11.

Maher, A.B., Salmond, S.W., & Pellino, T.A. (2002). *Orthopaedic Nursing* (1st ed.). Philadelphia, PA: Saunders.

Majid, K. & Fischgrund, J. (2008). Degenerative lumbar spondylolisthesis: Trends in management. *Journal of American Academy of Orthopaedic Surgeons, 16*, 208-15.

Mostofi, S.B. (2009). *Rapid Orthopedic Diagnosis*. London, England, UK: Springer.

Peer, K.S. & Fascione, J.M. (2007). Spondylolysis: A review of treatment approaches. *Orthopaedic Nursing, 26*(2), 104-11.

Rodts, M. & Hickey, M. (2007). Spine. In *Core Curriculum for Orthopaedic Nursing* (6th ed.). Boston, MA: Pearson.

Sarwark, J.F. (2010). Spine. In *Essentials of Musculoskeletal Care* (4th ed.). Rosemont, IL: American Academy of Orthopaedic Surgeons.

Spivak, J.M., & Connolly, P.J. (Eds.). (2006). *Orthopaedic knowledge update: Spine 3.* Rosemont, IL: American Academy of Orthopaedic Surgeons.

Stedman, T.L. (2006) *Stedman's Medical Dictionary* (28th ed.). Philadelphia, PA: Lippincott Williams & Wilkins.

Thompson, G.H., Lenke, L.G., Akbarnia, B.A., McCarthy, R.E., & Campbell Jr., R.M. (2007). Early onset scoliosis: Future directions. *Journal of American Bone and Joint Surgery, 89*, 163-166.

Vaccaro, A.R. & Baron, E.M. (2008). *Spine Surgery*. Philadelphia, PA: Saunders/Elsevier.

Wick, J., Konze, J., Alexander, K., & Sweeney, C. (2009). Infantile and juvenile scoliosis: The crooked path to diagnosis and treatment. *AORN, 90*(3), 347-76.

Wood, P.R., Mahoney, P.F., & Cooper, J.P. (2009). *Trauma and Orthopedic Surgery in Clinical Practice*. London, England, UK: Springer.

Chapter 18
The Shoulder

Rebecca L. Buti, MS, ANP-C, ONP-C

Objectives

- List common conditions and injuries that occur in the shoulder.
- Identify the four types of impingement.
- Recall typical history and physical findings for patients with rotator cuff tears.
- Identify the surgical options for treatment of shoulder instability.
- Describe the mechanism of injury of various shoulder dislocations.
- Develop nursing diagnoses and interventions for patients with common shoulder conditions.

The shoulder is a ball-and-socket joint with the most mobility and least stability of all joints in the human body. The large humeral head (ball) sits on the shallow glenoid (socket) of the scapula like a golf ball sitting on a tee. The glenoid labrum, a fibrocartilage rim, deepens the socket and creates a vacuum effect to assist with centering of the humeral head within the glenoid, thereby improving stability. The rotator cuff muscles (supraspinatus, infraspinatus, teres minor, and subscapularis) keep the humeral head centered within the glenoid fossa during movement of the shoulder. Additional muscles of the shoulder girdle, including the scapular stabilizers, assist with the function and stabilization of the shoulder. The most important functional motion of the shoulder is that of forward elevation to enable the hand to function in front of the body. The versatile shoulder joint, with its inherent lack of stability, renders it susceptible to acute traumatic or chronic overuse injury.

Impingement Syndrome (Tendinitis)

Overview

Definition. Impingement syndrome is a constellation of symptoms caused by encroachment or abutment of the soft tissues against bony structures of the shoulder, resulting in progressive pain and impaired function. Four types of shoulder impingement have been theorized: primary, secondary, internal, and coracoid (Jobe, Coen, & Screnar, 2000). *Primary impingement* is a painful condition in which the bursal side of the supraspinatus and infraspinatus tendons and subacromial bursa become pinched between the undersurface of the acromion, coracoacromial ligament, or greater tuberosity, and the humeral head during forward arm elevation. *Secondary impingement* is a painful condition in which the rotator cuff becomes pinched in the region of the coracoacromial space due to anterior translation of the humeral head from microinstability. *Internal impingement* is a painful condition in which the articular side of the supraspinatus and infraspinatus become pinched against the posterosuperior glenoid rim when the shoulder is abducted 90 degrees and maximally externally rotated. *Coracoid impingement* is a painful condition in which the coracoid process impinges against the lesser tuberosity of the humeral head when the arm is flexed, adducted, and maximally internally rotated, which may result in tears of the undersurface of the subscapularis. (The last type of impingement is mentioned for completeness and will not be discussed in great detail because it is beyond the scope of this chapter.)

Etiology. Many factors may contribute to the development of the various types of impingement syndrome (see Table 18.1).

Figure 18.1. Acromial Morphology

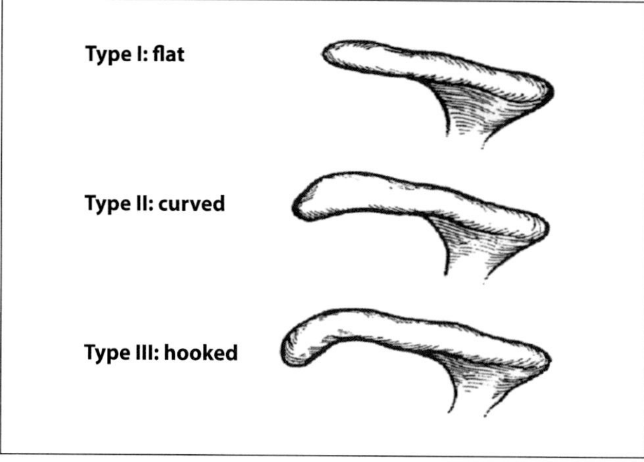

From "Shoulder Impingement Syndrome: Diagnosis, Radiographic Evaluation, and Treatment with a Modified Neer Acromioplasty" by C. Rockwood and F. Lyons, 1993, Journal of Bone and Joint Surgery, American, *75, p. 415. Reproduced with permission.*

Table 18.1. Contributing Factors of Impingement

Type	Causal Factors
Primary	• Overuse, muscle fatigue • Training errors • Abnormal acromion • Thickening of AC joint
Secondary	• Instability
Internal	• Repetitive overhead activities • Microinstability • SLAP lesions
Coracoid	• Humeral fracture nonunion • Congenital abnormalities • Degenerative changes

Pathophysiology and Incidence. Repeated pinching of the cuff tendons, by the anterior acromion, posterosuperior glenoid or coracoid, leads to pain and inflammation. An abnormally shaped acromion may contribute to impingement. Figure 18.1 describes three variations in the morphology of the acromion. Patients with a type II or III acromion are more likely to develop rotator cuff pathology. Figure 18.2 describes three stages of primary impingement. Rotator cuff and bicipital tendinitis, subacromial bursitis, and rupture of the long head of the biceps are possible consequences of repeated impingement of these soft tissue structures. There is no gender predilection for impingement syndrome. In the past, males have been more likely to engage in vocations or sports that require repetitive overhead use of the arm, which predisposed them to developing impingement syndrome compared to females; however, if females engage in those same activities, impingement syndrome affects both genders equally.

Figure 18.2.
Neer's Classification of the Progressive Stages of Impingement

Stage		
Stage I:	**Edema and Hemorrhage**	
	typical age	<25
	diff. diagnosis	subluxation, acromioclavicular arthritis
	clinical course	reversible
	treatment	conservative
Stage II:	**Fibrosis and Tendinitis**	
	typical age	25-40
	diff. diagnosis	frozen shoulder, calcium
	clinical course	recurrent pain with activity
	treatment	consider bursectomy, coracoacromial ligament division
Stage III:	**Bone Spurs and Tendon Rupture**	
	typical age	>40
	diff. diagnosis	cervical radiculitis, neoplasm
	clinical course	progressive disability
	treatment	anterior acromioplasty, rotator cuff repair

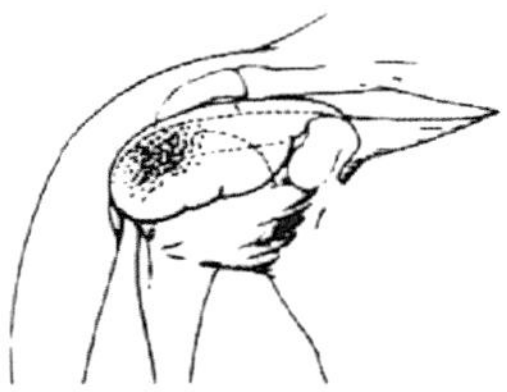

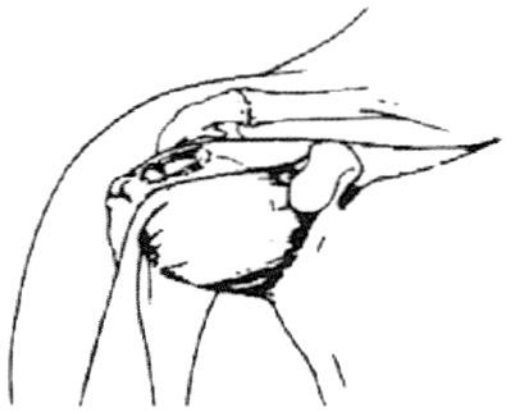

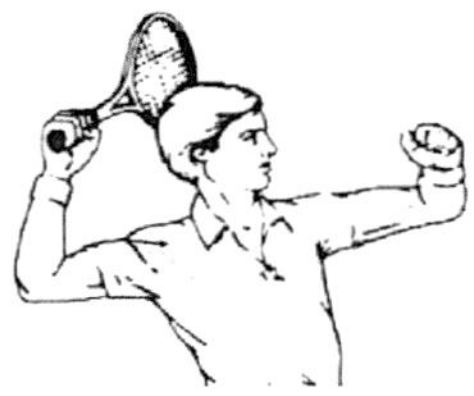

From "Impingement Lesions" by C. Neer, 1983, Clinical Orthopaedics and Related Research, *3, p. 70-77. Reprinted with permission.*

Risk Factors.

- Type II or Type III acromion, traction spurs of acromion or *os acromiale;*
- Repetitive overhead vocational or sporting activities;
- Anterior shoulder instability (even if subtle);
- Increasing age;
- Prior injury to rotator cuff or acromioclavicular (AC) joint;
- Adhesive capsulitis; and
- Malunited humerus fracture.

Complications. If the underlying cause is not addressed, impingement may recur and/or persist until cuff failure. Anterior shoulder instability, especially if subtle, may be overlooked as a possible cause of impingement and result in less-than-satisfactory outcomes if attempts are made to correct the impingement and not the instability. Despite all attempts at conservative treatment, patients with stage II or III impingement may go on to require surgical intervention. During an acromioplasty, all of the offending area of the undersurface of the anterior acromion must be resected to prevent recurrence of symptoms due to an inadequate subacromial decompression (SAD). Additionally, patients may develop recurrence of symptoms if they return to offending activities before adequate healing has occurred.

Preventive Strategies. Avoidance of symptom-provoking activities is prudent, shoulder motions above the horizontal plane (greater than 90 degrees of forward flexion) (Kierns & Whitman, 2009). Strength and flexibility of the shoulder girdle musculature should be maintained to prevent abnormal migration of the humeral head, leading to impingement. Athletes should utilize proper training techniques, wear proper protective equipment, and warm up adequately prior to physical activities.

Special Considerations. Impingement syndrome may occur at any age, but it is more likely to occur in younger patients, whereas cuff failure or tears are more common in patients with increased age. Progression of impingement to cuff degeneration, and subsequent tearing, may be asymptomatic.

Assessment

History. Patients with impingement syndrome are usually age 40-50, or younger if an athlete. Onset of pain is insidious. Pain is commonly located in the deltoid or front of the shoulder, and it may radiate down the arm. Pain is associated with shoulder use, although on occasion it may occur at rest. It is aggravated by overhead activities, such as combing hair or throwing a ball. Often times, the pain awakens the patient at night. Difficulty lying on the affected shoulder due to pain is common. Crepitus (cracking, popping, or crunching) is a common complaint.

Patients with bicipital tendinitis usually describe the pain as aching, and there may be tenderness in the area of the bicipital groove. Onset of pain is often insidious and aggravated by activities that require shoulder or elbow flexion and forearm supination, especially against resistance. Less commonly, the patient may give a history of a direct blow to the front of the shoulder. Increased warmth and redness in the region of the bicipital groove may be present. Younger patients and athletes should be questioned about any sensations of instability, as this implies an underlying instability that may be contributing to impingement symptoms.

Physical Exam. As with the physical examination of all joints, perusal of the shoulder joint should be systematic. Both shoulders should be examined, starting with the unaffected side first. Examination of the neck and elbow should also be included. Inspection, palpation of bony and soft tissue structures, measurement of range of motion (ROM), strength testing, neurovascular assessment, and performance of special tests are all part of a thorough examination of the shoulder. (For a detailed discussion on physical examination of the shoulder, please refer to Chapter 3—Musculoskeletal Assessment.)

Usually, there is little to no muscle wasting observed with impingement syndrome. When present, obvious muscle wasting of the supraspinatus and infraspinatus is suggestive of late stage III impingement or a chronic full-thickness rotator cuff tear. Tenderness over the humeral head, bicipital groove, subacromial region, AC joint, or coracoid process may be evident upon palpation of these structures, and implies their likely involvement in the impingement process. Decreased end-ROM in flexion (especially active) may be present. Limited internal rotation is a common finding among throwing athletes with internal impingement. Many special physical examination tests are available to confirm or negate the diagnosis of impingement syndrome, including the painful arc sign, Apley Scratch test, Hawkins-Kennedy test, Neer's impingement sign and injection test, drop arm test, and Jobe's (empty can) test.

Diagnostic Tests. The diagnosis of impingement syndrome may be made by history and physical examination alone; however, additional imaging modalities may be used to confirm the diagnosis and aid in treatment considerations. Plain x-rays are often normal in impingement syndrome, although over time, bony adaptive changes (acromial spurs) may readily be seen on plain x-rays (Rockwood & Lyons, 1993). Impingement series x-rays of the shoulder include a true anteroposterior (AP) view in the scapular plane, scapular outlet ("Y") view, axillary view, and 30 degree caudal tilt AP view. Ultrasound (US) may be used to evaluate the integrity of the rotator cuff tendons (Moosikasuwan, Miller, & Burke, 2005). Magnetic resonance imaging (MRI) scans provide the most extensive soft-tissue detail of the shoulder than any other imaging modality (Deutsch, Ramsey, & Iannotti, 2007). Computerized tomography (CT) scans provide high-quality images of bone. Shoulder arthrography (injection of contrast, and sometimes air, into the joint) may be combined with MRI or CT scans to provide enhanced images of the intra-articular structures. Lastly, diagnostic arthroscopy is the gold standard for evaluation of the shoulder joint, as it allows for direct visualization of any pathology within the shoulder and enables surgical intervention.

Common Therapeutic Modalities

Nonsurgical Management. Treatment of all types of impingement syndrome may be categorized into either conservative or surgical. Conservative measures may include PT, medications, and subacromial corticosteroid injections. PT is the mainstay of treatment for most shoulder conditions and is no exception for impingement syndrome or tendinitis. Patients with stage I impingement syndrome will most likely achieve complete relief of symptoms with physical therapy (PT), including gentle stretching, strengthening, and posture improvement. Patients with stage II impingement may have mixed outcomes with conservative measures, and ultimately require surgical intervention. Patients with stage III impingement syndrome will most likely fail conservative measures and require surgery. In any case, a trial of conservative measures should be attempted for at least 3 to 6 months before surgery is considered. Exercises that bring the patient's arm above 90 degrees should be avoided, along with any exercise that causes pain or reproduces symptoms. Joint and soft tissue mobilization techniques have been proven to enhance the effects of exercise programs in relieving symptoms of impingement syndrome, but therapeutic ultrasound has not (Kuhn, 2009).

Oral non-steroidal anti-inflammatory drugs (NSAIDs) are commonly prescribed to alleviate inflammation, pain, and swelling. Acetaminophen may also be used to relieve pain. On occasion, narcotics may be required to relieve severe pain and may be an indication of a rotator cuff tear or other shoulder pathology. Corticosteroid and anesthetic injected into the subacromial bursa is commonly used to decrease pain, inflammation, and swelling, and thus, improve gliding of the affected tissues and halt impingement. If impingement symptoms improve after the injection, it is generally considered to be a predictor of a positive outcome, should a SAD be considered in the future. To date, there has been no conclusive evidence to suggest whether corticosteroid injections are efficacious or not; however, they continue to be a common treatment modality with good anecdotal results. Corticosteroid injections are not without side effects, which include weakening and rupture of tendons and ligaments, atrophy of subcutaneous tissues, septic arthritis, hemarthroses, and hyperglycemia in diabetics.

Surgical Management. Surgery may be indicated for those patients in whom conservative measures fail. Depending on the condition of the rotator cuff, morphology of the acromion, and etiology of the impingement, an arthroscopic subacromial decompression (ASD), open anterior acromioplasty, or an arthroscopic or open rotator cuff repair may be performed. Secondary or internal impingement may be improved by procedures that address instability. Lastly, if severe arthritis of the AC joint is contributing to impingement, resection of the distal clavicle may be beneficial.

An ASD may be considered the gold standard for surgical treatment of impingement syndrome in patients with an intact rotator cuff (Leggin & Kelley, 2007). An ASD includes removal of the undersurface of the anterior third of the acromion, excision of the subacromial bursa, and release of the coracoacromial ligament, if needed. The goal of an ASD is to remove the structures causing mechanical enchroachment of the subacromial space, thereby preventing or postponing degeneration and tearing of the rotator cuff. Impingement syndrome can also be addressed by an open acromioplasty, which comes with it an incision and scarring, more postoperative pain, and a longer recovery than the arthroscopic approach.

Nursing Considerations

Nursing Diagnoses. Nursing diagnoses for this condition are expanded upon in the Appendix.

- Activity intolerance.
- Coping, ineffective.
- Disuse syndrome, risk for.
- Infection, risk for.
- Knowledge deficit.
- Mobility: physical, impaired.
- Noncompliance.
- Pain, acute.
- Pain, chronic.
- Role performance, ineffective.
- Self-care deficit: bathing/hygiene, dressing/grooming, feeding, toileting.

Interventions. *Preventing/minimizing complications:* Elimination of impingement will halt repetitive trauma to the rotator cuff and, hopefully, prevent or delay progression to a tear. Patients need to be encouraged to comply with PT and continue a home exercise program (HEP).

Activity/positioning: Repetitive overhead activities, or those that require the arm to be above 90 degrees of flexion, should be avoided. Activities that aggravate or reproduce impingement should also be avoided. Patients should not return to normal, unrestricted activities prematurely because adequate time is required for healing of the tissues. Patients with occupations that require repetitive overhead activities, who experience recurrent and disabling impingement symptoms, may want to consider changing occupations, if feasible.

Emotional support: Patients may benefit from emotional support if they are no longer able to continue their chosen vocation or sport. Similarly, patients may require continued encouragement to comply with the prescribed HEP indefinitely.

Patient teaching:

- Avoid or limit repetitive overhead activities.
- Perform your HEP as prescribed. If you have pain performing any of the exercises, stop doing the exercise and notify your doctor.
- NSAIDs should be taken with food to avoid developing peptic ulcer disease. If you develop stomach pain or dark or bloody stool after taking an NSAID, stop the medication immediately and notify your doctor.
- If you are diabetic and have received a subacromial corticosteroid injection, monitor your blood sugars carefully because corticosteroids, even when given within a joint, will elevate your blood sugars higher than usual.
- If you have had surgery, follow all incision care instructions provided to you by your surgeon. In general, once the surgical dressing has been removed, it is okay to shower; however, you should not take a bath or go swimming.
- Monitor your incision for signs and symptoms of infection, including redness, increased pain, swelling, heat, purulent drainage, or fevers. If you develop any of these signs or symptoms, call your surgeon immediately.

Rotator Cuff Tears

Overview

Definition. A rotator cuff tear is characterized by shoulder pain and weakness due to tearing of one or more of the rotator cuff tendons, and is often associated with inflammation of the subacromial bursa. The rotator cuff consists of four muscles (supraspinatus, infraspinatus, teres minor, and subscapularis) that wrap their tendinous insertions onto the humeral head like fingers gripping a baseball. The rotator cuff muscles are often referred to as the "SITS" muscles, which is a popular acronym used to describe their order of attachment. The main function of the rotator cuff as a whole is to maintain the humeral head within the glenoid fossa, providing strength and stability to the shoulder joint during a wide range of arm motions.

Etiology, Mechanism of Injury, and Pathophysiology. Multiple factors have been implicated in the development of rotator cuff tears. Factors may be subdivided into those of extrinsic or intrinsic origin. *Intrinsic factors* are age-related diminished blood supply to the tendon, age-related disuse, and intra-tendinous degeneration. Age-related diminished blood supply may contribute to tendon degeneration because of a decreased ability to heal or repair itself, even from microtears. Age-related disuse and degeneration of the substance of the tendon fibers also contribute to attrition of the rotator cuff tendons macroscopically. *Extrinsic factors* are numerous, and may include acromial abnormalities, separations, impingement syndrome, overuse, instability, and fractures, to name a few. Neer's theory of impingement

(1970) has been widely accepted as a plausible cause of rotator cuff tears; however, no one single factor has been implicated. More than likely, the etiology of rotator cuff disease is multifactorial.

Incidence. "Rotator cuff tears increase in frequency with age, are more common in the dominant arm, and asymptomatic tears may be present in the opposite arm" (AAOS, 2007, p. 2). The supraspinatus is the most commonly torn tendon of all the rotator cuff tendons. Over time, propagation of the tear may involve the infraspinatus tendon, biceps tendon anchor, and subscapularis tendon. There is no gender predilection for rotator cuff tears. Manual laborers and individuals who engage in repetitive overhead activities are more likely to sustain a cuff tear.

Risk Factors. Risk factors for sustaining a rotator cuff tear are the same as those for impingement syndrome (see above).

Complications. Pain (intermittent to constant), loss of motion, persistent weakness, shoulder stiffness, frozen shoulder, tear propagation, and functional limitations are possible complications of rotator cuff tears. Complications from a rotator cuff repair are procedure-dependent, vary in severity, and may include infection, thromboembolism, stiffness, neurovascular injuries from traction or portal placement, iatrogenic muscle and tendon injury, and implant failure.

Preventive Strategies. Once a rotator cuff tear is diagnosed, either partial or full-thickness, a PT program should be implemented. A shoulder with a stable platform with which to function upon is less likely to place further strain on a torn rotator cuff tendon, but a weak shoulder girdle may cause more strain and presumably extend the size of the tear.

Special Considerations. There is no known predilection of rotator cuff disease in any one race. The predominance of rotator cuff disease between genders is equal. Rotator cuff tears increase in frequency with age, and they are often asymptomatic.

Assessment

History. Rotator cuff tears may present with similar signs and symptoms as those found with impingement syndrome. An insidious onset of pain is common, but a patient may report a sudden onset of pain as a result of an acute injury. The pain is usually described as aching and may vary in intensity. Pain is commonly localized to the deltoid area. Pain that awakens the patient at night is common, as well as difficulty lying on the affected shoulder. Pain is worse with use of the arm, especially overhead. Loss of motion, especially in internal rotation and adduction, may be reported by the patient. Arm weakness may be experienced with motions above 90 degrees.

Physical Exam. Physical examination of the shoulder joint should be systematic and bilateral, with inclusion of the neck and elbow. The unaffected shoulder should be examined first, followed by the affected shoulder. Inspection, palpation of bony and soft tissue structures, ROM measurement, strength testing, neurovascular assessment, and performance of special tests are all part of a thorough examination of the shoulder. Muscle wasting of the supraspinatus and infraspinatus muscles may be present, especially with chronic, full-thickness rotator cuff tears. Tenderness to palpation may be present when the rotator cuff defect is palpated. There may be crepitus. Decreased end-ROM in flexion may be present, especially active. Weakness of rotation, both internal and external, and loss of motion will be evident.

Many special tests are helpful in confirming the diagnosis of a rotator cuff tear and are the same tests used to evaluate impingement syndrome. A painful arc will be present, usually between 60 and 120 degrees, and is indicative of subacromial impingement, whereas, pain toward the end of 180 degrees of full abduction points to AC joint pathology (Kessel & Watson, 1977). The Apley Scratch test will be positive. The Hawkins-Kennedy test and Neer's impingement sign are often positive in patients with rotator cuff tears. If a positive impingement sign has been observed, a Neer's impingement injection test may be used to confirm that the pain is originating from the subacromial region. The drop arm test and Jobe's (empty can) test may be positive, which is indicative of a full-thickness rotator cuff tear. The lift-off test may be used to assess for a tear in the subscapularis tendon. The patient will usually have negative instability tests. Yergason's and Speed's tests are expected to be negative unless there is associated bicipital pathology.

Many classification systems have been devised to describe rotator cuff tears. A commonly used method is to classify the tear based on its depth. Partial-thickness tears may be described as either articular or bursal-sided. No single classification system is superior to others, and choice is likely based on familiarity by a particular user.

Diagnostic Tests. The diagnosis of a rotator cuff tear may be made by history and physical examination alone, including, at times, an estimate of the size of the tear. Imaging studies may be utilized to provide details about the pathoanatomy of the various soft tissue and bony structures of the shoulder, and may assist with diagnostic and treatment considerations. Plain radiographs for the evaluation of rotator cuff tears should include a true AP view in the scapular plane, scapular outlet ("Y") view, axillary view, and 30 degree caudal tilt AP view. Plain radiographs of the shoulder are often negative when evaluating patients with an acute rotator cuff tear. Additionally, discovery of a rotator cuff tear on imaging studies may not be the source of the patient's pain because many patients, especially those of increased age, have asymptomatic rotator cuff tears. Ultrasonography may be used to evaluate the integrity of the rotator cuff and confirm the diagnosis of clinically or radiographically suspected rotator cuff tears. MRI scans are good for detecting full-thickness rotator cuff tears. MRI arthrography is superior to MRI alone at visualizing any partial defect in the cuff tendon. Diagnostic arthroscopy is the gold standard for providing a systematic diagnostic examination of the shoulder joint, including probing of cuff tendons from the bursal and articular side. The methylene blue color test, the suture marking technique for articular tears, and the "bubble sign" for intra-tendinous tears may be performed during a diagnostic shoulder arthroscopy to assist in diagnosing a rotator cuff tear.

Common Therapeutic Modalities

Nonsurgical Management. Conservative measures for the treatment of a rotator cuff tear include PT (supervised with progression to a HEP), medications, rest, avoidance of aggravating activities, and occasional subacromial corticosteroid injections. PT should be attempted in all patients with rotator cuff tears, regardless of tear size. As always, any activity or exercise that causes pain or reproduces symptoms should be avoided.

Surgical Management. Surgical management of a rotator cuff tear is indicated after an appropriate trial of conservative measures has failed. The choice of surgical technique (open, mini-open, or arthroscopic repair) depends on several factors, including the size and location of the tear, quality of the tendon and bone, anatomy, the patient's desire for a particular technique and expectations, and the surgeon's preference, familiarity, and expertise. The goal of surgical repair of a rotator cuff tear is to reattach the tendon to the bone, and hold the tendon securely in place until healing of the tendon onto the bone has occurred. An arthroscopic rotator cuff repair is less invasive and results in less postoperative pain, smaller incisions, and a quicker recovery time than the open or mini-open approach. According to the AAOS (2007), certain factors decrease the likelihood of a satisfactory outcome after a rotator cuff repair: poor tissue quality, large or massive tears, poor compliance with postoperative rehabilitation and restrictions, patient age (older than age 65), and Workers' Compensation claims. There are instances when a chronic, massive rotator cuff tear cannot be repaired by any means. In these cases, muscle transfers or debridement may be performed alternatively.

Nursing Considerations

Nursing Diagnoses. Nursing diagnoses for this condition are expanded upon in the Appendix.

- Activity intolerance.
- Coping, ineffective.
- Disuse syndrome, risk for.
- Infection, risk for.
- Knowledge deficit.
- Mobility: physical, impaired.
- Noncompliance.
- Pain, acute.
- Pain, chronic.
- Role performance, ineffective.
- Self-care deficit: bathing/hygiene, dressing/grooming, feeding, toileting.

Interventions. *Preventing/minimizing complications:* Patients who fail conservative therapy may want to consider rotator cuff repair sooner rather than later because cuff tears usually do not heal; instead, they become larger over time and may result in an irreparable tendon if repair is prolonged for many years. Proper patient selection will help limit or avoid complications. Patients with certain conditions should not be selected for rotator cuff repairs, including shoulder infection, inability or unwillingness to wear a sling and participate in PT postoperatively, or an irreparable rotator cuff tendon. Finally, it is imperative to ensure that the patient and/or caregiver understand the discharge instructions and adhere to them after discharge to decrease the complication rate.

Activity: Activities will be limited or restricted for several months. A sling or abduction pillow will need to be worn postoperatively, with the length of time varying based on procedure performed and surgeon preference. PT is prescribed postoperatively for at least 3 months, depending on the patient's expectations (i.e., return to sport) and demands placed on the shoulder. Athletes are not allowed to return to sports for up to 6 months, depending on the sport.

Emotional support: Patients may benefit from emotional support after rotator cuff surgery because of feelings of discouragement and helplessness due to the need for assistance from others to perform activities of daily living (ADLs). Postoperative pain may increase the risk of developing depression. Reassuring the patient of the temporary nature of the current situation may improve the patient's morale and help them cope as they recover.

Patient Teaching. *Positioning:* Patients often find it uncomfortable to lie flat in bed after undergoing a rotator cuff repair and may be more comfortable sleeping in a recliner. An alternative to sleeping in a recliner is to lay supine in bed and prop the operative arm up with one to two pillows.

Nutrition: A higher incidence of malnutrition may exist among patients undergoing rotator cuff repairs because of the associated malnutrition often found in the elderly population in general, and the higher prevalence in rotator cuff tears in the elderly. Malnutrition adversely affects wound and tendon healing, and increases the risk of developing complications. Malnourished patients, or those at risk, should be counseled to increase their protein and caloric intake, and perhaps take wound-healing vitamins (vitamin A, C, E, and zinc sulfate).

Practice Setting Considerations. *Office/outpatient:* Most rotator cuff repairs are performed as an outpatient procedure or 23-hour stay. This means that the majority, if not all, of the postoperative care will be provided and coordinated in the outpatient setting. All incisions need to be assessed for signs of infection or delayed healing. Generally, the incisions are kept covered with a dressing for 10 to 14 days, at which time any staples or sutures are removed. During each postoperative office appointment, the patient's level of pain should be assessed. Outpatient PT will also be prescribed.

Home care: Emphasis should be placed on patient compliance with activity modifications to maintain the integrity of the repair and allow for tendon healing. Patients may benefit from an occupational therapy consultation to assist with performance of ADLs and the use of any assistive devices. Patients will usually begin passive ROM exercises by postoperative day one, followed by formal PT.

Arthritis

Overview

Definition. Arthritis is the inflammation of a joint. Osteoarthritis of the shoulder may be synonymously referred to as degenerative joint disease (DJD) of the shoulder, glenohumeral arthritis, or shoulder arthritis. Osteoarthritis is characterized by an irreversible, slowly progressive erosion of the smooth outer covering of the hyaline articular cartilage of bone from degenerative "wear and tear." Rheumatoid arthritis is a systemic autoimmune disorder characterized as a chronic polyarthritis, resulting in inflammation of the joint lining (synovium), and usually affects multiple joints symmetrically. (Also see Chapter 13—Arthritis and Connective Tissue Disorders.)

Etiology. There is no known cause of primary (idiopathic) osteoarthritis of the shoulder. Osteoarthritis of the shoulder is more prevalent with increasing age, and affects males and females equally (Matsen & Warme, 2009). Prior shoulder injury and overuse have been suggested as contributing factors for the development of osteoarthritis (Matsen & Warme, 2009). Similarly, the exact reason the immune system begins to turn against itself and attack the body in rheumatoid arthritis is not known; however, genetic, environmental, and hormonal factors have been implicated (National Institute of Arthritis and Musculoskeletal and Skin Diseases [NIAMS], 2009).

Pathophysiology. Primary osteoarthritis involves slow, progressive erosion of the articular cartilage, with eventual exposure of the underlying subchondral bone and joint line osteophyte formation. The cartilage is able to repair itself, but the repair is inferior to that of the original. Bone remodeling also occurs, leading to sclerosis and abnormal mechanics. Rheumatoid arthritis is an autoimmune disorder that manifests itself primarily as an inflammatory disorder of the synovium of joints. The exact sequence of events leading up to the first attack of rheumatoid arthritis or a flare-up has not been determined. It has been postulated that a gene increases the susceptibility to environmental triggers, such as infection, which then triggers the onset of disease (Mayo Foundation for Medical Education and Research [MFMER], 2009). The thickened synovitis resembles that of granulation tissue and is known as a "pannus," as it drapes over the articular cartilage of the joint. Progression of inflammation causes erosion of surrounding bone, tendon, and ligaments, leading to subluxation and rupture of tendons or ligaments. Fibrosis of the synovial joint capsule is the end result of inflammation and limits joint motion.

Incidence. Primary osteoarthritis is the most common type of arthritis that affects the shoulder joint. Osteoarthritis affects men and women equally; however, it is more prevalent in men younger than age 50 and women older than age 50. Its incidence increases with age, and the shoulder is the site with the oldest average age of onset (Collins, 2007). It is estimated that 20% of the elderly population suffer from the pain and disability of shoulder osteoarthritis. The shoulder, after the knee and hip, is the third most common joint to require a joint arthroplasty (Matsen & Warme, 2009). Rheumatoid arthritis affects approximately 1% of the world's population (Gupta & Baghia, 2010). There is an approximately 3:1 female predominance of rheumatoid arthritis, with the peak age of onset between ages 35 and 45 (Wheeless, 2010a); however, rheumatoid arthritis may affect a person at any age. Of those affected with rheumatoid arthritis, 65%-90% report shoulder symptoms (Thomas, Noël, Goupille, Duquesnoy, & Combe, 2006).

Risk Factors. The main risk factor for the development of primary osteoarthritis is aging. A family history of osteoarthritis has been suggested as a risk factor. Participation in vocations and sports that require repetitive overhead motion increases the risk of developing shoulder osteoarthritis. Risk factors for the development of rheumatoid arthritis include female gender and 40 to 60 years of age. A family history of rheumatoid arthritis may lead to a predisposition to inheriting this disease. Lastly, smoking cigarettes doubles one's likelihood of developing rheumatoid arthritis.

Complications. The mere progression of osteoarthritis should be considered a complication because it results in progressive limitations in motion, decreased shoulder function, disabling pain, and difficulty or inability to perform ADLs. Rheumatoid arthritis of the shoulder may also be accompanied by systemic manifestations of disease, in addition to the polyarticular manifestations. Any delay in the diagnosis of rheumatoid arthritis will result in more erosion and permanent joint damage. By the time there is radiographic evidence of rheumatoid arthritis, the irreversible damage has been done. Patients with rheumatoid arthritis of the shoulder may be plagued by fatigue, depression, and/or anxiety from living with chronic, often debilitating, pain.

Overall, complications from shoulder arthroplasty are rare. The most common complication after shoulder arthroplasty is instability, with a reported rate of 2% to 5%, and is often the result of technical error (Lazarus, 2008). Component loosening, periprosthetic fractures, persistent pain, rotator cuff tears, infection, nerve injury, and deltoid dysfunction are some of the more common complications of shoulder arthroplasty. Patients with rheumatoid arthritis who undergo a total shoulder arthroplasty are more likely to require a revision than patients undergoing the same procedure for osteoarthritis. Moreover, patients with rheumatoid arthritis are more at risk of getting a postoperative wound infection due to a compromised immune system.

Preventive Strategies. The exact cause of osteoarthritis is unknown, and there remains no known cure. For this reason, risk factor modification remains the preventive strategy of choice. Unfortunately, aging is not a modifiable risk factor; however, limiting the "wear and tear" placed upon the shoulder is modifiable. There are no effective strategies for the prevention of rheumatoid arthritis because there is no known cause or cure.

Special Considerations. "In the United States, all races appear equally affected by osteoarthritis" (Shiel, 2010, paragraph 1). Primary osteoarthritis becomes more prevalent with aging and is more common in older women compared to men. Osteoarthritis found in persons younger than age 45 is most often from a secondary cause, such as trauma or instability.

Assessment

History. Pain is the most common presenting complaint of patients with primary osteoarthritis. The onset of pain is insidious and progressively worsens. The pain is described as a deep aching that may be concentrated posteriorly. The pain is aggravated by motion and may linger after the offending activity has ceased. In advanced cases, the pain may be constant. Night pain, along with difficulty lying on the affected shoulder, is common. Stiffness, crepitus, decreased ROM, pain, limited function, and difficulty performing ADLs may also be reported. Joint involvement in rheumatoid arthritis is always symmetrical. The pain may be intense, even before x-ray evidence of severe joint damage from rheumatoid arthritis is present. Loss of function may occur early in the disease process. Systemic manifestations of rheumatoid arthritis may include, fatigue, malaise, generalized morning stiffness that may last hours, fever, loss of appetite, decreased energy, weight loss, and vague arthralgias and myalgias.

Physical Exam. Physical examination of the shoulder joint should be performed in a systematic, comprehensive, and comparative manner. The contralateral shoulder, cervical spine, and elbow should be included in the examination. Decreased ROM in external rotation and abduction, crepitus, and posterior joint line tenderness are common physical findings in patients with shoulder osteoarthritis. Patients often have a fixed posterior humeral head subluxation, which leads to an anterior capsular contracture, limited external rotation, and abnormal "wear and tear" of the posterior glenoid. Disuse muscle atrophy may be present. Physical exam findings associated with rheumatoid arthritis will be symmetric in affected joints and may include tenderness, crepitus, erythema, warmth, edema, limited motion, deformities, and contractures. Rheumatoid nodules may be present.

Diagnostic Tests. Primary osteoarthritis may be diagnosed by obtaining a comprehensive history and physical examination, along with plain radiographs. The true AP and axillary views are obtained when evaluating glenohumeral osteoarthritis to demonstrate the amount of joint space and any irregularities of the joint surfaces. Osteophytes will most commonly be located along the inferior glenoid and humeral head. Bone erosion or loss due to a chronic, fixed posterior subluxation will commonly be seen along the posterior glenoid.

The diagnosis of rheumatoid arthritis of the shoulder is made by history, physical examination, and laboratory testing for the presence of rheumatoid factor or anti-citrullinated protein antibodies (ACPAs). Rheumatoid factor (RF) is present in the serum and synovial fluid within several months after the onset of rheumatoid arthritis, and it is positive in more than half of adults with rheumatoid arthritis. Numerous other medical conditions may also cause an increased RF, (including cancer, diabetes mellitus, and infectious mononucleosis, just to name a few), and an increased RF may also be present in persons older than age 60 without rheumatoid arthritis. Up to 10% of healthy individuals will have an elevated RF (Magrey & Abelson, 2010). Because RF is not very specific, it should not be relied upon as the primary diagnostic indicator of disease. Several other laboratory tests are commonly ordered to assess for other causes of arthritis, including a synovial fluid analysis, erythrocyte sedimentation rate (ESR), C-reactive protein (CRP) level, complete blood count, renal function tests, liver enzymes, antinuclear antibody (ANA) test, lupus anticoagulant, and a ferritin level. In rheumatoid arthritis, plain x-rays may show soft tissue swelling, juxta-articular osteopenia, marginal glenoid erosions, and uniform narrowing of the joint space from articular cartilage thinning, as opposed to central thinning in osteoarthritis. Serial x-rays are often used to monitor the effects of treatment as well. In 2010, the American College of Rheumatology (ACR) and European League Against Rheumatism (EULAR) updated the 1987 diagnostic criteria for establishing a diagnosis of rheumatoid arthritis. Patients must meet 6 of 10 ACR/EULAR criteria and have confirmed synovitis in at least one joint without an alternate diagnosis to substantiate the diagnosis of synovitis with rheumatoid arthritis (ACR/EULAR, 2010).

Common Therapeutic Modalities

Nonsurgical Management. The goals of conservative management for primary shoulder osteoarthritis involve measures to control pain, maintain ROM, and preserve function for as long as possible. Common modalities include the use of medications, injections, PT, rest, ice, heat, activity modification, and the use of assistive/adaptive devices. NSAIDs are commonly prescribed to help alleviate the pain and inflammation associated with osteoarthritis. Narcotics may be required for advanced cases of osteoarthritis or exacerbation of pain. Nutritional supplements, such as glucosamine and chondroitin, have anecdotal evidence of the ability to improve symptoms of osteoarthritis in the shoulder. Intra-articular corticosteroid injections may be used in advanced cases, or during episodes of recalcitrant pain, to provide temporary relief of pain and inflammation. PT for osteoarthritis should incorporate the same principles of therapy used for treatment of most other shoulder maladies. If a specific position, stretch, or exercise causes discomfort, it should not be forced nor continued because the pain may be due to bony impingement from osteophytes and will only result in worsening of symptoms. An occupational therapist can provide the patient with assistive/adaptive devices and instruct on the proper techniques to use them appropriately and safely to maximize function, increase independence, decrease pain and joint stress, and conserve energy.

The goals of conservative management of rheumatoid arthritis are to alleviate symptoms and modify or slow the progression of disease and, therefore, joint destruction and disability. The ACR recommends early, aggressive treatment with the use of a disease modifying anti-rheumatic drug (DMARD) for all patients, with combination therapy reserved for those patients with more aggressive disease (Singh et al., 2012). Specifically, DMARDs (gold salts, methotrexate) are used to provide a respite from symptoms, decrease the rate of joint destruction, and postpone or halt disease progression. DMARDs should be prescribed as soon as shoulder synovitis and pain are suspected. Corticosteroids may be taken orally, or an intra-articular shoulder injection may be given. Biologic response modifiers are also used for treatment of rheumatoid arthritis. Many other drugs are also available to treat the symptoms of rheumatoid arthritis, but none are curative. PT for rheumatoid arthritis should incorporate the use of moist heat and gentle stretching for the stiff, painful shoulder. Caution should be used during gentle stretching of the shoulder, as ligaments and tendons may subluxate secondary to joint deformity and destruction. PT goals should include prevention and correction of deformities, if possible. Cryotherapy, instead of heat, should be used during periods of inflammation. An occupational therapist may be beneficial for the patient with rheumatoid arthritis to provide them with the knowledge, skills, and assistive/adaptive devices to improve function, independence, and the ability to perform ADLs.

Surgical Management. If all conservative measures have failed to treat osteoarthritis or rheumatoid arthritis of the shoulder, surgical intervention may be appropriate. The goals of surgery are pain relief, improvement in motion and strength, restoration of function, and joint stabilization. Arthroscopy, shoulder arthroplasty (hemiarthroplasty, total shoulder arthroplasty, or reverse total shoulder arthroplasty), humeral head or glenoid resurfacing, arthrodesis, partial synovectomy, tendon reconstruction or transfers, osteotomy, and resection arthroplasty are all surgical procedures available to treat the arthritic shoulder. Shoulder arthroscopy may be used in the arthritic shoulder to "clean up" the shoulder joint until a shoulder arthroplasty is indicated. An arthroscopic partial synovectomy may be performed to remove overabundant inflamed synovial tissue found in the rheumatoid shoulder (Parsons, Weldon, Titelman, & Smith, 2004). Shoulder arthroscopy is indicated for patients with severe shoulder osteoarthritis who are not good candidates for shoulder arthroplasty due to young age, activity level, participation in contact or collision sports, poor general medical health making major elective surgery too risky, or the desire to avoid major surgery.

A hemiarthroplasty of the shoulder is the replacement of the humeral head only with a prosthetic metal implant, and is indicated for patients with severe osteoarthritis of the humeral head with no glenoid involvement or severe avascular necrosis of the humeral head (Williams & Iannotti, 2007). An intact rotator cuff is not mandatory for patients undergoing a hemiarthroplasty. Hemiarthroplasty is the procedure of choice for the arthritic shoulder with cuff tear arthropathy (Parsons et al., 2004). In contrast, a total shoulder arthroplasty replaces the humeral head with a prosthetic metal implant, and the glenoid with a plastic prosthetic cup (either cemented or cementless). A total shoulder arthroplasty is generally reserved for patients older than age 50, while a hemiarthroplasty may be recommended for patients between ages 40 and 50 (Williams & Iannotti, 2007). Patients with rheumatoid arthritis have more friable tissue, weaker tendons and ligaments, and brittle bones when compared to patients with osteoarthritis. For these reasons, extra caution is required when performing a shoulder arthroplasty on a rheumatoid shoulder. Recent septic arthritis and acute osteomyelitis of the glenohumeral joint are both contraindications for either a total shoulder arthroplasty or hemiarthroplasty. Revision arthroplasty is a more complex procedure than a primary arthroplasty, and each subsequent surgery becomes increasingly more complex. More skill and expertise is required of the surgeon, more bone stock is lost, and more scar tissue is formed each time a revision arthroplasty is undertaken. Lastly, the outcomes of revision arthroplasty are not as predictable or favorable as those of primary arthroplasty (Codsi & Iannotti, 2007).

Shoulder resurfacing of the surface of the humeral head and/or glenoid is an option for younger patients, and for those with irreparable rotator cuff tears or rotator cuff arthropathy (Krishnan, Harkins, & Burkhead, 2007). Resurfacing may be performed using synthetic or biologic materials. Shoulder resurfacing has the advantage of preserving bone stock to enable the patient to undergo a total shoulder arthroplasty in the future, if needed.

An arthrodesis (fusion) of the glenohumeral joint results in a strong, stable, and functioning shoulder, but all rotation through the glenohumeral joint is sacrificed with this procedure. Since the advent of arthroplasty, an arthrodesis is rarely indicated as a primary procedure for the shoulder, but it still remains an excellent salvage procedure.

Nursing Considerations

Nursing Diagnoses. Nursing diagnoses for this condition are expanded upon in the Appendix.

- Activity intolerance.
- Disuse syndrome, risk for.
- Coping, ineffective.
- Family coping, compromised.
- Family process, interrupted.
- Home maintenance, impaired.
- Infection, risk for.
- Knowledge deficit.
- Mobility: physical, impaired.
- Noncompliance.
- Pain, acute.
- Pain, chronic.
- Role performance, ineffective.
- Self-care deficit: bathing/hygiene, dressing/grooming, feeding, toileting.
- Self concept, readiness for enhanced.

Interventions. *Preventing/minimizing complications:* Choosing the correct implant size and version, achieving the correct amount of soft tissue tensioning, and ensuring adequate, healthy bone stock are all important factors to be considered by the orthopaedic surgeon to prevent or minimize complications and achieve excellent outcomes. Likewise, the patient has the responsibility of following all postoperative/discharge instructions, such as complying with lifting limitations, to allow time for healing of soft tissues and bony ingrowth of the implant.

Activity/positioning: Activity and positional restrictions will vary. Patients may require immobilization, which is dependent upon the type of procedure performed as this will dictate the length of time immobilization is required. Most patients undergoing arthroscopic procedures, as well as shoulder arthroplasty, are started on a rehabilitation regimen by postoperative day one. ROM exercises of the elbow and hand are always begun early (postoperative day zero) to prevent stiffness.

Emotional support: Patients with osteoarthritis and rheumatoid arthritis may be able to better cope with the effects of the disease by reducing the demands placed upon the shoulder. Family, friends or coworkers may assist with performing tasks that involve pushing, pulling, lifting, and reaching. Sleeping in a recliner may decrease nocturnal shoulder pain and decrease insomnia. Chronic pain may result in fatigue, depression, and anxiety, which may be more pronounced in patients with rheumatoid arthritis because of the accompanying deformities of the hands and upper extremities. Patients with rheumatoid arthritis of the shoulder may have an altered self-image due to the deformities.

Patient Teaching. *Nutrition:* Eating a well-balanced diet is important for overall well-being, especially tissue and wound healing after surgery. As mentioned previously, older patients often have poor nutrition, which contributes to poor wound healing. Even though patients undergoing shoulder procedures for treatment of arthritis are often younger than their cohorts undergoing a total knee or hip arthroplasty, their nutritional status should still be addressed. If a patient is found to have poor eating habits or malnutrition, a well-balanced diet should be encouraged, and a multivitamin and/or wound-healing vitamin regimen should be started.

Activity/restrictions: Patients with either osteoarthritis or rheumatoid arthritis of the shoulder need to "listen" to their shoulder. If activities aggravate the shoulder, they should be avoided. It may take several days to weeks for the pain and inflammation to subside after engaging in offending/aggravating activities. Chronic pain is often accompanied by fatigue, which makes rest periods an important part of daily living.

Patients who undergo total shoulder arthroplasty or hemiarthroplasty will wear a sling at all times for at least 2-3 weeks, except during bathing, PT, or unless otherwise specified by their surgeon. After a shoulder arthroplasty, patients are instructed not to lift anything heavier than a cup of coffee for 6 weeks. Patients need to be educated about vocational or recreational activities that are contraindicated after shoulder arthroplasty, such as repetitive pushing, pulling, jerking maneuvers, heavy lifting, repetitive impact, or vibration because they may contribute to premature implant failure and the need for early revision. Likewise, after shoulder arthroplasty, participation in contact sports or vocations that place a heavy strain on the shoulder must be discontinued because it will lead to early failure of the prostheses.

Incisional care: All incisions need to be kept clean and dry. After removal of the initial surgical dressing by the surgeon, subsequent dressing changes should be performed based on his or her instructions. The sutures and staples are usually removed 10-14 days after surgery; thereafter, the incision(s) may be left open to air. Most often, patients are instructed to sponge bathe until the sutures/staples are removed; however, showering may be allowed depending on surgeon preference. Depending on the procedure performed, a surgical drain may be in place for a couple of days. If a patient is discharged home with a drain, they will require education regarding how to care for the drain until it is removed, and home health care visits by a nurse may be arranged.

Practice Setting Considerations. *Office/outpatient:* Patients with osteoarthritis and rheumatoid arthritis of the shoulder will most likely be followed in an outpatient setting until the decision is made to proceed with surgery. In the interim, patients may receive pharmacologic therapy and/or PT in an effort to alleviate and manage the symptoms of arthritis. For patients with rheumatoid arthritis, pharmacologic therapies need to be evaluated on a regular basis to determine their effectiveness and assess if any changes in the current regimen are necessary. These patients will also have serial x-rays to monitor the effectiveness of therapy.

Hospital: Arthroscopic procedures are usually performed on an outpatient basis, allowing patients to go home the same day. Patients undergoing a shoulder arthroplasty, arthrodesis, resurfacing, or osteotomy will require hospital admission after surgery, and the length of stay will vary. Management of postoperative pain is essential. Drains are usually removed by the second postoperative day, unless the output remains high. In this case, the patient will be sent home with the drain. Deep vein thrombosis (DVT) prophylaxis is commonly started for patients undergoing shoulder surgery and will be continued until the patient is ambulatory and the risk of developing a DVT has diminished. Patients will also be encouraged to ambulate frequently. A continuous passive motion (CPM) machine may be used to gently begin ROM of the operative shoulder to prevent the formation of adhesions, scar tissue, and stiffness. Before discharge, a physical therapist should instruct the patient on how to perform gentle ROM exercises, which will be followed by formal PT. Patients are discharged home once the pain is controlled with oral pain medications, the incision is clean and dry, the patient is able to perform gentle ROM exercises, and their home support system is in place for a safe discharge. Upon discharge, it is important to ensure that the patient and/or caregiver understand the discharge instructions, including which signs and symptoms should prompt an immediate phone call to the surgeon or a visit to the emergency department. Ideally, patients should have their first postoperative appointment already scheduled prior to discharge.

Home: Ancillary services, such as home health care, PT and occupational therapy should be arranged to continue in the patient's home after discharge. A home health nurse will monitor the patient's incisions, medications, and overall transition to being at home. A physical therapist will provide supervised therapy visits, in addition to encouragement and positive reinforcement for the patient to continue with the HEP and comply with any functional restrictions. An occupational therapist will assist the patient with adaptation to enable functioning within the prescribed shoulder restrictions by using assistive/adaptive devices, if needed.

Shoulder Instability

Overview

Definition. "Laxity is the normal, asymptomatic, and necessary passive translation of the humeral head on the glenoid that allows normal shoulder motion" (Sher, Levy, Iannotti, & Williams, 2007, p. 339). Hyperlaxity may be present in some individuals, but remains asymptomatic, and therefore, not pathologic. On the other hand, instability is both pathologic and symptomatic. Glenohumeral (shoulder) instability is defined as the inability to maintain the humeral head centered within the glenoid fossa (Matsen, Lippitt, Bertlesen, Rockwood, & Wirth, 2009). It is characterized according to degree, direction, frequency, volition, and the associated circumstances in which the instability occurs. The degree of shoulder instability may range from apprehension to dislocation. Apprehension is the fear, or sensation, that the shoulder will subluxate or dislocate. Glenohumeral subluxation is defined as a symptomatic, excessive translation of the humeral head onto the glenoid rim with partial separation of the articular surfaces. Subluxations are usually transient, with spontaneous reduction of the humeral head within the center of the glenoid. During a dislocation, there is translation of the humeral head out of the glenoid with complete separation of the articular surfaces, which may spontaneously reduce or require manual reduction.

Etiology. During shoulder instability, the direction of humeral head translation may be anterior, inferior, posterior, multidirectional, and (very rarely) superior. Shoulder instability may be acute, recurrent, or chronic. For all patients with shoulder instability, it should be determined whether the instability is involuntary or voluntary. If the patient is unable to control the instability, it is considered involuntary. On the contrary, some patients are able to voluntarily subluxate or dislocate their shoulder by contraction of select muscle groups and/or positioning. Voluntary dislocators may intentionally subluxate or dislocate their shoulder because of emotional and/or psychiatric problems, or perhaps, financial gains. In these instances, a psychiatric consultation should be strongly considered because there is no surgery that can fix the urge to voluntarily dislocate, and they tend to have poor outcomes after surgical intervention. Associated circumstances that contribute to shoulder instability include congenital anomalies, neuromuscular disorders, and repetitive overhead activities (either in sport or vocation).

Mechanism of Injury, Pathophysiology, and Incidence. Shoulder instability may be subtle, as is seen in a throwing athlete who experiences pain during pitching or in a patient with multidirectional instability who experiences shoulder pain while carrying a heavy bag of groceries. On the other hand, instability may be obvious, as is seen with an acute traumatic anterior dislocation. Shoulder dislocations account for approximately 45% of all dislocations (Matsen et al., 2008). Anterior shoulder dislocations are the most common of the glenohumeral dislocations and account for up to 85-95% of cases (Afsari, A., 2011). Anterior shoulder dislocations may further be subdivided into subcoracoid (most common), subglenoid, subclavian, and intrathoracic. Various mechanisms of injury (Table 18.2) are responsible for the different types of shoulder instability and their associated pathophysiology (Table 18.3).

Table 18.2. Shoulder Dislocation—Types and Mechanisms of Injury

Type (subtype)	Mechanism
Anterior (subcoracoid, subglenoid, subclavicular intrathoracic, retroperitoneal)	• Forceful blow to front of arm in abduction, hyperextension & external rotation • Forceful abduction & external rotation • Direct blow to back of arm • Fall on outstretched hand (FOOSH)
Posterior (subacromial, subglenoid, subspinous)	• Axial load to arm in adduction & internal rotation • Violent muscle contraction (electrical shock, grand mal seizure, fall)
Superior	• Extreme forward & upward force to adducted arm
Inferior (luxatio erecta)	• Hyperabduction or upward force to arm
Multidirectional Instability	• Minimal force (such as, combing hair, carrying groceries, or turning over in bed)

Table 18.3. Shoulder Dislocation—Humeral Head Displacement and Pathophysiology

Type	Direction of Humeral Head Displacement	Pathophysiology
Anterior	• Anterior to glenoid, inferior to coracoid (subcoracoid) • Anteroinferior to glenoid fossa (subglenoid) • Medial to coracoid, inferior to clavicle (subclavicular) • Between ribs and thoracic cavity (intrathoracic) • Within abdominal cavity (retroperitoneal)	• Avulsion of AIGHL • Bankart lesion • Capsular stretching • Bony Bankart lesion • Hill-Sachs lesion • Glenoid bone loss
Posterior	• Humeral head posteroinferior to acromion (subacromial) • Humeral head medial to acromion & inferior to spine of scapula (subspinous)	• Impaction fracture • Reverse Bankart lesion • Reverse Hill-Sachs lesion
Superior	• Humeral head forced through rotator cuff (superior to acromion)	• Fractures of acromion, coracoid or clavicle • Biceps tendon Disruption
Inferior	• Humeral head faces inferiorly (inferior to glenoid fossa)	• Arm locked overhead (110-160 degrees of adduction)
Multi-Directional Instability	• Anterior & inferior (most common) • Posterior & inferior	• Ligamentously lax are unable to keep humeral head centered in glenoid and develop inferior translation

Risk Factors. Risk factors for the development of shoulder instability include:

- Generalized ligamentous laxity ("double jointed");
- History of previous subluxation/dislocation of the shoulder;
- Young persons (younger than age 20);
- Overhead or throwing athletes (baseball, tennis); and
- Athletes in contact sports (football, hockey, wrestling, lacrosse, rugby) (Slaney & Wahl, 2009).

Complications. Overall, recurrent instability and redislocation are the most common complications. Patients who sustain their first anterior shoulder dislocation at a younger age (younger than age 20) have up to a 90% chance of recurrent instability, with most redislocations occurring within 2 years of the initial dislocation (Matsen et al., 2009). In patients older than age 40, the incidence drops sharply to 10%-15% (Matsen et al., 2009). The easier the initial dislocation occurred, the easier it will recur. Recurrence rates tend to be higher in athletes than nonathletes, and in men more than women. Hand dominance does not seem to affect recurrence rates. Recurrent instability may cause excessive wear of the glenoid rim, potentially leading to further instability and/or arthritic changes. Stretching and elongation of the joint capsule occurs during episodes of shoulder instability. Fractures may frequently be associated with traumatic dislocations. Rotator cuff tears may accompany anterior and inferior dislocations. Neurovascular complications often accompany traumatic anterior dislocations because of the nearby proximity of the brachial plexus and axillary artery and vein. Severe inferior dislocations may present with the humeral head projecting through a wound in the axilla, and may also result in pulmonary and abdominal complications.

Postoperative complications after open shoulder stabilization procedures include infection, hematoma, neurovascular injury, stiffness, subscapularis rupture, arthrosis, hardware failure, recurrent instability, and capsular necrosis. Osteoarthritis may develop in some shoulders after a shoulder dislocation regardless of whether or not surgery is performed, and there is limited long-term evidence that shoulder surgery for instability prevents osteoarthritis (Gamradt, Williams, & Warren, 2009). Stiffness after shoulder stabilization surgery is a result of over-tightening of the soft tissues, accompanied by postoperative immobilization. Nonanatomic shoulder stabilization repairs, such as the Putti-Platt procedure, are more apt to lead to osteoarthritis than anatomic repairs. Complications caused by arthroscopic suture anchors, or chondrolysis after thermal capsulorrhaphy, may also contribute to the development of osteoarthritis of the shoulder. Absorbable suture anchors can migrate, dislodge, break, or cause chondral injury or synovitis.

Preventive Strategies. The single most effective measure to prevent recurrence of shoulder instability is to avoid provocative arm positions or motions. Compliance with, and continuity of, PT is integral to achieving and maintaining a stable shoulder and preventing recurrence.

Special Considerations. Age at the time of the initial dislocation is a strong predictor of redislocation. Patients who experience their first dislocation prior to the age of 20 are more likely to redislocate. Patients older than age 40, who sustain a shoulder dislocation, are less likely to redislocate and more likely to have an associated rotator cuff tear.

Assessment

History. "The degree to which the shoulder was 'torn loose' as opposed to 'born loose' or just 'worn loose' is critical in determining the best management strategy" (Matsen et al., 2009, p. 651). The circumstances surrounding each episode of shoulder instability, including the initial event and any recurrences, should be obtained. Voluntary dislocators should be identified through careful questioning. The age at onset of shoulder instability should be determined, as the younger the patient is at the onset, the worse the prognosis is for achieving a stable shoulder, and the more likely the symptoms will recur. Obtaining the details about the mechanism of instability will aid in classifying the type of instability and devising an appropriate treatment strategy. The acronyms TUBS and AMBRII may be useful for classifying most cases of shoulder instability (Table 18.4).

Table 18.4. Acronyms for Classification of Shoulder Instability

***T**raumatic*	***A**traumatic*
***U**nidirectional*	***M**ultidirectional*
***B**ankart lesion may be present*	***B**ilateral (often)*
***S**urgery most often effective treatment*	***R**ehab most often effective treatment*
	***I**nferior shift and rotator*
	***I**nterval closure (if surgery indicated)*

Arm position at the time of the initial event, including any recurrent episodes, severity of symptoms, and frequency will assist in determining the direction of instability, and thus, type. The characteristics of pain should be obtained. Pain associated with shoulder instability is usually described as a deep, dull ache within the joint and may be concentrated anteriorly, posteriorly, or inferiorly. Traumatic anterior dislocations cause severe pain until the shoulder is relocated. Positional shoulder pain may occur. A patient may experience pain only and no sensation of instability, while others may complain

CHAPTER 18

of the sensation that their shoulder is about to "pop out" or "slip out" of the joint. Painful clicking or clunking with arm movement may be present. Finally, the details about any prior treatment(s) for shoulder instability should be known, including the type and duration of immobilization, the need for manual reduction or self-reduction, availability of pre- and post-reduction x-ray films, type and duration of rehabilitation, and any prior surgical stabilization procedures. If a prior shoulder stabilization procedure has been performed, it should be determined if the instability symptoms are the same as before surgery with the arm in the same position, or an altogether different one. Finally, the effectiveness of all prior treatments, including surgery, is needed.

Table 18.5. Physical Examination Pearls in Shoulder Dislocations

Type	Arm Position	Visible Deformity
Anterior	Neutral	■ Anteroinferior fullness
Posterior	Adduction/ Internal Rotation	■ Posterior fullness ■ Rounding of back of shoulder ■ Flattening of front of shoulder ■ Prominent coracoid process
Superior	Adduction/ Internal Rotation	■ Fullness above acromion ■ Arm appears shorter ■ Abnormal dimpling/depression (sulcus sign)
Inferior	Overhead	■ Arm locked in 110-160 degrees of adduction ■ Axilla wound with visible humeral head (possible)

Physical Exam. Physical examination of the shoulder should be systematic and comprehensive, incorporating inspection, palpation, ROM measurements, muscle strength testing, neurovascular evaluation, and specialized tests, with comparison to the contralateral side. The surrounding skin should be inspected for any prior surgical or traumatic scars. Detection of abnormalities about the shoulder, by palpation of the soft tissue structures and bony prominences, will aid in narrowing the differential diagnoses and provide insight into the type of shoulder instability, if not readily apparent (Table 18.5).

During palpation, tenderness or decreased muscle tone may be evident. Generalized ligamentous laxity should be evaluated using the Beighton scale (Hypermobility Syndrome Association [HSA], 2011), which assesses the presence of hypermobility by assigning one point for each of the following maneuvers: ability to bend forward at the waist and place palms flat on the floor without bending knees, ability to bend each knee backwards (hyperextension), ability to bend each elbow backwards, ability to bend each thumb to touch the forearm, and ability to bend each little finger backwards greater than 90 degrees. A total score of 9 points is possible if all maneuvers are performed. A score of 5 or more is considered an indicator of hypermobility (HSA, 2011). Manual muscle strength testing should be performed in a pain-free ROM. Several special tests should be performed to evaluate for shoulder instability, including the apprehension test, relocation test, anterior and posterior drawer tests of the shoulder, sulcus sign, and load-and-shift test. A neurovascular assessment of the upper extremities should be performed, including pre- and post-reduction after a manual reduction. Any neurovascular compromise of the affected arm in a patient with a locked dislocation is a medical emergency. Moreover, any neurovascular compromise of the affected extremity is a contraindication to performing a manual reduction, and warrants immediate consultation with an orthopaedic surgeon.

Diagnostic Tests. During the initial evaluation of the shoulder, standard plain radiographs should be obtained: a true AP, axillary, and scapular outlet "Y" views. The West Point and Stryker-notch views may also be beneficial. Plain x-rays allow for evaluation of fractures, including a Hill-Sachs lesion, and the location of the humeral head. MRI scans provide excellent visualization of soft tissue pathology in the unstable shoulder, and numerous studies have shown MRI to be superior to other imaging modalities at defining labral and capsuloligamentous pathology (Sher et al., 2007). Diagnostic arthroscopy may be warranted if the history and physical exam findings are suggestive of pathology that is not well visualized on imaging modalities and may require surgical intervention. Examination under anesthesia (EUA) should be performed prior to a diagnostic arthroscopy, which affords an examination of a completely relaxed shoulder without any muscular inhibition or guarding secondary to patient apprehension or pain. During the EUA, the amount of humeral head translation may be more pronounced than in the awake patient, instability may be appreciated in more than one direction, and subtle instability may be detected.

Common Therapeutic Modalities

Nonsurgical Management. Nonsurgical management is the mainstay of treatment for shoulder instability, whether it manifests as a subluxation or dislocation, traumatic or atraumatic, or acute or recurrent. The initial treatment of an acute dislocation is early manual reduction. A delay in reducing a traumatic dislocation will result in the need to overcome powerful muscle spasms, making reduction more difficult. A neurovascular examination of the affected arm is required before and after manual reduction. Ideally, a manual reduction is performed after plain radiographs of the shoulder have ruled out fractures, as they are a contraindication to performing a manual reduction. The most common methods used for reduction are the traction-countertraction method and the Stimson's technique. Postprocedural x-rays should be obtained to confirm that the reduction was successful and to assess for any fractures. Immobilization is prescribed after reduction of a dislocation, but there is no concensus as to what type of immobilization or arm position is best. The length of time required for immobilization is also controversial, and dependent on the extent of any associated injuries, such as fractures, and the age of the patient. Generally, teenagers and young adults are at increased risk of recurrence and are consequently immobilized for at least 3-6 weeks. Older patients (those older than age 50) may be immobilized for a short period of time (or not at all) because the risk of recurrence in this age group is minimal, but the chance of developing stiffness with prolonged immobilization is great.

PT begins with modalities to reduce pain, inflammation, and swelling. Strengthening of the rotator cuff is essential to maintaining shoulder stability because the compressive force applied to the humeral head by the rotator cuff constrains the humeral head within the glenoid. It is difficult to achieve and maintain a stable shoulder if the treatment is being undermined by a psychiatric condition that compels a patient to repeatedly dislocate the shoulder; therefore, patients who voluntarily dislocate their shoulder may benefit from a psychiatric evaluation and are not surgical candidates for shoulder stabilization of any kind. Rather, PT is the mainstay of treatment for voluntary dislocators. Finally, medications may be prescribed to alleviate pain and inflammation associated with shoulder instability.

Surgical Management. Shoulder stabilization procedures should only be considered if a patient fails an attempt at conservative measures for at least 3-6 months, and they are not a voluntary dislocator. Indications for surgical intervention include an irreducible, open, or recurrent dislocation; failed non-operative treatment; young patient age; or failed procedures with significant glenoid or humeral bone defects (Miniaci, Haynes, Williams, & Iannotti, 2007). The decision to treat shoulder instability using an arthroscopic or open approach is dependent upon the patient's age, pathology, number and type of prior surgical attempts at stabilization, the patient's preference, and the surgeon's experience and expertise.

Shoulder stabilization techniques may be classified into anatomic and non-anatomic procedures. Anatomic reconstruction focuses on restoring the normal anatomy of the shoulder with particular attention to the "hammock-like" mechanism of the inferior glenohumeral ligament complex. Anatomic procedures (such as the Bankart repair, capsular shift or capsulorrhaphy, and capsular plication) address the joint capsule by tightening the capsule and decreasing the joint volume. Nonanatomic shoulder reconstruction procedures create a physical obstacle to humeral head translation and may be classified into three different types: subscapularis muscle alteration or tightening (Putti-Platt and Magnusen-Stack), suspensory (Nicola and Gallie), and bone block (Bristow and Latterjet) procedures. The Putti-Platt and Magnusen-Stack procedures are rarely performed today because of the pronounced loss of external rotation. The Bristow and Laterjet procedures are no longer popular because of the increased incidence of degenerative joint disease and the risk of hardware failure.

Nursing Considerations

Nursing Diagnoses. Nursing diagnoses for this condition are expanded upon in the Appendix.

- Activity intolerance.
- Disuse syndrome, risk for.
- Coping, ineffective.
- Family coping, compromised.
- Family process, interrupted.
- Home maintenance, impaired.
- Infection, risk for.
- Knowledge, deficit.
- Mobility: physical, impaired.
- Noncompliance.
- Pain, acute.
- Pain, chronic.
- Role performance, ineffective.
- Self-care deficit: bathing/hygiene, dressing/grooming, feeding, toileting.

Interventions. *Preventing/minimizing complications:* Recurrence is a major complication of shoulder instability, which may significantly be minimized by patient compliance. Complications related to reduction of a dislocation may be minimized by obtaining plain radiographs and performing a neurovascular examination pre- and post-reduction. Contraindications to performing a manual reduction should always be considered. Lastly, manual reduction of the dislocated shoulder should be performed gently and expeditiously to decrease the incidence of complications.

Activity/positioning. Provocative arm positions and instability-provoking activities should be avoided. For immobilized patients older than age 50, stiffness is a concern. Patient compliance with the prescribed type and duration of immobilization (when prescribed) and PT will improve the chance of preventing recurrence of instability.

Emotional support: All patients will benefit from emotional support and encouragement throughout the extended rehabilitation process. This is especially true for patients younger than age 20 who have a tendency to become disenchanted with the need to participate in PT and a

HEP. Voluntary dislocators may benefit from a psychiatric evaluation and psychological counseling in an effort to curtail their desire to voluntarily dislocate and sabotage their treatment for secondary gains.

Patient Teaching. *Activity/restrictions:* Patients should be educated on the importance of avoiding provocative arm positions and activities, as recurrence rates can be dramatically reduced by making these adjustments. Patients should also be informed of the deleterious effects of recurrent instability on the shoulder, including the increased likelihood of developing osteoarthritis.

Incisional care: Postoperatively, patients need to be educated on proper incision care. The incision(s) need to be kept clean and dry until the first postoperative appointment, and the dressing should not be removed unless instructed by the surgeon.

Practice Setting Considerations. *Playing field/sidelines:* The playing field (or sidelines) is a likely location where a shoulder dislocation may be encountered that requires manual reduction by a health care provider. Any dislocation that develops under these circumstances should be safely and expeditiously reduced on the playing field (or sidelines) because the more time that elapses without reduction, the more challenging it will become, and the risk of neurovascular compromise and damage to bone and soft tissues may increase with time elapsed. Shoulder dislocations associated with fractures, neurovascular compromise, or the inability to reduce the shoulder on the sidelines, will require evaluation and treatment in the emergency department.

Hospital: The hospital is an ideal setting to obtain pre- and post-reduction x-rays and administer sedation safely for manual reduction of difficult dislocations. Evaluation of a dislocation in the emergency department also allows an orthopaedic surgeon to be consulted for irreducible dislocations, and possible associated fractures that may require an immediate trip to the operating room.

Adhesive Capsulitis (Frozen Shoulder)

Overview

Definition. Adhesive capsulitis is used synonymously with "frozen shoulder" or "stiff shoulder" to describe a condition "characterized by the spontaneous onset of pain with significant restriction of both active and passive range of motion of the shoulder" (Cuomo & Holloway, 2007, p. 541).

Etiology and Mechanism of Injury. Adhesive capsulitis may be classified as primary or secondary. Primary adhesive capsulitis (most common) is an idiopathic, progressive, painful loss of active and passive shoulder motion. Secondary adhesive capsulitis is clinically identical to that of the primary type, but has identifiable, contributing factors, which may be systemic, intrinsic, or extrinsic. Intrinsic factors contributing to adhesive capsulitis include rotator cuff tears, osteoarthritis, fractures, and dislocations, to name a few. Extrinsic factors may be systemic or non-systemic, and include stroke, Parkinson's disease, diabetes mellitus, thyroid disease, trauma, prolonged immobilization, bedrest, or surgery. The exact etiology of adhesive capsulitis is unknown.

Pathophysiology. In 1934, Codman concluded that frozen shoulder is "difficult to define, difficult to treat and difficult to explain from the point of view of pathology" (p. 216). Many theories have attempted to explain the pathological process of adhesive capsulitis. Adhesive capsulitis has been found to histologically resemble that of Dupuytren's disease. Despite the common occurrence of adhesive capsulitis, the pathophysiology of this disease still remains elusive to date.

Incidence. Adhesive capsulitis affects approximately 3%-5% of the general population and up to 20% of diabetics (Manske & Prohaska, 2008). Patients with comorbid conditions, such as Parkinson's disease, thyroid disorders, diabetes mellitus, and cardiac disease have an associated increased incidence of adhesive capsulitis. Adhesive capsulitis is "most frequently found in patients between the fourth and sixth decades of life, and it is more common in women than men" (Cuomo & Holloway, 2007, p. 544). There is an increased incidence of adhesive capsulitis in the non-dominant arm. The reported increased incidence in the non-dominant arm may be related to the ability to function and perform ADLs with pain, limited motion, and disuse of the non-dominant arm as opposed to the dominant one. Adhesive capsulitis is more common in sedentary persons. Lastly, adhesive capsulitis has been described as a self-limiting condition that resolves in 1 to 3 years; however, between 20% and 50% of patients suffer long-term ROM deficits that may last up to 10 years (Manske & Prohaska, 2008).

Risk Factors. Risk factors for the development of adhesive capsulitis include female gender, ages 40-60, and the presence of comorbid conditions. Patients who have experienced adhesive capsulitis in the past are at an increased risk of developing adhesive capsulitis in the contralateral shoulder; however, it has not been found to recur in the same shoulder.

Complications. Residual stiffness and pain may linger despite treatment, which is more likely to occur if there is a delay in the correct diagnosis of adhesive capsulitis. Disuse of the affected arm may lead to osteopenia and osteoporosis, and an increased risk of fracture. Patients commonly self-treat shoulder pain and may not notice the associated loss of motion until the pain becomes severe. This delay in seeking medical attention results in the initial presentation at a later stage in the disease process and potentially adversely affects the outcomes of treatment.

Treatment of adhesive capsulitis is not without risk. Common treatments include PT, medications, intra-articular corticosteroid injections, manipulation under anesthesia (MUA), arthroscopic capsular release, hydrodilation, and open capsular release (not routinely performed in the United States). A complication of PT is exacerbation of pain, which may prohibit the patient from participating in this treatment option. NSAIDs or oral cortiosteroids may be prescribed, neither of which is devoid of adverse effects. Patients undergoing MUA may have an increase in pain postoperatively, which may limit the ability to begin early ROM and PT. Meanwhile, early ROM and PT help to maintain the gained ROM, and prevent the development of adhesions and scar tissue that may restrict motion. Possible complications from MUA of the shoulder include proximal humeral or shaft fractures, glenoid rim fractures, labral tears, shoulder dislocation, hemarthrosis, tears of the rotator cuff or joint capsule, traction injury to nerves, increased pain, and instability (rarely). The risk of fracture after MUA is increased in osteopenic and osteoporotic bones, as well as in the elderly. Complications of arthroscopic or open capsular release are rare, but include excessive or inadequate release of the capsule, damage to prior surgical repairs of the shoulder, and damage to the axillary nerve.

Preventive Strategies. There is no known specific strategy to prevent adhesive capsulitis as the cause is unknown. It seems logical that preventive strategies should include keeping the shoulder mobile. Prompt diagnosis and treatment of adhesive capsulitis are essential to prevent permanent disability.

Special Considerations. Stiffness of the shoulder may be caused by many shoulder conditions, such as rotator cuff tears and osteoarthritis, although none of these causes of shoulder stiffness are associated with the limitations of capsular motion as is seen with adhesive capsulitis. Lastly, adhesive capsulitis is more difficult to treat in diabetic patients.

Assessment

History. Patients with idiopathic adhesive capsulitis will describe an insidious onset of progressive pain and stiffness in the affected shoulder. There is often no known precipitating event, or only a minor trauma may be recalled. The hallmark of adhesive capsulitis is pain and stiffness that results in limited passive and active ROM (especially passive external rotation). The patient will often complain of shoulder pain during the night and difficulty sleeping on the affected shoulder. The pain is usually described as a diffuse, dull ache; however, severe stabbing pain that lasts several minutes can occur when the arm is taken near the extremes of motion. Because of the slowly progressive nature of adhesive capsulitis, patients often do not seek medical attention until the pain and stiffness have become severe enough to impact their ability to function and perform ADLs. They will often attempt self-treatment of the shoulder pain, not realizing that limitations in shoulder motion coexist. Patients with secondary adhesive capsulitis are more likely to notice the pain and stiffness after an inciting event because the pain from the inciting event improves, but the limited motion does not.

Physical Exam. The diagnosis of adhesive capsulitis may be determined by history and physical examination alone, and is often a diagnosis of exclusion. Examination will reveal a significant reduction in both passive and active ROM, compared to the unaffected shoulder. Tenderness may be diffuse or localized to the deltoid insertion. Disuse muscle atrophy may be seen. Provocative special tests of the shoulder should be included in the examination, depending on the history and clinical findings. The examiner should be mindful of the different stages of adhesive capsulitis during the physical exam because appropriate treatment is dependent on the accurate identification of the stage at the time of presentation. A hallmark of adhesive capsulitis is the early loss of external rotation with normal rotator cuff strength. The use of an intra-articular injection of anesthetic will help determine the stage of adhesive capsulitis. Patients in stage I will have early loss of external rotation, with a progressive loss of motion in forward flexion, abduction, and internal rotation. Identification of stage I adhesive capsulitis is not straightforward and is often confused with rotator cuff pathology due to the similarity of symptoms. In stage I, the anesthetic injection relieves the pain, and motion is significantly improved to normal or near normal. In stage II, motion remains restricted in forward flexion, abduction, and rotation (internal and external) with no, or very little, improvement in motion once the pain is relieved from an injection. In stage III, marked restriction in motion will be evident, with a firm "end feel" upon capsular stressing. An anesthetic injection given during this stage will not improve the ROM. Lastly, in stage IV, the ROM gradually improves, but residual restrictions of motion may remain; however, the patient usually does not report any limitations.

Diagnostic Tests. Adhesive capsulitis may be diagnosed by a comprehensive history and physical examination alone; however, plain x-rays are routinely obtained in any patient with shoulder stiffness (Neviaser & Hannafin, 2010). Disuse osteopenia may be seen on plain x-rays. A MRI scan is not essential for the diagnosis of adhesive capsulitis, and laboratory tests are not useful. Shoulder arthrography may be used to diagnose adhesive capsulitis; however, it is not helpful in determining the type or extent of healing (Cuomo & Holloway, 2007).Arthrographic findings of adhesive capsulitis include a decreased joint volume, obliteration of the axillary fold of the joint capsule, and abnormalities in filling of the bicipital tendon sheath. Lastly, a diagnostic arthroscopy may be performed, with the advantage of having the option to surgically intervene, if needed. Arthroscopic findings will vary depending on which stage of adhesive capsulitis is present at the time of arthroscopy (Table 18.6).

Table 18.6. Common Arthroscopic Findings in Each Stage of Adhesive Capsulitis

Stage	Arthroscopic Findings
I	• Diffuse hypervascular glenohumeral synovitis
II	• Thickened hypervascular synovitis • Early loss of axillary fold from scar formation & capsular fibroplasias
III	• Loss of axillary fold • Remnants of synovitis
IV	• Well-formed, mature adhesions

From "The Frozen Shoulder: Diagnosis and Management: by R. J. Neviaser & T. J. Neviaser, 1987, Clinical Orthopaedics and Related Research, *223, p. 60. Reproduced with permission.*

Common Therapeutic Modalities

Nonsurgical Management. Conservative measures for the treatment of adhesive capsulitis may include NSAIDs, intra-articular corticosteroid injections, hydrodilation, suprascapular nerve block, and PT. Determination of appropriate treatment strategies is dependent upon the stage of disease and clinical symptoms at the time of diagnosis. Patients in stage I generally respond better to NSAIDs or an intra-articular corticosteroid injection, rather than PT, because the pain is often severe and limits the ability to tolerate even gentle stretching. Patients in stage II or III are better served with PT with the adjunctive use of NSAIDs or intra-articular corticosteroid injections, if necessary. Hydrodilation, also referred to as capsular distension or brisement, has been used as an alternative to surgery and involves injecting a liquid into the joint, under local anesthesia, to increase the intracapsular pressure and capsular volume until capsular rupture occurs. The suprascapular nerve has been found to innervate the joint capsule of the shoulder and may be responsible for the pain in patients with adhesive capsulitis. The hypothesis behind the use of a suprascapular nerve block is that temporary disruption of efferent and afferent pain signals may allow "normalization" of the pathological and neurological processes perpetuating pain and disability, which may lead to better shoulder function (Neviaser & Hannafin, 2010). (Efferent pain signals travel away from the shoulder to the brain or spinal cord; afferent pain signals travel from the brain or spinal cord to the shoulder.)

Physical Therapy is a common nonsurgical treatment for adhesive capsulitis. For stage I, the focus of PT is reduction of pain and inflammation only. For all other stages, therapy begins with gentle pendulum exercises and progresses to passive, then active-assisted stretches in four planes. Forceful, vigorous stretching should be avoided because it will increase pain and inflammation, possibly leading to further stiffness and limitations in motion. Better outcomes are achieved if gentle stretching is performed up to 4-5 times a day on a daily basis. Conservative measures should be attempted for at least 3 months prior to considering surgical options. The majority of patients will have significant improvement after 3 months of PT. Approximately 10% of patients may not respond to conservative treatment, and may need to consider surgical intervention (Neviaser & Hannafin, 2010).

Surgical Management. Surgical options for the treatment of adhesive capsulitis include MUA or capsular release (open or arthroscopic), and are indicated after an attempt of at least 3 months of PT. Contraindications for MUA include the inflammatory phase (stage I) of adhesive capsulitis, significant osteopenia, failed prior MUA, concomitant rotator cuff tear, recent shoulder dislocation, generalized ligamentous laxity, and recent soft tissue surgery about the shoulder. MUA should be avoided in diabetics because this patient population has been known to have a high failure rate after this procedure. Risks of MUA may include: fracture, dislocation, subscapularis rupture, recurrent stiffness, nerve injury, and increased pain following the procedure. "The reported cumulative risk of an adverse event after MUA is less than 1%" (Endres, El Hassan, Higgins, & Warner, 2009, p. 1419).

Arthroscopic capsular release allows for evaluation of the glenohumeral joint and subacromial space for concomitant pathology, and the ability to perform a partial synovectomy. Arthroscopic capsular release is indicated in cases where MUA has previously failed or is contraindicated. After a diagnostic arthroscopy is performed, the capsule is released in a systematic fashion. Extreme care should be taken not to injure the brachial plexus or blood vessels in the vicinity. An open capsular release is not routinely performed, given the availability of the arthroscopic technique. However, an open procedure may be indicated if there is an extra-articular cause of a stiff shoulder, if an arthroscopic approach is not practical, if dense scar tissue is adhered to neurovascular structures, or, on occasion, if the shoulder is too stiff to enable safe introduction of the arthroscope.

Nursing Considerations

Nursing Diagnoses. Nursing diagnoses for this condition are expanded upon in the Appendix.

- Activity intolerance.
- Coping, ineffective.
- Disuse syndrome, risk for.
- Family coping, compromised.
- Family process, altered.
- Home maintenance, impaired.
- Infection, risk for.
- Knowledge, deficit.
- Mobility: physical, impaired.
- Noncompliance.
- Pain, acute.
- Pain, chronic.
- Role performance, ineffective.
- Self-care deficit: bathing/hygiene, dressing/grooming, feeding, toileting.

Interventions. *Preventing/minimizing complications.* By achieving adequate pain control, the patient is able to concentrate their focus on improving ROM and decreasing stiffness, thereby improving function and limiting the chance of developing permanent disability. Delays in diagnosis should be minimized, or avoided all together, if possible. Disuse of the arm should be discouraged because of the risk of osteopenia and fractures. Stretching exercises should not be performed with vigor. Gentle ROM stretches should be performed as prescribed to prevent recurrence of stiffness. Any reluctance or fears the patient may have with beginning early movement of the operative arm should be allayed. Patients undergoing MUA should be appropriately screened for any contraindications to undergoing this procedure to minimize or prevent complications from occurring.

Activity/positioning: After MUA, or capsular release (arthroscopic or open), the operative arm is not immobilized. Gentle stretching in 4 planes should be performed several times a day. The affected arm should be used to perform ADLs as tolerated, with increases in activity level as the pain abates.

Emotional support: Patients may be easily disappointed and discouraged due to the perceived chronicity of adhesive capsulitis, which could take several weeks to months to notice marked improvement, and months to years to resolve. Frequent encouragement and positive reinforcement to perservere and comply with the PT regimen is essential. Lastly, reassurance should be given to the patient that adhesive capsulitis is a self-limiting disease.

Patient Teaching. *Nutrition.* Patients, both women and men, should be educated about the importance of an adequate daily calcium intake, especially since adhesive capsulitis frequently affects women between the ages of 40 to 60 years of age. Menopausal women have an increased risk of osteoporosis, and disuse of the arm may further contribute to the development of significant osteopenia, osteoporosis, and fracture in this population. Additionally, surgical patients should be educated about the importance of eating a well-balanced, healthy diet to promote wound healing.

Activity: Proper technique when performing gentle stretching in 4 planes should be taught. Patients should also be aware of the deleterious effects that immobilizing or guarding the affected arm has on recovery. Lastly, patients should be informed that vigorous exercise or excessive stretching of the arm is counterproductive.

Restrictions: The patient with adhesive capsulitis should be taught that "no restriction is the only restriction" for use of the affected arm. The affected arm should be used to perform ADLs, but vigorous exercising should be postponed until the pain has resolved and full ROM has been restored.

Practice Setting Considerations. *Office/outpatient:* Patients need to have close, frequent monitoring of their progress as they regain motion. Setbacks may be identified and strategies taken to overcome any obstacles to recovery as they may arise. Interval ROM measurements should be obtained, and pain should be assessed at each office visit.

Hospital: It is imperative that patients fully understand how to perform the prescribed stretches, and how often, before being discharged from the hospital or outpatient surgery center. Also, the patient's pain should be adequately controlled to enable the patient to willingly perform the stretches as prescribed once home.

Fractures of the Shoulder

Overview

Definition. A shoulder fracture is a complete or incomplete break in a bone. This may occur in the proximal humerus, clavicle, and scapula.

Etiology and Mechanism of Injury. The most common cause of a *proximal humerus fracture* is a fall on an outstretched arm (Zuckerman & Sahajpal, 2007). In elderly patients, a fall from a seated position may result in a proximal humerus fracture, especially if the bones are osteoporotic. In children, falling backwards onto an outstretched hand, with the elbow in extension and the wrist in dorsiflexion, is a common mechanism, such as a fall while skateboarding (Zuckerman & Sahajpal, 2007). Other causes of proximal humerus fractures may include motor vehicle crashes, falls from heights, seizures, a direct blow to the shoulder, electrical shock, pathologic, and electroconvulsive therapy without the use of muscle relaxants. The most common mechanism of injury to sustain a *clavicle fracture*, in both children and adults, is a moderate or high energy traumatic injury, such as a fall from a height, a fall onto the shoulder, seat-belt injuries, stress fractures in athletes, pathologic incidents, and a direct blow to the clavicle with an object (Andermahr, Ring, & Jupiter, 2007). The mechanism of injury for a *scapular fracture* requires a high-energy impact, such as a motorcycle or motor vehicle crash or falling from a significant height (AAOS, 2007).

Pathophysiology. Neer (1970) devised a classification system for proximal humeral fractures, which remains the most widely used system in clinical practice today (Figure 18.3). This system divides the humeral head into four anatomic segments: articular, greater tuberosity, lesser tuberosity, and proximal shaft beginning at the surgical neck. The presence of displacement of one or more of the four segments determines fracture type; a segment is considered displaced if there is either displacement of more than 1 cm or angulation of more than 45 degrees from its anatomic position (Neer, 1970).

Salter and Harris (1963) defined five types of epiphyseal plate injuries, based on pathoanatomic and radiographic patterns. The mnemonic device "**SALTR**" has been used to help remember the types of Salter-Harris fractures: **S** is for slipped growth plate, type I. **A** is for above: the fracture lies above the growth plate (metaphyseal), type II. **L** is for lower: the fracture is lower than (below) the growth plate (epiphyseal), type III. **T** is for through: the fracture is through the growth plate (including the metaphysis and ephiphysis), type IV. **R** is for rammed: when the growth plate has been rammed or ruined (crushed), the physis suffers from a compression injury, type V. Clavicle fractures may be categorized as those occurring in the proximal, middle, or distal third of the clavicle. Lastly, fractures of the scapula are categorized according to the anatomic area of the fracture (scapular body or spine, glenoid neck or cavity, and coracoid or acromial process).

Incidence. "Proximal humeral fractures account for 4% to 5% of all fractures in adults and less than 1% of children's fractures" and for more than 75% of humerus fractures in patients older than age 40 (Zuckerman & Sahajpal, 2007). After age 50, women have a much higher incidence of proximal humerus fractures than men, which increases substantially after menopause due to osteoporotic fractures. Up to 85% of all proximal humerus fractures are one-part (nondisplaced or minimally displaced) fractures, and 15% to 20% are four-part (displaced) (Zuckerman & Sahajpal, 2007). Avascular necrosis is very common with displaced proximal humeral fractures. Proximal humeral epiphyseal plate fractures most commonly occur in adolescents between ages 10 and 16 due to sports participation, followed by neonates who sustain birth trauma. Salter-Harris type I and II fractures of the proximal humerus are the most common in children younger than age 17. More specifically, type I fractures are seen in newborns and type II fractures in teens.

Figure 18.3. Displaced Fractures

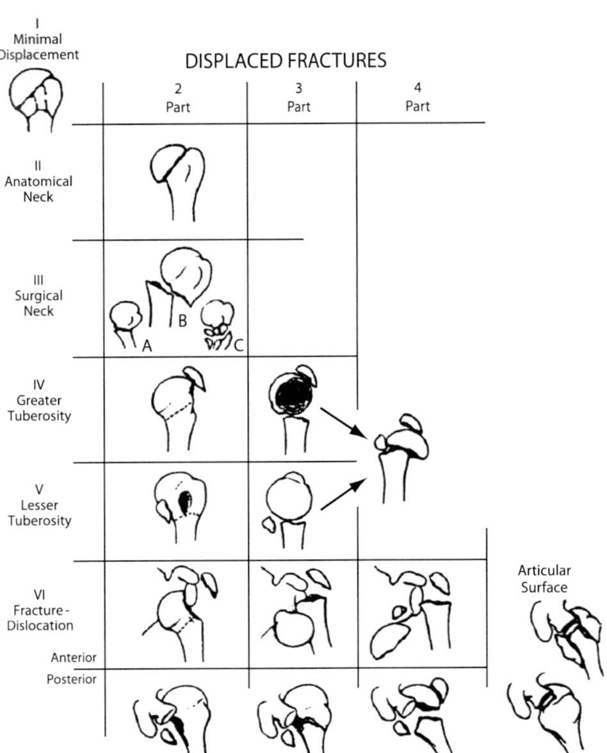

From "Displaced Proximal Humeral Fractures: Part I. Classification and Evaluation" by C. Neer, 1970, Journal of Bone and Joint Surgery, American, 52, *p. 1079. Reproduced with permission.*

Clavicle fractures involving the middle third of the clavicle are the most common in adults and children, and account for approximately 80% of all clavicle fractures. Fractures of the distal third of the clavicle account for approximately 10% to 15% of all clavicle fractures. Also, distal clavicle fractures are associated with a high incidence of nonunion, but most remain asymptomatic. Of the distal clavicular fractures with nonunion, only a small number are severe enough to require surgery. Lastly, fractures of the medial (proximal) third of the clavicle account for 5% of all clavicle fractures (Wheeless, 2010b).

Risk Factors.

- Unsteady gait;
- Falls, including from heights, skateboarding, bicycling;
- Osteopenia, osteoporosis;
- Sports participation, especially contact;
- Motor vehicle crash;

- Neoplasm; and
- Infection, tuberculosis.

Complications. Complications of bone healing include delayed union, malunion, or nonunion. Hardware complications may include pin or plate migration, loosening, breakage, encroachment on nearby neurovascular structures, or infection of the pin tracts or plate. Neurovascular injuries may occur early or late. Early neurovascular injuries are directly related to trauma from the initial injury. Neurovascular injuries may present later, if a large callus or malunion develops and compresses nearby neurovascular structures, or from a missed diagnosis at initial presentation. Fracture-specific complications include avascular necrosis in proximal humeral fractures, which is more prevalent in the elderly, osteoporotic bones, and four-part (displaced) fractures. Nonunion of the clavicle may result in neurovascular complications. Refracture of the clavicle may occur from a premature return to activities, such as contact sports. Complications of scapular fractures themselves are relatively uncommon. Although quite rare, nonunion of scapular fractures is possible, and generally well-tolerated except for some patients who experience painful crepitus with scapulothoracic movements. On the other hand, malunion of scapular fractures involving the glenoid cavity (articular surface) may contribute to premature degenerative joint disease. The most common complications related to scapular fractures are the associated injuries to nearby structures, including rib fractures (25% to 45%), pulmonary injuries (15% to 55%), humeral fractures (12%), brachial plexus and peripheral nerve injuries (5% to 10%), skull fractures (about 25%), cerebral contusions (10% to 40%), tibial and fibular fractures (11%), splenic rupture (8%), and death (2%) (Goss & Owens, 2007).

Procedure-specific complications, as in any procedure, do exist. The most common complication of percutaneous pinning of proximal humerus fractures is pin migration. The literature has reported a wide range in the incidence of superficial pin tract infections from 0% to 16% (Galatz & Kim, 2007). Similarly, incidence rates of 0% to 16% have been reported in the literature for avascular necrosis after closed reduction with percutaneous pin fixation of proximal humerus fractures (Galatz & Kim, 2007). The "figure 8" strap (if used) may lie directly over the fracture fragment and cause discomfort, compromise to underlying skin, and chronic deformity. Neurovascular compression and displacement of fracture fragments have been reported from inattentive placement of external immobilization devices. Wires and pins used for reduction of clavicular fractures have an uncanny ability to migrate and may ultimately be found in the ascending or abdominal aorta, pericardium, pulmonary artery, mediastinum, heart, lungs, or the spinal canal (Andermahr, et al., 2007). Plates used for fixation of clavicular fractures may break. Debilitating pain, limitations in ROM, and loss of function may be the consequence of complications from fractures about the shoulder.

Preventive Strategies. Key strategies for the prevention of fractures about the shoulder involve risk factor modification. For sports participation, especially contact sports such as football, all protective equipment should be of correct size and fit. Also, the protective equipment should be worn and not left sitting on the sidelines. Persons with gait disturbances, or extremes of age, should not climb ladders under any circumstance, or stairs unless assistance is available. They may benefit from physical therapy to improve balance and coordination, and decrease the risk of falls.

Special Considerations. Multiple fractures in a child, in various stages of healing, are a red flag for child abuse. It is mandated by law that all cases of suspected child abuse be reported to the local authorities. Nurses, physicians, and social workers are among the professionals obligated by law to report suspected abuse. Similarly, multiple fractures (in various stages of healing) in adults may be the result of domestic violence or elder abuse and should also warrant prompt reporting of the findings to the authorities.

Assessment

History. A careful history should be obtained, as previously described in this chapter. With proximal humeral and clavicular fractures, the patient may report a history of a FOOSH, a fall onto the lateral shoulder, a fall from a height, or a direct blow to the shoulder. A history of minimal or no trauma may be given if the fracture is pathologic. The onset of pain is sudden and severe. Pain, grinding, or crepitus with arm movement may be present. A palpable deformity or "bump" over the fracture site may be evident. The inability to lift the affected arm may occur with fractures of the proximal humerus or clavicle. Patients may also report progressive swelling and bruising, which may extend to the chest wall and hand. Scapular fractures are associated with severe pain, tenderness localized to the fracture site, swelling, bruising, and crepitus. A history of severe trauma, such as a rollover motor vehicle crash, may be given with a scapular fracture. Significant trauma, including life-threatening internal injuries, may mask the signs and symptoms of a scapular fracture and cause a delay in diagnosis.

Physical Exam. The shoulder area may be visibly deformed with proximal humeral fractures and clavicle fractures. Sagging of the affected shoulder may be seen. Scapular fractures will usually not result in visible deformities due to the overlying muscles of the back. Palpation of the fracture site will be tender. Patients will usually resist any movement of the affected arm due to pain. The elbow, wrist, hand, and rib cage should also be examined for any injuries, including associated fractures. Any opening in the skin should be evaluated for the possibility of an open (compound) fracture. Proximal humeral fractures should be assessed for stability by rotating the lower arm (humeral shaft) and observing if it moves as one unit with the humeral head, which implies a stable fracture. Crepitus is a sign of an unstable fracture. A neurovascular examination of the fractured arm, or ipsilateral arm in the case of a clavicle or scapula fracture, is essential.

Diagnostic Tests. Obtaining plain x-rays in the newborn are often difficult due to motion artifact, and requires an assistant to wear lead and hold the newborn still. Alternatively, ultrasonography has become a commonly used diagnostic tool for diagnosing birth fractures of the humerus or clavicle in the newborn. Shoulder trauma series x-rays should be obtained in any patient suspected of a fracture about the shoulder, and include a true AP in the scapular plane, a scapular "Y" view, and an axillary lateral view. If the patient is unable to tolerate passive abduction of the affected arm for an axillary lateral view, a Velpeau axillary view is an excellent alternative and may be obtained with the patient's arm in a sling. If intra-articular involvement is suspected with a clavicle or scapula fracture, a CT or MRI scan should be obtained. An emergent arteriogram of the upper extremity should be performed if there is any concern of a vascular injury. Most nerve injuries are neuropraxias due to a traction injury and resolve over time.

Common Therapeutic Modalities

Nonsurgical and Surgical Management. The majority of proximal humeral fractures are minimally displaced, stable fractures that require no surgical intervention. Patients are immobilized in a sling for 7-10 days, with a gradual increase in movement. The integrity of the skin under the sling, and in the axilla, should be checked on a regular basis. Additionally, the joints distal to the fracture should be actively taken through their full ROM several times a day to prevent stiffness and decrease swelling. PT begins within 2 weeks. Weekly plain x-rays are performed to monitor fracture healing and evaluate for any interval progression of displacement or angulation. The arm should remain immobilized for a total of 4-6 weeks, or until clinical and early radiographic evidence of union is evident. Patients often achieve good to excellent results with this method of fracture treatment.

Approximately 20% of proximal humerus fractures are comminuted or displaced and may require surgical intervention by means of closed reduction with splinting, percutaneous fixation, open reduction with internal fixation (ORIF), or hemiarthroplasty (Bohsali & Wirth, 2009). The patient's age, health status, medical comorbidities, activity level/physical demands, bone quality, and condition of the rotator cuff are all important factors to consider when choosing between non-surgical and surgical treatment of a proximal humerus fracture. Absolute contraindications to closed reduction and percutaneous pinning include severe comminution of the fracture fragments and osteopenia. Multiple methods of ORIF for proximal humerus fractures are available, and include plate-and-screw fixation, blade or locking plates, tension banding, nailing, or combinations of suture and metallic implant fixation (Bohsali & Wirth, 2009).

Nonsurgical treatment is the general rule of thumb for treatment of clavicle fractures in children. Newborns with clavicular birth fractures usually only require comfort measures due to the tremendous bone remodeling that accompanies rapid growth of the newborn. The newborn's arm may be gently bound to the chest by merely securing the sleeve of a long-sleeve shirt to the chest. Care should be used when swaddling the newborn as well. Healing usually occurs within 1-2 weeks in the newborn. In older children, nondisplaced or greenstick clavicle fractures may be treated with a sling (Choi, Chan, Skaggs, & Flynn, 2009). Use of a "figure 8" strap may prove to be uncomfortable, frustrating, and a burden, for both the child and parents. A Velpeau bandage has been used for treatment of clavicle fractures, which is similar to a sling and swathe, but the arm is held across the chest with the affected hand resting on the contralateral shoulder. Use of a sling, and possibly a swathe for added comfort, is also an acceptable treatment for most clavicle fractures in the adult. When indicated, a number of fixation methods are available for treatment of clavicle fractures using plate fixation, intramedullary pins or nails, or cerclage sutures.

Most fractures of the scapula (scapular body and spine or coracoid and acromial process) may be treated conservatively with the use of a sling for immobilization, followed by progressive ROM and PT. Most fractures of the glenoid neck and cavity may be successfully treated non-operatively as well; however, if there is significant displacement of a glenoid neck fracture, surgery should be considered because of the risk of developing malunion or nonunion with resultant bony impingement, degenerative joint disease of the glenohumeral joint, chronic shoulder pain, decreased function, and loss of motion.

Nursing Considerations

Nursing Diagnoses. Nursing diagnoses for this condition are expanded upon in the Appendix.

- Anxiety.
- Coping, ineffective.
- Disuse syndrome, risk for.
- Family coping, compromised.
- Fear.
- Growth and development, delayed.
- Home maintenance, impaired.
- Infection, risk for.
- Mobility: physical, impaired.
- Noncompliance.

- Pain, acute.
- Pain, chronic.
- Parenting, impaired.
- Role performance, ineffective.
- Self-care deficit: bathing/hygiene, dressing/ grooming, feeding, toileting.
- Self-concept, readiness for enhanced.
- Skin integrity, impaired.

Interventions. *Preventing/minimizing complications:* Methods to help minimize complications of bone healing (delayed union, malunion, and nonunion) include elimination of any gross movement of the fracture fragments by ensuring that patients comply with immobilization. The device must be worn correctly, and for the designated length of time, to allow for bone healing to occur. Activity modification is required to minimize the chance of refracture. Confirmation of fracture healing should be made both clinically and radiographically before activity restrictions are lifted. Frequent skin assessments, including the area of skin under the immobilization devices, are crucial to preventing skin breakdown, especially in the elderly. Meticulous wound care is also mandatory to prevent infections, and includes pin care, incision care, and local wound care of any abrasions or lacerations.

Activity/positioning: The length of time required for immobilization and activity modification is dependent upon the patient's age and the fracture type. With newborns, no immobilization is required for normal bone healing to occur in 1-2 weeks. Adults may require up to 8 weeks (or longer) of immobilization for bone healing to occur. For most fractures about the shoulder, gentle pendulum exercises are allowed within 2 weeks. Thereafter, progression of exercises is dependent upon fracture type and evidence of bone healing. Return to full, unrestricted activities usually occurs at 3 months.

Patient Teaching. *Activity restrictions/immobilization:* The importance of adherence to activity restrictions, to allow time for fracture healing, should be stressed. Patients should also receive an age-appropriate explanation of the importance of wearing the prescribed immobilization device. Athletes should be strongly discouraged from any efforts to shorten the length of time they are required to be sidelined as this may result in refracture, with further prolongation of time away from play.

Pain control: Patients—and their parents in the case of minors—should be educated about the importance of taking pain medications as prescribed and only when needed. The pain medication is more effective when it is taken when the pain is still in the mild range, rather than waiting until the pain is severe. Also, ice should be used to relieve pain, decrease swelling, and inflammation. Ice packs should not be placed directly on the patient's skin due to the risk of thermal burns.

Pin care/incision care: Patients and/or parents need to be instructed on how to properly perform pin and incision care, including the frequency and duration of such care. The surgical dressing should be kept clean, dry, and intact until the first postoperative visit. Thereafter, the dressing should be changed per the surgeon's instructions.

Practice Setting Considerations. Office/outpatient: In addition to weekly x-rays, a physical examination of the shoulder needs to be performed at each office visit to assess for clinical evidence of bone healing, which will be apparent prior to detectable callus formation on plain x-rays.

Hospital: Pain should be adequately controlled with oral analgesics prior to a patient's discharge from the hospital or outpatient surgery center. Also, the patient and/or parents need to understand all discharge instructions, including activity restrictions, the use of immobilization devices, and any pin or incision care, if indicated.

Sprains, Strains, Contusions, and Separations

Overview

Definition. Ligaments are fibrous bands of connective tissue that attach bone to bone and function as joint stabilizers and checkreins with motion of the arm. A sprain is a stretched or torn ligament. Tendons are rope-like fibrous connective tissue structures that attach muscles to bone. A strain is a stretched or torn muscle, usually at the musculotendinous junction. A contusion is an injury to the skin and underlying soft tissue with resultant bruising, and if severe, a hematoma may form. The acromioclavicular (AC) ligament attaches the acromion to the clavicle. The coracoclavicular ligament attaches the coracoid process to the clavicle. An AC joint separation represents a spectrum of injury from inflammation to dislocation. Similarly, a sternoclavicular (SC) separation may range from inflammation to a dislocation of the ligament that attaches the manubrium of the sternum to the clavicle.

Etiology and Mechanism of Injury. Shoulder sprains may occur from a FOOSH, a direct blow, errors in training, or overuse. Shoulder strains may result from a sudden stretch or overload of a contracted muscle, a FOOSH, a direct blow, a sudden increase or change in activity, errors in training, or overuse. Shoulder contusions are the result of a direct blow to the shoulder. AC separations may be caused by a fall or blow to the lateral aspect of the shoulder, or less commonly a FOOSH. SC separations may be caused by a direct blow to the medial clavicle or a fall onto the lateral aspect of the shoulder, especially if combined with an anteriorly or posteriorly directed force.

Pathophysiology. Sprains and strains are graded according to severity. A grade I injury is microscopic tearing of the ligament or tendon fibers without macroscopic elongation of the ligament or tendon. A grade II injury is a partial tear of the ligament or tendon. With grade I and II sprains or strains, the injury causes pain, but there is no dysfunction of the ligament or tendon. A grade III injury is a complete tear of the ligament or tendon, with resultant inability to perform its function. During a contusion, the force of the direct blow causes rupture of the smaller blood vessels and capillaries, with bleeding into the tissues and swelling. AC joint separations are classified into 6 types (Table 18.8).

Table 18.7. Types of AC Joint Separations

Type	Characteristics
I	Sprain of AC ligament only
II	Torn AC (acromioclavicular) ligament, disruption of AC joint & sprain of CC (coracoclavicular) ligament
III	Type II + CC interspace wider than normal, detachment of deltoid & trapezius from clavicle & inferior displacement of shoulder complex
IV	Type III + posterior displacement of clavicle through trapezius
V	Disruption of AC & CC ligaments, AC joint dislocation, gross displacement between clavicle & scapula, & detachment of deltoid & trapezius muscles
VI	Disruption of AC & CC ligaments, detachment of deltoid & trapezius muscles & distal clavicle inferior to acromion or coracoid process

From "Acromioclavicular Joint Injuries" by A. Tom, A. Mazzocca, and C. Pavlatos, 2009, The Athlete's Shoulder, p. 304, Philadelphia, PA: Saunders Elsevier. Reproduced with permission.

Incidence. The shoulder is not the most commonly sprained or strained joint; however, shoulder sprains and strains are more common in athletes, especially those who participate in contact or overhead sports. Contusions often go unreported and underdiagnosed. "Acromioclavicular joint dislocations represent 12% of all dislocations of the shoulder girdle and 8% of all joint dislocations in the body" (Collins, 2009, p. 474). The incidence of sternoclavicular joint dislocations is 3%, according to Cave and colleagues (as cited in Rockwood, et al., 2009).

Risk Factors. Risk factors for sustaining a sprain, strain, contusion, or shoulder separation include sports participation, poor physical conditioning, improper warm-up prior to physical activities, fatigue, improper use or ill-fitting protective equipment, and previous shoulder injuries, to name a few.

Complications. Complications of sprains and strains may include the inability of the damaged tissue to heal, resulting in chronic pain, instability, prolonged weakness, tightness, or recurrent injury. Also, heterotopic bone may form in soft tissues. Shoulder contusions may result in a hematoma, with the potential to compress nearby neurovascular structures or become infected. Complications of AC joint separations include persistent pain and weakness, an undesirable cosmetic deformity, re-injury, and skin breakdown underneath immobilization devices. Posterior displacement of the clavicle from a SC joint separation may have potentially lethal complications, such as pneumothorax, brachial plexus injury, esophageal fistula, and injury to nearby major blood vessels.

Preventive Strategies. Many strategies may be used to minimize the risk of shoulder sprains, strains, and separations, such as a proper warm-up prior to physical activities and use of properly fitting protective equipment.

Special Considerations. Sprains, strains, contusions, and separations occur more commonly in athletes, and have been reported to occur more frequently in males.

Assessment

History. With a shoulder sprain or strain, a patient may report a sudden onset of shoulder pain after a FOOSH or direct blow to the shoulder. A popping or snapping sensation may be heard and felt, and the shoulder may feel unstable. Patients with shoulder contusions will report a history of a direct blow to the shoulder with pain, soreness, decreased motion (both active and passive), bruising, and swelling. A history of physical abuse or bleeding disorders should be ascertained any time there is a contusion or hematoma. Patients with shoulder separations will describe mild to severe pain and tenderness localized to the affected AC or SC joint. Posterior SC joint dislocations, although rare, may have associated symptoms that affect swallowing and breathing, which should be considered a medical emergency.

Physical Exam. Localized swelling, bruising, visible deformities, asymmetry, and guarding of the affected shoulder may be detected in patients with a shoulder sprain, strain, contusion, or separation. Palpation may reveal areas of tenderness overlying a tendon, muscle, ligament, or the AC or SC joint. If present, a hematoma will be tender to palpation and firm to touch. A deformity or gapping overlying the AC or SC joint may be palpable. With strains, a defect may be palpable over a muscle belly or musculotendinous junction. Both active and passive ROM will be limited in varying amounts, depending on the severity of the injury. Muscle strength may be normal, minimally decreased, or severely limited with a strain, depending on severity. Routine special tests for the shoulder should be performed to assess the integrity of the tendinous and ligamentous structures. Finally, several pain-provoking maneuvers may be performed to localize the pain to the AC joint, such as the cross-body adduction test.

Diagnostic Tests. Plain x-rays should be obtained in any patient who has sustained a sprain, strain, or contusion of the shoulder to rule out fractures or dislocations. Advanced imaging studies may be necessary to further evaluate soft tissue or bone injuries. When shoulder separations are suspected, plain x-rays are obtained to evaluate for deformities of the AC or SC joint and the severity of the separation. CT scan is the imaging modality of choice for evaluating pathology of the SC joint.

Common Therapeutic Modalities

Nonsurgical Management. The mainstay of conservative treatment for shoulder sprains, strains, and contusions is use of rest, ice, compression, and elevation, which has been popularized by the acronym R.I.C.E. Heat may be initiated in a few days, once swelling has subsided. NSAIDs and acetaminophen may help decrease inflammation and pain, respectively. Immobilization may be used for comfort, along with activity modification to protect the injured shoulder and allow time for healing. Surgical intervention may be indicated for grade III sprains or strains of the shoulder. PT may not be necessary for treatment of grade I sprains or strains, or mild contusions, but is recommended for more severe injuries to prevent chronic disability or recurrence. Treatment of type I and II AC joint separations is conservative, and consists of immobilization with a sling, rest, ice, and activity modification. Once pain has subsided, the sling may be discontinued and activities resumed as tolerated. Avoidance of forceful maneuvers with the arm, as well as contact or collision sports, is recommended for up to 12 weeks to avoid the risk of further, more serious injury while the ligaments heal (Collins, 2009). In type III AC joint separations, the conservative approach is also the preferred method of treatment. After reduction of the AC joint dislocation, the arm is immobilized in a sling. Once pain has subsided, PT is begun to restore motion and strength. Outcomes of nonoperative treatment have been reported to be comparable to, if not better than, those for operative treatment with respect to pain, ROM, and strength (Collins, 2009).

Surgical Management. Generally, surgical intervention is necessary for treatment of type IV, V, and VI AC joint separations. Heavy manual laborers, patients younger than age 25, athletes, and persons who frequently require the ability to use their arms overhead should also be considered for surgical repair (Collins, 2009). Otherwise, inactive persons and those with extremely low physical demand, such as the elderly, should not be considered for surgical repair because significant gains may not be attainable when compared to those achievable by non-operative means in this subset of patients (Collins, 2009). Non-operative treatment of SC joint dislocations involves reduction of the displaced head of the clavicle. A "figure 8" strap may be applied post reduction and worn for 4-6 weeks.

Nursing Considerations

Nursing Diagnoses. Nursing diagnoses for this condition are expanded upon in the Appendix.

- Anxiety.
- Coping, ineffective.
- Disuse syndrome, risk for.
- Fear.
- Home maintenance, impaired.
- Infection, risk for.
- Mobility: physical, impaired.
- Noncompliance.
- Pain, acute.
- Pain, chronic.
- Role performance, ineffective.
- Self-care deficit: bathing/hygiene, dressing/ grooming, feeding, toileting.
- Skin integrity, impaired.

Interventions. *Preventing/minimizing complications:* Allowing for adequate time to heal after shoulder sprains, strains, and separations is of utmost importance to prevent chronic pain and disability, recurrent injury, instability, arthritis, and deformity. The skin should be assessed underneath any immobilization device, especially any device with a strap traversing across the clavicle, such as a "figure 8" strap. Lastly, all patients with a suspicion of a posterior SC joint dislocation need to undergo a thorough examination for associated, potentially lethal complications so that they may be identified promptly and appropriate treatment rendered.

Immobilization/activity: When immobilization is recommended, the typical method used is an arm sling, except for SC joint separations, which are customarily held in a reduced position with a "figure 8" strap. Resumption of full, unrestricted activities should not be hastened due to the risk of a chronically unstable AC or SC joint.

Patient Teaching. *Activity restrictions:* Patients with grade I shoulder sprains or strains, or type I AC joint separations need to be instructed to modify their activities until the pain subsides and motion improves, followed by a gradual return to activities. Similarly, patients with grade II or III sprains or strains, or type II AC joint separations need to be instructed to gradually resume activities once the pain and tenderness has subsided, and motion returns to normal.

Medications: Patients taking any pain medication should be instructed to take the medication before the pain becomes severe to achieve better pain control. Also, any patient who is prescribed a narcotic pain medication should be cautioned about the risk of potential abuse, addiction, and withdrawal.

Incisional care. The surgical dressing should be kept clean, dry, and intact until the first postoperative appointment. Once the sutures and staples are removed on postoperative day 10-14, the patient is usually allowed to shower.

Practice Setting Considerations. *Office/outpatient:* The skin underneath immobilization devices should be assessed at each office visit and by the patient at home. After the skin assessment, it is an opportune time to watch the patient don the sling or "figure 8" strap to assess for proper application and positioning. Assist and correct the patient's application and positioning as needed.

Sprengel's Deformity

Overview

Definition and Etiology. Sprengel's deformity, also known as congenital elevation of the scapula, is a rare congenital anomaly of the shoulder girdle. Normally, at approximately 5 weeks gestation, the scapula develops opposite the fourth to sixth cervical vertebrae, and begins its downward migration between the ninth and twelfth week to its usual thoracic position between the second and seventh ribs (Grogan, Stanley, & Bobechko, 1983). In patients with Sprengel's deformity, this normal descent of the scapula does not occur. The exact cause of Sprengel's deformity is unknown.

Pathophysiology. Failure of normal descent of the scapula results in one that is elevated, malrotated, and misshapen, with resultant cosmetic and functional implications. The abnormality is almost always unilateral, and the scapula is smaller, broader, and flatter than normal. Because of abnormal medial rotation, the superior angle of the scapula causes a noticeable lump in the web space of the neck, making the neck appear shorter and fuller on the affected side. Occasionally, the superomedial pole of the scapula may curve over the top of the rib cage. The trapezius, levator scapulae, and rhomboids may be hypoplastic or absent. Sometimes, the pectoralis major, latissmus dorsi, or sternocleidomastoid muscles may also be underdeveloped. An omovertebral bone is present in 25-40% of cases in the reported literature (McMurtry, Bennet, & Bradish, 2004). An omovertebral bone is a trapezoidal or rhomboid (wedge)-shaped structure of bone and cartilage, extending from the superomedial border of the scapula to the spinous or transverse process of the cervical spine, causing limited shoulder elevation and abduction on the affected side. Several associated anomalies may be present, and include congenital scoliosis with a hemivertebra, spina bifida, rib abnormalities, chest wall asymmetry, Klippel-Feil syndrome, and multiple other anomalies involving other organ systems, including the eyes, heart, and kidneys.

Incidence. Sprengel's deformity seems to affect girls three times more often than boys. There is no consensus as to whether the deformity predominantly affects the left or right shoulder. Sprengel's deformity is considered a sporadic mutation. There have been a few cases of Sprengel's deformity documented among multiple members within a single family suggesting a hereditary tendency, but this is a rare occurrence (Engel, 1943).

Assessment

History. The presenting complaint may be a parent's concern that his or her child's shoulder looks abnormal or too high, and the child may be having difficulty lifting the affected shoulder. Sometimes, Sprengel's deformity may not be diagnosed until adolescence because it tends to be painless or misdiagnosed as scoliosis. An associated congenital scoliosis may mask or exaggerate the deformity. A detailed account of the child's family, perinatal, and developmental history should be obtained. Lastly, the child's psychosocial history is also important because children may be the victim of teasing or feel self-conscious.

Physical Exam. Sprengel's deformity is a problem of cosmesis and function. Functional limitations and the degree of cosmetic disfigurement will vary, with some children afflicted by both. Cavendish (1972) developed a grading system to aid in describing the severity of Sprengel's deformity to guide treatment by ranking the severity of the deformities as follows:

Grade 1 (very mild)—shoulder joints are level, and deformity is invisible (or almost so) when patient fully dressed;

Grade 2 (mild)—shoulder joints are level or almost level, but deformity is visible when patient fully dressed as a lump in the web of the neck;

Grade 3 (moderate)—shoulder joint is elevated 2-5 cm, and the deformity is easily visible; and

Grade 4 (severe)—shoulder very elevated with the superior angle of the scapula near the occiput with or without neck webbing or brevicollis.

Physical examination of the shoulder should include inspection, palpation, and measurement of ROM, including scapulothoracic and glenohumeral motion in abduction. The unaffected shoulder should be examined first, followed by the affected side. The cervical and thoracic spine should also be examined. The affected shoulder will usually have normal passive glenohumeral motion with limitations in active forward flexion and abduction, and the inability to abduct the shoulder more than 90 to 100 degrees. If an omovertebral bone is present, there will be severe functional limitations, including decreased scapulothoracic movement.

Diagnostic Tests. Plain x-rays should be obtained, including an AP view of both shoulders with the arms in abduction and adduction, scapula lateral and oblique views, and a lateral view of the cervical and thoracic spine. The AP view is used for measuring the degree of abduction radiographically. The scapular views are helpful when evaluating restrictions of movement, especially if an omovertebral bone is present. Lastly, cervical and thoracic views will aid in determining the presence of scoliosis or other associated anomalies. CT scan with 3-D reconstructions provides an excellent depiction of the morphopathology of the scapula, and is invaluable for surgical planning.

Common Therapeutic Modalities

Nonsurgical Management. The main objectives of any form of treatment for Sprengel's deformity are to improve cosmesis and function. The cosmetic goal is for the deformity to be undetectable when the child is fully dressed. From a functional standpoint, the goal is for the child to have improved ROM and function of the shoulder. PT is the mainstay of treatment for all patients with a Cavendish grade 1 deformity. A trial of PT should also be attempted for Cavendish grade 2 deformities because some of these children will achieve enough of a functional improvement to avoid surgery. Surgical intervention is usually required for Cavendish grade 3 and grade 4 deformities.

Surgical Management. The most popular techniques performed to correct Sprengel's deformity are the Woodward and Green procedures. The ideal surgical candidate is between ages 3 and 8. Unfortunately, no surgical procedure will create a normal-appearing shoulder because the scapula itself is hypoplastic. Similarly, the goal of surgery is not to attempt relocation of the hypoplastic scapula to a symmetric position because this is not feasible, and overcorrection may lead to brachial plexus palsy. On average, 30 degrees of abduction may be gained postoperatively.

Complications. The most common complications of surgery to correct Sprengel's deformity are widened, keloid scar formation of the upper thoracic portion of the scar, no improvement or worsening of the deformity, recurrence of the deformity later in life due to re-growth of bone, scapular winging, and neurovascular injury.

Nursing Considerations

Nursing Diagnoses. Nursing diagnoses for this condition are expanded upon in the Appendix.

- Anxiety.
- Coping, ineffective.
- Disuse syndrome, risk for.
- Family coping, compromised.
- Family process, interrupted.
- Fear.
- Growth and development, delayed.
- Home maintenance, impaired.
- Infection, risk for.
- Mobility: physical, impaired.
- Pain, acute.
- Pain, chronic.
- Parenting, impaired.
- Role performance, ineffective.
- Self-care deficit: bathing/hygiene, dressing/grooming, feeding, toileting.
- Self-concept, readiness for enhanced.
- Skin integrity, impaired.

Interventions. *Preventing/minimizing complications:* Great care is usually taken during closure of the upper thoracic portion of the incision in an effort to minimize excessive scarring and a poor cosmetic outcome. Even with meticulous closure, it is possible that the upper thoracic portion of the incision will not heal as nicely as the distal portion, resulting in an aesthetically unpleasing scar. The parents and child (if age-appropriate) should be informed of this prior to surgery, and reassured that every effort will be made to achieve a cosmetically aesthetic result. An unfortunate complication of surgical correction of Sprengel's deformity is the risk of no improvement or worsening of the deformity, which may be minimized by careful patient selection.

Emotional support: Once children begin school, they may become the victim of teasing or bullying by their peers, resulting in feelings of shame, embarrassment or being different. A referral to a school counselor, child/family counselor, or child psychologist may help the child cope. Educating the child's peers about Sprengel's deformity may give them a better understanding, and perhaps more compassion and empathy for others who appear different. Additionally, the parents may have feelings of guilt and difficulty coping with the fact that their child has a congenital deformity, and should also be referred to counseling, as needed.

Child and Parent Teaching. The parent and child (if age-appropriate) should be educated about the goals of treatment. Improvement in the cosmetic appearance of the shoulder is the primary focus, but the scapula will never look normal due to its smaller size. The secondary goal is to improve function.

Practice Setting Considerations. *Office/outpatient:* At each office visit, the parents and child should be interviewed to ascertain whether the child appears comfortable, is eating, and playing normally. Also, the parents and child should be asked if they have any questions or concerns.

Hospital. All efforts should be made to ensure that the child has adequate pain control prior to discharge home. All discharge instructions should be reviewed with both parents (if possible), especially the parent who will be providing postoperative care to the patient. Written and verbal discharge instructions should be given to the parents at the time of discharge. The phone number of the surgeon's office should be given in case the parents have any questions or concerns after discharge, or if any problems arise.

Congenital Dysplasia or Hypoplasia of the Glenoid

Overview

Definition and Etiology. The terms congenital dysplasia or hypoplasia of the glenoid, primary glenoid dysplasia, shallow glenoid, and dysplasia or hypoplasia of the scapular neck have all been used synonymously to describe a congenital anomaly of the scapula characterized by incomplete ossification of the lower two thirds of the glenoid and adjacent scapular neck. The exact etiology of congenital glenoid hypoplasia remains uncertain. However, it may be due to obstetrical trauma, failure (maldevelopment) of ossification of the inferior glenoid, infection, muscular dystrophy, arthrogryposis (a congenital disorder characterized by multiple joint contractures, muscle weakness and fibrosis) or inheritance (Wirth, Lyons, & Rockwood, 1993).

Pathophysiology. In congenital glenoid hypoplasia, the lower two thirds of the glenoid and adjacent scapular neck are underdeveloped or absent. The hypoplastic glenoid appears concave or flat, with either a smooth or irregular (dentate) surface, which may contribute to glenohumeral joint instability. The scapular neck is usually shortened. Other common features include hypoplasia of the humeral head, a prominent, angulated coracoid process, and an enlarged acromion.

Incidence. Congenital glenoid dysplasia is a rare anomaly, with the exact incidence unknown. Fewer than 80 cases have been reported in the literature (Smith & Bunker, 2001). Congenital glenoid hypoplasia is often found incidentally during a work-up for another medical condition. Patients may remain asymptomatic or present with shoulder pain and dysfunction. Of those patients who present with shoulder pain and dysfunction, there appears to be two predominant age groups: in the late adolescent years and in the fifth to sixth decades of life (Lintner, Sebastianelli, Hanks & Kalenak, 1992). Congenital glenoid hypoplasia affects males more often than females and occurs bilaterally in the vast majority of cases. Only five reported cases of unilateral involvement have been reported in the literature (Trout & Resnick, 1996; Wirth et al., 1993). Glenoid hypoplasia has been found in multiple members of the same family suggesting an inheritable tendency in some cases (Kozlowski, Colavita, Morris, & Little, 1985).

Risk Factors. There appear to be no known risk factors for the development of congenital glenoid hypoplasia because the exact cause remains elusive; however, obstetrical trauma, maldevelopment, muscular dystrophy, arthrogryposis and inheritance have been implicated.

Complications. Complications of congenital glenoid hypoplasia may include glenohumeral joint instability, (frank dislocation is rare), secondary osteoarthritis, chronic pain, and shoulder dysfunction. PT tends to be less effective the older the patient is, possibly due to more pronounced glenohumeral joint osteoarthritis than in their younger cohorts. Total shoulder arthroplasty for treatment of congenital glenoid hypoplasia is more technically challenging and may have a higher risk of complications than for primary osteoarthritis.

Preventive Strategies. There is no known strategy to prevent congenital glenoid hypoplasia. Early identification of this congenital anomaly may be beneficial to allow for initiation of PT at a younger age as conservative measures are less effective the older the patient is, presumably because secondary glenohumeral osteoarthritis is more advanced with age. Therefore, one would have to surmise that if congenital glenoid hypoplasia is found incidentally, a patient would benefit from a shoulder strengthening program to decrease the deleterious effects of instability and prevent progression of osteoarthritis.

Special Considerations. Congenital glenoid hypoplasia has no predilection for any one ethnic group. As mentioned previously, males seem to be affected more commonly than females. Symptomatic patients predominantly present at two different age groups: in the late teens and in the fifth to sixth decades of life. It has been postulated that the younger cohorts present in their teens because of sports participation, and the latter cohort due to osteoarthritis.

Assessment

History. In asymptomatic children, congenital glenoid hypoplasia is usually discovered incidentally. On the other hand, symptomatic adults may present with the complaint of an insidious onset of shoulder pain, which may increase with activities, especially those involving overhead movements. Stiffness, limited motion (especially in abduction), instability, and premature osteoarthritis may also be present. The characteristics of pain should be obtained. Lastly, the patient's past medical, surgical, family, and birth history should be documented to determine if the anomaly may possibly be an inheritable disorder or the result of a birth injury.

Physical Exam. A systematic, comprehensive physical examination of the shoulder should be performed, including inspection, palpation, ROM measurements, muscle strength testing, instability testing, and administration of the Beighton scale. The most common clinical findings of congenital glenoid hypoplasia are painful, limited motion (mostly in abduction), and localized tenderness. Shoulder instability may be present due to deficient inferior glenoid bone stock; however, no laxity will be evident upon ligamentous testing, and the Beighton scale will be normal. Associated findings may include webbing of the axilla, spina bifida, thoracic hemivertebra, and cervical ribs.

Diagnostic Tests. Plain x-rays will suffice for evaluation of the presence and severity of congenital glenoid hypoplasia. Wirth, et al. (1993) devised a grading system to classify the severity of the radiographic features found in congenital glenoid hypoplasia. A grade of "mild" describes a shallow (possibly dentate) glenoid fossa with slight irregularity and underdevelopment of a portion of the scapular neck and glenoid rim. A "moderate" grade describes shoulders with absence of the inferior aspect of the glenoid rim and scapular neck, along with an irregular, elongated-appearing glenoid. Lastly, a "severe" grade involves extensive hypoplasia of the inferior glenoid, which appears to be contiguous with the lateral scapular border, flattening and varus angulation of the humeral head, inferior joint irregularity, hooked distal clavicle, enlarged, angulated acromion, and a prominent coracoid process (p. 1176). A CT scan with 3-D reconstructions is an invaluable diagnostic study for preoperative planning.

Common Therapeutic Modalities

Nonsurgical Management. Conservative measures used to treat congenital glenoid hypoplasia include PT, NSAIDs, cryotherapy and/or heat, and activity modification. Patients should avoid activities that cause pain or reproduce symptoms.

Surgical Management. A total shoulder arthroplasty is a surgical option for the treatment of congenital glenoid hypoplasia if the patient has exhausted all conservative measures and still remains symptomatic. There are three options available for treatment of the deficient bone during a total shoulder arthroplasty, including bone grafting in conjunction with placement of a glenoid component, bone grafting or osteotomy in conjunction with a hemiarthroplasty, and a glenoid component reinforced inferoposteriorly with additional metal to fill in the defect (Sperling, Cofield, & Steinmann, 2002). Shoulder arthroplasty remains more technically challenging in the hypoplastic glenoid shoulder due, in part, to the limited number of patients from which to gain knowledge and expertise.

Nursing Considerations

Nursing Diagnoses. Nursing diagnoses for this condition are expanded upon in the Appendix.

- Activity intolerance.
- Coping, ineffective.
- Disuse syndrome, risk for.
- Infection, risk for.
- Knowledge deficit.
- Mobility: physical, impaired.
- Noncompliance.
- Pain, acute.
- Pain, chronic.
- Role performance, ineffective.
- Self-care deficit: bathing/hygiene, dressing/grooming, feeding, toileting.

Interventions. *Preventing/minimizing complications:* The sooner congenital glenoid hypoplasia is diagnosed, the earlier PT and activity modification may be initiated in an effort to prevent or slow the progression of secondary osteoarthritis. Please refer to the subsection "Preventing/minimizing complications" in the section on Arthritis of the Shoulder in this chapter for additional information.

Activity/positioning: The rationale for activity modification in patients with congenital glenoid hypoplasia is to slow the progression of secondary osteoarthritis as previously mentioned. Moreover, some patients with a hypoplastic glenoid may also have instability due to lack of bone stock, which may warrant additional modification of activities; specifically, repetitive overhead use of the arm, along with contact or collision sports, should be avoided. Likewise, any activities or positions that aggravate symptoms or cause pain should be avoided.

Emotional support: Patients may appreciate emotional support and reassurance if they are no longer able to continue with their current vocation because of progression of symptoms. Athletes may benefit from emotional support, as they may need to change or decrease their training routine, miss practice or competition/games, or stop participating in their chosen sport altogether.

Patient Teaching. *Activity/restrictions:* Patients should be strongly encouraged to comply with all activity modifications and restrictions. The importance of adhering to the shoulder rehabilitation program, in addition to continuation of a HEP long-term, should be stressed.

Medications: NSAIDs, acetaminophen, and narcotics may be prescribed to alleviate pain and/or inflammation. As with any medication, patients should be instructed on their proper use, including indications, dosage, frequency, side effects, and when to stop the medication and call the prescribing provider.

Incisional care: Please refer to the subsection "Incision care" in the section on Arthritis of the Shoulder in this chapter for information on patient education after total shoulder arthroplasty.

Referred Visceral Somatic Pain

Overview

Definition and Etiology. The term "referred pain" is used to describe pain that is localized to a different site than its origin, but remains within the same nerve root distribution. Referred pain may be either visceral or somatic. "Visceral pain" is a term used to describe pain originating from the viscus. The term "somatic pain" is often referred to as musculoskeletal pain. Both visceral and somatic pain may be referred to the shoulder (Figure 18.4).

Pathophysiology. Visceral nociceptors are innervated by afferent fibers of the autonomic nervous system and respond to mechanical stimuli and chemical irritation. At the onset, visceral pain is usually described as aching, grawing, or cramping, and is poorly localized in the midline of the body. Over time, the pain becomes sharp and localized to a somatic structure. Referred visceral pain is thought to be the result of the lack of a dedicated sensory pathway in the brain for visceral signals. The sensory neurons from the viscera converge in the brain with sensory pathways carrying somatic signals, which causes the signals to mix. Consequently, the brain misinterprets the signals from the viscera as those coming from the skin, muscles, and joints.

Incidence. The exact incidence of referred shoulder pain is unknown, given the many medical conditions with the potential to refer pain to the shoulder region.

Risk Factors. Risk factors for the development of referred shoulder pain are dependent upon the predisposition to, or presence of, medical conditions that have the potential to refer pain to the shoulder.

Complications. The most serious complication of referred shoulder pain (either visceral or somatic) is when the source of pain is overlooked or misdiagnosed, with potentially life-threatening consequences. Another complication of referred shoulder pain is the phenomenon of lingering shoulder pain even though the pain at the origin has resolved, which results in chronic pain and disability.

Preventive Strategies. There is no specific strategy to prevent referred pain to the shoulder, other than avoidance of the medical conditions that are capable of referring pain to the shoulder.

Special Considerations. Advancing age seems to coincide with an increased propensity to develop pathological conditions involving the viscera. In the elderly, the presentation of pain from any source is often atypical and accompanied by an increased pain threshold; therefore, shoulder pain may be the only complaint in an elderly person, who could have a potentially life-threatening problem.

Assessment

History. A thorough history of the referred shoulder pain, including the characteristics and any associated symptoms, should be elicited from the patient. The mnemonic device "OPQRST" is helpful to use when gathering details about the history of shoulder pain: Onset, Provocation/palliation, Quality, Region/radiation, Severity, and Timing. The presence of associated symptoms is not a common finding with intrinsic shoulder conditions and should trigger the exploration of an alternate source of the pain. Lastly, the presence of shoulder pain prior to the onset of associated symptoms suggests that the pain is originating from an extrinsic visceral or somatic source rather than the shoulder itself, and has the potential to linger long after the cause of the referred pain has resolved.

Figure 18.4.
Referred Shoulder Pain

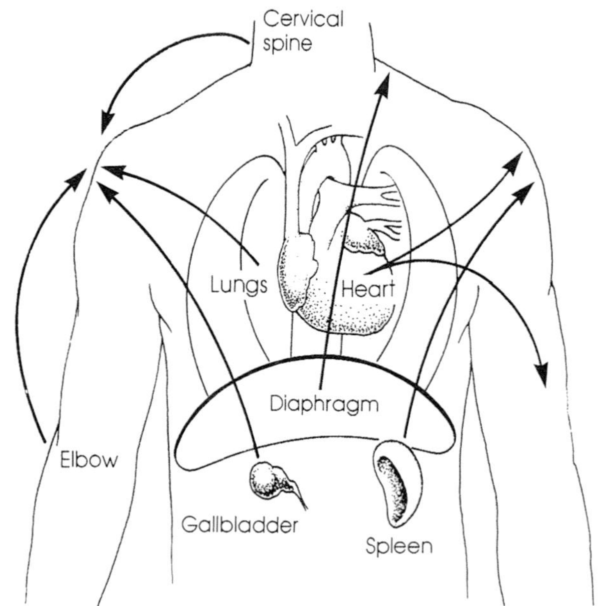

From Orthopedic Physical Assessment *(2nd ed., p. 125), by D. Magee, 1992, Philadelphia, PA: W.B. Saunders. Reproduced with permission.*

Physical Exam. A comprehensive physical examination of the shoulder is a requisite to establishing the correct etiology of shoulder pain, which holds true even if there is a strong suspicion that no intrinsic shoulder pathology exists. Physical examination of the shoulder will essentially be normal, or near normal, if the pain is referred from elsewhere.

Diagnostic Tests. Plain x-rays are the imaging modality of choice for the initial evaluation of shoulder pain. A general rule of thumb when obtaining plain x-rays of the shoulder is to obtain two views perpendicular to each other. A true AP view, along with either an axillary or lateral scapular view, will satisfy this criteria and serve as a screening tool to rule out intrinsic shoulder pathology as the cause of pain.

Common Therapeutic Modalities

The source of referred shoulder pain must be correctly identified to devise an effective treatment plan for eradication of the pain at the shoulder and at its source. Referred pain at the shoulder may be treated symptomatically with conservative modalities. Unfortunately, the shoulder pain may linger and require continued treatment after the source of the pain has resolved.

Nursing Considerations

Nursing Diagnoses. Nursing diagnoses for this condition are expanded upon in the Appendix.

- Anxiety.
- Coping, ineffective.
- Disuse syndrome, risk for.
- Family coping, compromised.
- Family process, interrupted.
- Fear.
- Home maintenance, impaired.
- Mobility: physical, impaired.
- Noncompliance.
- Pain, acute.
- Pain, chronic.
- Role performance, ineffective.
- Self-care deficit: bathing/hygiene, dressing/grooming, feeding, toileting
- Self-concept, readiness for enhancement.

Interventions. *Preventing/minimizing complications:* Proper diagnosis and treatment of the underlying cause of referred shoulder pain is crucial to preventing morbidity and mortality related to the origin of pain, such as myocardial ischemia. Ideally, treatment of the underlying medical condition will result in concomitant resolution of the shoulder pain.

Activity/positioning: There are no specific activity restrictions or positioning recommendations for referred shoulder pain, other than the avoidance of activities or positions that cause pain or aggravate symptoms.

Patient Teaching. *Activity:* As mentioned above, patients should be instructed to avoid all activities that cause shoulder pain or exacerbate symptoms. Activities that do not cause an exacerbation of pain or symptoms, including ADLs and sports, may be continued. In fact, guarding a painful shoulder may increase the likelihood of developing a frozen shoulder or disuse osteopenia.

Medications: NSAIDs, acetaminophen, and rarely narcotics may be prescribed for symptomatic relief of referred shoulder pain. An intra-articular injection of corticosteroids should not be used for treatment of referred shoulder pain due to the absence of intrinsic shoulder pathology.

Practice Setting Considerations. *Office/outpatient:* A patient who presents to the office with referred shoulder pain may require a referral for evaluation and management of the origin (source) of pain. Patients may present to the office with fulminant signs and symptoms of a very serious, potentially life-threatening medical condition, which requires activation of the local EMS or "911" or immediate treatment in the nearest emergency department.

Summary

Forward elevation of the shoulder enables the hand to function in front of the body. To accomplish this important functional motion, the shoulder joint has the most mobility and least stability of all joints, making it vulnerable to acute traumatic or chronic overuse injuries. The shoulder may also be afflicted by a number of rare congenital conditions. Prompt recognition, diagnosis, and treatment are essential to caring for the patient with a shoulder complaint, no matter what the condition. The goal of shoulder treatment is to prevent altogether, or at least lessen, the chance of developing chronic shoulder pain, dysfunction, and disability.

References

Afsari, A. (2011). *Anterior glenohumeral instability.* Retrieved October 25, 2011, from http://emedicine.medscape.com/article/1262004-overview.

American Academy of Orthopaedic Surgeons (AAOS). (2007). *Fracture of the shoulder blade (Scapula).* Retrieved August 25, 2010, from http://www.orthoinfo.aaos.org

American Academy of Orthopaedic Surgeons (AAOS). (2007). *Rotator cuff tears and treatment options.* Retrieved August 25, 2010, from http://www.orthoinfo.aaos.org

American College of Rheumatology/European League Against Rheumatism Collaborative Initiative. (2010). 2010 Rheumatoid arthritis classification criteria. *Arthritis & Rheumatism, 62*(9), 2569-2581.

Andermahr, J., Ring, D.C., & Jupiter, J.B. (2007). Fractures of the clavicle. In J. P. Iannotti & G.R. Williams Jr. (Eds.), *Disorders of the Shoulder: Diagnosis & Management* (2nd ed.,Vol. 2, pp. 943-976). Philadelphia, PA: Lippincott Williams & Wilkins.

Basamania, C.J. & Rockwood Jr., C.A. (2009). Fractures of the clavicle. In C.A. Rockwood & F.A. Matsen III (Eds.), *The shoulder* (4th ed.,Vol. 1, pp. 295-332). Philadelphia, PA: Saunders Elsevier.

Bohsali, K.I. & Wirth, M.A. (2009). Fractures of the proximal humerus. In C.A. Rockwood & F.A. Matsen III, (Eds.), *The shoulder* (4th ed.,Vol. 1, pp. 295-332). Philadelphia, PA: Saunders Elsevier.

Cavendish, M. (1972). Congenital elevation of the scapula. *Journal of Bone and Joint Surgery, British, 54-B*(3), 395-408.

Choi, P.D., Chan, G., Skaggs, D. L., & Flynn, J. M. (2009). Fractures, dislocations, and acquired problems of the shoulder in children. In C.A. Rockwood & F.A. Matsen III, (Eds.), *The shoulder* (4th ed., Vol. 1, pp. 583-616). Philadelphia, PA: Elsevier Saunders.

Codman, E.A. (1934). *The shoulder: Rupture of the supraspinatus tendon and other lesions in or about the subacromial bursa.* Boston, MA: Thomas Todd Company.

Codsi, M.J., & Iannotti, J.P. (2007). Techniques for revision arthroplasty: Management of bone and soft tissue loss. In J.P. Iannotti & G.R. Williams Jr. (Eds.), *Disorders of the Shoulder: Diagnosis & Management* (2nd ed.,Vol. 2, pp. 773-790), Philadelphia, PA: Lippincott Williams & Wilkins.

Collins, D.N. (2007). Pathophysiology, classification, and pathoanatomy of glenohumeral arthritis and related disorders. In J.P. Iannotti & G.R. Williams (Eds.), *Disorders of the Shoulder: Diagnosis & Management* (2nd ed.,Vol. 1, p. 595). Philadelphia, PA: Lippincott, Williams & Wilkins.

Collins, D.N. (2009). Disorders of the joint. In C.A. Rockwood & F.A. Matsen III, (Eds.), *The shoulder* (4th ed.,Vol. 1, pp. 453-514). Philadelphia, PA: Saunders Elsevier.

Cuomo, F. & Holloway, G. (2007). Diagnosis and management of the stiff shoulder. In J.P. Iannotti & G.R. Williams (Eds.), *Disorders of the Shoulder: Diagnosis & Management* (2nd ed.,Vol. 1, pp. 541-559). Philadelphia, PA: Lippincott Williams & Wilkins.

Endres, N.K., El Hassan, B., Higgins, L.D., & Warner, J.J. (2009). The stiff shoulder. In C.A. Rockwood & F.A. Matsen III, (Eds.), *The shoulder* (4th ed.,Vol. 2, pp. 1405-1435). Philadelphia, PA: Saunders Elsevier.

Engel, D. (1943). The etiology of the undescended scapula and related syndromes. *Journal of Bone & Joint Surgery, American, 25*(3), 613-625.

Galatz, L., & Kim, H. (2007). Minimally invasive techniques for proximal humeral fractures. In J.P. Iannotti & G.R. Williams Jr. (Eds.), *Disorders of the Shoulder: Diagnosis & Management* (2nd ed.,Vol. 2, pp. 873-888). Philadelphia, PA: Lippincott Williams & Wilkins.

Gamradt, S.C., Williams III, R.J., & Warren, R.F. (2009). Shoulder arthroscopy: Arthroscopic treatment of shoulder instability. In C.A. Rockwood & F.A. Matsen III, (Eds.), *The shoulder* (4th ed., Vol. 2, pp. 940-960). Philadelphia, PA: Saunders Elsevier.

Goss, T.P. & Owens, B.D. (2007). Fractures of the scapula: diagnosis and treatment. In J.P. Iannotti & G.R. Williams (Eds.), *Disorders of the Shoulder: Diagnosis & Management* (2nd ed.,Vol. 2, pp. 793-840). Philadelphia, PA: Lippincott Williams & Wilkins.

Grogan, D.P., Stanley, E.A., & Bobechko, W.P. (1983). The congenital undescended scapula: Surgical correction by the Woodward procedure. *Journal of Bone & Joint Surgery, British, 65-B*(5), 598-605.

Gupta, K. & Bhagia, S.M. (2010). *Rheumatoid arthritis.* Retrieved August 3, 2010, from http://emedicine.medscape.com/article/305417

Hypermobility Syndrome Association (HSA). (2011). *Beighton score.* Retrieved October 27, 2011, from http://www.hypermobility.org/beighton.php

Jobe, C.M., Coen, M.J., & Screnar, P. (2000). Evaluation of impingement syndromes in the overhead-throwing athlete. *Journal of Athletic Training, 35*(3), 293-299.

Kessel, L. & Watson, M. (1977). The painful arc syndrome. *Journal of Bone & Joint Surgery, British, 59*(2), 166-172.

Kierns, M.A. & Whitman, J.M. (2009). Nonoperative treatment of shoulder impingement. In K.E. Wilk, M.M. Reinhold, & J.R. Andrews (Eds.), *The Athlete's Shoulder* (2nd ed., pp. 527-544), Philadelphia, PA: Saunders Elsevier.

Kozlowski, K., Colavita, N., Morris, L., & Little, K.E.T. (1985). Bilateral glenoid dysplasia (report of 8 cases). *Australasian Radiology, 29*(2), 174-177.

Krishnan, S.G., Harkins, D.C., & Burkhead Jr., W.Z. (2007). Alternatives to replacement arthroplasty for glenohumeral arthritis. In J.P. Iannotti & G.R. Williams Jr. (Eds.), *Disorders of the Shoulder: Diagnosis & Management* (2nd ed.,Vol. 1, pp. 655-673), Philadelphia, PA: Saunders Elsevier.

Kuhn, J.E. (2009). Exercise in the treatment of rotator cuff impingement: A systematic review and a synthesized evidence-based rehabilitation protocol. *Journal of Shoulder and Elbow Surgery, 18*, 138-160.

Lazarus, M.D. (2008). *Glenohumeral arthritis.* Retrieved August 1, 2010, from http://emedicine.medscape.com/article/1261152

Leggin, B.G. & Kelley, M.J. (2007). Disease-specific methods of rehabilitation. In J.P. Iannotti & G.R. Williams Jr. (Eds.), *Disorders of the Shoulder: Diagnosis & Management* (2nd ed.,Vol. 2, pp. 1265-1294), Philadelphia, PA: Lippincott Williams & Wilkins.

Lintner, D.M., Sebastianelli, W.J., Hanks, G.A., & Kalenak, A. (1992). Glenoid dysplasia: A case report and review of the literature. *Clinical Orthopaedics and Related Research, 283*, 145-148.

Magee, D.J. (1992). *Orthopedic physical assessment* (2nd ed., p. 125). Philadelphia, PA: W.B. Saunders.

Magrey, M. & Abelson, A. (2010). *Laboratory evaluation of rheumatic diseases.* Retrieved October, 25, 2011, from http://clevelandclinicmeded.com/medicalpubs/diseasemanagement/rheumatology/laboratory-evaluation-rheumatic-diseases/.

Manske, R.C. & Prohaska, D. (2008). Diagnosis and management of adhesive capsulitis. *Current Reviews of Musculoskeletal Medicine, 1*(3-4), 180-189.

Matsen III, F.A., Lippitt, S.B., Alexander, B., Rockwood Jr., C.A., & Wirth, M.A. (2009). Glenohumeral instability. In C.A. Rockwood & F.A. Matsen III, (Eds.), *The shoulder* (4th ed., Vol. 1, pp. 617-770). Philadelphia, PA: Saunders Elsevier.

Matsen III, F.A. & Warme, W.J. (2009). *Shoulder arthritis: Osteoarthritis, chondrolysis, rheumatoid arthritis, degenerative joint disease arthritis after shoulder surgery.* Retrieved September 1, 2010, from http://www.orthop.washington.edu/uw/shoulderarthritis.

Mayo Foundation for Medical Education and Research (MFMER). (2009). *Rheumatoid arthritis.* Retrieved August 5, 2010, from http://www.mayoclinic.com/health/rheumatoid-arthritis/DS00020.

McMurtry, I., Bennet, G.C., & Bradish, C. (2005). Osteotomy for congenital elevation of the scapula (Sprengel's deformity). *Journal of Bone & Joint Surgery, 87-B*(7), 986-989.

Miniaci, A., Haynes, D.E., Williams Jr., G.R., & Iannotti, J.P. (2007). Anterior and anteroinferior instability: Open and arthroscopic management. In J.P. Iannotti & G.R. Williams Jr. (Ed.), *Disorders of the Shoulder: Diagnosis & Management* (2nd ed., Vol. 1, pp. 369-399). Philadelphia, PA: Lippincott Williams & Wilkins.

Moosikasuwan, J.B., Miller, T.T., & Burke, B.J. (2005). Rotator cuff tears: Clinical, radiographic, and US findings. *RadioGraphics, 25*(6), 1591-1607.

National Institute of Arthritis and Musculoskeletal and Skin Diseases (NIAMS). (2009). *What is rheumatoid arthritis?* Retrieved August 3, 2010, from www.niams.nih.gov.

Neer, C.S. II (1983). Impingement lesions. *Clinical Orthopaedics and Related Research, 3*(173), 70-77.

Neer, C.S. II (1970). Displaced proximal humeral fractures: Part I. Classification and evaluation. *Journal of Bone and Joint Surgery, American, 52*(6), 1077-1089.

Neviaser, R. & Hannafin, J. (2010). Adhesive capsulitis: A review of current treatment. *American Journal of Sports Medicine, 38*(11), 2346-56.

Neviaser, R.J. & Neviaser, T.J. (1987). The frozen shoulder: Diagnosis and management. *Clinical Orthopaedics and Related Research*, 223, 59-64.

Parsons IV., I.M., Weldon III., E.J. Titelman, R.M., & Smith, K.L. (2004). Glenohumeral arthritis and its management. *Physical Medicine and Rehabilitation Clinics of North America, 15*, 447-474.

Rockwood, C.A. & Lyons, F.R. (1993). Shoulder impingement syndrome: Diagnosis, radiographic evaluation, and treatment with a modified Neer acromioplasty. *Journal of Bone and Joint Surgery, American, 75*(3), 409-424.

Salter, R.B. & Harris, W.R. (1963). Injuries involving the epiphyseal plate. *Journal of Bone and Joint Surgery, American, 45*(3), 587-622.

Sher, J.S., Levy, J.C., Iannotti, J.P., & Williams Jr., G.R. (2007). Diagnosis of glenohumeral instability. In J.P. Iannotti, & G.R. Williams Jr. (Eds.), *Disorders of the Shoulder: Diagnosis and Management* (2nd ed., Vol. 1, pp. 339-367). Philadelphia, PA: Lippincott Williams & Wilkins.

Shiel, J.W. (2010). *Osteoarthritis.* Retrieved September 6, 2010, from http://www.medicinenet.com/osteoarthritis/article.htm

Singh, J.A., Furst, D.E., Bharat, A., Curtis, J.R., Kavanaugh, A.F., Kremer, J.M., ...Saag, K.G. (2012). 2012 Update of the 2008 American College of Rheumatology recommendations for the use of disease-modifying antirheumatic drugs and biologic agents in the treatment of rheumatoid arthritis. *Arthritis Care & Research, 64*(5), 625-639.

Slaney, S.L. & Wahl, C.J. (2009). *Arthroscopic shoulder surgery for shoulder dislocation, subluxation and instability: Why, when and how it is done.* Retrieved September 14, 2010, from http://www.orthop.washington.edu/shoulderscope.

Smith, S. & Bunker, T. (2001). Primary glenoid dysplasia. *Journal of Bone and Joint Surgery, British, 83-B*(6), 868-872.

Sperling, J.W., Cofield, R.H., & Steinmann, S.P. (2002). Shoulder arthroplasty for osteoarthritis secondary to glenoid dysplasia. *Journal of Bone and Joint Surgery, American, 84-A*(4), 541-546.

Thomas, T., Noel, E., Goupille, P., Duquesnoy, B., & Combe, B. (2006). The rheumatoid shoulder: Current consensus on diagnosis and treatment. *Journal of Joint, Bone and Spine, 73*(2), 139-143.

Tom, A., Mazzocca, A.D., & Pavlatos, C.J. (2009). Acromioclavicular joint injuries. In K.E. Wilk, M. M. Reinold, & J.R. Andrews (Eds.), *The Athlete's Shoulder* (2nd ed., pp. 303-313). Philadelphia, PA: Saunders Elsevier.

Trout, T. & Resnick, D. (1996). Glenoid hypoplasia and its relationship to instability. *Skeletal Radiology, 25*(1), 37-40.

Wheeless, C.R. (2010a). *RA: Clincial aspects.* Retrieved September 3, 2010, http://www.wheelessonline.com

Wheeless, C.R. (2010b). *Clavicle fractures.* Retrieved August 24, 2010, from http://wheelessonline.com

Williams Jr., G.R. & Iannotti, J.P. (2007). Unconstrained prosthetic arthroplasty for glenohumeral arthritis with an intact or repairable rotator cuff: Indications, techniques, and results. In J.P. Iannotti & G.R. Williams Jr. (Eds.), *Disorders of the Shoulder: Diagnosis and Management* (2nd ed., Vol. 2, pp. 697-726), Philadelphia, PA: Lippincott Williams & Wilkins.

Wirth, M., Lyons, F., & Rockwood, J.C. (1993). Hypoplasia of the glenoid. A review of sixteen patients. *Journal of Bone and Joint Surgery, American*, 75-A(8), 1175-1184.

Zuckerman, J.P. & Sahajpal, D.T. (2007). Fracture of the proximal humerus: Classification, diagnosis, and nonoperative Management. In J.P. Iannotti & G.R. Williams Jr. (Eds.), *Disorders of the Shoulder: Diagnosis and Management* (2nd ed., Vol. 2, pp. 841-866). Philadelphia, PA: Lippincott Williams & Wilkins.

Chapter 19
The Elbow

Rebecca A. Perz, MSN, NP-C, ONP-C

Objectives

- Recognize common interventions to provide safety and prevent injury for patients with elbow conditions.
- Describe the pathophysiology of common elbow conditions.
- List the potential life-changing and limiting consequences of elbow conditions.
- Identify assessment criteria for each elbow condition or injury.
- Identify key subjective components in obtaining the history of the elbow condition.
- Select common tests to establish definitive diagnoses.
- List potential differential diagnoses related to elbow conditions.
- Describe outcome criteria for patients with elbow conditions.
- Develop nursing diagnoses and interventions for patients with elbow problems.

The elbow joint is one of the most useful joints in the body. It allows for basic functions such as eating, grooming, and other self-care activities, as well as allowing the individual to push, pull, or lift objects. Full function of the elbow is particularly important when the injury or condition pertains to the individual's dominant arm.

The elbow may be injured or dislocated in both children and adults. It is susceptible to injury due to repetitive use such as with manual laborers or those participating in sports activities (especially tennis players, golfers, and baseball pitchers). As the elbow is essential for full function of the arm, the patient who sustains an injury must not only heal the injured area but attempt to regain range of motion (ROM) as soon as possible in order to achieve the best possible outcomes. This often requires sound decision making on the part of the provider caring for the patient, a team approach to care including therapists, and motivation and understanding of the potential severity and complications of elbow injuries by the patient. Team efforts are needed to coordinate this patient care. This includes prehospital and first aid care, emergency/urgent care, and follow-up care in the hospital such as an orthopaedic unit or in the outpatient clinic setting. Most injuries to the elbow benefit from physical and occupational therapy to promote the highest level of functioning possible for these patients.

Care of the elbow has changed significantly in recent years. Elbow replacements (whether full or partial), arthroscopy, suture anchors for repair of tendon rupture, and other elbow-specific hardware have all made an impact in the care of the patient with an elbow injury.

Anatomy and Key Points Related to the Elbow

It is important to understand the anatomy of the joint to better clarify the potential problems that can arise from an injured or diseased elbow. The elbow is a hinge joint, consisting of the distal humerus (including medial epicondyle and lateral epicondyle), proximal ulna, olecranon, proximal radius, and radial head (see Figure 19.1). Each of these bones has significant muscular attachments that allow the entire joint to flex, extend, supinate, and pronate. The shoulder and wrist muscles are both connected at the elbow, and this partnership of anatomy needs to be disrupted as little as possible. Elbow injuries will thus affect the joints above and below them significantly, with associated weakness, stiffness, atrophy, and other problems.

The elbow is stabilized by the coronoid process and the radial head, preventing posterior displacement, and by the olecranon, preventing anterior displacement. The articulation of these bones allows the greatest ROM, and provides medial and lateral stability.

Figure 19.1. Elbow Anatomy

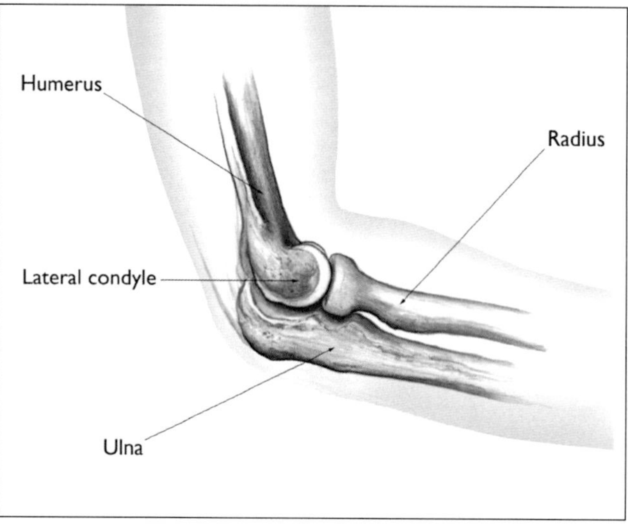

From The 2003 Body Almanac *by the American Academy of Orthopaedic Surgeons, 2003. Reprinted with permission.*

When radiographs are taken of the elbow, two views should always be obtained: anteroposterior (AP) and lateral. Elbow fractures may not be visible when the patient presents to be seen. It is important to always look for a "fat pad sign" on the lateral x-ray, which may be noted on the anterior and posterior aspects of the humerus (see Figure 19.2). It arises when the adipose tissue overlaying the joint capsule displaces if there is an effusion or hemarthrosis due to fracture (Egol, Koval, & Zuckerman, 2010). A positive fat pad sign is generally

Figure 19.2. Lateral X-Ray Image of Positive Fat Pad Sign

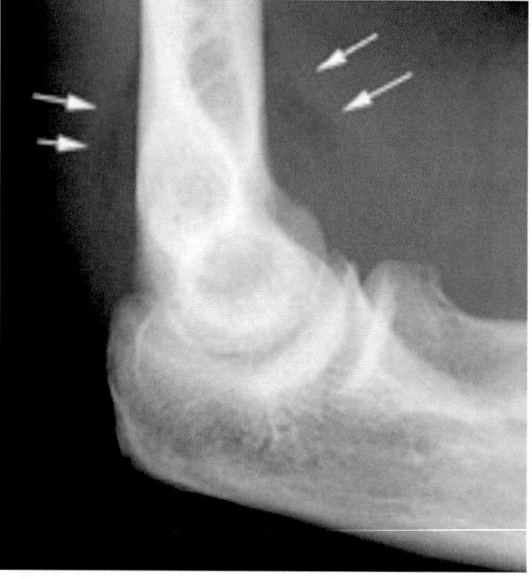

From "Interactive Atlas of Signs in Musculoskeletal Radiology" by A. Gentili, M. Beller, S. Masih, and L. Seeger, http://www.gentili.net/signs/images/400/Elbowsfatpadarrow.jpg. Reproduced with permission.

CHAPTER 19

Figure 19.3.
X-Ray Image of MO of the Elbow

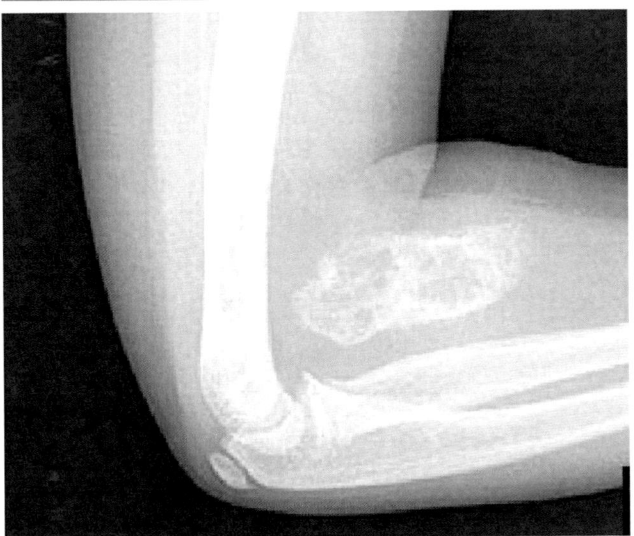

From "Myositis Ossificans Mimicking Compartment Syndrome of the Forearm" by E. Melamed and D. Angel, 2008, Orthopedics, 31 *(12). orthosupersite.com/view.asp?rID=32936. Reproduced with permission.*

indicative of fracture, and the patient should be treated as having a fracture until proven otherwise.

Any patient with an elbow injury, whether pediatric or adult, has the potential to develop heterotopic bone, also known as myositis ossificans (MO). (See Figure 19.3.) Incidence of MO can be as high as 30% in elbow fracture-dislocations (Strauss et al., 2011). In these cases, injured muscles changes into heterotopic bone, which causes capsular tightness and often leads to a significant loss of function in the elbow as the muscles lose their ability to stretch (Berg, 2000; Egol et al., 2010). This will be noted on subsequent x-rays after a crush injury, dislocation, or fracture with associated soft tissue trauma. It occurs in 3% of dislocations, and 18% when associated with fracture/dislocations (Egol et al., 2010). It is seen more often in patients under the age of 30, and men are more affected than women (Reiser, Baur-Melnyk, & Glaser, 2008). Treatment for MO is aimed at prophylaxis, i.e., avoiding prolonged muscle trauma in reducing dislocations (particularly if the reduction was attempted several times), using ice after muscle trauma, and treating with either non-steroidal anti-inflammatories (NSAIDs) to prevent development. Indomethacin 75mg SR (given once or twice daily, pending surgeon preference) is often the drug of choice, but in the pediatric population, ibuprofen or other NSAIDs may be used. If MO develops, careful monitoring of functioning, early mobilization, and occasionally surgical removal of the heterotopic bone may be performed (Berg, 2000; Reiser et al., 2008).

Research on the use of radiation therapy for elbow trauma is inconclusive. One recent retrospective study noted that patients who received a single prophylactic dose of radiation therapy within the first day after surgery, in addition to NSAIDS, had significantly smaller incidence and amount of MO. The amount of MO did not impair the patients, and no adverse side effects were noted from the single dose of radiation therapy. This may be considered an adjunct of therapy in high-risk patients (Strauss et al., 2011). Another study evaluating the use of radiation therapy in prophylaxis of MO after elbow trauma, however, noted an increased incidence of nonunion in the patients. The significance of nonunion of these fractures was high enough that the study was terminated (Hamid et al., 2010). Because of these conflicting results, treatment at this time will most likely continue with use of NSAIDS.

Common Elbow Treatment Modalities

Physical therapy (PT) and occupational therapy (OT) are essential for maximizing healing for the patient after injury, surgery (from minor releases to major surgery such as replantation), and other trauma sustained to the elbow. Essential orthopaedic care includes therapy to regain joint function, control pain, maximize healing, and manage wound care. Many soft tissue sprains can be treated with the **PRICEMM** acronym: **P**rotection, **R**est, **I**ce, **C**ompression, **E**levation, **M**edications, **M**odalities (see Chapter 20—The Wrist).

Edema Reduction. Therapy can reduce edema by many modalities, including use of compressive dressings, early range of motion, splints, and passive ROM.

Wound Management. Physical and occupational therapists will examine the healing wound for different stages of healing. Different modalities, including use of whirlpool, ultrasound, medications and debridement may be used to manage the wound and optimize healing.

Scar Management. Therapy may reduce the development of hypertrophic scars, keloids, and disorganized collagen depositions, which alter the cellular matrix for healing. Scar management is also managed with massage and exercises such as pressure therapy with use of splints.

Range of Motion. Therapy will assist with active as well as passive ROM, allowing for earlier tendon strength, healing and preventing joint contracture. Skilled therapists will begin tendon glides and other means to increase ROM, but will follow protocols to prevent too early aggressive motion, which may cause rupture of the tendon repair.

Desensitization and Sensory Re-education. The nervous systems signals to the affected extremity are disrupted, and the stimuli received by the injured extremity need to be redirected so the central nervous system does not interpret these signals as painful or noxious stimuli. Desensitization uses different textures and surfaces to stimulate healing, including massage, contrast baths, fluid therapy, exposure to different textures, such as towels, rice, sand, and dried beans, to decrease hypersensitivity.

Other Modalities. Other modalities used by physical and occupational therapists include soft-tissue mobilization, strengthening, work hardening, and conditioning. The therapist may use different techniques in addition to the above described contrast baths and ultrasound, which include fluidotherapy, cryotherapy, continuous passive motion, phonophoresis, iontophoresis, transcutaneous electrical nerve stimulation, and neuromuscular electrical stimulation.

Lateral and Medial Epicondylitis

Overview

Definitions. *Lateral epicondylitis* is irritation and inflammation of the extensor tendons that originated from the lateral epicondyle of the distal humerus. *Medial epicondylitis* is irritation and inflammation of the common flexor origin at the medial epicondyle of the distal humerus. The pain is at the flexor/pronator origin at the distal humerus.

Etiology. The common name for lateral epicondylitis is "tennis elbow" because this irritation comes from repetitive wrist motion in supination and extension (particularly repetitive backhand strokes for tennis players). The tendon gets inflamed and eventually develops microscopic tears, which is quite painful. The common name for medial epicondylitis is "golfer's elbow" because this irritation comes from repetitive activity in pronation (necessary for golf swings).

Pathophysiology. The extensor carpi radialis longus (ECRL) and extensor carpi radialis brevis (ECRB) originate at the lateral epicondyle. This tendon develops microscopic tears in lateral epicondylitis from repetitive trauma. The common flexor pronator (the common flexor origin) originates at the medial epicondyle and sustains a similar injury (Abrahams, Marks, & Hutchings, 2003; McMahon & Skinner, 2003). Cadaveric studies note that the tendons tear longitudinally, not intrasubstance but at the musculotendinous junction or avulsion fractures off the bone (Bunata, Brown, & Capelo, 2007).

Incidence. Lateral and medial epicondylitis are seen more frequently in patients who play tennis and golf, as suggested by the common names. In addition, patients who work in industries that involve significant repetitive squeezing activities of the hand are more susceptible to these tears and injuries. Examples of these activities include using hammers, trigger or spray guns, power washers, and paint guns (Garberina, Fagelman, & Getz, 2008a).

Complications. Complications of either lateral or medial epicondylitis are related to prolonged treatment or severe conditions. Either condition can be treated simply if caught early, but if not caught early, the treatment can be prolonged and may require surgery to repair. The patient may experience ongoing pain or functional limitations, including flexion contractures (Wise, Owens, & Binkley, 2011).

Assessment

History. Determine the mechanism of injury, repetitive use, and dominance of hand. It is important to note occupational and recreational/hobby activities that may precipitate development of either syndrome. Determine what treatment measures the patient has already tried, what relieves the symptoms, and what exacerbates the symptoms. Ascertain if the patient has a history of neck injury or pain, as some of the symptoms may be related to cervical radiculopathy (Garberina, et al., 2008a).

Physical Exam. Test the strength of the affected extremity compared to the nonaffected extremity, including biceps and triceps strength. Assess for neurovascular symptoms distal to the elbow, particularly if there is numbness or tingling noted. Assess ROM. Palpate along the lateral epicondyle and/or the medial epicondyle. Patients will often complain of significant pain with light or deep palpation of the area.

Diagnostic Tests. Two-view radiographs may be taken if there is concern of an avulsion injury to the elbow. Calcium deposits may be noted if calcific tendinitis has developed (McMahon & Skinner, 2003). On occasion, an electromyelogram may be performed if there is subsequent numbness, tingling, or other neurological symptoms distal to the elbow.

Common Therapeutic Modalities

Conservative treatment measures should be attempted first, but in spite of vigorous care and therapy, it is noted that 5%-10 % of individuals fail conservative treatment (Wise et al., 2011).

Decreasing Risk Factors. The first line treatment is generally avoidance of the repetitive activity and rest of the affected extremity.

Pain Management. Generally, NSAIDs will be given as analgesics. Ice may be used for pain control, applying 20 minutes at a time every 2 hours while awake, using a cross-friction massage technique.

Tennis Elbow Band or Wrist Extension Splint. Use of a tennis elbow band will displace the tissues on the proximal forearm, thus reducing the inflammation and pain along the extensor tendons. The wrist extension splint has been found to relieve pain in patients with tennis elbow (Getz, Parsons, & Ramsey, 2011).

PT/OT. Stretching and exercises can be effective in reducing pain and inflammation. Iontophoresis, a small electric charge that delivers medication through the skin (needle-less injection), is also a possible therapy modality.

Corticosteroids. Corticosteroid injections may also reduce pain and inflammation; however, weakening and possible degradation of the tendons may occur (Wise et al., 2011). The patient must be educated that the steroid injection does not make the problem go away or help the area heal; it only treats the symptoms. Time, removing the irritating source, and stretching and other exercises will help the area heal.

Surgical. Surgical treatment modalities for lateral epicondylitis are generally a last resort. The success rate of the surgery is often met with mixed results, and patients need to know that the symptoms may not completely disappear with surgery. The patient will require splinting, rest, and postoperative therapy. There will be lifting and repetitive activity restrictions for several months. There are different surgical measures for treatment of tennis elbow, involving the release of the common extensor origin (ECRB and ECRL) (McMahon & Skinner, 2003) or possibly the debridement of the tendon's degenerative areas. In the case of medial epicondylitis, the tendon is reattached to the medial epicondyle, instead of just releasing it, as the common flexor origin is an important stabilizer in the elbow (McMahon & Skinner, 2003).

Nursing Considerations

Nursing Diagnoses. Nursing diagnoses for this condition are expanded upon in the appendix.

- Body image, disturbed.
- Infection, risk for.
- Injury, risk for.
- Knowledge deficit.
- Pain, acute.
- Self-care deficit: bathing/hygiene, dressing/grooming, toileting, feeding.

Pitcher's Elbow

Overview

Definition. Pitcher's elbow arises from partial or complete tears of the ulnar collateral ligament (UCL). These tears are associated with repetitive injuries, such as seen with pitchers, particularly in youth.

Etiology. When pitching, the shoulder is in maximum external rotation. During the pitching motion, the pitcher must suddenly stop the elbow going backwards and throw the ball forward under a great deal of torque, in order to propel the ball with velocity. Frequent repetitive action of this nature causes microtrauma in the UCL, which can continue to tear and cause further damage if not allowed to rest or not treated appropriately.

Pathophysiology. Children have open growth plates, less developed muscles, and more lax ligaments. This repetitive forcing can cause avulsion fractures along the growth plate or near the insertion of the UCL (Fleisig, Weber, Hassell, & Andrews, 2009).

Incidence. Young adolescent males are at greatest risk for this injury. Statistics have shown that those who pitch more than "85 pitches per game, more than 9 months out of a year, or with arm fatigue" are more likely to require surgery and have significant problems with the elbow (Fleisig et al., 2009, p. 250).

Assessment

History. Assess when symptoms started. Often the pitcher may have had issues for several months or even years, in that pain was noted after a game, but these issues were not determined to be significant enough to warrant treatment. The duration of repetitive trauma may affect the outcome of this injury.

Physical Exam. Assess the elbow for swelling, pain and ecchymosis. Ask the patient to mimic the throwing motion, and assess for pain, swelling, and scar tissue. Establish hand dominance.

Diagnostic Tests. Two-view radiographs of the elbow may be obtained to rule out occult fracture or calcium deposits. On occasion, a computerized tomography (CT) scan or magnetic resonance imaging (MRI) of the elbow will be obtained to evaluate the medial ulnar collateral ligament (MUCL) for the extent of damage and integrity of the ligament itself.

Common Therapeutic Modalities

Conservative. The initial treatment is rest. The pitcher needs to not only rest between games but also have a limit to the number of pitches per game and total games played. Therapy is directed toward strengthening the arm, decreasing inflammation, teaching proper throwing/pitching techniques, strengthening the flexor pronator, and addressing thickening of the MUCL (Ahmad & ElAttrache, 2006).

Surgical. If the MUCL is instable, which will be determined by physical exam and valgus stress x-rays (an opening of >3mm is diagnostic of valgus instability), a surgical reconstruction of the elbow may be performed

(Ahmad & ElAttrache, 2006). The reconstruction will consist of tendon harvest, graft fixation, screw fixation, or a combination of these techniques.

Nursing Considerations

Nursing Diagnoses. Nursing diagnoses for this condition are expanded upon in the Appendix.

- Body image, disturbed.
- Infection, risk for.
- Injury, risk for.
- Knowledge deficit.
- Pain, acute.
- Self-care deficit: bathing/hygiene, dressing/grooming, toileting, feeding.

Olecranon Bursitis

Overview

Definition. Olecranon bursitis is inflammation of the olecranon bursal sac on the posterior aspect of the elbow, overlying the olecranon of the ulna. It is the only bursal sac on the elbow. The bursal sac gets inflamed and fills with fluid. As the sac gets fuller, pressure accumulates in the synovium and causes pain (Garberina, Fagelman, & Getz, 2008b).

Etiology. Bursitis can develop due to a direct blow to the elbow, or from repetitive trauma or use (such as constant leaning on the area), which causes the bursal sac to remain inflamed. Generally, it is a noninfectious process, and only 20% of cases are septic (Aaron, Patel, Kayiaros, & Calfee, 2011).

Incidence. Risk factors associated with this include age between 40 and 60 years, and increased incidence in those with chronic renal failure, gout, pseudogout, and rheumatoid arthritis. Approximately 3 out of every 1,000 outpatient visits are related to bursitis (Aaron et al., 2011; Garberina et al., 2008b). Patients receiving hemodialysis have a predisposition to developing bursitis on the extremity with the shunt (Aaron et al., 2011).

Complications. Complications related to bursitis include infection, chronicity of the bursal sac being inflamed, pain, and limitation of activity with subsequent elbow stiffness.

Assessment

History. Ask the patient when the symptoms started and whether there was any precipitating or repetitive trauma. Note any current or past fever, chills, or warmth around the elbow, as well as any changes in ROM since the symptoms began. Past medical history is important to ascertain, including renal disease, autoimmune disease, prior history of bursitis, and any bursitis treatment that the patient has already sought.

Physical Exam. Examine the patient's elbow for redness, swelling, or warmth. Generally it will be tender to palpate and sore upon attempting full ROM. Fluctuance will be noted over the olecranon. If stiffness or deformity is present, it may be due to underlying disease such as osteoarthritis or rheumatoid arthritis. Determine if the patient has constitutional symptoms such as fever, chills, or malaise, which may be indicative of infection, or septic bursitis.

Diagnostic Tests. Two-view x-rays of the elbow, AP and lateral, may be obtained to rule out any occult fracture (particularly if there is a trauma history), determine if a fat pad sign is evident, or note any calcium deposits. Aspiration of the bursal sac may be performed (Garberina et al., 2008b). If an aspiration is performed, fluid should be sent for white blood cell count to rule out infection and a fluid analysis to assess for crystals (such as gouty crystals).

Common Therapeutic Modalities

Conservative. The initial treatment for olecranon bursitis includes elbow rest, ice, anti-inflammatories, and compressive dressings. In addition, avoidance of the repetitive activity and rest of the affected extremity are important. The elbow may be placed in a posterior splint or sling to rest while waiting for the symptoms to abate.

Pain Management. Generally, NSAIDs will be given as analgesics. Ice may be used for pain control, applying 20 minutes at a time every 2 hours while awake, using a cross-friction massage technique.

Aspiration. An aspiration may be performed to remove the fluid from the sac. A compressive dressing should be placed on the elbow to prevent re-accumulation of fluid in the bursal sac. After the aspiration, occasionally a cortisone injection will be given into the bursal sac to reduce inflammation and reduce pain. If the aspirate appeared infected, the clinical exam of the bursa was suspicious for infection, or the cultures come back positive, antibiotics should be prescribed. Generally, dicloxacillin 500mg 4 times a day (or ciprofloxacin 750 mg twice a day for patients with penicillin allergy) is administered for 2 weeks (Garberina et al., 2008b). Follow-up is essential to ensure that the infection has resolved. If an infection is suspected, corticosteroids should not be administered.

Surgical. Rarely, the bursal sac may need to be excised in the operating room (OR), either via open incision or arthroscopically. After surgery, the patient will be placed in a posterior splint at 90 degrees to protect the area and prevent hematoma formation. Satisfactory outcomes are generally noted in patients who undergo surgical care (Aaron et al., 2011), but surgery is not performed as first line treatment.

Nursing Considerations

Nursing Diagnoses. Nursing diagnoses for this condition are expanded upon in the Appendix.

- Body image, disturbed.
- Infection, risk for.
- Injury, risk for.
- Knowledge deficit.
- Pain, acute.
- Self-care deficit: bathing/hygiene, dressing/ grooming, toileting, feeding.

Distal Biceps Tendon Rupture

Overview

Definition. A distal biceps tendon rupture is defined as a detachment of the distal biceps tendon from the radial tuberosity. This usually occurs as the result of a "sudden eccentric load placed on a flexed and supinated forearm" (Geaney & Mazzocca, 2009, p. 374), generally with overhead motion and lifting or sudden force.

Pathophysiology. The distal biceps tendon anchors the biceps muscles to the radial tuberosity. This provides for supination of the elbow and assists in flexion of the elbow.

Incidence. The incidence of rupture is more common in men, smokers, individuals in the 4th and 5th decades of life, and anabolic steroid users (Freeman, McCormick, Mahoney, Baratz, & Lubahn, 2009; Geaney & Mazzocca, 2009).

Complications. If the distal biceps is completely torn, the complications arise from loss of supination and strength in the affected extremity. The patient will lose strength and supination if this occurs. One study noted that supination strength was significantly different in operated individuals compared to those who did not have surgery. Flexion strength was not greatly affected by the lack of surgical repair (Freeman et al., 2009; Miyamoto, Elser, & Millett, 2010).

Assessment

History. Ascertain the mechanism of injury. Generally the patient will report a specific incident that caused the pain in the elbow. Once the initial pain resolves, chronic pain will ensue (Miyamoto et al., 2010). Weakness will be reported by the patient. The patient will often recall a "pop" or a sudden tearing pain in the inner aspect of the elbow.

Physical Exam. The patient will have weakness in the affected extremity. If the patient extends both arms, the affected arm will display a "Popeye" deformity in which the biceps retracts toward the humerus, causing a swelling just above the crease. There may be a palpable defect noted at the antecubital fossa where the distal biceps has separated from the radial tuberosity. In the acute phase, there will be ecchymosis and swelling in the anterior elbow.

Diagnostic Tests. Two-view (AP and lateral) x-rays will be taken of the elbow to look for fracture fragments from an avulsion fracture. A complete tear can be diagnosed by clinical exam, but a MRI will often be ordered to assess the biceps tendon and determine if the tear is partial or complete. If the date of the injury is indeterminate, it is much more important to have a MRI to evaluate retraction of the tendon and amenability to repair.

Common Therapeutic Modalities

Nonoperative Repair. This is rarely a chosen option. It is "reserved for sedentary patients who do not require elbow flexion and supination strength and endurance or for patients who are not medically fit for operative treatment" (Miyamoto et al., 2010, p. 2133). This conservative treatment consists of pain control, temporary splinting, and therapy for strengthening, ROM, and pain control, particularly if this becomes a chronic problem (Freeman et al, 2009; Miyamoto et al.; Sutton, Dodda, Ahmad, & Sethi, 2010).

Surgical Repair. A complete distal biceps tendon rupture needs to be repaired in the OR as soon as possible. Generally there is a 2-week window of time to do the repair before the tissue starts to shrink and travel up into the upper arm and becomes harder to repair. There are several different methods for fixation that include

Figure 19.4.
X-Ray of Proximal Radius

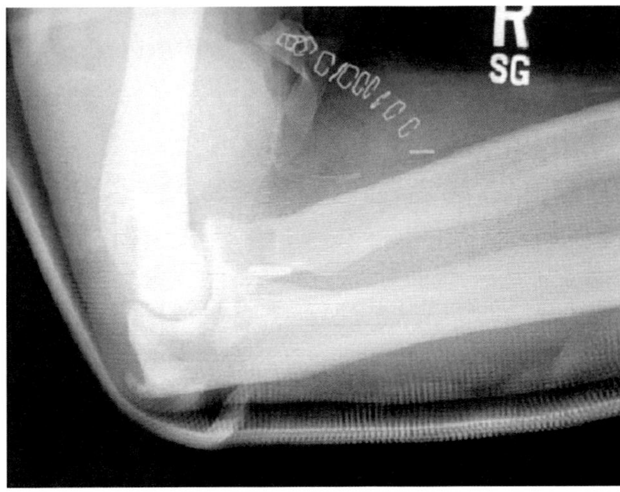

Author creation. Reproduced with permission.

CHAPTER 19

suture repair and/or use of specialized instruments to repair. Figure 19.4 shows one such method of repair, a biotenodesis interference screw with button-type anchor used to repair the distal biceps tendon.

The patient will need postoperative immobilization for several weeks to promote complete tendon-to-bone healing. The patient will usually be in a posterior splint for 1-2 weeks. As the healing occurs, the posterior splint will get changed to a hinged splint, initially set at 90 degrees of flexion. This prevents the patient from inadvertently stretching the elbow too much and rupturing the new repair. Strengthening will begin on or about 8 weeks after surgical repair (Sutton et al., 2010).

Nursing Considerations

Nursing Diagnoses. Nursing diagnoses for this condition are expanded upon in the Appendix.

- Body image, disturbed.
- Infection, risk for.
- Injury, risk for.
- Knowledge deficit.
- Pain, acute.
- Self-care deficit: bathing/hygiene, dressing/ grooming, toileting, feeding.

Radial Head, Monteggia, Coronoid Process, and Olecranon Fractures

Overview

Definitions. A *radial head fracture* is a fracture of the proximal radius. It is the "most common bony injury to the adult elbow" (Tashijian & Katarincic, 2006). A *Monteggia fracture* is a combination injury with a fracture of the ulna and disruption of the radiohumeroulnar joint. The radial head is typically dislocated (and sometimes fractured), allowing the compression forces to break the ulna. A *coronoid fracture* is a fracture of the coronoid process. This can be associated with elbow dislocation, radial head fracture, and instability. An *olecranon fracture* is a fracture of the olecranon on the proximal ulna. Olecranon fractures are almost always intra-articular, as the joint is involved due to the nature of the anatomy of the olecranon. Olecranon fractures are typically considered unstable fractures.

Etiology. Most elbow fractures are the result of trauma, typically from landing on the elbow in a fall or in a motor vehicle accident, or with an outstretched hand (Egol et al, 2010). In the elderly, the trauma may be secondary due to a medical reason for a fall such as a stroke, diabetes, or heart attack.

Pathophysiology. During an impact on the elbow joint, the bones absorb the weight from the fall, and fracture. Because the patient often tries to protect him-/herself in a fall, the arm is often outstretched, and the forces impact the elbow.

Incidence. Most radial head and neck fractures occur in patients between ages 30 and 40, and are more commonly seen in women (2:1) (Garberina, Fagelman, & Getz, 2008c; Reiser et al., 2008).

Complications. All elbow fractures, regardless if treatment is conservative or surgical, have the risk of decreased ROM after healing. The elbow gets stiff very easily, and these fractures require sustained immobilization for healing. It is imperative that the patient is able to attend therapy when the time is appropriate to decrease the incidence of this complication. For those patients who require a surgical repair, the risk of infection is also present. As with most elbow injuries, MO is also a possible complication (see Figure 19.3).

Assessment

History. Ascertain the mechanism of injury. Establish dominance of the patient's upper extremity. Assess whether the patient also injured another extremity in the fall. Determine the reason for the fall, particularly in the elderly, as the elbow injury may be minor compared to the reason for the fall.

Physical Exam. Palpate the elbow for pain. Examine for ecchymosis and swelling. Determine if the patient is able to flex, extend, supinate, and pronate. Compare the upper extremities for changes in appearance and musculature. Assess neurovascular status distal to the injury.

Diagnostic Tests. To correctly diagnose all of these four fractures, a two-view x-ray of the elbow (AP and lateral) will be obtained. In addition, a two-view x-ray of the wrist will also be obtained, as these types of fractures are often accompanied by wrist injuries. A CT scan may be obtained to determine the extent of the fracture and what type of surgical intervention may be needed.

Common Therapeutic Modalities

Conservative. *Radial head, nondisplaced:* A nondisplaced radial head fracture will be treated in a posterior splint and a sling for several weeks. Once callous formation is noted on the x-rays, the patient will begin a gentle ROM program.

Radial head, displaced: A displaced radial head fracture will be treated intraoperatively (see next section), as well as fractures with comminuted fragments.

Monteggia: Depending on the accompanying injury to the ulna, a Monteggia fracture is treated either conservatively or surgically. It is important to assess for the potential of this additional injury to the radial head when an individual has an injury to the ulna, as this can change the type of treatment performed (Egol et al., 2010).

Coronoid: A coronoid fracture may be treated nonsurgically if less than 15% of the coronoid process is involved, elbow instability is not noted, and the fracture does not occur in a pure transverse fashion (Steinmann, 2008). If there is an accompanying radial head fracture or lateral collateral ligament (LCL) injury, the patient will be treated surgically.

Olecranon: An olecranon fracture may be treated conservatively with splinting, but most often this will require a tension band or plating in the OR (see Figure 19.5 and Figure 19.6). If splinting is used, the patient will be in a splint or long-arm cast with the elbow in 45 to 90 degrees of flexion. ROM will be started after approximately 7 days (Egol et al., 2010).

Surgical. Surgical intervention is the treatment of choice for most elbow fractures. Common surgical care, including preventing infection, immobilization, neurovascular checks, and routine postoperative care, are necessary for any patient undergoing an open reduction internal fixation (ORIF).

Radial head, displaced: A radial head fracture with significant comminution will be treated with miniplates or with a metallic radial head replacement. If the radial head is absent, the elbow will lose 30% of valgus stability, so this is important to take into consideration in repair (Tashjian & Katarincic, 2006).

Coronoid: A coronoid fracture may be repaired with suture fixation, plates, and screw, and occasionally accompanied by radial head replacement (Steinmann, 2008).

Olecranon: An olecranon fracture can be treated with plates and screws if it is in a stable position, and the fracture is more distal on the ulna (see Figure 19.5). If the fracture is displaced, or occurs more proximally, generally a wire and tension band fixation (see Figure 19.6) will be used (Egol et al., 2010).

Nursing Considerations

Nursing Diagnoses. Nursing diagnoses for this condition are expanded upon in the Appendix.

- Body image, disturbed.
- Infection, risk for.
- Injury, risk for.
- Knowledge deficit.
- Pain, acute.
- Self-care deficit: bathing/hygiene, dressing/grooming, toileting, feeding.

Subluxation/Nursemaid's Elbow (Pediatric)

Overview

Definition. A subluxation of the elbow occurs when the annular ligament displaces, enabling the radial head to dislocate. This is called a "nursemaid's elbow," as this type of injury occurs when a child's hand is being held and a babysitter, or "nursemaid", tries to pull the child back by grabbing the hand with the arm in extension. As the elbow is extended and pronated at the same time, this causes the elbow to dislocate (Brown, 2009).

Pathophysiology. The radioulnar joint is stabilized by the annular ligament. The pediatric ligament is weak and doesn't get strong enough to prevent this dislocation until about age 5 (Egol et al., 2010).

Incidence. Nursemaid's elbow is common between ages 2 and 5, and accounts for 1% of all youth visits to the emergency department; in 2006, there were nearly 200,000 emergency room visits due to this condition (Brown, 2009). The male-to-female ratio is 1:2, with the left elbow being injured 70% of the time (Egol et al., 2010).

Complications. Complications are rare with this type of injury. The primary goal is to prevent this from

Figure 19.5.
a: Olecranon Fracture
b: Repair of Olecranon Fracture with Plates and Screws (Lateral View)
c: Same Repair (AP View)

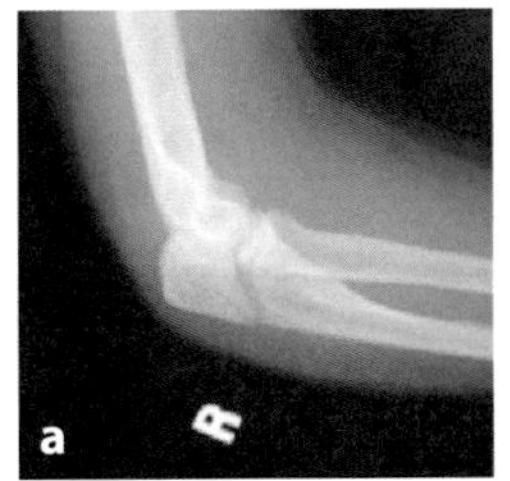

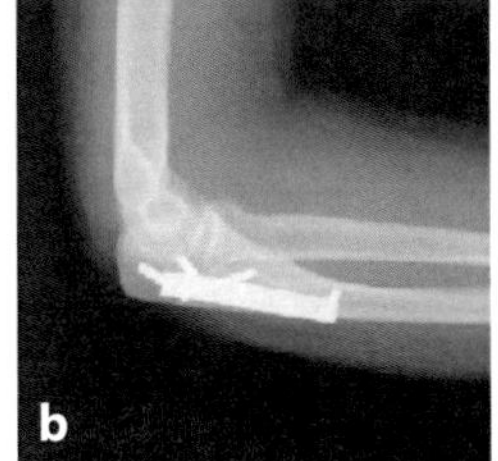

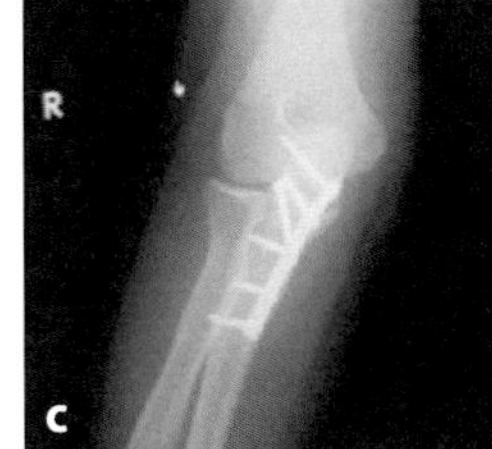

Author creation. Reproduced with permission.

Figure 19.6.
a: Olecranon Fracture
b: Same Fracture After Tension Band Repair

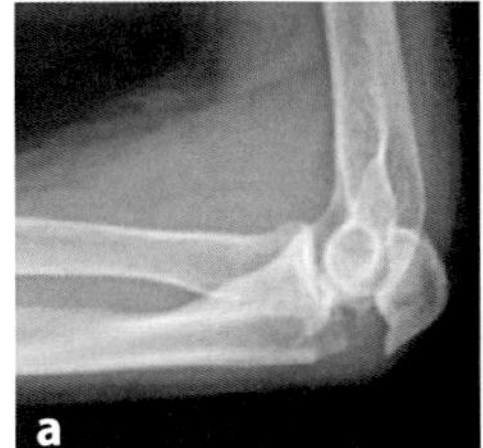

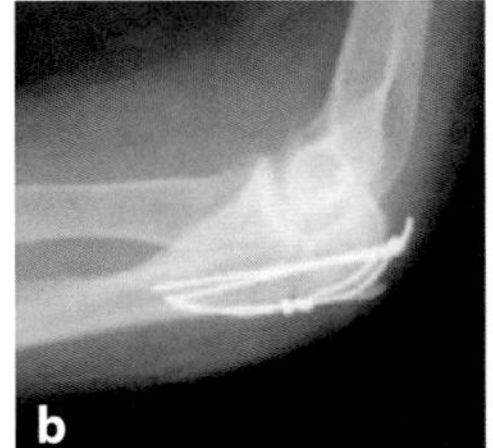

Author creation. Reproduced with permission.

CHAPTER 19

recurring by explaining the mechanism of injury to the parents or care providers. On occasion, the mechanism of injury may be related to child abuse, but this is rare. Parents or siblings may need to be consoled due to feelings of guilt at having caused this injury to the child (Rodts, 2009).

Assessment

History. Carefully identifying the mechanism of injury will almost always confirm the diagnosis. In addition, the child will often come in crying, holding onto the arm in a partially flexed position, refusing to move the arm or hand.

Physical Exam. Palpate the child's elbow for pain. Examine for ecchymosis and swelling. Examine the fingers for swelling. Determine neurovascular status.

Diagnostic Tests. If the history is "classic," as described above, a reduction will often be performed without x-rays (Rodts, 2009). If there is any doubt in the clinician's mind, however, a two-view x-ray of the affected elbow may be obtained. On occasion, post-dislocation reduction x-rays will also be obtained. When the radiologic technician obtains the x-ray, the arm is typically placed in extension and supination. When the arm is placed into flexion for the lateral film, with pressure on the radial head, the radial head may fall back into position. Otherwise, the same technique is used to reduce the dislocation.

Common Therapeutic Modalities

Reduction. The elbow will be reduced. The child may be kept in a sling for 1-2 weeks to allow scar tissue to form, to assist in preventing this dislocation from recurring. Most children feel better once the reduction has been performed, and they begin to use their elbow as tolerated without further problem; however, the recurrence rate is 5%-30% (Egol et al., 2010; Rodts, 2009).

Education. The best way to prevent dislocation from happening or recurring is to educate the caregivers on the mechanism of injury.

Nursing Considerations

Nursing Diagnoses. Nursing diagnoses for this condition are expanded upon in the Appendix.

- Body image, disturbed.
- Fear.
- Infection, risk for.
- Injury, risk for.
- Knowledge deficit.
- Pain, acute.
- Self-care deficit: bathing/hygiene, dressing/grooming, toileting, feeding.

Supracondylar/Distal Humerus Fractures

Overview

Definition. Supracondylar fractures, or distal humerus fractures, involve the distal third of the humerus. In children, the epicondyles get fractured, and these are more common than distal humerus fractures.

Etiology. In younger adults, most distal humerus fractures are related to accidents (such as motor vehicle crashes) or sporting incidents (such as bicycle injuries, skateboarding, and inline skating falls). The patient puts an arm out for protection and lands on the elbow or an outstretched arm. If the wrist doesn't break in the fall, often the impact of the fall will transmit up the arm and cause the fracture in the distal humerus. In the elderly, most of these fractures are "low-energy," meaning the fall came from a standing height (Egol et al., 2010; Reiser et al., 2008).

Pathophysiology. Supracondylar fractures occur frequently in the pediatric population as the ligaments are more lax, which makes the elbow more prone to dislocation and injury. Because the anterior capsule is thicker and stronger than the posterior capsule, the olecranon can become impinged in the olecranon fossa, which then puts added forces on the humerus, leading to fracture.

Incidence. The incidence of fractures is equally distributed among males and females, with peak incidence occurring in males ages 12 to 19 and females ages 80 and older (Egol et al., 2010). Adult distal humerus fractures only account for approximately 2% of all fractures. In children, supracondylar fractures are the most common elbow fracture in children (Hart, Turner, Albright, & Grottkau, 2011). These fractures occur most often between ages 5 and 8, with a slight male predilection (3:2) (Egol et al., 2010).

Complications. Complications related to this type of fracture are displacement, poor healing, and, more commonly, stiffness. Even in children, there is a risk of stiffness occurring with this type of fracture as it heals because it involves the elbow joint. The distal humerus needs a period of immobilization to heal that may last 3-6 weeks, during which time the elbow will get stiff. Occupational therapy is often needed to regain function and mobility of the elbow. Delayed union or nonunion of lateral condyle fractures is also possible in children due to the repeated exposure to synovial fluid (Hart et al, 2011). Due to the mechanics of the elbow joint, the site of a distal humerus/supercondylar fracture is more prone to developing arthritis due to the disruption of the cartilage in the joint.

Assessment

History. As mentioned above, the usual mechanism of injury is a fall; however, be sure to verify the actual mechanism of injury and determine if anything else was injured at the same time. Ascertain dominance of hand. Inquire whether the patient has ever been injured before and if there were limitations in motion of the elbow/shoulder/wrist before the injury. Check for numbness or tingling distal to the injury.

Physical Exam. Assess for deformities, associated lacerations, abrasions, and contusions. Observe swelling, as this can be significant with this type of fracture. Verify that the patient can flex, extend, supinate, and pronate the elbow. If the patient has obvious instability, or is very reluctant to move the arm, do not try to bend the arm until x-rays have been taken because of the potential for neurovascular compromise with this type of injury. Check the pulses distal to the injury, and verify that the patient has appropriate neurologic function. Because significant arterial and neurovascular anatomy is located in the elbow, it is important to determine this. If the fracture is comminuted, there is the potential for this to change, i.e., go from a strong pulse to pulseless. Always assess the joints above and below the elbow.

Figure 19.7.
a: Distal Humerus Fracture on a 5-Year-Old Female
b: Healing Visible on Same Fracture 6 Weeks Later

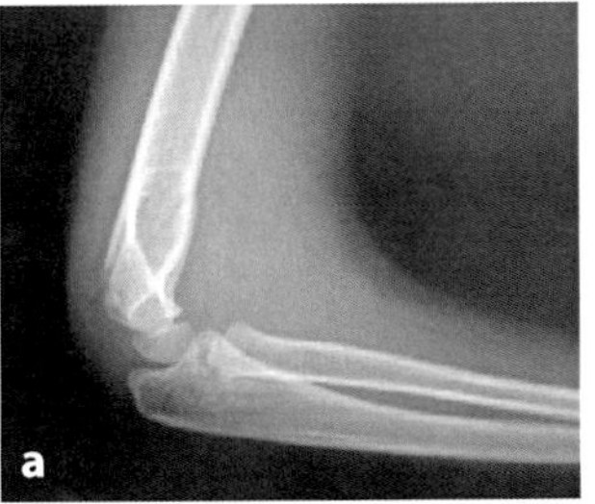

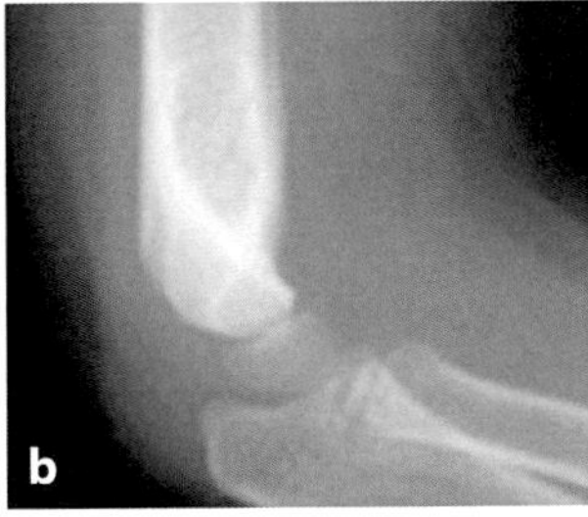

Author creation. Reproduced with permission.

Figure 19.8.
Supracondylar Humeral Fracture, Treated with Kirschner Wires

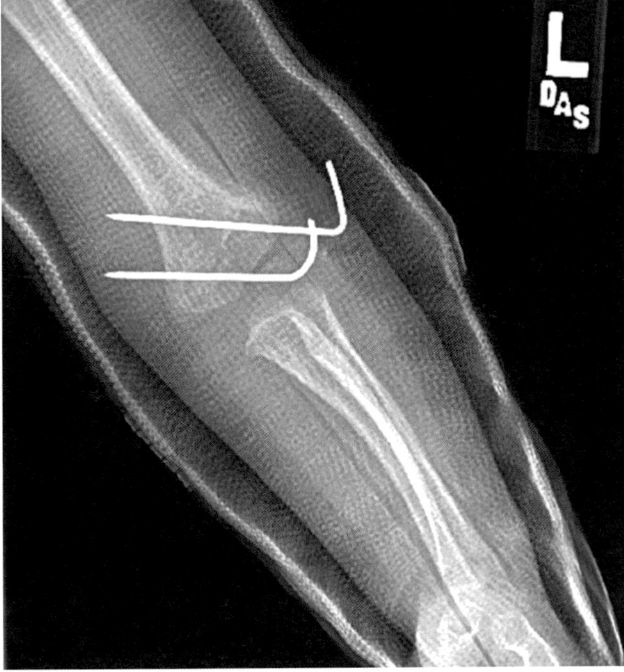

From "Common Pediatric Elbow Fractures" by E. Hart, A. Turner, M. Albright, M., and D. Grottkau, 2011, Orthopaedic Nursing, 30 *(1), p. 13. Reproduced with permission.*

Diagnostic Tests. Two-view x-rays of the elbow should be obtained, if possible. Often it is difficult to get a true AP x-ray once the patient has sustained a fracture to the distal humerus because the pain makes it difficult to extend the elbow. A fracture may not be easily seen, particularly if it is nondisplaced. On occasion, a CT scan may be ordered to evaluate the fracture, particularly if there is comminution in adults. This evaluation may determine whether the fracture should be treated conservatively or surgically.

Common Therapeutic Modalities

Splinting. Nondisplaced fractures or fractures with displacement of less than 2 mm (Sullivan, 2006) will be placed in a posterior long-arm splint for 2-3 weeks for immobilization. At the 2- or 3-week mark, the splint will either be replaced with a hinged brace (with adults) or be removed several times daily (with children) to allow early ROM of the elbow. Serial x-rays will often be taken at week 1, week 2, and possibly week 3 to ensure that the fracture has not displaced (Figure 19.7).

Pain Management. Patients will need NSAIDs or narcotic pain medications to treat the fracture pain, typically for 2-3 weeks. If there is concern of MO, the patient may be placed on indomethacin or NSAIDs prophylactically for 3-6 weeks to prevent the development of this potential complication (see "Anatomy" and Figure 19.3).

Surgical. If the fracture is significantly displaced, an ORIF will be required. The patient will only have temporary immobility, and early ROM will be started to prevent stiffness and loss of motion. If K-wires are used to repair the fracture, they will be removed 3-4 weeks after surgery (Figure 19.8). If the elbow is significantly comminuted, a total elbow arthroplasty may be required (Egol et al., 2010).

Nursing Considerations

Nursing Diagnoses. Nursing diagnoses for this condition are expanded upon in the Appendix.

- Body image, disturbed.
- Infection, risk for.
- Injury, risk for.

- Knowledge deficit.
- Pain, acute.
- Peripheral neurovascular dysfunction, risk for.
- Self-care deficit: bathing/hygiene, dressing/grooming, toileting, feeding.

Elbow Dislocation

Overview

Definition. An elbow dislocation is when the hinge joint of the elbow comes "out of place."The elbow is generally considered a very stable joint, with forces surrounding it from the anterior and posterior sides, as well as the inherent "lock"of the olecranon in the trochlea of the humerus. It takes a significant fall, generally a fall on an outstretched hand (or "FOOSH"), to cause this dislocation.

Etiology. The elbow is usually dislocated as described above in a FOOSH, which causes the locked olecranon to displace from the trochlea. Because of the anatomy of the elbow, most dislocations occur posteriorly. In order for the elbow to dislocate anteriorly, a force must be applied to the elbow when in a flexed position (Egol et al., 2010).

Incidence. A population of 100,000 sees approximately 6-8 cases per year of elbow dislocations (Egol et al., 2010). There is a higher incidence in 10- to 20-year-olds due to sports injuries. The dislocations may be simple (ligament disruption only) or complex (associated with fracture).

Complications. Complications with a simple dislocation are not common but may include neurovascular damage that occurs at the time of injury, MO, and, rarely, recurrence. A significant complication occurs if the injury has occluded the arteries, leaving the patient pulseless in the distal forearm. This is a true orthopaedic emergency and must be reduced as soon as possible to prevent further problems. If the patient has sustained a fracture dislocation and requires surgical intervention, associated risks of surgery are present.

CHAPTER 19

Figure 19.9.
a: Posterior Dislocation Pre-Reduction
b: Same Dislocation Post-Reduction

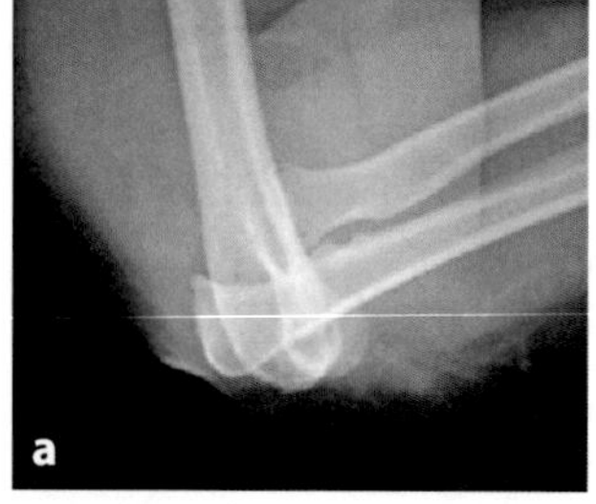

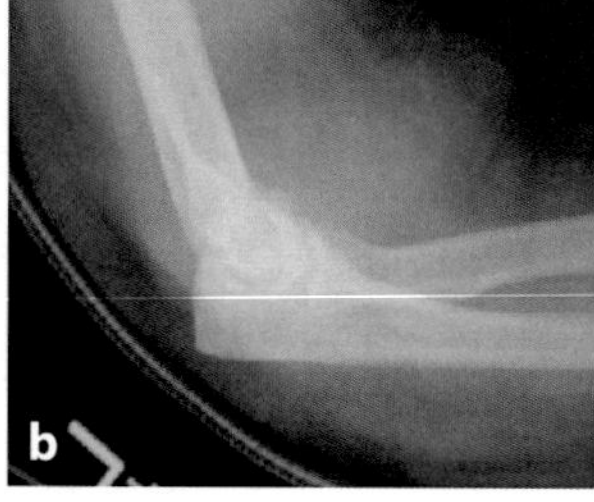

Author creation. Reproduced with permission.

Assessment

History. Ascertain how the injury occurred, and if the injury was with the elbow outstretched or flexed. Establish dominance of hand. Check for numbness and tingling distal to the elbow. Determine any treatment already attempted, such as "I tried to put my elbow back into place."

Physical Exam. Examine the elbow for swelling and deformity. Evaluate pulses. Assess neurovascular status (this should be done prior to x-rays). Check for any breaks in the skin, significant swelling, or ecchymosis.

Diagnostic Tests. If the patient is neurovascularly intact, two-view x-rays (AP and lateral) of the affected extremity will be obtained. In the case of fracture-dislocation, a CT scan may be obtained to better characterize the fracture and determine the type of surgical intervention required.

Common Therapeutic Modalities

Conservative. A dislocated elbow will be reduced back into place (Figure 19.9). If the patient is seen relatively soon after the dislocation, this can be done under sedation in the emergency room. If the patient suffered significant other trauma, the swelling is significant, or more time has elapsed since the injury, the reduction will need to be done in the OR. Once the dislocation was reduced, the patient will be placed in a posterior splint, encompassing the wrist (including an ulnar gutter portion of the wrist) to prevent supination and pronation of the forearm. The splint will be removed after 10 days to 2 weeks to allow early guarded ROM of the elbow. Often, the patient will need therapy to strengthen the elbow. It may take 3-6 months to gain full functional recovery in strength and ROM after a dislocation (Egol et al., 2010).

Pain Management. The patient will be provided narcotic medications for postoperative pain for 2-3 weeks. The patient who sustained a dislocation with closed reduction will also need medications to prevent MO, as dislocations are more prone to this condition than any other elbow injury.

Monitoring the Healing. Radiographs will need to be taken at regular intervals for the surgical patient. Even the patient who did not require an ORIF will need to have x-rays to evaluate for MO in the musculature of the elbow.

Nursing Considerations

Nursing Diagnoses. Nursing diagnoses for this condition are expanded upon in the Appendix.

- Body image, disturbed.
- Infection, risk for.

- Injury, risk for.
- Knowledge deficit.
- Pain, acute.
- Peripheral neurovascular dysfunction, risk for.
- Self-care deficit: bathing/hygiene, dressing/ grooming, toileting, feeding.

Nerve Entrapments

Overview

Definitions. Nerve entrapments encompass cubital tunnel syndrome, radial tunnel syndrome, posterior interosseous nerve syndrome, and pronator syndrome. *Cubital tunnel syndrome* (CUTS) is compression of the ulnar nerve, *radial tunnel syndrome* (RTS) is compression of the radial nerve, and *posterior interosseous nerve syndrome* (PINS) is compression of the radial nerve where it divides into the posterior interosseous nerve. *Pronator syndrome* is due to compression of the median nerve in the forearm and differs from carpal tunnel syndrome, which is compression of the median nerve in the wrist (see Chapter 20—Hand and Wrist).

Pathophysiology. These four syndromes are related to nerve compression as the nerves travel through the related bony and soft tissue areas, resulting in parasthesias, pain, and weakness. Nerve entrapment, compression, or traction injury may be secondary to congenital anomalies, soft tissue constriction, bone spurs, space-occupying lesions, elbow fracture or dislocation, cysts, direct blow, local swelling from metabolic or endocrine diseases (Adams & Steinman, 2006; Schoen, 2002) or swelling seen from overuse (such as weight training using a flexed elbow to pull an abdominal crunch machine).

CUTS (or ulnar nerve entrapment) is the most common upper extremity nerve entrapment condition following carpal tunnel syndrome (Darowish, Lawton, & Evans, 2009). The ulnar nerve passes through a soft tissue tunnel that is posterior to the medial epicondyle of the elbow. When the elbow is flexed, the ulnar nerve becomes become taunt and flattened against the medial epicondyle, which can cause irritation. Recently, this has been coined "cell phone elbow" for prolonged periods of cell phone use (Darowish et al., 2009).

The radial nerve may be entrapped in two separate components, causing either RTS or PINS. The radial nerve travels over the lateral epicondyle, then over the anterior aspect of the proximal radius and under the arcade of Froshe where it divides. The deep radial nerve becomes the posterior interosseous nerve at the proximal supinator muscle (Schoen, 2002). Compression along the radial tunnel is thought to cause pain, whereas compression of the posterior interosseous nerve causes motor weakness.

Etiology. CUTS can be brought on by blunt trauma, contact sports, and sports that involve throwing. RTS is found in masons, carpenters, power lifters, and those who play racket sports. Medical conditions such as rheumatoid arthritis, lipomas, hemangioma, nonunion of fractures, and cysts can predispose individuals to these syndromes. On occasion, an inebriated person may fall asleep unaware that he/she is lying on an area compressing the nerve, causing the symptoms (also noted as "Saturday night palsy") (Elhassan & Steinman, 2007).

Complications. Complications of these entrapment syndromes are related initially to discomfort of the nerve, causing numbness, tingling, and pain. Eventually, muscle weakness, atrophy, loss of strength, loss of function, and chronic pain occur. Patients with "Saturday night palsy" may wake up with wrist drop that can last for up to 4-6 weeks, due to radial nerve palsy (Devitt, Baker, Ahmed, Menzies, & Synnott, 2011).

Assessment

History. Patients with problems related to nerve entrapment usually have a history of parasthesias, fasciculations, pain, and muscle weakness in the area of the affected nerve. Patients with CUTS may feel like they hit their "funny bone," have a decreased sensation in the small finger, or complain of a deep ache (Alhassan & Steinman, 2007; Schoen, 2002) When a patient presents with RTS or PINS, it is often with a complaint of weakness in the wrist or in finger extension, or of pain. This is similar to that of lateral epicondylitis, and it is important to differentiate between the two problems. Patients with RTS may describe pain that radiates up the arm or down to the wrist, whereas pain with lateral epicondylitis is localized.

Physical Exam. Determine hand dominance. Compare the affected to the unaffected extremity. Observe for forearm atrophy and decreased wrist ROM, and complete a neuromuscular exam. Compare strength of both extremities. Patients with CUTS will notice weakness in flexion of the proximal interphalangeal joint, and abduction of small and ring fingers. The ulnar nerve distribution of the ring and small fingers will have reduced 2-point discrimination, a simple test where two objects (such as a caliper or bent paper clip) touch the skin simultaneously. In a normal neurological exam, the patient will be able to discern that two areas are being touched; in an abnormal exam, the patient will often only note one area of sensation. Ulnar deviation may also be noted (Elhassan & Steinman, 2007).

Provocative tests of the ulnar nerve include the elbow flexion test, Tinel's sign, and Froment's sign. The elbow flexion test pronates the forearm and flexes the elbow to apply maximum tension on the ulnar nerve through the cubital tunnel and reproduce symptoms. Tinel's sign is conducted by tapping the elbow over the medial posterior aspect of the elbow. Tingling down the forearm to the small finger denotes a positive exam. A positive Froment's sign is noted when a patient is asked to hold a piece of paper between the thumb and radial side of the index finger proximal phalanx. If the adductor pollicus muscle is weak (which is innervated by the ulnar nerve), the thumb interphalangeal joint flexes, instead of staying straight. It is best to compare both hands when doing this test (American Society for Surgery of the Hand, 1990; Elhassan & Steinman, 2007; Schoen, 2002).

Diagnostic Tests. Two-view radiographs of the elbow, forearm, and wrist should be obtained to rule out tumors, occult fractures, or underlying bony abnormality that is causing the nerve compression. MRIs may be ordered to evaluate soft tissue swelling and rule out sarcoma, lesions, or underlying pathology that is compressing the nerve. MRIs of the elbow often take an hour or more, however, and the patient may have difficulty maintaining the required position of the elbow during the exam. Electromyelograms (EMGs) are used to assess nerve and muscle patency strength and entrapment syndromes. The EMG assists in determining the severity of the problem, which will help the health care team advise the patient if surgical intervention is needed. On occasion, ultrasound will be used to assess fluid collection and other abnormalities. In addition to avoiding radiation exposure, ultrasound is a helpful additional diagnostic tool because the elbow can be evaluated in flexion as well as extension, whereas MRI only evaluates the elbow in extension.

Common Therapeutic Modalities

Conservative. Prevention strategies are aimed at reducing compression of nerves by avoiding pressure on the medial elbow, leaning on elbows, or sleeping with elbows flexed. Padding used during contact sports may also be helpful. Rest of the extremity is encouraged. Splints, anti-inflammatories, and occupational therapy may help with stretching, ROM, pain control, and edema reduction. For patients with "cell phone elbow," use of headsets can reduce symptoms.

CHAPTER 19

Surgical. If conservative treatment fails, surgical intervention may be required. There are several options for surgery, including release, grafting, debridement, and ulnar nerve transposition (Adams & Steinman, 2006; Elhassan & Steinman, 2007). The first option includes decompression of the nerve, which essentially removes all tissue that is causing compression on the ulnar nerve. A medial epicondylectomy may be performed, in which the flexor pronator origin is reattached to the periosteum with the elbow in extension. Another option is an ulnar nerve transposition. The ulnar nerve is released proximal to distal, and a new fascial sling is made to house the ulnar nerve and protect it from trauma. The ulnar nerve may be moved more medially and anteriorly, and tissue anchors may be used to secure the flexor-pronator group into a new position, thus decreasing compression and subsequent pain on the ulnar nerve (Elhassan & Steinman, 2007).

Nursing Considerations

Nursing Diagnoses. Nursing diagnoses for this condition are expanded upon in the Appendix.

- Body image, disturbed.
- Infection, risk for.
- Injury, risk for.
- Knowledge deficit.
- Pain, acute.
- Self-care deficit: bathing/hygiene, dressing/grooming, toileting, feeding.

Patient education is important with any of these syndromes. Some patients may experience symptoms for a long time, and the symptoms can even be permanent. Caution patients about exposure to extreme heat, cold, or sharp objects or otherwise injuring the elbow, as these potential injuries may not be noted due to decreased nerve sensation. Patients with these syndromes may want to use gloves to help protect the digits from injury. If any symptoms worsen, the patient should notify the provider, as conservative therapy may be failing, and surgical intervention may be required.

Osteochondritis of the Capitellum

Overview

Definition. Osteochondritis dissecans (OCD) of the capitellum is a lesion of the cartilage along the capitellum, associated with frequent repetitive activity such as with throwing. OCD affects young, skeletally immature athletes. Panner's disease similarly affects the capitellum, but it is not related to trauma, generally affects males younger than age 10, and involves osteochondrosis of the entire capitellum of the elbow (Ruchelsman, Hall, & Youm, 2010).

Etiology. OCD primarily affects those with repetitive trauma, such as pitchers and gymnasts.

Pathophysiology. Repetitive microtrauma to the cartilage of the capitellum may lead to fracture and damage to the microcirculation, which in turn causes resorption and cartilage damage. Eventually this cartilage damage causes separation of the cartilage, which may break off into the joint with loose pieces (Ruchelsman et al., 2010).

Incidence. The average age of incidence is 12 to 14 years, with males more commonly injured than females. The dominant arm is usually affected. Athletes who develop OCD of the capitellum often participate in sports such as gymnastics, baseball, tennis, weightlifting, and cheerleading (Ruchelsman et al., 2010).

Complications. If treated early, positive outcomes can be obtained simply through rest, particularly in children with open capitellar physes. If treated after symptoms have been present for a while, however, patients who are treated nonsurgically have poorer outcomes than those treated surgically (Ruchelsman et al., 2010).

Assessment

History. Patients with OCD of the capitellum typically report pain with movement, repetitive activity, or throwing. The pain is often relieved with rest. As the symptoms progress, mechanical symptoms such as locking and catching may occur, as well as nocturnal pain (Ruchelsman et al., 2010).

Physical Exam. Examine the elbow for stiffness, swelling, and effusion. Typically, the pain will be elicited with palpation of the radiocapitellum articulation. Lack of extension may occur, sometimes from 15 to 30 degrees less than the unaffected extremity.

Diagnostic Tests. Two-view x-rays should be obtained. Occasionally comparative films of the unaffected extremity will be obtained also. A defect may or may not be noted radiographically. If there is an index of suspicion of the problem, a MRI should be obtained for a more definitive diagnosis, particularly with the condition of the cartilage. A false positive reading on an MRI will sometimes be noted due to the normal anatomy of the capitellar cleft (Ruchelsman et al., 2010).

Common Therapeutic Modalities

Conservative. Rest is recommended initially for patients diagnosed early in the disease process, as mentioned previously.

Surgical. Patients with OCD lesions of the capitellum will be treated with a variety of surgical interventions, including debridement, fragment excisions, intraoperative mosaicplasty, fragment fixation, osteotomy, and osteochondral autograft transplantation (Iwasaki et al., 2010; Ruchelsman et al., 2010). Intraoperative mosaicplasty was found to have significant clinical results in relieving pain and allowing patients to return to the competitive sports played before surgery (Iwasaki et al., 2010).

Nursing Considerations

Nursing Diagnoses. Nursing diagnoses for this condition are expanded upon in the Appendix.

- Body image, disturbed
- Infection, risk for
- Injury, risk for
- Knowledge deficit.
- Pain, acute.
- Self-care deficit: bathing/hygiene, dressing/ grooming, toileting, feeding.

Elbow Arthroplasty

Overview

Definition. Arthroplasty is a partial or total replacement of the joint surface, with metal and polyethylene plastic or silicone. Pain relief and restoration of function, although often limited, is often the main reason for this procedure

Etiology. Total elbow arthroplasty (TEA) is performed on patients with end-stage inflammatory or rheumatoid arthritis (15%-45% of cases), and to manage trauma such as nonunion or comminuted fractures of the distal humerus (50%-60% of cases) (Kim, Mudgal, Konopka, & Jupiter, 2011).

Pathophysiology. Patients with underlying inflammatory arthritis have erosion of the joint and cartilage, which causes pain and instability. Medications can treat the inflammatory condition, which often treats the underlying problem and delays (or even eliminates) the need for elbow replacement. Ongoing inflammation will affect the cartilage and capsule, causing articular changes, pain, and loss of joint function. In osteoarthritis, the cartilage and joint space may be preserved, but formation of osteophytes and contraction of the joint capsule lead to pain, weakness, and stiffness (Cheung, Adams, & Morrey, 2008). More commonly, failed union of distal humerus fractures requires the need for a TEA in order to restore function of the elbow.

Incidence. Primary osteoarthritis of the elbow is rare, affecting less than 2% of the population (Cheung et al., 2008).

Complications. As noted by Kim et al. (2011), complications related to elbow arthroplasty include implant failure and/or loosening, infection, nerve palsy, periprosthetic fracture, and triceps insufficiency. There are more complications associated with elbow arthroplasty than other types of joint replacements, in part because patients who need TEA are often undergoing treatment with medications that impair healing (such as rheumatoid agents) and because TEA patients have often undergone previous surgery (due to trauma) that failed, leaving poorer tissue to work with in the secondary surgery (Sanchez-Sotelo & Morrey, 2011).

Preventive Strategies. Because most elbow replacements are related to trauma, avoiding risk-taking activities that lead to higher incidence of trauma may decrease the incidence of total elbow replacements.

Assessment

History. Determine if the patient has had prior elbow surgery. Establish hand dominance. Assess the pain: what the symptoms are, when the joint hurts, and what exacerbates and relieves the pain. Check for other affected joints, as well as any constitutional symptoms such as fever, chills, fatigue, malaise, or weakness. Ascertain a family history of arthritis or joint replacement. Determine when the patient was diagnosed with arthritis. In patients with rheumatoid arthritis, past treatments, medication plans, and progression of disease are important factors to ascertain. (See Chapter 13—Arthritis.)

Physical Exam. Assess the joint involved, as well as the joints above and below the affected joint. Assess active and passive ROM. Compare the affected extremity to the unaffected extremity. Check the neurovascular status of the affected extremity. Examine the skin for any breakdown, lesions, or sores.

Diagnostic Tests. Radiographs (AP, lateral, and oblique) should be obtained of the affected extremity. Joint narrowing, osteophytes, sclerosis, and other problems may be noted.

Common Therapeutic Modalities

Injections. Intra-articular corticosteroid injections may be considered to reduce mild pain in the elbow. Hyaluronic acid injections have not proven as effective for the elbow (Cheung et al., 2008).

Medications. Analgesics are often used for pain. NSAIDs are a typical choice.

PT/OT. Therapy is often used to increase ROM, instruct patients on adaptive techniques to reduce stress on the elbow, and maintain strength.

Surgical interventions. Elbow arthroscopy may be performed to debride the joint, remove loose pieces, and debride spurs. A capsulectomy may also be performed. These procedures may be open or arthroscopic. Resurfacing techniques may be attempted. Decompression or transposition of the ulnar nerve may be attempted to reduce pain, particularly if ulnar neuritis exists (Cheung at al., 2008). There are other treatment options, such as linked or unlinked prostheses, but use of these is controversial in orthopaedic literature. TEA can be performed, but often the more conservative options will have been attempted first.

Nursing Considerations

Nursing Diagnoses. Nursing diagnoses for this condition are expanded upon in the Appendix.

- Bleeding, risk for.
- Body image, disturbed.
- Infection, risk for.
- Injury, risk for.
- Knowledge deficit.
- Pain, acute.
- Self-care deficit: bathing/hygiene, dressing/ grooming, toileting, feeding
- Sensory perception, tactile, disturbed.
- Skin integrity, impaired.

Nursing care of the patient with an arthroplasty will focus on routine postoperative care (dressing, splint, elevation). Strategies should be identified for strengthening, preventing infection, improving ROM with use of therapy, and identifying preventable risk factors that may have precipitated the need for an arthroplasty. This may include activity modification, medical control of rheumatology concerns, or preventing trauma that may have precipitated the event.

Summary

The elbow is a unique joint that is essential to many everyday activities. Due to its anatomy, it is prone to specific injuries that must be noted. Orthopaedic nurses must understand the proper care, assessment, and interventions in caring for individuals with elbow injury, trauma, or deformity, in order to promote proper healing, prevent complications, and return the individual to the highest possible level of functioning. It is essential to have clear communication with all health care team members, including surgeons, nurse practitioners, clinical nurse specialists, physician assistants, therapists, radiologists, pharmacists, emergency staff, and surgical team members. Each team member brings unique knowledge and care delivery to the patient, and understanding and respecting that care will enhance patient care and facilitate the best possible outcomes in these injuries.

References

Aaron, D., Patel, A., Kayiaros, S., & Calfee, R. (2011). Four common types of bursitis. *Journal of the American Academy of Orthopaedic Surgeons, 19*(6), 359-367.

Abrahams, P., Marks, S.C., Jr., & Hutchings, R. (2003). *McMinn's Color Atlas of Human Anatomy* (5th Ed). New York, NY: Mosby.

Adams, J. & Steinman, S. (2006). Nerve injuries about the elbow. *Current Opinion in Orthopedics, 17*, 348-354.

Ahmad, C. & ElAttrache, N. (2006). Elbow valgus instability in the throwing athlete. *Journal of the American Academy of Orthopaedic Surgeons, 14*(12), 693-700.

American Academy of Orthopaedic Surgeons (AAOS). (2003). *The 2003 body almanac: Your personal guide to bone and joint health*. Rosemont, IL: AAOS.

American Society for Surgery of the Hand (1990). *The hand: Examination and diagnosis* (3rd ed.). New York, NY: Churchill Livingstone.

Berg, E. (2000). Deep muscle contusion complicated by myositis ossificans, (a.k.a. heteroptic bone). *Orthopaedic Nursing, 19*(6), 66-67.

Brown, D. (2009). Emergency department visits for nursemaid's elbow in the United States, 2005-2006. *Orthopaedic Nursing, 28*(4), 161-162. doi:10.1097/NOR.Ob013e3181ada779

Bunata, R., Brown, D., & Capelo, R. (2007). Anatomic factors related to the cause of tennis elbow. *Journal of Bone and Joint Surgery, 89*(9), 1955-1963. doi:10.2106/JBJS.F.00727

Cheung, E., Adams, R., & Morrey, B. (2008). Primary osteoarthritis of the elbow: Current treatment options. *Journal of the American Academy of Orthopaedic Surgeons, 16*(2), 77-87.

Darowish, M., Lawton, J., & Evans, P. (2009). What is cell phone elbow and what should we tell our patients? *Cleveland Clinic Journal of Medicine, 76* (5), 306-308. doi:10.3949/ccjm.76a.08090

Devitt, B., Baker, J., Ahmed, M., Menzies, D., & Synnott, K. (2011). Saturday night palsy or Sunday morning hangover? A case of alcohol-induced Crush Syndrome. *Archives of Orthopaedic and Trauma Surgery, 131*(1), 39-43.

Dorf, E., Blue, C., Smith, B., & Koman, L. (2010). Therapy after injury to the hand. *Journal of the American Academy of Orthopaedic Surgeons, 18*(8), 464-473.

Egol, K., Koval, K., & Zuckerman, J. (2010). *Handbook of Fractures* (4th ed., pp. 214-269). Philadelphia, PA: Lippincott, Williams & Wilkins.

Elhassan, B. & Steinman, S. (2007). Entrapment neuropathy of the ulnar nerve. *Journal of the American Academy of Orthopedic Surgeons, 15*, 672-681.

Fleisig, G., Weber, A., Hassell, N., & Andrews, J., (2009). Prevention of elbow injuries in youth baseball pitchers. *Current Sports Medicine Reports, 8*(5), 250-254.

Freeman, C., McCormick, K., Mahoney, D., Baratz, M., & Lubahn, J. (2009) Nonoperative treatment of distal biceps tendon ruptures compared with a historical control group. *Journal of Bone and Joint Surgery, 91*(10), 2329-2334. doi:10.2106/JBJS.H.01150

Garberina, M., Fagelman, M., & Getz, C. (2008a). Lateral epicondylitis. In P.A. Lotke, J.A. Abboud, & J. Ende (Eds), *Lippincott's Primary Care Orthopedics* (pp. 235-241). Philadelphia, PA: Lippincott, Williams & Wilkins.

Garberina, M., Fagelman, M. & Getz, C. (2008b). Olecranon bursitis. In P.A. Lotke, J.A. Abboud, & J. Ende (Eds.), *Lippincott's Primary Care Orthopedics* (pp. 242-246). Philadelphia, PA: Lippincott, Williams & Wilkins.

Garberina, M., Fagelman, M. & Getz, C. (2008c). Radial head and neck fractures. In P.A. Lotke, J.A. Abboud, & J. Ende (Eds.), *Lippincott's Primary Care Orthopedics* (pp. 247-252). Philadelphia, PA: Lippincott, Williams & Wilkins.

Geaney, L. & Mazzocca, A. (2009). Distal biceps brachii tendon rupture: What do we do with these? *Current Orthopedic Practice, 20*(4), 374-381.

Gentili, A., Beller, M., Masih, S., & Seeger, L. (n.d.). *Interactive atlas of signs in musculoskeletal radiology*. Retrieved from http://www.gentili.net/signs/images/400/Elbowsfatpadarrow.jpg

Getz, C., Parsons, B., & Ramsey, M. (2011). What's new in shoulder and elbow surgery. *Journal of Bone and Joint Surgery, 93*, 1176-1181. doi.10.2106/JBJS.K.00384

Hamid, N., Ashraf, N., Bosse, M., Connor, P., Kellam, J., Sims, S.,… Lowe, T. (2010). Radiation therapy for heterotopic ossification prophylaxis acutely after elbow trauma. *Journal of Bone and Joint Surgery, 92*, 2032-2038. doi:10.2106/JBJS.I.01435

Hart, E., Turner, A., Albright, M., & Grottkau, D. (2011). Common pediatric elbow fractures. *Orthopaedic Nursing, 30*(1), 11-17.

Iwasaki, N., Kato, H., Ishikawa, J., Masuko, T., Funakoshi, T. & Minami, A. (2010). Osteochondritis dissecans of the elbow in teenage athletes: Surgical technique. *Journal of Bone and Joint Surgery, 92*(1), 208-216. doi:10.2106/JBJS.J.00214

Kim, J., Mudgal, C., Konopka, J., & Jupiter, J. (2011). Complications of total elbow arthroplasty. *Journal of the American Academy of Orthopaedic Surgeons, 19* (6), 328-339.

McMahon, P. & Skinner, H. (2003). Sports medicine. In H.B. Skinner (Ed.), *Current Diagnosis and Treatment in Orthopedics* (3rd ed., p. 155-204). New York, NY: Lange Medical Books/McGraw-Hill.

Melamed, E. & Angel, D. (2008). Myositis ossificans mimicking compartment syndrome of the forearm. *Orthopedics, 31*(12), 1237. Retrieved from http://www.orthosupersite.com/view.aspx?rid=32936

Miyamoto, R., Elser, F., & Millett, P. (2010). Distal biceps tendon injuries. *Journal of Bone and Joint Surgery, 92* (11), 2128-2138. doi:10.2106/JBJS.1.01213

Reiser, M., Baur-Melnyk, A., & Glaser, C. (2008). *Musculoskeletal Imaging*. Stuttgart, Germany: Thieme.

Rodts, M. (2009). Nursemaid's elbow: A preventable pediatric injury. *Orthopaedic Nursing, 28*(4), 163-166.

Ruchelsman, D., Hall, M., & Youm, T. (2010). Osteochonridits dissecans of the capitellum: Current concepts. *Journal of American Academy of Orthopaedic Surgeons, 18*(9), 557-567.

Sanchez-Sotelo, J. & Morrey, B. (2011). Total elbow arthroplasty. *Journal of the American Academy of Orthopaedic Surgeons, 19*(2), 121-125.

Schoen, D. (2002). Upper extremity nerve entrapments. *Orthopaedic Nursing, 21*(2), 15 – 31.

Steinmann, S. (2008). Coronoid process fractures. *Journal of the American Academy of Orthopaedic Surgeons, 16*(9), 519-529.

Strauss, J., Wysock, R., Shah, A., Chen, S., Sha, A., Abrams, A., & Cohen, M. (2011). Radiation therapy for heterotopic ossification prophylaxis after high-risk elbow surgery. *The American Journal of Orthopedics, 40*(8), 400-405.

Sullivan, J. (2006). Fractures of the lateral condyle of the humerus. *Journal of the American Academy of Orthopaedic Surgeons, 14*(1), 58-62.

Sutton, K., Dodds, S. Ahmad, C., & Sethi, P. (2010). Surgical treatment of distal biceps rupture. *Journal of American Academy of Orthopaedic Surgeons, 18*(3), 139-148.

Tashjian, R. & Katarincic, J. (2006). Complex elbow instability. *Journal of the American Academy of Orthopaedic Surgeons, 15*(5), 278-286.

Wise, S., Owens, D., & Binkley, H. (2011). Rehabilitating athletes with medial epicondylalgia. *Strength and Conditioning Journal, 33*(2), p. 84-91.

Chapter 20
The Hand & Wrist

Rebecca Perz, MSN, NP-C, ONP-C

Objectives

- Recognize common interventions to provide safety and prevent injury for patients with hand/wrist conditions.
- Describe the pathophysiology of common hand conditions.
- Discuss the potential life-changing and limiting consequences of hand/wrist conditions.
- Identify assessment criteria for each hand/wrist condition or injury.
- Identify key subjective components in obtaining the history of the hand/wrist condition.
- Select common tests to establish definitive diagnoses.
- Outline potential differential diagnoses related to the hand/wrist conditions.
- Discuss outcome criteria for patients with hand/wrist conditions.

The hand and wrist are essential to everyday activities. Imagine not being able to wash, brush teeth, manage toileting, eat independently, use the computer, text-message family and friends, operate a remote control, or pour a morning cup of coffee due to a limiting injury or condition in the hand. This is particularly important when the injury or condition pertains to the individual's dominant hand.

There are many work-related injuries to the hand and wrist. Following the back, the hand and fingers are the most common sites of traumatic injuries sustained at work. Lacerations to the fingers are most commonly noted, but the injuries range from tendonitis and carpal tunnel syndrome to fracture and amputation. Hand and wrist injuries account for approximately 30% of all work-related injuries. It is estimated that time off work is 30 days for a fracture, 21 days for treatment of carpal tunnel, and 15 days for a musculoskeletal injury to the hand or wrist (Bureau of Labor Statistics, 2010). Knowledge of the care of these types of injuries is paramount for patient healing, emotional and physical well-being, and to allow patients to return to prior levels of activity and productivity – on both a personal level and a level that affects society as a whole.

Team efforts are needed to coordinate this patient care. This includes prehospital and first aid care, emergency/urgent care, follow-up care in the hospital, such as an orthopaedic floor, and in outpatient clinic settings after the injury sustained. Most injuries to the hand and wrist benefit from occupational therapy as well, to promote the highest level of functioning possible for these patients.

Table 20.1. Treatment of Soft Tissue Sprains Using the PRICEMM Acronym

Many soft tissue sprains can be treated with this acronym:	
P	Protection by altering ROM, modifying sport/work/activities by way of splint/support
R	Rest of injured joint to decrease stress loading and allow tissue repair
I	Ice/cold compresses to decrease swelling and relieve pain
C	Compression with tape/splint to control edema, provide support/comfort/stability
E	Elevate hand to decrease swelling by mobilization of post inflammatory fluid
M	Medications such as non-steroidal anti-inflammatory medications (NSAIDs) to decrease the effects of the local inflammatory mediators, decrease swelling/pain; narcotics for pain relief
M	Modalities such as physical therapy (PT)/occupational therapy (OT) after sufficient time in splint to gently mobilize joints, regain mobility/flexibility/strength

Common Hand and Wrist Treatment Modalities

Occupational Therapy

Occupational therapy or hand therapy will be essential for maximizing healing for the patient after injury and surgery (from minor releases to major surgery such as replantation), as well as other trauma sustained to the hand. The following areas related to hand therapy were noted by Dorf, Blue, Smith, and Koman (2010) and apply to many injuries, whether acute or chronic, to the hand, wrist, and fingers. Essential orthopaedic care will include therapy for not only regain of function, but for pain control, maximizing healing, and wound management. Table 20.1 includes a helpful mnemonic device to remember protocol for treating soft tissue injury.

Edema Reduction. Therapy can reduce edema by many modalities, including use of compressive dressings, early and passive range of motion (ROM), and splints.

Wound Management. Therapists will examine the healing wound for different stages of healing. Different modalities, including use of whirlpool, ultrasound, medications, and debridement may be used to manage the wound care and optimize healing.

Scar Management. Therapy may reduce the development of hypertrophic scars, keloids, and disorganized collagen deposition, which alters the cellular matrix for healing. Scar management is also optimized with massage, use of gloves, and exercises such as pressure therapy with use of splints.

Range of Motion. Hand therapy will assist with active and passive ROM, allowing for earlier flexor tendon strength, healing, and preventing joint contracture. Skilled therapists will begin tendon glides and other means to increase ROM but will follow protocols to prevent a prematurely aggressive ROM, which may cause rupture of the tendon repair.

Desensitization and Sensory Re-education. This is extremely important for the patient who has experienced an amputation. The nervous system's signals to the affected digit are disrupted, and the stimuli received by the hand need to be redirected so the central nervous system does not interpret these signals as painful or noxious stimuli. Desensitization uses different textures and surfaces to stimulate the healing digit and decrease hypersensitivity, including massage, contrast baths, fluid therapy, and exposure to different textures such as towels, rice, sand, and dried beans.

Other Modalities. Other modalities used by therapists for treatment of the hand and wrist include soft-tissue mobilization, strengthening, work hardening, and conditioning. The therapist may use different techniques in addition to the above described contrast baths and ultrasound, which include fluidotherapy, cryotherapy, continuous passive motion, phonophoresis, iontophoresis, transcutaneous electrical nerve stimulation, and neuromuscular electrical stimulation.

HAND

Mallet Finger

Overview

Definition. Mallet finger is a deformity of the finger resulting from an open or closed tendon injury of the distal extensor apparatus of the distal interphalangeal (DIP) joint (Childs, 2007).

Etiology. This type of injury is commonly noted during sports-related injuries, being struck by a ball, skiing, jamming the finger, or pulling at a jersey of another player, i.e., "jersey finger." It is also seen with falls, as well as environmental or occupational activities (Childs, 2007; Leinberry, 2009). If left untreated, it can lead to finger dysfunction.

Pathophysiology. When the digit is suddenly forced into flexion or extension, this can cause disruption of the insertion of the flexor/extensor apparatus onto the dorsal/volar base of the DIP. This can also cause a fragment of bone to break off, as in an avulsion fracture.

Incidence. This is more commonly noted in the dominant hand. It affects the DIP joint only and accounts for 18% of finger sprains (Childs, 2007). Young to middle-aged males have a higher incidence of this type of injury (Bendre, Hartigan, & Kalainov, 2005). It is difficult to avoid, but once mallet finger is diagnosed, appropriate treatment is as important as preventive measures.

Complications. Delayed treatment and/or avulsion fractures can cause loss of function of the digit. The joint will appear cosmetically different. If the tendon is completely disrupted, this can cause significant disability related to the deformity of the finger if not treated. If surgical intervention is chosen as the treatment, there is a risk of pin site infection. Skin maceration, splint-related pain, and ulceration may also occur during treatment (Childs, 2007; Bendre et al., 2005).

Assessment

History. Determine the mechanism of injury, and assess how much pain the patient is having. Has there been a similar injury in the past, particularly in the last 6 weeks (possible re-injury?)

Physical Exam. Examine the finger for deformity, pain, tenderness, ecchymosis, and swelling. Evaluate active and passive ROM. Assess neurovascular status. Note any open lesions that may suggest an open fracture.

Diagnostic Tests. Radiographs (three views – anterior/posterior (AP), lateral, and oblique) will be obtained of the affected digit to evaluate for fracture.

Common Therapeutic Modalities

Open Reduction. If the DIP is dislocated, splinting is generally the treatment of choice for relocation. Alternatively, pinning with a Kirschner (K)-wire may be done for 6-8 weeks, particularly if the individual displays high potential for noncompliance or has an occupation that would be quite difficult to perform with an external splint, such as musicians or surgeons (Bendre et al., 2005).

Finger Splint. There are many types of splints that can be used to treat mallet finger. The importance of maintaining the use of the splint at all times must be stressed to the patient, and patient compliance is essential for proper healing with this type of injury (Leinberry, 2009). The splint will be used, in extension, continuously for 6 – 8 weeks and then may be used at nighttime for an additional 2 weeks. If, at any time during treatment of this injury, the DIP is allowed to flex, the timing of splinting starts over (Bendre et al., 2005).

Open Injury. Administer tetanus prophylaxis and antibiotic treatment. Apply dry sterile dressing.

Nursing Considerations

Nursing Diagnoses. Nursing diagnoses for this condition are expanded upon in the Appendix.

- Body image, disturbed.
- Infection, risk for.
- Injury, risk for.
- Knowledge deficit, ready for enhanced learning.
- Pain, acute.
- Self-care deficit, bathing/dressing/feeding/toileting.

Patients need to be taught – and thoroughly comprehend – the importance of continuous use of the splint, and the importance of not flexing the finger when readjusting the splint, as this is paramount to the time involved in healing. Regardless of whether the fracture was treated with a splint or pinning, patients must be aware of a probable slight extension lag and/or "bump" on the end of the finger (Leinberry, 2009). (See Figure 20.1.)

Figure 20.1.
Example of Extension Lag of a Mallet Finger

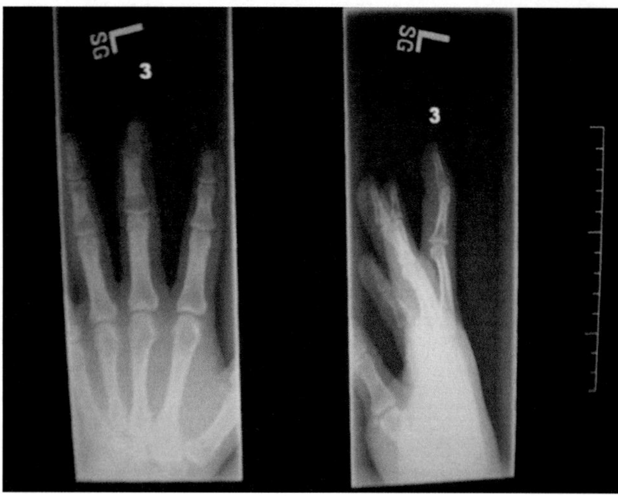

This patient was treated with K-wires for 4 weeks, followed by an extension splint for 4 weeks. The patient was not able to attend therapy and didn't use the splint full-time, leaving the noted deformity.

Author creation. Reproduced with permission.

Boutonniere and Swan Neck Deformities

Overview

Definition. A boutonniere deformity results from either a laceration or a rupture of the extensor tendon mechanism of the finger. This occurs over the proximal interphalangeal (PIP) joint, which flexes and shortens the extension of the finger, causing hyperextension of the DIP joint (ASSH, 1990a; Mortiere, 2004). A swan neck deformity is one in which the PIP joint is in hyperextension, with the DIP in flexion (the opposite of the boutonniere deformity).

Etiology. A boutonniere deformity is generally a result of trauma or a laceration, whereas a swan neck deformity is generally related to a chronic condition, such as rheumatoid arthritis, an old mallet finger deformity that has worsened or was not treated appropriately, or an old volar plate injury (ASSH, 1990a). The injury may be open or closed. The pathophysiology is as noted above, i.e., it is related to injury to the central slip of the extensor tendon of the finger. In patients with rheumatoid arthritis who have a swan neck deformity, the thumb is most commonly involved (50 – 74% of cases) (Silva, Lombardi, Breitschwerdt, Araujo, & Natour, 2008).

Incidence. When related to injury, this can occur in all age groups, as a result of a fall or laceration to the finger. When related to rheumatoid arthritis, there is a greater incidence in middle-aged women.

Complications. Complications are related to lack of or improper treatment. The affected finger needs to be treated appropriately and for the correct amount of time, or deformity can result (see Figure 20.2 for an improperly treated partial extensor tendon laceration – the index finger on the right has a boutonniere's deformity). If the deformity is associated with an open injury, potential for infection exists also.

Figure 20.2.
Boutonniere Deformity of Right Index Finger

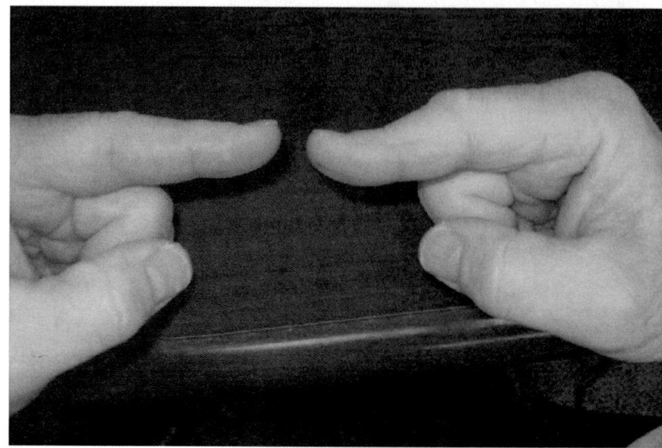

Author creation. Reproduced with permission.

Preventive Strategies. Prevention is aimed at avoiding trauma, such as wearing gloves when using a saw or hand tools. Keeping an open wound clean is important for preventing infection. With rheumatoid arthritis, preventive strategies also involve maintaining mobility and keeping pain under control. When the arthritis leads to deformities, splints may allow the affected individual to have more control of the digit, experience less pain, and prevent a worsening deformity.

Assessment

History. If related to trauma, ask the patient how the trauma occurred. Is there an open wound? What initial treatment was performed? If there is an open cut, ascertain if the item that cut the patient was clean or dirty, or contaminated with an item that may cause significant risk for tenosynovitis (dirty knives, grease-filled tools, pet-related cleanup with fecal or other contamination). Determine the patient's tetanus status.

Physical Exam. Assess the finger for swelling, ecchymosis, and deformity. Evaluate neurovascular status. Ascertain the ability to flex or extend the finger. If there an open wound, is there debris involved? If the tendon is exposed, is a partial or full cut visible?

Diagnostic Tests. Three-view radiographs (AP, lateral, and oblique) may be taken of the affected finger. In cases of rheumatoid arthritis, an x-ray of the entire hand may be taken to observe for underlying pathology possibly developing in other fingers.

Common Therapeutic Modalities

Open Injury. Splinting is generally the treatment of choice for DIP dislocation, but a repair of the tendon may be necessary if there was an open wound. Administer tetanus prophylaxis, if necessary, and antibiotic treatment. Apply dressing.

Finger Splint. As with mallet finger, there are many types of splints that can be used. The importance of maintaining the use of the splint at all times (for injury-related boutonniere's deformity) must be stressed to the patient, as patient compliance is essential for proper healing of this type of injury. The splint will be used continuously, in extension, for 6 – 8 weeks and then may be used at nighttime for an additional 2 weeks. If, at any time during treatment of this injury, the finger is allowed to flex, the timing of splinting starts over. In cases of rheumatoid arthritis, the splint is used for comfort as well as for maintaining dexterity in the extremity (Silva et al., 2008).

Nursing Considerations

Nursing Diagnoses. Nursing diagnoses for this condition are expanded upon in the Appendix.

- Body image, disturbed.
- Infection, risk for.
- Injury, risk for.
- Knowledge deficit, enhanced for learning.
- Pain, acute.
- Self-care deficit, bathing/dressing/feeding/toileting.

Interventions. Patients need to be taught dressing or wound care, as well as the importance of the use of the splint for the determined amount of time. The patient also needs to understand the potential for a deformity of the finger, with possible associated decreased function, even if treated appropriately. In practices where patients with rheumatoid arthritis are managed, these patients need to maintain mobility and be aware of changes that may occur in other digits.

Gamekeeper's Thumb

Overview

Definition. Gamekeeper's thumb, or skier's thumb, is the "partial or complete rupture of the ulnar collateral ligament of the thumb at the metacarpophalangeal joint" (Mortierre, 2004, p. 80).

Etiology. This type of injury was historically known as gamekeeper's thumb, as it affected individuals who were pulling the heads off birds or rabbits for butchering. Injury would occur primarily to the dominant hand. Today, it is more commonly seen in skiers, who catch their thumb on the ski pole. It can occur to anyone who falls forcefully on the thumb, stressing the metacarpal of the thumb in abduction. This injury is quite painful; patients often feel as though their thumb is broken (ASSH, 1990b; Lackey & Sutton, 2008; Mortierre, 2004).

Pathophysiology. As mentioned in the definition, the hallmark of this injury is the instability at the MCP of the affected thumb due to the avulsion or tear of the ulnar collateral ligament. The ligament may tear intrasubstance, or it may be associated with an avulsion fracture of the proximal phalanx. Because of the tear and/or fracture, the thumb may sublux fairly easily in a radial deviation (ASSH, 1990b). This also causes weakness in the grip strength of the thumb.

Complications. The main complication of this injury is decreased thumb strength/pincer ability. Joint stiffness can occur. Rarely injury to the radial nerve can occur. Chronic joint instability may also occur, even with properly treatment (Lackey & Sutton, 2008).

Preventive Strategies. Manufacturers are now making ski gloves that help to prevent this injury from occurring (Lackey & Sutton, 2008). Early recognition and treatment of the injury to prevent chronic instability are also very important.

Assessment

History. Determine the mechanism of injury. Has the individual injured the thumb before? What is the dominant hand? How long ago did the injury occur? Was any initial treatment performed?

Physical Exam. Examine the hand for deformity, swelling, and ecchymosis. Stability of the thumb will be checked by radial and ulnar deviation of the thumb, while flexing the MCP and interphalangeal (IP) joints in partial (10 to 20 degrees) and full flexion (ASSH, 1990b; Lackey & Sutton, 2006; Mortierre, 2004). Test for neurologic deficits. Compare the affected to the non-affected thumb.

Diagnostic Tests. Three-view radiographs (AP, lateral, and oblique) will be taken of the affected thumb. The radiographs will show if there is an avulsion fracture, but in cases of partial tear of the ligament, the radiographs will often be negative.

Common Therapeutic Modalities

Splinting or Thumb Spica Cast. A thumb spica splint or cast will be used for 4 – 6 weeks to allow the ulnar collateral ligament to heal, when there is minimal instability noted. The use of splint versus cast will often depend on the instability noted, surgeon preference, and determination of patient compliance.

Open Reduction. If there is significant instability, an open reduction may need to be performed to evaluate if the ligament is trapped, which will prevent closed reduction and satisfactory healing. In addition, reconstruction, repair, or re-attachment of the tendon will be performed (Hand, 1990b; Mortierre, 2004).

Nursing Considerations

Nursing Diagnoses. Nursing diagnoses for this condition are expanded upon in the Appendix.

- Body image, disturbed.
- Infection, risk for.
- Injury, risk for.
- Knowledge deficit, enhanced for learning.
- Pain, acute.
- Self-care deficit, bathing/dressing/feeding/toileting.

Interventions. Patients need to be cautioned that any reduced fracture or dislocation has the potential to lose position. Appropriate timing and use of splints is important. Monitoring for infection needs to be maintained. The affected thumb will be stiff after immobilization, with or without surgical repair, and will require occupational therapy to regain as much functionality as possible.

Nail Bed Injuries

Overview

Definition. A nail bed injury may or may not damage the underlying nail matrix. The injury may be associated with a laceration, in addition to the crush injury that is often the cause for this type of trauma.

Pathophysiology. The fingers have a significant vascular and neurologic anatomy. When an extremity is crushed and affects the nail bed, there is often significant bleeding; if there is no open wound, the blood will accumulate under the nail itself, forming a subungal hematoma. This will cause severe, throbbing pain. Treatment for nail bed injuries will vary depending on whether or not the germinal matrix (the part of the matrix that is under the skin, from which the nail grows) is affected (ASSH, 1990b).

Complications. Infection can result, depending on the mechanism of injury. Improper healing and abnormal growth of the nail will occur if the germinal matrix has been involved. Nail fragments can remain, which can catch on dressings and clothing, causing significant pain.

Assessment

History. Ascertain how the injury occurred. Determine dominance of the hand. Discover if the patient experienced prior injury to the hand or fingers.

Physical Exam. Examine the patient's affected finger for deformity, ecchymosis, open wound, other injuries, and presence of subungal hematoma. Determine level of pain. Examine the nail matrix to see if that has been affected by this injury.

Diagnostic Tests. Three-view radiographs (A/P, lateral, and oblique) will be obtained, as often with nail bed injuries there are associated fractures, such as distal tuft or comminuted fractures of the distal phalanx. A wound culture may be taken.

Common Therapeutic Modalities

Splinting. Splinting will be initially done of the finger to reduce pain and maintain position of function.

Drainage of Subungal Hematoma. This will need to be performed if the nail was crushed and there is no opening for the blood to drain. The patient will have severe throbbing pain, and this will only be relieved if the blood has the ability to drain from the nail. There are many options to drain the hematoma, and these include twirling an 18-gauge needle on top of the nail until a hole is formed in the nail, heating the end of a paper clip to burn a hole in the nail, or using a battery-operated cautery to burn a hole in the nail. Any of these options will work. The patient will need to be prepared about what is happening, as it is often scary. Pain relief is near instantaneous once the blood is allowed to evacuate (ASSH, 1990b).

Repositioning of Nail if Partially Attached. This will be re-attached via suture or by gently putting back into place. If the nail has been put into place, it acts as a template for the new nail to grow. Removing the nail is also considered a treatment option; if this is done, the underlying tissue needs to be protected (ASSH, 1990b).

Treatment of Open Injury. If there is an open wound, irrigate the wound, cover with a dry sterile dressing, and confirm tetanus status. Oral or parenteral antibiotic therapy may be initiated, pending mechanism of injury.

Nursing Considerations

Nursing Diagnoses. Nursing diagnoses for this condition are expanded upon in the Appendix.

- Infection, risk for (open wound).
- Injury, risk for.

- Knowledge, deficient, care for wound.
- Pain, acute.
- Self-care deficit, bathing/dressing/feeding/toileting.
- Sensory perception: tactile, disturbed.
- Skin integrity, impaired.

Nursing care for application of dry sterile dressing and monitoring for signs of infection is important. The patient will need to be instructed that he/she may lose the nail. Further care may need to be sought to monitor the new nailbed as infection or ingrown nails may occur during the healing process.

Thumb Fractures – Bennett's and Rolando's

Overview

Definition. A Bennett's fracture is an oblique intra-articular fracture of the first metacarpal (MCP) of the thumb (ASSH, 1990a). A Rolando's fracture is also an oblique intra-articular fracture of the first MCP of the thumb, but it contains more comminuted fracture fragments.

Etiology. A thumb fracture will occur from a direct axial loading onto the affected digit. It generally occurs from falling forward on an outstretched hand (generally the dominant hand) while the thumb is stuck in abduction during axial compression (as in stretching out the hand to protect oneself). These injuries can occur during a fall, contact sports, motor vehicle crash, and other events (Childs, 2007).

Pathophysiology. During axial loading, or forced abduction, the bone will split at the main portion of the metacarpal. The ulnar portion of the metacarpal on the palmer surface has a significant ligament structure that stabilizes the joint. This portion of the metacarpal will be separated from the larger distal fragment as the abductor pollicus longus (APL) tendon pulls the fragment away. There is obvious deformity to the thumb. If comminution occurs, the fracture changes from a Bennett's fracture to a Rolando's fracture (Childs, 2007; ASSH, 1990a).

Complications. If left untreated, these fractures will affect grip strength, pinch strength, and movements. Secondary arthritis will occur, as well as decreased ability to perform activities of daily living (ADLs). Subsequent instability will also result at the first metacarpal (Childs, 2007).

Preventive Strategies. Common strategies in the elderly include home safety tips such as securing throw rugs, moving cords out of the way, proper lighting to prevent falls, and appropriate traffic patterns.

Assessment

History. Ascertain how the injury occurred. Determine dominance of the hand. Discover if the patient experienced prior injury to the hand or fingers.

Physical Exam. Examine the patient's thumb and base of thumb with active and passive ROM. Determine if the patient is able to abduct or adduct the finger. Evaluate for swelling, ecchymosis, and neurovascular status. Assess for crepitus noted at the fracture or obvious deformity.

Diagnostic Tests. Three-view radiographs (A/P, lateral, and oblique) will be obtained. Comparative x-rays will be taken in pediatric and adolescent patients. A computerized tomography (CT) scan may be necessary (Childs, 2007).

Common Therapeutic Modalities

Splinting. Splinting will be initially done of the hand to reduce pain and maintain position of function.

Reduction of Fracture. This will be performed if necessary.

Treatment of Open Fracture. If there is an open wound, irrigate the wound, cover with a dry sterile dressing, and confirm tetanus status. Oral or parenteral antibiotic therapy may be initiated (Childs, 2007).

Stabilization of Fracture. This will be treated with a thumb spica cast, percutaneous pinning (K-wire), or open reduction internal fixation.

Nursing Considerations

Nursing Diagnoses. Nursing diagnoses for this condition are expanded upon in the Appendix.

- Infection, risk for (open wound).
- Injury, risk for.
- Knowledge, deficient, care for wound.
- Pain, acute.
- Self-care deficit, bathing/dressing/feeding/toileting.
- Sensory perception: tactile, disturbed.
- Skin integrity, impaired.

Nursing care includes monitoring for neurovascular status before and after reduction of the fracture. Follow routine cast care instructions. Pin site care may need to be performed at cast change. Monitor for complications, such as nonunion, infection, loss of motion, and contractures (Egol, Koval, & Zuckerman, 2010).

Boxer's Fracture

Overview

Definition. A boxer's fracture is a fracture of the fourth or fifth metacarpal (MCP), which sometimes involves the head of the metacarpal.

Etiology. This fracture often occurs when the patient strikes an object, such as a wall or another person, with a closed fist. This may occur in sports, occupational injuries, or in a fight.

Pathophysiology. In this type of fracture, there are longitudinal forces distributed down the long axis of the MCP. The base of the MCP remains articulated with the hamate, and the remaining section of the MCP subluxes proximally and dorsally, which generally causes a spiral fracture of the MCP. The fracture itself may be rotated, shortened, or angulated due to traction exerted by the musculature and flexor tendons (Childs, 2007).

Incidence. This is the second-most common fracture of the hand, often seen in fights (hence the term "boxer's fracture"). It is most commonly found on the dominant hand. Risk factors for this type of fracture are primarily related to the mechanism of injury (hitting another person or a wall).

Complications. Complications related to improper healing include cosmetic deformity, malunion or nonunion, or decreased grip strength. Standard post-surgical risk of infection and hematoma are possible. If the injury occurred from a laceration or bite (from hitting another individual in the face), and the skin was broken, there is a significantly higher risk of complications. Suppurative tenosynovitis is possible, as well as deep space wounds that require incision, drainage, and/or antibiotic therapy. An open wound with a bite over the MCP is treated as an orthopaedic emergency to prevent soft tissue complications or osteomyelitis.

Preventive Strategies. Avoidance of trauma is the primary preventive measure. Once the fracture has been sustained, the main strategies to prevent complications include preventing infection and ensuring proper healing.

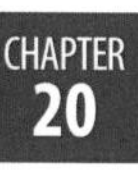

Assessment

History. Obtain thorough history as to mechanism of injury, time of injury, and any treatment done already. Determine if prior injury had occurred to the same hand. Establish hand dominance.

Physical Exam. Assess the hand for deformity, pain, swelling, and ecchymosis. Determine if the patient is able to make a fist. Is any MCP deformity noted? Generally, a loss of prominence of the MCP will be noted. If the patient flexes at the MCP joint, is rotation noted along the fingers? What is the neurovascular status distal to the injury? Determine if the patient has suppurative tenosynovitis by examining for Kanavel's signs. These include: "1) symmetrical swelling along the flexor tendon sheath, 2) tenderness and erythema along the flexor tendon sheath, 3) a semiflexed posture of the involved finger, and 4) severe pain on passive extension of the distal interphalangeal joint (DIP)" (ASSH, 1990b, p. 82). The most important sign is number 4, as this aids in diagnosis of involvement of the flexor tendon sheath.

Diagnostic Tests. Three-view radiographs (A/P, lateral, and oblique) of the affected finger/hand are obtained. Rarely, a CT scan will be used to enhance diagnosis.

Common Therapeutic Modalities

Splinting and Reduction of the Fracture. An ulnar gutter splint will be applied initially. Closed reduction may need to be done prior to the splinting, but the hand can be splinted and the reduction may wait until the patient can be seen by the orthopaedic surgeon. Boxer's fractures involving the fifth MCP alone have more mobility due to the carpal articulation, and acceptable function can still be noted with up to 30-40 degrees of angulation (ASSH, 1990b).

Routine Cast and/or Splint Care. The fracture site, as well as the area over the ulner styloid, should be sufficiently padded to prevent irritation from the cast. The fingers should be well-padded with absorbent padding placed between to prevent maceration due to sweating.

Pain Management. Generally, NSAIDs will be given as analgesics. Ice may be used as a modality for pain control, with precautions to keep the cast/splint dry. Narcotic analgesics may be used for pain control, but these need to be used sparingly for the first 24 hours if the mechanism of injury is related to intoxicant use.

Wound Management. In case of open fracture, irrigation of the wound and dressing management will be managed. Tetanus status will be monitored as well.

Surgical Intervention. On occasion, percutaneous pinning will be required with routine postoperative care.

Nursing Considerations

Nursing Diagnoses. Nursing diagnoses for this condition are expanded upon in the Appendix.

- Body image, disturbed.
- Infection, risk for (open wound).
- Injury, risk for.
- Knowledge deficit, care for wound, need for enhanced learning.
- Pain, acute.

- Self-care deficit, bathing/dressing/feeding/toileting.
- Skin integrity, impaired.

Interventions. Routine postoperative care, as well as routine cast care, will be monitored. Pain should be assessed. Open wounds will be monitored for signs of infection. Neurovascular status and function of the fingers should be noted.

Replantation

Overview

Definition. Replantation is the re-attachment of severed body parts. See Table 20.2 for the individual definitions of the specific types of replantation.

Etiology. Generally amputations are the result of vehicular trauma, occupational hazards (industry, mechanics, farming injuries, such as power take-off (PTO), and home accidents (lawn mowers, power tools such as chainsaws and circular/radial saws).

Table 20.2. Definitions of Replantation

Total replantation	The microvascular surgical procedure to restore the hand/digit to its original site.
Revascularization	The term for reconstruction of the microcirculation that has been damaged to prevent ischemic tissue from becoming necrotic. This also refers to restoration of an incomplete amputation, which is technically more demanding than a total replant.
Complete amputation	The digit or extremity has been totally severed from the body. An incomplete or partial amputation is one in which the digit or extremity has been partially severed from the body with part of the neurovascular structures remaining intact.
Warm ischemia time	The amount of time since the amputated part was severed (without adequate cooling). A replantation needs to be performed as rapidly as possible due to ischemia time (irreversible after 6 hours of warm ischemia time) and to inhibit bacterial growth.
Cool ischemia time	The amount of time the severed part was maintained on ice.
Total ischemia time	The sum of the warm and cold ischemia times or the time elapsed from the loss of blood flow to the amputated tissue to the beginning of the surgical intervention.

Data from "Hand and Wrist" by S. Childs, 2007, NAON Core Curriculum for Orthopedic Nursing *(6th ed.). Boston, MA: Pearson.*

Pathophysiology. Replantation consists of re-attachment of partially or completely severed parts. This complex process usually involves microsurgery to re-establish the neurovascular structures, as well as surgery to promote function and appearance, with reattachment of tendons, ligaments, and often skin grafts. Digital distal parts may be replaced beyond the amputation site.

Incidence. The upper extremity is most commonly involved. Digital viability and distal replants have a higher success rate, with return of function at approximately 85%. Digits have less muscle mass and decreased metabolic needs, with microcirculation that enhances the ability to heal. Digit replantation time can extend longer (24-36 hours), depending on tissue viability and total ischemia time. Proximal replants with large muscle mass have higher failure and lower function rates because of increased ischemia, higher metabolic demands, poor re-innervation, and decreased sense of proprioception, but proximal replants at the palm and wrist generally result in good hand function (Childs, 2007).

Risk Factors. Amputations typically occur in a traumatic setting and are at great risk for infection. In addition, if the amputation occurs during a motor vehicle crash or farm injury, there may be transportation issues that affect the time of ischemia for the amputated part.

Complications. *Arterial occlusion (thrombosis):* Occlusion will be treated with heparin, fibrinolytic agents, and vasodilators. The area will need to be surgically revised.

Venous congestion: This common complication can be treated with manual massage, occupational therapy, lymphedema treatment, and medicinal leech therapy. Medicinal leech therapy "secretes hirudin, an enzyme with anticoagulant properties that assists in vascular patency causing the wound to ooze 50 ml of blood for 24-48 hours after detachment" (Childs, 2007, p. 494). Each leech will remove approximately 5 ml of blood.

Functional Limitations: Limitations including contractures, loss of sensation, and proprioception may occur. Patients may need serial surgeries to regain maximal function. Decreased tolerance to cold is a common occurrence.

Donor Site Morbidity: Special considerations must be taken into account if the patient is receiving a donor organ. The donor site may be susceptible to infection, tissue necrosis, poor/inefficient wound healing, and scarring.

Other Issues: Patients undergoing replantation may suffer from systemic complications such as sepsis, acute renal failure due to systemic inflammatory response, and shock. Complex regional pain syndrome can occur, which may be very difficult to treat. Patients who have had an amputation, with or without replantation, will often have psychological issues to overcome due to cosmetic deformity, post-traumatic stress disorder, change in lifestyle, or ability to be gainfully employed in prior occupation, etc.

Preventive strategies: Industrial sites have long had safety measures in place to prevent these injuries, from requiring gloves to installing automatic stops on saws. Common sense occasionally prevails, but newer equipment such as lawn mowers turn off if the handle is let go to prevent injuries due to reaching into the blade mechanism. Educating consumers on equipment at time of purchase, as well as encouraging gloves, safety glasses, and other protective measures, is also important.

Special considerations: This type of injury can occur in all age groups, but it is less common in children. When replantation is successful, children have better ability to re-innervate and adapt. The digit will usually grow to 80% of the expected adult length. Attempts will be made to re-attach even the more severe injuries in order to accommodate children's developmental needs (Childs, 2007).

In elderly patients, careful attention needs to be paid to the patient's co-morbidities in terms of ability to heal, ability to withstand the lengthy surgical time and anesthesia, and the metabolic demands for healing (Childs, 2007). This puts the elderly population at greater risk for amputation with revision, versus replantation.

Assessment

History. It is very important to determine the type of injury and how it occurred. Clean-cut (guillotine) amputations have the best prognosis. Severely crushed limbs are not replanted because the tissue viability is poor due to nerve stretching, massive soft tissue and vascular bed damage, contamination, comminuted fracture segments, and often missing pieces. Does the patient have other illnesses, such as diabetes, peripheral vascular disease, or neuropathy, that will impair healing? Does the patient smoke, which will make healing at the microcirculatory level difficult?

Emergency Assessment at the Scene. Initially the patient's airway, breathing, and circulation (ABCs) will need to be assessed, including an assessment of the amputated part and injury to any other organs. Blood loss needs to be estimated. Treatment for shock should be administered per protocols. Bleeding needs to be controlled, and topical debris should be removed if possible. Direct pressure needs to be applied; tourniquets are not used to control bleeding unless the patient is hemorrhaging. If so, then the tourniquet should be placed as proximally as possible to prevent further tissue ischemia.

Recovery of Amputated Tissue and Part(s). Any amputated parts that can be found should be covered with slightly moistened normal saline or dry gauze, and placed in a watertight sealed container. The part(s) should not be immersed in solution directly, nor placed directly on ice due to frostbite risk. The sealed container should be placed on ice, with time noted (very important to determine cold ischemia time). If the part is partially amputated, ice will be placed on the distal extremity, and splints are applied to prevent further movement of the tissue, ensure immobilization of the fracture, and avoid stretching of the nerves and vessels. The part(s) should be transported with the patient to the nearest emergency department. The replantation needs to be performed as rapidly as possible due to ischemia time (irreversible after 6 hours of warm ischemia time) and bacterial growth.

Emergency Department/Preoperative Care. Continue prior treatment, as well as basic and advanced life support care. Continue to assess the affected limb. Clean gross contaminants. Further debridement will be performed by the operating surgeon. Administer medications as needed, including tetanus update, antibiotics as indicated, analgesics, and any life-supporting medications and IV fluids. The patient should ingest nothing by mouth (NPO) until surgery.

Family and Patient Emotional Care and Support. This will be an extensive portion of the patient's care. The patient and family will often be devastated about the injury, as well as the decisions for further care and operations. If the trauma was due to an accident, potential blame, guilt, anger, and hostility can all contribute adversely to the patient's and family's healing and psychological well-being.

Diagnostic Tests. Radiographs will be taken of the amputated part(s) and the proximal stump. Arteriograms may be performed to determine patency of vessels. Depending on the type of trauma sustained (multi-system), type and cross match, chemistry panels, electrocardiogram, and others tests may be ordered, as determined by trauma protocols.

Common Therapeutic Modalities

Short-Term Care. Cares for this injury have been described under assessment, as this type of care need to happen simultaneously with the assessment. Certain short-term needs to be considered, such as tissue viability, avoiding infection, appropriate therapeutic clotting times, and advanced life support cares, were noted above.

Long-Term Functional Outcomes. The functional outcomes depend on several factors, including the success of the replantation, the patient's motivation and ability to use the extremity, emotional stability of patient and family, job requirements, and support of family and friends during this lengthy rehabilitation process.

Nursing Considerations

Nursing Diagnoses. Nursing diagnoses for this condition are expanded upon in the Appendix.

- Bleeding, risk for.
- Body image, disturbed.
- Coping, ineffective.
- Coping, readiness for enhanced.
- Family processes, interrupted.
- Fear.
- Grieving.
- Infection, risk for.
- Knowledge deficient, care for wound.
- Pain, acute
- Perioperative positioning injury, risk for.
- Role performance, ineffective.
- Self-care deficit, bathing/dressing/feeding/toileting.
- Sensory perception, disturbed, tactile.
- Skin integrity, impaired.
- Tissue perfusion: peripheral, ineffective.

The patient will require significant emotional support, as the patient may have significant disability and needs to understand that success of replantation is unpredictable. True hand or limb function may not be determined for several years. If the injury occurred in the work force, there will be workers' compensation issues to consider.

Home Care. The patient will need to avoid direct trauma to the limb, from collision, temperature extremes, restrictive clothing, etc. Avoid vasoconstriction by avoiding use of nicotine or alcohol. The limb needs to be constantly protected.

Outpatient Setting. Occupational or physical therapy will be needed for regaining function and desensitization. Vocational rehabilitation may need to be considered to gain employment. The patient may need to rethink occupations, as well as consider lifestyle changes and economic changes, in order to adapt to this injury. Community services may need to be utilized.

Dupuytren's Contracture

Overview

Definition. Dupuytren's contracture is a progressive thickening of the palmar aponeurosis (fascia) between the skin and flexor tendons in the distal palm and fingers. It most commonly affects the ring and small fingers at the level of the metacarpal (MCP) (American Society for Surgery of the Hand (ASSH, 1990a).

Etiology. This disease is most commonly seen in middle-aged Caucasians (rarely seen in patients of Asian or African descent), with a male-to-female frequency of 7:1. It tends to run in families, as it is an autosomal dominant trait. It is considered a middle-aged to elderly disease but has also been seen in younger persons in their twenties (ASSH, 1990a; Childs, 2007). Middle-aged to elderly Caucasian males are at greatest risk for the disease (Childs, 2007; Hughes, Mechcrefe, Littler & Akelman, 2003). It affects about 2% of the United States population.

Pathophysiology. Dupuytren's begins at the cellular level, as fibroblasts and myofibroblasts proliferate within the palmar aponeurosis (fascia), which causes thickening and fibrosis. The fascia consists of connective tissue that covers the tendons in the hand to the digits. These fibers become inflamed, which slowly leads to fibrous bands in the palmar fascia. This subsequently causes nodules to form and leads to flexion contractures of the digits. Function will get more limited due to the further worsening contractures, if not treated (ASSH, 1990a; Childs, 2005; Hughes et al., 2003).

Risk Factors. Dupuytren's has been associated with excessive alcohol use, diabetes, epilepsy, and use of repetitive vibrating equipment, such as jackhammers. The correlation to alcohol and smoking has not been directly related, however, and is controversial (Hughes, et al, 2003; Watt, Curtin, & Hintz, 2010).

Complications. Dupuytren's is associated with skin breakdown due to moisture in the contracted tissue. The nodules will eventually cause contractures, which are the major complication as these limit ROM. After surgical treatment, there is risk of recurrence in the same area or on other digits. Neurovascular damage at the time of surgery is a risk. Postoperative complications associated with orthopaedic surgery include infection, hematoma, scarring, and incomplete release of the contracture.

Preventive Strategies. These strategies are limited but primarily associated with lifestyle changes related to alcohol use (again, questionable etiology) or manual labor precipitating the inflammatory process. Modifications of job and/or lifestyle, as well as the use of braces to prevent repetitive gripping or tension, may also help reduce the incidence of Dupuytren's.

Assessment

History. Generally there is no history of trauma. Patients will often complain of progressive thickening of the palm or gradual contractures of the digits in the hand (see Figure 20.3). The disease is generally associated with mild pain or dull aches. Patients usually seek medical attention due to functional limitations, not pain.

Physical Exam. Palpate the palmar crease over the affected finger(s) and note the thickening. Determine the patient's ROM. Compare to the unaffected extremity. Dimpling or nodules are often palpated along the hand. Observe the condition of the skin, particularly between digits if more than one digit is affected; there will often be evidence of maceration. Note neurovascular status of the hand (Childs, 2007).

Figure 20.3.
Example of DuPuytren's Contracture

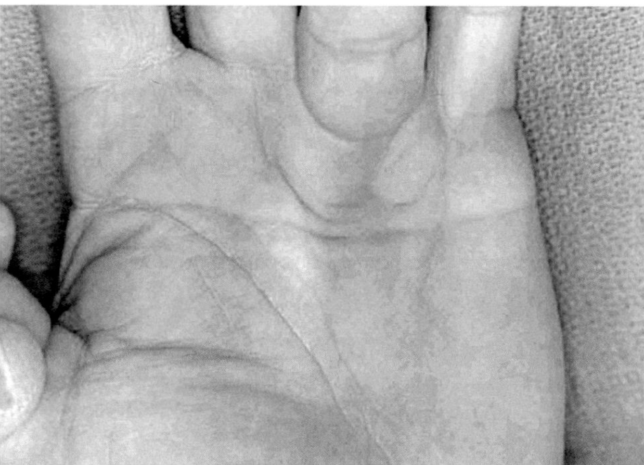

From the American Society for Surgery of the Hand, www.assh.org. Reproduced with permission.

Diagnostic Tests. A three-view x-ray of the hand may be obtained to rule out bony mass or tumor. Rarely an MRI is ordered to determine other soft tissue abnormalities.

Common Therapeutic Modalities

Therapy. Occupational therapy is often considered the first line of treatment in early Dupuytren's to maintain flexibility and mobility of the hand. This will be limited based on the progression of the disease. Often therapy is used postoperatively to regain ROM, prevent or decrease scar formation and development of adhesions, and reduce edema.

Enzymatic Fasciotomy. This consists of injecting a collagenase material into the fascia. Studies have shown that this initially decreases the thickened fascia significantly in initial treatment. The contractures can recur but tend to be milder after long-term recurrence (Watt et al., 2010).

Surgery. Surgery is the treatment of choice. The thickened palmar fascia will be excised as an outpatient procedure, generally under regional anesthesia. A bulky dressing will remain place for 5 – 7 days, allowing the hand to rest after surgery. Sutures remain for 10 – 14 days. Occupational therapy is often begun several days after surgery and may continue for several months (Childs, 2007; Hughes et al, 2003).

Nursing Considerations

Nursing Diagnoses. Nursing diagnoses for this condition are expanded upon in the Appendix.

- Body image, disturbed.
- Infection, risk for.
- Injury, risk for.
- Self-care deficit, bathing/dressing/feeding/toileting.
- Skin integrity, impaired.

Interventions. Specific nursing interventions apply to the post-surgical care of the wound, as there is often a z-shaped (Z-track or Brunner) incision. These types of incisions tend to have thin subcutaneous tissue due to the disease itself, and management of the incision can be challenge (Hughes et al., 2003).

Patient Teaching. Patients must understand post-surgical care instructions to keep the area clean, dry, and protected until healed after surgery. Specific incisional care will be determined by the attending physician as to parameters when sutures are removed, or if use of antibiotic salve or oils for scar massage is indicated. Patients need to monitor for sign of infection (erythema, drainage, and increasing pain) during healing.

Trigger Thumb or Finger

Overview

Definition. Trigger thumb or finger is a locking or snapping of the digit in a flexed position due to thickening of the tendon sheath.

Etiology. Trigger thumb or finger is often caused by repetitive movements, whether related to occupational or non-occupational exposure. It also may be related to trauma of the tendon sheath.

Pathophysiology. The affected tendon sheath gets inflamed and often develops a nodule. This inflammation causes the tendon sheath to stenose, making movement into extension more difficult. The tendon will catch, and the "pop" or "trigger" occurs as the tendon is released back into extension. The A1 pulley at the MCP head is involved in this pathology (Childs, 2007). Overall, there is too much volume in the tendon sheath. Recent studies have noted more of a degenerative versus inflammatory change as the primary cause of triggering (McAuliffe, 2010).

Incidence. There is a 6:1 female-to-male ratio for incidence of trigger thumb or finger. It tends to occur in all ages, though more common in the 40s, 50s, and early 60s (Fleisch, Spindler, & Lee, 2007). Infants may have this, most commonly in the thumb (Childs, 2007). Triggering tends to occur in the dominant hand, and often more than one digit is involved. A systematic review noted that trigger finger, as well as tendon problems, tends to occur more in those older than age 40, with a body mass index (BMI) greater than 30, and employed in jobs that have high shoulder ratings (McAuliffe, 2010).

Risk Factors. Diabetics have a fourfold increased chance of developing trigger finger. There is also an increased chance of this condition for those with rheumatoic arthritis, gout and metabolic disorders (ASSH, 1990a; Childs, 2007; Fleisch et al., 2007).

Complications. Even though 30% of trigger fingers will resolve on their own, persistent untreated triggering can worsen over time. Most complications are related to injection side effects (infection, injection of the tendon instead of the sheath, fat necrosis, skin depigmentation from steroids) or post-surgical complications (transection of the A2 pulley, incomplete release of the A1 pulley, hematoma, and/or infection) (Childs, 2007; McAuliffe, 2010).

Preventive Strategies. Diabetics should make every effort to keep sugars under control. Splinting and rest may help early in the disease.

Assessment

History. The patient will often complain of pain in the finger, particularly the proximal interphalangeal joint. Trigger fingers often lock during the night, and the patient wakes up with a "locked" finger that can be quite painful. Determine co-morbidities, prior history of trigger finger, familial tendencies for triggering, and occupational exposure. Identify if the patient has any neurovascular deficits (Childs, 2007; ASSH, 1990a).

Physical Exam. Compare the affected hand to the unaffected hand. Palpate over the tendon and at the metacarpal head for a nodule. Attempt to flex/extend the finger or thumb; triggering should be noted, or a popping sound will be heard. Edema or fluid may be palpated over the tendon sheath. Assess neurovascular status.

Diagnostic Tests. Radiographs may be taken to rule out bony pathology and to differentiate diagnosis from hypoplastic and arthrogrypotic thumb (Childs, 2007).

Common Therapeutic Modalities

Ice. Ice may be applied for 20 minutes at a time every 4 – 6 hours to reduce pain and swelling.

NSAIDS. These medications are to be taken as directed to reduce inflammation.

Therapy/Exercises. Therapy is often used to increase ROM, but it will not affect the mechanics of the disease unless iontophoresis of steroid patches is added to the treatment regimen.

Corticosteroids. Corticosteroids and local anesthetic may be injected into the tendon sheath. These injections are usually limited to two lifetime injections of the triggering area (ASSH, 1990), to prevent adverse effects of cortisone causing degradation of the tendon sheath. Diabetic patients should be instructed that corticosteroid injections are not as successful (McAuliffe, 2010). Systematic review of four randomized controlled trials provided relief in 57% of patients (Fleish et al., 2007).

Splinting. A custom-made splint may be used to decrease the patient's symptoms. A recent study showed success, in spite of lack of patient full compliance with its use, in decreasing symptoms. Longevity of this type of treatment has not been determined however (Colbourn, Heath, Manary, & Pacifico, 2008).

Surgical Decompression. Generally, the conclusive treatment for trigger thumb or trigger finger is a surgical decompression performed on an outpatient basis. The surgery involves an incision over the affected pulley, and the pulley itself is transected to allow free movement of the affected tendon. Inflammatory or degenerative changes are occasionally noted, but rarely is the tissue submitted for pathology. The surgery is considered safe and effective, and recent studies note near-complete long-term resolution of triggering (ASSH, 1990b; McAuliffe, 2010).

Nursing Considerations

Nursing Diagnoses. Nursing diagnoses for this condition are expanded upon in the Appendix.

- Injury, risk for.
- Pain, acute/chronic.
- Self-care deficit, bathing/dressing/feeding/toileting.

Nursing interventions are related to the care of the post-operative patient, including wound care, patient teaching, and preventive strategies. Orthopaedic aftercare is considered the primary learning need of patients with this type of problem. Patients need to understand that triggering may return in other fingers and can recur in a finger that was not surgically treated.

WRIST

De Quervain's

Overview

Definition. De Quervain's is a painful tenosynovitis (inflammation) of the extensor pollicis brevis and abductor pollicus longus tendons and surrounding sheath, which are located in the 1st dorsal compartment of the wrist (Childs, 2007).

Etiology. Typically seen in persons between 30 and 50 years of age, the disease is often referred to as "mother's thumb" due to repetitive lifting and carrying of an infant. It is primarily caused by repetitive and forceful exertion of the hand and thumb (Childs, 2007).

Pathophysiology. Awkward, forceful, and repetitive movements of the thumb cause inflammation, fatigue, and accumulation of waste products along the tendon sheath (Childs, 2007).

Incidence. This is more commonly seen in women, in the dominant hand. It is also noted in weekend athletes and in new mothers. De Quervain's as a work-related musculoskeletal disorder accounts for 56% of all occupational injuries (Child, 2007).

Complications. If left untreated, de Quervain's can cause permanent scarring in the first dorsal compartment, which may lead to decreased thumb motion.

Preventive Strategies. Avoid repetitive activities or known triggers. Use a thumb spica splint to allow the thumb to rest.

Assessment

History. The patient will often experience pain with lifting or abducting the thumb. This may often be quite severe. The patient may complain of difficulty holding a coffee mug or using a hairbrush as the area becomes inflamed. Determine what movements exacerbate the condition. Assess job functions, as well as non-occupational functions such as those with "weekend warriors." Evaluate duration and intensity of pain, as well as current treatment methods.

Figure 20.4.
Demonstration of Finkelstein Test

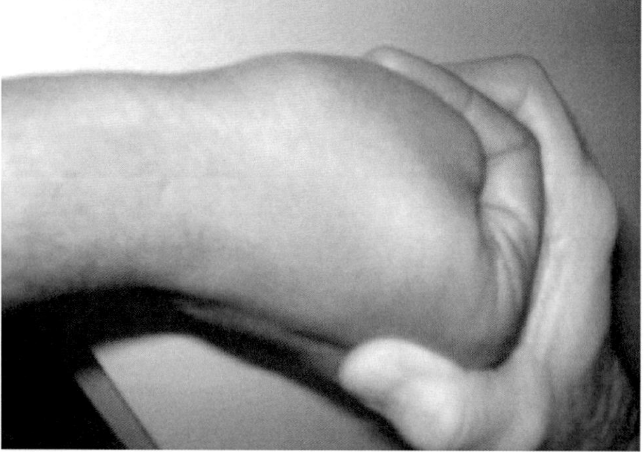

Author creation. Reproduced with permission.

Physical Exam. Assess the patient for an area of swelling along the dorsum of the wrist, particularly on the radial (thumb) side. A Finkelstein test will be performed, which involves flexing the thumb against the palm, then applying ulnar deviation to the wrist (see Figure 20.4). The patient will have pain along the first dorsal compartment.

Diagnostic Tests. The Finkelstein's test will be performed, as described above. Radiographs may be taken to rule out carpal metacarpal arthrosis of the thumb, unless trauma precipitated symptoms.

Common Therapeutic Modalities

Occupational Therapy. The therapist will review job functions and ergonomics to prevent repetitive movements, as well as use splints.

Immobilization. Use of splints during activity and at bedtime can help decrease inflammation.

NSAIDS. NSAIDs are used as anti-inflammatory, either on a scheduled or as-needed basis. Ice. Typical use in orthopaedic hand conditions is 20 minutes at a time, every 4 hours while awake, during acute flare-ups of pain.

Cortisone Injection. A short-acting steroid such as Triamcinolone acetonide (Kenalog) may be injected into the tendon sheath for inflammation and pain control.

Surgical Intervention. A surgical decompression of the first dorsal compartment is generally the last modality for treatment of De Quervains. This will open up the sheath and decrease symptoms, allowing for free movement of the tendon.

Nursing Considerations

Nursing Diagnoses. Nursing diagnoses for this condition are expanded upon in the Appendix.

- Injury, risk for.
- Pain, acute.
- Self-care deficit, bathing/dressing/feeding/toileting.

Ganglion Cyst

Overview

Definition. This benign cystic structure is found adjacent to a joint or tendon sheath.

Etiology. Cyst formation is generally related to repetitive stress that causes synovial herniation in the joint capsule. The ligament or capsule then heals, and the fluid has no place to secrete to, so it secretes into a cyst that develops under the skin. On occasion, the cyst reabsorbs and then re-forms, and patients may note that the cyst "comes and goes." They can develop after trauma to a joint. Ganglion cysts may be associated with rotary subluxation of the scaphoid (RSS) (Childs, 2007; ASSH, 1990a).

Pathophysiology. Ganglion cysts are typically found on the radial side of the wrist, either volar or dorsal. Seed ganglia may erupt on dorsal DIP or palmer surface of digits. The cysts contain a clear, jelly-like substance. They are benign.

Incidence. Ganglion cysts are more commonly found in women than men (3:1). They typically present in patients from ages 30 – 60. Ganglion cysts often recur, after spontaneous popping or even after surgical excision. They are rarely seen in the elderly population. Repetitive use, particularly after trauma, may precipitate formation.

Complications. Generally a ganglion cyst is benign. If the cyst begins to push on a nerve, however, it is generally recommended to have it excised as a pan control measure. After excision, the risk of infection or hematoma development is present.

Preventive Strategies. Avoiding repetitive stress to the affected extremity is the only known preventive strategy.

Assessment

History. The cyst may develop over time or abruptly. It may often be post-traumatic. Ask the patient if a cyst was present before (many cysts can grow back after injection or aspiration; there is an 80% recurrence rate after aspiration) (Thommasen, 2006). Is there any associated numbness, weakness, or tingling? Is there any loss of function?

Physical Exam. Determine the patient's dominant hand. Assess for pain and weakness over the area of the cyst. Have the patient dorsiflex and extend the joint to assess pain and any numbness. The cyst itself typically will feel smooth, fairly tense, and movable. On occasion, the cyst can be quite hard.

Diagnostic Tests. Radiographic studies (A/P, lateral, and oblique) of the hand and wrist will rule out additional pathology. Ultrasound and MRI may be ordered to facilitate imaging to determine depth, size, and location (Thomassen, 2006).

Common Therapeutic Modalities

Reassurance. Ganglion cysts usually resolve without treatment.

Aspiration. Aspiration of the cyst can be performed in the office under local anesthetic. This will remove the fluid but not eliminate the source of the problem. Patients who choose this option must know the likelihood of recurrence of the cyst.

Excision. This will be performed as an outpatient procedure under regional anesthesia. A compressive surgical dressing will be placed postoperatively, to be left in place for 7 – 14 days. Immobilization with use of a splint may be used also, particularly with ganglion excision over the dorsum of the wrist, to allow rest and healing (ASSH, 1990b; Childs, 2007).

Nursing Considerations

Nursing Diagnoses. Nursing diagnoses for this condition are expanded upon in the Appendix.

- Body image, disturbed.
- Infection, risk for.
- Injury, risk for.
- Knowledge deficit, care of wound.
- Self-care deficit, bathing/dressing/feeding/toileting.
- Skin integrity, impaired.

Routine nursing care of the postoperative patient is followed. Education regarding the potential recurrence of the cyst, even after operative intervention, should be reviewed with the patient. Patients often need reassurance that this type of cyst is generally benign, without long-term complications.

Arthroplasty

Overview

Definition. Arthroplasty is a partial or total replacement of the joint surface, with metal and polyethylene plastic or silicone. The purpose of replacement is for pain relief, and to improve function, flexibility, and mobility of the hand, fingers, and/or wrist. Pain relief is often the main reason for this procedure.

Etiology. The surgery is performed on patients with osteoarthritis or rheumatoid arthritis. It may also be ordered after trauma, nonunion of fractures, or tumors.

Pathophysiology. Patients with underlying disease such as rheumatoid arthritis, psoriatric arthritis, osteoarthritis, systemic lupus erythematosus, and ankylosing spondylitis have erosion of the joint and cartilage, which causes pain and instability. Inflammation will affect the cartilage and capsule, causing articular changes, pain, and loss of joint function. Often joint space narrowing, crepitus, osteophytes, and sclerosis are noted. Many mediators of inflammation are noted, which include "bioactive lipids (prostaglandins, leukotrienes, lipoxegenase products, platelet activating factors, thromboxane), complement components, cytokines (interleukins, tumor necrosis factor, colony stimulating factors, growth promoting factors), coagulation factors, proteinases, activated platelets, oxygen-derived free radicals (super-oxide anion, hydrogen peroxide and hydroxyl radical)" (Childs, 2007, p. 500).

Complications. Complications related to joint arthroplasty include infection, lack of function post-operatively, and pain while healing.

Preventive Strategies. Avoidance of repetitive activities may decrease the pain that precipitates the need for joint replacement.

Assessment

History. Determine if the patient has had prior hand or wrist surgery. What is the dominant hand? What are the symptoms? When does the joint hurt? What exacerbates the pain? Does anything relieve the pain? Are there other symptoms or joints affected? Does the patient have any constitutional symptoms, such as fever, chills, fatigue, malaise, or weakness? Is there a family history of arthritis or joint replacement?

Physical Exam. Assess the joint involved, as well as the joints above and below the affected joint. Evalute active and passive ROM. Compare the affected extremity to the unaffected extremity. Are any nodes (Heberden's and Bouchard's) noted? What is the neurovascular status of the affected extremity? Determine if there are any skin breakdowns, lesions, or sores. Is there deviation of the wrist that may lend suspicion to a joint disease of multiple joints versus an isolated joint?

Diagnostic Tests. Radiographs will be obtained in multiple views of the affected extremity. Joint narrowing, osteophytes, sclerosis, and other problems may be noted.

Common Therapeutic Modalities

Injections. Intra-articular injections may be considered of either corticosteroids or hyaluronic acid for decreasing inflammation and providing a smoother articulating surface.

Medications. Analgesics are often used for pain. NSAIDs can also be considered.

Splinting. Splints may be utilized to provide pain control and to limit movement of the affected extremity. These may be used pre- and postoperatively. These splints are often used in combination with physical or occupational therapy.

Nursing Considerations

Nursing Diagnoses. Nursing diagnoses for this condition are expanded upon in the Appendix.

- Bleeding, risk for.
- Body image, disturbed.
- Infection, risk for.
- Knowledge deficient, care for wound.
- Pain, acute.
- Perioperative positioning injury, risk for.
- Self-care deficit, bathing/dressing/feeding/toileting.
- Sensory perception: tactile, disturbed.
- Skin integrity, impaired.

Nursing care of the patient with an arthroplasty will focus on routine postoperative care, as well as strategies for strengthening, preventing infection, improving ROM through therapy, and identifying preventable risk factors that may have precipitated the need for an arthroplasty. This may include activity modification, medical control of gout or rheumatology concerns, or preventing trauma that may have precipitated the development of osteoarthritis.

Scaphoid Fracture

Overview

Definition. A scaphoid fracture involves a fracture of the scaphoid (navicular) bone in the wrist.

Etiology. This common fracture occurs as a result of trauma, generally a fall, on an outstretched hand (FOOSH). It is known for increased incidence of non-union.

Pathophysiology. A scaphoid fracture occurs from forceful hyperextension of the wrist. There are several areas of the scaphoid that can be injured (waist, proximal, distal, and tubercle), depending on the position of the forearm at the time of injury. A fracture through the waist or proximal portion of the scaphoid is the most serious, as this threatens the bone's distal blood supply, which can lead to avascular necrosis of the proximal fragment (Childs, 2007; Mortiere, 2004).

Incidence. This is the most common carpal bone fracture (68%) and is most often seen after falls. It is more common in females ages 20 - 40 (Childs, 2007; Egol et al., 2010).

Risk Factors. Risk factors are related to failure to properly diagnose the fracture, as well as delayed union or non-union of the fracture, which can cause significant pain and impairment, particularly of the thumb, later on in life.

Complications. If misdiagnosed, the patient may be predisposed to chronic wrist pain, delayed union or non-union, and avascular necrosis. This can lead to loss of ROM, decreased grip strength, and cosmetic deformity. If surgery is required to reduce the fracture, common postoperative complications can include infection, pain, or loss of reduction of the fracture (Childs, 2007).

Assessment

History. Determine mechanism of injury for the presenting complaint of pain and/or deformity. Establish hand dominance of the patient. Ascertain if the patient has pain at rest or while gripping objects, or if there is loss of ROM.

Physical Exam. The patient may or may not complain of pain at the anatomic snuffbox of the radial aspect of the wrist. Examine the wrist for swelling, ecchymosis, neurovascular status of the hand, and ROM of the thumb. Assess if axial compression of the thumb along with radial deviation of the wrist elicits pain (Childs, 2007).

Diagnostic Tests. Radiographs of the wrist (A/P, lateral, oblique, and navicular/scaphoid) will be obtained. Comparison x-rays to the unaffected extremity may be needed. Please note that initial radiographs may not indicate the fracture. A bone scan may be performed to assist with diagnosis of the fracture.

Common Therapeutic Modalities

Splinting. Any patient who presents with the possibility of a scaphoid fracture should be treated as a confirmed fracture until proven otherwise. The patient should be placed, at minimum, in a long-arm (or short-arm pending physician preference) thumb spica splint until repeat radiographs or bone scan confirm the presence or absence of a fracture.

Medications. Generally, NSAIDs are used for anti-inflammatory purposes. Analgesics, with or without narcotics, will be used for pain.

Casting. If fracture is confirmed (at either the initial visit or subsequent visits), a thumb spica short- or long-arm cast will be placed. Immobilization will be for 6 – 8 weeks.

Surgical Intervention. An open reduction internal fixation with placement of screws and/or bone graft may be required. In cases of non-union, further surgeries may be needed, which may include arthrodesis of the wrist or carpectomy.

Bone Stimulators. Bone stimulators, either by electrical impulses or ultrasound, may be needed to promote increased blood supply to the affected bone in cases of delayed union.

Nursing Considerations

Nursing Diagnoses. Nursing diagnoses for this condition are expanded upon in the Appendix.

- Infection, risk for (if open wound).
- Injury, risk for.
- Knowledge deficit, care of wound, cast care.
- Pain, acute.
- Self-care deficit, bathing/dressing/feeding/toileting.
- Skin integrity, impaired.

Patient Teaching. Routine cast care, neurological exams, and management of patient postoperative needs, such as pain management and teaching of hygiene and personal care with the use of one hand, will be necessary. As this type of fracture is notorious for mal-union or delayed union, it is imperative that patients understand the need for close follow-up of this type of fracture. Frequent x-rays to monitor healing and possibly CT scans may be utilized to determine this.

Distal Radius Fractures – Colles' and Smith's Fractures

Overview

Definition. A fracture of the distal radius may or may not involve the articular surface. The fracture can be simple or comminuted. Often the fracture will also involve the ulna, as the two bones work together with flexion and extension of the wrist. There are two common distal radius fractures, a Colles' fracture and a Smith's fracture. A Colles' fracture generally has dorsal angulation and will occur within 2 cm of the distal radius (Altizer, 2008). A Smith's fracture has volar angulation and tends to be very unstable.

Figure 20.5.
Common Position of Hand During a Fall

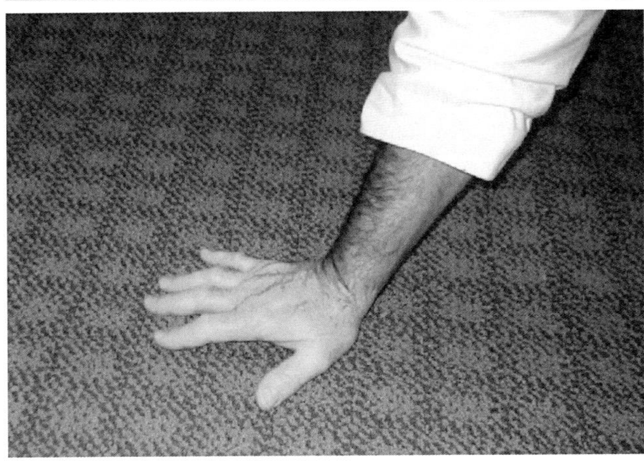

Author creation. Reproduced with permission.

Etiology. Both of these fractures generally occur due to a fall, when the patient puts his or her hand out to catch him- or herself, and the blow causes the wrist to break. These fractures can also be associated with objects landing on the wrist, or if the wrist gets placed into a forceful hyperextension. (See Figure 20.5 for an example of hand position during a fall, causing a Smith's or Colles' fracture.)

Pathophysiology. The distal radius and ulna articulate with the bones of the wrist. A forceful injury to the radius can cause displacement of the other soft tissues or the triangular fibrocartilage complex (TFCC), which can also cause an ulnar styloid fracture. There are many classification systems defining the specific type of fractures, angulation patterns, comminution, etc., but the

Figure 20.6a.
AP View of Smith's Fracture

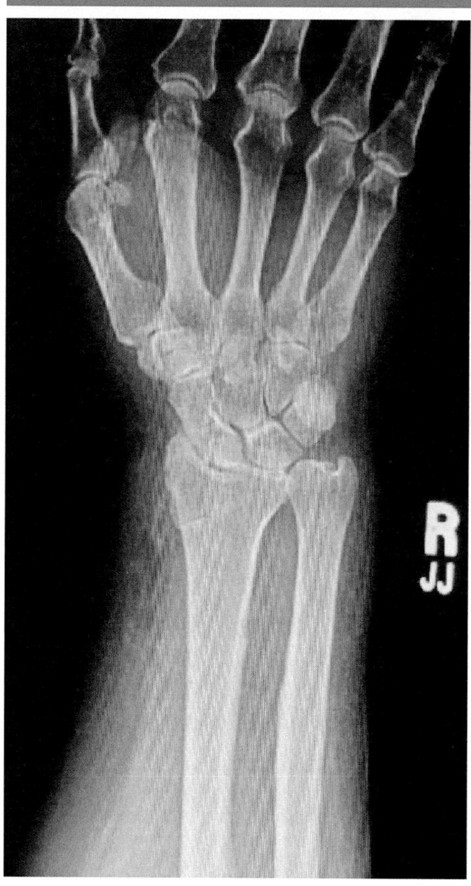

Figure 20.6b.
Lateral view of Smith's Fracture

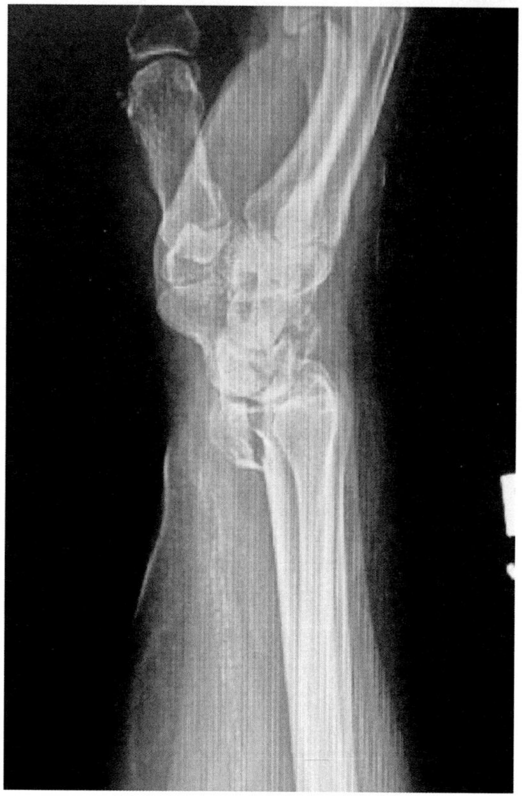

Note volar displacement of fracture.
Author creations. Reproduced with permission.

most important areas to define are the stability of the fracture, the density of the bone, and if there is articular involvement of the fracture. The median nerve lies in the carpal bones and is susceptible to stretching, tearing, or compression following these fractures.

Incidence. Distal radius fractures occur at any age, but they are more significant in both severity and incidence in the elderly population. This is primarily due to delayed reaction times, sensory losses that increase the chance of falling, and osteopenic or osteoporotic bone. Distal radius fractures are the most common fracture of the upper extremity, with 650,000 fractures occurring annually in the United States (Egol et al., 2010).

Complications. Complications can vary from pain, infection if there is an open fracture, poor or delayed healing, mal-union, articular involvement with predisposition for development of arthritis in the wrist, damage to the median nerve, or loss of ROM or function, particularly if the dominant hand is involved. Compartment syndrome can occur due to significant swelling in the wrist, and an emergent carpal tunnel release may be necessary to prevent permanent damage to the median nerve.

Preventive Strategies. Fractures sustained due to falls, or from accidents such as with bicyclists, are difficult to prevent. There is generally a higher incidence of these fractures in the winter in climates with ice. Prompt removal of snow and ice, good-soled shoes, and proper lighting may help decrease the incidence of these types of fractures.

Assessment

History. How was the injury sustained? Was any treatment performed before arrival? Does the patient have a history of prior injury? Which is the dominant hand?

Physical Exam. The wrist will often be deformed. Assess the skin for open areas, ecchymosis, tenting of the skin, and bleeding. Does the patient complain of numbness or tingling to the fingers? This is particularly important to assess, given the proximity of the median nerve to the fracture. Movement of the fingers and edema is important to assess. Any jewelry should be removed from the hand at the time of injury due to the swelling that will occur.

Diagnostic Tests. Three-view radiographs (AP, lateral, and oblique) will be taken of the affected extremity (see

Fibure 20.6a and 20.6b). On occasion, comparative views of the other extremity or a reconstructive CT scan may be ordered to help the surgeon determine if an open reduction needs to occur, and if use of both volar plates and possibly dorsal screws or fixation is needed.

Common Therapeutic Modalities

Splinting. Initially, a sugar-tong splint will be used to stabilize the fracture until the swelling has receded enough for a cast to be placed. The fracture may be reduced during splint placement via a gentle "nudge" by the orthopaedic surgeon, after a hematoma block or conscious sedation by anesthesia.

Medications. Pain medications will be used. If the fracture was open, antibiotic therapy may be instituted.

Casting. Casts will be placed, either long- or short-arm depending on the stability of the fracture and surgeon preference, after the initial swelling has gone down.

Surgical Intervention. Surgical intervention will be required for fractures with a tendency to displace, such as seen with osteopenic bone, elderly, comminuted fractures, and fractures with significant angulation or radial shortening. Surgical intervention will include the use of a volar plate (either locked or unlocked), a dorsal plate (less common), or percutaneous pins with use of external fixator or casting (Egol et al., 2010). Figures 20.7a and 20.7b show fracture repair.

Nursing Considerations

Nursing Diagnoses. Nursing diagnoses for this condition are expanded upon in the Appendix.

- Infection, risk for (if open wound).
- Injury, risk for.
- Knowledge deficit, need for enhanced learning.
- Pain, acute.
- Self-care deficit, bathing/dressing/feeding/toileting.
- Skin integrity, impaired.

Patient Teaching. Standard postoperative instructions, cast and wound care, and the importance of follow-up appointments will be reviewed with the patient. Adjusting to completing activities of daily living with an impaired extremity during treatment, as well as beginning occupational therapy after casting, will be started. The patient will need education regarding complications such as infection, compartment syndrome, and median nerve damage.

Figure 20.7a.
Lateral View of Smith's Fracture After Repair

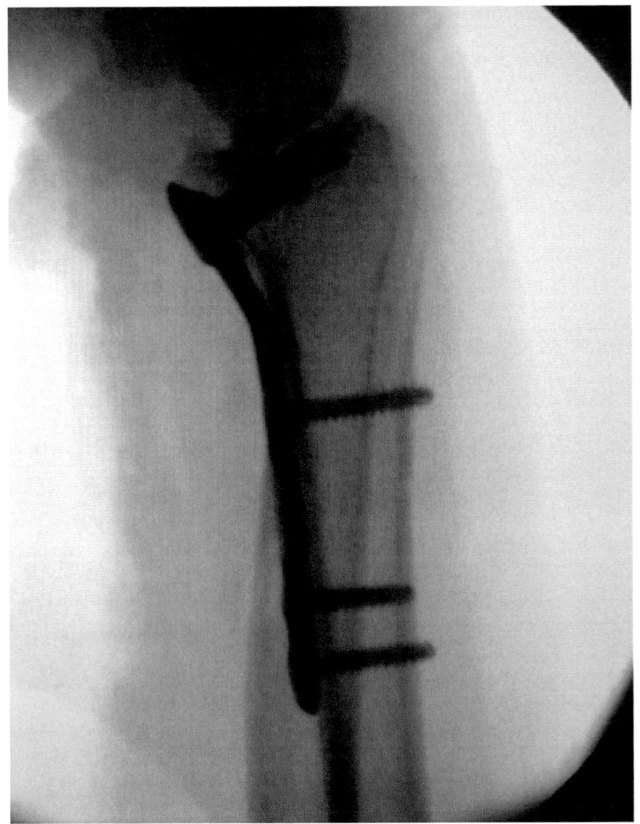

Figure 20.7b.
PA View of Smith's Fracture After Repair

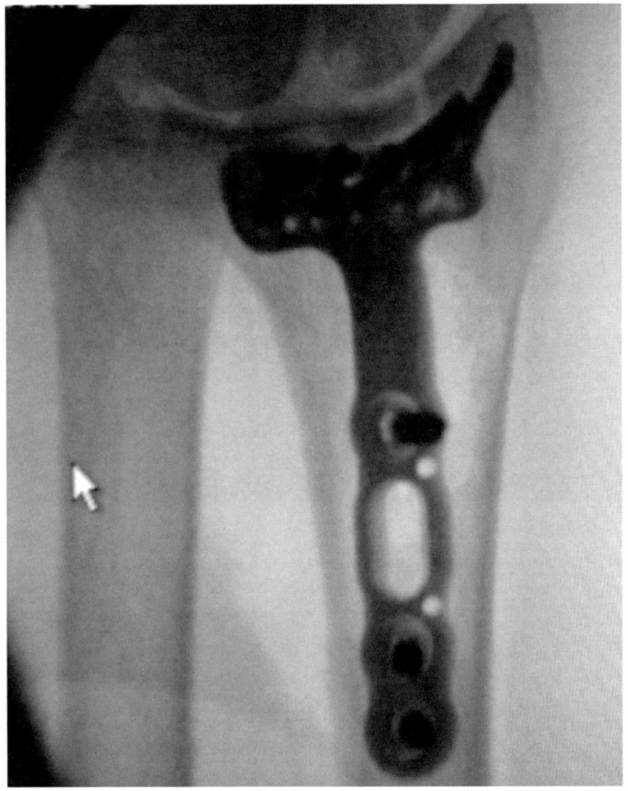

Author creations. Reproduced with permission.

Carpal Tunnel Syndrome

Overview

Definition. Carpal tunnel syndrome is an entrapment of the median nerve, which becomes compressed beneath the transverse carpal ligament of the wrist, with subsequent pressure and decreased function (Childs, 2007; Keith, Masear, Chung, et al., 2009).

Etiology. It is the most common nerve entrapment of the upper extremity. It is seen with arthritis and lipomas, and may be related to repetitive or sustained occupational exposure, though recent studies are questioning the validity of that. It is seen more commonly in diabetics and in those with thyroid dysfunction.

Pathophysiology. The carpal tunnel consists of the transverse carpal ligament and the carpal bones. The median nerve travels over the carpal bones and under the ligament. As the ligament thickens, it presses on the median nerve, causing numbness and pain.

Incidence. Carpal tunnel syndrome is more common in women and those with diabetes and thyroid imbalance. It is more often noted on the dominant hand.

Risk Factors. This affliction is associated with pregnancy, menopause, and repetitive work and/or squeezing the mechanism of injury.

Complications. If left untreated, carpal tunnel syndrome can progress from numbness and tingling to pain. Eventually, muscle wasting will occur in the thenar and hypothenar eminence, and permanent nerve damage is likely, particularly with fine motor skills. Complications seen postoperatively include infection, hematoma, neurovascular injury, incomplete transaction of the transverse carpal ligament, and temporary nerve paresthesias.

Preventive Strategies. Once symptoms start, patients can try to avoid activities that exacerbate their symptoms. Use of a carpal tunnel splint, particularly, at bedtime is helpful to reduce symptoms. NSAIDs can reduce inflammatory symptoms but will generally not reverse the thickening of the ligament that has occurred.

Assessment

History. The patient will often present with a history of numbness, tingling, or "sleepiness" in the thumb, index finger, and middle and radial side of the ring finger. Occasionally, the symptoms can radiate to the forearm and shoulder. Often patients will shake the affected extremity to "wake up" the nerve and decrease the symptoms. Repositioning may decrease the symptoms. Positions that increase pain and numbness are associated with gripping, vibration, and hyperextension, which can be related to certain occupational professions such as computer operators, carpenters, paint sprayers, writers, etc. The patient will often present once the pain worsens or when function begins to get affected such as dropping small objects, difficulty grasping large or heavy objects, etc. Ascertain if the pain radiates to specific areas of the body. What are the patient's occupation and hobbies? Does the pain seem to get worse with certain activity? (Childs, 2007; Keith, Masear, Chung, et al., 2009).

Physical Exam. The affected hand should be compared to the non-affected hand. Atrophy of the thenar and hypothenar eminence is often noted, as well as decreased grip strength. Classic tests for carpal tunnel syndrome include the Phalen's and Tinel's tests. The Phalen's test consists of maintaining the wrist in flexion for 60 seconds. It is considered positive if symptoms are reproduced. In a Tinel's test, the examiner percusses the volar aspect of the wrist. A positive test elicits symptoms in the median nerve distribution. Two-point discrimination, and for neuropathy testing, and muscle testing will be performed (Keith, Masear, Chung, et al., 2009).

Diagnostic Tests. A radiograph may be taken (A/P and lateral of wrist) to rule out bony abnormalities. An electromyelogram (EMG) is often performed to rule out decreases in muscle and nerve conduction. The EMG will grade the severity of the syndrome, as well as note lesions related to the median nerve or from upper extremity or cervical radiculopathy.

Common Therapeutic Modalities

Treatment of Underlying Cause. The patient may be instructed in ergonomic positioning. In pregnancy, the symptoms may persist until the pregnancy ends.

Splinting and Rest of the Affected Extremity. Use of splints at nighttime and during occupational exposure may reduce symptoms, particularly if this begins early in treatment.

Corticosteroid. Short-acting corticosteroids, such as Triamcinolone Acetonide (Kenalog), may be injected to reduce inflammation of the carpal tunnel ligament. If this does not significantly reduce the patient's symptoms, another treatment option should be considered, such as surgery (Keith, Masear, Amadio, et al., 2009).

NSAIDs. NSAIDs are used as anti-inflammatory, either on a regular schedule or as needed.

Occupational Therapy. Therapy may look at ergonomics and treatment modalities such as splinting, ice, exercises, ultrasound, and massage. Therapy can be used alone or as an adjunct to pre- and postoperative care.

Surgical Decompression. The surgical treatment varies from endoscopic to open decompression of the transverse carpal tunnel ligament (flexor retinaculum).

Generally, a dressing and splint will be used for the first 7 – 14 postoperative days, and then use of the splint at bedtime as needed. The patient will be allowed to use the fingers as tolerated immediately following surgery, then the wrist as tolerated once the splint is discontinued. In endoscopic decompression, splinting is rarely used, and the patient may return to work or full function several days after surgery. Therapy, as described above, may be used postoperatively for edema reduction, pain control, strengthening, and increasing ROM (Keith, Maesar, Amadio, et al., 2009).

Nursing Considerations

Nursing Diagnosis. Nursing diagnoses for this condition are expanded upon in the Appendix.

- Body image, disturbed.
- Infection, risk for.
- Knowledge deficit, enhanced learning.
- Self-care deficit, bathing/dressing/feeding/toileting.
- Skin integrity, impaired.

Patient Teaching. Patient teaching will be tailored toward postoperative care of the surgical patient. The patient may or may not need therapy postoperatively but should be encouraged to use the fingers and hand to reduce edema and stiffness. If an EMG is ordered as part of the diagnostic studies, the patient should have the procedure explained to him/her prior to arriving for the exam.

Summary

As noted throughout this chapter, the hand and wrist are essential to everyday activities. It is imperative that the orthopaedic nurse understand the proper care, assessment, and interventions in caring for individuals with injury, trauma, or deformity of the hand and wrist to promote proper healing, prevent complications, and return the individual to the highest level of functioning possible in order to return to the previous quality of life and productivity. Productivity is defined not only in terms of employment means and making a living, but also in the activities that give the patient pleasure and a source of comfort. These may include computer work, sewing, scrapbooking, embroidery, woodwork, and other types of crafts, all involving intricate use of the hand and wrist. Working as a team, the surgeons, nurse practitioners, clinical nurse specialists, physician assistants, therapists, radiologists, pharmacists, emergency staff, and surgical team members must use clear communication and show mutual respect for the knowledge that each team member brings to the care of the patient. This will enhance the care of these patients and facilitate the best possible outcomes in these injuries.

References

Altizer, L. (2008). Colles' fracture. *Orthopaedic Nursing, 27*(2), pp. 140-145. doi:10.1097/01.NOR.0000315631.30676.2b

American Society for Surgery of the Hand (1990a). *The hand: Examination and diagnosis* (3rd ed.). New York, NY: Churchill Livingstone.

American Society for Surgery of the Hand (1990b). *The hand: Primary care of common problems* (2nd ed). New York, NY: Churchill Livingstone.

Bendre, A., Hartigan, B., & Kalainov, D. (2005). Mallet finger. *Journal of the American Academy of Orthopedic Surgeons, 13*(5), 336-344.

Childs, S. (2007). Hand and wrist. In NAON's *Core Curriculum for Orthopedic Nursing* (6th ed., pp. 483-506). Boston, MA: Pearson Custom Publishing.

Childs, S. (2005). Dupuytren's disease. *Orthopaedic Nursing, 24*(2), 160-165.

Colbourn, J., Heath, N., Manary, S., & Pacifico, D. (2008). Effectiveness of splinting for the treatment of trigger finger. *Journal of Hand Therapy, 21*(4), 336-343. doi:10.1197/j.jht.2008.05.001

Dorf, E., Blue, C., Smith, B., & Koman, L. (2010). Therapy after injury to the hand. *Journal of the American Academy of Orthopaedic Surgeons, 18*(8), 464-473.

Egol, K., Koval, K., & Zuckerman, J. (2010). Hand. Wrist. Distal radius. In *Handbook of Fractures* (4th ed., pp. 269-323). Philadelphia, PA: Lippincott, Williams and Wilkins.

Fleisch, S., Spindler, K., & Lee, D. (2007). Corticosteroid injection in the treatment of trigger finger: A level 1 and 2 systematic review. *Journal of the American Academy of Orthopaedic Surgeons, 15*(3), 166-171.

Hughes, T., Jr., Mechrefe, A., Littler, W., & Akelman, E. (2003). Dupuytren's disease. *The Journal of Hand Surgery, 3*(1), 27-40. doi:10.1053/jssh.2003.50005

Keith, M., Masear, V., Amadio, P., Andary, M., Barth, R., Graham, B., …McGowan, R. (2009). Treatment of carpal tunnel syndrome. *Journal of the American Academy of Orthopedic Surgeons, 17*(6), 397-405.

Keith, M. Masear, V., Chung, K., Maupin, K., Andary, M., Amadio, P., …Wies, J. (2009). Diagnosis of carpal tunnel syndrome. *Journal of the American Academy of Orthopaedic Surgeons, 17*(6), 389-396.

Lackey, E., & Sutton, R. (2006). The diagnosis of gamekeeper's thumb. *General Practitioner.* Retrieved from http://www.gponline.com/Clinical/article/586033/diagnosis-gamekeepers-thumb/

Leinberry, C. (2009). Mallet finger injuries. *The Journal of Hand Surgery, 34*(9), 1715-1717. doi:10.1016/j.jhsa.2009.06.018

McAuliffe, J. (2010). Tendon disorders of the hand and wrist. *The Journal of Hand Surgery, 35A*, 846-853.

Mortiere, M. (2004). Common orthopedic injuries of the hand. In M.D. Mortiere's *Principles of Primary Wound Management* (2nd ed., pp. 79-82). Fairfax, VA: Clifton Publishing.

Silva, P., Lombarid, I., Jr., Breitschwerdt, C., Araujo, P., & Natour, J. (2008). Functional thumb orthosis for type 1 and 2 boutonniere deformity on the dominant hand in patients with rheumatoid arthritis: a randomized controlled study. *Clinical Rehabilitation, 22,* pp. 684-689.

Tendon trouble in the hands: de Quervain's tenosynovitis and trigger finger (2010). *Harvard Women's Health Watch, 17*(8), 4-5.

Thommasen, H., Johnston, C., & Thommasen, A. (2006). Management of the occasional wrist ganglion. *Canadian Journal of Rural Medicine, 11*(1), 51-53.

U.S. Department of Labor, Bureau of Labor Statistics. (2010). *Nonfatal occupational injuries and illnesses requiring days away from work.* Retrieved March 1, 2011 from http://www.bls.gov/news.release/archives/osh2_11092010.pdf

Watt, A., Curtin, C. & Hentz, V. (2010). Collagenase injection as nonsurgical treatment of Dupuytren's disease: 8 year follow up. *The Journal of Hand Surgery, 25*(4), 534-539.doi:10.1016/j.jhsa.2010.01.003

Chapter 21
The Hip, Femur, & Pelvis

Barbara Kahn-Kastell, RN, ONC

Objectives

- Identify different options for surgical treatment of hip arthritis.
- Explain the different prosthetic implants used for hip replacements.
- Classify different actions of the hip and pelvis.
- Compare and contrast the differences between inflammatory arthritis, osteoarthritis, and avascular necrosis.
- Explain the indications, pre- and postoperative management, and complications associated with hip arthroscopy.
- Define femeroacetabular impingement.
- Differentiate between cam-type and pincer-type procedures.
- Identify risk factors for pelvic, femoral, and hip fractures. Discuss the different nursing considerations for each.

There are many diagnoses associated with trauma or disease of the hip, femur, and pelvis. The care of patients sustaining such disorders is complex; therefore, it is imperative to have proficient and extensive knowledge in orthopedic nursing when caring for these patients. Falls are the primary cause of injuries to those ages 65 or older; in the United States, more than 11 million falls are expected annually within this patient population, with more than 60% occurring in the home (Cleveland Clinic Foundation, n.d.).

Hip Fractures

Overview

Hip fracture is defined as a break or disruption in the continuity of the proximal portion of the femur. Lateral rotation injury can occur when the head of the femur is fixed in the acetabulum; the femoral neck rotates and buckles, causing a fracture. Stress fractures may occur spontaneously or secondary to trauma. In patients with prosthetic hips, the tensile load from the bone displaces to the area below or between the prosthesis due to a stress riser that occurs at the interface, resulting in weakness and fracture vulnerability. Hip muscles tend to displace fracture fragments and are responsible for some clinical signs of hip fracture, including internal rotation and shortening. Vascular supply to the femoral head consists of arteries that enter at the junction of the femoral head and femoral neck. Fractures may tear the blood vessels, which may cause moderate to severe blood loss or avascular necrosis.

There are three types of hip fractures:

1. Intracapsular: Located within the joint capsule and include femoral neck and subcapital fractures (see Figure 21.1). Intracapsular fractures can also be categorized as displaced or nondisplaced.
2. Extracapsular: Located outside the joint capsule and include intertrochanteric (between trochanters) and subtrochanteric (below lesser trochanters) fractures. Extracapsular fractures are more common in males and more active elderly, and are usually related to greater trauma/force and increased physical activity.
3. Periprosthetic: Located within the area below or between replaced joints (see Figure 21.2). Periprosthetic fractures occur below the femoral stem of a hip prosthesis or between the femoral stem and the femoral component of a knee replacement.

Although falls are the major cause of hip fractures, vehicular accidents and pathology such as osteoporosis, metastatic disease, and Paget's disease can also be causative reasons for fracture. Surgical intervention can be very successful when treating these patients. Unfortunately, only 25% of hip fracture patients will have a complete recovery, 40% will require admission to a skilled nursing facility, and 24% of patients older than age 50 will die within 1 year of hip surgery (American Academy of Orthopaedic Surgeons [AAOS], n.d.). Complications to

Figure 21.1.
Intracapsular Femoral Neck Fracture

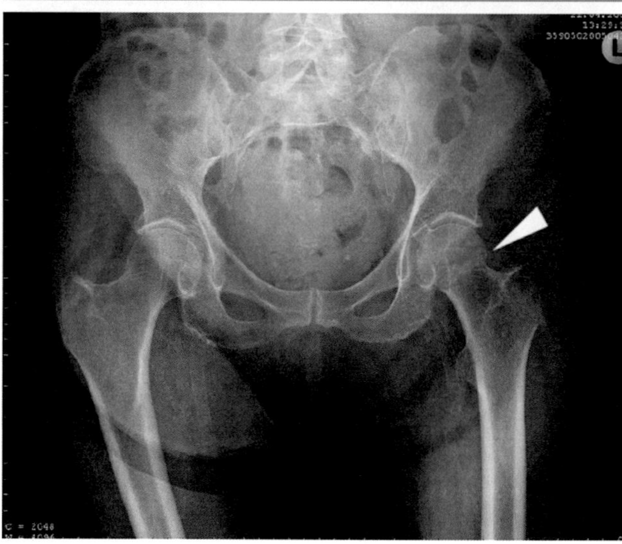

From "Anonymisierte Röntgenaufnahme einer medialen Schenkelhalsfraktur ohne Dislokation" by Sjoehest, 2005, http://en.wikipedia.org/wiki/File:Shf_ohne_dislokation_medial_ap.jpg. Reproduced with permission.

Figure 21.2.
Periprosthetic Fracture of the Lesser Trochanter

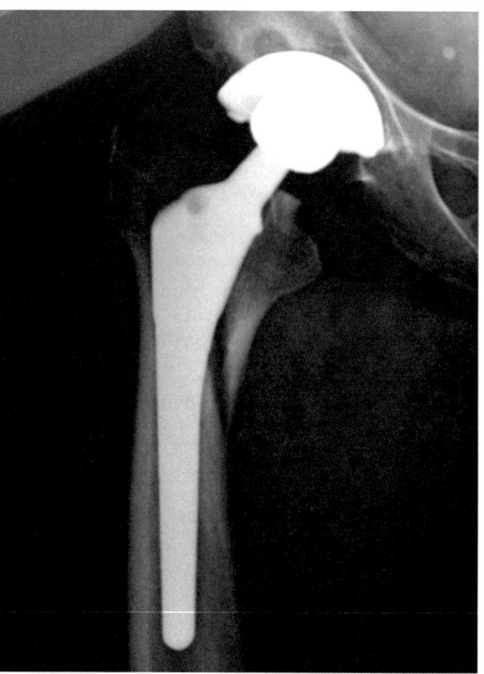

From Dr. Douglas Padgett—Hospital for Special Surgery, 2011. Reproduced with permission.

hip surgery can include delayed union/nonunion, avascular necrosis, pulmonary embolism/thrombophlebitis, and postoperative infections (Theis & Kahn, 2007).

Hip fracture is an acute event that results in a crisis for the patient and caregivers. Postfracture lifestyle changes can affect multiple family members. It is important to identify special risk factors and prevent further harm. Safety in the home, weight-bearing exercise programs, and routine testing for osteoporosis should be emphasized to patients at risk for hip fractures.

Assessment

History and Physical Exam. There are several factors to consider when assessing a hip fracture patient. It is important to know the circumstances of the accident, time between when the injury occurred and care was sought, the patient's prior level of function, the patient's home environment and support system, and the patient's chronic health problems. When conducting a physical exam, movement of the joints on the injured leg should be kept to a minimum due to severe pain in the hip and leg. These patients often hold the affected extremity in a position of comfort rather than anatomic alignment. They are typically unable to walk, or bend and move the injured leg when lying supine. Hip fracture patients will present with several physical symptoms, including the following:

- shortening of the affected leg;
- pain in the affected extremity;
- pressure over the greater trochanter;
- external or internal rotation of the injured leg (external is most common);
- swelling around the site of the injury; and
- discoloration of the surrounding tissues, extending into the groin or down the affected thigh.

Neurovascular assessment of the affected leg should be conducted and compared to the unaffected leg for a baseline. (See Chapter 3—Musculoskeletal Assessment). Bony prominences on the hip and leg should be assessed for skin breakdown or bruising.

Diagnostic Tests. Laboratory diagnostics to assess hip fractures should include complete blood count (CBC), metabolic panel, Protime/INR, and type and crossmatch. Radiographs typically include anteroposterior (AP) and lateral views of the hip, along with chest x-rays for surgery if indicated. Bone scans may be ordered if there is a suspicion of a fracture that does not appear on plain x-rays.

Common Therapeutic Modalities

Conservative. Conservative treatment modalities may be chosen if a patient has dementia, resides in extended care, was not ambulatory prefracture, or has a poor prognosis to return to a functional level of mobility (Theis & Kahn, 2007). A patient with severe osteoporosis, for example, could end up with a nonunion of the fracture. Medical compromise could result in death if an operation is performed. In addition, nondisplaced, stable, or impacted hip fractures may not need surgical repair.

Surgical. Preoperative therapeutic modalities include the following:

- Buck's traction to decrease muscle spasm and immobilize the leg;
- IV fluids as ordered;
- NPO per anesthesia protocol;
- Pain management with a goal of optimum pain relief without over sedation;
- Skin care;
- Repositioning (between back and side-lying on the unaffected extremity, keeping legs abducted with a pillow);
- Relieve patient anxiety and answer questions; and
- Complete surgical preparation and obtain consents.

Surgery should be scheduled within 24 hours of the patient's arrival in the emergency department. The goal of surgery is to repair the fracture and return the patient to prefracture functional levels. Operative choices are based on the type of fracture:

- Intracapsular or femoral neck fractures may require threaded pins, compression hip screws, femoral head replacement, primary total hip replacement, or hemiarthroplasty (less invasive than total replacement, often used in low-demand, elderly, and medically unstable patients).
- Intertrochanteric fractures repaired with open reduction and internal fixation may require nails, pins, and compression hip screws.
- Subtrochanteric fracture repairs require open reduction and internal fixation with intermedullary nail, sliding nail plate, or fixed plate.
- Periprosthetic fractures require revision of the component to a larger stemmed prosthesis that bypasses the fracture site. Plates, cables, and/or strut grafting may also be used if additional strength of the bone is needed.

The type of fracture, bone integrity, and stability of repair will dictate postoperative weight-bearing status. Internal fixation may limit weight-bearing for up to 6 months, while hemiarthroplasty or primary total hip replacement will allow for a more rapid progression with weight-bearing (Theis & Kahn, 2007).

Nursing Considerations

Nursing Diagnoses. Nursing diagnoses for this condition are expanded upon in the Appendix.

- Activity intolerance.
- Anxiety.
- Caregiver role strain, risk for.
- Confusion, acute.
- Constipation, risk for.
- Coping, ineffective.
- Disuse syndrome, risk.
- Falls, risk for.
- Family processes, interrupted.
- Fear.
- Gas exchange, impaired.
- Hopelessness.
- Infection, risk for.
- Knowledge deficit.
- Loneliness, risk for.
- Mobility: physical, impaired.
- Nutrition, imbalanced: risk for less than body requirements.
- Pain, acute.
- Post-trauma syndrome, risk for.
- Powerlessness.
- Self-care deficit: bathing/hygiene, dressing/grooming, feeding, toileting.
- Surgical recovery, delayed.
- Skin integrity, risk for impairment.
- Tissue perfusion: cardiac, risk for decreased.
- Tissue perfusion: peripheral, ineffective.

Interventions and Outcomes. A return to prefracture living arrangements, with support from family and friends, is ideal and can be accomplished when patients are involved in discharge planning. Home care arrangements and support systems should be assessed during discharge planning. Patient/caregiver discussions determine the level of care after the acute hospital stay. The nurse, together with the case manager or discharge planner, needs to assist the patient/caregivers in reviewing options for home care, rehabilitation facility, community-based residential facility (CBRF), or subacute facility, and communicate all plans with the physician. It is essential to discuss several options in discharge planning, as individualized care will depend on the patient's level of function at the time of discharge. Supporting the patient/caregivers in decision-making and coping with potential lifestyle changes is highly important as well (Theis & Kahn, 2007).

Patients who have undergone treatment for hip fractures face a significant risk for complication. Nonunion or malunion of the fracture may occur with hip pinning. Leg length shortening, leading to altered gait and balance, can also be seen. Loosening of the prosthesis after hemiarthroplasty or total hip replacement to fix femoral neck fractures can be an issue, as well as dislocation of the femoral stem from the acetabular cup (Ossendorf, Scheyerer, Wanner, Simmen, & Werner, 2010). Avascular necrosis is a complication after femoral neck fractures are pinned due to the compromised blood supply to the head of the femur. Patients must be anticoagulated to prevent deep vein thrombosis (DVT) and thromboembolic events.

Infection is a major concern for the practitioner caring for a hip fracture patient. Many patients are frail or confused. Aspiration pneumonia, pneumonia from prolonged bed rest and ineffective deep breathing, urinary tract infection, and skin breakdown can cause significant morbidity in this patient group (Theis & Kahn, 2007).

Hip Arthroplasty

Overview

Hip arthroplasty (HA) refers to the surgical removal of the hip joint, including the femoral head and surrounding tissue structures, and replacing the joint with artificial components (see Figure 21.3). These components can be made from metal alloys and titanium, plastic, zirconium oxide, or ceramic materials. HA may be a partial replacement (as in a hemiarthroplasty, bipolar, or hip resurfacing procedure), or it may be a total hip replacement (THR) in which the entire joint is replaced with artificial surfaces that articulate against each other. Revision arthroplasty is

Figure 21.3.
Components of Total Hip Replacement In Situ

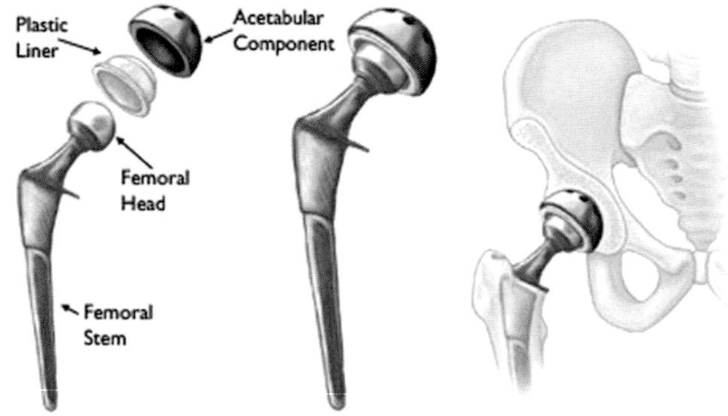

From "Total Hip Replacement" by the American Academy of Orthopaedic Surgeons, 2011, OrthoInfo, http://orthoinfo.aaos.org/topic.cfm?topic=A00377. Reproduced with permission.

Figure 21.4.
Arthritic Hip with Joint Space Obliteration and Superior Migration of the Femur

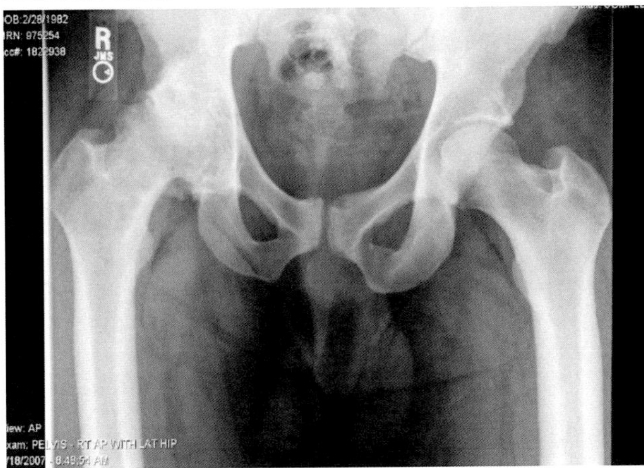

From The Department of Radiology—Hospital for Special Surgery, 2011. Reproduced with permission.

a procedure for a loosened, infected, or mechanically failed prosthesis. This is done by removing the original components, debriding the bone and soft tissue structures, and inserting new components into the hip. A revision may be partial or complete, depending on the severity of the underlying problem.

The use of conservative measures such as activity modification, weight loss programs when indicated, NSAIDs, intraarticular injections, acupuncture, and physical therapy (PT) may delay the need for surgical intervention. Arthroscopy and femoral neck debridement may also eliminate or prolong the need for HA. HA is most commonly performed to alleviate the pain and dysfunction caused by severe degenerative changes of the hip joint after conservative measures have been exhausted (see Figure 21.4) (Sandiford, Muirhead-Allwood, Skinner, & Hua, 2010).

Indications for THR include severe, constant joint pain, inability to sleep, impairment in activities of daily living (ADLs) such as the ability to put shoes/socks on, loss of balance due to joint stiffness and leg length inequality, inflammatory arthritis, post-traumatic degenerative joint disease, avascular necrosis, congenital deformities (hip dysplasia, perthes disease, slipped femoral-capital epiphysis), and femoral neck or pathologic fractures (Theis & Kahn, 2007).

There are certain instances where THR is not the recommended treatment for hip disorders mentioned in the previous section. Acute or chronic systemic infection or osteomyelitis is a contraindication for THR due to the increased risk of bacteria infecting the replaced hip. Along the same line, chronic venous stasis ulcerations, open sores or lesions, and decubiti are also considered to be too risky for THR in terms of infection. Only under certain conditions, a surgeon may choose to do a THR in a patient who receives dialysis or has severe lymphadema of the involved extremity. Patients who are compromised prior to the surgery face a greater risk of infection in the replaced joint. Decreased verbal understanding and cognitive impairment may contraindicate THR if the patient is unable to remember or understand the hip precautions. Metabolic bone disorders such as multiple myeloma or Gaucher's disease may also be contraindicated as these conditions weaken the strength of the bone and have increased risk of fracturing (Theis & Kahn, 2007).

For those patients whose situations contraindicate THR but still require surgical intervention, the surgeon and patient/caregivers will explore other options to ensure that the correct prosthesis will be used. This is especially important in younger patients, obese patients, those who participate in high-impact or aggressive sports or physical activity, and those employed in physically demanding jobs. Alternatives to THR that alleviate pain and restore function of the hip joint include hemiarthroplasty, hip arthroscopy, or hip resurfacing.

If the best option for the patient is THR, the patient needs to be educated as to hip maintenance across the lifespan. In a younger patient, a revision of a partial or total hip prosthesis may be required later in life due to the longevity of the prosthesis. Activity and employment modification, along with appropriate body weight maintenance, should be stressed. The patient should also be counseled on the potential complications following THR and hemiarthroplasty, including the following:

- Dislocation or loosening of the prosthetic components;
- Instability and suluxation of components;
- Prosthetic joint wear (adhesive/abrasive/corrosive surface wear);
- Wound infection;
- Hematoma;
- Thromboembolism;
- Periprosthetic fracture;
- Calcar resorption;
- Heterotrophic ossification; and
- Peroneal nerve palsy/foot drop.

Assessment

History and Physical Exam. Progressive degeneration of the hip commonly results in a Trendelenburg gait, abductor tilt or lurch, or flexed hip gait (see Chapter 3—Musculoskeletal Assessment and Table 3.8). Passive ROM of the joint can exacerbate the symptoms. Shortening of the affected extremity can occur due to erosion of the joint and muscle contractures. Muscle atrophy may be present due to disuse and decreased ROM. The patient may present with any of the following common conditions:

- Groin or anterior thigh pain radiating towards the knee that presents along the major nerve pathway
- Pain at night that impedes sleeping on the affected side. There is often difficulty rising from a seated position or getting out of a car.
- Pain is generally insidious, increasing over a period of months and associated with a variety of activities.
- Decreased range of motion (ROM) of the joint. Many patients complain that they can no longer put their socks on or cut their toenails, and that ADLs have become increasingly more difficult.
- Gait change to accommodate loss of joint motion and pain.

Diagnostic Tests. Laboratory tests should include CBC, metabolic panel, Protime/INR, type and crossmatch, urinalysis, and culture and sensitivity (if indicated), and EKG. Radiographs of the hip should include AP and lateral views to evaluate joint space, articular surfaces, osteophyte and cyst formation, and subchondral collapse; chest x-ray; and MRI to stage avascular necrosis. CT scan is indicated for patients with juvenile rheumatoid arthritis, history of severe hip trauma, or any other instance where a customized prosthesis may be necessary. CT allows for evaluation of bone thickness and bone dimensions to assure that the prosthesis will fit inside the femur and that there is enough bone on the acetabulum to support the component.

Common Therapeutic Modalities

There are several different fixation options for the patient considering THR. For the first option, the entire prosthesis may be ingrowth, where there is no cement used on either the femoral or pelvic component to keep the prosthesis in place. The prosthesis itself is porous, with thousands of microbeads that the bone grows between. With this type of replacement, patients are usually placed on 50% weight-bearing for 6 weeks while the bone ingrowth occurs. This noncemented technique is used for the younger, more active patient with robust bone quality (Bozic et al., 2009). Hybrid replacements, a second option, are commonly used in lower-demand but still active, older patients (older than age 65). With this technique, cement is placed around the femoral stem within the bone, but ingrowth occurs between the acetabular component and the pelvis. Allowing full weight-bearing stimulates the osteoblastic formation within the bone. A third option is to cement both the femoral and pelvic components into the bone. This is usually done in sedentary or inactive patients with extremely poor bone quality.

Different bearing surfaces are available on the prosthesis, along with the different fixation techniques. The bearing surface is the ball or head attached to the femoral stem and its articulation with the lining of the acetabular component. There are three main bearing surface types, each with its own pros and cons. First, a metal head attached to the femoral component articulating with a low molecular polyethylene (LMP) liner inside the acetabular component is currently the standard used in THR (Bozic et al., 2009). While strong, the metal head articulating with LMP may cause microabrasion of the surfaces, which causes debris within the hip joint. This debris may lead to premature loosening of the prosthesis. Second, a ceramic head on a LMP or a ceramic head with a ceramic liner is a newer option in the younger patient population. The ceramic head articulating with the LMP or ceramic liner is thought to decrease scratching and therefore reduce debris produced. The disadvantage is that ceramic can crack or fracture with impact activity, and "squeaking" noises have been reported (Schroder et al., 2010). Third, a metal head in a metal liner is another option for the younger, higher-demand patient, as these materials are supposed to reduce the amount of scratching and wear debris over time (Bozic et al., 2009). It is possible, however, that the debris that does occur over time may cause metalosis or become a carcinogen for the patient. It is not advisable to use this type of prosthesis for women of childbearing age (Zywiel, Sayeed, Johnson, Schmalzried, & Mont, 2010).

The choice of fixation technique and the type of bearing surface utilized are based on the factor of wear of the prosthesis, which may lead to loosening over time. Regardless of the type of prosthesis used or the surgical technique, hip replacements may develop significant wear or loosening. If the wear of the liner becomes severe, the hip may become painful or dislocate from a change in the way the femoral component articulates with the acetabular component (Zywiel et al., 2010). With the loosening of the prosthesis, there is usually significant thigh pain if the femoral component loosens or significant groin pain if the acetabular component loosens. In either event, a revision of one or both components will be necessary.

The goal of surgery is to provide a functional, pain-free joint. The type of surgical approach will determine postoperative considerations. After an anterolateral procedure, the patient must avoid external rotation, abduction, and hip hyperextension. Posterolateral patients must avoid internal rotation, adduction, and hip hyperflexion postoperatively. Whichever position is used by the surgeon, ROM considerations must be established and implemented postoperatively to avoid complications.

Table 21.1. Advantages and Disadvantages of Minimally Invasive Hip Surgery

Potential Benefits
■ Minimal soft tissue trauma with less muscle and tendon resection intraoperatively. ■ Less postoperative pain. ■ Shorter hospital stay and quicker recovery. ■ Increased patient satisfaction due to the cosmetic appearance of a smaller incision.
Potential Disadvantages/Complications
■ Decreased intraoperative visualization. ■ Component malpositioning. ■ Intraoperative fracture. ■ Sciatic or femoral nerve palsy. ■ Leg length discrepancy. ■ Damage to muscle or skin from excessive retraction. ■ Difficult for inexperienced surgeons, with a high learning curve.

Minimally invasive procedures use standard positioning and require accurate placement of the incision, specialized retractors/instruments, and an experienced surgeon. This procedure is done through a smaller incision (8cm) or the two-incision technique that is fluoroscopically guided. See Table 21.1 for the advantages and disadvantages of minimally invasive surgery.

Bone grafting may be necessary when there is inadequate bone stock to support the implant components. Bone grafts can be allograft or morselized (ground femoral head) femoral head grafting and autograft. Bone grafts are most often necessary for patients with:

- rheumatoid arthritis;
- congenital dislocated/subluxed hip;
- nonunion of acetabular fracture;
- previous unsuccessful surgery requiring a revision arthroplasty;
- previous infection; or
- steroid-induced or disuse osteoporosis.

During surgery, the extremity is evaluated intraoperatively for length, motion, and stability, and the joint is put through ROM. Radiographs are done to verify prosthesis placement and alignment. Surgical technique may be different and surgical time longer with a revision arthroplasty for many reasons. Blood loss from revision arthroplasty is usually greater. The surgical method may not be the same as the original surgery, as it depends on the reason the prosthesis needed to be revised such as a mechanical failure, amount/type of bone stock lost, type of original prosthesis, signs of infection, and patient age. Outcomes may not be as good as with primary arthroplasty.

Nursing Considerations

Nursing Diagnoses. Nursing diagnoses for this condition are expanded upon in the Appendix.

- Activity intolerance.
- Anxiety.
- Caregiver role strain, risk for.
- Confusion, acute.
- Constipation, risk for.
- Coping, ineffective.
- Falls, risk for.
- Family processes, interrupted.
- Fear.
- Gas exchange, impaired,
- Hopelessness.
- Infection, risk for.
- Knowledge deficit.
- Loneliness, risk for.
- Mobility: physical, impaired.
- Pain, acute.
- Post-trauma syndrome, risk for.
- Powerlessness.
- Self-care deficit: bathing/hygiene, dressing/grooming, feeding, toileting.
- Skin integrity, risk for impairment.
- Surgical recovery, delayed.
- Tissue perfusion: cardiac, risk for decrease.
- Tissue perfusion: peripheral, ineffective.

Interventions and Education. Postoperative interventions include teaching the patient to properly use assistive devices (walker, crutches, cane) independently. Maintaining joint function using postoperative precautions and the importance of these restrictions should be reinforced. Patients should be instructed on correct weight-bearing status, based on the prosthetic components. Cemented or hybrid components allow full weight-bearing with assistive device unless bone grafting was used; that may require protected weight bearing. Cementless components allow partial or full weight-bearing per surgeon instruction with assistive exercises. Patients should be taught/reinforced hip precautions (see Table 21.2) and isometric exercises:

- Quadriceps setting;
- Gluteal setting;
- Dorseflexion/plantar flexion (ankle pumps);
- Ankle circumduction exercises; and
- Therapy will instruct in additional exercises.

Table 21.2. Postarthroplasty Positioning and Mobility Considerations

Arthroplasty

Total hip replacement (THR): replacement of both the femoral head and resurfacing of the acetabulum.

1. Can be cemented or cementless.
2. Patient prone to dislocation may be placed in a spica cast or abductor brace.

Hip hemiarthroplasty: replacement of femoral component.

Positioning and Mobility Considerations

Prevent dislocation through proper positioning:

1. Abduct operative hip using abductive devices.
   a. Abduction pillows.
   b. Regular pillows.
   c. Skin traction.
   d. Abduction slings.
   e. Splints.
2. Maintain hip in abduction, neutral rotation, or slight external rotation.
3. Avoid hip flexion over 60-90 degrees per surgeon.
4. Avoid adduction.
5. Avoid internal rotation.
6. General policy is to turn to non-operative side only.
7. Maintain abduction with pillows.
8. Move extremity gently when transferring or turning in bed.

Assess for symptoms of dislocation:

1. Acute groin pain
2. Shortened extremity in external rotation (usually).
3. Patient may hear or feel a "popping" sensation.

Positioning considerations:

1. Maintain good body alignment in abduction devices.
2. Turn with pillows or supports to maintain abduction.
3. Have patient lie flat several times per day to prevent hip flexion contractures.
4. Head of bed generally not raised more than 45-60 degrees based on surgeon preference.

Activity/exercise regimen:

1. Out of bed to chair.
2. Orthopaedic high chair and elevated toilet seat to prevent excessive flexion.
3. Do not elevate the affected extremity when sitting in chair.

From Core Curriculum for Orthopaedic Nursing *(6th ed., p. 544) by National Association of Orthopaedic Nurses (NAON), 2007, Boston, MA: Pearson. Reproduced with permission.*

Because of the risk for postoperative infection, patients must be assessed for incisional or joint infection. Strict sterile technique should be maintained in the OR, and circulating particles in the air should be reduced using a low traffic policy and/or laminar flow (Theis & Kahn, 2007). Nurses should administer IV antibiotics as ordered pre- and postoperatively. Signs and symptoms of infections should be assessed and indwelling catheters removed as soon as possible. Sterile dressing changes should be performed and patients instructed in appropriate wound care. The patient must be instructed in lifelong hip care. It is important to emphasize the need for the patient to continue taking prophylactic antibiotics as instructed by the surgeon, inform physicians and dentists of the arthroplasty, and notify the physician if infection is suspected.

Outcomes. The patient will graduate to unassisted ambulation when instructed to do so by the surgeon, based on progression with PT. Additionally, the patient will remain free of infection by following prophylactic antibiotic guidelines and verbalizing an understanding of the significance of avoiding infection. Ultimately, the patient's goal is to return to desired activity levels.

Practice Setting Considerations. *Office/outpatient setting:* Patients/caregivers should be assisted in evaluating discharge needs. Advance directives should be reviewed and discussed prior to surgery, and patients should be assisted in obtaining necessary equipment. Nurses should provide preoperative teaching materials, coordinate appointments with the preadmission center or joint class, and identify infections prior to surgery. The floor and office nurses should assist with postoperative follow-up care and monitor lab tests as ordered, especially with anticoagulants.

Hospital setting: Postoperative care is provided per protocol. Hip precautions are taught to the patient and caregivers, and should be continually reinforced. The nurse assists the case manager and social worker in the coordination of discharge plans. Some THR/arthroplasty patients are not able to go home after acute care. Depending on their postsurgery progress, they may be candidates for an alternative level of care such as acute inpatient rehabilitation or short-term skilled care. Factors to consider include level of endurance, functional capacity, amount of support at home, and any co-morbidities.

Home setting: Furniture arrangement, guardrails, accessibility to the bathroom and bedroom, and overall safety need to be evaluated prior to surgery. Support systems also need to be evaluated at that time. Home discharges should be reassessed for safety and functional ability. Physical therapists/occupational therapists will make recommendations depending on the patient's level of function and progress towards independence. Mobility and exercise plans will be reinforced and lab values or medications monitored. The patient and caregivers are taught home ADL management. The nurse needs to monitor/assist with and teach the patient incision care.

Hip Resurfacing Arthroplasty

Overview

Hip resurfacing (or surface replacement) is designed to be a preservation procedure when advanced osteoarthritis or avascular necrosis (AVN) has been diagnosed in a younger patient. The success of this procedure is directly related to choosing patients who meet the criteria for hip surface replacement (McMinn, Daniel, Ziaee, & Pradhan, 2010). These criteria include younger patients with excellent bone quality who have advanced osteoarthritis of the hip joint. Inflammatory disease, advanced AVN, congenital hip malformation, and history of infection or osteoporosis are contraindications. The goal of surface replacement is to restore function, increase hip motion, and reduce pain, while preserving as much bone as possible (Sandiford et al., 2010).

Hip resurfacing involves a mushroom-shaped prosthesis (see Figure 21.5). A thin, short stem attached to a hollow dome is driven into the femoral head through to the level of the trochanter. The femoral head is altered surgically to accommodate the dome or base portion of the implant. The diameter of the dome is fairly large to decrease the chance of dislocation. The acetabulum has a press-fit cap that fits around the dome and articulates with it. Both implants are metal, and the fixation is hybrid with cementing of the femoral implant underneath the dome, leaving only the stem available for ingrowth. Partial hip resurfacing (or hemi-resurfacing) is another option, in which bone preservation is maintained. With this procedure, only the femur has a device implanted. The acetabular surface is preserved, and it articulates directly with the femoral component (McMinn et al., 2010).

Figure 21.5.
Components Used in Hip Resurfacing

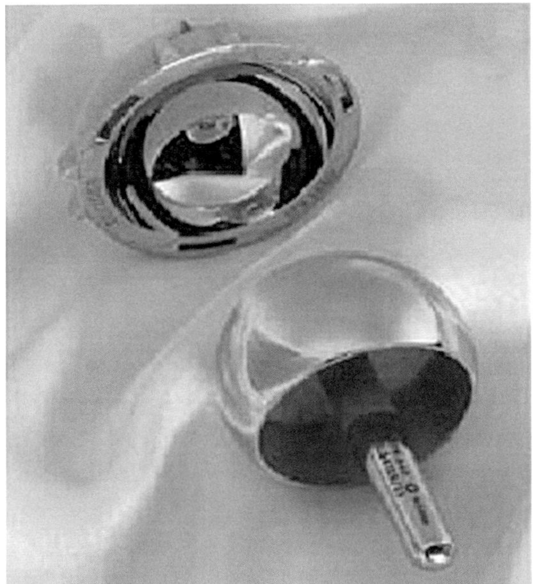

From Stryker, 2011. Reproduced with permission.

Indications for hip resurfacing are similar to those of total hip arthroplasty (THA). There are a few exceptions. The patient cannot have a current or previous femoral neck fracture or neoplastic disease. Sepsis is contraindicated, as with any prosthetic implant. Significant AVN of the femoral head is contraindicated because the bone around the surface replacement may break down or not support the resurfacing (McMinn et al., 2010). Surface replacement in female patients has been controversial because, once in the system, metal ions aren't necessarily absorbed and/or excreted. This is a concern for those interested in becoming pregnant, as the ions in the system can cross the placenta (McMinn, et al., 2010). Metal ion debris is a concern for both male and female patients, as the ions are released in the urine. Patients with impaired renal function, who require dialysis, or have had kidney transplants would not be candidates for surface replacements. Another potential problem associated with metal debris is the potential for metalosis or carcinogens. Chromium and cobalt ions are measurable in the blood of patients with metal-on-metal prosthesis. At this time, there is no evidence to support an increase in cancer or other diseases as it relates to metal ion release, but safety levels for these materials has not yet been determined (Desouza et al., 2010).

Femoral neck fracture after surface replacement is a complication that has been reported at 1-2% (Garbuz, Tanzer, Greidanus, Masri, & Duncan, 2009). Nerve injury can also occur with surface replacement just as with THR or hemiarthroplasty. Infection of the incision site, as well as the replaced joint, may be seen postoperatively. Every precaution should be taken to avoid infection in a patient with hip resurfacing. Failure of the prosthesis can be attributed to loosening, infection, postoperative AVN, or femoral neck fracture. Since this procedure tends to be done in younger, more active patients, failure is a significant concern as the patient will most likely outlive the longevity of the device.

Following a failed surface replacement, revision to a THR is required. If the patient is very young (younger than age 45), a total hip prosthesis may also fail during the patient's lifetime. A revision hip replacement would then be necessary. With each procedure, more bone will be compromised. Surface replacement may, therefore, be a good option in a younger patient to attempt to preserve bone for future procedures (Cordingley, Kohan, & Ben-Nissan, 2010).

Surface replacements are done through a posterolateral incision. The length of the incision is longer than that for THR, as a full capsular resection is done. The visual field required for surface replacement needs to be larger because the femoral head is dislocated but not resected. There is a higher incidence of vascular compromise because the anterior capsule is cut for this procedure. Intraoperative infection and nerve injuries can occur, similarly to those seen with THR.

Assessment

History and Physical Exam. Refer to the history and physical exam section in Hip Arthroplasty and inclusion criteria for surface replacements.

Diagnostic Tests. Refer to the diagnostic testing section for Hip Arthroplasty.

Common Therapeutic Modalities

Just like hip arthroplasty, surface replacements are elective procedures. Patients must decide if this is something that will be beneficial and suitable to their needs. A patient may elect to continue with conservative management to include activity alterations, anti-inflammatory and narcotic pain medications, intra-articular injections, and use of assistive devices.

Nursing Considerations

Nursing Diagnoses. Nursing diagnoses for this condition are expanded upon in the Appendix.

- Activity intolerance.
- Caregiver role strain, risk for.
- Constipation, risk for.
- Coping, ineffective.
- Family processes, interrupted.
- Fear.
- Gas exchange, impaired.
- Infection, risk for.
- Knowledge deficit.
- Mobility: physical, impaired.
- Nutrition, imbalanced: risk for less than body requirements.
- Pain, acute.
- Post-trauma syndrome, risk for.
- Powerlessness.
- Self-care deficit: bathing/hygiene, dressing/ grooming, feeding, toileting.
- Surgical recovery, delayed.
- Tissue perfusion: cardiac, risk for decreased.
- Tissue perfusion: peripheral, ineffective.

Interventions and Education. The length of hospital stay for surface replacement is 2-3 days. Patients are weight-bearing as tolerated. Hip restrictions are based on the surgeon's preference and take into account the quality of the bone, supporting tissues, and musculature. The femoral component of the prosthesis has a larger head than that used for THR, lowering the rate of dislocation substantially. Nevertheless, the capsular resection is extensive, so hip ROM restrictions may be utilized for up to 6 weeks. Patients without a prior history of DVT can be anticoagulated using an enteric-coated aspirin twice a day for 4-6 weeks. Because patients tend to be mobile quickly, home care services are usually unnecessary as patients can attend physical therapy at a facility outside the home. Patients should be taught/ reinforced hip precautions and isometric exercises such as quadriceps setting, gluteal setting, dorseflexion/ plantar flexion (ankle pumps), and ankle circumduction exercises. Therapists will instruct in additional exercises per patient tolerance.

Patients are at risk for infection and must remain free of incisional or joint infection. Strict sterile technique must be maintained in the OR, and circulating particles in the air should be reduced using a low traffic policy and/or laminar flow. As per physician orders, the nurse should administer antibiotics pre- and postoperatively. Signs and symptoms of infections should be assessed and indwelling catheters removed as soon as possible. Sterile dressing changes should be performed and patients instructed in appropriate wound care.

Prior to discharge, patients must be taught and then be able to verbalize lifelong joint care for infection control. Lifelong care of the resurfaced hip joint emphasizes the following points:

- Taking prophylactic antibiotics as instructed by the surgeon;
- Informing physicians and dentists of arthroplasty;
- Notifying the physician if infection is suspected; and
- Return to physical activity as directed by surgeon.

Outcomes. The patient will ambulate as tolerated and return to more strenuous activity when instructed to do so by the surgeon. Additionally, the patient will remain free of infection by following prophylactic antibiotic guidelines. Ultimately, the goal for the patient is to return to prior level of function without pain or dislocation.

Practice Setting Considerations. *Office/outpatient setting:* Patients/caregivers should be assisted in evaluating discharge needs. Nurses should provide preoperative teaching materials, coordinate appointments with the preadmission center or joint class, and identify infections prior to surgery. The floor and office nurses should assist with postoperative follow-up care and monitor lab tests as ordered, especially with anticoagulants.

Hospital setting: Postoperative care is provided per protocol. The nurse assists the case manager and social worker in the coordination of discharge plans.

Home setting: Furniture arrangement, guardrails, accessibility to the bathroom and bedroom, and overall safety need to be evaluated prior to surgery. Support systems also need to be evaluated at that time. Home discharges should be reassessed for safety and functional ability. Physical therapists/occupational therapists will make recommendations depending on the patient's level of function and progress towards independence. Mobility and exercise plans will be reinforced and lab values or medications monitored. The patient and caregivers are taught home ADL management. The nurse needs to monitor/assist with and teach the patient incision care.

Hemiarthroplasty/Bipolar Replacement

Overview

Hemiarthroplasty (unipolar) or bipolar replacement is done in select patients who have suffered a femoral neck fracture, osteoarthritis, or AVN. This procedure addresses the femur only, leaving the pelvic acetabulum preserved. The metal prosthetic component is either cemented or press-fit into the femur, and it articulates with the acetabulum. These patients commonly have compromised bone stock, and they tend to be high-risk patients due to age and comorbidities (Theis & Kahn 2007). Patients who are sedentary, older than age 70, and have coexisting conditions such as poor health, Parkinson's disease, altered mental status, or shortened life expectancy may be indicated for hemiarthroplasty rather than THA (Ossendorf et al., 2010).

Hemiarthroplasty is not recommended for younger, active patients or those who exhibit degeneration of the articular cartilage within the acetabulum. Additionally, a hemiarthroplasty cannot be done if the patient has an infection or osteomyelitis of the involved femur. Hemiarthroplasty/bipolar replacement may cause deterioration of the acetabular articular cartilage. If this occurs, revision to a total hip replacement will be necessary. Complications are similar to those seen with THA and include the following:

- Component malpositioning;
- Intraoperative fracture;
- Periprosthetic fracture;
- Hematoma;
- Sciatic or femoral nerve palsy;
- Heterotrophic ossification;
- Leg length discrepancy;
- Damage to muscle or skin from excessive retraction;
- Loosening of the prosthesis;
- Articular cartilage wear of the acetabulum; and
- Infection.

Assessment

History and Physical Exam. Similar to hip arthroplasty, progressive degeneration of the hip commonly results in a Trendelenburg gait, abductor tilt, or lurch or flexed hip gait (see Chapter 3—Musculoskeletal Assessment and Table 3.8). As with assessment of hip arthroplasty, passive ROM of the hip joint can exacerbate the symptoms. Shortening of the affected extremity can occur due to erosion of the joint and muscle contractures. Muscle atrophy may be present due to disuse and decreased ROM. See Table 21.3 for symptoms differentiating the surgical need based on cause.

Diagnostic Tests. Laboratory tests should include CBC, metabolic panel, Protime/INR, type and crossmatch, urinalysis, culture and sensitivity (if indicated), and EKG). Radiographs should include AP and lateral views of the hip to evaluate joint space, articular surfaces, osteophyte and cyst formation, and subchondral collapse, chest x-ray, and MRI to stage avascular necrosis. Potential hemiarthroplasty or bipolar arthroplasty candidates may need additional medical testing, depending on their ability to give an accurate medical history, overall cognitive abilities, and noted physical comorbidities.

Table 21.3. Presenting Symptoms Based on Cause

Hip Fracture	AVN / Osteoarthritis
Leg length shortening.	Groin or anterior thigh pain radiating toward knee that presents along the major nerve pathway.
Pain in the affected extremity.	Pain at night that alters sleeping on the affected side. There is often difficulty rising from a seated position or getting out of a car.
Inability to walk or bend/move the injured leg when lying supine.	Pain is generally insidious, increasing over a period of months and associated with a variety of activities.
Extremity in a position of comfort rather than anatomical alignment.	Decreased joint ROM. Many patients complain that they can no longer put their socks on or cut their toenails and that ADLs have become increasingly more difficult.
External or internal rotation.	Gait change to accommodate loss of joint motion and pain.

The patient requires routine preoperative testing and medical clearance. The operative time and intraoperative blood loss is less with hemiarthroplasty/bipolar replacement than with THR, and the patient is not required to donate autologous blood in preparation for surgery. Additionally, this is often an emergent procedure, rendering the patient unable to donate prior to surgery. Associated traumas may need to be addressed preoperatively. An anemic patient may require a pre- or postoperative blood transfusion.

Common Therapeutic Modalities

The hemiarthroplasty (unipolar) procedure consists of a metal stem implanted into the femur, with a metal head or ball snapped onto the proximal end. The prosthesis components are modular, and the head should be large enough to accommodate the diameter of the acetabulum. The patient is made full weight-bearing after surgery. If the prosthesis is noncemented, the patient may be kept partial weight-bearing for at least 6 weeks.

A bipolar replacement is similar to the hemiarthroplasty, but there is an additional piece or pocket snapped onto the head of the prosthesis. This component consists of a thin metal shell with a polyethylene liner. The logic behind this design is that the erosion and protrusion of the acetabulum would be reduced because motion is present between the metal head and polyethylene socket (inner bearing), as well as between the metallic cup and the acetabulum (Bhattacharyya & Koval, 2009). The bipolar prosthesis is designed so loading of the hip causes the metallic cup to rotate outward instead of inward, avoiding fracture of the polyethylene insert and dislocation.

Nursing Considerations

Nursing Diagnoses. Nursing diagnoses for this condition are expanded upon in the Appendix.

- Activity intolerance.
- Caregiver role strain, risk for.
- Constipation, risk for.
- Coping, ineffective.
- Family processes, interrupted.
- Fear.
- Gas exchange, impaired.
- Infection, risk for.
- Knowledge deficit.
- Mobility: physical, impaired
- Nutrition: imbalance, risk for less than body requirements.
- Pain, acute.
- Post-trauma syndrome, risk for.
- Powerlessness.
- Self-care deficit: bathing/hygiene, dressing/grooming, feeding, toileting.
- Surgical recovery, delayed.
- Tissue perfusion: cardiac, risk for decreased.
- Tissue perfusion: peripheral, ineffective.

Interventions and Education. Postoperatively, patients are able to ambulate a functional distance with the use of an assistive device such as a walker or cane. Although patients are placed in hip motion restrictions for the first 6 weeks after surgery, dislocation of the prosthesis from the acetabulum is rare following this procedure. Patients should be instructed on correct weight-bearing status. Cemented or hybrid components allowed full weight-bearing with an assistive device, unless bone grafting was used or other trauma/fracture prevents full weight-bearing. In that case, they may require protected weight-bearing status until surgeon approval. Patients should be taught/reinforced hip precautions and isometric exercises such as quadriceps setting, gluteal setting, dorseflexion/plantar flexion (ankle pumps), and ankle circumduction exercises. Therapists will instruct in additional exercises as needed and/or as tolerated.

Patients are at risk for infection and must remain free of incisional or joint infection. Strict sterile technique must be maintained in the OR, and circulating particles in the air should be reduced using a low traffic policy and/or laminar flow. If the surgeon orders preoperative antibiotics, the nurse should administer as ordered. Signs and symptoms of infections should be assessed and indwelling catheters removed as soon as possible. Sterile dressing changes should be performed and patients instructed in appropriate wound care. Prior to discharge, patients must be taught and then be able to verbalize lifelong joint care for infection control. Lifelong care of the resurfaced hip joint emphasizes the following points:

- Taking prophylactic antibiotics as instructed by the surgeon;
- Informing physicians and dentists of arthroplasty;
- Notifying the physician if infection is suspected; and
- Return to physical activity as directed by surgeon.

Outcomes. The patient will progress to unassisted ambulation when instructed to do so by the surgeon. Additionally, the patient will remain free of infection by following prophylactic antibiotic guidelines. Ultimately, the patient's goal is to return to prior level of functioning without pain.

Practice Setting Considerations. *Office/outpatient setting:* Patients/ caregivers should be assisted in evaluating discharge needs. Nurses should provide preoperative teaching materials, coordinate appointments with the

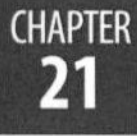

preadmission center or joint class, and identify infections prior to surgery. The floor and office nurses should assist with postoperative follow-up care and monitor lab tests as ordered, especially with anticoagulants.

Hospital setting: Postoperative care should be provided per protocol. Hip precautions should be reinforced. The nurse should assist in coordinating discharge plans.

Home setting: Furniture arrangement, guardrails, accessibility to the bathroom and bedroom, and overall safety need to be evaluated prior to surgery. Support systems also need to be evaluated at this time. Home discharges should be assessed for safety and functional ability. Mobility and exercise plans should be reinforced and lab values or medications monitored. Patients/caregivers should be taught home ADL management. The nurse should monitor/assist with and teach the patient incision care. Case management works with the patient and family in discharge planning and assessing the most appropriate level of care for post acute discharge. Factors to consider include current function levels, the ability to care for self safely in the home setting, and level of support. A patient may be eligible for acute inpatient rehabilitation, skilled care, or assisted living until able to return to home. Preservation of autonomy and safety are key factors to address.

Hip Arthroscopy

Overview

Hip pathology and life-altering hip conditions are not simply a problem of the aging population. Hip pain in recreational athletes can result from acute injury or high-demand, repetitive activities across the lifespan. Football, jogging, tennis, golf, and dancing are some of the activities associated with hip injuries. Usually, the structures sustaining the damage include the acetabular labrum, the joint capsule, and the chondral surfaces. Patients mostly present with groin pain and loss of motion.

Hip arthroscopy replaces conservative management or arthrotomy of the hip in many situations. Labral tears and frayed articular cartilage can be debrided, femeroacetabular impingement can be minimized, and microfracture procedures can be performed less invasively. In the past, open surgical procedures, including joint replacement and osteotomy, would have been the standard of surgical care for treating hip conditions (Botser, Smith, Nasser, & Domb, 2011). Advances in hip arthroscopy over the past 15 years have paved the way for arthroscopic-assisted open procedures, as well as arthroscopy alone, as surgical solutions for hip conditions.

Because the hip is a ball-and-socket joint, traction must be applied during hip arthroscopy to avoid damaging intracapsular structures with surgical instruments. Fluoroscopic guidance is required to assure proper placement of instruments within the joint at the start of the procedure. Two small incisions will require suturing at the end of the procedure.

Complications. The most frequent complications associated with hip arthroscopy are related to patient positioning and fluid management. Careful positioning of the lower extremity with adequate padding is very important. Intraoperative traction may not exceed 2-hour periods (Ilizaliturri, 2009). Palsy of the pudendal, femoral, sciatic, and obturator nerves can occur, yet these frequently resolve spontaneously during the recovery period (Ilizaliturri, 2009). Neurovascular status must be checked frequently but won't return to normal until after the epidural block wears off. Patients usually go home on the day of surgery, so they must be taught how to recognize signs of infection and nerve damage. Intra-abdominal fluid extravasation can occur from high concentration of fluids under significant pressure (Ilizaliturri, 2009). DVT is rarely seen but must be considered if severe swelling and calf pain ensue.

Assessment

History and Physical Exam. Patients undergoing hip arthroscopy usually experience pain that is not relieved by rest, anti-inflammatory medications, or PT. There may be locking or restricted mobility of the hip joint.

Diagnostic Tests. MRI of the hip is usually performed to evaluate the integrity of the hip structures. Radiographic evaluation, to include AP and lateral views, is necessary to visualize joint space and articular surfaces. Preoperative chest x-ray may be necessary as part of the standard precautionary preoperative testing.

Common Therapeutic Modalities

Conservative. Prior to undergoing hip arthroscopy, the patient and medical team should consider nonsurgical management of the hip condition/pain. This would include rest, changes in athletic activities, and PT for strengthening, stretching, and conditioning. Therapeutic modalities of heat, ice, TENS unit ultrasound, and massage are also key treatment options. Anti-inflammatory medications may be helpful in decreasing pain, swelling, and inflammation. Intra-articular injections of cortisone and/or hyulauronic acid may also be useful alternatives to arthroscopic surgery.

Surgical. Arthroscopic surgery of the hip is done under epidural anesthesia. Patients leave the hospital on crutches for comfort. They are full weight-bearing and can usually return to work in 7-10 days. Sutures need to be removed 10-14 days postoperatively, and PT begins at that time. Most patients can return to full activity in 6-8 weeks, although patients should be cautioned that discomfort may persist for 3-6 months (Stalzer, Wahoff, & Scanlon, 2006).

Nursing Considerations

Nursing Diagnoses. Nursing diagnoses for this condition are expanded upon in the Appendix.

- Activity intolerance.
- Anxiety.
- Caregiver role strain, risk for.
- Constipation, risk for.
- Coping, ineffective.
- Falls, risk for.
- Family processes, interrupted.
- Fear.
- Infection, risk for.
- Knowledge deficit.
- Mobility: physical, impaired.
- Pain, acute.
- Self-care deficit: bathing/hygiene, dressing/grooming, feeding, toileting.
- Surgical recovery, delayed.
- Skin integrity, risk for impaired.
- Tissue perfusion: peripheral, ineffective.

Interventions and Education. Patients ambulate immediately, which decreases the risk of blood clots and altered skin integrity. Narcotics are given for pain, but most patients will not require these medications for extended periods. Because patients leave the hospital on the day of their surgery, postoperative teaching is of major importance. Assessment of home arrangements and support systems are necessary for recovery. It is critical that the patient is able participate in PT. If unable to attend PT on an outpatient basis, the patient may need to arrange in-home therapy services. The patient and family members may have difficulty coping with childcare issues, absence from work, and decreased activity levels. Expected outcomes would include returning to work, family obligations, ADLs, driving, and athletic/recreational activities as directed by the orthopedic surgeon.

Femoro-Acetabular Impingement

Overview

Femoro-acetabular impingement (FAI) occurs when the head of the femur does not have full ROM within the acetabulum. Impingement is the premature and improper collision or impact between the head and/or neck of the femur and acetabulum. This causes a decreased range of hip joint motion, in addition to pain. In a FAI hip joint, the extra bone on the femoral head and/or neck hits the rim of the acetabulum, causing damage to the cartilage and labrum that line the acetabulum.

FAI is a result of excess bone that has formed around the head and/or neck of the femur, otherwise known as cam-type impingement. The extra bone that impedes motion is often the result of normal bone growth and development. Cam-type impingement is when such development leads to the abnormal bump of bone on the femoral head and/or neck (Fritz, Reddy, Meehan, & Jamali, 2010).

FAI also commonly occurs due to overgrowth of the acetabular (socket) rim. This is known as pincer-type impingement, when the socket is angled in such a way that abnormal impact occurs between the femur and the rim of the acetabulum. It can also occur with a protrusio-type hip deformity (penetration of the femoral head and acetabulum into the pelvis) and with retroversion of the femur (Fritz et al., 2010).

Impingement usually presents between the ages of 18 and 35 (Hart, Metkar, Rebello, & Grottkau, 2009). Extra bone can appear on x-rays as a seemingly very small bump. Over time, however, when the bump repeatedly rubs against the cartilage and labrum (which serve to cushion the impact between the ball and socket), the cartilage and labrum can fray or tear, resulting in pain. As more cartilage and labrum is lost, the bone of the femur will articulate with the bone of the pelvis. Tears of the labrum can also fold into the joint space, further restricting motion of the hip and causing additional pain. This is similar to what occurs in the knee of someone with a torn meniscus.

Hip trauma can also lead to impingement. The tears of the labrum and/or cartilage are often the result of athletic activities that involve repetitive pivoting movements or repetitive hip flexion.

Assessment

History & Physical Exam. Many patients first realize a pain in the front of their hip (groin) after prolonged sitting and walking. Climbing uphill may be difficult, and ROM may become restricted. Another presenting symptom may be catching or locking of the joint with or without pain. The pain can be a consistent dull ache, or a catching and/or sharp, popping sensation. Pain can also be felt along the side of the thigh and in the buttocks.

Diagnostic Tests. Medical imagery in the form of x-ray and MRI is crucial for diagnosing FAI. X-ray can reveal an excess of bone on the femoral head, neck, or acetabular rim. An MRI can reveal fraying or tears of the cartilage and labrum.

Common Treatment Modalities

Conservative. Nonsurgical treatment should be the first line of treatment for FAI, as it often resolves with rest, activity modification, PT, and/or anti-inflammatory medications. It is often necessary to differentiate between pain radiating from the hip joint versus the lower back or abdomen. The way in which most surgeons differentiate the location of the pain is by injecting the hip with a steroid and analgesic. If the pain indeed stems from the hip joint as a result of FAI, the injection provides the patient with pain relief. Secondly, the injection serves to confirm the diagnosis as coming from the hip joint and not from the back.

Surgical. Surgical management to correct FAI is typically in the form of femoral head debridement. This procedure used to be performed as an open procedure, but many physicians are now doing the entire procedure arthroscopically or arthroscopically-assisted (Botser et al., 2011). (See the separate section on Hip Arthroscopy). With the open technique, the femoral head is manually dislocated by the surgeon, and the anteromedial aspect of the femoral neck is debrided. It may be necessary to trim or remove degenerative pieces of the labrum as well. Arthroscopically, the femoral head remains within the acetabulum, and the entire procedure is done through two small portal incisions. Both procedures are done under regional anesthesia, and preoperative lab work includes PT/INR, PTT, CBC, BMP, and urinalysis. EKG and chest x-ray prior to the surgical procedure is dependent on past medical history and hospital policy (Botser et al, 2011).

Nursing Considerations

Nursing Diagnoses. Nursing diagnoses for this condition are expanded upon in the Appendix.

- Activity intolerance.
- Anxiety.
- Caregiver role strain, risk for.
- Constipation, risk for.
- Coping, ineffective.
- Falls, risk for.
- Family processes, interrupted.
- Fear.
- Infection, risk for.
- Knowledge deficit.
- Loneliness, risk for.
- Mobility: physical, impaired.
- Pain, acute.
- Self-care deficit: bathing/hygiene, dressing/grooming, feeding, toileting.
- Skin integrity, risk for impaired.
- Surgical recovery, delayed.
- Tissue perfusion: peripheral, ineffective.

Interventions and Education. Management of the patient undergoing femoral neck debridement to correct FAI includes assessment for joint and wound infection, hematoma, DVT, and neurovascular deficits. Pain management is also an important consideration. NSAIDs may be prescribed to decrease inflammation and potential formation of heterotrophic bone. Drug interactions and side effects of NSAIDs need to be reviewed with the patient.

Patients are usually released full weight-bearing with crutches for balance and comfort. If the procedure is done through "traditional" arthrotomy, total hip precautions must be maintained for 4-6 weeks. This is due to the fact that the femur was dislocated and the surrounding structures weakened during the surgery. If the procedure is done arthroscopically, femoral neck debridement is an outpatient surgery. Education is crucial for these patients, as they need to be instructed on how to bathe, dress, care for the incision, and take medications. Signs and symptoms of adverse events or complications must be reinforced.

Complications. Several complications may be seen after femoral neck debridement and hip arthroscopy, and have the potential to evolve into long-term sequellae. The most common is continued degeneration of the hip joint, leading to advanced osteoarthritis. Pudendal and lateral femoral cutaneous nerve damage can occur, as well as abdominal, peroneal, or genital trauma (Botser et al., 2011). AVN may occur following the "traditional" open procedure, secondary to disruption in blood flow to the femoral head when the hip is temporarily dislocated. Bony islands within muscles or tendons, known as heterotrophic ossification, may form and lead to decreased ROM and hip stiffness. While there is greater joint visualization with the open and arthroscopic-assisted techniques, these two methods involve more invasive surgery with potentially more complications and a longer recovery period (Botser et al., 2011).

Hip Dislocation

Overview

Hip dislocation is a traumatic injury in which displacement of the femur from the acetabulum causes the articulating surfaces to lose contact (see Figure 21.6). Postarthroplasty dislocations occur in approximately 2% of patients and are more likely to occur in the first 8 postoperative weeks (Theis & Kahn, 2007). Following hip arthroplasty, positions of extreme flexion, adduction, or internal rotation are the least stable related to surgical muscle

Figure 21.6.
Dislocated Hip Arthroplasty with Superior Migration of Femur

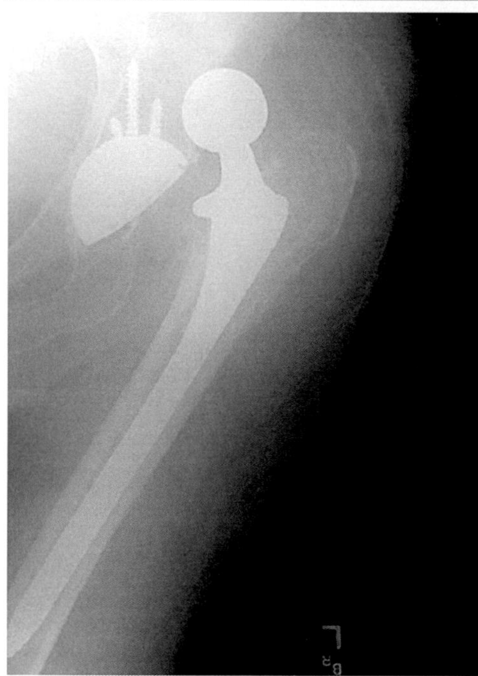

From "Dislocated Hip Replacement" by B. Rhodes, 2008, http://en.wikipedia.org/wiki/File:Dislocated_hip_replacement.jpg. Reproduced with permission.

damage and need to rebuild periarticular muscle tone. *Posterior dislocation* is most common (Theis & Kahn, 2007). This can happen from force along the shaft of the femur when the hip is flexed and adducted such as with a fall or dashboard injury in a motor vehicle accident (MVA). *Anterior dislocation* is rare and occurs when the hip is extended, abducted, and externally rotated. Central dislocation can occur with a severe blow to the lateral aspect of the hip, especially if the hip is abducted (Theis & Kahn, 2007). Nerve injuries, loss of motion, and AVN (if the dislocation is traumatic in a nonreplaced joint) are some complications that can arise from a nonoperative hip dislocation.

Assessment

History and Physical Exam. During the physical examination, it is important to inspect the extremity for shortening or external leg rotation, ROM, and the patient's ability to stand/bear weight on the affected leg. Neurovascular status of the extremity must be evaluated as well. The patient may complain of feeling a "pop" or hearing a cracking sound. Pain is usually intense. The surgeon should be notified immediately.

Diagnostic Tests. Diagnostic tests to consider a hip dislocation include AP and lateral radiographs of the hip to determine joint condition, type of dislocation, and any fractures. Pelvis x-ray or CT may be needed to clearly view some central dislocations associated with an acetabular fracture. CT anteversion studies are often ordered to view the angulation of the femoral component in relation to the acetabular component. Laboratory tests may be required if the patient is a surgical candidate.

Common Therapeutic Modalities

Conservative. Conservative treatment includes closed reduction with analgesia and muscle relaxant. Reduction should be done as quickly after the injury as possible to minimize potential nerve damage, alleviate pain, and restore function. Reduction is followed by a brace to hold the hip in desired alignment based on type of dislocation. A hip spica cast or buck skin traction may be used for patients who haven't had joint replacements, simply to keep the reduced hip in place.

Surgical. If the hip is unable to be reduced, an open reduction is performed surgically. Traction or bracing is sometimes needed to keep the hip from dislocating again after the open reduction. A hip spica cast, buck skin traction, skeletal traction, or internal fixation (if fractures occurred during the trauma) are used with dislocations of nonreplaced joints. For recurrent dislocation, the surgeon may choose to do anteversion studies to see the angle of the femoral component in relation to the acetabular component. The patient may also need to return to the operating room for a larger prosthetic femoral head on the femoral shaft or for a constrained polyethylene liner. The larger head provides greater stability, and the constrained liner has a ring around it to capture the femoral portion of the prosthesis during movement, thus keeping it in proper alignment.

Nursing Considerations

Nursing Diagnoses. Nursing diagnoses for this condition are expanded upon in the Appendix.

- Activity intolerance.
- Caregiver role strain, risk for.
- Constipation, risk for.
- Coping, ineffective.
- Falls, risk for.
- Family processes, interrupted.
- Fear.
- Knowledge deficit.
- Mobility: physical, impaired
- Pain, acute.
- Self-care deficit: bathing/hygiene, dressing/grooming, feeding, tioleting.
- Skin integrity, risk for impaired.
- Tissue perfusion: peripheral, ineffective.

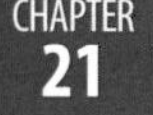

Interventions and Education. Hip dislocation after arthroplasty or trauma is an acute injury that is very painful and frightening to the patient and their support system. These patients must be brought to the hospital via ambulance and often need 911 assistance. The orthopaedic team, including the residents, physician assistants, admission department, and office nurse, must be notified to coordinate care. Medical and surgical history needs to be available to all involved caretakers to expedite treatment.

The nurse should assist with the hospital admission process, and provide emergency and postprocedure care. The nurse should reinforce mobility and activity restrictions and instruct patients on the proper use of the assistive devices that they are issued, including an elevated toilet seat, reacher, sock aid, and abduction pillows. Sometimes braces are indicated postoperatively, typically a knee immobilizer brace or abduction brace, to keep hip flexion minimized.

If a brace is given, patients need to be taught how to use the brace and to watch for skin irritation or breakdown. In order to avoid component dislocation, patients maintain abduction pillows between their legs while supine. They are also taught total hip precautions that instruct the patients to avoid adduction, internal rotation, and flexion past 90 degrees. These restrictions stay in place for a minimum of 6 weeks or at the surgeon's discretion.

Hip Girdlestone Pseudarthrosis

Overview

Girdlestone pseudarthrosis, also referred to as resectional arthroplasty, is a surgical procedure to totally or partially excise a joint, lengthen soft tissues, and develop new articulating surfaces. Hip girdlestone pseudarthrosis involves creation of a new false hip joint. Prior to the advent of modern hip implants, hip girdlestone pseudarthrosis was used occasionally to manage the pain of severe arthritis. More frequent use of this procedure was for chronic joint infections or tuberculosis (Theis & Kahn, 2007). Current orthopaedic techniques use this procedure almost exclusively as a last resort for salvage of failed THA or severe infection of a hip arthroplasty.

Failed THA can result from the body's inability to retain a prosthetic implant due to a lack of adequate bone stock to hold the prosthesis. Fracture below a prosthesis with a resulting nonfunctional repair or multiple hip arthroplasty revisions that remain unsuccessful with poor function and severe pain are also common causes of THA failure. Unresolved infected THA may require hip girdlestone pseudarthrosis after all antibiotic possibilities are tried without success. With the advances in modern medicine, however, current antibiotic combinations rarely necessitate the procedure for an infected arthroplasty anymore (Theis & Kahn, 2007).

Positive outcomes of hip girdlestone pseudarthrosis include eradication of osteomyelitis and subsequent infections, and greatly decreased pain. Because of the number of significant side effects and resulting complications, however, hip girdlestone pseudarthrosis is done very infrequently and usually as a final option. This procedure greatly impedes ambulation ability because of leg length inequality and instability related to absence of the joint. In removing the joint, a fibrous pseudarthrosis is formed between the ilium and femur, and the affected leg is significantly shortened. Consequently, patients will ambulate with the leg in external rotation with a severe abductor lurch. An external shoe lift will be necessary in order to walk (Theis & Kahn, 2007). This has the potential for altered body image issues for the patient. In the elderly, these complications of immobility may necessitate being wheelchair-bound or bedridden, depending on ambulation/transfer ability or learning ability if confused. In addition, recurrent infection is also a risk with any surgery.

Assessment

History and Physical Exam. It is important to know a detailed patient history of infection. If the patient is chronically immunosuppressed or immunocompromised, a girdlestone procedure may be the only alternative. If the patient has had multiple infections in the same joint that recur after antibiotic therapy and removal of the prosthesis has been completed, this information must be given to the surgeon and an infectious disease specialist experienced in joint infections and osteomyelitis. Multiple unresolved infections in a replaced joint have a higher rate of recurrent reinfection that are resistant to antibiotic therapies. A patient who has had a girdlestone procedure will have a significantly shorter leg length on the affected side. Flailing of the lower extremity is noted with ambulation and all other movements regarding this extremity because there is no longer a joint (Theis & Kahn, 2007).

Diagnostic Tests. Diagnostic tests to determine if hip girdlestone pseudarthrosis is necessary include radiographs of AP and lateral hip views. CT/MRI for more detailed definition of the joint space and femoral shaft may be necessary. Hip aspirations and culture results from the laboratory, along with ESR, CRP, synovial fluid analysis and white blood cell (WBC) count, are necessary preoperatively to confirm and classify an infection.

Common Therapeutic Modalities

Conservative. Continued courses of intravenous antibiotic therapy may be administered or suppressive antibiotics may be given to try and keep the infecting organism from proliferating.

Surgical. During surgery, the femoral head and neck are resected, which results in the shortening of the femur by 2 inches or more. Pseudarthrosis forms between the wing of the ilium and the proximal femur. Muscle spasm is common following the procedure. Skeletal traction is used postoperatively to reduce muscle spasm and provide alignment for the fibrous pseudarthrosis to form. Weight-bearing is restricted for up to 6 months for healing to occur (Thies & Kahn, 2007).

Nursing Considerations

Nursing Diagnoses. Nursing diagnoses for this condition are expanded upon in the Appendix.

- Activity intolerance.
- Anxiety.
- Body image, altered.
- Caregiver role strain, risk for.
- Constipation, risk for.
- Coping, ineffective.
- Falls, risk for.
- Family processes, interrupted.
- Fear.
- Infection, risk for.
- Knowledge deficit.
- Mobility: physical, impaired
- Pain, acute.
- Self-care deficit: bathing/hygiene, dressing/ grooming, feeding, toileting.
- Skin integrity, risk for impaired.
- Surgical recovery, delayed.
- Tissue perfusion: peripheral, ineffective.

Interventions and Education. Because of impaired physical mobility following hip girdlestone pseudarthrosis, the patient must use assistive devices for ambulation. Physical and occupational therapists will work closely with the patient to issue or make recommendations on the appropriate equipment for home use. The nurse should instruct and reinforce the ongoing permanent use of these assistive devices for ambulating and work with occupational /physical therapy, as needed, to obtain necessary ADL devices and home equipment. The nurse should assess the patient for body image/self-esteem issues and coordinate counseling as appropriate.

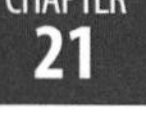

Practice Setting Considerations. The nurse should provide postoperative care per protocol and assist in coordinating discharge plans. Support systems and patient safety are very important. The patient may not be able to manage in the home setting, and an alternative level of care should be considered. Some patients need to go to skilled care for therapy until able to return to home. There must be adequate support at home for the patient to return safely to that setting. The patient and caregivers should be taught home ADL management. The nurse should reinforce mobility instructions and assist with/teach incisional care. Driving restrictions must also be addressed, especially if the procedure was done on the right side.

Proximal Femoral Osteotomy

Overview

Proximal femoral osteotomy (PFO) realigns the femoral neck and is indicated in early hip arthritis, usually caused by congenital malformation, if conservative measures have failed. PFO provides greater coverage of the femoral head by the acetabulum and increases joint space. This procedure alters the weight-bearing axis so that a nonarthritic area of the femoral head is structured to bear the weight.

PFO is indicated for younger patients to provide an alternative to immediate THR. It is also used in patients whose activities, occupations, or lifestyles make them less-than-ideal candidates for joint replacement (Theis & Kahn 2007). PFO, successful in approximately 80% of patients, is generally a temporary alternative for up to 10 years (Theis & Kahn, 2007). By 10 years after an osteotomy procedure, one half to three quarters of patients require further surgery, including joint replacement.

Complications from PFO include nonunion or malunion, thromboembolism, wound infection, and under or overcorrection. Internal hardware is used to maintain fixation, and this may become painful. Because of these complications, PFO has become a fairly infrequent procedure, especially now that other treatment options such as resurfacing and FAI are readily available (Ilizaliturri, 2009).

Assessment

For history, physical exam, and diagnostic tests, refer to the sections on Total Hip Arthroplasty or Hip Resurfacing Arthroplasty earlier in this chapter.

Common Therapeutic Modalities

During the PFO surgery, a wedge of bone is removed from the proximal femur, usually near the lesser trochanter. The angle of the femoral neck relative to the femoral shaft is realigned, and a plate and screws are used to fix the proximal femur. Approximately 3 months of partial weight-bearing is necessary for complete healing (Theis & Kahn, 2007).

Nursing Considerations

Nursing Diagnoses. Nursing diagnoses for this condition are expanded upon in the Appendix.

- Activity intolerance.

- Anxiety.
- Caregiver role strain, risk for.
- Constipation, risk for.
- Coping, ineffective.
- Falls, risk for.
- Family processes, interrupted.
- Fear.
- Infection, risk for.
- Knowledge deficit.
- Mobility: physical, impaired.
- Pain, acute.
- Self-care deficit: bathing/hygiene, dressing/grooming, feeding, toileting.
- Skin integrity, risk for impaired.
- Surgical recovery, delayed.
- Tissue perfusion: peripheral, ineffective.

Interventions and Education. The need for 3 months of non-weight-bearing may be the biggest concern for these patients. If the right leg is involved, the patient will not be able to drive for this extended period of time. Also, patients require postoperative anticoagulation to prevent DVT. If the surgeon's preference is for warfarin/coumadin, a system of monitoring will need to be set up, and patient teaching must include signs and symptoms of bleeding, dietary considerations, and medication interactions. If other anticoagulants are being used, the patient/caregivers must learn injection technique, syringe disposal, and rotation of sites appropriate to the type of anticoagulant. Family routines may be interrupted, as this procedure is usually done in young or middle-aged patients.

Outcomes. The goal of a successful proximal femoral osteotomy is to relieve pain and allow for more vigorous activities with fewer restrictions. Healing in the correct position during the 3-month period is critical to obtain the optimal result.

Femoral Shaft Fractures

Overview

Femoral shaft fractures occur between the subtrochanteric and supracondylar areas. Shaft fractures may be open or closed, comminuted or noncomminuted, and displaced or nondisplaced. They can occur when the bone is subjected to more stress than it can absorb and may be caused by direct or indirect force, stress, or pathologic process. Femoral shaft fractures usually result from tremendous forces and may cause a loss of 1-2.5 liters of blood volume (Theis & Kahn, 2007). Amount of force required to fracture the femur varies with the quality of the bone. As age increases, the force required to result in a fracture decreases. Bone that is weakened from disease requires less stress to become fractured. High-risk activities or recreation may predispose the younger adult to a higher incidence of femoral shaft fractures (Theis & Kahn, 2007).

Complications from femoral shaft fractures include fat embolism, pulmonary embolism, DVT, compartment syndrome, shock, nonunion, malunion, wound infection and osteomyelitis, pin tract infections with external fixation devices, impaired mobility, and limb length discrepancy in children. (Refer to Chapter 15—Trauma for early interventions for femoral fractures.)

Assessment

History and Physical Exam. When assessing femoral shaft fracture patients, it is important to note the mechanism of injury and any presenting symptoms that can include pain, deformity, leg length discrepancy, inability to move the extremity, complaints of altered neurovascular status to the affected extremity, and an open wound related to an open fracture. Altered hemodynamic status related to extensive soft tissue damage and considerable blood loss from fracture site may be seen.

Physical examination of the extremity should assess appearance, position, and neurovascular function. The extremity may be swollen, bruised, have open wounds, or be deformed. The extremity may be rotated externally, shortened, and malaligned compared to the opposite extremity. Vital signs should be assessed for shock due to blood loss. A general physical examination will be necessary for operative preparation.

Diagnostic Tests. Radiographs (AP and lateral views of the femur) will evaluate the degree of fracture to determine management, and laboratory tests appropriate to trauma work-up or preoperative requirements will be ordered.

Common Therapeutic Modalities

Conservative. The goal of treatment is adequate fracture reduction with return to full mobility.

Conservative therapeutic modalities would include skin traction, skeletal traction, cast brace, or hip spica cast. Casting is the preferred treatment for children up to approximately age 10. Skeletal traction may be used short-term (for several days) to medically stabilize the patient prior to surgery, to reduce edema if there is extensive soft tissue swelling, or to provide better alignment of fracture fragments. Skeletal traction may also be used as the entire treatment modality; however, this requires 4-6 weeks of traction with associated potential complications of immobility (Theis & Kahn, 2007).

Surgical. Surgery is the preferred choice of treatment because it allows for early mobilization and ambulation. The surgeon will need to determine the patient's weight-bearing restrictions once the surgery is complete, based on the fracture itself and the fixation method. Internal fixation requires intermedullary rods, strut grafting, and plate and screws. External fixation may be chosen with an open fracture.

Open femur fractures are treated as an emergency and require certain considerations. Soft tissue damage generally has priority over fracture treatment. All open femur fractures are considered contaminated; therefore, antibiotic therapy is automatically initiated. Wounds may have primary closure or delayed closure, depending on the extent of the wound, the need for grafting, and the potential for compartment syndrome.

Nursing Considerations

Nursing Diagnoses. Nursing diagnoses for this condition are expanded upon in the Appendix.

- Activity intolerance.
- Anxiety.
- Caregiver role strain, risk for.
- Constipation, risk for.
- Coping, ineffective.
- Falls, risk for.
- Family processes, interrupted.
- Fear.
- Infection, risk for.
- Knowledge deficit.
- Mobility: physical, impaired.
- Pain, acute.
- Self-care deficit: bathing/hygiene, dressing/grooming, feeding, toileting.
- Surgical recovery, delayed.
- Skin integrity, risk for impaired.
- Tissue perfusion: peripheral, ineffective.

Interventions and Education. Femoral shaft fractures can require prolonged rehabilitation and thus an altered lifestyle/occupation, especially for the younger patient. In children, fractures through the shaft of a long bone stimulate growth; therefore, to avoid limb length discrepancy due to overgrowth, the fracture ends may be set in a slight overlap (Theis & Kahn 2007). The prolonged bed rest typically required for a child recovering from a femoral shaft fracture can be very challenging for children and adolescents; the nurse should assist caregivers in developing age-appropriate diversional activities. In elderly patients with very osteoporotic bone, internal fixation can be more difficult related to poor bone stock.

The nurse should reinforce the importance of mobility once weight-bearing is approved. Mobility helps in the healing process by avoiding medical complications associated with immobility such as DVT, PE, infiltrates, and overall deconditioning. The nurse should monitor incision care and teach pin site care if external fixation is in place. Patient education includes signs and symptoms of infection, compartment syndrome, DVT, and anticoagulation. Comorbidities related to other injuries must also be addressed, and this is often a team approach with the trauma surgeon and any other physicians participating in the care of these patients.

Pelvic Fracture

Overview

Pelvic fractures are generally caused by severe trauma, including motor vehicle accidents, falls from great heights, or crushing injuries. In the elderly, pelvic fractures occur after falls onto the buttocks. Pelvic fractures occur in the ilium, ischium, or pubic bone. Sacral fractures occurring with pelvic ring fractures increase the severity of pelvic fractures (Theis & Kahn 2007). Pelvic fractures may be stable or unstable. The location and amount of fractures in the pelvic ring determines the stability of the pelvis. Displacement of fracture fragments can lead to shifting of the pelvic ring and instability.

Because major blood vessels are located in the pelvic region (the common iliac and femoral arteries, and femoral and greater saphenous veins), pelvic fractures can result in a high volume of blood loss. Severe damage to these major vessels can cause hemorrhagic shock. Major nerve damage can also occur related to the location of lumbar and sacral plexus. With severe fractures, additional abdominal pain is likely (Theis & Kahn, 2007). It is also important to be aware of bladder injury or injury to the internal organs in the abdominal cavity.

Pelvic fractures require prolonged rehabilitation because of the key role the pelvis plays in supporting the abdominal cavity, spine, and lower extremities. Pelvic fractures alter the lifestyle of the adult related to recreation, work, and ADLs. The resulting extended immobility increases the potential for altered skin integrity and DVT. In the pediatric patient, prolonged immobility or altered activity requirements will be more challenging to manage because of the patient's lower level of understanding and the need for creativity with diversional activities.

Complications of pelvic fractures include hemorrhagic shock, nerve damage, thromboembolism, malunion, nonunion, and complications of immobility (Theis & Kahn, 2007). (Refer to Chapter 15—Trauma for initial assessment and intervention for pelvic fractures.)

Assessment

History and Physical Exam. When assessing pelvic fracture patients, the mechanism of injury must be considered. Presenting symptoms may include bruising, deformity, pain, an open wound related to an open fracture, and signs of hemorrhagic shock. Severe back pain may indicate retroperitoneal bleeding (Theis & Kahn, 2007). The lower extremities should be assessed for any alterations in neurovascular status. Pelvic fractures can involve other organs (including abdomen, bladder, intestines, and rectum), depending on the position of the pelvis during the trauma, as well as the force and mechanism of injury.

Physical examination of the abdomen and pelvis can reveal swelling, bruising, deformity, and open wounds (Theis & Kahn, 2007). The type, location, and amount of pain are important considerations. Any crepitus of pelvic bones should be noted and movement avoided until radiologic assessment is complete. Assessment of vital signs for shock due to blood loss is important. Neurovascular assessment of bilateral lower extremities and peripheral pulses is important. An absence of peripheral pulses may indicate a major artery tear (Theis & Kahn, 2007).

Diagnostic Tests. Radiographs and laboratory tests are essential. Radiographs should include a complete pelvic series and CT scan to assess for abdominal injuries. Always suspect and look for fractures on radiographs in the pelvic ring, as its circular construction predisposes it to shifting and resulting instability (Theis & Kahn, 2007). Laboratory tests should be ordered as appropriate for trauma work-up or preoperative requirements. Sometimes an exploratory laparotomy is performed to assess peritoneal trauma and fluid collection within the abdominal cavity following a pelvic fracture.

Common Therapeutic Modalities

Choice of treatment for a pelvic fracture will depend on the type, location, stability versus instability of the fracture(s), and surgeon preference. Other factors include the patient's current status, comorbidities, and overall prefracture health. A combination of conservative and surgical options may be used.

Conservative. Conservative treatment can include bed rest, progressing to ambulation with restricted weight-bearing for stable fractures, skeletal traction, and pelvic sling traction. Depending on the fracture, the patient may need external fixation to stabilize the pelvic ring.

Surgical. Surgical treatment would be an open reduction internal fixation. Adequate fracture reduction with a stable pelvis using plates, pins, and screws is the typical surgical procedure for pelvic fractures. A external fixator frame may be applied in the immediate trauma period to stabilize the fracture and align the fracture fragments. Sometimes the frame is applied while other medical conditions stabilize in the trauma patient, until more definitive surgery can be performed. Surgical treatment of comorbidities is based on the severity of injury and optimal interventions as decided by the trauma team and associated physicians involved in the patient's care.

Nursing Considerations

Nursing Diagnoses. Nursing diagnoses for this condition are expanded upon in the Appendix.

- Activity intolerance.
- Anxiety.
- Caregiver role strain, risk for.
- Constipation, risk for.
- Coping, ineffective.
- Falls, risk for.
- Family processes, interrupted.
- Fear.
- Infection, risk for.
- Knowledge deficit.
- Mobility: physical, impaired.
- Pain, acute.
- Self-care deficit: bathing/hygiene, dressing/grooming, feeding, toileting.
- Skin integrity, risk for impaired.
- Surgical recovery, delayed.
- Tissue perfusion: peripheral, ineffective.

Interventions and Education. In pelvic fracture patients, pain control is paramount, with frequent assessment and monitoring. Interventions include log-rolling, per physician order, to maintaining pelvic alignment. Exercise programs, as instructed by physical therapists, should be reinforced. Nurses should help patients/caregivers obtain assistive devices for ambulating prior to discharge and should teach proper use of the devices. Nurses should ensure that patients/caregivers understand the weight-bearing status and restrictions. If there is an external fixator, the patient/caregivers must learn pin care and incision care.

The nurse assists with postoperative care and monitoring. Posttrauma and postoperative care should be provided per protocol. The patient's home situation needs to be assessed for safety and functional ability. Mobility restrictions must be reinforced until the patient verbalizes understanding. Patients/caregivers are instructed in wound care, incision care, and ADL management.

Summary

Hip replacement surgery can significantly improve the quality of life in patients with advanced hip arthritis. Younger patients are now suffering from degenerative joint disease at earlier stages in their lives. This has led to new demands in treatment from both the patient and the medical team, including faster recoveries and quicker returns to desired activity levels. Older patients are living longer, more active lifestyles, and this too has changed the standard of care for this patient population. It has also driven the technology in developing improved surgical practices and devices to return patients to their preinjury physically active lives.

Recent advances in technology afford the orthopedic surgeon many new treatment options to offer patients. For hip replacement and hip resurfacing, the minimization of debris from wear with highly cross-linked polyethylene or ceramic and metal surfaces has shown to improve outcomes and patient satisfaction (Garbuz et al., 2010). Along with these new approaches, there remain those treatments and procedures that are the standard practices in the fixation of pelvic, femur, and extraarticular hip fractures. Triage for traumatic injuries, medical comorbidities, and postoperative complications has seen little change, yet the standard of care remains at a very high level.

As with any lower extremity impairment, a plethora of potential and actual nursing diagnoses may occur. The orthopedic nurse plays a vital role in assisting patients and their caregivers with teaching, emotional support, safety needs, development of support systems, and supplemental care while managing medical well-being and decreasing medical risks and injury.

References

American Academy of Orthopaedic Surgeons (AAOS). (n.d.). *Falls and hip fractures.* Retrieved November 24, 2010, from http://orthoinfo.aaos.org/topic.cfm?topic=A00121

American Academy of Orthopaedic Surgeons (AAOS). (2011). *Total hip replacement.* Retrieved from http://orthoinfo.aaos.org/topic.cfm?topic=A00377.

Bhattacharyya, T. & Koval, K.J. (2009). Unipolar versus bipolar hemiarthroplasty for femoral neck fractures: Is there a difference? *Journal of Orthopedic Trauma, 23*(6), 426-427.

Botser, I.B., Smith, T.W., Nasser, R., & Domb, B.G. (2011). Open surgical dislocation versus arthroscopy for femoroacetabular impingement: A comparison of clinical outcomes. *Journal of Arthroscopy and Related Research, 27*(2), 270-278.

Bozic, K.J., Kurtz S., Lau E., Ong K., Chiu V., Vail T.P.... Berry D.J. (2009). The epidemiology of bearing surface usage in total hip arthroplasty in the United States. *Journal of Bone and Joint Surgery, American, 91*(7), 1614-1620.

Cleveland Clinic Foundation. (n.d.). *Hip fractures in the elderly.* Retrieved December 13, 2010, from http://my.clevelandclinic.org/disorders/osteoporosis/hic_hip_fractures_in_the_elderly.aspx

Cordingley, R., Kohan, L., & Ben-Nissan, B. (2010). What happens to femoral neck bone mineral density after hip resurfacing surgery? *Journal of Bone and Joint Surgery, British, 92*(12), 1648-1653.

Desouza, R.M., Parsons, N.R., Oni, T., Dalton, P., Costa, M., & Krikler, S. (2010). Metal ion levels following resurfacing arthroplasty of the hip: Serial results over a ten-year period. *Journal of Bone and Joint Surgery, British, 92*(12), 1642-1647.

Fritz, A.T., Reddy, D., Meehan, J.P., & Jamali, A.A. (2010). Femoral neck exostosis: A manifestation of CAM Pincer combined femoroacetabular impingement. *Arthroscopy, 26*(1), 121-127.

Garbuz, D.S., Tanzer, M., Greidanus, N.V., Masri, B.A., & Duncan, C.P. (2010). Metal-on-metal hip resurfacing versus large-diameter head metal-on-metal total hip arthroplasty. *Clinical Orthopaedics and Related Research, 468*(2), 318-325.

Hart, E.S., Metkar, U.S., Rebello, G.N., & Grottkau, B.E. (2009). Femoroacetabular impingement in adolescents and young adults. *Orthopaedic Nursing, 28*(3), 117-124.

Ilizaliturri, V.M. (2009). Complications of femoroacetabular impingement treatment: A review. *Clinical Orthopaedics and Related Research, 467*(3), 760-768.

McMinn, D.J., Daniel, J., Ziaee, H., & Pradhan, C. (2011). Indications and results of hip resurfacing. *International Orthopaedics, 35*(2), 231-237.

National Association of Orthopadic Nurses (NAON). (2007). *Core curriculum for orthopaedic nursing* (6th ed.). Boston, MA: Pearson.

Ossendorf, C., Scheyerer, M.J., Wanner, G.A., Simmen, H.P., & Werner, C. (2010). Treatment of femoral neck fractures in elderly patients over 60 years of age: Which is the ideal modality of primary joint replacement? *Patient Safety in Surgery, 4*(1), 16.

Rhodes, B. (2008). *Dislocated Hip Replacement.* Retrieved from http://en.wikipedia.org/wiki/File:Dislocated_hip_replacement.jpg

Sandeford, N.A., Muirhead-Allwood, S.K., Skinner, J.A., & Hua, J. (2010). Metal-on-metal hip resurfacing versus uncemented custom total hip replacement: Early results. *Journal of Orthopedic Surgery and Research, 5*, 8.

Schroder, D., Bornstein, L., Bostrom, M.P., Nestor, B.J., Padgett, D.E., & Westrich, G.H. (2010). Ceramic-on-ceramic total hip arthroplasty: Incidence of instability and noise. *Clinical Orthopaedics and Related Research, 469*(2), 437-442.

Sjoehest. (2005). Anonymisierte Röntgenaufnahme einer medialen Schenkelhalsfraktur ohne Dislokation. Retrieved from http://en.wikipedia.org/wiki/File:Shf_ohne_dislokation_medial_ap.jpg

Stalzer, S., Wahoff, M., & Scanlon, M. (2006). Rehabilitation following hip arthroscopy. *Clinics in Sports Medicine, 25*(2), 337-357.

Theis, L. & Kahn, B. (2007). The hip, femur and pelvis. In NAON, *Core Curriculum for Orthopaedic Nursing* (6th ed., 534-554). Boston: Pearson.

Zywiel, M.G., Sayeed, S.A., Johnson, A.J., Schmalzreid, T.P., & Mont, M.A. (2011). Survival of hard-on-hard bearings in total hip arthroplasty: A systemic review. *Clinical Orthopaedics and Related Research, 469*(6), 1536-1546.

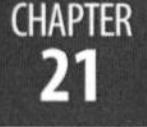

Chapter 22
The Knee

Jack Davis, MSN, RN, ONC & Penny Saulog-Wendel, BSN, RN, ONC

Objectives

- Discuss five common nonsurgical therapeutic modalities in the management of the patient with osteoarthritis of the knee.
- Identify three surgical options for the patient with osteoarthritis of the knee.
- Identify three pediatric knee conditions.
- Describe five types of meniscal tears.
- Identify three goals of physical therapy following ACL injury.
- Identify three common nursing diagnoses, outcomes, and interventions for patients with knee pathology.
- Identify three postoperative management considerations for patients with knee pathology.
- Identify three office practice considerations related to management of patients with knee pathology.

The knee is a complex joint consisting of four bones: the femur, the tibia, the fibula, and the patella. The femur is the large bone in the thigh, attached by ligaments and a capsule to the tibia (or shinbone). The fibula runs parallel to the tibia. The patella (or knee cap) slides on the knee joint as the knee bends. (See Figure 22.1.)

Figure 22.1.
Anatomy of the Knee

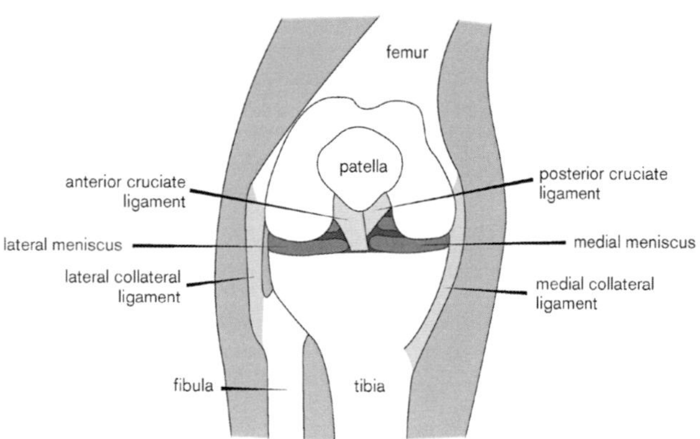

From Cynthia Conklin, 2011, Hospital for Special Surgery Digital Media Center. Reproduced with permission.

The muscle groups attached to the knee joint, the quadriceps and hamstrings, enable joint movement. Knee motion includes bending (flexion), straightening (extension), and slight rotation. The quadriceps muscles are anterior and hamstrings are posterior to the knee. Ligaments and tendons provide joint stability. The two cruciate ligaments located in the center of the knee joint, the anterior cruciate ligament (ACL) and the posterior cruciate ligament (PCL), are the major stabilizing ligaments of the knee. The ACL prevents the femur from sliding backwards on the tibia, and the PCL prevents the femur from sliding forward on the tibia. The collateral ligaments (medial [MCL] and lateral [LCL]) work with the cruciate ligaments to add stabilization of the knee joint during rotation (Flandry & Hommel, 2011).

Articular (or hyaline) cartilage is an extremely smooth, hard material that lies on a bone's articulating surfaces (those surfaces that come into contact with other bones). Its function is to allow for the smooth interaction between two bones in a joint. Menisci are semilunar-shaped cartilage pads between the long bones of the lower extremity and function as cushions for shock absorption during weight-bearing activities. The purpose of the menisci is to protect the articular cartilage that covers the ends of the tibia and femur from injury and to act as spaces to stabilize the knee. There is a medial and a lateral meniscus.

All of these structures together are critical to the patient's performance of activities of daily living (ADLs). The nurse should consider the activities of sitting, standing, kneeling, ambulating, and other mobility when understanding the implications of lower extremity injuries and how they impact patients' daily activities. Significant disability can result in both the short and long term due to associated injuries, deformities, and lost range of motion (ROM). Before initiating treatment, the care providers should take into account a variety of practice considerations discussed in Table 22.1.

Table 22.1.
Common Office Practice Considerations

A. Assist with patient flow and scheduling.
B. Take history and perform physical examination.
C. Provide telephone triage.
D. Support insurance certification issues.
E. Communicate effectively.
F. Assist with patient/family education. 1. Pre-procedure. 2. Post-procedure.
G. Assist with clinical procedures. 1. Injections/aspirations. 2. Suture/staple removal.
H. Monitor treatment effectiveness.
I. Track medications and effects.
J. Assist with outcomes data collection and management.

Osteoarthritis of the Knee

Overview

Definition. Osteoarthritis (OA) is degenerative or wear-and-tear arthritis, classified as primary/idiopathic (unknown cause) or secondary (known cause). Each class exhibits different patterns of onset and risk factors. Primary OA is a process in which articular degeneration occurs in the absence of any obvious underlying abnormality. Secondary OA results from either an abnormal concentration of force across an articulation with normal articular matrix or a normal concentration of force across an abnormal joint. Secondary OA is often the result of injury or repetitive motion, such as found in certain occupations, but it can also result from congenital conditions and systemic disease or various inflammatory disorders. Post traumatic arthritis can result from trauma to the joint including tibial plateau fractures, fractures of the femoral condyles, nonunion fractures of the femoral condyles and tibial plateau, and ligamentous injuries that cause joint instability. (Also see Chapter 13—Arthritis.)

Pathophysiology. OA is more prevalent in weight-bearing joints, such as the knee. Approximately four times the body weight is transmitted through the joints during normal walking. The medial compartment of the knee is the most frequently affected.

Incidence. OA of the knee is one of the five leading causes of physical disability and morbidity in the United States. It has been estimated that 59.4 million Americans, or 18.2 % of the population, will carry a diagnosis of arthritis by the year 2020 (Huddleston et al., 2009). Franks and Mor (2006) described the evolving etiology and prevalence of various inflammatory disorders affecting the knee to also include Lyme disease, human immunodeficiency virus (HIV)-associated arthritis, and hepatitis C. Avascular necrosis, osteonecrosis, and bone infarction are used synonymously to define the spontaneous or traumatic death in situ of a segment of bone. This diagnosis can also lead to OA. Other predisposing factors for knee OA are chronic patella dislocations, severe varus and valgus deformity, and chondromalacia patella.

Assessment

History and Physical Exam. Pain is the predominant symptom of OA of the knee and the main reason patients seek medical attention. Synovitis is a prime source of pain because the synovium is richly innervated. Patients with early OA may not show much evidence of synovial inflammation. Synovial inflammation leads to release of inflammatory mediators, thus sensitizing nociceptive cells and directly damaging cartilage (Hungerford, Khanuja, & Hungerford, 2006). Subjective pain can be measured and is currently the best criterion for evaluating potential therapy. Clinical examination often reveals pain on active and passive motion (Luyten, Westhovens, & Taelman, 2006). The pain, typically mechanical in nature and described as "aching," is one way by which OA is differentiated from inflammatory arthropathies. Night pain or pain at rest may occur with disease progression. Pain may also increase with the fall in barometric pressure that precedes inclement weather. The experience of pain is not necessarily related to other evidence of disease but reflects the individual client's pain threshold and his or her use of the affected joint. A visual analogue scale can be used with the initial assessment to gauge the client's current pain. Tenderness may be present along the joint line, even in the absence of overt inflammation. Joint enlargement may result from effusion, popliteal fullness, synovial hyperplasia, or osteophytes. Bakers cysts, otherwise known as popliteal cysts, are the most common synovial cyst. These typically manifest as a distended bursa, produced either by herniation of the synovial membrane through the capsule or escape of fluid and communication with the bursa around the knee. Patients with popliteal cysts typically present with a tender, swollen area in the posterior knee. They must be differentiated from vascular thrombosis or soft tissue tumor. Cysts are typically translucent. Osteophytes may be palpated as irregular bony masses. Crepitus (or a crackling sound) may occur with movement of the knee. It is important to note the presence of patellofemoral crepitus throughout ROM. Patients may complain of trouble with kneeling, climbing stairs, and getting in and out of a chair. Locking of the knee may result from loose bodies in the joint. Morning stiffness is common but usually lasts less than 30 minutes (Paget, Gibofsky, Beary, & Sculco, 2006).

The clinician should grossly evaluate leg alignment, contour, and gait pattern with the patient standing and walking. A valgus deformity (knock-knee) indicates destruction of the lateral knee compartment and is usually associated with MCL laxity. A varus deformity (bowleg) indicates pathology in the medial knee compartment and may be associated with LCL laxity. It is common that knee arthritis, particularly of the medial compartment, is associated with a flexion deformity. These patients typically also have posterior capsule thickening and contracted hamstring tendons. An additional deformity is recurvatum or hyperextension, which can result from weakness of the extensor mechanism (quadriceps) or posterior capsular laxity. Check stability of the knee to assess the laxity of the MCLand LCL. Varus and valgus stability is best performed by cradling the knee with one hand and, with the knee in extension, applying a medial or lateral knee stress. A jog of motion is suggestive of instability. The presence of any muscle atrophy should be noted (Paget et al., 2006). The degree of pain and the extent of any related functional disability should be evaluated. History of injury is important as a possible precipitating factor in the appearance or increase of pain.

Diagnostic Tests. Radiography should be performed while the patient is in the standing position (anteroposterior [AP] and lateral views) to demonstrate joint space narrowing (see Figure 22.2). Tangential patellar views (merchant views) are obtained to assess the patellofemoral compartment. A tunnel view is obtained to assess the intercondylar notch. Screening blood tests such as CBC, ESR, Rheumatoid factor, and biochemistry profile should be performed if systemic disease is suspected. Aspiration of synovial fluid for analysis of cells and crystals is helpful to rule out rheumatoid arthritis (RA), gout, and pseudogout. Culture and sensitivity are definitive in infectious arthritis. A bone scan or magnetic resonance imaging (MRI) may be helpful to demonstrate early osteonecrosis when radiographic findings are still normal.

Common Therapeutic Modalities

Conservative Management. Appropriate treatment of knee OA starts with correct diagnosis of the underlying disease and identification of the causes of the condition. Wellness promotion and disease prevention focuses on reducing the factors that contribute to excessive joint loading. Patients should be counseled on body mechanics, orthotics to correct and support pronated feet, workplace modifications, weight reduction, and gait training with

Figure 22.2.
Standing AP Radiograph: Severe Osteoarthritis

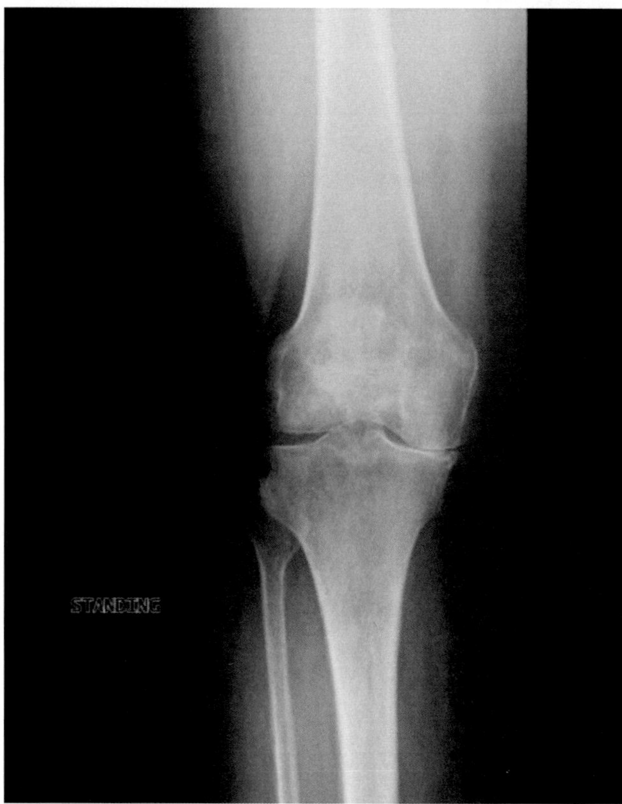

From Thomas Sculco, 2011, Hospital for Special Surgery. Reproduced with permission.

assistive device if indicated. Every one-pound weight loss translates to a three- to four-pound reduction in load across the joint. The use of bracing and splinting for support and compartment unloading should be considered. The five following treatment modalities address the typical symptoms of pain, swelling, and loss of motion:

1. Physical therapy (PT): The beneficial effect of PT, coupled with absence of side effects, argues for a prominent role for these modalities. OA typically leads to a rapid loss of muscle strength and function. Hungerford et al. (2006) found that 30% of muscle atrophy can occur in 1 week. PT often consists of multiple modalities, including bracing, orthoses, educational plans, adjunctive treatments like transcutaneous electrical nerve stimulation (TENS), ultrasound, cryotherapy, and whirlpool and aquatic therapy. These modalities are usually supported with an exercise program designed to increase muscle strength, endurance, and ROM as part of a daily routine to improve joint function, reduce joint pain, and decrease swelling. A secondary goal is to prevent disability and poor health related to inactivity and decreased mobility. Care should be taken with inflamed joints because passive ROM exercise or repetitive joint motion has been shown to increase joint inflammation (Hungerford et al., 2006).
2. Non-steroidal anti-inflammatory drugs (NSAIDs): The use of NSAIDS should be considered for patients with moderate to severe pain. NSAIDs are the most common drugs used to treat knee OA. NSAIDs inhibit cyclooxygenase-1 or -2 (COX- 1-or-2) and provide an anti-inflammatory and analgesic benefit for patients. NSAIDs can be associated with unwanted gastrointestinal side effects. There is no definitive evidence to suggest that one NSAID is better than another in relieving the pain associated with OA of the knee. COX 2 selective inhibitors have no greater efficacy than selective NSAIDs do for the treatment of OA. They may offer some gastrointestinal safety advantage for patients who are at increased risk, but the adverse cardiovascular, renal, and thrombotic effects should be considered.
3. Corticosteroids: Cortisone injections are useful if there is a significant inflammatory component to OA, but they are not as useful if OA is advanced and symptoms are largely associated with mechanical findings. A cortisone injection is frequently combined with a local anesthetic to provide short-term relief. Adverse effects related to intra-articular injections of corticosteroids are post-injection flare, long-term joint damage, and serious infection (McGarry & Daruwalla, 2010). Aspirations, as well as joint irrigation of acute or recurrent knee effusion, combined with the instillation of corticosteroids may offer significant relief (Franks & Mor, 2006).
4. Intra-articular hyaluronan derivative: Hyaluronic acid (HA) is a key constituent of both cartilage ground substance and synovial fluid. HA injections have become a common tool for the management of OA of the knee, and the number of randomized controlled trials on the efficacy and safety of this treatment is expanding. Treatment with HA is indicated for patients with inadequate pain relief from oral medications, exercise, and PT, and for patients who have gastrointestinal or renal intolerance to NSAIDs (Divine, Zazulak, & Hewett, 2007). Hungerford et al. (2006) reported on the beneficial effect of an intra-articular hyaluronan derivative on knee pain for selected patients with OA. It is generally well-tolerated, yet infrequent problems may arise. Infection is a small risk and, though not specifically reported, may be assumed of the same magnitude as reported for corticosteroid injection. A series of three to five weekly injections is a drawback for some patients. Divine et al. (2007) reported that there are five injectable formulations of HA approved by the United States Food and Drug Administration: Hyalgan® (Sanofi

Synthelabo, Inc, New York, NY), Nufflexa® (Sanient Pharmaceuticals, East Brunswick, NJ), Orthovisc® (Anika Therapeutics Inc, Woburn, MA), Supartz® (Seikagaku Corp, Tokyo, Japan), and Synvisc® (Genzyme Corp, Cambridge, MA). HA preparations are dispensed in 2ml vials or 2ml syringes. The recommended injection cycles are one injection per week for 3 weeks for Synvisc and 3-5 weeks for Hyalgan, Supartz, Orthovisc, and Euflexxa. Recently, Synvisc introduced a new preparation known as Synvisc –One. As the name implies, this cycle consist of a single injection (Benke & Shaffer, 2009).

5. Chondroitin/Glucosamine: Several other amino sugars or glycosaminoglycans are commercially available for the treatment of OA. They are thought to be useful in all stages of OA, as these agents may alter the course of OA progression. Adverse reactions to glucosamine and or chondroitin are infrequent and relatively benign, consisting primarily of gastrointestinal disturbances easily reversed after discontinuation of treatment.

Surgical Management. Surgical techniques have made significant advances in the past 3 decades. Technology has allowed surgeons to replace the surfaces of the entire anatomical knee joint (total) or replace either the medial or lateral portions of the knee (unicondylar/unicompartmental). Minimally invasive surgery and high flex knee prostheses are just two of the most recent technological advancements (Cahill & Kosman, 2006).

Total knee arthroplasty (TKA) is considered the gold standard treatment of advanced arthritis of the knee. More than 542,000 TKAs are performed annually in the United States, and it is estimated that 1.5 million primary TKA surgeries will be performed by 2015 (Parker, 2011). The rationale for TKA surgery is to reestablish a movable functioning joint by removing portions of the distal femur and the proximal tibial plateau and replacing them with metal, ceramic, and/or plastic components. Most implants are made of a titanium alloy or a chrome-cobalt alloy and a high-density polyethylene. Traditionally, polymethylmethacrylate bone cement has been used as a grout between the implant and the bone. Cemented fixation is the gold standard in total knee arthroplasty. Meticulous technique—including careful soft tissue balancing, bone preparation, and cement handling—all are fundamental to implant longevity. Cemented TKA is particularly indicated in patients with inflammatory conditions such as RA. Antibiotic-impregnated cement may be advisable for certain group of patients, including those undergoing revision arthroplasty, those with diabetes mellitus, and those taking immunosuppressive medications.

The goal is to restore soft tissue balance, optimize biomechanics of the knee, maximize function, and relieve pain (Cahill & Kosman, 2006). Indications for TKA include severe OA that persists after conservative treatments (medication, PT, intra-articular injections, weight reduction, and activity modification), disabling pain with activity, post traumatic injury/arthritis, inflammatory arthritis, significant varus/valgus deformity, osteonecrosis, and failed peri-articular osteotomies (see Figure 22.3). TKA is contraindicated for patients who place very high stress demands on the knee, are a young age, have morbid obesity, live a very active lifestyle, have prior osteomyelitis about the knee, experience ongoing subclinical infection, suffer severe peripheral vascular disease, and have any medical condition that may seriously risk the patient's ability to withstand the surgery. Strict and absolute contraindications include active sepsis of the knee, solid painless surgical arthrodesis, significant genu recurvatum, and inability to carry out and maintain active extension.

Less invasive TKA is categorized as a procedure through a smaller incision. The mini-midvastus technique uses an arthrotomy that minimizes quadriceps damage and avoids patella eversion (Schroer, Diesfeld, Reedy, & LeMarr, 2008). The incision with the traditional medial parapatellar approach is generally carried proximally to the end of the split in the quadriceps tendon, while the less invasive approach uses a midline incision from the

Figure 22.3.
AP Radiograph: Right Knee s/p Total Knee Replacement

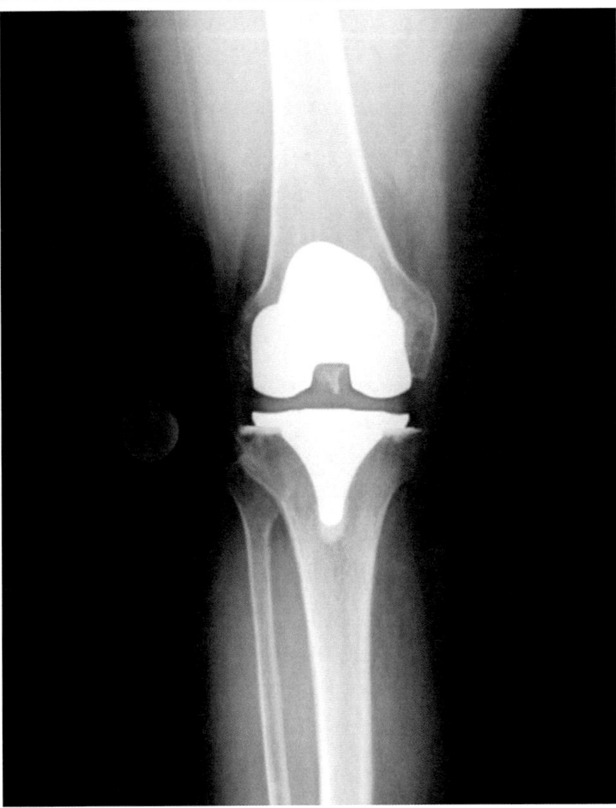

From Thomas Sculco, 2011, Hospital for Special Surgery. Reproduced with permission.

superior pole of the patella to the tibial tubercle. TKA can be safely and accurately performed through an 8.5-12 cm skin incision with improved instrumentation. In theory, this approach enhances patellofemoral stability, increases postoperative quadriceps control, and decreases scarring in the quadriceps mechanism, should revision surgery be required. The technique also intends to enhance patient recovery, reduce pain, and improve cosmesis without compromising the radiographic position of the implants (Haas, Mannita, & Burdick, 2006). Patient selection for less invasive TKA is determined by several key assessment points. Clinical examination should focus on the patient's size, although it is the actual girth of the knee that affects the surgical difficulty and not the overall size of the patient. The preoperative ROM should be greater than 110 degrees, and the surgeon should be sure to assess for presence of prior surgical scars, deformity of the extremity, and neurovascular status of the limb. Radiographs are interpreted for deformity, bone loss, presence of patella baja, and overall bone quality (Haas et al., 2006).

Unicondylar knee arthroplasty (UKA) involves resurfacing only one compartment of the knee joint, while the other compartments remain untouched. Berend and Lombardi (2007) describe UKA in patients who have degeneration either in the lateral or medial compartments of the knee but not both compartments simultaneously. Another traditional indication is osteonecrosis of the femoral condyle (Ahlbaeck's disease). Proper patient selection is key. UKA is an excellent, conservative procedure that can produce satisfactory results with a minimal complication rate in properly selected patients. If there is destruction of articular cartilage in other compartments, however, the UKA will have less satisfactory results because of deterioration of the non-replaced compartment. Patients exceeding 80 kg in weight, patients engaged in demanding sports activities, patients with a fixed varus or valgus deformity more than 5-10 that cannot be corrected easily without soft tissue releases, patients with patellofemoral degeneration, and patients with excessive varus/valgus deformities are poor candidates for UKA. The advantages of UKA include keeping the cruciate ligaments intact, sparing bone, and a potential faster recovery. It also shows excellent postoperative ROM, with the average flexion reported between 105 and 120 degrees or more. (See Figure 22.4.)

Surgical debridement has been shown to slow the progression of degenerative disease by eliminating intra-articular irritants. Arthroscopic debridement is indicated for young patients with mild degenerative disease,

Figure 22.4.
Total Knee Arthroplasty and Unicompartmental Knee Arthroplasty

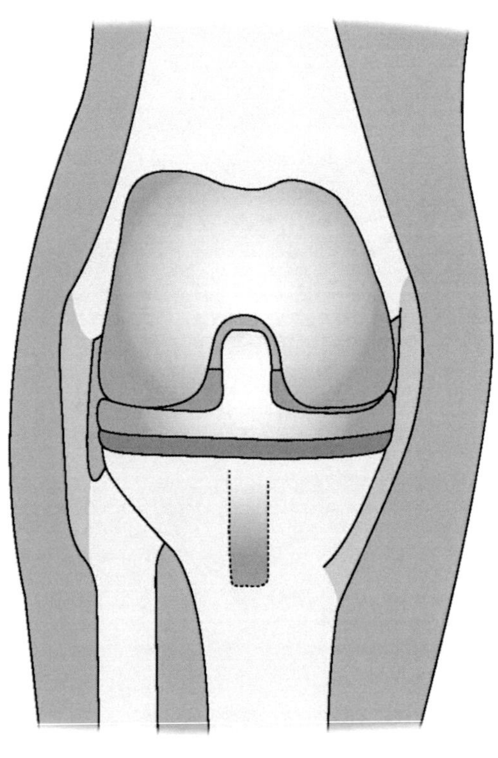

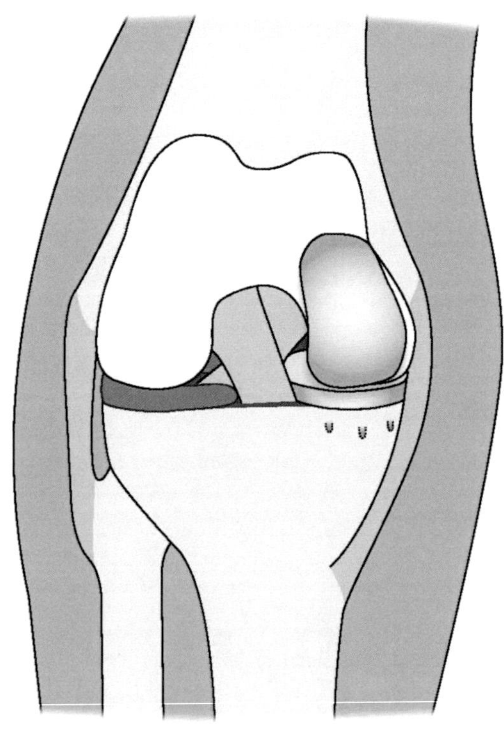

From Cynthia Conklin, 2011, Hospital for Special Surgery Digital Media Center. Reproduced with permission.

early onset OA, acute onset of crystalline-induced inflammation, and symptoms secondary to mechanical derangements. Contraindications include patients with advanced arthritis, history of long duration of symptoms, and malalignment of the knee. The role of arthroscopy in the treatment of knee OA has been subject to continuous change, and continues to evolve, as equipment and arthroscopic techniques are refined.

Minimally invasive patellofemoral arthroplasty is an attractive option for the treatment of debilitating isolated patellofemoral arthritis and diffuse grade IV patellofemoral chondromalacia. The pain relief resulting from patellofemoral arthroplasty is superior to other patellofemoral-specific treatment strategies like patellectomy and tibial tubercle unloading procedures (Lonner, 2010). Patellofemoral arthroplasty should be avoided in patients with considerable patellar maltracking or malalignment, unless these conditions are corrected preoperatively. Other contraindications include inflammatory arthritis, chondrocalcinosis involving the menisci or tibiofemoral chondral surfaces, and diffuse pain. Patellofemoral arthroplasty is most effective in patients younger than age 55 with isolated anterior compartment arthrosis. It is less predictable in elderly patients who may be better off undergoing TKA.

A *proximal tibial valgus osteotomy* is designed to realign the distal articular surface of the knee, distribute the weight more evenly within the knee joint, and relieve pain due to varus deformities and medial compartment osteoarthritis. The best candidates for proximal tibial osteotomy are young, healthy, highly active patients with isolated varus gonarthrosis and severe pain. Osteotomy is indicated for someone whose life expectancy far exceeds the expected survival of the knee implant, and who demonstrates less than 10 degrees of fixed flexion and greater than 90 degrees of active flexion (Dettoni et al., 2010) This procedure is contraindicated for patients with significant chondral degeneration in other compartments, subluxation of the tibiofemoral articulation, and ACL insufficiency, unless the surgeon plans a second-stage procedure that includes ACL reconstruction.

A *distal femoral varus osteotomy* is designed to realign the proximal weight-bearing surfaces of the knee joint as a result of valgus deformity with a lateral gonathrosis. It is indicated for larger valgus deformities associated with lateral tibiofemoral osteoarthritis.

Arthrodesis, or knee fusion, is one of the last options to obtain a stable, painless knee for severe disability and a damaged knee joint. Indications include chronic sepsis, failed TKA, and periarticular tumor. If both knees are affected, arthrodesis of the more disabled knee occasionally may be indicated to relieve the other knee of some of its burden of weight-bearing. The expected outcomes of arthrodesis include pain relief and improved function, and may reduce the need for additional future knee surgery (MacDonald, Agarwal, Lorei, Johanson, & Freiberg, 2006).

Synovectomy is a procedure that can be performed arthroscopically or open for a variety of disorders, including pigmented villonodular synovitis (PVNS), synovial chondromatosis, hemophilia, and adult or juvenile RA. The surgical removal of an inflamed synovial membrane offers rapid pain relief and a diminished associated swelling. The basic indication for synovectomy in RA is failure of the disease to respond to appropriate medical treatment after 6 months. Late synovectomy performed on knees with advanced arthritic changes has an unacceptably high failure rate and is not recommended.

Nursing Considerations

Nursing Diagnoses. Nursing diagnoses for this condition are expanded upon in the Appendix.

- Constipation, risk for.
- Falls, risk for.
- Fluid volume, deficient.
- Gastointestinal motility: risk for dysfunctional.
- Infection, risk for.
- Knowledge deficit, managing degenerative arthritis disease.
- Mobility, impaired.
- Pain, acute.
- Pain, chronic.
- Self-care deficit: bathing/hygiene, dressing/grooming, feeding, toileting.
- Skin integrity, risk for impaired.
- Tissue perfusion: peripheral, ineffective.

Interventions. Specific issues related to nursing management of the patient with OA of the knee are largely dependent on the interventions and course of treatment. Patient teaching should include discussion and evaluation of patient understanding on topics related to common therapeutic modalities: pain medications, NSAIDs, cold therapy, rest, compression, bracing, elevation, gait training, use of assistive devices for ambulation, and other conservative treatments. Surgical intervention warrants additional, more detailed, specific-patient instructions related to the surgical procedure and should include directions related to postoperative management that prevent or minimize surgical complications. Patients recovering from knee surgery should be taught to recognize untoward events and communicate with their physician expeditiously if they exhibit signs and symptoms of infection, experience venous thromboembolic events (VTEs), are unable to flex or extend the knee, have excessive bleeding, or feel pain that is unrelieved by pain medication. Although complication rates of knee arthroplasty surgery are relatively low, preventing infection and VTE is a main concern and requires preoperative risk assessment, special consideration, and appropriate preventive strategies. Talmo, Robbins, and Bono (2010) describe complication rates with infection from 0.2% to 2.5%, pulmonary embolism at 0.7%, and deep vein thrombosis (DVT) at 1.5% following TKA. Nursing care strategies to prevent infection include attention to other potential infective sources, frequent handwashing, 24-hour intravenous antibiotic coverage, wound care monitoring, observation, and patient and family teaching.

Prophylaxis to prevent VTE is universally recommended. Commonly used strategies are often multimodal and include a combination of medications, mechanical compression, and early mobilization. Rehabilitation treatment plans are tailored to include various muscle strengthening and ROM exercises, and require routine communication with other members of the health care team. Expectations regarding the return of knee function and ROM should be clearly defined, reported, and communicated to the physician on a routine basis.

Overuse Syndromes of the Knee

Overview

Knee pain is a common complaint and often associated with patients who participate in various repetitive exercise activities that may lead to acute ligamentous sprains or overuse injuries. Kodali, Islam, and Andrish (2011) describe anterior knee pain (AKP) as a broad clinical entity that includes all causes of pain in the anterior aspect of the knee. The specific diagnosis is extensive and should be narrowed by a good history and physical examination.

Chondromalacia

Definition. Chondromalacia patella is a general term that is often referred to as patellofemoral pain syndrome. It describes knee disorders that result from excessive pressure on the patellar cartilage and the subsequent softening and fibrillation of the articular surface. It is a common cause of AKP in young females. The diagnosis is only truly confirmed by visual inspection and palpation during an open or arthrosopic surgical procedure.

Assessment. Chondromalacia patella causes AKP with activities related to deep knee flexion, stair and hill ascent and descent, and prolonged sitting. Common sports that are associated with chondromalacia patella, as they may cause overloading of the patellofemoral joint, include jogging, basketball, gymnastics, and dancing. Patients with true chondromalacia patella will often demonstrate a knee effusion, crepitus, and tenderness on the undersurface of the patella. Hypermobility of the patella with medial or lateral subluxation may be present. Prior evidence of trauma to the anterior knee may also be present (O'Keefe, Hogan, Eustace, & Kavanagh, 2009).

Diagnostic Tests. Initial studies that are useful in discerning the cause of AKP include plain x-rays of the knee. The most helpful views are standing AP, lateral, and Merchant or sunrise views. The Merchant view is very specific to detect patella pathology. It can visualize the patellofemoral articulation and the degree of joint space narrowing. Advanced studies such as magnetic resonance imaging (MRI), computed tomography (CT), and bone scan are rarely indicated especially during the early assessment.

Common Therapeutic Modalities. The patient should avoid activities that exacerbate pain. Quadriceps muscle strengthening is the single most important objective. This is accomplished through quadriceps exercises or through straight leg raises. In some cases, NSAIDs may be helpful to control acute pain. Other interventions that may be helpful include patellar taping (i.e., McConnell taping) or patellar bracing.

Tendinitis/Bursitis

Tendinitis and bursitis are the inflammation of the tendon and bursae, respectively. Many bursae surround the knee, and any of these can become inflamed and cause pain. The pain may be acute and secondary to trauma, or it may be chronic and secondary to prolonged microtrauma. Sepsis should always be ruled out as a possible cause of the bursitis (Abbate & Davis, 2007). The three most common bursae associated with clinical symptomatology are prepatellar, anserine, and infrapatellar bursae.

Prepatellar Bursitis

Definition. Prepatellar bursitis (or Housemaid's Knee) is the most common form of knee bursitis and occurs when the bursa located between the patella and the shin becomes inflamed. It is often associated with patients who spend a lot of time kneeling (i.e., maids, carpet installers, and wrestlers).

Assessment. *History and physical exam:* As with all knee conditions, a detailed history of acute or chronic trauma or infection should be taken. Patients usually present with a history of frequent kneeling and trauma to the knee. A complaint of redness and swelling is also common. Walking and climbing activities may exacerbate the symptoms. The classic finding is tenderness over the prepatellar bursa.

Diagnostic tests: Plain radiographs and examination that reveals localized tenderness and activity-exacerbated pain may guide the diagnosis. If swelling and warmth is noted, septic bursitis should be suspected. Bursal fluid should be aspirated and sent for gram stain, culture, and white blood cell analysis. Poor response to initial treatment modalities may indicate an MRI study to look for a thickened tendon consistent with tendinosis.

Common Therapeutic Modalities. The treatment of non-septic bursitis consists of rest, topical analgesics, NSAIDs, ice, and PT. Steroid and anesthetic injections may be used to relieve pain and inflammation. Septic bursitis should be treated with appropriate antibiotics. Common pathogens include Staphylococcus aureus and Streptococcus. These pathogens can be treated empirically and then more specifically based on the results of the fluid culture and sensitivity.

Pes Anserinus Bursitis

Definition. Pes anserinus bursitis is an irritation of the bursa often associated with repetitive flexion and extension of the knee. The anserine bursa is one of 13 bursa found around the knee and is in close proximity to the primary flexors of the knee with a secondary influence on the internal rotation of the tibia (Helfenstein & Kurimoto, 2010).

Assessment. *History and physical exam:* Patients often present with pain in the anteromedial aspect of the knee with point tenderness and a palpable boggy fullness to the inflamed bursa. It is commonly seen in long-distance runners, overweight females with OA of the knee with valgus deformity, and patients with diabetes mellitus (Helfenstein & Kurimoto, 2010).

Diagnostic tests: Diagnosis is based primarily on symptoms of medial knee pain with stair climbing and sensitivity to palpation on the area of muscle insertion. An MRI, rather than x-ray, can help determine the etiology of pain along the medial side of the tibia and differentiate from mensical and other pathology.

Common Therapeutic Modalities. Initial treatment for pes anserinus bursitis involves rest and avoidance of activities that contribute to symptoms and irritation. In addition, a stretching and conditioning program may be initiated, beginning with isometric exercises and electrical muscle stimulation, incorporating resistive exercises as symptoms allow. The use of cryotherapy and NSAIDs therapy has shown to be beneficial. Further treatment modalities can include ultrasound, phonophoresis, iontophoresis, and deep tissue transverse friction massage. The use of neoprene sleeves and properly fitted orthotics may help provide support and address mechanical deformities. Corticosteroid injections have also been successful in treating the symptoms. For chronic cases of pes anserinus bursitis, a bursectomy may be indicated.

Patella Tendinitis

Definition. Patella tendinitis is also known as "Jumper's Knee" and is typically a result of an overuse injury of the knee extensor muscles. Patients often participate in jumping or kicking sports. The patella tendon inserts into the tibial tuberosity and enables the quadriceps to extend the lower leg. Overuse tendon injuries account for 40% of knee injuries in volleyball players and are numerous in athletes who run and jump during basketball, soccer, and dancing. Patella tendon overuse is also seen in military recruits and weightlifters (Rutland et al., 2010).

Assessment and Diagnostic Tests. Patients are typically younger than age 40 and present with anterior knee pain. The pain is exacerbated by stair-climbing, squatting, and participating in sports. The hallmark examination finding is point tenderness over the inferior pole of the patella and quadriceps tendon that reproduces the patient's symptoms. Resisted knee extension may also reproduce symptoms. Patients may complain of a "giving way" sensation under load.

Common Therapeutic Modalities. Avoidance of jumping or running, relative rest, cryotherapy, and PT form the cornerstones of treatment. PT utilizes modalities, soft tissue mobilization, and stretching and strengthening exercises. NSAIDs and topical analgesic creams are often helpful, particularly in the acute phase of the injury. Steroid injections are not advised because they may lead to tendon rupture. The knee should not be immobilized because further stiffening of the joint and atrophy of the muscles may result (Cooper & Herrera, 2008).

Nursing Considerations for All Overuse Syndromes

Nursing Diagnoses. Nursing diagnoses for this condition are expanded upon in the Appendix.

- Diversional activity, deficient.
- Infection, risk for.
- Knowledge deficit, managing care.
- Mobility, impaired.
- Pain, acute.
- Pain, chronic.
- Self-care deficit: bathing/hygiene, dressing/grooming, feeding, toileting.
- Self-health management, ineffective.

Interventions. Specific issues related to nursing management of the patient with overuse syndromes of the knee are largely dependent on the interventions and course of treatment. Patient teaching should include discussion and evaluation of patient understanding on topics related to common therapeutic modalities: pain medications, NSAIDs, cold therapy, rest, compression, bracing, avoidance of specific activity, and other conservative treatments. Rehabilitation treatment plans are tailored to include various muscle strengthening and ROM exercises, and require routine communication with all members of the health care team. Expectations regarding the return of knee function and ROM should be clearly defined, and progress should be reported and communicated to the physician on a routine basis.

Trauma and Soft Tissue Injuries of the Knee

Overview

In addition to overuse syndromes, soft tissue injuries to the various support structures and degenerative wear can lead limited knee function that interferes with ADLs and participation in sports activity. Correction of underlying soft tissue injury to maintain joint stability is crucial to prevent end-stage joint destruction.

Meniscal Tears

Definition. Meniscal tears are defined as a tearing of the menisci within the knee joint. The primary function of the meniscus is to distribute loads across the knee joint, acting as a cushion for shock absorption between the bones during weight-bearing activities. The menisci serve a variety of functions such as to protect the underlying articular surface, guide rotation, and stabilize translation (Flandry & Hommel, 2011). The pathophysiology of meniscal tears is numerous and can be classified as either acute or degenerative. The tear should also be described by location, morphology, stability, and respect of vascularity, as this will determine treatment.

Menisco-capsular separation is where the meniscus is separated from its insertion at the capsule. A bucket handle tear is a tear in the body of the meniscus that appears like a bucket handle. Bucket handle tears frequently cause locking of the knee as the "handle" catches in joint and prevents extension. A flap tear is when part of the meniscus has torn and flipped up, causing a locking sensation; this is rarely repairable. A linear tear is the most common type of tear and in general is not repairable. A cleavage tear in the body of meniscus is repairable, but usually not full thickness. Degenerative tears are unrelated to a traumatic episode, frequently associated with articular cartilage wear, and not repairable (Figure 22.5).

Assessment, Physical Exam, and Diagnostic Tests. A detailed history, including mechanism of injury and whether it occurred during torsion, squatting, direct impact, or without trauma, is helpful because traumatic lesions are most commonly caused by rotation and axial loading of the flexed knee. Symptoms often include medial or lateral joint line pain on compression, position-related joint line pain when walking or twisting the knee, and swelling. A locking sensation in extension or flexion is associated with larger tears. Provocative maneuvers performed during the examination can be used to help diagnose a torn meniscus. The McMurray test is performed with the patient lying supine with the hip and knee flexed to about 90 degrees. One hand holds the foot and turns it from external to internal rotation, while the other hand applies compression to the knee. If positive, the meniscus will be trapped and produce a pop or click that can be felt by the examiner. An MRI can provide great diagnostic accuracy of meniscal pathology.

Common Therapeutic Modalities. Treatment of meniscal injuries can be surgical and nonsurgical. Nonsurgical management includes attempts to reduce pain and swelling with NSAIDs and cryotherapy, and PT to restore motion and maintain quadriceps and hamstring strength. Bracing may be indicated as patients slowly return to sports activities (Abbate & Davis, 2007).

Figure 22.5.
Common Tears (ACL and Meniscus)

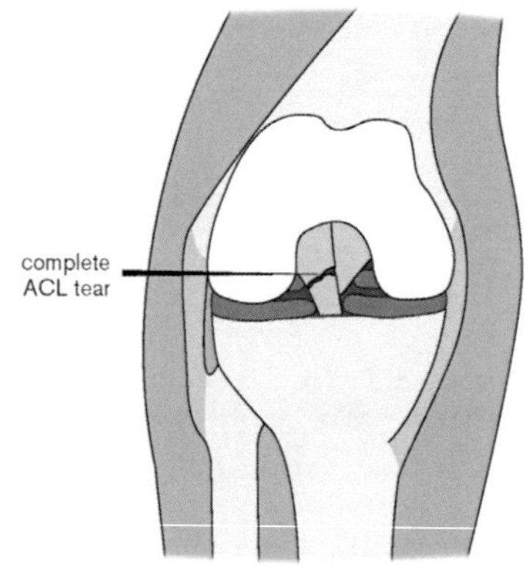

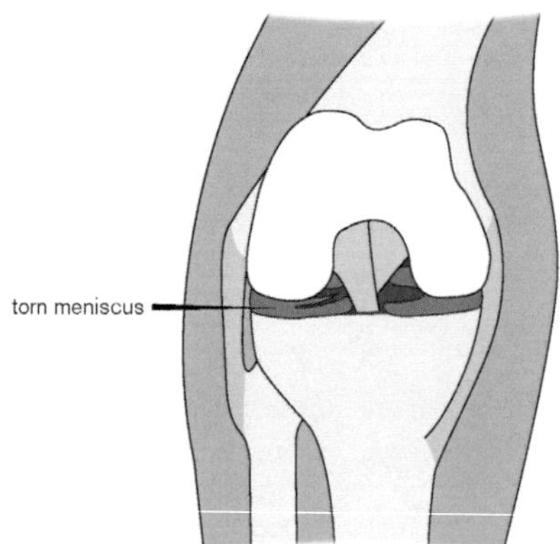

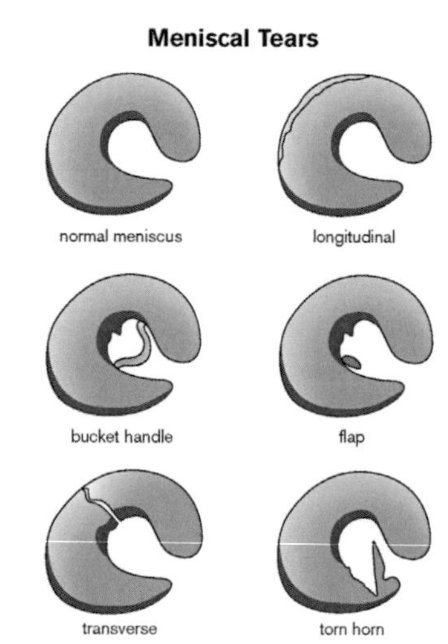

From Cynthia Conklin, 2011, Hospital for Special Surgery Digital Media Center. Reproduced with permission.

Surgical intervention for meniscal tears includes repair of vascularized portions and removal of portions in avascularized zones as the general rule. Additional strategies may include newer surgical procedures such as meniscal transplantation or partial meniscus replacement.

Ligament Injuries

Anterior Cruciate Ligament. The ACL is a rope-like ligamentous structure that inserts at the tibial spine and posterolaterally in the femur. The ACL function is to prevent excessive rotation of the knee, as well as excessive anterior translation of the tibia on the femur. The ACL and PCL crisscross in the center of the knee and provide for front-to-back and rotational stability of the knee. ACL injuries are usually the result of a non-contact twisting injury. The prevalence of ACL injury, with approximately 250,000 to 300,000 patients per year sustaining a complete tear and an increasing number of young people sustaining these injuries, is based on multiple factors, including increased female participation and increased exposure to higher-risk sports on a year-round basis (Schub & Saluan, 2011). ACL tears are identified as partial and complete tears.

ACL Assessment. Assessment includes describing the mechanism of injury and performing various physical examination maneuvers and tests. The mechanism of most ACL tears is non-contact. Examples of ACL injury causes include ski activity when a slow, twisting fall occurs when bindings do not release; a running injury during lacrosse, soccer, or football when the foot gets planted or stuck on the ground and the body continues to accelerate; or a basketball injury when a leap in the air results in landing on one foot off balance and the body falls the other way. A patient often describes hearing or feeling a pop with severe pain.

ACL Physical Exam. The physical examination includes observation of swelling, as torn muscle fibers bleed in the knee joint. This can often lead to limited ROM, and use of a knee immobilizer may be indicated for stabilization. A baseline examination of the contralateral knee is performed for comparison. A Lachman test (see Chapter 3—Musculoskeletal Assessment for other diagnostic maneuvers) is performed to assess ligament tension. The knee is flexed between 15 and 30 degrees, the femur is stabilized, and the tibia is pulled anteriorly. A positive Lachman test is when the tibia moves forward and the infra-patellar tendon slope disappears. A pivot shift test is performed with the knee in full extension and applying a valgus and internal stress. A reverse pivot shift test is performed with the knee in flexion and applying and external rotation and valgus stress

An anterior drawer test is performed by placing the patient in a supine position and flexing the affected knee to 90 degrees and placing the foot on the examination table. Sit on the foot to stabilize the leg, cup your hands around the knee and place your fingers in the area of the popliteal fossa (insertion of medial and lateral hamstrings). Place your thumbs along the lateral and medical joint line, and pull the head of the tibia toward you so that it glides on the femoral condyles. A positive anterior drawer test is if the tibia slides more than one centimeter forward; that is a sign that the ACL may be torn. This should also be done to the contralateral knee for comparison.

A posterior drawer test is performed in a similar fashion as the anterior drawer test, but instead of pulling the head of the tibia toward you, push the head of the tibia away from you. A positive posterior drawer sign is if the tibia slides one centimeter backward on the femoral condyles, indicating PCL damage.

ACL Diagnostic Tests. A partial tear is when 30% to 40% of the ligament is torn and can be diagnosed on examination when the knee feels loose, as compared to the opposite knee, but an endpoint can be felt. A complete tear is when most of the fibers are torn, the knee feels grossly loose on examination, and the knee is unstable during pivoting or lateral motion. 50% of ACL injuries have corresponding meniscal tears, with the lateral meniscus more frequently torn in acute injury and medial meniscus tears more commonly associated with chronic ACL tears. Other diagnostic tests include radiographs to assess any bony injury, MRI to evaluate ligament and cartilage injury, and a KT-1000 Biodex (a computerized dynamometer for neuromuscular testing) to assess degree of ligament tearing.

Common ACL Therapeutic Modalities. Conservative management is often recommended for individuals who do not plan on returning to aggressive pivotal or rotational sports. Initial treatment is aimed to reduce pain and swelling. Cryotherapy, elevation of extremity, and aspiration of blood from the knee may be indicated. NSAIDs and mild narcotics can be used to manage pain. Bracing for compression and support may be indicated for isolated ACL and meniscal tears. If the injury includes the MCL and posterolateral corner, more significant immobilization may be required. Crutches can be helpful for activity if weight-bearing is poorly tolerated. Restoration of joint motion is the priority, and PT to maintain muscle tone and knee motion often includes quadriceps strengthening exercises. Hamstring strengthening exercises are recommended to pull the tibia backward on femur for those with deficient cruciate ligaments.

Surgical treatment is advocated for young adults who wish to return to aggressive sport activity or where conservative measures have failed and symptoms continue to impact daily activities. Patients with concurrent meniscal tears or posterolateral corner injuries are also recommended for surgical reconstruction (Abbate & Davis, 2007).

Posterior Cruciate Ligament. The PCL is one of the main stabilizing ligaments of the knee and attaches at the posterior surface of the tibia and inserts at the lateral intracondylar notch surface of the medial femoral condyle. PCL injuries usually result from falling directly on the flexed knee, where the tibia is forced backward, or when there is a direct blow to the anteromedial aspect of the knee with the leg extended. The incidence of PCL injuries is lower than that of ACL injuries and occurs in approximately 3.4% to 20% of all knee ligament injuries (Chen, 2007).

PCL Assessment, Physical Exam, and Diagnostic Tests. The history of mechanism of injury is a very helpful diagnostic tool of PCL injury. Swelling is often less than with ACL tears. ROM may not be significantly compromised, and patients frequently do not realize the extent of the injury. Injuries to the PCL are less common and more subtle than other knee ligament injuries. PCL injuries often occur with other concomitant ligament injuries. Patients describe a feel of unsteadiness when descending slopes or bearing weight on a bent knee. A positive posterior sag sign can be observed from the side as the tibia sags backward. The examination and initial assessment is similar to those for ACL injury. X-rays to assess for bony avulsion from the femur or tibia may be helpful.

Common PCL Therapeutic Modalities. Initial treatment for PCL injury is designed to reduce swelling, pain, and inflammation and includes cyrotherapy, elevation, NSAIDs, mild analgesics, and compressive or hinged bracing. Conservative management may include refraining from sports activity for 6-12 weeks with further evaluation. Many PCL tears are partial and tend to heal with conservative management. Surgical treatment may include primary repair or the use of a tissue graft to reconstruct the knee in the case of combined injuries.

Medial Collateral Ligament and Lateral Collateral Ligament. The MCL is a structure that attaches to the medial femoral condyle proximally and the medial tibial plateau distally. The LCL forms a connection between the femur and fibula head. MCL and LCL injuries usually result from a blow to the outside of the knee during contact sports. The LCL is most commonly injured in sports by a direct impact to the inner surface of the knee joint, such as by a rugby or a football tackle. Injuries of this type are less common than those affecting the MCL, which usually occur as a result of trauma to the outer surface of the knee joint. In addition, the LCL is not connected to the lateral menicus and so, unlike MCL injuries, LCL injuries are not normally associated with meniscal tears. Due to the nature of the injury, however, the ACL or PCL may also be involved. The major functions of the MCL are to resist valgus rotation of the knee and control sideways motion. MCL disruption is usually partial, but the ligament can be completely ruptured from the femoral insertion.

MCL/LCL Assessment, Physical Exam, and Diagnostic Tests. MCL and LCL injuries are often classified as "sprains" and are graded for levels of severity. A grade 1 sprain indicates mild damage or slightly stretched, but it still has capacity to stabilize the knee joint. A grade 2 sprain is described as stretching the ligament to the point where it becomes loose, and it is often referred to as a partial ligament tear. A grade 3 sprain is often referred to as a complete ligament tear that destabilizes the knee joint.

Common MCL/LCL Therapeutic Modalities. Initial treatment for MCL and LCL injury is designed to reduce swelling, pain, and inflammation and includes cyrotherapy, elevation, NSAIDs, mild analgesics, and compressive or hinged bracing. Conservative management may include refraining from sports activity for 6-12 weeks with further evaluation. Surgical treatment may include primary repair or the use of a graft.

Nursing Consideration for All Knee Trauma and Soft Tissue Injuries

Nursing Diagnoses. Nursing diagnoses for this condition are expanded upon in the Appendix.

- Diversional activity, deficient.
- Infection, risk for.
- Knowledge deficit, managing care.
- Mobility, impaired.
- Pain, acute.
- Pain, chronic.
- Self-care deficit: bathing/hygiene, dressing/grooming, feeding, toileting.
- Self-health management, ineffective.

Interventions. Specific issues related to nursing management of the patient with trauma and soft tissue injuries of the knee are largely dependent on the interventions and course of treatment. Patient teaching should include discussion and evaluation of patient understanding on topics related to common therapeutic modalities: pain medications, NSAIDs, cold therapy, rest, compression, bracing, avoidance of specific activity, and other conservative treatments. Rehabilitation treatment plans are tailored to include various muscle strengthening and ROM exercises, the use of brace support and assistive devices, and weight-bearing status. Effective rehabilitation requires routine communication with all members of the health care team. Expectations regarding the return of knee function and ROM should be clearly defined, and progress should be reported and communicated to the physician on a routine basis.

Surgical intervention warrants additional, more detailed, patient-specific instructions related to the indicated surgical procedure and should include directions related to postoperative management that prevent or minimize surgical complications. Patients recovering from knee surgery should be taught to recognize untoward events and communicate with their physician expeditiously if they exhibit signs and symptoms of infection, experience VTE, are unable to flex or extend the knee, have excessive bleeding, or experience pain that is unrelieved by pain medication. Although complication rates of knee arthroscopy surgery are relatively low, prevention of infection is a main concern and requires preoperative risk assessment, special consideration, and appropriate preventive strategies. The postoperative infection rate for arthroscopic knee procedures is reported at below 0.2%; this low rate is attributed to the surgical approach, lavage, and short duration of surgery (Marmor, Farman, & Lortat-Jacob, 2009). Nursing care strategies to prevent infection include attention to other potential infective sources, frequent handwashing, prophylactic antibiotic coverage, wound care monitoring, observation, and patient and family teaching.

Pediatric Knee Conditions

Discoid Lateral Meniscus

Overview. Discoid lateral meniscus is an intra-articular knee lesion in children and describes the cartilage pad formed in a disc shape rather than the normal c-shape found in most individuals. Discoid lateral meniscus can be classified as Type I (complete), Type II (incomplete), or Type III (Wrisberg variant), and has an incidence estimated to be 1% to 3% in the pediatric population (Hart et al., 2008). Initially, discoid lateral meniscus was believed to be a failure of the embryological degeneration of the center of the meniscus, but it may simply represent a congenital anomaly. There is also a genetic or familial factor and a greater overall incidence in Asian populations, with up to 17% of patients from Korean and Japanese descent (Hart et al., 2008).

Assessment, History, and Physical Exam. Some patients with discoid lateral meniscus may be asymptomatic, but the thickening irregularity is more prone to tear as the child develops. Children between ages 5 and 10 often exhibit the classic findings: joint line tenderness, popping, effusion, and decreased ROM. It also is referred to as the "snapping knee syndrome." In children with stable discoid lateral menisci, symptoms often present when an associated tear is present. Signs and symptoms of acute meniscal tear often include pain, swelling, catching, locking, difficulty with weight-bearing, and limited motion.

Diagnostic Tests. Plain radiographs (AP and lateral views) are often normal but may show subtle widening of the lateral joint space, with flattening and a tilt of the articular surface on the lateral femoral condyle. MRI is often a more definitive modality to confirm diagnosis of discoid lateral meniscus and may also reveal tears or other meniscal abnormalities. Some diagnosis of discoid lateral meniscus need to be confirmed through visualization with arthroscopy.

Common Therapeutic Modalities. Conservative treatment with NSAIDS, PT, and/or observation is indicated for asymptomatic discoid lateral menisci. In symptomatic patients with a stable, complete, or incomplete discoid menisci tear, meniscal repair, partial meniscectomy, or "saucerization" is the treatment of choice. These have shown satisfactory results.

Osteochondritis Dissecans

Overview. Osteochondritis dissecans (OCD) is a condition of unclear etiology in which bone and overlying articular cartilage separate from the medial or lateral condyle. Theories of etiological factors include ischemia, repetitive microtrauma, genetics and familial predisposition, endocrine imbalance, epiphyseal abnormalities, accessory centers of ossification, growth disorders, and osteochondral fracture (Polousky, 2011). It is a relatively common cause of knee pain and dysfunction in children and adolescents.

Assessment, History, and Physical Exam. Most patients with a stable lesion complain of aching and activity-related knee pain localized to the anterior aspect of the knee. Children with unstable OCD lesions may walk with a slight antalgic gait, may have an effusion, and may experience crepitus during ROM. Pain is often associated in the lateral aspect of the medial femoral condyle and is more commonly associated in males (Polousky, 2011).

Diagnostic Tests. Most OCD lesions can be diagnosed on plain radiographs to include AP, lateral tunnel, and merchant views. MRI is currently the preferred modality to determine the size of the lesion and the status of cartilage in the subchondral bone.

Common Therapeutic Modalities. Nonoperative or conservative management is the treatment of choice for skeletally immature children and for stable-appearing joint lesions. Azar and Canale (2008) describe conservative management that includes modified activity, coupled with immobilization via casting, bracing, and other standard knee splinting. The patients should maintain partial weight-bearing in slight flexion during ambulation to minimize shear while preserving a limited amount of compression across the lesion. Operative treatment should be considered for patients approaching skeletal maturity with unstable and/or detached lesions, and when the lesion has not resolved with an appropriate period of nonoperative management. Arthroscopic drilling for a stable lesion with an intact articular surface promotes revascularization and healing. Surgical fixation is indicated for unstable lesions. Postoperative management may include non-weight-bearing activity for 4-6 weeks, full-range exercises, no bracing, and avoidance of progressive resistance exercise for the initial 6 weeks (Polousky, 2011).

Congenital Knee Dislocation

Overview. Congenital knee dislocation (CKD) is a very rare condition, with an incidence estimated at 1 per 100,000 live births (Cheng & Ko, 2010). CKD can be diagnosed in the prenatal period using ultrasound. The condition is not genetic, although congenital dislocation is seen frequently in association with other hereditary conditions (e.g., Larsen's syndrome). Multiple etiological theories involving intrauterine events include abnormal fetal position of hyperextension, congenital absence of the cruciate ligaments, fibrosis of quadriceps, and intrauterine ischemia causing compartment syndrome-like fibrosis. Those unfamiliar with the deformity may describe the extremity as having "the knee on backwards" because of the unstable excessive hyperextension.

Common Therapeutic Modalities. Nonoperative treatment includes serial manipulation and splinting in increasing flexion until the knee will flex more than 90 degrees, at which time a removable plastic splint can be used to maintain reduction while allowing some active motion. Forceful manipulation is contraindicated because of the risk of pressure damage to cartilaginous epiphyses or fracture-separation of the proximal tibial physis.

Surgical treatment, indicated for patients not responding to nonoperative means, has been advocated for infants as young as 6 months of age. The classic surgical treatment of CDK is reduction/flexion with a femoral shortening procedure. The procedure typically involves an extensive V-Y quadriceps tendon lengthening to gain flexion and hence reduction of the joint. Early and direct closed reduction within 24 hours of birth has shown positive outcomes (Cheng & Ko, 2010).

Osgood-Schlatter Disease

Overview. Osgood-Schlatter disease (OSD) (or tibial tubercle apophysitis) is a traction apophysitis of the tibial tubercle. It represents the most frequent occurrence of overgrowth injury and generally occurs in girls between the age of 8 and 13 years and in boys between 10 and 15 years (de Lucena, dos Santos Gomez, & Guerra, 2011). (See Chapter 11—Pediatrics.)

Assessment and Diagnostic Tests. Patients often present with a painful localized bump at the insertion point of the patella tendon into the tibial tubercle. Diagnosis is often made during physical assessment when tenderness, swelling, and pain is described with kneeling and other activities that involves quadriceps contraction. Pain on palpation of the tubercle, and with resisted knee extension, is almost always present. Radiography often shows a displaced ossicle of bone anterior to the tubercle within the tendinous insertion (Kodali et al., 2011).

Common Therapeutic Modalities. The patient's pain usually resolves when the ossicle fuses with the underlying tibia. Conservative treatment includes monitoring the activity level until the ossicle fuses. Depending on the severity of the pain, some or all impact athletic activity should be discontinued. Swimming or cycling may be allowed. Supportive bracing for 4-6 weeks may be necessary. NSAIDs therapy may be used during the acute phase (Kodali et al., 2011).

Nursing Consideration for All Pediatric Conditions of the Knee

Nursing Diagnoses. Nursing diagnoses for this condition are expanded upon in the Appendix.

- Development, risk for delayed.
- Diversional activity, deficient.
- Family processes, interrupted.
- Infection, risk for.
- Knowledge deficit, managing care.
- Mobility, impaired.
- Pain, acute.
- Pain, chronic.
- Self-care deficit: bathing/hygiene, dressing/grooming, feeding, toileting.
- Self-esteem: situational low, risk for.
- Self-health management, ineffective.

Interventions. Specific issues related to nursing management of the pediatric patient with knee conditions are largely dependent on the interventions and course of treatment. Patient teaching should include discussion and evaluation of patient and parent understanding on topics related to common therapeutic modalities: pain medications, NSAIDs, cold therapy, rest, compression, bracing, avoidance of specific activity, and other conservative treatments. Rehabilitation treatment plans are tailored to age-appropriate growth and development and include various muscle strengthening and ROM exercises, the use of brace support and assistive devices, and weight-bearing status. Successful recovery requires routine communication with all members of the health care team. Expectations regarding the return of knee function and ROM should be clearly defined, and progress should be reported and communicated to the physician on a routine basis.

Surgical intervention warrants additional, more detailed, patient-specific instructions related to the selected surgical procedure and should include directions related to postoperative management that prevents or minimizes surgical complications. Pediatric patients and their parents should be taught to recognize untoward events and communicate with their physician expeditiously if they exhibit signs and symptoms of infection, experience VTE, are unable to flex or extend the knee, have excessive bleeding, or experience pain that is unrelieved by pain medication. Although complication rates of pediatric knee surgery are relatively low, prevention of infection is a main concern and requires preoperative risk assessment, special consideration, and appropriate preventive strategies. Nursing care strategies to prevent infection include attention to other potential infective sources, frequent handwashing, prophylactic antibiotic coverage, wound care monitoring, observation, and patient and family teaching.

Summary

The knee is a complex joint. As such, it is subject to numerous associated conditions and injuries. Assessment of the knee involves a detailed history and physical examination, with emphasis on identifying a hierarchy of probable causes to direct the subsequent evaluation. Knowledge of onset of symptoms—whether it is an acute or chronic condition—and mechanism of injury can conserve valuable time. A focused assessment can lead to a proper diagnosis while maximizing patient comfort during examination. Additional diagnostic tests often include weight-bearing radiographs in multiple views, MRI, and ultrasound. Aspiration and other laboratory testing can provide more specific support.

Patient age is a significant factor when considering treatment options. Both surgical and nonsurgical options are available for many knee pathologies. Cryotherapy, NSAIDs, and compressive bracing can often reduce pain and swelling during the initial treatment phase. Many knee injuries require an exercise program or PT to maintain and restore motion and strength. Surgical interventions require pre- and postoperative management related to pain management, wound care, and mobility (see Table 22.2).

Table 22.2.
Management of the Patient with Knee Surgery

A. Interdisciplinary communication with health care team

1. MD and nurse to review plan of care and update report of progress
2. Pharmacists to track and monitor medication usage
3. Physical therapists to outline specific plan and provide progress reports

B. Patient and family teaching

1. Report to MD if any of the following occur:
   a. Signs and symptoms of infection
   b. Inability to flex or extend the knee
   c. Excessive bleeding
   d. Pain unrelieved by pain medications
2. Signs and symptoms of surgical site infection
   a. Fever
   b. Wound drainage
   c. Erythema
   d. Swelling
   e. Increased pain
3. DVT/PE prophylaxis
   a. Observe for signs and symptoms:
      (1) Calf pain
      (2) Severe lower extremity swelling
      (3) Chest pain
      (4) SOB
   b. Medications:
      (1) Aspirin
      (2) Coumadin
      (3) Low molecular weight heparin
   c. Laboratory monitoring as indicated
   d. Activity, rest, and exercise
4. Pain Management
   a. Encourage elevation and cold therapy-3 times a day to reduce swelling, bleeding, and bruising
   b. Analgesics, opioids, and NSAIDs
      (1) Explain dosage and frequency
      (2) Monitor for side effects – nausea, constipation, addiction, and potential bleeding
      (3) Encourage half hour before therapy
      (4) Observe pain levels and behavioral changes
5. Postsurgical follow-up
   a. Schedule timely appointments
   b. Discuss antibiotic prophylaxis (hardware/implant) for invasive procedures – dental/urological
6. Bracing and support
   a. Compression sleeve
   b. Splint/immobilizer
   c. Hinged brace
   d. Cane, crutch, or walker

C. Physical/Occupational Therapy

1. Review muscle strengthening and ROM exercises as ordered
2. Gait training with assistive devices (cane, crutches, or walker)
3. Promote return to ADLs
4. Facilitate continuous passive motion machines as indicated

References

Abbate, N. & Davis, J. (2007). The Knee. In National Association of Orthopaedic Nursing *Core Curriculum for Orthopaedic Nursing* (6th ed., pp. 555-575). Boston, MA: Pearson.

Azar, F. & Canale, T. (2008). Osteocondritis dessicans of the knee. In G. Cooper & J. Herrera (Eds.), *Manual of Musculoskeletal Medicine* (1st ed., p. 189). Philadelphia, PA: Lippincott, Williams and Wilkins, p. 189.

Benke, M. & Shaffer, B. (2009). Viscosupplementation treatment of arthritis pain. *Current Pain and Headache Reports*, 13(6), 440-446.

Berend, K. & Lombardi, A. (2007). Liberal indications for minimally invasive oxford unicondylar arthroplasty provide rapid functional recovery and pain relief. *Surgical Technology International 16*, 193-197.

Cahill, J. & Kosman, L. (2006). Total knee arthroplasty. In J. Cioppa-Mosca, J. Cahill, J. Cavanaugh, D. Corradi-Scalise, H. Rudnick, A. Wolff, & C. Young-Tucker (Eds.), *Postsurgical Rehabilitation Guidelines for the Orthopaedic Clinician*. (pp. 17-28). St. Louis, MO: Mosby.

Chen, C. (2007). Surgical treatment of posterior cruciate ligament injury. *Chang Gung Medical Journal*, 30(6), 480-491.

Cheng, C. & Ko, J. (2010). Early reduction for congenital dislocation of the knee within twenty-four hours of birth. *Chang Gung Medical Journal, 33*(3), 266-273.

Conklin, C. (2011). *Knee graphics and illustrations.* Hospital for Special Surgery, Digital Media.

Cooper, G. & Herrera, J. E. (2008). *Manual of Musculoskeletal Medicine.* Philadelphia, PA: Wolters Kluwer Lippincott Williams & Wilkins.

De Lucena, G., dos Santos Gomez, C. & Guerra, R. (2011). Prevalence and associated factors of Osgood-Schlatter syndrome in a population-based sample of Brazilian adolescents. *American Journal of Sports Medicine, 39*(2), 415-420.

Dettoni, F., Bonasia, D., Castoldi, F., Bruzzone, M., Blonna, D., & Rossi, R. (2010). High tibial osteotomy versus unicompartmental knee arthroplasty for medial compartment arthrosis of the knee: a review of the literature. *Iowa Orthopaedic Journal, 30*, 131-140.

Divine, J., Zazulak, B., & Hewett, T. (2007). Viscosupplementation for knee osteoarthritis: A systematic review. *Clinical Orthopaedics and Related Research, 455*, 113-122.

Flandry, F. & Hommel, G, (2011). Normal anatomy and biomechanics of the knee. *Sports Medicine and Arthroscopy Review, 19*(2), 82-92.

Franks, Jr., A. & Mor, A. (2006). Inflammatory arthritis of the knee. In N.W. Scott (Ed.), *Insall and Scott Surgery of the Knee* (4th ed.). Philadelphia, PA: Churchill Livingstone, pp. 734-737.

Haas, S., Manitta, M., & Burdick, P. (2006). Minimally invasive total knee arthroplasty: The mini-midvastus approach. *Clinical Orthopaedics and Related Research, 452*, pp.112-116.

Hart, E., Kalra, K., Grottkau, B., Albright, M., & Shannon, E. (2008). Discoid lateral meniscus in children. *Orthopaedic Nursing, 27*(7), 174-179.

Helfenstien, M. & Kuromoto, J. (2010). Anserine syndrome. *Brasilian Journal of Rheumatology, 50*(3), 313-327.

Huddleston, J. Maloney, W., Yun, W., Verzier, N., Hunt, D., & Herndon, J. (2009). Adverse events after TKA a national Medicare study. *Journal of Arthroplasty [Supplement 1], 24*(6), pp. 95-100.

Hungerford, M., Khanuja, H., & Hungerford, D. (2006). Non-operative treatment of knee arthritis. In N. Scott (Ed.), *Surgery of the Knee* (4th ed., pp. 329-349). Philadelphia, PA: Churchill Livingstone.

Johansson, N. & Pellicci, P. (2006). Knee Pain. In S. Paget, A. Gibofsky, J. Bearry, & T. Sculco (Eds.) *Hospital for Special Surgery Manual of Rheumatology and Outpatient Orthopedic Disorders: Diagnosis and Therapy* (5th ed.), pp. 169-173. Philadelphia, PA: Lippincott Williams & Wilkins.

Kodali, P., Islam, A., & Andrish, J. (2011). Anterior knee pain in the young athlete diagnosis and treatment. *Sports Medicine Arthroscopy Review, 19*(1), 27-33.

Leone, J. & Hanssen, A. (2006). Osteotomy about the knee: American perspective. In N. Scott (Ed.), *Surgery of the Knee* (4th ed.). Philadelphia, PA: Churchill Livingstone.

Lonner, J. H. (2010). Patellofemoral arthroplasty. *Instructional Course Lectures, 59*, 67-84.

Luyten, F., Westhovens, R., & Taelman (2006). Arthritis of the knee: Diagnosis and management. In J. Bellmans, J. Victor & M. Ries (Eds.) *Total Knee Arthroplasty: A Guide to Better Performance.* (pp. 3-13). New York, NY: Springer.

MacDonald, J., Agaral, S., Lorei, M., Johanson N., & Freiberg, A. (2006). Knee arthrodesis. *Journal American Academy of Orthopaedic Surgeons 14*(30), 154-163.

Marmor, S., Farman, T., & Lortat-Jacob, A. (2009). Joint infection after knee arthroscopy: *Medicolegal aspects. Orthopaedics & Traumatology: Surgery & Research, 95*(4), 278-283.

McGarry, J. & Daruwalla, Z. (2010), The efficacy, accuracy and complications of corticoid injections of the knee joint. *Knee Surgery Sports Traumatology and Arthroscopy*, Published online ahead of print. doi:10.1007/s00167-010-1380-I

O'Keefe, S., Hogan, B., Eustace, S., & Kavanagh, E. (2009). Overuse injuries of the knee. *Magnetic Resonance Imaging Clinic of North America 17*(4), 725-39.

Paget, S., Gibofsky, A., Bearry, J., & Sculco, T. (2006). *Hospital for Special Surgery Manual of Rheumatology and Outpatient Orthopedic Disorders: Diagnosis and Therapy* (5th ed.). Philadelphia, PA: Lippincott Williams & Wilkins.

Parker, R. (2011). Evidence-Based Practice: Caring for a patient undergoing total knee arthroplasty. *Orthopaedic Nursing, 30*(1), 4-8.

Polousky, J. (2011). Juvenile ostechodritis dissecans. *Sports Medicine Arthroscopic Review, 19*(1), 56-63.

Rutland, M., O'Connell, D., Brismee, J., Sizer, P., Apte, G., & O'Connell, J. (2010). Clinical commentary: Evidence-supported rehabilitation of patellar tendinopathy. *North American Journal of Sports Physical Therapy, 5*(3), 166-178.

Schroer, W., Diesfeld, P., Reedy, M., & LeMarr, A. (2008). Mini-subvastus approach for total knee Arthroplasty. *Journal of Arthroplasty, 23*(1), 19-25.

Schub, D. & Saluan, P. (2011). Anterior cruciate ligament injuries in the young athlete: Evaluation and treatment. *Sports Medicine Arthroscopy Review, 19*(1), 34-43.

Sculco, T. (2011). Knee radiographs. Hospital for Special Surgery.

Talmo, C., Robbins, C., & Bono, J. (2010). Total joint replacement in the elderly patient. *Clinics of Geriatric Medicine 26*(3), 517-529.

Chapter 23
The Foot & Ankle

Kate Hill, RN & Marianne K. Ostrow, RN, MSN, ONC

Objectives

- List the most common foot and ankle injuries.
- Name five key components in assessing foot and ankle injuries.
- Identify the nonsurgical treatment for foot and ankle conditions.
- Discuss the surgical treatment related to foot and ankle pathologies.
- Select the nursing interventions for patients with foot and ankle injuries.
- Identify home care needs for the patient with foot and ankle problems.

The foot and ankle together make up one of the most complex structures of the human skeleton and provide two main functions: weight-bearing and propulsion. Because of the complexity and importance of the structure, it is susceptible to a wide range of acute and chronic afflictions. Throughout a lifetime, most people will experience some kind of problem with a toe, foot, or ankle. Normal body movements do not cause these problems; however, it is not surprising that symptoms can develop from everyday wear and tear, overuse, or poor footwear choices. Toe, foot, or ankle problems can also occur from trauma, the natural process of aging, disease, or congenital disorder. Whatever the cause, normal function can be disrupted.

A stable foot and ankle structure supports a person's full body weight in motion. The goal of treatment is to restore the foot and or ankle to the fullest function possible, thereby restoring quality of life and returning the individual to desired activities.

Ankle Sprains

Overview

Ankle sprains usually occur when the foot is planter flexed, adducted, and inverted. They account for nearly one in 10 emergency room visits. Additionally, nearly half of all athletic injuries consist of ankle sprains (Lotke, 2008). Some 5 million ankle injuries occur annually in the United States, with ankle sprains accounting for 40% of sports injuries (Smalls, 2009).

An ankle sprain is an injury to the ligaments that hold the bones of the ankle joint together and provide stability. These ligaments prevent excessive twisting or turning of the ankle. Ankle ligaments can stretch; however, there is a limit. The sprain occurs as ligaments stretch beyond their capabilities. In severe sprains, the ligaments can be actually torn. As the fibers of the ligament tear, an inflammatory response is initiated that causes pain and swelling. Depending on the extent of the tear, bleeding may occur and stability of the joint may be compromised. Ankle sprains are divided into 3 grades (see Table 23.1).

Lateral ankle sprains are the most common injury in sports, especially in cross county running, dance, and ballet. Ankle sprains account for 45% of all injuries in basketball and up to 31% in soccer (Coughlin, Mann, & Salzman, 2007). The incidence of ankle sprains decreases with age. The same ligamentous injury in a young person can often result in a fracture in an older person. Repetitive ankle sprains can lead to ankle instability, osteochondral injuries, or early osteoarthritis.

Prevention of ankle sprains involves five main components: strength conditioning, coordination, proprioception, stretching, and external support (Delee, Drez, & Miller, 2010). Taping of the ankle is the most widely used prophylactic method for preventing ankle sprains.

Assessment

A thorough history should be taken from the patient to determine if this is a chronic problem. Ask where, when, and how the injury occurred. Ankle sprain assessment should include observation of the ankle for swelling, discoloration, and deformity; compare both ankles. Obtain the level of pain, stability, mobility, ability to bear

Table 23.1. Ankle Sprain Classifications

Grading	Definition	Signs & Symptoms	Treatment
One	Partial tear of ligament	1. Minimal pain 2. No instability 3. Early symptom resolution 4. Mild tenderness and swelling 5. Ecchymosis mild to moderate	1. RICE (Rest, Ice, Compression, Elevation) 2. Use joint as normally as possible 3. Weight bearing as tolerated (WBAT)
Two	Incomplete tear of a ligament, with moderate functional impairment	1. Tenderness over involved structure 2. Some loss of motion and function 3. Pain with weight bearing	1. RICE 2. Support/splint 3. Gentle ROM 4. WBAT. May need assistive device
Three	Complete ligament rupture	1. Severe pain initially 2. Loss of function and motion, inability to bear weight 3. Swelling 4. Ecchymosis 5. Often associated with bony injury	1. RICE 2. Immobilize 3. Possible surgery 4. Protected weight bearing

From Core Curriculum for Orthopaedic Nursing (6th Ed., p. 581), by the National Association of Orthopaedic Nurses (NAON), 2007, Boston, MA: Pearson. Reproduced with permission.

Table 23.2. Imaging Studies of the Foot and Ankle		
Test	**Technique**	**Purpose**
X-ray radiographs	A high electromagnetic wave that penetrates solid matter and projects in onto film. 1. Common views of the ankle are: anterior-posterior, lateral, and mortise. 2. Common views of the foot are: anterior-posterior, lateral, and oblique. Usually done weight bearing.	1. Assesses for fractures, tumors, arthritis and joint integrity. 2. May involve stress views to asses ankle ligaments.
CAT/CT scan (computerized axial topography)	Transverse planes of tissue are swept by a pinpoint radiographic beam and then reproduced by computer analysis.	1. Helps diagnose fractures difficult to assess or evaluate with traditional x-ray. 2. Assists with assessment of soft tissue tumors or injury.
MRI (magnetic resonance imaging)	A magnetic field and radio waves are used to delineate the hydrogen density of tissues in the body. The image differentiates the differing hydrogen contents among tissue.	1. Assesses high water content tissues such as ligament, tendons, and bone marrow (osteomyelitis, tumor, etc.). 2. Able to detect avascular necrosis earlier than traditional x-rays.
Arthogram	X-ray/CT of a joint after injection of a radio-opaque dye into the joint space.	1. Assesses joint integrity by visualizing the dye-filled joint space. 2. Is invasive. 3. May result in hypersensitivity reaction.
Bone scan	A radioisotope is injected into the blood and concentrated in areas of increased bone activity. A gamma camera picks up the emitting rays and identifies "hot spots" that may indicate abnormalities.	1. Detects osteoblastic changes only (stress fracture, infection, arthritis, certain cancers). 2. Results are usually verified by additional testing.

From Core Curriculum for Orthopaedic Nursing (6th Ed., p. 580), by the National Association of Orthopaedic Nurses (NAON), 2007, Boston, MA: Pearson. Reproduced with permission.

weight, and any changes in sensation. If possible, observe gait pattern. Assess foot and ankle range of motion (ROM). Palpate the three ankle ligaments (the anterior talofibular ligament [ATFL], the posterior talofibular ligament [PTFL], and the calcaneofibular ligament [CFL]), the base of the 5th metatarsal, and the proximal fibula.

The anterior drawer test is performed to assess the stability of the ligaments. The anterior drawer test is performed to evaluate the integrity of the ATFL. Have the patient sit with the knee flexed on the end of the exam table with the foot dangling, stabilize the tibia with one hand and try to anteriorly push the foot forward grasping the heel with the other hand. The test is done with the ankle in both neutral and plantar flexion positions (Delee et al., 2010). To evaluate the CFL, the test is performed with the ankle in dorsiflexion. A positive test will produce pain and demonstrate instability of these ligaments. A skin dimple will appear in the anterolateral joint from suction.

The talar tilt test is also performed while sitting. Support the lower leg with one hand and grasp the heel with the other hand and an inversion force is applied to produce talar tilt. As with the anterior drawer test, the ankle is in neutral and plantar positions for the ATFL and in dorsiflexion for the CFL. Both tests are performed on the contralateral side as well for comparison. These may not be tolerated in the acute phase of injury. Radiographs are obtained to assess for fractures and joint integrity.

The Ottawa Ankle Rules are useful criteria to determine the necessity of obtaining radiographs. Based on the Ottawa criteria, radiographs are required only for patients with tenderness at the posterior edge or the tip of the medial or lateral malleolus, inability to bear weight initially or at presentation (four steps in the emergency room), or pain at the base of the fifth metatarsal (Lotke, 2008).

Standard x-rays of the ankle include weight-bearing anteroposterior (AP), mortise, and lateral views. If a grade III or chronic injury is suspected, the x-rays may involve stress views to assess ankle stability. Magnetic resonance imaging (MRI) helps to diagnose soft tissue injuries and is not usually done in the acute phase of injury. (See Table 23.2.)

Common Therapeutic Modalities

Treatment of a grade 1 ankle sprain is initially R.I.C.E. (rest, ice, compression, and elevation), followed by gentle stretching and protected weight-bearing as inflammation subsides. Home exercises include ROM stretching, strengthening, and proprioceptive training. Grade 2 and 3 sprains are treated with R.I.C.E., along with a short-leg cast or boot for 6-8 weeks to allow for healing. Weight-bearing is as tolerated. Early stretching and motion can be done to prevent excessive stiffness. Patients in both categories can take non-steroidal anti-inflammatory drugs (NSAIDs) for pain control if there are no contraindications. Physical therapy is often added for grade 2 and 3 sprains to restore function and decrease risk for subsequent re-injury following the sprain or prolonged immobilization.

Surgery is indicated when the patient has failed a well-designed nonoperative treatment plan (Coughlin et al., 2007). Treatment for the patient with chronic ankle instability may be nonsurgical or surgical, depending on several factors, including the age and activity level of the patient, the relative severity of the ankle instability, and the presence of any concomitant injuries or co-morbidities (Pinzur, 2008).

Nursing Considerations

Nursing Diagnoses. Nursing diagnoses for this condition are expanded upon in the Appendix.

- Activity intolerance.
- Mobility: physical, impaired.
- Pain, acute or chronic (as in sinus tarsi syndrome).

Interventions. External support can be in the form of various ankle braces, high top shoes, orthotics, or taping of the ankle joint. Cold therapy, along with relative rest, compression, and elevation are key in the treatment of ankle sprains. Activity restrictions are often self-imposed, given the degree of discomfort; however, it is important to maintain ankle joint mobility.

Achilles Tendinitis

Overview

The Achilles (or calcaneal) tendon connects the large calf muscles (gastrocnemius and soleus) to the heel (calcaneus) and is responsible for the push-off phase of the gait cycle in walking and running. Achilles tendinitis is defined as an inflammation of the tendon or paratenon from repetitive overuse or extension of the Achilles tendon, or tendinosis (non-inflammatory) with atrophic degeneration of the tendon, or both. Tendinitis is classified as insertional or noninsertional. It commonly occurs in athletes, especially runners, and is mostly associated with adults ages 20-30.

Risk factors that predispose someone to Achilles tendinitis include weak or tight gastrocnemius or soleus muscles, decreased ankle mobility, decreased vascularity, excessive foot pronation, and normal aging. Extrinsic factors include sudden increases in training intensity (such as distance, speed, and inclines), less recovery time between workouts, and improper footwear (Delee et al., 2010). Complications that can occur include tendon thickening and chronic tendon rupture.

Some preventive strategies to decrease risk of tendinitis include stretching before exercising, warming up the Achilles tendon before running, wearing proper shoes for the activity being done, using inserts to correct pronation, and icing for 10-15 minutes after running.

Assessment

A thorough history and physical examination are key to the accurate assessment of Achilles tendinitis. Complaints of a gradual onset of pain over a few days, especially at the beginning of activity, are noted, but this pain often dissipates after warm-up and rest. There may be reports of a recent change in training schedule. The physical exam will reveal tenderness with palpation usually at the attachment of the Achilles tendon to the calcaneus (insertional) or 4cm above the heel (noninsertional). Some localized soft tissue swelling and crepitus may be present.

In chronic tendinitis, the pain will occur over weeks or months, and patients will complain of pain throughout the activity, especially with hills or steps. They may give a history of morning and start-up pain, as well as stiffness and inability to run without pain. Physical examinations may show tendon thickening and tenderness on palpation.

Diagnostic tests are not usually necessary. Routine AP and lateral radiographs of the foot should be done to rule out any bony problems such as Haglund's deformity or calcification in the Achilles tendon. An MRI is useful to evaluate for partial or complete rupture. (See Table 23.2.)

Common Therapeutic Modalities

Noninvasive modalities are the mainstay of Achilles tendinitis treatment, especially rest and anti-inflammatory medication. Activity modification and cross training are suggested, using the pain as a guide to indicate the need to decrease running or sporting activity. Avoidance of uneven surfaces and inclines, along with a decrease in pace, is suggested in the early portion of rehabilitation. Proper stretching prior to activity is crucial, especially focusing on the Achilles, as well as the gastrocnemius and soleus muscles. Cold therapy is extremely important after activity to decrease pain and inflammation, with a goal of reducing soft tissue swelling and internal bleeding.

Another modality utilized in the treatment of chronic noninsertional Achilles tendinitis is application of topical glyceryl trinitrate (GTN) 1.25mg/24hours to the involved portion of the tendon. This is found to be effective in reducing Achilles tendon tenderness and pain (Paoloni & Murrell, 2007). The mechanism of action for GTN is thought to be related to the fibroblastic stimulation of collagen and increased blood supply to the region from local vaso-dilation to help clear local inflammatory substances (Paolini, 2007). GTN has both an analgesic and healing effect on the tendon, and the most common side effect reported is headaches.

Heel lifts or wedges can be useful in the acute phase to take the stress off the tendon. Inserts or orthotics may be beneficial to correct any pronation, and appropriate shoes for the activity need to be worn.

Steroid injections are used infrequently because of the possibility of tendon rupture. Physical therapy may provide relief through ultrasound or iontophoresis incorporating steroids to decrease inflammation. Eccentric strengthening/stretching programs can be included into the patient's therapy treatment plan (Andres & Murrell, 2008). The goal of eccentric strengthening is to produce less force than the load placed on the muscle. Eccentric muscle-tendon load contracts the muscle while being lengthened at the same time. An example of this type of exercise is eccentric heel raises. The exercise is performed by positioning the foot on a step so that the ball of the foot is on the step and the heel is hanging off. Rise up on tip-toe on the uninjured leg and slowly lower until a stretch is felt on the back of the leg. Repeat three sets of 15 repetitions twice daily.

Stretching exercises are used to increase ROM and flexibility at the ankle joint. An example of this is the gastroc and soleus stretches. The gastroc stretch is performed by placing both hands on the wall keeping back leg straight, with the heel on the floor and turned slightly outward, lean into the wall until a stretch is felt in the calf. The soleus stretch is done with both knees bent and the involved foot back, gently lean into the wall until the stretch is felt in the lower calf.

The Graston technique is a relatively new technique used in therapy to promote healing and improve function. This technique requires stainless steel instruments for cross-fiber massage and soft tissue mobilization. This initiates the inflammatory cascade to start the healing process by increasing fibroblast formation (DeLuccio, 2006).

If symptoms are severe enough, immobilization for 7-10 days may be warranted to rest the tendon. Extracorporeal shock wave therapy, sclerosing therapy, and growth factors are modalities that can be utilized in the treatment of chronic Achilles tendinopathy. These are treatment options for people who failed conventional conservative treatment prior to surgical intervention. More long-term clinical studies need to be performed to advocate the overall efficacy with some of these treatment options (Andres & Murrell, 2008). The use of platelet-rich plasma therapy containing growth factors, which promote tissue healing and repair, has shown promising results in treating chronic Achilles tendinopathy (Diehl, 2011).

Surgery is usually unnecessary unless symptoms persist for 3-6 months and should only be considered after exhausting all nonoperative treatment options (Irwin, 2010).

Nursing Considerations

Nursing Diagnoses. Nursing diagnoses for this condition are expanded upon in the Appendix.

- Diversional activity, deficient.
- Knowledge deficit.
- Pain, acute or chronic.

Interventions. Preventing Achilles tendinitis through patient education and support is important. The need for proper interval training and appropriate footwear should be emphasized, and the routine practice of stretching and icing should be encouraged. If pain occurs, modified activities and incorporation of various therapeutic modalities are needed. If symptoms persist, patients should be encouraged to seek medical help.

Achilles Tendon Rupture

Overview

Achilles tendon rupture is the disruption of the fibers within the tendon and can be classified as partial or complete. The Achilles tendon can rupture from degeneration of the tendon (chronic) or an acute sudden event usually associated from pushing off the toes and forceful dorsiflexion of the foot. The Achilles tendon ruptures because the rapid loading force applied to the area is greater than the elasticity of the tendon.

As the body ages, tendons (like other tissues in the body) become less flexible and more rigid, thus becoming more susceptible to injury. Achilles tendon ruptures occur across the life span from the second to the eighth decades, with a peak incidence between the third and fifth decades (Coughlin et al., 2007). Males outnumber females 5:1 in tendon rupture occurrence, and most susceptible are recreational athletes who normally lead relatively sedentary lifestyles. Rupture of the left Achilles is more common because of the higher prevalence of right hand dominance, thus push-off with the left foot (Cretnik, Kosir, & Kosanovic, 2010).

Risk factors associated with Achilles tendon rupture include prior history of Achilles tendinitis, previous cortisone injections in the area, and systemic inflammatory arthritis (such as gout or rheumatoid arthritis). The use of fluoroquinolone antibiotics has also been implicated.

Complications include re-ruptures of the tendon (with a higher incidence in cases of nonoperative treatment), loss of power and strength, and an abnormally long tendon that decreases functionality.

Assessment

History often shows a sudden sharp pain in the back of the leg; there may have been an audible crack or pop associated with this (Coughlin et al., 2007). Patients will demonstrate weakened plantar flexion, difficulty walking, and an inability to stand on tiptoe.

On physical examination, a palpable gap at the rupture site may be felt. There may be swelling and ecchymosis in the ankle region or heel. If there is complete rupture, a positive Thompson's test will occur. The Thompson's test (or calf squeeze) is done with the patient lying prone on the table with the feet over the edge of the table. The examiner's thumb and forefingers squeeze the calf muscles in the middle third of the calf just below the widest area, causing the foot to flex. A positive test, indicating a rupture, is when there is no foot movement. Standard radiographs are usually not helpful in determining Achilles tendon rupture. MRI and ultrasound are the recommended diagnostic tools to evaluate the extent and location of injury, especially with large amounts of soft tissue swelling present. (See Table 23.2.)

Common Therapeutic Modalities

Partial or complete Achilles tendon ruptures can be treated conservatively or surgically. Nonsurgical treatment is casting or using a hinged walking boot. The cast or boot is applied with the foot and ankle in gravity equinus. The rationale for this conservative care is that placing the foot in dorsiflexion brings the ends of the tendon into apposition to reduce the gap. Generally, 8 weeks of cast immobilization is followed by a custom-molded brace (in more sedentary patients or those with comorbidities), a cam walker, or stirrup brace for another 4 weeks. There is controversy in the literature on the length and duration of the casting (Coughlin et al., 2007), as well as on the use and type of bracing. Heel lifts may be utilized in the shoe to remove undue tension on the tendon. The patient will perform ROM exercises, followed by active exercises for several weeks after injury.

Operative treatment is usually indicated for acute complete rupture, large partial rupture, or re-ruptures of the tendon. Surgery is recommended for athletes and more active persons, as a lower re-rupture rate has been demonstrated (Coughlin et al., 2007). Immobilization is for several weeks after surgery, with the goal of getting the foot into a neutral position. Once the cast is removed, ROM exercises are started followed by stretching and strengthening exercises.

Nursing Considerations

Nursing Diagnoses. Nursing diagnoses for this condition are expanded upon in the Appendix.

- Knowledge deficit.
- Mobility: physical, impaired.
- Pain, acute or chronic.

Interventions. Patient education should be focused on safe ambulation with an assistive device, maintaining non-weight-bearing status. The patient should be able to demonstrate cast care and appropriately perform a home exercise program. Many patients will require formal physical therapy in conjunction with their home program.

Fractures

Overview

A fracture is, by definition, a break in the continuity of the bone, which occurs when the force or impact on the bone is greater than the bone can withstand. Approximately 10% of all fractures occur in the foot. The fractured ankle is the most common intra-articular fracture of a weight-bearing joint (Coughlin et al., 2007). These fractures are most often associated with trauma and frequently have a soft tissue component. A fracture can also occur as the result of overuse (stress fracture) or weakening of the bone due to a systemic disease such as osteoporosis or diabetes.

Fracture complications include vascular injury; damage to surrounding tissue, nerves, or skin; compartment syndrome; infection; malunion or nonunion; or post traumatic arthritis. The incidence of ankle fractures has increased since 1950, and there has been an increasing trend toward operative intervention, although there is sound evidence that stable fractures can successfully be treated nonoperatively (Pakarinen, Flinkila, Ohtonen, & Ristiniemi, 2011).

The most common types of fractures in the foot and ankle are those in the distal fibula (called a lateral malleolus fracture) and the distal tibia (called a medial malleolus fracture) (Reddy & Okereke, 2008). When both bones of the ankle are involved, it is a bimalleolar fracture. A trimalleolar fracture is a fracture of the lateral malleolus, and the medial and posterior malleoli of the tibia. When an ankle fracture extends into the tibiotalor joint, it is known as a pilon fracture.

"Fractures or dislocations of the talus are often associated with disruption in the blood supply and thus pose potential problems for the healing and integrity of the talus" (Coughlin et al., 2007). Calcaneal fractures are often associated with axial loading, such as occurs after falling from a height.

In the metatarsals, the most commonly fractured is the fifth metatarsal. A Jones fracture is a fracture at the metaphyseal-diaphyseal junction in the region of or just distal to the articulation between the fourth and fifth metatarsals. The Jones fracture is associated with a high incidence of non union. Another fracture in the metatarsals, which is at high risk for poor outcomes, is the Lisfranc fracture dislocation, which interrupts the arch and therefore the stability of the tarsometatarsal joint.

Fracture of the phalanges are usually simple fractures and easily treated, sometimes as simply as taping toes together unless open, significantly displaced, or crushed. Bleeding under the nail should raise suspicion of an open fracture of the phalanx.

A final type of fracture to be aware of in the foot and ankle is the stress fracture. Stress fractures occur most often as a result of overuse. Findings on x-ray are often subtle, and fracture lines may not be visible initially on plain x-rays. The elderly may be at higher risk because of decreased strength and soft tissue elasticity. While the elderly are more susceptible to stress fractures, however, the young and active are at risk due to the nature of their activities. Specifically, groups such as military recruits, athletes involved in high-impact sports, dancers, and women with hormonal imbalances are more at risk. Patients with impaired mobility may require special considerations to avoid complications such DVT, PE, or pneumonia.

Assessment

A complete history is necessary to assess the nature of the fracture. When, where, and how the fracture occurred all are factored into the treatment. On physical exam, the patient often has pain, swelling, deformity, ecchymosis, and guarding. The patient's weight-bearing ability may be affected. Observation of skin integrity should include assessment for fracture blisters, which are commonly seen with lower extremity fractures. Careful assessment must be made of the neurovascular status.

Most fractures are diagnosed by radiographic evaluation utilizing three views, most commonly the AP, lateral, and mortise (an oblique view with the foot internally rotated). Despite the importance of weight-bearing x-rays, this is the one instance where weight-bearing films should not be obtained.

In the case of stress fractures, the patient may report a gradual onset of pain and a history of overuse. The diagnosis of stress fractures may require an MRI or bone scan, especially in areas at higher risk for nonunion, such as the navicular, the talar neck, or the proximal fifth metatarsal. (See Table 23.2.) MRI is also useful in persons who need to return to early activity or who are not progressing as expected. If symptoms are mild, conservative treatment with repeat x-rays 10-14 days later could be done to assess for bone callous formation (Pinzur, 2008).

Common Therapeutic Modalities

Given that the foot and ankle support the body's entire weight, most fractures in this area are treated with some kind of immobilization or support. Treatment for all fractures starts with resting the bone, usually 6-8 weeks (depending on location). Taping, splinting, bracing, or special fracture shoes are all employed, depending on the fracture location. For those fractures that require non-weight-bearing, crutches or knee walkers are employed. Some patients need to use a wheelchair if there are extenuating circumstances.

Surgical intervention may be necessary for intra-articular, open, comminuted, or displaced fractures. Surgical treatment can utilize internal fixation, such as plates, screws or nails, or external fixation. After surgical intervention, most patients will initially be non-weight-bearing. Surgery is considered when an open procedure will provide superior results to closed treatment (Coughlin et al., 2007).

Nursing Considerations

Nursing Diagnoses. Nursing diagnoses for this condition are expanded upon in the Appendix.

- Falls, risk for.
- Infection, risk for.
- Mobility: physical, impaired.
- Pain, acute.
- Skin integrity, risk for impaired.

Interventions. Once a fracture has occurred, it is important to keep the patient safe from further injury, which may be caused by impaired mobility or even by the immobilization device itself, as in skin breakdown. Awareness of the risk of falls, proper crutch or kneewalker use, potential for infection, and skin integrity are all aspects of patient teaching. Cast care must be taught from the start, showing the patient what to look for, what sensations to be aware of, and when to call the health care provider. If an external fixation device has been employed, pin care must be taught per protocol.

Some patients may require home care for dressing changes, pin care, or ADL assistance. Home health aides, physical therapists, or visiting nurses may provide services. Some patients may even require a short-term stay in a rehabilitation facility before returning home.

Plantar Fasciitis

Overview

Heel pain affects millions of people annually and is one of the most frustrating problems for both the patient and the orthopaedic care provider. The most common cause of heel pain is proximal plantar fasciitis (Pinzur, 2008).

Plantar fasciitis is degeneration and inflammation of the plantar fascia and periosteum at the fascial insertion site of the calcaneus. It may be caused by overuse (such as running or jumping activities) and/or overloading due to obesity or sudden weight gain. It can also be caused by mechanical factors such as flat foot deformity (pes planus), a tight gastrosoleal complex, or a very high arch (pes cavus). The typical patient is between ages 40 and 70, is affected bilaterally approximately 8-13% of the time, has a history of recent weight gain, or may report a recent change in activity level. Males and females are generally affected equally (Craig, 1999). Resolution of symptoms occurs in the majority of patients within 10 months; however, about 10% of people go on to have chronic pain (DiGiovanni et al., 2006).

The plantar fascia is a thick band of tissue (like ligament) that runs from the toes to the heel under the skin and acts as a support to the longitudinal arch. Plantar fasciitis is caused by repetitive trauma, producing micro-trauma to the plantar fascia; this leads to the body's attempted repair of the area and chronic inflammation. Heel pad atrophy occurs naturally with aging from loss of collagen and elastin, or from poorly placed steroid injections, thus increasing an individual's risk for developing plantar fasciitis.

Assessment

Obtain a thorough history and physical examination. The patient will complain of pain, typically at the plantar medial tuberosity of the calcaneus. It is often worse first thing in the morning, or upon taking the first few steps or after rest, known as "start-up pain." Pain will usually improve throughout the day but worsens by nighttime. Patients will have a difficult time walking barefoot, especially on hard surfaces.

Pain is described as sharp and burning. The patient may complain of a throbbing pain that radiates into the arch or forefoot. Physical examination reveals point tenderness to palpation of the plantar fascia at its origin on the plantar medial turbercle of the calcaneal tuberosity (League, 2008). Pain may be reproduced with passive dorsiflexion of the toes or foot. The Achilles tendon should be evaluated for any tightness, which can contribute to heel pain by overloading the foot. Inspect for any heel pad atrophy, and perform a squeeze test on the tuberosity and calcaneal walls to rule out a calcaneal stress fracture.

Standing full weight-bearing radiographs of the heel and foot should be taken. AP and lateral views will provide information about the biomechanics or position of the foot, such as normal, planus, or cavus deformity. Small calcaneal spurs may be seen in approximately 50% of patients, but this is not the cause of their pain (Coughlin et al., 2007). An MRI or bone scan may be ordered to rule out a calcaneal stress fracture or plantar fascial tear. (See Table 23.2.)

Common Therapeutic Modalities

The majority of patients with plantar fasciitis will improve with nonoperative treatment. This begins with patient education about the pathology of the disease process, which allows them to understand the chronic nature of this problem. Initial options for conservative care include NSAIDs with proper precautions; stretching exercises for the plantar fascia, gastrocnemius, and soleus; heel pad or cup; night splint; shoe modification; activity modification; weight reduction; ice and/or heat; and rest. If pain continues, an orthosis, physical therapy utilizing ultrasound, phonophoresis or iontophoresis, steroid injection, or immobilization can be incorporated into the treatment plan.

Almost all patients with plantar fasciitis will respond to a combination of the conservative modalities if compliant with the treatment plan. Complete resolution of pain may take several months to a year. Orthotripsy or extracorporeal shockwave therapy (ESWT) may be used if the pain is unresponsive to nonoperative management prior to surgery. ESWT administers high-pressure sound waves to injured tissue to provide pain relief (Ibrahim, Donatelli, Schmitz, Hellman, & Buxbaum, 2010). Surgery is rarely required unless conservative care for more than a year has failed. If required, surgery can be done open or endoscopically, and both have potential complications of posterior tibial nerve injury, arch collapse, or persistent pain (League, 2008).

Nursing Considerations

Nursing Diagnoses. Nursing diagnoses for this condition are expanded upon in the Appendix.

- Knowledge deficit.
- Mobility, impaired.
- Pain, acute or chronic.

Interventions. Patient education concerning the etiology of plantar fasciitis and its treatment modalities is required so that they have a good understanding of the chronic nature of this problem. This will aid the patient in identifying and modifying any risk factors associated with heel pain. Instruct the patient on the proper stretching exercises, and provide them with written material. Reinforce the need to be consistent when performing exercises, especially first thing in the morning. Patients need to understand the importance of proper shoe wear and know how to use any assistive appliance, such as a night splint.

Pes Planus

Overview

Pes planus, commonly known as flat foot, generally refers to loss of the normal medial longitudinal arch. The head of the talus is displaced medially and in a plantar direction away from the navicular, stretching the ligaments and the posterior tibial tendon causing the foot to be flattened. Pes planus can be rigid or flexible. This flat foot deformity, which can be seen from birth to adulthood, can be either congenital or acquired. The acquired type of deformity can be caused by rupture of the posterior tibial tendon, traumatic midfoot fracture dislocation or Charcot arthropathy of the midfoot (discussed in detail in its own section of this chapter), which is the progressive destruction of bones and soft tissues often associated with diabetes and peripheral neuropathy causing the fracture dislocation and collapse of the midfoot. Pes planus can be present without any need for treatment. When treatment is required, it runs from simple shoe wear adjustments to complex surgical intervention.

According to Buchannan (2009), progressive pes planus deformity in adults is a common entity. Despite the significant incidence of this condition, the pathophysiology is still debated and often multifactorial. Clinical presentation, progression, and severity of adult-acquired flat foot deformity can be extremely variable; a multitude of conservative and surgical options are available for this common entity. Complications include pain, no toe-off, or a change in gait.

Assessment

A thorough history and physical examination will provide a family history to ascertain if the flat foot has been present since birth or has been acquired. Observe the patient sitting and standing, and observe them from behind to see the position of the heel in varus or valgus. Ask the patient to stand on their toes, first on both feet and then each foot individually. A patient with posterior tibial tendon dysfunction or insufficiency will be unable to do a single limb heel rise. Note should be made of the patient's level of pain. On palpation, the patient may have pain along the posterior tibial tendon. On inspection of the foot, look for any callous formation over the navicular or on bony prominences, especially in the diabetic or Charcot patient.

Weight-bearing radiographs are necessary to evaluate the severity of the deformity and to evaluate the longitudinal arch. These radiographs show the relationship of the involved bones to each other. This gives the clinician a clear picture of the degree of involvement. (See Table 23.2.)

Common Therapeutic Modalities

There are two schools of thought on the treatment of pes planus in children: some argue that the continuous use of molded orthosis over an extended period of time can result in the improvement of the arch, while others contend that shoes and inserts worn for 3 years do not influence the course of flat foot in children (Coughlin et al., 2007). Physical therapy can be employed to strengthen the foot and leg.

In the adult population, the nonsurgical treatment options include bracing and physical therapy. Many times an ankle foot orthosis (AFO) or brace is prescribed. If conservative treatment is not successful, procedures to correct acquired flat foot deformity range from osteotomies and tendon transfers to fusion, depending on the degree and severity of the deformity.

Nursing Considerations

Nursing Diagnoses. Nursing diagnoses for this condition are expanded upon in the Appendix.

- Activity intolerance.
- Anxiety.
- Mobility, impaired.
- Pain, chronic.

Interventions. The goal of treatment is to allow the patient to ambulate without symptoms. Nonoperative treatment may provide patients with significant relief. Physical therapy to stretch tight muscles and strengthen weak muscles may provide early relief. Orthotics with extra-depth shoes to offload bony prominences and prevent rubbing of the toes may improve symptoms. Whether that is done surgically or non-surgically depends on the degree of involvement and the degree of symptoms. With pes planus in children, parents need to be educated to understand that this condition is often a developmental issue that children can outgrow. This will reassure the parent and allay anxiety.

Pes Cavus

Overview

Pes cavus is a deformity of the foot characterized by an abnormally high arch, which never flattens on weight bearing. This results in a decreased plantar weight-bearing surface. Its incidence may be congenital, traumatic, or most commonly from a neuromuscular disease. Charcot-Marie-Tooth (CMT) is the most common cause of the cavus foot. CMT is an inherited demyelinating neuropathy characterized by the loss of muscle tissue and touch sensation in the extremities. It specifically affects the peripheal nerves resulting in atrophy of the corresponding muscles. The first nerve usually affected is the peroneal nerve, resulting in muscle weakness (Pinzur, 2008).

"The common thread in all forms of cavus foot is muscle imbalance" (Coughlin et al., 2007, p. 1129). Pes cavus is rarely idiopathic. This condition can be present without any need for treatment. When treatment is required, it ranges from footwear accommodation to surgical intervention. The main complications of pes cavus are stress fractures and pain.

Assessment

Obtain a detailed history from the patient or parent. Typically there will be a positive history of pes cavus or neuromuscular disease in the family. On physical exam, observe the patient sitting and standing. On standing, the arch with pes cavus remains high, and more pressure is placed on the metatarsal heads and lateral foot. Often painful callosities or stress fractures are seen in these areas because of the added weight-bearing load. When sitting, the patient may exhibit general weakness of the muscles in the foot and ankle and have ankle instability. Observe them walking from behind, and note the position of the heel and toes during the stance phase, as the heel may position in varus and this should be noted. During the swing phase, observe for any signs of foot drop.

Standing radiographs of the foot are necessary to evaluate the degree of deformity. These radiographs show the relationship of the involved bones to each other. This gives the clinician a clear picture of the degree of involvement and defines the treatment plan. If an unknown neurological condition is suspected, a full neurological evaluation is required. MRI of the spine may be necessary to determine any diseases of the spinal cord. Electromyography and nerve conduction studies are also helpful in detecting abnormalities of lower extremity muscle imbalance. (See Table 23.2.)

Common Therapeutic Modalities

Initial nonoperative treatment for pes cavus starts with a comprehensive rehabilitation program for joint mobilization and bracing to prevent or treat deformity. Other nonoperative options include custom orthotics, extra depth shoes, or lateral wedges in the shoe. These devices increase comfort but do not correct the deformity. Again, the degree of deformity dictates the treatment. Surgical options can range from soft tissue realignments to complicated bony procedures, even fusions.

Surgical treatment is done to provide a plantigrade foot. No single procedure is appropriate for all patients, and multiple individual procedures are often needed. Tendon transfers and osteotomies can provide correction of the deformity without requiring an arthrodesis; however, arthrodesis may be warranted if arthritic changes are observed in the joints. Some of the more common procedures are plantar fascia release, mid-foot osteotomy, calcaneal osteotomy, various tendon transfers, and even triple arthrodesis. Recovery is long, with as much as 12 weeks of immobilization.

Nursing Considerations

Nursing Diagnoses. Nursing diagnoses for this condition are expanded upon in the Appendix.

- Activity intolerance.
- Mobility: physical, impaired.
- Pain, chronic.

Interventions. Given the multiple causes and degrees of deformity, as well as the range of procedures to correct pes cavus, the interventions can be highly varied. Postoperative patient teaching, again depending on the degree of surgical intervention, is important. If therapy is employed, it must be stressed that consistency of the therapy is necessary to get worthwhile results. If footwear adjustments are added, consistency is again important.

Foot Drop

Overview

Foot drop is the inability to dorsiflex the foot. It is one of the most disabling disorders, affecting one's gait and thus interfering with quality of life (Elsner, Barg, Stufkens, & Hinterman, 2010). The disability can progress over time as a result of generalized muscle weakness or damage. Foot drop can be the result of trauma, idiopathic incident, or systemic disease. The nerve injury can be local or peripheral, usually affecting the common peroneal nerve in adult foot drop. Central nerve injuries that can cause foot drop include spinal cord injury, herniated lumbar disk, L5 radiculopathy, cauda equina, and stroke. Diseases such as polio, CMT, and cerebral palsy are conditions commonly associated with foot drop.

Complications related to foot drop revolve around gait abnormalities due to the muscle weakness. It is described as a steppage gait, with slapping of the forefoot. The patient will often stub the front of the foot during the gait cycle because the foot does not dorsiflex and prevents the forefoot to clear. Shortening of the Achilles tendon can occur. There may be pain from overloading the lateral forefoot. Callosities or pressure ulcers can develop, especially when there is associated diminished sensation.

Table 23.3. Footwear Guidelines	
Suggestion	**Rationale**
Have both feet measured before trying on shoes. Select the shoe that fits the largest foot.	1. Foot size changes with age. 2. Most people have one foot larger than the other. 3. Sizes vary among brands and styles.
Try on shoes at the end of the day.	1. Feet are largest and widest after being on them all day.
Select a style that conforms to the shape of the foot so that the ball of the foot fits comfortably into the widest part of the shoe.	1. Prevents toe constriction. Shoes that are no more than 1/4" narrower than the foot yield the lease problems. 2. Prevents pressure points. 3. Optimizes biomechanics of the foot.
When standing there should be 3/8" to 1/2" between the longest toe and the end of the shoe.	1. Prevents blisters, callus, and deformities to toes. 2. Allows air circulation.
Avoid high heels.	1. High-heeled shoes usually have triangular toe boxes causing constriction. 2. As the height of the heel rises the pressure on the forefoot increases. A 3" heel exerts 76% more pressure than a flat heel. Heel height is recommended 1/2" to 1".
Avoid shoes with seams stitched over prominent areas of the foot.	1. Prevents blisters or calluses.
Shoe material should be breathable (leather or canvas not plastic or nylon).	1. Allows air circulation. 2. Minimizes abrasion, maceration, and microbial growth.
Do not plan to "break in" shoes.	1. It implies improper fit. The shoe should fit comfortably when it is first worn. 2. The foot conforms more often than the shoe.
Walk in the shoe before buying it.	1. Tests the comfort and fit.

From Core Curriculum for Orthopaedic Nursing (6th Ed., p. 586), *by the National Association of Orthopaedic Nurses (NAON), 2007, Boston, MA: Pearson. Reproduced with permission.*

Assessment

A thorough medical background needs to be obtained, including birth, family, and any trauma history. The key to the examination is assessing the gait cycle. Observations during the stance phase include limited ankle dorsiflexion, an overload of the lateral border of the foot (varus deformity), and instability. During the swing phase, observe drop foot with foot clearance problems, excessive hip and knee flexion to help clear the foot, and the slap of the forefoot making contact first as opposed to the heel strike first in normal walking.

On further examination, the patient may exhibit medial and lateral tibial-talar instability, progressive hindfoot varus, and a supination deformity of the forefoot (Elsner et al., 2010). Perform a neurological exam, and assess for any muscle atrophy. Assess the skin for callosities, ulcers, or pressure areas, especially in the lateral forefoot.

Diagnostic tests that are beneficial include weight-bearing radiographs of the foot and ankle, electromyography, and nerve conduction velocity studies. (See Table 23.2.)

Common Therapeutic Modalities

Orthoses and proper footwear stabilize and protect the foot and are the mainstay of conservative treatment. The most common is the AFO, which helps to keep the ankle in a dorsiflexed position. These are accommodative not corrective devices; they function by exerting a force on the foot and ankle in a controlled manner to transfer pressure and restrict motion. These must be worn in a shoe. Padding or cushioning may be added to help unload the pressure areas. The goals of surgical treatment are to restore normal foot function and create a plantigrade foot (Pinzur, 2008).

Nursing Considerations

Nursing Diagnoses. Nursing diagnoses for this condition are expanded upon in the Appendix.

- Body image, disturbed.
- Falls, risk for.
- Injury, risk for.
- Mobility: physical, impaired.

Interventions. Patients need to understand that the purpose of orthoses and footwear modifications is to protect the foot and aid in walking. Reinforce safety issues: never wear the AFO without shoes because the surface is slippery and the brace could crack. Frequent skin checks are required to evaluate skin integrity. Instruct the patient in shoe selection: increase shoe size by one size to accommodate the brace. Shoes with laces are better, and custom-molded shoes are often necessary. Footwear and bracing issues can be challenging for the female or younger patients. (See Table 23.3.)

Hallux Valgus

Overview

Hallux valgus, commonly known as a bunion, is the lateral deviation of the proximal phalanx of the great toe on the first metatarsal head (metatarsalphalangeal joint). It is one of the most common forefoot deformities seen. A bunion refers to the enlargement of the medial eminence of the first metatarsalphalageal joint, which can become inflamed and erythematous, causing "bump pain" or joint pain because of abnormal positioning of the joint.

Stability of the toe is maintained through the fan-shaped collateral ligaments from the head of the metatarsal to the base of the proximal phalanx medially and laterally. There are no actual muscle insertions in the head of the first metatarsal. The capsular ligamentous sling and the shape of the joint provide the stability, thus failure of the supporting structures will lead to deviation. The proximal phalanx of the great toe will deviate laterally, and the metatarsal head will deviate medially, creating a prominent medial eminence, the bunion. Symptoms and deformity of a bunion may be mild to severe.

There are various extrinsic and intrinsic factors that play a role in the development of a symptomatic hallux valgus. Extrinsic factors are those that exert their influence from the outside, and include narrow restrictive footwear and high-heeled shoes. Intrinsic factors that can contribute to hallux valgus formation are incompetent soft tissues, ligamentous laxity, instability of the first metatarsocunieform joint, Achilles tendon contracture, pes planus deformity, and genetic pre-disposition.

According to Coughlin, Mann, and Salzman (2007), the incidence of hallux valgus is seen in a female-to-male ratio of 9-1, usually in the 30-50 year age range, and is often bilateral. This rationale supports the theory that footwear is a major factor in hallux valgus formation. There is a 60% genetic predisposition associated with bunion deformity (Coughlin et al., 2007). It is important to consider that feet widen as the body ages, and there is an increase in soft tissue laxity. Complications are pain and deformity.

Assessment

The history and physical exam must evaluate the patient sitting and standing, as the hallux valgus deformity will be more pronounced with weight-bearing and lesser toe deformities may be observed, such as a second crossover toe from the lateral deviation of the first toe. Obtain a family history, as there is a strong genetic predisposition. Find out about their pain. Usually there is an increase in pain when wearing shoes and none or mild pain when walking barefoot. Examine the foot for any callouses or corns, check the ROM of the MTP joint, and note any abnormal motion of the MTC joint. Normal first MTP joint motion is at least 65 degrees of dorsiflexion and 15 degrees of plantar flexion (Hart, DeAsla, & Grottkau, 2008). Examine the type of shoes they wear. Have the patient stand on a piece of white paper and trace the foot; place their shoe on top of the paper to assess shoe size relative to foot size.

Weight-bearing AP, lateral, and oblique radiographs of the foot need to be taken to evaluate joint congruity and arthritis. Several measurements must be taken to provide information as to the level of deformity, all of which will determine the appropriate treatment plan (Hart et al., 2008). The most common angular measurements are the hallux valgus angle (HVA), the intermetatarsal angle (IMA), and the distal metatarsal articular angle (DMAA). The HVA normal angle is less than 15 degrees, mild deformity is less than 20 degrees, moderate deformity is 20-40 degrees, and severe deformity is greater than 40 degrees. The IMA normal angle is less than 9 degrees, mild deformity is 11 degrees or less, moderate deformity is greater than 11 degrees and less than 16 degrees, and severe is greater than 16 degrees. The DMAA normal is 6 degrees or less of lateral deviation (Coughlin et al., 2007). Positioning of the sesamoids is also noted.

Common Therapeutic Modalities

Conservative management starts with educating the patient about the negative effects of improper shoes, which is often met with resistance. Comparing an outline of the patient's foot to his or her footwear assists in conveying this point. Nonsurgical treatment includes the use of sufficiently wide footwear to accommodate the deformity. Provide guidelines for properly fitting shoes. They should be wide, low-heeled, have an extra depth toe box, and be made of soft leather to help alleviate pressure and reduce painful symptoms. Adaptive devices such as night bunion splint, toe spacers, padding, and inserts all may help to diminish symptoms.

After conservative management, if the patient continues to have pain and deformity that interferes with their lifestyle, surgery can be performed. The goal of surgery is to create a painless, plantigrade, shoeable foot (Craig, 1999). Cosmesis and the desire to wear high-fashion footwear is a poor indicator for surgery. Bunion surgery should not be taken lightly, and appropriate preoperative planning and decision-making should include the patient's expectations, athletic interests, occupation, physical exam, and radiographs. The type of surgical repair will vary, depending on the severity of the deformity, whether the joint is congruent or incongruent, and if there is arthritis present. Postoperatively, patients will have to restrict their activities, wear a special postoperative shoe or boot, and be on limited weight-bearing status. If the right foot is involved, no driving is allowed for a limited period of time. Ice and elevation are important to help control postoperative swelling and pain. Cold therapy systems are very beneficial because they are placed on the patient at the time of surgery and provide immediate cold therapy as early as the recovery room. The patient should be educated that the cold system needs to be cycled, just as if they were using ice at 20-minute intervals, as frostbite can result. Most patients will need to be out of work while recovering from surgery. The type of work they do will dictate how long they will be out, usually anywhere from 2-8 weeks.

Nursing Considerations

Nursing Diagnoses. Nursing diagnoses for this condition are expanded upon in the Appendix.

- Infection, risk for.
- Knowledge deficit.
- Pain, acute.

Intervention. Patient education regarding proper shoe modification is very important, both in providing relief of symptoms and in understanding the relationship between footwear and the deformity. (See Table 23.3.) Assist the patient in having realistic expectations after surgery regarding activity restrictions, driving, work, dressing changes, pain management, and assistive devices.

Interdigital Neuroma

Overview

A neuroma results from the compression of the interdigital nerve at the level of the metatarsal head. A neuroma can develop in the common digital nerve as a result of direct trauma or from an extrinsic pressure against the nerve. The nerve is tethered under the metatarsal heads and the metatarsal ligament, as the toes are dorsiflexed during the normal gait cycle. Tight-fitting and high-heeled shoes force plantar flexion of the metatarsal heads and hyper-dorsiflexion of the MTP joints. This causes recurrent trauma to the nerves and entrapment neuropathy beneath the transverse metatarsal ligament. For this reason, a neuroma is more common in women, usually 8-10 times more often than in men (Lotke, 2008). The third web space has the highest incidence of neuroma formation. It is attributed to the common digital nerve being thicker because it has branches from the lateral and medial plantar, nerve thus being subjected to trauma. There is more mobility in the third web space, thus resulting in more motion to the nerve. The second and third web spaces are much narrower than the first and fourth, making them more susceptible to a neuroma formation (Pinzur, 2008). Pain and web space dysesthesias are the most common complications. Preventive strategies include wearing proper-fitting shoes that are wide and supportive.

Assessment

On physical examination, the patient will complain of pain localized to the plantar aspect of the foot between the metatarsal heads of the involved area. They will describe the pain as burning, stabbing, tingling, or electrical in nature, with radiation to the toes. Shoes, especially narrow high heels, aggravate pain. The patients are symptom-free when resting or walking barefoot. When palpating the interspace, there will be fullness and possible tenderness. Simultaneous medial and lateral compression of the metatarsal heads while palpating the plantar web space may create a palpable click (Mulder's Sign) that reproduces the patient's symptoms (Pinzur, 2008).

Diagnostic testing should include weight-bearing foot radiographs to rule out any osseous abnormality. MRI and ultrasound have been utilized but remain controversial. Selective injections of a local anesthetic into the web space can be a useful diagnostic tool for detecting neuromas.

Common Therapeutic Modalities

Initial treatment of interdigital neuroma is to relieve the compression on the nerve. Shoes that have include soft leather, a wide toe box, and a low heel will allow splaying of the metatarsal heads to reduce pressure on the nerve. Metatarsal pads or bars placed right below or just proximal to the metatarsal heads, depending on the location of the neuroma, will offload and reduce the traction on the nerve. Ultrasound-guided steroid injections with a local anesthetic have been beneficial in controlling symptoms, and placement is more specific. Complications associated with steroid injections include fat pad atrophy, discoloration of the skin, and disruption of the joint capsule causing deviation of the toe. Two other modalities that have been successful in treating neuromas are radiofrequency ablation and alcohol-sclerosing therapy. Radiofrequency ablation uses an electrical current produced by a radio wave to heat up a small area of nerve tissue, which causes an interuption in the pain signal thereby reducing pain in the treated area. An ultrasound guided radiofrequency probe is placed in the nerve under local anesthesia and the electrical stimulation heats the surrending tissue. Alcohol-sclerosing therapy is a procedure using a combination of ethanol and a long-acting anesthetic, injected around the nerve under ultrasound guidance to decrease nerve impulses. The ethanol produces a chemical neurolysis through dehydration, necrosis, and precipitation of protoplasm (Hughes, Ali, Jones, Kendall, & Connell, 2007). Multiple injections are usually required to achieve the desired results.

If pain persists after all conservative management options have been exhausted, surgery can be performed. An interdigital neuroma can be excised through either a dorsal or a plantar approach. The dorsal approach will prevent scar tissue from developing on the bottom of the foot.

Recurrent neuromas following surgery can occur from either inadequate resection of the nerve or from a bulb neuroma that develops beneath a metatarsal head. Symptoms may occur within the first 12 months after surgery to as far out as 4 years (Coughlin et al., 2007). The pain is often described as electric-like and localized on the plantar aspect of the foot. Treatment options are the same as a primary neuroma. Re-exploration should be carefully considered and patient expectations thoroughly discussed prior to any surgery.

Nursing Considerations

Nursing Diagnoses. Nursing diagnoses for this condition are expanded upon in the Appendix.

- Knowledge deficit.
- Pain, acute.

Interventions. As in most foot conditions and deformities, having the patient understand the relationship of the problem and shoe choice is very important. Provide shoe modification guidelines and instructions on proper application of any metatarsal pads. (See Table 23.3.)

LESSER TOE DEFORMITIES

Lesser toe deformities can develop as the result of trauma, inflammatory conditions, neurologic disorders, or poor fitting shoes, or they may have a congenital origin. The lesser toes are important for balance and pressure distribution on the plantar surface of the foot. Treatment goals are to restore function to the lesser toes, alleviate pain, and allow the use of various types of footwear. The most common lesser toe deformities are hammertoes, mallet toes, and claw toes.

Hammertoe Deformity

Overview

A hammertoe deformity is the most common of all lesser toe deformities. It is a plantar flexion deformity of the PIP joint, the middle phalanx is flexed on the proximal phalanx, and the DIP joint is not involved. There may be hyperextension of the MTP joint. Hammertoes can result from tight, ill-fitting shoes. They can also be caused by a muscle imbalance from neuromuscular diseases such as CMT, cerebral palsy, multiple sclerosis, or degenerative disk disease. Other conditions that can lead to a hammertoe deformity are diabetes causing insensate feet, inflammatory arthritis such as rheumatoid or psoriatic arthritis, and hallux valgus deformity. Trauma such as a tibia fracture or compartment syndrome can also lead to hammertoe deformity. The frequency of the deformity increases with the age of the patient, peaking in the fifth to seventh decades, and is more common in women (Coughlin et al., 2007). Hammertoes can occur in all toes; however, it is most frequently seen in the second toe. Complications as a result of hammertoe deformity are painful callosities, ulcerations, nail deformities, and rarely a traumatic boutonniere deformity can develop (see Chapter 20—The Hand and Wrist). Proper footwear may help to prevent to hammertoe deformity.

Assessment

A thorough history needs to be obtained to see if any underlying medical condition is causing the hammertoe deformity, such as diabetes or neuromuscular disease. As in all examinations, the patient needs to be observed sitting and standing. The patient will complain of pain over the dorsum of the PIP joint. They will have a callus or ulceration on the dorsal aspect of the PIP joint from pressure on the shoe when they walk. Intractable plantar keratoses may develop on the plantar aspect of the foot under the metatarsal head. Evaluate whether it is a fixed or flexible deformity. If the deformity is flexible, the toe can be passively corrected to a neutral position. In rigid or fixed deformities, the contracture will not permit passive correction. The position of the first MTP joint must also be evaluated, especially if the second toe is involved because a hallux valgus deformity may be occupying the toe's space. Diagnostic tests include weight-bearing AP and lateral radiographs of the foot.

Common Therapeutic Modalities

Wide, soft shoes with an adequate toe box to accommodate the deformity is the initial treatment for hammertoe deformities. Elastic splints, felt pads, toe cradles, toe caps, or sleeves may all be used to help alleviate pain by reducing friction from footwear. Over time, however, even with appropriate care, most deformities become fixed and require surgical intervention. If surgery is required, appropriate planning is necessary, as the surgery is selected based on the specific cause and type of deformity. For flexible deformity, a flexor tendon transfer can be performed to realign the toe. The rigid hammertoe deformity requires a more involved procedure that includes proximal phalanx condylectomy, collateral ligament release, possible FDL tenotomy, and insertion of a Kirschner wire for stabilization. If there is deformity of the first MTP joint as well as a second hammertoe, surgical correction of this deformity must also be considered.

Mallet Toe Deformity

Overview

A mallet toe is a flexion deformity of the distal interphalangeal joint of the toe on the middle phalanx, with no deformity at the proximal interphalangeal joint or metatarsal phalangeal joints. The deformity may be classified as flexible or fixed. The most common deformity is fixed, but it may be flexible in the younger patient. Symptoms develop when the tip of the toe strikes the ground, resulting in a painful callus or ulcer. The primary cause of a mallet toe is a tight, narrow shoe with a constricting toe box. It can also develop as a result of trauma, following a hammertoe repair, or from inflammatory arthritis. The second toe is involved most often because it is the longest ray. Women are affected more than men, which again demonstrates the effect of ill-fitting shoes on the foot (Craig, 1999). Complications that are associated with mallet toes are painful callosities, ulcerations, and nail deformities. Proper footwear may help to prevent mallet toe deformity.

Assessment

Perform the physical exam with the patient sitting and standing to observe the deformity with weight-bearing. The patient will complain of pain over the dorsal aspect of the DIP joint and the tip of the toe when it strikes the ground. They will have callus or ulceration at the tip of the toe. Determine if the flexion contracture is flexible (passively correctable) or a fixed deformity (not passively correctable). They may also demonstrate tightness in the flexor digitorium longus tendon. In young children, a tight flexor digitorum longus can cause a flexion deformity in the PIP and DIP joints. In pediatrics, this is known as a curly toe and is often asymptomatic. Standard weight-bearing radiographs of the foot will confirm the diagnosis.

Common Therapeutic Modalities

Shoes with a wide and deep toe box are the foundation to conservative care. There are numerous appliances that can aid in padding and protecting the toes. Metatarsal pads, lambswool, and toe cradles all help to reduce pressure on the toe. Taping techniques and stretching exercises are also incorporated in treatment, especially if the deformity is flexible. If nonoperative care fails, surgery can be performed. Surgical planning is dependent on the type of deformity. A flexible mallet toe can be corrected by a flexor digitorum longus tenotomy. The fixed deformity, which is more common, requires a condylectomy of the middle phalanx, FDL tenotomy, and stabilization with Kirschner wire.

Claw Toe Deformity

Overview

A claw toe deformity combines a hammertoe deformity and dorsiflexion (hyperextension) deformity at the MTP joint. The causes of claw toe deformities are associated with the same neuromuscular diseases, arthritic conditions, diabetes, or trauma as the hammertoe deformity; however, many of these deformities have no clear cause. Claw toes are frequently bilateral, involve multiple toes, and are commonly associated with cavovarus foot deformities or an underlying neuromuscular condition (Coughlin et al., 2007) (See Figure 23.1). It is felt that weakness from the intrinsic muscles that cause a muscular imbalance of the foot may contribute to claw toe formation (Craig, 1999).

Figure 23.1.
Claw Toe Deformity

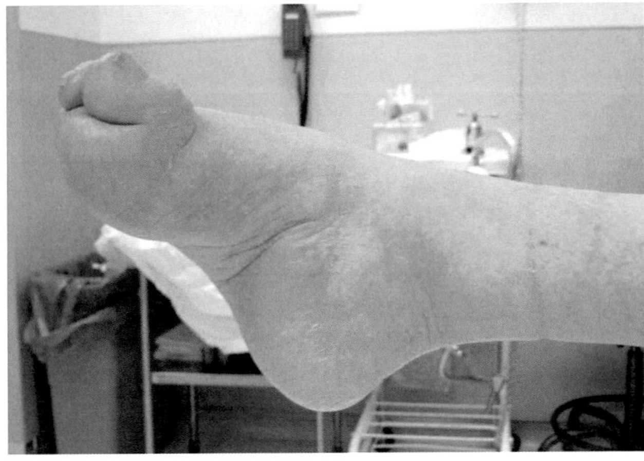

From Keith L. Wapner, MD. Reproduced with permission.

As with the other lesser toe deformities, the claw toe can be classified as flexible or fixed. The deformity seems to develop slowly over time, and the incidence increases with age, peaking in the sixth and seventh decades. Complications associated with claw toes are similar to those of hammertoe and mallet toe: callosities, ulceration, pain, and nail deformities. Gait may also be altered, especially if there is an underlying medical condition.

Assessment

Evaluation must include a thorough medical history, especially neurological aspects. As with the other lesser toe deformities, the patient must be observed sitting and standing. Patients with claw toe deformities will have similar complaints as those with hammertoe deformity: pain or discomfort at the dorsal aspect of the PIP joint where a callosity develops from hitting the shoe while walking. On the plantar aspect, they will develop a painful callus at the metatarsal head. Typical findings associated with claw toe deformity include multiple toe involvement, metatarsophalangeal joint subluxation or dislocation, and a cavus foot deformity. Assess whether the deformity is flexible or rigid. If there is no clawing of the toes when the ankle is in plantar flexion, but present with dorsiflexion of the ankle joint, a flexible claw toe deformity is present.

Diagnostic tests to confirm claw toe deformity, especially to determine the presence of MTP subluxation or dislocation, are the standard weight-bearing AP and lateral foot radiographs. (See Table 23.2.)

Common Therapeutic Modalities

As with the other two lesser toe deformities, treatment for claw toe begins with shoe modification. A wide, soft, low-heeled shoe with a deep toe box to accommodate the deformity is the foundation of nonsurgical treatment. Any associated medical condition should also be treated if necessary. Assistive devices such as metatarsal pads, toe cradles, toe sleeves, and cushioned inserts may all be used to relieve pressure and protect bony prominences. Surgery is dependent on the underlying condition. The goal of surgery is to realign the toe. A flexor tendon transfer corrects a claw toe flexible deformity. Soft tissue release, tendon lengthening, and condylectomy of the PIP joint are used to correct the rigid deformity.

Nursing Considerations for All Three Lesser Toe Deformities

Nursing Diagnoses. Nursing diagnoses for all lesser toe deformities (hammertoe, mallet toe, and claw toe) are expanded upon in the Appendix.

- Infection, risk for.
- Knowledge deficit.
- Pain, acute or chronic.

Interventions. Patients diagnosed with any of the three lesser toe deformities need to understand the rationale for shoe modification and protection of bony prominences, especially if they have an insensate foot. Remind patients, when applying any assistive appliance to the toes or foot, that more space will be needed in the shoe to accommodate both the deformity and the appliance. They should also monitor for any irritation from the assistive devices. (See Table 23.3.)

Postoperative care for any lesser toe deformity procedure requires 4-6 weeks in a special shoe or boot and weekly (routine) visits for wound checks and dressing changes. Educate the patient that lesser toe deformity correction frequently results in stiffness at either the IP or MTP joint, and remind them that swelling can persist for several months following surgery.

Corns

Overview

A corn is a hyperkeratotic lesion that forms over a bony prominence on the lesser toes because of excessive pressure and friction on the skin. Corns occur most frequently over the lateral dorsum of the fifth toe, where the shoe exerts an extrinsic pressure on the bony prominence (O'Connor & Schaller, 2001). Corns are classified as hard or soft, depending on their location. Hard corns are typically seen on the dorsal aspect of the IP or DIP joints and are often associated with lesser toe deformities. Soft corns, also known as interdigital corns or interdigital clavus, develop in the web space and form over a condyle of the phalanx between the toes from pressure and rubbing. The hyperkeratosis becomes macerated from moisture and is often confused with a fungal infection. The fourth web space is the most common area for an interdigital corn (Coughlin et al., 2007). Tight-fitting shoes are generally the cause of these lesions. The callosity usually develops over time on the bony prominence. Occasionally, if pressure is applied rapidly, skin breakdown or ulceration may occur instead. This can be particularly problematic for a patient who has an insensate foot.

Complications associated with corns are infection, pain, and ulceration, especially in patients with diabetes. The key to preventing corns is proper footwear. The elderly and patients with diabetes are at-risk populations because they often have trouble self-administering foot care due to decreased visual acuity and difficulty reaching their foot.

Assessment

Obtain a history of any previous corns, ulcerations, and treatment. Assess the patient while sitting and standing. Observe for any lesser toe deformities. Evaluate the patient's footwear, and examine the relationship between the corn location and the fit of the shoe. The curvature of the outer border of shoes often causes direct pressure on the lateral aspect of the fifth toe and results in corn development. The patient will complain of pain or discomfort when wearing shoes. The toe will be tender when palpating the area of the corn. The corn can be hard or soft, wet or dry, depending on location: the skin will be hardened, thickened, and dry if the corn is on the dorsal aspect of the joint or thickened, white, macerated, and moist if in the web space.

Diagnostic tests include standard weight-bearing radiographs of the foot. Bony prominences are identified, and if prolonged ulceration is present, assessment for possible osteomyelitis is done.

Common Therapeutic Modalities

Palliative measures are aimed at reducing the hyperkeratotic formation by alleviating the pressure and friction on the toes. Changing the patient's footwear to a wide toe, soft sole, and low heel with a deep toe box is the most important step in providing symptomatic relief. Corn pads, toe sleeves, lambs wool, and padding in the affected area to relieve pressure will also decrease symptoms. Many patients can also use a pumice stone after bathing to pare down the callus. Avoid this in patients who have an insensate foot. Paring down of the callus buildup with a #17 blade (a rounded, sharp podiatric blade that allows for safe and effective trimming) will provide relief of symptoms; however, a bruised sensation may persist. The area needs to be padded to protect from further pressure. Interdigital corns can also be treated with a desiccating agent such as Carbolfuchsin (Carfusin®), an antifungal and astringent, or rubbing alcohol to heal the macerated area (Coughlin et al., 2007).

Surgical treatment is recommended for patients whose conservative management options have failed. Surgery consists primarily of excising the prominent exostosis and condylectomy. If the corn/callus formation is a result of a lesser toe deformity, once this is corrected, the callus will stop accumulating because the pressure will be removed.

Nursing Considerations

Nursing Diagnoses. Nursing diagnoses for this condition are expanded upon in the Appendix.

- Infection, risk for.
- Knowledge deficit.
- Pain, acute or chronic.

Interventions. Provide footwear guidelines with appropriate shoe modification with rationale. (See Table 23.3.) Teach patients how to trim down the callus, or, if unable, refer them to a professional health care provider. Encourage diabetic patients to seek medical care as soon as possible when they notice callus formation to avoid breakdown or ulcer formation. Patients who have an interdigital corn need to watch for any signs of infection and seek medical care if this develops.

Verruca Plantaris

Overview

Warts are viral benign skin growths caused by the human papilloma virus (HPV). The HPV types 1 and 2 cause verruca plantaris, commonly known as plantar warts. The incubation period may last for several months, and the virus can survive without being contagious. Warts are characterized as benign epithelial proliferation of the outer layer of the epidermis. Warts are the most common infectious skin lesions seen on the feet, as well as the entire body, especially in children and young adults. The incidence is higher in children ages 12-16 and people who share common bathing areas, such as dormitories, swimming pools, and gyms (Cole, 2010).

Risk factors include a weakened immune system, skin breakdown, and multiple exposures to the virus. The virus is encountered on contaminated surfaces and attacks the skin through direct contact, entering through cuts or abrasions on the foot. The virus thrives in moist environments like the foot, although the wart may not appear for several weeks or months.

To prevent plantar warts, avoid direct contact with warts, keep feet clean and dry, and avoid walking barefoot especially in public places. Children should not share shoes or socks, and these should be changed daily. In public bathing or changing areas, flip-flops or water shoes should be worn.

Assessment

On history, the patient may report recent activity in a public bathing area or gym. Some patients may provide a history of a cut or puncture wound in the last month or so prior to observing the growth. On physical examination, the patient will present with a keratotic patch that forms on the plantar surface of the foot not usually associated with a weight-bearing bony prominence. The lesions can range from 1-2 mm to several centimeters in size. There may be solitary or multiple growths. Patients may have a mosaic pattern, which is a large wart surrounded by several smaller lesions. These lesions differ from painful callosities because they will be very tender when squeezed, and the central core contains capillaries that are thrombosed and appear as multiple black dots.

Unlike a callus, a wart will cause a disruption of the dermal ridges of the skin. Careful paring of the lesion with a #17 blade may be necessary to distinguish a wart from a foreign body reaction. Because of the wart's vascularity, bleeding will occur with trimming of the lesion. Diagnostic tests are not normally required, except occasionally a culture or biopsy of the lesion is obtained if unusual in appearance to rule out skin cancer commonly seen in the feet, such as Bowen's disease or verrucous squamous cell carcinoma.

Common Therapeutic Modalities

There is no simple single treatment to eradicate plantar warts. Prior to beginning any therapy for plantar warts, it is important to remember that many warts can resolve on their own without treatment, especially in children. The average life span of a wart is approximately 2 years (Coughlin et al., 2007). Treatment is usually initiated because of pain and interference with activities.

Chemical therapy using topical agents such as Cantharidin (Canthrone®), ascetic acid, or salicylic acid can be used in conjunction with paring down the lesion. The lesion is trimmed as much as the patient can tolerate, then the agent is applied to the lesion followed by applying an occlusive dressing. This is repeated every few days. Multiple treatments are required, and resolution may take up to 6 weeks. Chemical therapy is about 50% effective (O'Connor & Schaller, 2001). Salicylic acid can be purchased over the counter, and this treatment is often initiated at home before seeking medical assistance. Other agents, such as Efudex (2-Fluorouracil®), bleomycin, and 40% trichloroacetic acid, have also shown to be effective in the treatment of warts.

Electrical removal or burning of warts with electrocautery has been used to treat recalcitrant warts. Disadvantages to this therapy are that it is painful, requiring a local anesthetic, it leaves a hole, requiring wound care, and it may take several weeks to heal and may result in scar tissue.

Liquid nitrogen or cryotherapy is a treatment commonly used by dermatologists. This requires several applications and cycles of treatment. The liquid nitrogen is applied to the wart under pressure, and it freezes, burns, or vaporizes the growth. A blister forms, then peels away in layers, removing the wart. This form of treatment is painful, and the blistering may require the use of antibiotic ointment.

Laser therapy has also been used in treating plantar warts. It burns the wart off and eradicates the virus. This requires local anesthesia and is expensive.

Surgical excision is rarely used in the plantar surface of the foot because of excessive scarring and pain.

Immunotherapy involves injecting the wart with interferon, a drug that boosts the immune system, and then injecting an antigen to stimulate the immune system. This therapy tries to use the body's natural rejection system to destroy the wart and virus (Mayo Clinic, 2010). Recently, candida albicans has been used in the treatment of warts by injecting a diluted protein from the yeast into the wart, which triggers the immune system to respond and fight back the virus.

Nursing Considerations

Nursing Diagnoses. Nursing diagnoses for this condition are expanded upon in the Appendix.

- Infection, risk for.
- Knowledge deficit.
- Pain, acute or chronic.

Interventions. Patients need to be educated concerning the treatment and causes of plantar warts. More than 50% will resolve on their own, without treatment, within 2 years. If treatment is required because of pain and trouble walking, there are multiple options to choose from. Simple home remedies, such as silver duct-taping, can be just as effective in treating small lesions as some of the chemicals. Treatment can be time-consuming and expensive, and carries a high recurrence rate. When administering treatment, remind patients to wash hands frequently, use a pumice stone to help debride, (use a separate stone on other healthy tissue), avoid picking at warts, and use occlusive dressing over any chemicals used. Children must remember not to share shoes or socks, and these should be changed regularly. Wear flip-flops in public bathing and changing areas.

Onychocryptosis

Overview

Onychocryptosis, or ingrown toenail infection, results from impaction of the nail into the surrounding tissue, often caused by improper nail trimming or the inherent shape of the nail (Pinzur, 2008). The normal space between the nail margin and the nail groove is approximately 1mm. Extrinsic forces, such as narrow shoes and tight stockings, cause a pressure to develop on the nail plate, fold, or lip. This eliminates the normal space, causing constant irritation and swelling and leading to hyperplasia of the soft tissue surrounding the nail. It is most common in the great toe and in the young active population. Some of the causes are shoes that are too tight or too short, improper nail cutting, and toe deformities. Some cases are congenital: the nail is just too large or incurvated for the toe. Trauma, such as stubbing the toe or having the toe stepped on, may also cause an ingrown toenail. The tissue can become hot and painful. Infection occurs when the traumatized tissue is invaded by local bacteria (paronychia and onychia). Ingrown toenails are seen often in teenagers and middle-aged women. To prevent ingrown toenails, the patient should be instructed in proper footwear, use of loose-fitting stockings or hose, and proper nail-cutting procedure.

Assessment

The history and physical exam of the patient should include a close examination of the foot, noting color and temperature, along with a complete history of nail deformities. A careful look at their shoes may provide some hint to the cause of the ingrown toenail.

Careful examination of the involved foot is important. Given that the foot is usually in a closed environment, there are more issues than in the hand. Most toenail problems are easily diagnosed by simple inspection. The skin around the nail will be red and inflamed, and there may be drainage present. The area will be painful and sensitive to the touch. Culture and sensitivity testing may be done if drainage is noted.

Common Therapeutic Modalities

At first, the toenail may be tender but not infected. A piece of cotton under the nail, just after a shower when the nail is soft, trains the nail in the way it should grow. This, followed by proper nail trimming, can often be the end of the problem. Left untreated, the soft tissue can become infected. Warm water soaks and antibiotics can often treat early infections. For more advanced infections, incision and drainage of the infection, along with a course of antibiotics, is needed. If there is a pattern of ingrown toenails, surgical removal of part of the nail may be necessary. Loose-fitting stockings and wide toe-box shoes can aid in prevention. There are several surgical procedures for the treatment of ingrown toenails; however, postoperative recurrence is common (Coughlin et al., 2007).

Nursing Considerations

Nursing Diagnoses. Nursing diagnoses for this condition are expanded upon in the Appendix.

- Infection, risk for.
- Knowledge deficit.
- Pain, acute.

Interventions. Patients must be taught the proper technique to trim their toenails, including cutting straight across and not over-trimming at the corners. Proper fitting footwear is also important, especially the use of wide toe shoes. (See Table 23.3.)

Onychomycosis

Overview

Onychomycosis is a variety of fungal infections of the toenails, causing destruction of the normal tissue. This condition is very common, with approximately 20% of the US population affected. The prevalence may be much higher in patients older than age 60; some sources quote as high as 75% of the population (Coughlin et al., 2007). Men are more commonly affected than women (Coughlin et al., 2007). It manifests as a progressive thickening of the nails with yellow debris under them, splitting, pitting, or ridging of the nail can also occur.

Risk factors include family history, advancing age, poor health, trauma, warm climate, bathing in communal showers, and wearing shoes that cover the toes completely and don't allow any airflow. Complications can include permanent nail scaring and advanced infection within the toe. Treatment can be long, expensive, and does not always solve the problem.

Assessment

Physical examination of the foot can quickly identity onychomycosis. The nail plate will be thickened, brittle, discolored, and sometimes deformed. There may be a build-up of chronic debris under the nail bed that caused the nail plate to detach. The patient may complain of painful pressure under the nail. Careful history may reveal other risk factors, such as those related to footwear. A culture is necessary to identify which type of fungus is involved and to assist in diagnosing other causes, such as psoriasis.

Common Therapeutic Modalities

Treatment is usually chemical, both topical and oral, with surgery in rare instances. Debridement of the fungus aids in relieving the pressure under the nail. Terbinafine (Lamisil®), fluconazole (Diflucan®) and griseofulvin (Vulvicin®) are the most common oral agents used to treat this condition. Liver studies must be done while on most of these drugs. Topical therapy is prolonged, and has a high relapse rate. Combination of oral, topical, and surgical therapy can reduce the risk of recurrence. Treatment of footwear with antifungals is often recommended if treatment is pursued.

Nursing Considerations

Nursing Diagnoses. Nursing diagnoses for this condition are expanded upon in the Appendix.

- Body image, disturbed.
- Infection, risk for.
- Knowledge deficit.

Interventions. Patient teaching must include education on the common side effects of these oral agents, which include hypersensitivity, liver toxicity, gastrointestinal disorders, and cardiovascular effects. Patients will be taught to inspect their feet regularly. Proper nail care and the prevention of infection are also important. As always, education on proper footwear is key (see Table 23.3). Shoes with a large toe box with plenty of circulation are vital. It is important to encourage patients to verbalize feelings about the appearance of their toenails.

Amputations

Overview

Amputation is the removal of a body part as a result of disease (systemic or vascular), mutilating trauma, infection, or lack of function. As a surgical measure, it is used to control pain or a disease process in the affected limb, such as gangrene or malignancy. It may also occur as a result of injury. For some patients with a long history of disease, this is the first step on the road to restored or renewed function (Coughlin et al., 2007). No matter what the reason, this is a major consequence of any disease process, and care must be taken to address the patient's physical and psychological needs. More than half of all non-traumatic lower limb amputations occur in people with diabetes (Coughlin et al., 2007). Preservation of limb length correlates with decreasing energy expenditure during ambulation (Myerson, 2000).

Complications of amputation include infection, poor healing, phantom pain, neuroma formation, or the need for another higher amputation. The patient may struggle with a poorly fitting prosthesis, emotional adjustment, inadequate family support, or lack of the needed energy to ambulate with the prosthesis.

Assessment

Prior to the amputation, a complete history and physical will reveal the mechanism of injury or disease process that brought the patient to the point of amputation. Also important are concurrent diseases such as diabetes, which is common in these cases. A complete neurovascular and skin assessment are critical to final healing. X-rays, vascular studies (including venogram and arteriogram), and lab studies (including serum glucose and hemoglobin A1C) are all part of this evaluation prior to the surgery. Adequate circulation is a prerequisite for primary healing of the wound, whereas sensitivity will save the residual limb from future breakdown (Bohne, 1999). Adequate padding, residual circulation, and residual sensitivity become key elements in preoperative surgical planning. In the preoperative planning phase, special attention must be given to the psychological and social needs of the patient.

Common Therapeutic Modalities

The goal of amputation surgery is to reach the best soft tissue possible to provide pressure relief and wound healing. A team approach should be incorporated for the best outcome. Amputations around the foot and ankle can be as simple as a toe excision or as complex as removal of the entire foot. (See Figure 23.2.)

Figure 23.2. Levels of Partial Foot Amputation

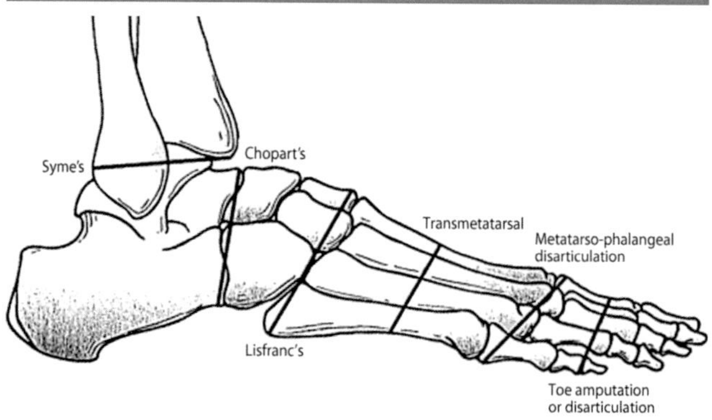

From Surgery of the Foot and Ankle (8th ed., Vol II, p. 1370), by M.J. Coughlin, R.A. Mann, & C.L. Saltzman, 2007, Philadelphia, PA: Mosby Elsevier. Reproduced with permission.

Toe removals, commonly seen in diabetics, do not require prosthesis. With adequate skin coverage, the patient can do quite nicely in a normal shoe if there are no other problems.

The metatarsal ray amputation involves the toe and complete or partial removal of the metatarsal. This procedure changes the width of the foot and also the amount of weight-bearing surface. Extra-depth shoes and custom orthosis can accommodate these changes.

Midfoot amputations include transmetatarsal and Lisfranc amputation. The transmetatarsal amputation ("transmet") is the last level that allows the patient to walk without assistive devices. An AFO with a long footplate, with a toe filler or stiff-soled shoe, is necessary to accommodate walking. The Lisfranc amputation cuts through the talonavicular and calcaneal cuboid joints, so it is more involved than the transmet and will require some form of prosthesis.

In the hindfoot, the amputation is called a Chopart procedure. This removes the forefoot and midfoot, leaving only the calcaneus and the talus. This also will require prosthesis after postoperative casting.

Lastly, the Symes procedure is removal of the entire foot, using the distal tibia and fibula as the weight-bearing surface. This is the last chance to create a weight-bearing stump below the knee. A prosthesis is needed to ambulate after postoperative casting.

Nursing Considerations

Nursing Diagnoses. Nursing diagnoses for this condition are expanded upon in the Appendix.

- Body image, disturbed.
- Falls, risk for.
- Infection, risk for.
- Mobility: physical, impaired.

- Pain, acute.
- Self-esteem, risk for situational low.
- Sensory perception, disturbed.
- Transfer ability, impaired.

Interventions. The amputee is dealing with both physical and psychological issues. Once healing and pain issues are addressed, ambulation becomes the focus. Physical therapy will be involved to teach the patient safe ambulation. The prosthetist will work with the patient to provide a well-fitting prosthetic device. Family members are an important part of this team. The patient is encouraged to care for himself and return as closely as possible to life before the amputation. Depending on the level of amputation, some patients may not be able to return to their previous work. Job training or adjustments may be necessary.

Osteoarthritis

Overview

Osteoarthritis (OA), also known as degenerative arthritis, is a group of mechanical abnormalities involving degradation of joints, including articular cartilage and subchondral bone. It affects more than 27 million people, making it a leading cause of disability in American adults (Monti, 2010). Nearly half of the elderly population of the US is estimated to have some form of arthritis involving the foot or ankle, with osteoarthritis the most common type. (Also see Chapter 13—Arthritis.)

Heredity, age, and gender are all factors that play a role in developing OA. These, of course, are beyond direct control. Other controllable factors that can influence the onset of OA are obesity, overuse, and posture. Since OA tends to run in families and is directly related to the "wear and tear" on the body, the longer an individual practices healthy living, the longer he may be able to delay its development. OA is equally common in men and women before age 55. After the age of 55, women have significantly higher rate of occurrence (Monti, 2010). People who have had injuries or fractures in the past have a higher probability of developing OA. A variety of causes—hereditary, developmental, metabolic, and mechanical—may initiate processes leading to loss of cartilage. When bone surfaces become less well-protected by cartilage, bone may be exposed and damaged. All areas of the foot and ankle can be involved: the ankle, the hindfoot, the midfoot, or the forefoot. Primary OA is rarely seen in the ankle; secondary OA related to trauma is the most common cause of ankle OA, as opposed to the hip or knee (Coughlin et al., 2007). Complications can include sleep disorders due to pain, a sedentary lifestyle, and reduced productivity.

Assessment

A complete history and physical are essential to the diagnosis. The patient will complain of joint pain, tenderness, stiffness, locking, and sometimes effusion. Other symptoms include decreased ROM swelling, and deformity. The physical should also include examination of the patient's knees and observation of overall gait. Question the patient to determine if changes in lifestyle have occurred as a result of pain. A particular focus on a possible correlation of pain and external circumstances will be helpful to the diagnosis. Observe for deformity, pain, callus formation, and difficulty ambulating. Standard weight-bearing radiographs of the foot and ankle need to obtained to determine the degree of arthritis. (See Table 23.2.)

Common Therapeutic Modalities

Treatment generally involves a combination of exercise, lifestyle modification, and analgesics. The patient's activity level, expectations, and co-morbidities will also influence the health care choices.

Braces, orthotics, and footwear modifications are all used in the nonsurgical treatment of osteoarthritis of the foot or ankle. These, combined with medications, can often delay the need for surgery or, in some cases, eliminate the need for surgery altogether. An AFO can control motion and alignment, thereby relieving pain.

Surgery for OA patients can range from simple to extremely complex. The goal of surgery is to decrease motion and relieve pressure on bony prominences. A fusion of the joint will do just that, whether it is in the ankle, midfoot, or forefoot. To maintain motion, a joint replacement can be done, thereby replacing the deformed parts.

Nursing Considerations

Nursing Diagnoses. Nursing diagnoses for this condition are expanded upon in the Appendix.

- Activity intolerance.
- Infection, risk for.
- Knowledge deficit.
- Mobility, impaired.
- Pain, acute or chronic.

Interventions. For nonsurgical patients, changes in footwear, non-steroidal medications, and local application of heat can help to alleviate most of the symptoms. The chronic nature of the disability must be addressed with each patient. Preventing postoperative infections is key for the surgical patient. Once the postoperative pain is gone, they often have relief from their original pain.

Charcot Foot

Overview

Charcot foot, otherwise known as Charcot's arthropathy, is the progressive destruction of the bones and soft tissue in the foot or ankle. There are two theories regarding the etiology. The first is neurotraumatic destruction, as a result of repetitive trauma to the insensate foot. The second theory is that it is due to neurovascular destruction, characterized by bone resorption and ligament loosening related to a vascular reflex (Pinzur, 2008). Usually a complication of diabetes, it is always associated with nerve damage. These patients present with a wide variety of symptoms and sequellae. "Many say that the Charcot joint is the most dramatic manifestation of diabetic peripheral neuropathy" (Coughlin et al., 2007, p. 1333). Any patient with an insensate foot is at risk to develop Charcot's arthropathy.

According to the American Diabetes Association (2011), 60%-70% of people with diabetes develop mild to severe peripheral nerve damage that can lead to Charcot foot. The disorder occurs at the same rate in men and women, and 30% of the cases are bilateral (Pinzur, 2008).

The involvement may manifest as fractures, dislocations, fracture-dislocations, and subluxations proximal to the metatarsal shafts. Complications include deformity, infections, ulcers, and amputations. Prevention is a challenge because most Charcot joints manifest with a history that includes trauma and impaired sensation caused by the neuropathy (Coughlin et al., 2007).

Assessment

Obtain a complete medical history from the patient, including diabetes, glucose control, previous ulcer history, changes in sensation, and overall foot health. The patient will generally present with a painless swelling of the lower extremity or foot. Often they cannot recall any injury or precipitating event leading up to the swelling (Houston, 2001). Perform a complete examination of the patient sitting and standing. Sensation is monitored by using a 5.07 Semmes Weinstein monofilament, the standard tool for assessing protective sensation. This simple tool is used in the office to assess the degree of sensory deficit in the patient; typically, the patient will not be able to detect this size of monofilament. Assess for pulse rate, skin temperature, callosities and ulcerations.

The Charcot foot may be in an acute, subacute, or chronic stage. The acute stage mimics cellulitis or a deep vein thrombosis. On physical exam, the foot or ankle will be swollen, warm to touch, and often red in color. Radiographs show fractures, joint subluxation, and fragmentation. Persistent swelling is the most consistent finding of a Charcot foot. In the subacute stage (also known as coalescence), there are varying degrees of bony deformity and new bone formation, as seen on x-ray. The foot is usually wider than normal and may have a classic "rocker bottom" look to it. Swelling will still be present but with a decrease in warmth and redness. Once the disease has progressed, it is easy to recognize radiographically. The chronic stage is characterized by consolidation of the bones, as seen on x-ray, with frequent deformity and resolution of the inflammatory response. In all these stages, pain is less than expected and never commensurate with the destructive changes. (See Figure 23.3.)

Figure 23.3. Charcot Foot

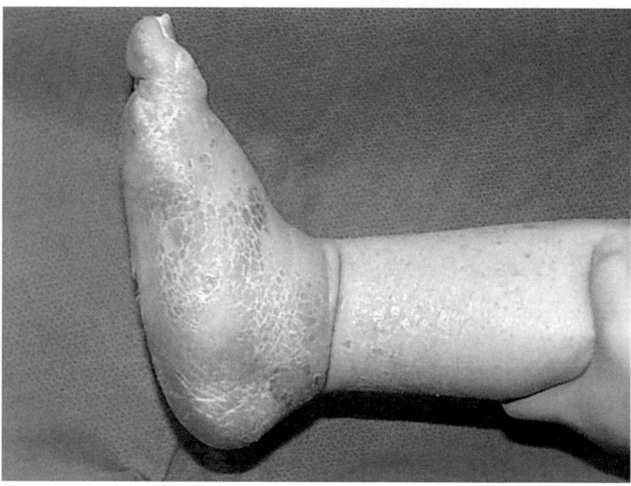

From Keith L. Wapner, MD. Reproduced with permission.

Common Therapeutic Modalities

The goal of treatment is to maintain a stable foot that can be placed in a shoe or brace. Treatment of the Charcot foot in the acute stage begins with immobilization (for example with a diabetic total contact cast) and elevation to control swelling. Weight-bearing status is dependent on each physician's protocol. In the sub-acute stage, a total contact brace is most often utilized. A Charcot restraint orthotic walker (CROW) or a molded AFO and a diabetic shoe are used to support the foot in the consolidation stage. The diabetic patient requires careful, regular maintenance and evaluation. Many Charcot patients need vascular and bony reconstruction. It is not uncommon for ulcers to develop, given the changing pressures on weight-bearing. Deformity may be so advanced that surgery is necessary, even to get the foot into a shoe. Surgery is generally warranted if there is severe biomechanical deformity, recurrent ulceration, or unmanageable instability (Houston, 2001). Surgery may involve excision of bony prominences, fusion, or realignment of bones. This can be accomplished by internal or external fixation.

Nursing Considerations

Nursing Diagnoses. Nursing diagnoses for this condition are expanded upon in the Appendix.

- Health behavior, risk-prone.
- Infection, risk for.
- Knowledge, deficit.
- Peripheral neurovascular dysfunction, risk for.
- Sensory perception: tactile, disturbed.
- Skin integrity, impaired.
- Walking, impaired.

Interventions. Patient education is critical with diabetic Charcot patients, as they are an at-risk population. Constant reinforcement of the signs and symptoms of Charcot is essential when working with this patient population. (See "The Diabetic Foot" in this chapter for a detailed discussion of proper foot care techniques for the diabetic patient.) The need for vigilant foot care is crucial in maintaining foot health. Patients must be instructed to check their feet daily, keep their feet clean and dry, and never walk barefoot given the possibility of injury from the lack of sensation. They should always wear appropriate shoes and seek treatment for any skin breaks as soon as possible. (See Table 23.3.)

The Diabetic Foot

Overview

The diabetic foot is one of the most challenging of all foot and ankle entities. Diabetic neuropathy is one of the most common complications of diabetes (Pinzur, 2008). Approximately 85% of diabetic patients who have an amputation have foot ulcers (Laborde, 2010). The effects of the diabetes extend to the sensory, motor, peripheral vascular, and autonomic systems. The sensory neuropathy of diabetes deprives the patient of early warning signs of pain or pressure from footwear, inadequate soft tissue padding, or infection. This neuropathy appears in a stocking-glove distribution in the feet and hands. The patient often complains of burning pain, usually bilateral and affects both hands and feet (Lotke, 2008).

The combination of peripheral vascular disease and autonomic neuropathy allows the skin to become contaminated and infected by normally nonpathogenic organisms. The duration of diabetes strongly affects the occurrence of neuropathy (Pinzur, 2008). Two percent of people with diabetes develop a Charcot joint (Lotke, 2008).

The structural deformity leads to areas of increased pressure that, when combined with lack of sensation, can lead to ulcers at advanced stages before they are even noticed. Risk factors include poor glycemic control, duration of diabetes, and advancing age (Burton & Tierney, 2007). Further risk factors include trauma, repetitive stress, thermal trauma, vascular occlusion, skin and nail conditions, gender, and social situations. Obesity and alcohol both have a negative effect on the diabetic foot (Coughlin et al., 2007). Many diabetic patients may have chronic health problems that further complicate their treatment. A team approach is very helpful in managing the diabetic patient. Some who may be included are the orthopedic surgeon, podiatrist, physiatrists, neurologists, primary care provider, endocrinologist, infectious disease, physical therapist, orthotist, wound care specialists, and the patient's family.

It is extremely important to educate patients on the importance of checking their feet twice a day. Glycemic control is the most important preventive strategy. Exercise is often encouraged to the level of the patient's ability.

Assessment

Included in the history and physical should be a very careful assessment of the foot to evaluate for deformity, such as hammertoes or claw toes, and history of foot pain or changes in sensation, previous ulcers, and infection. Specific questions should be asked regarding the care of their feet. Note should be taken regarding the glucose control, as well as a vascular and neurologic assessment. Evaluate for arterial insufficiency, such as claudication. The patient may complain of burning or searing pain in the foot, which is generally worse in the evening. The skin assessment will generally show allodynia and dry, scaly, thin skin. The loss of protective sensation is measured best with a 5.07 Semmes Weinstein monofilament test. Note should be made of the stocking-glove distribution. If ulcers are present, measurement should be obtained and wound care treatment established. Meggit and Wagner's classification for grading diabetic foot ulcers is widely used (see Table 23.4). Brodsky proposed a depth-ischemia classification that separates the two components of ulceration and ischemia (Myerson, 2000) (see Table 23.5).

Table 23.4. Meggit-Wagner Ulcer Classification

0	Preulceration lesions, healed ulcer, or bony deformity
1	Superficial ulcer; no subcutaneous tissue involvement
2	Full-thickness, ulcer; may expose bone, tendon, ligament, or joint capsule
3	Osteitis, abscess, or osteomyelitis
4	Gangrene of toe
5	Gangrene of foot

From Core Curriculum for Orthopaedic Nursing (6th Ed., p. 600), *by the National Association of Orthopaedic Nurses (NAON), 2007, Boston, MA: Pearson. Reproduced with permission.*

Table 23.5. University of Texas Staging System			
Under this system, a wound is assigned a stage based on the presence or absence of infection and ischemia, and a grade based on the depth of the wound. The higher the grade and stage, the greater the risk of amputation.			
Stage A	Clean wound	Grade 0	Preulcerative or postulcerative lesion, completely epithelized
Stage B	Nonischemic infected wounds	Grade I	Superficial wound, not involving tendon, capsule or bone
Stage C	Ischemic noninfected wounds	Grade II	Wound penetrating to bone and joint
Stage D	Ischemic infected wounds	Grade III	Wound penetrating to bone or joint

From Core Curriculum for Orthopaedic Nursing (6th Ed., p. 601), by the National Association of Orthopaedic Nurses (NAON), 2007, Boston, MA: Pearson. Reproduced with permission.

Some patients complain of weakness and issues of lack of coordination and poor balance. Evaluate for tendon imbalance, especially Achilles and gastrocnemius-soleus tightness. This imbalance can cause increased stress in the foot, thus callus or ulceration may develop (Laborde, 2010).

Standing radiographs will document the degree of deformity present. Nerve conduction studies will show the degree of neuropathy. The ankle-brachial index will detect commonly associated peripheral vascular disease.

Common Therapeutic Modalities

Treatment is centered on management of pain and sensory neuropathy. If an ulcer is present, the first and foremost concern is to offload that foot. Knee walker devices, wheelchairs, walkers, or crutches are all possibilities for this patient. There are a variety of off-loading shoes that may be appropriate. Shoes may need to be a full size larger than previously, due to the changes in the shape of the foot. Total contact casting is an effective treatment in skilled hands. This casting places a well-molded, minimally padded cast that maintains total contact with the entire foot and lower leg, effectively distributing the pressure evenly over the entire plantar surface. This method usually reduces edema. Frequent cast changes are required as the cast loosens. The total contact cast also protects the foot from further trauma. As swelling lessens, the patient may wear custom shoes or orthoses. A removable cast walker can be helpful, as it allows inspection of the feet.

The goal of surgical intervention, if needed, is to relieve pain and restore or improve function. This can be done by incision, debridement and drainage, or a reconstructive procedure to get the foot into some kind of shoe. Another form of surgical treatment is tendon lengthening, which is done to offload stress from the foot, thus promoting ulcer healing (Laborde, 2010). The surgery will create a plantar grade foot and stabilize the foot and ankle. Consideration must be given to the patient's ability to heal postoperatively. The risks of surgery must be weighed against the benefits. Will the quality of life be

Table 23.6. ADA Recommendations for Foot Health	
Check your feet every day.	Look at your bare feet for red spots, cuts, swelling, and blisters. If you cannot see the bottoms of your feet, use a mirror or ask someone for help
Be more active.	Plan your physical activity program with your health team.
Ask you doctor about Medicare coverage.	Speak with your doctor about coverage for special shoes.
Keep your skin soft and smooth.	Rub a thin coat of skin lotion over the tops and bottoms of your feet, but not between your toes. Read more about skin care.
Trim your toenails.	If you can see and reach your toenails, trim them straight across, and file the edges with an emery board or nail file
Wash your feet every day.	Dry them carefully, especially between the toes.
Wear shoes and socks at all times.	Never walk barefoot. Wear comfortable shoes that fit well and protect your feet. Check inside your shoes before wearing them. Make sure the lining is smooth and there are no objects inside.
Protect your feet from hot and cold.	Wear shoes at the beach or on hot pavement. Don't put your feet into hot water. Test water before putting your feet in it just as you would before bathing a baby. Never use hot water bottles, heating pads, or electric blankets. You can burn your feet without realizing it.
Keep the blood flowing to your feet.	Wiggle your toes and move your ankles up and down for 5 minutes, 2-3 times a day. Don't cross your legs for long periods of time. Don't smoke.
Get started now.	Begin taking good care of your feet today. Set a time every day to check your feet.

From "Take Care of Your Feet for a Lifetime" by the American Diabetes Association (ADA), 2011, http://www.cdc.gov/diabetes/pubs/estimates11.htm#13

improved after the surgery, including an extended non-weight-bearing period? Surgical risks include nonunion, malunion, wound healing problems, failure of fixation due to poor quality bone, infection, osteomyelitis, and vascular compromise leading to amputation.

Nursing Considerations

Nursing Diagnoses. Nursing diagnoses for this condition are expanded upon in the Appendix.

- Infection, risk for.
- Injury, risk for.
- Knowledge, deficit.
- Mobility, impaired.
- Peripheral neurovascular dysfunction, risk for.
- Sensory perception: tactile, disturbed.
- Skin integrity, impaired.
- Sleep pattern, disturbed.

Interventions. The prevention of diabetic foot disorders begins with the proper screening of patients and providing education concerning complication of risk factors (Pinzur, 2008). All care providers must be involved, including the family, to have a positive outcome. Screening must be frequent, and regular foot examinations are key. Patients must be educated on foot care and the need for consistency. Instruct the patient on safe ambulation to prevent falls. Share with the patient the recommendations on good foot health from the American Diabetes Association (ADA, 2011) (see Table 23.6).

Summary

Foot and ankle conditions occur across the life span. The causes can be rooted in systemic disease, trauma, or improper footwear. These conditions run the gamut, from skin lesions (such as plantar warts) to complete bony destruction of the foot (as seen in Charcot's arthropathy). These conditions affect mobility, thus causing even the simplest concern to influence lifestyle.

References

American Diabetes Association (ADA). (2011). *Take care of your feet for a lifetime* (A Publication of the National Diabetes Education Program). Retrieved April 29, 2011, from http://www.cdc.gov/diabetes/pubs/estimates11.htm#13

Andres, B.M. & Murrell, G.A. (2008). Treatment of tendinopathy: What works, what does not, and what is on the horizon. *Clinical Orthopaedic and Related Research, 466*(7), 1539-1554.

Bohne, W.H. (1999) Amputations around the foot and ankle. In E. Craig (Ed.), *Clinical Orthopedics* (pp. 955-962). Philadelphia, PA: Lippincott, Williams, Wilkins.

Buchanan, M. (2009, February). Pes planus. Retrieved May 2, 2011, from emedicine.medscape.com/article

Burton, N. & Tierney, C. (2007). Foot and ankle. In National Association of Orthopaedic Nurses (NAON). *Core Curriculum for Orthopaedic Nursing* (6th ed., pp. 577-599). Boston, MA: Pearson Publishing.

Cole, G. (2010, August). *Plantar Warts.* Retrieved April 20, 2001, from http:www.emedicinehealth.com

Coughlin, M.J., Mann, R.A., & Salzman, C.L. (2007). *Surgery of the Foot and Ankle* (8th ed.). Philadelphia, PA: Mosby.

Craig, E.V. (1999). *Clinical Orthopaedics*. Philadelphia, PA: Lippincott, Williams, Wilkins.

Cretnik, A., Kosir, R., & Kosanovic, M. (2010). Incidence and outcome of operatively treated achilles tendon rupture in the elderly. *Foot and Ankle International, 31*(1), 14-17.

Delee, J.C., Drez, D. Jr., & Miller, M.D. (2010). *Orthopedic Sports Medicine, Principals and Practice* (3rd ed.). Philadelphia, PA: Saunders Elsevier.

Diehl, J.W. (2011), Platelet-rich plasma therapy in chronic achilles tendinopathy. *Techniques in Foot and Ankle Surgery, 10*(1), 2-6.

DiGiovanni, B.F., Nawoczenski, D.A., Malay, D.A., Graci, P.A., Williams, T.T., Wilding, G.E., & Baumhauer, J.F. (2006). Plantar fascia-specific stretching exercise improves outcomes in patients with chronic plantar fasciitis: A prospective clinical trial with two-year follow-up. *Journal of Bone and Joint Surgery, 88*(8), 1775-1781.

Deluccio, J. (2006). Instrument assisted soft tissue mobilization utilizing graston technique: A physical therapist's perspective. *Orthopaedic Physical Therapy Practice, 18*(3), 32-34.

Elsner, A., Barg A., Stufkens, S.A., & Hinterman, B. (2010). Lambrinudi arthrodesis with posterior tibialis transfer in adult drop-foot. *Foot and Ankle International, 31*(1), 30-37.

Hart, E.S., DeAsla, R.J., & Grottkau, B.E. (2008). Current concepts in the treatment of hallux valgus. *Orthopaedic Nursing, 27*(5), 274-280.

Houston, D.S. & Curran, J. (2001) Charcot Foot. *Orthopedic Nursing, 20*(1), 11-15.

Hughes, R., Ali, K., Jones, H., Kendall, S. & Connell, D. (2007). Treatment of Morton's neuroma with alcohol injection under sonographic guidance: Follow-up of 101 cases. *American Journal of Roentgenology, 188*(6), 1535-1539.

Ibrahim, M.I., Donatelli, R.A., Schmitz, C., Hellman, M.A., & Buxbaum, F. (2010), Chronic plantar faciitis treated with two sessions of radial extracorporeal shock wave therapy. *Foot and Ankle International, 31*(5), 391-397.

Irwin, T.A. (2010). Current concepts review; Insertional achilles tendonopathy. *Foot and Ankle International, 31*(10), 933-939.

Laborde, J.M. (2010). Tendon lengthening for neuropathic foot problems. *Orthopedics, 33*(5), 319-326.

League, A.C. (2008). Current concepts review: Plantar faciitis. *Foot and Ankle International, 29*(3), 358-366.

Mayo Clinic. (2010). *Common Warts*. Retrieved May 2, 2011, from www.mayoclinic.com

Myerson, M.S. (2000). *Foot and Ankle Disorders*. Philadelphia, PA: WB Saunders Co.

National Association of Orthpaedic Nurses (NAON). (2007). *Core Curriculum for Orthopaedic Nursing* (6th ed.). Boston, MA: Pearson Publishing.

O'Connor, P.L. & Schaller, T.N. (2001) *Footworks II: The patient's guide to the foot and ankle*. Portage, MI: O'Connor.

Pakarinen, H.J., Flinkila, T., Ohtonen, P., & Ristiniemi, J.Y. (2011). Stability criteria for nonoperative ankle fracture management. *Foot and Ankle International, 32*(2), 141-147.

Paoloni, J.A. & Murrell, G.A.C. (2007). Three-year follow-up study of topical glyceryl trinitrate treatment of chronic noninsertional achilles tendinopathy. *Foot and Ankle International, 28*(10), 1064-1068.

Pinzur, M.S. (2008). *Orthopaedic Knowledge Update Foot and Ankle*. Rosemont, IL: American Academy of Orthopaedic Surgeons.

Reddy, S. & Okereke, E., (2008). Fractured fibula; Nondisplaced avulsion fracture. In P.A. Lotke, J.A. Aboud, J. Ende, J. (Eds.) *Lippincott's Primary Care Orthopaedics* (pp. 137-145). Philadelphia, PA: Lippincott Williams & Wilkins.

Smalls, K. (2009). Ankle sprains and fractures in adults. *Orthopedic Nursing, 28*(6), 314-320.

Thordarson, D.B. (2004) *Orthopaedic Surgery Essentials, Foot & Ankle*. Philadelphia, PA: Lippincott Williams & Wilkins.

Chapter 24

The Orthopaedic Nursing Certification Exams: Strategies for Success

Jan Foecke, MS, RN, ONC

Objectives

- Describe the benefits of orthopaedic nursing certification.
- Identify strategies for certification examination preparation and success.
- Define resources to prepare for an orthopaedic certification examination.
- Review methods of reducing test anxiety.

According to the American Nurses Credentialing Center (ANCC, 2010a), "Certification is the process by which a nongovernmental agency or an association grants recognition to an individual who has met certain predetermined qualifications" (p. 4). Nurses achieve certification credentials through specialty education, specific hours of specialty experience, and successful completion of a qualifying exam. Many specialty nursing organizations also have certification bodies that grant certification credentials to nurses. The American Board of Nursing Specialties (ABNS) provides consumer protection by establishing and maintaining standards for professional specialty nursing certification (Orthopaedic Nursing Certification Board [ONCB®], 2010d). The robust and extensive test development process results in fair and accurate measurement of professional competency through certification examination (ANCC, 2010a).

Benefits of Certification

Certification in orthopaedic nursing is a formal process by which the Orthopaedic Nursing Certification Board (ONCB®) validates an orthopaedic nurse's knowledge, skills, and abilities in a specific role based on predetermined standards. According to the ONCB® (2010b), the decision to take one of the orthopaedic nursing certification examinations represents significant progress in career advancement and a personal commitment toward providing quality orthopaedic nursing care. Specialty nursing certification has become more essential, according to goals listed in the ANCC Magnet Recognition Program® (2010b), for individual nurses as well as for facilities that are pursuing the Malcolm Baldrige National Quality Award, Joint Commission accreditation, or grant funding (ANCC, 2010c).

Additionally, successful completion of an orthopaedic certification examination yields many potential benefits, such as those compiled from the ABNS (2005), ANCC (2010c), and the ONCB® (2010c):

- Elevated level of orthopaedic nursing knowledge.
- Enhanced confidence in one's orthopaedic clinical practice.
- Increased sense of pride and professional accomplishment.
- Improved readiness to meet the specialty demands of the patient.
- Higher quality patient care, professional credibility.
- Recognition from peers and other health care clinicians.
- Professional position security.
- Career advancement.
- Financial rewards and discounts.
- Advancement of the nursing profession through recognition of professional achievement.

Orthopaedic Nursing Knowledge

Knowledge development occurs through various methods of study (education) and experience. Successfully passing a certification exam requires specific nursing knowledge, valuable test-taking skills, and self-knowledge. A wide array of orthopaedic nursing knowledge is required to achieve an orthopaedic certification credential.

The ONCB® (2010a; 2010c) lists eligibility requirements to take orthopaedic nursing certification exams in several documents. Those requirements are listed in Table 24.1. There is also an exam candidate handbook available from the ONCB® website (2010c) and a Frequently Asked Questions document (2010a) that provides additional information about the exams and orthopaedic nursing certification.

Self-Assessment

Take an inventory of your orthopaedic nursing knowledge and experience to guide your study plan. Assess specific learning needs by reviewing test blueprints on the ONCB® website (found at www.oncb.org), which provides the distribution of test content areas and objectives to direct study topics. The test blueprint matrix displays the sample distribution of test items on the exam. Avoid spending significant time thoroughly reviewing a topic if just a few topic questions will be on the exam. Instead, spend the most time studying areas in which you may have limited knowledge or experience and that comprise a considerable number of questions on the exam (ONCB®, 2009). Study in short bursts and take breaks (Hazard & Millonig, n.d.; ONCB®, 2009).

Study Timeline

ONCB® (2009) suggests developing a study timeline to offer an at-a-glance view of topics for review in chronological order. Develop an effective timeline by working backward from the intended exam date and noting a visual study plan on a calendar. A timeline can assist to prioritize those topics in need of extra attention (Davis et al., 2004). Checking off topics and their dates can yield a sense of accomplishment as one works toward the successful completion of a certification exam.

Getting Organized

The Orthopaedic Nurses Certification (ONC®), Orthopaedic Clinical Nurse Specialist Certification (OCNS-C®), and Orthopaedic Nurse Practitioner Certification (ONP-C®) examinations should be given serious preparation planning in order to ensure successful completion and subsequent recognition as a certified orthopaedic nurse, orthopaedic clinical nurse specialist, or orthopaedic nurse practitioner. There are numerous strategies to plan for certification success (Ludwig, 2004; Martinez, 2010; ONCB®, 2009; 2010b). A study group can offer interactivity for enhanced learning and anxiety reduction. The group can be initiated through contacts with fellow orthopaedic nurses, local National Association of Orthopaedic Nurses (NAON) chapter members, or other NAON members via the online NAON discussion forums. Group study can occur via face-to-face meetings, telephone conference calls, e-mails, or electronic virtual meetings. Some prefer individual study methods (Davis, Gonzales, Hawk, Rourke, & Roberts, 2004). Those methods include reading the *Orthopaedic Nursing* journal and taking CE tests, attending orthopaedic conferences, reviewing NAON products, participating in a review course, taking a practice exam, and conversing with expert orthopaedic nurses about difficult practice questions.

Hazard and Millonig (n.d.) suggest the following for study preparation: 1) create a quiet, undisturbed environment to set the stage for valuable study; 2) organize study materials; 3) rank content for areas of personal strengths or weaknesses; 4) develop a study plan; and 5) use time wisely. Use of current study resources (described later in this chapter) aids in overall orthopaedic nursing content retention. Take notes to review highlights at a later date (ONCB®, 2009). Take a practice exam to increase understanding about test format. Consult with orthopaedic nursing experts to clarify content areas that may be difficult to fully understand. Participate in a review course to reinforce knowledge about familiar topics and offer new knowledge about less familiar ones. Keep study materials close at hand for review while stuck in traffic, waiting for appointments, or even during television commercial breaks (ONCB®, 2009). Find a method of reward for adhering to the identified study plan and timeline.

Table 24.1. Eligibility Requirements for Taking Orthopaedic Nursing Certification Exams

ONC® Exam	OCNS-C® and ONP-C Exams®
Licensed registered nurse.	Licensed registered nurse.
Practice of at least 2 years.	Practice of at least 3 years.
1000 practice hours in orthopaedics within the last 3 years.	Master's degree with qualifications for APN licensure within the state of practice.
	1,500 practice hours for the APN with the ONC® credential.
	2,500 practice hours for the APN with no ONC® credential.

Test-Taking Strategies

Hazard and Millonig (n.d.) note the following effective test-taking strategies:

- Read the test directions carefully.
- Identify the purpose of the question.
- Recognize the parts of the question.
- Acknowledge the key words in the question.
- Distinguish the item type.
- Determine an educated guess.
- The ONCB® certification exams are offered by computer method only. Benefits to computer testing include flexibility of when to take the exam and earlier delivery of test results.

Returning to a question is allowed on the ONCB® exams. It may be best to answer all the easy questions first and then go back to the ones that require additional consideration (Martinez, 2010). Keep track of time in order to answer every question (Davis et al., 2004; Martinez, 2010), and focus on one question at a time (Davis et al., 2004). The ONCB® (2009) considers it safe to allow 1 minute per test item and notes that higher scores are achieved by those who answer all questions on an exam. Test-takers will not know which questions are experimental and not counted in the overall exam score (Davis et al., 2004). The ONCB® uses experimental questions on the orthopaedic certification exams (2009). Some items are considered experimental after they are validated with reputable references and inserted into the exam. The items are answered by the test-taker, but not counted in scoring. The results of those pilot questions are analyzed for test statistic purposes. The items are reviewed and may be discarded or added to the exam in the future. This process keeps the exam current with changes in practice, technology, and knowledge (ONCB®, 2009). Table 24.2 lists additional test-taking strategies.

Table 24.2. Additional Test-Taking Strategies

Mentally answering each question before reading the options may prevent confusion related to the answer options.	Ludwig, 2004; Martinez, 2010; ONCB®, 2009
Rephrasing a difficult question may be helpful as long as the meaning does not change.	Martinez, 2010
Remember that a question may contain more information than actually needed to answer the question, thus eliminating the distracting information in the question is useful. Review all answer options before selecting a final choice.	Ludwig, 2004; Martinez, 2010; Davis et al., 2004
Generally, words such as never, always, only, best, worst, all of the above, and none of the above are not used in a question stem, but if they are, select the answer option while carefully considering those type of words	Ludwig, 2004; Martinez, 2010, Davis et al., 2004
Using qualifiers in an answer option such as never, always, only, best, worst, all of the above, and none of the above usually means that it is the wrong answer.	Davis et al., 2004
It may be helpful to turn a multiple choice option into a true or false statement for option elimination.	Davis et al., 2004
It is likely that one answer option is correct in a pair of options that have opposite meanings.	Davis et al., 2004.
It may be safest to select the answer option that causes the other to happen.	ONCB®, 2009.
Usually, the longer, more inclusive answer is often the correct one when forced to guess about the answer options.	Martinez, 2010; Davis et al., 2004.
Repeating key words in the stem and in an option may signify the correct answer.	Davis et al., 2004
Resist the urge to change an answer unless there is certainty of its inaccuracy because the answer that first comes to mind is often the correct one.	Martinez, 2010
Changing an answer is recommended only if the reason for the change is known.	ONCB® (2009)

Self-Knowledge

The Stanford Encyclopedia of Philosophy (2008) describes self-knowledge as "knowledge of one's particular mental states, including one's beliefs, desires, and sensations." Recognizing personal characteristics can be very helpful in reducing anxiety about one's approach to taking an exam. Only the individual can change his or her own attitude. Let's examine methods of reducing anxiety and investigate how specific test-taking personalities affect the exam experience and success.

Test-Taking Personality

Hazard and Millonig (n.d.) believe that each of us has developed a certain set of behaviors related to taking tests. Some behaviors are obstructive, and others are beneficial. Identify desirable and undesirable behaviors in order to improve overall test performance. Make a list of how to address the problematic behaviors, and implement those actions during exam preparation and completion. Obstructive behaviors include ineffective studying related to procrastination, rushing through the exam, progressing through the exam too slowly, personalizing exam questions and/or answer options, over-analyzing exam questions, second-guessing exam answer options, and reading too much into the exam question or answer option (Hazard & Millonig, n.d.).

Anxiety Reduction

Reducing anxiety is very important for a successful certification exam outcome (Hazard & Millonig, n.d.). Some methods of anxiety reduction are simple, and others are more complex. Table 24.3 displays some anxiety reduction techniques that may be useful before and during exams.

Table 24.3. Sample Anxiety Reduction Techniques for Taking Certification Exams

Anxiety Reduction Strategy	Source
Create an item checklist of what to bring.	Ludwig, 2004
Get a good night's sleep.	Davis et al., 2004; Ludwig, 2004; Martinez, 2010; ONCB®, 2009
Select a healthy diet the day before and morning of the exam.	Davis et al., 2004; Ludwig, 2004; ONCB®, 2009
Wear comfortable clothing.	Ludwig, 2004; ONCB®, 2009
Bring necessary items.	Ludwig, 2004; ONCB®, 2009
Arrive to the testing site early	Martinez, 2010; ONCB®, 2009
Practice relaxation breathing, visualization.	Davis et al., 2004; Ludwig, 2004
Use positive self-talk.	Ludwig, 2004; Hazard & Millonig, n.d.; ONCB®, 2009

Filling the car with gas (if driving to the exam) may seem simple, but running out of gas would be a dreadful occurrence on the day of the exam. Making a checklist of all items to do before the exam and what to take along to the exam can be invaluable. Items to take along may include those such as two forms of identification (Martinez, 2010) including a photo ID, exam permit, payment for parking and the exam, a watch, ear plugs, eye glasses, two pens/pencils, chewing gum, tissues, medications, and a bottle of water. Do not bring electronic devices into the testing room (ONCB®, 2009). Relaxing the evening before the exam should be a priority, without late studying to ensure a good night's sleep. Allow for exam room temperature fluctuations. Eat a meal that facilitates energy, including vegetables and a source of protein. Use positive visualization and remember that past clinical experience can aid in successfully answering exam questions.

Study Resources

Visit the ONCB® website (www.oncb.org) for information about exam description, eligibility, fees, application/testing sites, and preparation, as well as recommended study resource lists. The *ONC® Online Practice Module* is a diagnostic tool used to assess strengths and areas for improvement related to orthopaedic nursing knowledge. It is a 50-item multiple choice practice test that is similar in content and level of difficulty to the orthopaedic nursing certification examination. The ONC OR/Peds/Neuromuscular/Congenital Module is another 50-item multiple choice practice test that can be used to prepare for the exam. The *Examination Preparation Guide* (2009)/*Test-Taking Strategies CD* (Davis et al., 2004) combination packet can assist the test-taker related to content, structure, preparation for the orthopaedic nursing certification examination, and strategies for question analysis that result in successful answers.

NAON (2010) offers a variety of study resources related to orthopaedic nursing certification exams via the Online Store (www.orthonurse.org). The *Core Curriculum for Orthopaedic Nursing* (7th ed.) was specially designed as a comprehensive review text for orthopaedic nursing certification examinations. There are online review questions that accompany the *Core* to test knowledge of its content. The *Orthopaedic Nursing Self-Assessment CD* (3rd ed.), a compilation of case studies and nearly 600 questions and answers about all major musculoskeletal disorders, was created to prepare those who wish to take an orthopaedic nursing certification exam. The *Orthopaedic Operating Room Manual* (2nd ed.) is a thorough reference for novice to expert orthopaedic operating room nurses. For an overview of basic musculoskeletal anatomy, common adult orthopaedic conditions, and appropriate nursing assessment and care, *An Introduction to Orthopaedic Nursing* (4th ed.) manual is a good choice. There are corresponding online questions to test its content knowledge. *Orthopaedic Core Competencies: Across the Lifespan* (3rd ed.) can be

Figure 24.4. Study Resources
Agency for Healthcare Research and Quality. (2011). *Evidence-based practice*. Retrieved from http://www.ahrq.gov/clinic/epcix.htm#reports
Hodgson, B.B., & Kizior, R.J. (2011). *Saunders nursing drug handbook 2012*. St. Louis, MO: Elsevier Saunders. OR EQUIVALENT GENERAL REFERENCE
Kurkowski, C. (Ed.). (2003). *Orthopaedic operating room manual* (2nd ed.). Pitman, NJ: Anthony J. Jannetti.
Kunkler, C. (Ed.). (2012). *Orthopaedic nursing core competencies: Across the lifespan* (3rd ed.). Chicago, IL: National Association of Orthopaedic Nurses.
Mosher, C. (Ed.). (2010). *Introduction to orthopaedic nursing* (4th ed.). Chicago, IL: National Association of Orthopaedic Nurses.
National Association of Orthopaedic Nurses. (2012). *Core curriculum for orthopaedic nursing* (7th ed.). Boston, MA: Pearson.
National Association of Orthopaedic Nurses. (2009). *Orthopaedic nursing self-assessment CD* (3rd ed.). Chicago, IL: National Association of Orthopaedic Nurses.
Orthopaedic Nurses Certification Board. (2008). *ONC® online practice module*. Columbia, SC: Orthopaedic Nurses Certification Board.
Orthopaedic Nurses Certification Board. (2009). *Examination preparation guide/Test-taking strategies CD*. Columbia, SC: Orthopaedic Nurses Certification Board.
Orthopaedic Nurses Certification Board. (2011). ONC OR/peds/neuromuscular/congenital module. Columbia, SC: Orthopaedic Nurses Certification Board.
Orthopaedic Nursing Journal (2008-2011). Hagerstown, MD: Lippincott Williams & Wilkins.
Polit, D.F., & Beck, C.T. (2009). *Essentials of nursing research: Methods, appraisal, and utilization* (6th ed.). Philadelphia: Lippincott Williams & Wilkins.
Sarwark, J.F. (Ed.). (2010). *Essentials of musculoskeletal care (4th ed.)*. Rosemont, IL: American Academy of Orthopaedic Surgeons and Elk Grove Village, IL: American Academy of Pediatrics.
The Joint Commission. (2011). *National patient safety goals*. Retrieved from http://www.jointcommission.org/patientsafety/nationalpatientsafetygoals/
The National Quality Forum (2011). *NQF-endorsed® standards*. Retrieved from http://www.qualityforum.org/Measures_List.aspx
Weinstein, S.L. & Buckwalter, J.A. (2005). *Turek's orthopaedics: Principles and their application* (6th ed.). Philadelphia: Lippincott Williams & Wilkins.

NAON publications are available from the online store (www.orthonurse.org) or 800.289.6266; ONCB® publications are available from the eStore (www.oncb.org) or 888.561.6622.

Contact NAON to enroll in an orthopaedic nursing or advanced orthopaedic nursing review course. Review courses are offered at the NAON Annual Congress, at regional locations, and online.

used to assess proficiency in major orthopaedic clinical topics, including pediatrics, complications, and topics for advanced practice nurses.

Articles from the last several years in the *Orthopaedic Nursing* journal can be used to obtain timely information about orthopaedic nursing research and literature findings. The Joint Commission National Patient Safety Goals, the National Quality Forum-Endorsed Standards, and the Agency for Healthcare Research and Quality's Evidence-Based Practice Reports help to guide priorities related to orthopaedic patient care.

Specific to the ONC® exam is the *Saunders Nursing Drug Handbook 2011*, which provides detailed coverage such as IV drug administration, nursing considerations, fixed combinations, and guidance for clinical priorities and prescription decisions.

Several additional resources are meant to assist those preparing to take the OCNS-C and ONP-C exams. One is the online *AAOS Clinical Guidelines*, which enhances the diagnosis and treatment of musculoskeletal conditions. Another resource is *Essentials of Nursing Research: Methods, Appraisal, and Utilization* (6th ed.) that can be used to better read, understand, analyze, and evaluate research reports in nursing practice and read, interpret, and critique systematic reviews related to evidence-based practice. *Essentials of Musculoskeletal Care* (4th ed.) provides clinical information to make confident decisions related to patient diagnosis and management for many musculoskeletal conditions. Finally, Turek's *Orthopaedics: Principles and Their Application* (6th ed.) completes the list of study aids that are specific to the advanced practice exams, offering a general overview of pediatric and adult orthopaedics. See Figure 24.4 for a listing of ONCB exam study resources.

Summary

A successful test-taker knows how to prepare for and take an exam (Hazard & Millonig, n.d.). Martinez (2010) believes that preparing, practicing, following through, and relaxing are the key steps to successful testing. Additional strategies are helpful. Organize study materials and space. Make use of the many study resources that are available. Recognize how you best study and take an exam. Develop an attainable timeline. Enhance orthopaedic nursing knowledge. Create better test taking skills and ways to reduce anxiety.

After sitting for the exam, celebrate! Reward for completing the exam and accepting congratulations upon achieving the desired certification credential is important. Reward signifies a positive outcome and is deserved for a job well done (Ludwig, 2004). If a second attempt at an exam is necessary, remember that it is not the end of the world. Rather, it is an opportunity to further increase orthopaedic nursing knowledge through additional study. Successfully passing the next exam and attaining the desired certification credential will have even more meaning.

References

American Board of Nursing Specialties. (2005). *Value of certification survey executive summary*. Retrieved from http://www.nursingcertification.org/pdf/executive_summary.pdf

American Nurses Credentialing Center. (2010a). *An overview of ANCC nursing certification*. Silver Spring, MD: American Nurses Credentialing Center.

American Nurses Credentialing Center. (2010b). *Magnet recognition program® FAQ: Data and expected outcomes*. Retrieved from http://nursecredentialing.org/FunctionalCategory/FAQ/DEO-FAQ.aspx

American Nurses Credentialing Center. (2010c). *Why certify?* Silver Spring, MD: American Nurses Credentialing Center.

Davis, D., Gonzales, C., Hawk, D., Rourke, K., & Roberts, D. (2004). *Getting rid of the "fear factor": Test-taking strategies for the ONC Exam*. Presentation at NAON®'s 24th Annual Congress in Nashville, TN.

Hazard, N. & Millonig, V. (n.d.). *Test taking strategies and techniques*. Retrieved from http://www.resptrec.org/resources/Test_Strategies.pdf

Ludwig, C. (2004). *Preparing for certification: Test-taking strategies*. Retrieved from http://findarticles.com/p/articles/mi_m0FSS/is_2_13/ai_n17206929/?tag=content;col1

Martinez, A. (2010). *Test taking strategies*. Retrieved from http://www.gocertify.com/article/strategies.shtml

National Association of Orthopaedic Nurses. (2010). *NAON® orders information*. Retrieved from https://www.orthonurse.org/eOrders/tabid/235/Default.aspx

Orthopaedic Nurses Certification Board. (2009). *ONC® examination preparation guide*. Columbia, SC: Orthopaedic Nurses Certification Board.

Orthopaedic Nurses Certification Board. (2010a). *Exam FAQs*. Retrieved from http://www.oncb.org/images/FAQ2010.doc

Orthopaedic Nurses Certification Board. (2010b). *Exam preparation*. Retrieved from http://www.oncb.org/onccertification/exampreparation.html

Orthopaedic Nurses Certification Board. (2010d). *ONCB and ABNS*. Retrieved from http://www.oncb.org/aboutoncb.html

Stanford's Encyclopedia of Philosophy. (2008). Retrieved from http://plato.stanford.edu/entries/self-knowledge/

Appendix

Christina Kurkowski, MS, ONC, CNOR, ANP-C, ONP-C

Nursing Diagnosis (NANDA): Activity Intolerance; Activity Intolerance, Risk for		
Orthopaedic Conditions*	**Nursing Intervention Classifications (NIC)**	**Nursing Outcome Classifications (NOC)**
Chapter 8: Orthopaedic Complications Hemorrhage/Significant Blood Loss **Chapter 9: Orthopaedic Infections** Osteomyelitis Septic Arthritis Prosthetic Joint Infections Bone and Joint/Extrapulmonary Tuberculosis Skin and Soft Tissue Infection **Chapter 10: Therapeutic Modalities** Braces/Orthotics/Orthoses **Chapter 11: Pediatrics** Duchene's Muscular Dystrophy **Chapter 13: Arthritis and Connective Tissue Disorders** Juvenile Arthritis Rheumatoid Arthritis Osteoarthritis Polymyalgia Rheumatica Rheumatic Fever **Chapter 15: Orthopaedic Trauma** Spine Fractures Pelvic Fractures Amputations **Chapter 16: Tumors of the Musculoskeletal System** Benign Lesions Primary Malignant Tumors **Chapter 17: The Spine** Scoliosis Kyphosis Herniated Nucleus Pulposus Degenerative Disc Disease Spinal Stenosis Spondylosis Spondylolithesis Failed Back Surgery Syndrome Spinal Fractures **Chapter 18: The Shoulder** Impingement Syndrome Rotator Cuff Tears Arthritis Shoulder Instability Adhesive Capsulitis Glenoid Hypoplasia *(continued next page)*	**Body Mechanics Promotion:** Facilitating the use of posture and movement in daily activities to prevent fatigue and musculoskeletal strain or injury **Energy Management:** Regulating energy use to treat or prevent fatigue and optimize function **Environmental Management:** Manipulation of the patient's surroundings for therapeutic benefit, sensory appeal, and psychological well-being **Environmental Management:** Comfort: Manipulation of the patient's surrounding the promotion of optimal comfort **Environmental Management:** Home Preparation: Preparing the home and safe and effective delivery of care **Exercise Promotion:** Facilitation of regular physical activity to maintain or advance to a higher level of fitness and health **Exercise Promotion:** Stretching: Facilitation of systematic slow stretch-and-hold muscle exercises to induce relaxation, prepare muscles/joints for more vigorous exercise, or increase total-body flexibility **Exercise Therapy:** Ambulation: Promotion of and assistance with walking to maintain or restore autonomic and voluntary body functions during treatment and recovery from illness or injury **Exercise Therapy:** Balance: Use of specific activities, postures, and movements to maintain, enhance, or restore balance **Exercise Therapy:** Joint Mobility: Use of active or passive body movement to maintain or restore joint flexibility **Exercise Therapy:** Muscle Control: Use of specific activity or exercise protocols to enhance or restore controlled body movement **Home Maintenance Assistance:** Helping the patient/family to maintain the home as a clean, safe, and pleasant place to live **Pain Management:** Alleviation of pain or reduction in pain to a level of comfort that is acceptable to the patient **Self-Care Assistance:** Assisting another to perform activities of daily living **Self-Care Assistance:** IADL: Assisting in instructing a person to perform instrumental activities of daily living (IADL) needed to function in the community **Teaching:** Prescribed Activity/Exercise: Preparing a patient to achieve and/or maintain a prescribed level of activity	**Activity Tolerance:** Physiologic response to energy-consuming movements with daily activities **Endurance:** Capacity to sustain activity **Energy Conservation:** Personal actions to manage energy for initiating and sustaining activity **Fatigue Level:** Severity of observed or reported prolonged generalized fatigue **Physical Fitness:** Performance of physical activities with vigor **Psychomotor Energy:** Personal drive and energy to maintain activities of daily living, nutrition, and personal safety **Rest:** Quantity and pattern of diminished activity for mental and physical rejuvenation **Self-Care: Activities of Daily Living:** Ability to perform the most basic physical tasks and personal care activities independently with or without assistive device **Self-Care: Instrumental Activities of Daily Living (IADL):** Ability to perform activities need to function in the home or community independently with or without assistive device

Nursing Diagnosis (NANDA): Activity Intolerance; Activity Intolerance, Risk for *(continued)*		
Orthopaedic Conditions*	**Nursing Intervention Classifications (NIC)**	**Nursing Outcome Classifications (NOC)**
Chapter 21: The Hip, Femur & Pelvis Hip Fractures Hip Arthroplasty Hip Resurfacing Arthroplasty Hemiarthroplasty/Bipolar Replacement Hip Arthroscopy Femoro-Acetabular Impingement Hip Dislocation Hip Girdlestone Psuedoarthrosis Femoral Shaft Fractures Pelvic Fracture **Chapter 23: The Foot & Ankle** Ankle sprains Pes Planus Pes Cavus Osteoarthritis	*(see page 620)*	*(see page 620)*

Nursing Diagnosis (NANDA): Airway Clearance, Ineffective		
Orthopaedic Conditions*	**Nursing Intervention Classifications (NIC)**	**Nursing Outcome Classifications (NOC)**
Chapter 6: Immobility Respiratory Issues **Chapter 8: Orthopaedic Complications** Hospital Acquired Pneumonia	**Airway Management:** Facilitation of patency of air passages **Airway Suctioning:** Removal of airway secretions by inserting a suction catheter into the patient's oral airway and/or trachea **Aspiration Precautions:** Prevention or minimization of risk factors in the patient at risk for aspiration **Cough Enhancement:** Promotion of deep inhalation by the patient with subsequent generation of high intrathoracic pressures and compression of the underlying lung parenchyma for forceful expulsion of air **Positioning:** Deliberate placement of the patient or body part to promote physiological and/or psychological well-being **Respiratory Monitoring:** Collection and analysis of patient data to ensure airway patency and adequate gas exchange **Ventilation Assistance:** Promotion of an optimal spontaneous breathing pattern that maximizes oxygen and carbon dioxide exchange in the lungs	**Aspiration Prevention:** Personal actions to prevent the passage of fluid and solid particles into the lung **Respiratory Status: Airway Patency:** Open, clear tracheobronchial passages for air exchange **Respiratory Status: Ventilation:** Movement of air in and out of the lungs

Nursing Diagnosis (NANDA): Anxiety		
Orthopaedic Conditions*	**Nursing Intervention Classifications (NIC)**	**Nursing Outcome Classifications (NOC)**
Chapter 8: Complications Venous Thromboembolism Fat Emboli Syndrome **Chapter 11: Pediatrics** Achondroplasia Arthrogryposis Multiplex Congenita Blount's Disease Cerebral Palsy Clubfoot Developmental Dysplasia of the Hip Genu Valgum/Genu Varum Legg-Calve-Perthes Disease Metatarsus Adductus Neurofibromatosis Osgood-Schlatter Diease Osteogenesis Imperfecta Slipped Capital Femoral Epiphysis Torsional Issues **Chapter 15: Orthopaedic Trauma** Amputations Soft Trauma Dislocations/Subluxations Strains Sprains **Chapter 16: Tumors of the Musculoskeletal System** Benign Lesions Primary Malignant Tumors **Chapter 17: The Spine** Scoliosis Kyphosis **Chapter 18: The Shoulder** Fractures of the Shoulder Sprains, Strains, Contusions, Separations Sprengel's Deformity Referred Visceral Somatic Pain **Chapter 21: The Hip, Femur & Pelvis** Hip Fractures Hip Arthroplasty Hip Arthroscopy Femoro-Acetabular Impingement Hip Girdlestone Psuedoarthrosis Proximal Femoral Osteotomy Femoral Shaft Fractures Pelvic Fracture **Chapter 23: The Foot & Ankle** Pes Planus	**Active Listening:** Attending closely to and attaching significance to a patient' s verbal and nonverbal messages **Anticipatory Guidance:** Preparation of patient for an anticipated developmental and/or situational crisis **Anxiety Reduction:** Minimizing apprehension, dread, foreboding, or uneasiness related to an unidentified source of anticipated danger **Calming Technique:** Reducing anxiety in a patient experiencing acute distress **Coping Enhancement:** Assisting patient to adapt to perceived stressors, changes, with friends which interfere with meeting life demands and roles **Emotional Support:** Provision of reassurance, acceptance, and encouragement during times of stress **Presence:** Being with another, both physically and psychologically, during times of need **Relaxation Therapy:** Use of techniques to encourage and elicit relaxation for the purpose of decreasing undesirable signs and symptoms such as pain, muscle tension, or anxiety	**Anxiety Level:** Severity of manifested apprehension, tension or uneasiness arising from an unidentifiable source **Anxiety Self-Control:** Personal actions to eliminate or reduce feelings of apprehension, tension, or uneasiness from an unidentifiable source **Concentration:** Ability to focus on a specific stimulus **Coping:** Personal actions to manage stressors that tax an individual's resources

Nursing Diagnosis (NANDA): Aspiration, Risk for		
Orthopaedic Conditions*	**Nursing Intervention Classifications (NIC)**	**Nursing Outcome Classifications (NOC)**
Chapter 8: Orthopaedic Complications Hospital Acquired Pneumonia **Chapter 10: Therapeutic Modalities** Casts **Chapter 11: Pediatrics** Cerebral Palsy	**Airway Management:** Facilitation of patency of air passages **Aspiration Precautions:** Prevention or minimization of risk factors in the patient at risk for aspiration **Cough Enhancement:** Promotion of deep inhalation by the patient with subsequent generation of high intrathoracic pressures and compression of underlying lung parenchyma for forcible expulsion of air **Respiratory Management:** Collection and analysis of patient data to ensure airway patency and adequate gas exchange **Vomiting Management:** Prevention and alleviation of vomiting	**Airway Patency:** Open, clear tracheobronchial passages for air exchange **Aspiration Prevention:** Personal actions to prevent the passage of fluid and solid particles into the lung **Respiratory Status: Airway Patency:** Open, clear tracheobronchial passages for air exchange **Swallowing Status:** Safe passage of fluids

Nursing Diagnosis (NANDA): Bleeding, Risk for		
Orthopaedic Conditions*	**Nursing Intervention Classifications (NIC)**	**Nursing Outcome Classifications (NOC)**
Chapter 20: The Hand & Wrist Replantation Arthroplasty **Chapter 21: The Hip, Femur & Pelvis Hip** Femoral Shaft Fractures Pelvic Fractures	**Bleeding Precautions:** Reduction of stimuli that induce bleeding or hemorrhage in at-risk patients **Bleeding Reduction:** Limitation of the loss of blood volume during an episode **Bleeding Reduction: Wound:** Limitation of the blood loss from a wound that may be a result of trauma, incision, or placement of a tube or catheter **Blood Product Administration:** Administration of blood or blood products and monitoring of patient response **Incision Site Care:** Cleansing, monitoring, and promotion of a healing wound that is closed with sutures, clips, or staples **Thrombolytic Therapy Management:** Collection and analysis of patient data to expedite safe, appropriate provision of an agent that dissolves a thrombus	**Blood Coagulation:** Extent to which blood clots within normal period of time **Blood Loss Severity:** Severity of internal or external bleeding/ hemorrhage **Circulation Status:** Unobstructed, unidirectional blood flow at an appropriate pressure through large vessels of the systemic and pulmonary circuits **Compliance Behavior: Prescribed Medicine:** Personal actions to administer medication safely to meet therapeutic goals as recommended by a health professional **Fall Prevention Behavior:** Personal or family caregiver's actions to minimize risk factors that might precipitate falls in the personal environment **Knowledge: Fall Prevention:** Extent of understanding conveyed about prevention of falls **Knowledge: Medication:** Extent of understanding conveyed about the safe use of medication **Physical Injury Severity:** Severity of injuries from accidents and trauma

Nursing Diagnosis (NANDA): Body Image, Disturbed		
Orthopaedic Conditions*	**Nursing Intervention Classifications (NIC)**	**Nursing Outcome Classifications (NOC)**
Chapter 8: Orthopaedic Complications Delayed Union/Nonunion **Chapter 10: Therapeutic Modalities** Ambulatory Devices and Techniques Braces/Orthotics/Orthoses Casts External Fixators Traction Wheelchairs **Chapter 11: Pediatrics** Arthrogryposis Multiplex Congenita **Chapter 13: Arthritis & Connective Tissue Disorders** Juvenile Arthritis Rheumatoid Arthritis Osteoarthritis Ankylosing Spondylitis **Chapter 15: Orthopaedic Trauma** Pelvic Fractures **Chapter 17: The Spine** Scoliosis Kyphosis Spondylosis Spondylolithesis Failed Back Surgery Syndrome Spinal Fractures **Chapter 19: The Elbow** Lateral and Medial Epicondylitis Pitcher's Elbow Olecranon Bursitis Distal Biceps Tendon Rupture Radial Head/Monteggia/Coronoid Process/Olecranon Fractures Subluxation/Nursemaid's Elbow Supracondylar/Distal Humerus Fractures Elbow Dislocation Nerve Entrapments Osteochondritis of the Capitellum Elbow Arthroplasty **Chapter 20: The Hand & Wrist** Mallet Finger Boutonniere and Swan Neck Deformities Replantation Dupuytren's Contracture Ganglion Cyst Carpal Tunnel Syndrome Arthroplasty **Chapter 21: The Hip, Femur & Pelvis** Hip Girdlestone Pseudarthrosis **Chapter 23: The Foot & Ankle** Foot Drop Onychomycosis Amputations	**Anticipatory Guidance:** Preparation of a patient for an anticipated developmental and/or situational crisis **Body Image Enhancement:** Improving a patient's conscious and unconscious perceptions and attitudes toward own body **Coping Enhancement:** Assisting a patient to adapt to perceived stressors, changes, or threats that interfere with meeting life demands and roles **Developmental Enhancement: Adolescent:** Facilitating optimal physical, cognitive, social, emotional growth of individuals during the transition from childhood to adulthood **Developmental Enhancement: Child:** Facilitating or teaching parents/caregivers to facilitate the optimal gross motor, fine motor, language, cognitive, social, and emotional growth of preschoolers and school-aged children **Parent Education: Childrearing, Family:** Assisting parents to understand and promote the physical, psychological, and social growth and development of their toddler, preschooler, or school-aged child/children **Self-Esteem Enhancement:** Assisting a patient to increase his/her personal judgment of self-worth **Unilateral Neglect Management:** Protecting and safely reintegrating the affected part of the body while helping the patient adapt to disturbed perceptual abilities	**Adaptation to Physical Disability:** Adaptive response to a significant functional challenge due to a physical disability **Body Image:** Perception of own appearance and body functions **Child Development: Adolescent:** Milestones of physical, cognitive, and psychosocial progression from ages 12-17 **Child Development: Middle Childhood:** Milestones of physical, cognitive, and psychosocial progression from ages 6-11 **Heedfulness of Affected Side:** Personal actions to acknowledge, protect, and cognitively integrate body part(s) into self **Psychosocial Adjustment: Life Change:** Adaptive psychosocial response of an individual to a significant life change **Self-Esteem:** Personal judgment of self-worth

Nursing Diagnosis (NANDA): Body Temperature, Risk for Imbalance		
Orthopaedic Conditions*	**Nursing Intervention Classifications (NIC)**	**Nursing Outcome Classifications (NOC)**
Chapter 6: Immobility Neurosensory Issues	**Energy Management:** Regulating energy use to treat or prevent fatigue and optimize function **Environmental Management: Comfort:** Manipulation of the patient's surroundings for promotion of optimal comfort **Fluid Management:** Promotion of fluid balance and prevention of complications resulting from abnormal or undesired fluid levels **Fluid Monitoring:** Collection and analysis of patient data to regulate fluid balance **Infection Control:** Minimizing the acquisition and transmission of infectious agents **Infection Control: Intraoperative:** Preventing nosocomial infection in the operating room **Infection Protection:** Prevention and early detection of infection in the patient at risk **Malignant Hyperthermia Precautions:** Prevention or reduction of hypermetabolic response to pharmacological agents used during surgery **Temperature regulation: Intraoperative:** Attaining and/or maintaining body temperature within a normal range during a surgical procedure	**Activity Tolerance:** Physiologic response to energy-consuming movements with daily activities **Burn Healing:** Extent of healing of a burn site **Infection Severity:** Severity of infection and associated symptoms **Medication Response:** Therapeutic and adverse effects of prescribed medication **Thermoregulation:** Balance among heat production, heat gain, and heat loss

Nursing Diagnosis (NANDA): Breathing Pattern, Ineffective		
Orthopaedic Conditions*	**Nursing Intervention Classifications (NIC)**	**Nursing Outcome Classifications (NOC)**
Chapter 6: Immobility Respiratory Issues **Chapter 8: Orthopaedic Complications** Fat Emboli Syndrome **Chapter 13: Arthritis & Connective Tissue Disorders** Ankylosing Spondylitis Systemic Sclerosis	**Airway Management:** Facilitation of patency of air passages **Airway Suctioning:** Removal of airway secretions by inserting a suction catheter into patient's oral airway and/or trachea **Artificial Airway Management:** Maintenance of endotracheal and tracheostomy tubes and prevention of complications associated with their use **Aspiration Precautions:** Prevention or minimization of risk factors in the patient at risk for aspiration **Anxiety Reduction:** Minimizing apprehension, dread, foreboding, or uneasiness related to an unidentified source of anticipated or perceived danger Endotracheal Extubation: Purposeful removal of the endotracheal tube from the nasopharyngeal or oropharyngeal airway **Mechanical Ventilation:** Use of artificial device to assist a patient to breathe **Mechanical Ventilation Weaning:** Assisting the patient to breathe without the aid of a mechanical ventilator **Oxygen Therapy:** Administration of oxygen and monitoring of its effectiveness **Pain Management:** Alleviation of pain or a reduction in pain to a level of comfort that is acceptable to the patient Respiratory Monitoring: Collection and analysis of patient data to ensure airway patency and adequate gas exchange **Vital Signs Monitoring:** Collection and analysis of cardiovascular, respiratory, and body temperature data to determine and prevent complications	**Mechanical Ventilation Response: Adult:** Alveolar exchange and tissue perfusion are supported by mechanical ventilation **Mechanical Ventilation Weaning Response: Adult:** Respiratory and psychological adjustment to progressive removal of mechanical ventilation **Respiratory Status: Airway Patency:** Open, clear tracheobronchial passages for air exchange **Respiratory Status: Ventilation:** Movement of air in and out of the lungs **Vital Signs:** Extent to which temperature, pulse, respiration, and blood pressure are within normal range

Nursing Diagnosis (NANDA): Caregiver Role Strain; Caregiver Role Strain, Risk for		
Orthopaedic Conditions*	**Nursing Intervention Classifications (NIC)**	**Nursing Outcome Classifications (NOC)**
Chapter 13: Arthritis & Connective Tissue Disorders Juvenile Arthritis **Chapter 16: Tumors of the Musculoskeletal System** Primary Sarcoma Bone Metastasis Multiple Myeloma **Chapter 21: The Hip, Femur & Pelvis** Hip Fractures Hip Arthroplasty Hip Resurfacing Arthroplasty Hemiarthroplasty/Bipolar Replacement Hip Arthroscopy Femoro-Acetabular Impingement Hip Dislocation Hip Girdlestone Psuedoarthrosis Proximal Femoral Osteotomy Femoral Shaft Fractures Pelvic Fracture	**Caregiver Support:** Provision of the necessary information, advocacy, and support to facilitate primary patient care by someone other than a health care professional **Coping Enhancement**: Assisting a patient to adapt to perceived stressors, changes, or threats that interfere with meeting life demands and roles **Decision-Making Support:** Providing information and support for a patient who is making a decision regarding health care **Energy Management:** Regulating energy use to treat or prevent fatigue and optimize function **Health System Guidance:** Facilitating a patient's location and use of appropriate health services **Nutrition Management:** Assisting with or providing a balanced dietary intake of foods and fluids **Parenting Promotion:** Providing parenting information, support, and coordination of comprehensive services to high-risk families **Respite Care:** Provision of short-term care to provide relief for family caregiver **Role Enhancement:** Assisting a patient, significant other, and/or family to improve relationships by clarifying and supplementing specific role behaviors **Teaching: Disease Process:** Assisting the patient to understand information related to a specific disease process **Teaching: Prescribed Diet:** Preparing a patient to follow a healthful diet with adequate intake of nutrients to aid in recovery **Teaching: Prescribed Medication:** Preparing a patient to safely take prescribed medications and monitor for their effects	**Caregiver Emotional Health:** Emotional well-being of a family care provider while caring for a family member **Caregiver Lifestyle Disruption:** Severity of disturbances in the lifestyle of a family member due to caregiving **Caregiver Well-Being:** Extent of positive perception of primary care provider's health status and life circumstances **Caregiver-Patient Relationship:** Positive interactions and connections between the caregiver and care recipient **Caregiver Performance: Direct Care:** Provision by family care provider of appropriate personal and health care for a family member **Caregiver Performance: Indirect Care:** Arrangement and oversight by family care provider of appropriate care for a family member **Caregiver Physical Health:** Physical well-being of a family care provider while caring for a family member **Caregiver Role Endurance:** Factors that promote family care provider's capacity to sustain caregiving over an extended period of time **Parenting Performance:** Parental actions to provide a child with a nurturing and constructive physical, emotional, and social environment **Role Performance:** Congruence of an individual's role behavior with role expectations

Nursing Diagnosis (NANDA): Comfort, Impaired		
Orthopaedic Conditions*	**Nursing Intervention Classifications (NIC)**	**Nursing Outcome Classifications (NOC)**
Chapter 10: Therapeutic Modalities Wheelchairs **Chapter 13: Arthritis & Connective Tissue Disorders** Osteoarthritis Rheumatic Fever Reactive Arthritis **Chapter 14: Metabolic Bone Conditions** Osteomalcia Paget's Disease	**Anxiety Reduction:** Minimizing apprehension, dread, foreboding, or uneasiness related to an unidentified source of anticipated or perceived danger **Calming Technique:** Reducing anxiety in a patient experiencing acute distress **Culture Brokerage:** The deliberate use of culturally competent strategies to mediate between the patient's culture and the biomedical health care system **Dementia Management:** Provision of a modified environment for the patient who is experiencing a chronic confusional state **Environmental Management: Comfort:** Manipulation of the patient's surroundings for therapeutic benefit, sensory appeal, and psychological well-being **Environmental Management: Safety:** Monitoring and manipulation of the physical environment to promote safely **Positioning:** Deliberate placement of the patient or body part to promote physiological and/or psychological well-being **Relaxation Therapy:** Use of techniques to encourage and elicit relaxation for the purpose of decreasing undesirable signs and symptoms such as pain, muscle tension, or anxiety **Self-Efficacy Enhancement:** Strengthening an individual's confidence in his/her ability to perform a health behavior **Self-Modification Assistance:** Reinforcement of self-directed change initiated by the patient to achieve personally important goals **Spiritual Support:** Assisting the patient to feel balance and connection with a greater power **Support System Enhancement:** Facilitation of support to the patient by family, friends, and community	**Agitation Level:** Severity of disruptive physiological and behavioral manifestations of stress or biochemical triggers **Client Satisfaction: Physical Environment:** Extent of positive perception of living environment, treatment environment, equipment, and supplies in an acute or long-term care settings **Comfort Status:** Overall physical, psychospiritual, sociocultural, and environmental ease and safety of an individual **Comfort Status: Environment:** Environmental ease, comfort, and safety of surroundings **Comfort Status: Physical:** Physical ease related to bodily sensations and homeostatic mechanisms **Comfort Status: Psychospiritual:** Pscychospiritual ease related to self-concept, emotional well-being, source of inspiration, and meaning and purpose in one's life **Comfort Status: Sociocultural:** Social ease related to interpersonal, family, and societal relationships within a cultural context **Symptom Control:** Personal actions to minimize perceived adverse changes in physical and emotional functioning **Symptom Severity:** Severity of perceived adverse changes in physical, emotional, and social functioning.

Nursing Diagnosis (NANDA): Confusion, Acute; Confusion, Risk for Acute		
Orthopaedic Conditions*	**Nursing Intervention Classifications (NIC)**	**Nursing Outcome Classifications (NOC)**
Chapter 8: Orthopaedic Complications Delirium **Chapter 13: Arthritis & Connective Tissue Disorders** Systemic Lupus Erythemetosis **Chapter 15: Orthopaedic Trauma** Spine Fractures **Chapter 21: The Hip, Femur & Pelvis** Hip Arthoplasty	**Acid-Base Management:** Promotion of acid-base balance and prevention of complications resulting from acid-base imbalance **Cerebral Perfusion Promotion:** Promotion of adequate perfusion and limitation of complications for a patient experiencing or at risk for inadequate cerebral perfusion **Cognitive Stimulation:** Promotion of awareness and comprehension of surroundings by utilization of planned stimuli **Delirium Management:** Provision of a safe and therapeutic environment for the patient who is experiencing an acute confusional state **Delusion Management:** Promotion of the comfort, safety, and reality orientation of a patient experiencing false, fixed beliefs that have little or no basis in reality **Fluid/Electrolyte Management:** Regulation and prevention of complications from altered fluid and/or electrolyte levels **Fluid Management:** Promotion of fluid balance to prevent complications resulting from abnormal or undesired fluid levels **Fluid Monitoring:** Collection and analysis of patient data to regulate fluid balance **Hallucination Management:** Promotion of the safety, comfort, and reality orientation of a patient experiencing hallucinations **Infection Protection:** Prevention and early detection of infection in the patient at risk **Neurologic Monitoring:** Collection and analysis of patient data to prevent or minimize neurologic complications **Reality Orientation:** Promotion of the patient's awareness of personal identity, time, and environment	**Acute Confusion Level:** Severity of disturbance in consciousness and cognition that develops over a short period of time **Alcohol Abuse Cessation Behavior:** Personal actions to eliminate alcohol use that poses a threat to health **Cognition:** Ability to execute complex mental processes **Cognitive Orientation:** Ability to identify person, place, and time accurately **Concentration:** Ability to focus on a specific stimulus **Distorted Thought Self-Control:** Self-restraint of disruptions in perception, thought processes, and thought content **Electrolyte & Acid/Base Balance: Hydration:** Adequate water in the intracellular and extracellular compartments of the body **Infection Severity:** Severity of infection and associated symptoms **Information Processing:** Ability to acquire, organize, and use information **Neurological Status:** Consciousness: Arousal, orientation, and attention to the environment

Nursing Diagnosis (NANDA): Constipation, Risk for		
Orthopaedic Conditions*	**Nursing Intervention Classifications (NIC)**	**Nursing Outcome Classifications (NOC)**
Chapter 6: Orthopaedic Effects of Immobility Metabolic/Gastrointestinal Issues **Chapter 8: Orthopaedic Complications** Constipation **Chapter 10: Therapeutic Modalities** Casts Traction Wheelchairs **Chapter 15: Orthopaedic Trauma** Soft Trauma Dislocations/ Subluxations Strains Sprains **Chapter 17: The Spine** Kyphosis Herniated Nucleus Pulposus Degenerative Disc Disease Spinal Stenosis Spondylolysis and Spondylolisthesis Failed Back Syndrome **Chapter 21: The Hip, Femur & Pelvis** Hip Fractures Hip Arthroplasty Hip Resurfacing Arthroplasty Hemiarthroplasty/Bipolar Replacement Hip Arthroscopy Femoro-Acetabular Impingement Hip Dislocation Hip Girdlestone Psuedoarthrosis Proximal Femoral Osteotomy Femoral Shaft Fractures Pelvic Fracture **Chapter 22: The Knee** Osteoarthritis	**Bowel Management:** Establishment and maintenance of a regular pattern of bowel elimination **Bowel Training:** Assisting the patient to train the bowels to evacuate at specific intervals **Constipation/Impaction Management:** Prevention and alleviation of constipation/impaction **Electrolyte Management:** Promotion of electrolyte balance and prevention of complications resulting from abnormal or undesired serum electrolyte levels **Exercise Therapy: Ambulation:** Promotion and assistance with walking to maintain or restore autonomic and voluntary body functions during treatment and recovery from illness or injury **Fluid Management:** Promotion of fluid balance and prevention of complications resulting from abnormal or undesired fluid levels **Self-Care Assistance: Toileting:** Assisting another will elimination	**Bowel Elimination:** Formation and evacuation of stool **Gastrointestinal Function:** Extent to which foods (ingested or tube-fed) are moved from ingestion to excretion **Hydration:** Adequate water in the intracellular and extracellular compartments of the body **Immobility Consequences: Physiological:** Severity of compromise in physiological functioning due to impaired physical mobility **Self-Care: Toileting:** Ability to toilet independently with or without assistive device

Nursing Diagnosis (NANDA): Coping, Ineffective; Coping, readiness for enhanced		
Orthopaedic Conditions*	**Nursing Intervention Classifications (NIC)**	**Nursing Outcome Classifications (NOC)**
Chapter 10: Therapeutic Modalities External Fixators Traction Wheelchairs **Chapter 13: Arthritis & Connective Tissue Disorders** Rheumatoid Arthritis Osteoarthritis Polymyalgia Rheumatica Rheumatic Fever Fibromyalgia Syndrome **Chapter 15: Orthopaedic Trauma** Spine Fractures Pelvic Fractures Femur/Hip Fractures Amputations **Chapter 16: Tumors of the Musculoskeletal System** Benign Lesions Primary Malignant Tumors Primary Sarcoma Bone Metastasis Multiple Myeloma **Chapter 17: The Spine** Scoliosis Kyphosis Spondylosis Spondylolithesis Failed Back Surgery Syndrome Spinal Fractures **Chapter 18: The Shoulder** Impingement Syndrome Rotator Cuff Tears Arthritis Shoulder Instability Adhesive Capsulitis Fractures of the Shoulder Sprains, Strains, Contusions, Separations Sprengel's Deformity Glenoid Hypoplasia Referred Visceral Somatic Pain **Chapter 20: The Hand & Wrist** Replantation **Chapter 21: The Hip, Femur & Pelvis** Hip Fractures Hip Arthroplasty Hip Resurfacing Arthroplasty Hemiarthroplasty/Bipolar Replacement Hip Arthroscopy Femoro-Acetabular Impingement Hip Dislocation Hip Girdlestone Psuedoarthrosis Proximal Femoral Osteotomy Femoral Shaft Fractures Pelvic Fracture	**Anticipatory Guidance:** Preparation of patient for an anticipated developmental and/or situational crisis **Anxiety Reduction:** Minimizing apprehension, dread, foreboding, or uneasiness related to an unidentified source of anticipated danger **Behavioral Modification:** Promotion of a behavior change **Coping Enhancement:** Assisting a patient to adapt to perceived stressors, changes, or threats that interfere with meeting life demands and roles **Decision-Making Support:** Providing information and support for a patient who is making a decision regarding health care **Emotional Support:** Provision of reassurance, acceptance, and encouragement during times of stress **Health System Guidance:** Facilitating a patient's location and use of appropriate health services	**Acceptance: Health Status:** Reconciliation to significant change in health circumstances **Adaptation to Physical Disability:** Adaptive response to a significant functional challenge due to a physical disability **Caregiver Adaptation to Patient Institutional:** Adaptive response of family caregiver when the care recipient is moved to an institution **Child Adaptation to Hospitalization:** Adaptive response of a child from 3-17 years of age to hospitalization **Coping:** Personal actions to manage stressors that tax an individual's resources **Decision-Making:** Ability to make judgments and choose between two or more alternatives **Knowledge: Health Resources:** Extent of understanding conveyed about relevant health care resources **Psychosocial Adjustment: Life Change:** Adaptive physcosocial response of an individual to a significant life change

Nursing Diagnosis (NANDA): Development, Risk for Delayed		
Orthopaedic Conditions*	**Nursing Intervention Classifications (NIC)**	**Nursing Outcome Classifications (NOC)**
Chapter 10: Therapeutic Modalities Wheelchairs **Chapter 11: Pediatrics** Arthrogryposis Multiplex Congenita **Chapter 13: Arthritis & Connective Tissue Disorders** Juvenile Arthritis **Chapter 17: The Spine** Scoliosis Kyphosis **Chapter 18: The Shoulder** Fractures of the Shoulder Sprengel's Deformity **Chapter 22: The Knee** Pediatric Knee Conditions	**Behavior Modification: Social Skills Development:** Assisting the patient to develop or improve interpersonal social skills **Developmental Enhancement: Adolescent:** Facilitating optimal physical, cognitive, social, and emotional growth of individuals during the transition from childhood to adulthood **Developmental Enhancement: Child:** Facilitating or teaching parents/caregivers to facilitate the optimal gross motor, fine motor, language, cognitive, social and emotional growth of preschool an school-aged children **Environmental Management: Safety: Risk Identification:** Analysis of potential risk factors, determination of health risks, and prioritization of risk reduction strategies for an individual or group **Parent Education: Adolescent:** Assisting parents to understand and help their adolescent children	**Child Development: (age specific):** Milestones of physical, cognitive, and psychosocial progression by (age specific) **Social Interaction Skills:** Personal behaviors that promote effective relationships

Nursing Diagnosis (NANDA): Disuse Syndrome, Risk for		
Orthopaedic Conditions*	**Nursing Intervention Classifications (NIC)**	**Nursing Outcome Classifications (NOC)**
Chapter 6: Immobility Musculoskeletal Issues **Chapter 10: Therapeutic Modalities** Braces/Orthotics/Orthoses Traction **Chapter 11: Pediatrics** Duchene's Muscular Dystrophy **Chapter 17: The Spine** Scoliosis Kyphosis **Chapter 18: The Shoulder** Impingement Syndrome Rotator Cuff Tears Arthritis Shoulder Instability Adhesive Capsulitis Fractures of the Shoulder Sprains, Strains, Contusions, Separations Sprengel's Deformity Glenoid Hypoplasia Referred Visceral Somatic Pain **Chapter 21: The Hip, Femur & Pelvis** Hip Fractures	**Activity Therapy:** Prescription of and assistance with specific physical, cognitive, social, and spiritual activities to increase the range, frequency, or duration of an individual's (or group's) activity **Energy Management:** Regulating energy use to treat or prevent fatigue and optimize function	**Endurance:** Capacity to sustain activity **Immobility Consequences: Physiological:** Severity of compromise in physiological functioning due to impaired physical mobility

Nursing Diagnosis (NANDA): Diversional Activity, Deficient		
Orthopaedic Conditions*	**Nursing Intervention Classifications (NIC)**	**Nursing Outcome Classifications (NOC)**
Chapter 6: Immobility Psychosocial/Mental Status **Chapter 22: The Knee** Overuse Syndromes Pediatric Knee Conditions **Chapter 23: The Foot & Ankle** Achilles Tendinitis	**Activity Therapy:** Prescription of and assistance with specific physical, cognitive, social, and spiritual activities to increase the range, frequency, or duration of an individual's (or group's) activity **Recreation Therapy:** Purposeful use of recreation to promote relaxation and enhancement of social skills **Self-Modification Assistance:** Reinforcement of self-directed change initiated by the patient to achieve personally important goals **Self-Responsibility Facilitation:** Encouraging a patient to assume more responsibility for own behavior **Socialization Enhancement:** Facilitation of another person's ability to interact with others **Therapeutic Play:** Purposeful and directive use of toys and other material to assist children in communicating their perception and knowledge of their world and to help in gaining mastery of their environment	**Leisure Participation:** Use of relaxing, interesting, and enjoyable activities to promote well-being **Motivation:** Inner urge that moves or prompts an individual to positive action(s) **Play Participation:** Use of activities by a child ages 1-11 to promote enjoyment, entertainment, and development **Social Involvement:** Social interactions with persons, groups, or organizations

Nursing Diagnosis (NANDA): Falls, Risk for		
Orthopaedic Conditions*	**Nursing Intervention Classifications (NIC)**	**Nursing Outcome Classifications (NOC)**
Chapter 8: Orthopaedic Complications Delirium **Chapter 10: Therapeutic Modalities** Ambulatory Devices and Techniques Wheelchairs **Chapter 13: Arthritis & Connective Tissue Disorders** Anklosing Spondylitis **Chapter 14: Metabolic Bone Conditions** Osteoporosis Paget's Disease **Chapter 17: The Spine** Herniated Nucleus Pulposus Degenerative Disc Disease Spinal Stenosis Spondylosis Spondylolithesis Failed Back Surgery Syndrome Spinal Fractures **Chapter 21: The Hip, Femur & Pelvis** Hip Fractures Hip Arthroplasty Hip Arthroscopy Femoro-Acetabular Impingement Hip Dislocation Hip Girdlestone Psuedoarthrosis Proximal Femoral Osteotomy Femoral Shaft Fractures Pelvic Fracture *(continued next page)*	**Body Mechanics Promotion:** Facilitating the use of posture and movement in daily activities to prevent fatigue and musculoskeletal strain or injury **Delirium Management:** Provisions of escape and therapeutic environment for the patient was experiencing an acute confusional state **Dementia Management:** Provision of a modified environment for the patient who is experiencing a chronic confusional state **Exercise Therapy: Balance:** Use of specific activities, postures, and movements to maintain, enhance, or restore balance **Exercise Therapy: Muscle Control:** Use of specific activity or exercise protocols to enhance or restore controlled body movement **Environmental Management: Safety:** Monitoring and manipulation of the physical environment to promote safety **Fall Prevention:** Instituting special precautions for a patient at risk of injury from falling **Risk Identification:** Analysis of potential risk factors, determination of health risks, and prioritization of risk reduction strategies for an individual or group **Teaching: Prescribed Activity/Exercise:** Preparing a patient to achieve and/or maintain a prescribed level of activity	**Acute Confusion Level:** Severity of disturbance and consciousness and cognition that develops over a short period of time **Agitation Level:** Severity of disruptive physiological and behavioral manifestations of stress or biochemical triggers **Balance:** Ability to maintain body equilibrium **Client Satisfaction: Safety:** Extent of positive perception of procedures, information, and nursing care to prevent harm or injury **Cognition:** Ability to execute complex mental processes **Coordinated Movement:** Ability of muscles to work together voluntarily for purposeful movement **Fall Prevention Behavior:** Personal or caregiver actions to minimize risk factors that might precipitate falls in the personal environment **Falls Occurrence:** Number of falls in the past ______ (define period of time) *(continued next page)*

Nursing Diagnosis (NANDA): Falls, Risk for *(continued)*		
Orthopaedic Conditions*	**Nursing Intervention Classifications (NIC)**	**Nursing Outcome Classifications (NOC)**
Chapter 22: The Knee Osteoarthritis **Chapter 23: The Foot & Ankle** Fractures Foot Drop Amputations	*(see page 632)*	**Fatigue Level:** Severity of observed or reported prolonged generalized fatigue **Knowledge: Fall Prevention:** Extent of understanding conveyed about prevention of falls **Physical Injury Severity:** Severity of injuries from accidents and trauma **Sensory Function: Proprioception:** Extent to which the position and movement of the head and body are correctly sensed

Nursing Diagnosis (NANDA): Family Coping, Compromised		
Orthopaedic Conditions*	**Nursing Intervention Classifications (NIC)**	**Nursing Outcome Classifications (NOC)**
Chapter 13: Arthritis & Connective Tissue Disorders Juvenile Arthritis Polymyositis/Dermatomyositis Systemic Lupus Erythmatosis **Chapter 17: The Spine** Scoliosis Kyphosis Herniated Nucleus Pulposus Degenerative Disc Disease Spinal Stenosis **Chapter 18: The Shoulder** Arthritis Fractures of Shoulder Shoulder Instability Adhesive Capsulitis Sprengel's Deformity Referred Visceral Somatic Pain **Chapter 20: The Hand & Wrist** Replantation **Chapter 21: The Hip, Femur & Pelvis** Hip Fractures Hip Arthroplasty Hip Resurfacing Arthroplasty Hemiarthroplasty/Bipolar Replacement Hip Arthroscopy Femoro-Acetabular Impingement Hip Dislocation Hip Girdlestone Psuedoarthrosis Proximal Femoral Osteotomy Femoral Shaft Fractures Pelvic Fracture	**Caregiver Support:** Provision of the necessary information, advocacy, and support to facilitate primary patient care by someone other than a health care professional **Coping Enhancement:** Assisting a patient to adapt to perceived stressors, changes, or threats that interfere with meeting life demands and roles **Family Integrity Promotion:** Promotion of family cohesion and unity **Family Involvement Promotion:** Facilitation of family participation in the emotional and physical care of the patient **Family Presence Facilitation:** Facilitation of the family's presence and support of an individual undergoing resuscitation and/or invasive procedures **Family Process Maintenance:** Minimization of disruptive or adverse effects on the family process **Family Support:** Promotion of family values, interests, and goals **Health System Guidance:** Facilitation of a patient's location and use of appropriate health services **Learning Facilitation:** Promoting the ability to process and comprehend information **Normalization Promotion:** Assisting parents and other family members of children with chronic illnesses or disabilities in providing normal life experiences for their children and families **Respite Care:** Provision of short-term care to provide relief for family caregiver	**Caregiver Emotional Health:** Emotional well-being of a family care provider while caring for a family member **Caregiver-Patient Relationship:** Positive interactions and connections between caregiver and care recipient **Caregiver Performance: Direct Care:** Provision by family care provider of appropriate personal and health care for a family member **Caregiver Performance: Indirect Care:** Arrangement and oversight by family care provider of appropriate care for a family member **Caregiver Role Endurance:** Factors that promote a family care provider's capacity to sustain care over an extended period of time **Family Coping:** Family actions to manage stressors that tax family resources **Family Normalization:** Capacity of the family system to develop strategies for optimal function when a member has a chronic illness or disability

Diagnosis (NANDA): Family Processes, Interrupted		
Orthopaedic Conditions*	**Nursing Intervention Classifications (NIC)**	**Nursing Outcome Classifications (NOC)**
Chapter 13: Arthritis & Connective Tissue Disorders Systemic Erythymatosis Lupus **Chapter 17: The Spine** Scoliosis Kyphosis **Chapter 18: The Shoulder** Arthritis Shoulder Instability Adhesive Capsulitis/Frozen Shoulder Sprengel's Deformity Referred Visceral Somatic Pain **Chapter 20: The Hand & Wrist** Replantation **Chapter 21: The Hip, Femur & Pelvis** Hip Fractures Hip Arthroplasty Hip Resurfacing Arthroplasty Hemiarthroplasty/Bipolar Replacement Hip Arthroscopy Femoro-Acetabular Impingement Hip Dislocation Hip Girdlestone Psuedoarthrosis Proximal Femoral Osteotomy Femoral Shaft Fractures Pelvic Fracture **Chapter 22: The Knee** Pediatric Knee Conditions	**Coping Enhancement:** Assisting a patient to adapt to perceived stressors, changes, or threats that interfere with meeting life demands and roles **Family Integrity Promotion:** Promotion of family cohesion and unity **Family Involvement Promotion:** Facilitation of family participation in the emotional and physical care of the patient **Family Presence Facilitation:** Facilitation of the family's presence and support of an individual undergoing resuscitation and/or invasive procedures **Family Process Maintenance:** Minimization of disruptive or adverse effects on the family process **Family Support:** Promotion of family values, interests, and goals **Normalization Promotion:** Assisting parents and other family members of children with chronic illnesses or disabilities in providing normal life experiences for their children and families **Resiliency Promotion:** Assisting individuals, families, and communities in development, use, and strengthening of protective factors to be use din coping with environmental and societal stressors	**Family Coping:** Family actions to manage stressors that tax family resources **Family Functioning:** Capacity of the family system to meet the needs of its members during developmental transitions **Family Normalization:** Capacity of the family system to maintain routines and develop strategies for optimal functioning when a member has a chronic illness or disability **Family Resiliency:** Capacity of the family system to successfully adapt and function competently following significant adversity or crisis **Family Social Climate:** Supportive milieu as characterized by family member relationships and goals **Family Support During Treatment:** Family presence and emotional support for an individual undergoing treatment

Nursing Diagnosis (NANDA): Fatigue		
Orthopaedic Conditions*	**Nursing Intervention Classifications (NIC)**	**Nursing Outcome Classifications (NOC)**
Chapter 10: Therapeutic Modalities Wheelchairs **Chapter 13: Arthritis & Connective Tissue Disorders** Lyme Disease Fibromyalgia Syndrome **Chapter 14: Metabolic Bone Conditions** Osteomalacia	**Activity Therapy:** Prescription of and assistance with specific physical, cognitive, social, and spiritual activities to increase the range, frequency, or duration of an individual's (or group's) activity **Energy Management:** Regulating energy use to treat or prevent fatigue and optimize function **Environmental Management:** Manipulation of the patient's surroundings for therapeutic benefit, sensory appeal, and psychological well being **Exercise Therapy: Ambulation:** Promotion and assistance with walking to maintain or restore autonomic and voluntary body functions during treatment and recovery from illness or injury **Exercise Therapy:** Balance: Use of specific activities, postures, and movements to maintain, enhance, or restore balance **Exercise Therapy: Joint Mobility:** Use of active or passive body movement to maintain or restore joint flexibility **Exercise Therapy: Muscle Control:** Use of specific activity or exercise protocols to enhance or restore controlled body movement *(continued next page)*	**Activity Tolerance:** Physiologic response to energy-consuming movements with daily activities **Endurance:** Capacity to sustain activity **Energy Conservation:** Personal actions to manage energy for initiating and sustaining activity **Fatigue Level:** Severity of observed or reported prolonged generalized fatigue **Nutritional Status: Energy:** Extent to which nutrients and oxygen provide cellular energy *(continued next page)*

Nursing Diagnosis (NANDA): Fatigue *(continued)*		
Orthopaedic Conditions*	**Nursing Intervention Classifications (NIC)**	**Nursing Outcome Classifications (NOC)**
(see page 634)	**Exercise Promotion: Strength Training:** Facilitation of regular resistive muscle training to maintain or increase muscle strength **Exercise Promotion: Stretching:** Facilitation of systematic slow stretch-and-hold muscle exercises to induce relaxation, to prepare muscles/joints for more vigorous exercise, or to increase or maintain body flexibility **Mood Management:** Providing for safety, stabilization, recovery, and maintenance of a patient experiencing dysfunctionally depressed or elevated mood **Nutritional Management:** Assisting with or providing a balanced dietary intake of food and fluids	**Psychomotor Energy:** Personal drive and energy to maintain activities of daily living, nutrition, and personal safety

Nursing Diagnosis (NANDA): Fear		
Orthopaedic Conditions*	**Nursing Intervention Classifications (NIC)**	**Nursing Outcome Classifications (NOC)**
Chapter 6: Effects of Immobility **Chapter 18: The Shoulder** Fractures of the Shoulder Sprains, Strains, Contusions, Separations Sprengel's Deformity Referred Visceral Somatic Pain **Chapter 19: The Elbow** Subluxation/Nursemaid's Elbow **Chapter 20: The Hand & Wrist** Replantation **Chapter 21: The Hip, Femur & Pelvis** Hip Fractures Hip Arthroplasty Hip Resurfacing Arthroplasty Hemiarthroplasty/Biplolar Replacement Hip Arthroscopy Femoro-Acetabular Impingement Hip Disolocation Hip Girdlestone Pseudarthrosis (Resectional Arthroplasty) Proximal Femoral Osteotomy Femoral Shaft Fractures	**Anxiety Reduction:** Minimizing apprehension, dread, foreboding, or uneasiness related to an unidentified source of anticipated or perceived danger **Calming Technique:** Reducing anxiety in patient experiencing acute distress **Coping Enhancement:** Assisting a patient to adapt to perceived stressors, changes, or threats which interfere with meeting life demands and roles **Presence:** Being with another, both physically and psychologically, during times of need **Security Enhancement:** Intensifying a patient's sense of physical and psychological safety	**Fear Level:** Severity of manifested apprehension, tension, or uneasiness arising from an identifiable source **Fear Level:** Child: Severity of manifested apprehension, tension, or uneasiness arising from an identifiable source in a child ages 1-17 **Fear Self-Control:** Personal actions to eliminate or reduce disabling feelings of apprehension, tension, or uneasiness from an identifiable source

Nursing Diagnosis (NANDA): Fluid Volume, Deficient; Fluid Volume, Risk for Deficient; Fluid Volume, Risk for Imbalanced		
Orthopaedic Conditions*	**Nursing Intervention Classifications (NIC)**	**Nursing Outcome Classifications (NOC)**
Chapter 6: Immobility Cardiovascular Issues Neurosensory Issues **Chapter 8: Orthopaedic Complications** Postoperative Nausea and Vomiting **Chapter 15: Orthopaedic Trauma** Femur/Hip Fractures **Chapter 22: The Knee** Osteoarthritis **Chapter 17: The Spine** Scoliosis/Kyphosis Herniated Nucleus Pulposus Degenerative Disc Disease Spinal Stenosis Spondylolysis and Spondylolisthesis Failed Back Surgery Syndrome Spinal Fractures	**Acid-Base Management:** Promotion of acid-base balance and prevention of complications resulting from acid-base imbalance **Electrolyte Management:** Promotion of electrolyte balance and prevention of complications resulting from abnormal or undesired serum electrolyte levels **Fluid/Electrolyte Monitoring:** Collection and analysis of patient data to regulate fluid/electrolyte balance **Fluid/Electrolyte Management:** Regulation and prevention of complications from altered fluid and/or electrolyte levels **Hypovolemia Management:** Reduction in extracellular and/or intracellular fluid volume and prevention of complications in a patient who is fluid-overloaded **IV Insertion:** Insertion of a needle into a peripheral vein for the purpose of administering fluids, blood, or medications **IV Therapy:** Administration and monitoring of intravenous fluids and medications **Laboratory Data Interpretation:** Critical analysis of patient laboratory data in to assist with clinical decision making **Medication Administration:** Preparing, giving, and evaluating the effectiveness of prescription and nonprescription drugs **Medication Management:** Facilitation of safe and effective use of prescription and over-the-counter drugs **Nutrition Management:** Assisting with or providing a balanced dietary intake of foods and fluids **Shock Management: Volume:** Facilitation of the delivery of oxygen and nutrients to systemic tissue with removal of cellular waste products in a patient with severely altered tissue perfusion **Urinary Elimination Management:** Maintenance of an optimum urinary elimination pattern **Vital Signs Monitoring:** Collection and analysis of cardiovascular, respiratory, and body temperature data to determine and prevent complications	**Electrolyte and Acid/ Base Balance:** Balance of the electrolytes and nonelectrolytes in the intracellular and extracellular compartments of the body **Fluid Balance:** Water balance in the intracellular and extracellular compartments of the body **Hydration:** Adequate water in the intracellular and extracellular compartments of the body **Kidney Function:** Filtration of blood and elimination of metabolic waste products through the formation of urine **Nutrition Status: Food and Fluid Intake:** Amount of food and fluid taken into body over a 24-hour period

Nursing Diagnosis (NANDA): Fluid Volume, Excess; Fluid Volume, Risk for Excess; Fluid Volume, Risk for Imbalanced		
Orthopaedic Conditions*	**Nursing Intervention Classifications (NIC)**	**Nursing Outcome Classifications (NOC)**
Chapter 6: Immobility Cardiovascular Issues **Chapter 8: Orthopaedic Complications** Hemorrhage/Significant Blood Loss Compartment Syndrome (Acute and Crush Syndrome) Postoperative Nausea and Vomiting **Chapter 17: The Spine** Scoliosis/Kyphosis Herniated Nucleus Pulposus Degenerative Disc Disease Spinal Stenosis Spondylolysis and Spondylolisthesis Failed Back Surgery Syndrome Spinal Fractures **Chapter 22: The Knee** Osteoarthritis	**Acid-Base Management:** Promotion of acid-base balance and prevention of complications resulting from acid-base imbalance **Electrolyte Management:** Promotion of electrolyte balance and prevention of complications resulting from abnormal or undesired serum electrolyte levels **Fluid/Electrolyte Monitoring:** Collection and analysis of patient data to regulate fluid/electrolyte balance **Fluid/Electrolyte Management:** Regulation and prevention of complications from altered fluid and/or electrolyte levels **Hypervolemia Management:** Expansion of intravascular fluid volume in a patient who is volume-depleted **IV Insertion:** Insertion of a needle into a peripheral vein for the purpose of administering fluids, blood, or medications **IV Therapy:** Administration and monitoring of intravenous fluids and medications **Laboratory Data Interpretation:** Critical analysis of patient laboratory data in order to assist with clinical decision making **Medication Administration:** Preparing, giving, and evaluating the effectiveness of prescription and nonprescription drugs **Medication Management:** Facilitation of safe and effective use of prescription and over-the-counter drugs **Nutrition Management:** Assisting with or providing a balanced dietary intake of foods and fluids **Shock Management: Volume:** Facilitation of the delivery of oxygen and nutrients to systemic tissue with removal of cellular waste products in a patient with severely altered tissue perfusion **Urinary Elimination Management:** Maintenance of an optimum urinary elimination pattern **Vital Signs Monitoring:** Collection and analysis of cardiovascular, respiratory, and body temperature data to determine and prevent complications	**Electrolyte and Acid/Base Balance:** Balance of the electrolytes and nonelectrolytes in the intracellular and extracellular compartments of the body **Fluid Balance:** Water balance in the intracellular and extracellular compartments of the body **Fluid Overload Severity:** Severity of excess fluids in the intracellular and extracelluar compartments of the body **Kidney Function:** Filtration of blood and elimination of metabolic waste products through the formation of urine **Nutrition Status:** Food and Fluid Intake: Amount of food and fluid taken into body over a 24-hour period

Nursing Diagnosis (NANDA): Gas Exchange, Impaired		
Orthopaedic Conditions*	**Nursing Intervention Classifications (NIC)**	**Nursing Outcome Classifications (NOC)**
Chapter 8: Orthopaedic Complications Venous Thromboembolism Fat Embolism Syndrome Hospital Acquired Pneumonia **Chapter 9: Orthopaedic Infections** Healthcare-Associated Infections **Chapter 21: The Hip, Femur & Pelvis** Hip Fractures Hip Arthroplasty Hip Resurfacing Arthroplasty Hemiarthroplasty/Bipolar Replacement	**Airway Insertion and Stabilization:** Insertion or assistance with insertion and stabilization of an artificial airway **Airway Management:** Facilitation of patency of air passages **Airway Suctioning:** Removal of airway secretions by inserting a suction catheter into the patient's oral airway and/or trachea **Cough Enhancement:** Promotion of deep inhalation by the patient with subsequent generation of high intrathoracic pressures and compression of underlying lung parenchyma for forceful expulsion of air **Embolus Care: Pulmonary:** Limiting complications for a patient experiencing, or at risk for, occlusion of pulmonary circulation **Laboratory Data Interpretation:** Critical analysis of patient laboratory data in order to assist with clinical decision-making **Oxygen Therapy:** Administration of oxygen and monitoring of its effectiveness **Respiratory Monitoring:** Collection and analysis of patient data to ensure airway patency and adequate gas exchange	**Mechanical Ventilation Response:** Adult: Alveolar exchange and tissue perfusion are supported by mechanical ventilation **Respiratory Status: Gas Exchange:** Alveolar exchange of carbon dioxide and oxygen to maintain arterial blood gas concentrations **Respiratory Status: Ventilation:** Movement of air in and out of the lungs **Tissue Perfusion: Pulmonary:** Adequacy of blood flow through pulmonary vasculature to perfuse alveoli/capillary unit **Vital Signs:** Extent to which temperature, pulse, respiration, and blood pressure are within normal range

Nursing Diagnosis (NANDA): Gastrointestinal Motility: Dysfunctional; Gastrointestinal Motility: Risk for Dysfunctional		
Orthopaedic Conditions*	**Nursing Intervention Classifications (NIC)**	**Nursing Outcome Classifications (NOC)**
Chapter 8: Complications Constipation **Chapter 15: Orthopaedic Trauma** Soft Trauma Dislocations/Subluxations **Chapter 17: The Spine** Herniated Nucleus Pulposus Spinal Stenosis Degenerative Disc Disease Spondylolysis and Spondylolisthesis Failed Back Surgery Syndrome Spinal Fractures **Chapter 21: The Hip, Femur & Pelvis** Hip Fractures Hip Arthroplasty Hip Resurfacing Arthroplasty Hemiarthroplasty/Bipolar Replacement Hip Arthroscopy Femoro-Acetabular Impingement Hip Dislocation Hip Girdlestone Psuedoarthrosis Proximal Femoral Osteotomy Femoral Shaft Fractures Pelvic Fracture **Chapter 22: The Knee** Osteoarthritis	**Anxiety Reduction:** Minimizing apprehension, dread, foreboding, or uneasiness related to an unidentified source of anticipated or perceived danger **Bowel Management:** Establishment and maintenance of a regular pattern of bowel elimination **Exercise Therapy: Ambulation:** Promotion and assistance with walking to maintain or restore autonomic involuntary body functions during treatment and recovery from illness or injury **Gastrointestinal Intubation:** Insertion of a tube into the gastrointestinal tract **Risk Identification:** Analysis of potential risk factors, determination of health risks, and prioritization of risk reduction strategies for an individual or group **Surveillance:** Purposeful and ongoing acquisition, interpretation, and synthesis of patient data for clinical decision-making **Teaching: Prescribed Diet:** Preparing a patient to correctly follow a prescribed diet	**Bowel Elimination:** Formation and evacuation of stool **Compliance Behavior: Prescribed Diet:** Personal actions to follow food and fluid intake as recommended by health professional for a specific health condition **Gastrointestinal Function:** Extent to which foods (ingested or tube-fed) are moved from ingestion to excretion **Knowledge: Diet:** Extent of understanding conveyed about recommended diet

Nursing Diagnosis (NANDA): Grieving; Grieving, Complicated; Grieving, Complicated, Risk for;		
Orthopaedic Conditions*	**Nursing Intervention Classifications (NIC)**	**Nursing Outcome Classifications (NOC)**
Chapter 11: Pediatrics Achondroplasia Cerebral Palsy Duchenne's Muscular Dystrophy **Chapter 13: Arthritis & Connective Tissue Disorders** Ankylosing Spondylitis **Chapter 16: Tumors of the Musculoskeletal System** Primary Sarcoma Bone Metastasis Multiple Myeloma **Chapter 17: The Spine** Scoliosis Kyphosis **Chapter 20: The Hand & Wrist** Replantation	**Active Listening:** Attending closely to and attaching significance to a patient's verbal and nonverbal messages **Anxiety Reduction:** Minimizing apprehension, dread, foreboding, or uneasiness related to an unidentified source of anticipated or perceived danger **Coping Enhancement:** Assisting a patient to adapt to perceived stressors, changes, or threats which interfere with meeting life demands and roles **Family Integrity Promotion:** Promotion of family cohesion and unity **Grief Work Facilitation:** Assisting with the resolution of a significant loss **Role Enhancement:** Assisting a patient, significant other, and/or family to improve relationships by clarifying and supplanting specific role behaviors **Self-Awareness Enhancement:** Assisting a patient to explore and understand his/her thoughts, feelings, motivations, and behaviors	**Adaptation to Physical Disability:** Adaptive response to a significant functional challenge due to a physical disability **Anxiety Level:** Severity of manifested apprehension, tension, or uneasiness arising from an identifiable source **Comfort Status: Psychospiritual:** Psychospiritual ease related to self-concept, emotional well-being, source of inspiration, and meaning and purpose in one's life **Comfort Status: Sociocultural:** Social ease related to interpersonal, family, an societal relationships within a cultural context **Coping:** Personal actions to manage stressors that tax an individual's resources **Family Coping:** Family actions to manage stressors that tax family resources **Grief Resolution:** Adjustment to actual or impending loss **Psychosocial Adjustment: Life Change:** Adaptive psychosocial response of an individual to a significant life change **Role Performance:** Congruence of an individual's role behavior with role expectations

Nursing Diagnosis (NANDA): Growth and Development, Delayed		
Orthopaedic Conditions*	**Nursing Intervention Classifications (NIC)**	**Nursing Outcome Classifications (NOC)**
Chapter 10: Therapeutic Modalities Wheelchairs **Chapter 11: Pediatrics** Arthrogryposis Multiplex Congenita **Chapter 18: The Shoulder** Fractures of the Shoulder Sprengel's Deformity	**Body Mechanics Promotion:** Facilitation of the use of posture and movement in daily activities to prevent fatigue and musculoskeletal strain or injury **Exercise Promotion:** Facilitation of regular physical activity to maintain or advance to a higher level of fitness and health **Nutritional Management:** Assisting with or providing a balanced dietary intake of foods and fluids **Resiliency Promotion:** Assisting individuals, families, and communities in development, use, and strengthening of protective factors to be use in coping with environmental and societal stressors **Role Enhancement:** Assisting a patient, significant other, and/or family to improve relationships by clarifying and supplementing specific role behaviors **Self-Responsibility Facilitation:** Encouraging a patient to assume more responsibility for own behavior	**Growth:** Normal increase in bone size and body weight during growth years **Physical Aging:** Normal physical changes that occur with the natural aging process

Nursing Diagnosis (NANDA): Health Behavior, Risk-Prone		
Orthopaedic Conditions*	**Nursing Intervention Classifications (NIC)**	**Nursing Outcome Classifications (NOC)**
Chapter 13: Arthritis & Connective Tissue Disorders Reactive Arthritis **Chapter 14: Metabolic Bone Conditions** Paget's Disease **Chapter 23: The Foot & Ankle** Charcot Foot Diabetic Foot	**Anticipatory Guidance:** Preparation of a patient for an anticipated developmental and/or situational crisis **Coping Enhancement:** Assisting a patient to adapt to perceived stressors, changes, or threats that interfere with meeting life demands and roles **Counseling:** Use of an interactive helping process focusing on the needs, problems, or feelings of the patient and significant other to enhance or support coping, problem solving, and interpersonal relationships **Health Education:** Developing and providing instruction and learning experiences to facilitate voluntary adaptation of behavior conducive to health in individuals, families, groups, or communities **Mutual Goal Setting:** Collaborating with patient to identify and prioritize care goals, then developing a plan for achieving those goals **Patient Contracting:** Negotiating an agreement with an individual that reinforces a specific behavior change **Risk Identification:** Analysis of potential risk factors, determination of health risks, and prioritization of risk reduction strategies for an individual or group **Self-Efficacy Enhancement:** Strengthening an individual's confidence in his/her ability to perform a health behavior **Self-Responsibility Facilitation:** Encouraging a patient to assume more responsibility for own behavior **Values Clarification:** Assisting another to clarify her/his own values in order to facilitate effective decision-making	**Acceptance: Health Status:** Reconciliation to significant change in health circumstances **Adaptation to Physical Disability:** Adaptive response to a significant functional challenge due to a physical disability **Compliance Behavior:** Personal actions to promote wellness, recovery, and rehabilitation as recommended by a health professional **Coping:** Personal actions to manage stressors that tax an individual's resources **Health-Seeking Behavior:** Personal actions to promote optimal wellness, recovery, and rehabilitation **Motivation:** Inner urge that moves or prompts an individual to positive actions(s) **Psychosocial Adjustment: Life Change:** Adaptive psychosocial response of an individual to a significant life change **Risk Control:** Personal actions to prevent, eliminate, or reduce modifiable health threats

Nursing Diagnosis (NANDA): Health Maintenance, Ineffective		
Orthopaedic Conditions*	**Nursing Intervention Classifications (NIC)**	**Nursing Outcome Classifications (NOC)**
Chapter 10: Therapeutic Modalities Ambulatory Devices and Techniques Braces/Orthotics/Orthoses Continuous Passive Motion Machine External Fixators Traction Wheelchairs **Chapter 13: Arthritis & Connective Tissue Disorders** Reactive Arthritis **Chapter 14: Metabolic Bone Conditions** Osteoporosis Osteomalacia Paget's Disease	**Case Management:** Coordinating care and advocating for specified individuals and patient populations across settings to reduce cost, reduce resource use, improve quality of health care, and achieve desired outcomes **Decision-Making Support:** Providing information and support for a patient who is making a decision regarding health care Family Involvement Promotion: Facilitating family participation in the emotional and physical care of the patient **Financial Resource Assistance:** Assisting an individual/family to secure and manage finances to meet health care needs **Health Education:** Developing and providing instruction and learning experiences to facilitate voluntary adaptation of behavior conducive to health in individuals, families, groups, or communities **Health Literacy Enhancement:** Assisting individuals with limited ability to obtain, process, and understand information related to health and illness **Health System Guidance:** Facilitating a patient's location and use of appropriate health services **Mutual Goal Setting:** Collaborating with patient to identify and prioritize care goals, then developing a plan for achieving those goals **Risk Identification:** Analysis of potential risk factors, determination of health risks, and prioritization of risk reduction strategies for an individual or group **Self-Care Assistance:** Assisting another to perform activities of daily living **Self-Care Assistance: IADL:** Assisting and instructing a person to perform instrumental activities of daily living (IADL) needed to function in the home or community **Self-Efficacy Enhancement:** Strengthening an individual's confidence in his/her ability to perform a health behavior **Self-Responsibility Facilitation:** Encouraging a patient to assume more responsibility for own behavior **Support System Enhancement:** Facilitation of support to patient by family, friends and community **Teaching: Disease Process:** Assisting the patient to understand information related to a specific disease process **Teaching: Individual:** Planning, implementation, and evaluation of a teaching program designed to address a patient's particular needs **Teaching: Procedure/Treatment:** Preparing a patient to understand and mentally prepare for a prescribed procedure or treatment	**Client Satisfaction: Access to Care Resources:** Extent of positive perception of access to nursing staff, supplies, and equipment needed for care **Health Beliefs: Perceived Resources:** Personal conviction that one has adequate means to carry out healthy behavior **Health Promoting Behavior:** Personal actions to sustain or increase wellness **Health-Seeking Behavior:** Personal actions to promote optimal wellness, recover, and rehabilitation **Knowledge: Health Behavior:** Extent of understanding conveyed about the promotion and protection of health **Knowledge: Health Promotion:** Extent of understanding conveyed about information needed to obtain and maintain optimal health **Knowledge:** Health Resources: Extent of understanding conveyed about relevant health care resources **Knowledge:** Treatment Regimen: Extent of understanding conveyed about a specific treatment regimen **Participation in Health Care Decisions:** Personal involvement in selecting and evaluating health care options to achieve desired outcome **Self-Care Status:** Ability to perform basic personal care activities and household tasks **Self-Direction of Care:** Care recipient actions taken to direct others who assist with or perform physical tasks and personal health care **Social Support:** Perceived availability and actual provision of reliable assistance from others **Treatment Behavior: Illness or Injury:** Personal actions to palliate or eliminate pathology

Diagnosis (NANDA): Home Maintenance, Impaired		
Orthopaedic Conditions*	**Nursing Intervention Classifications (NIC)**	**Nursing Outcome Classifications (NOC)**
Chapter 10: Therapeutic Modalities Ambulatory Devices and Techniques Braces/Orthotics/Orthoses Continuous Passive Motion Machine External Fixators Traction Wheelchairs **Chapter 13: Arthritis & Connective Tissue Disorders** Rheumatoid Arthritis Reactive Arthritis **Chapter 15: Orthopaedic Trauma** Fractures Spine Fractures **Chapter 18: The Shoulder** Arthritis Shoulder Instability Adhesive Capsulitis Fractures of the Shoulder Sprains, Strains, Contusions, Separations Sprengel's Deformity Referred Visceral Somatic Pain	**Environmental Management: Safety:** Monitoring and manipulation of the worksite environment to promote safety and health of workers **Fall Prevention:** Instituting special precautions with patient at risk for injury from falling **Home Maintenance Assistance:** Helping the patient/family to maintain the home as a clean, safe, and pleasant place to live **Parenting Promotion:** Providing parenting information, support, and coordination of comprehensive services to high-risk families **Self-Care Assistance: IADL:** Assisting in instructing a person to perform instrumental activities of daily living (IADL) needed to function in the community **Surveillance: Safety:** Purposeful and ongoing collection and analysis of information about the patient and the environment for use in promoting and maintaining patient safety	**Safe Home Environment:** Physical arrangements to minimize environmental factors that might cause physical harm or injury in the home **Self-Care: Instrumental Activities of Daily Living:** (IADL): Ability to perform activities needed to function in the home or community independently with or without assistive device

Nursing Diagnosis (NANDA): Infection, Risk for		
Orthopaedic Conditions*	**Nursing Intervention Classifications (NIC)**	**Nursing Outcome Classifications (NOC)**
Chapter 8: Orthopaedic Complications Delayed Union/Nonunion Nosocomial Surgical Site Infections Hospital Acquired Pneumonia Pressure Ulcers Compartment Syndrome Postoperative Urinary Retention **Chapter 9: Orthopaedic Infections** Osteomyelitis Septic Arthritis Prosthetic Joint Infections Bone and Joint Tuberculosis Skin and Soft Tissue Infections Healthcare-Associated Infections **Chapter 10: Therapeutic Modalities** External Fixators Traction **Chapter 11: Pediatrics** Leg Length Discrepancies *(continued next page)*	**Amputation Care:** Promotion of physical and psychological healing before and after amputation of a body part **Incision Site Care:** Cleansing, monitoring, and promotion of healing in a wound that is closed with sutures, clips, or staples **Infection Control:** Minimizing the acquisition and transmission of infectious agents **Infection Control:** Intraoperative: Prevention of nosocomial infection in the operating room **Infection Protection:** Prevention and early detection of infection in a patient at risk **Skin Care: Donor Site:** Prevention of wound complications and promotion of healing at the donor site **Skin Care: Graft Site:** Prevention of wound complications and promotion of graft site healing **Skin Surveillance:** Collection and analysis of patient data to maintain skin and mucous membranes integrity **Suturing:** Approximating edges of a wound using sterile suture material and a needle **Wound Care:** Prevention of wound complications and promotion of healing **Wound Care: Closed Drainage:** Maintenance of the pressure drainage system at the wound site **Wound Irrigation:** Flushing of an open wound to cleanse and remove debris and excessive drainage *(continued next page)*	**Burn Healing:** Extent of healing of a burn site **Infection Severity:** Severity of infection and associated symptoms **Wound Healing: Primary Intention:** Extent of regeneration of cells and tissue following intentional closure **Wound Healing: Secondary Intention:** Extent of regeneration of cells and tissue in an open wound

Nursing Diagnosis (NANDA): Infection, Risk for *(continued)*		
Orthopaedic Conditions*	**Nursing Intervention Classifications (NIC)**	**Nursing Outcome Classifications (NOC)**
Chapter 13: Arthritis & Connective Tissue Disorders Polymyalgia Rheumatica Lyme Disease Psoriatic Arthritis Systemic Sclerosis Polymyositis and Dermatomyositis **Chapter 15: Orthopaedic Trauma** Spine Fractures Pelvic Fractures Femur/Hip Fractures Soft Trauma Dislocations and Subluxations Strains Sprains Amputations **Chapter 16: Tumors of the Musculoskeletal System** Multiple Myeloma **Chapter 18: The Shoulder** Impingement Syndrome/Tendinitis Rotator Cuff Tears Arthritis Shoulder Instability Adhesive Capsulitis Fractures of the Shoulder Sprains, Strains, Contusions, Separations Sprengel's Deformity Glenoid Hypoplasia **Chapter 19: The Elbow** Lateral and Medial Epicondylitis Pitcher's Elbow Olecranon Bursitis Distal Biceps Tendon Rupture Radial Head, Monteggia, Coronoid Process, and Olecranon Fractures Subluxation/Nursemaid's Elbow Supracondylar/Distal Humerus Fractures Elbow Dislocation Nerve Entrapments Osteochondritis of the Capitellum Elbow Arthroplasty **Chapter 20: The Hand & Wrist** Mallet Finger Boutonniere and Swan Neck Deformities Gamekeeper's Thumb Nail Bed Injuries Thumb Fractures—Bennett's and Rolando's Boxer's Fracture Replantation Dupuytren's Contracture Distal Radius Fractures—Colles' and Smith's Ganglion Cyst Carpal Tunnel Syndrome Arthroplasty Scaphoid Fracture *(continued next page)*	**Wound Care: Burns:** Prevention of wound complications due to burns and facilitation of wound healing	*(see page 642)*

Nursing Diagnosis (NANDA): Infection, Risk for *(continued)*		
Orthopaedic Conditions*	**Nursing Intervention Classifications (NIC)**	**Nursing Outcome Classifications (NOC)**
Chapter 21: The Hip, Femur & Pelvis Hip Fractures Hip Arthroplasty Hip Resurfacing Arthroplasty Hemiarthroplasty/Bipolar Replacement Hip Arthroscopy Femoro-Acetabular Impingement Hip Girdlestone Psuedoarthrosis Proximal Femoral Osteotomy Femoral Shaft Fractures Pelvic Fracture **Chapter 22: The Knee** Osteoarthritis Overuse Syndromes Trauma and Soft Tissue Injuries Pediatric Knee Conditions **Chapter 23: The Foot & Ankle** Fractures Toe Deformities Corns Verrunca Plantaris Onychocryptosis Onychomycosis Amputations Osteoarthritis Charcot Foot Diabetic Foot	*(see page 643)*	*(see page 643)*

Nursing Diagnosis (NANDA): Injury, Risk for		
Orthopaedic Conditions*	**Nursing Intervention Classifications (NIC)**	**Nursing Outcome Classifications (NOC)**
Chapter 8: Orthopaedic Complications Delirium **Chapter 10: Therapeutic Modalities** Ambulatory Devices and Techniques Braces/Orthotics/Orthoses Continuous Passive Motion Machine External Fixators Traction Wheelchairs **Chapter 13: Arthritis & Connective Tissue Disorders** Rheumatic Fever Polymyositis/Dermatomyositis **Chapter 14: Metabolic Bone Conditions** Osteoporosis Rickets **Chapter 15: Orthopaedic Trauma** Femur/Hip Fractures *(continued next page)*	**Bleeding Precautions:** Reduction of stimuli that may induce bleeding or hemorrhage in at-risk patients **Dementia Management:** Provision of a modified environment for the patient who is experiencing a chronic confusional state **Energy Management:** Regulating energy use to treat or prevent fatigue and optimize function **Environmental Management:** Safety: Monitoring and manipulation of the physical environment to promote safety **Fall Prevention:** Instituting special precautions with patient at risk for injury from falling **Sports-Injury Prevention: Youth:** Reducing the risk of sports-related injury in young athletes **Surveillance: Safety:** Purposeful and ongoing collection and analysis of information about the patient and the environment for use in promoting and maintaining patient safety	**Falls Occurrence:** Number of falls in the past _______ (define period of time) **Personal Safety Behavior:** Personal actions of an adult to control behaviors that cause physical injury **Balance:** Ability to maintain body equilibrium **Client Satisfaction: Safety:** Extent of positive perception of procedures, information, and nursing care to prevent harm or injury **Fall Prevention Behavior:** Personal or family caregiver actions to minimize risk factors that might precipitate falls in the personal environment *(continued next page)*

Nursing Diagnosis (NANDA): Injury, Risk for *(continued)*		
Orthopaedic Conditions*	**Nursing Intervention Classifications (NIC)**	**Nursing Outcome Classifications (NOC)**
Chapter 16: Tumors of the Musculoskeletal System Primary Malignant Tumors **Chapter 19: The Elbow** Lateral and Medial Epicondylitis Pitcher's Elbow Olecranon Bursitis Distal Biceps Tendon Rupture Radial Head, Monteggia, Coronoid Process, and Olecranon Fractures Subluxation/Nursemaid's Elbow Supracondylar/Distal Humerus Fractures Elbow Dislocation Nerve Entrapments Osteochondritis of the Capitellum Elbow Arthroplasty **Chapter 20: The Hand & Wrist** Mallet Finger Trigger Thumb/Finger DeQuervain's Ganglion Cyst Boutonniere and Swan Neck Deformities Gamekeeper's Thumb Nail Bed Injuries Dupuytren's Contracture Distal Radius Fractures—Colles' and Smith's Thumb Fractures—Bennett's and Rolando's Boxer's Fracture Scaphoid Fracture **Chapter 21: The Hip, Femur & Pelvis** Hip Fractures Hip Arthroplasty Hip Resurfacing Arthroplasty Hemiarthroplasty/Bipolar Replacement Hip Arthroscopy Femoro-Acetabular Impingement Hip Girdlestone Pseudarthrosis Proximal Femoral Osteotomy Femoral Shaft Fractures Pelvic Fracture **Chapter 22:The Knee** Osteoarthritis Overuse Syndrome Trauma and Soft Tissue Injuries Pediatric Knee Conditions **Chapter 23: The Foot & Ankle** Foot Drop	*(see page 644)*	**Fatigue Level:** Severity of observed or reported prolonged generalize fatigue **Cognitive Orientation:** Ability to identify a person, place, and time accurately **Physical Injury Severity:** Severity of injuries from accidents and trauma

Nursing Diagnosis (NANDA): Hopelessness		
Orthopaedic Conditions*	**Nursing Intervention Classifications (NIC)**	**Nursing Outcome Classifications (NOC)**
Chapter 10: Therapeutic Modalities Ambulatory Devices/Techniques Wheelchairs **Chapter 21: The Hip, Femur & Pelvis** Hip Fractures Hip Arthoplasty	**Cognitive Restructuring:** Challenging a patient to alter distorted thought patterns and view self and the world more realistically **Coping Enhancement:** Assisting a patient to adapt to perceived stressors, changes, or threats that interfere with meeting life demands and roles **Hope Inspiration:** Enhancing the belief in one's capacity to initiate and sustain positive or healthy actions **Mood Management:** Providing for safety, stabilization, recovery, and maintenance of a patient experiencing dysfunctionally depressed or elevated mood **Resiliency Promotion:** Assisting individuals, families, and communities in development, use, and strengthening of protective factors to be use din coping with environmental and societal stressors **Self-Modification Assistance:** Reinforcement of self-directed change initiated by the patient to achieve personally important goals	**Depression Level:** Severity of melancholic mood and loss of interest in life events **Depression Self-Control:** Personal actions to minimize melancholy and maintain interest in life events **Hope:** Optimism that is personally satisfying and life-supporting **Mood Equilibrium:** Appropriate adjustment of prevailing emotional tone in response to circumstances **Psychomotor Energy:** Personal drive and energy to maintain activities of daily living, nutrition, and personal safety **Quality of Life:** Extent of positive perception of current life circumstances **Will to Live:** Desire, determination, and effort to survive

Nursing Diagnosis (NANDA): Knowledge Deficit, (specify)		
Orthopaedic Conditions*	**Nursing Intervention Classifications (NIC)**	**Nursing Outcome Classifications (NOC)**
Chapter 8: Orthopaedic Complications Delayed Union/Nonunion **Chapter 10: Therapeutic Modalities** Ambulatory Devices and Techniques Braces/Orthotics/Orthoses Continuous Passive Motion Machine External Fixators Traction Wheelchairs **Chapter 13: Arthritis & Connective Tissue Disorders** Juvenile Arthritis Polymyalgia Rheumatica Gout Lyme Disease Reactive Arthritis Systemic Lupus Erythematosus *(continued next page)*	**Active Listening:** Attending closely to and attaching significance to a patient's verbal and nonverbal message **Admission Care:** Facilitating entry of a patient into a health care facility **Allergy Management:** Identification, treatment, and prevention of allergic responses to food, medications, insect bites, contrast material, blood, and other substances. **Analgesic Administration:** Use of pharmacologic agents to reduce or eliminate pain **Anticipatory Guidance:** Preparation of a patient for an anticipated developmental and/or situational crisis **Body Mechanics Promotion:** Facilitating the use of posture and movement in daily activities to prevent fatigue and musculoskeletal strain or injury **Discharge Planning:** Preparation for moving a patient from one level of care to another within or outside the current health care agency **Energy Management:** Regulating energy use to treat or prevent fatigue and optimize function **Environmental Management:** Manipulation of the patient's surroundings for therapeutic benefit, sensory appeal, and psychological well-being *(continued next page)*	**Client Satisfaction: Teaching:** Extent of positive perception of instruction provided by nursing staff to improve knowledge, understanding, and participation in care **Discharge Readiness: Independent Living:** Ability to walk from place to place independently with or without assistive device **Discharge Readiness: Supported Living:** Readiness of a patient to relocate from a health care institution to a lower level of supported living *(continued next page)*

Nursing Diagnosis (NANDA): Knowledge Deficit, (specify) *(continued)*		
Orthopaedic Conditions*	**Nursing Intervention Classifications (NIC)**	**Nursing Outcome Classifications (NOC)**
Chapter 14: Metabolic Bone Conditions Osteoporosis Osteomalacia Rickets Primary Hyperparathyroidism Secondary and Tertiary Hyperparathyroidism Hypoparathyroidism **Chapter 15: Orthopaedic Trauma** Spine Fractures **Chapter 16: Tumors of the Musculoskeletal System** Benign Lesions Primary Malignant Tumors Primary Sarcoma Bone Metastasis Multiple Myeloma **Chapter 17: Spine** Scoliosis/Kyphosis Herniated Nucleus Pulposus/ Degenerative Disc Disease Spinal Stenosis Spondylolysis and Spondylolisthesis Failed Back Surgery Syndrome Spinal Fractures **Chapter 18: The Shoulder** Impingement Syndrome Rotator Cuff Tears Arthritis Shoulder Instability Adhesive Capsulitis Fractures of the Shoulder Sprains, Strains, Contusions, Separations Sprengel's Deformity Glenoid Hypoplasia Referred Visceral Somatic Pain **Chapter 19: The Elbow** Lateral and Medial Epicondylitis Pitcher's Elbow Olecranon Bursitis Distal Biceps Tendon Rupture Radial Head, Monteggia, Coronoid Process, and Olecranon Fractures Subluxation/Nursemaid's Elbow Supracondylar/Distal Humerus Fractures Elbow Dislocation Nerve Entrapments Osteochondritis of the Capitellum Elbow Arthroplasty *(continued next page)*	**Exercise Promotion: Strength Training:** Facilitating regular resistive muscle training to maintain or increase muscle strength **Exercise Promotion: Stretching:** Facilitation of systematic slow stretch-and-hold muscle exercises to induce relaxation, to prepare muscles/joints for more vigorous exercise, or to increase or maintain body flexibility **Exercise Therapy: Ambulation:** Promotion and assistance with walking to maintain or restore autonomic and voluntary body functions during treatment and recovery from illness or injury **Exercise Therapy: Balance:** Use of specific activities, postures, and movements to maintain, enhance, or restore balance **Exercise Therapy: Joint Mobility:** Use of active or passive body movement to maintain or restore joint flexibility **Exercise Therapy: Muscle Control:** Use of specific activity or exercise protocols to enhance or restore controlled body movement **Fall Prevention:** Instituting special precautions with patients at risk for injury from falling **Health Education:** Developing and providing instruction and learning experiences to facilitate voluntary adaptation of behavior conducive to health in individuals, families, groups, or communities **Health System Guidance:** Facilitating a patient's location and use of appropriate health services **Infection Control:** Minimizing the acquisition and transmission of infectious agents **Infection Protection:** Prevention and early detection of infection in a patient at risk **Learning Facilitation:** Promoting the ability to process and comprehend information **Learning Readiness Enhancement:** Improving the ability and willingness to receive information **Medication Management:** Facilitation of safe and effective use of prescription and over-the-counter medications **Nutrition Counseling:** Use of an interactive helping process focusing on the need for diet modification **Pain Management:** Alleviation of pain or reduction in pain to a level of comfort that is acceptable to the patient **Patient-Controlled Analgesia (PCA) Assistance:** Facilitating patient control of analgesic administration and regulation **Patient Rights Protection:** Protection of health care rights of a patient, especially a minor, incapacitated, or incompetent patient unable to make decisions **Preparatory Sensory Information:** Describing in concrete and objective terms the typical sensory experiences and events associated with an upcoming stressful health care procedure/treatment *(continued next page)*	**Knowledge: Arthritis Management:** Extent of understanding conveyed about arthritis, its treatment, and the prevention of complications **Knowledge: Body Mechanics:** Extent of understanding conveyed about proper body alignment, balance, and coordinated movement **Knowledge: Cancer Management:** Extent of understanding conveyed about cause, type, progress, symptoms and treatment of cancer **Knowledge: Disease Process:** Extent of understanding conveyed about a specific disease process **Knowledge: Energy Conservation:** Extent of understanding conveyed about energy conservation techniques **Knowledge: Fall Prevention:** Extent of understanding conveyed about prevention of falls **Knowledge: Health Behavior:** Extent of understanding conveyed about the promotion and protection of health **Knowledge: Health Promotion:** Extent of understanding conveyed about information needed to obtain and maintain optimal health **Knowledge: Health Resources:** Extent of understanding conveyed about relevant health care resources **Knowledge: Illness Care:** Extent of understanding conveyed about illness-related information needed to achieve and maintain optimal health *(continued next page)*

Nursing Diagnosis (NANDA): Knowledge Deficit, (specify) *(continued)*		
Orthopaedic Conditions*	**Nursing Intervention Classifications (NIC)**	**Nursing Outcome Classifications (NOC)**
Chapter 20: The Hand & Wrist Mallet Finger Boutonniere and Swan Neck Deformities Gamekeeper's Thumb Nail Bed Injuries Distal Radius Fractures—Colles' and Smith's Ganglion Cyst Carpal Tunnel Syndrome Replantation Thumb Fractures—Bennett's and Rolando's Boxer's Fracture Scaphoid Fracture **Chapter 21: The Hip, Femur & Pelvis** Hip Fractures Hip Arthroplasty Hip Resurfacing Arthroplasty Hemiarthroplasty/Bipolar Replacement Hip Arthroscopy Femoro-Acetabular Impingement Hip Dislocation Hip Girdlestone Psuedoarthrosis Proximal Femoral Osteotomy Femoral Shaft Fractures Pelvic Fracture **Chapter 22: The Knee** Osteoarthritis Overuse Syndromes Trauma and Soft Tissue Injuries Pediatric Knee Conditions **Chapter 23: The Foot & Ankle** Achilles Tendinitis Achilles Tendon Rupture Plantar Fasciitis Hallux Valgus Interdigital Neuroma Toe Deformities Corn, Verruca Plantaris Onychocryptosis Onychomycosis Osteoarthritis Diabetic Foot Charcot Foot	**Risk Identification:** Manipulation of the patient's surroundings for therapeutic benefit, sensory appeal, and psychological well being **Teaching: Disease Process:** Assisting the patient to understand information related to a specific disease process **Teaching: Group:** Development, implementation, and evaluation of a patient teaching program for a group of individuals experiencing the same health condition **Teaching: Individual:** Planning, implementation, and evaluation of a teaching program designed to address a patient's particular needs **Teaching:** Preoperative: Assisting a patient to understand and mentally prepare for surgery and the postoperative recovery period **Teaching: Prescribed Activity/Exercise:** Preparing a patient to achieve and/or maintain a prescribed level of activity **Teaching: Prescribed Medication:** Preparing a patient to safely take prescribed medications and monitor for their effects **Teaching: Procedure/Treatment:** Preparing a patient to understand and mentally prepare for a prescribed procedure or treatment **Teaching: Psychomotor Skill:** Preparing a patient to perform a psychomotor skill **Weight Management:** Facilitating maintenance of optimal body weight and percent of body fat	**Knowledge: Infection Management:** Extent of understanding conveyed about infection, its treatment, and the prevention of complications **Knowledge: Medication:** Extent of understanding conveyed about the safe use of medication **Knowledge: Pain Management:** Extent of understanding conveyed about causes, symptoms, and treatment of pain **Knowledge: Personal Safety:** Extent of understanding conveyed about prevention of unintentional injuries **Knowledge: Prescribed Activity:** Extent of understanding conveyed about prescribed activity and exercise **Knowledge: Treatment Procedure(s):** Extent of understanding conveyed about procedure(s) required as part of a treatment regimen **Knowledge: Treatment Regimen:** Extent of understanding conveyed about a specific treatment regimen

Nursing Diagnosis (NANDA): Lifestyle, Sedentary		
Orthopaedic Conditions*	**Nursing Intervention Classifications (NIC)**	**Nursing Outcome Classifications (NOC)**
Chapter 10: Therapeutic Modalities Wheelchairs	**Activity Therapy:** Prescription of and assistance with specific physical, cognitive, social, and spiritual activities to increase the range, frequency or duration of an individual's (or group's) activity **Exercise Promotion:** Facilitation of regular physical activity to maintain or advance to a higher level of fitness and health **Exercise Promotion: Strength Training:** Facilitating regular resistive muscle training to maintain or increase **muscle strength** **Exercise Promotion: Stretching:** Facilitation of systematic slow stretch-and-hold muscle exercises to induce relaxation, to prepare muscles/joints for more vigorous exercise, or to increase or maintain body flexibility **Exercise Therapy: Joint Mobility:** Use of active or passive body movement to maintain or restore joint flexibility **Self-Modification Assistance:** Reinforcement of self-directed change initiated by the patient to achieve personally important goals **Self-Responsibility Facilitation:** Encouraging a patient to assume more responsibility for own behavior **Teaching: Prescribed Activity/Exercise:** Preparing a patient to achieve and/or maintain a prescribed level of activity **Weight Management:** Facilitating maintenance of optimal body weight and percent body fat	**Motivation:** Inner urge that moves or prompts an individual to positive action(s) **Physical Fitness:** Performance of physical activities with vigor

Nursing Diagnosis (NANDA): Loneliness, Risk for		
Orthopaedic Conditions*	**Nursing Intervention Classifications (NIC)**	**Nursing Outcome Classifications (NOC)**
Chapter 10: Therapeutic Modalities Wheelchairs **Chapter 21: The Hip, Femur & Pelvis** Hip Arthroplasty Hip Fractures Femoro-Acetabular Impingement	**Activity Therapy:** Prescription of and assistance with specific physical, cognitive, social, and spiritual activities to increase the range, frequency, or duration of an individual's (or group's) activity **Animal-Assisted Therapy:** Purposeful use of animals to provide affection, attention, diversion, and relaxation **Behavior Modification: Social Skills:** Assisting the patient to develop or improve interpersonal social skills **Caregiver Support:** Provision of the necessary information, advocacy, and support to facilitate primary patient care by someone other than a health care professional. **Emotional Support:** Provision of reassurance, acceptance, and encouragement during times of stress **Family Integrity Promotion:** Promotion of the family cohesion and unity **Family Process Maintenance:** Minimization of disruptive or adverse effects on the family process **Grief Work Facilitation:** Assisting with the resolution of a significant loss **Relocation Stress Reduction:** Assisting the individual to prepare for and cope with movement from one environment to another	**Adaptation to Physical Disability:** Adaptive response to a significant functional challenge due to a physical disability **Family Functioning:** Capacity of the family system to meet the needs of its members during developmental transitions **Family Integrity:** Family members' behaviors that collectively demonstrate cohesion, strength, and emotional bonding **Family Social Climate:** Supportive milieu as characterized by family member relationships and goals **Grief Resolution:** Adjustment to actual or impending loss **Leisure Participation:** Use of relaxing, interesting, and enjoyable activities to promote well-being **Loneliness Severity:** Severity of emotional, social, or existential isolation response **Psychosocial Adjustment: Life Change:** Adaptive psychological response of an individual to a significant life change Social Involvement: Social interactions with persons, groups, or organizations **Social Support:** Reliable assistance from others

Nursing Diagnosis (NANDA): Memory, Impaired		
Orthopaedic Conditions*	**Nursing Intervention Classifications (NIC)**	**Nursing Outcome Classifications (NOC)**
Chapter 8: Orthopaedic Complications Delirium	**Cerebral Perfusion Promotion:** Promotion of adequate perfusion and limitation of complications for a patient experiencing or at risk for inadequate cerebral perfusion **Delirium Management:** Provision of a safe and therapeutic environment for the patient who is experiencing an acute confusional state **Dementia Management:** Provision of a modified environment for the patient who is experiencing a chronic confusional state **Memory Training:** Facilitation of memory **Neurological Monitoring:** Collection and analysis of patient data to prevent or minimize neurologic complications **Reality Orientation:** Promotion of patient's awareness of personal identify, time, and environment	**Cognitive Orientation:** Ability to identify person, place and time accurately **Memory:** Ability to cognitively retrieve and report previous stored information **Neurological Status:** Ability of the peripheral and central nervous systems to receive, process, and respond to internal and external stimuli

Nursing Diagnosis (NANDA): Mobility: Physical, Impaired; Mobility: Bed, Impaired; Mobility: Wheelchair Impaired		
Orthopaedic Conditions*	**Nursing Intervention Classifications (NIC)**	**Nursing Outcome Classifications (NOC)**
Chapter 6: Immobility Musculoskeletal Issues **Chapter 8: Orthopaedic Complications** Venous Thromboembolism Delayed Union/Non-Union **Chapter 9: Orthopaedic Infections** Osteomyelitis Septic Arthritis Prosthetic Joint Infections Bone and Joint/Extrapulmonary Tuberculosis Skin and Soft Tissue Infections **Chapter 10: Therapeutic Modalities** Ambulatory Devices and Techniques Cast External Fixator Traction Wheelchairs **Chapter 11: Pediatrics** Arthrogryposis Multiplex Congenita Cerebral Palsy Developmental Dysplasia of the Hip Duchene's Muscular Dystrophy Leg Length Discrepencies Myelomenignocele Osteogenesis Imperfecta Pediatric Fractures Slipped Capital Femoral Epiphysis *(continued next page)*	**Analgesic Administration:** Use of pharmacologic agents to reduce or eliminate pain **Bed Rest Care:** Promotion of comfort and safety and prevention of complications for a patient unable to get out of bed **Body Mechanics Promotion:** Facilitating the use of posture and movement in daily activities to prevent fatigue and musculoskeletal strain or injury **Cast Care: Maintenance:** Care of a cast after the drying period **Cast Care: Wet:** Care of new cast during the drying period **Exercise Promotion: Strength Training:** Facilitate regular resistive muscle treating to maintain or increase muscle strength **Exercise Therapy: Ambulation:** Promotion and assistance with walking to maintain or restore autonomic and voluntary body functions during treatment and recovery from illness or injury **Exercise Therapy: Joint Mobility:** Use of active or passive body movement to maintain or restore joint flexibility **Exercise Therapy: Muscle Control:** Use of specific activity or exercise protocols to enhance or restore controlled body movement **Fall Prevention:** Instituting special precautions with patient at risk for injury from falling **Pain Management:** Alleviation of pain or a reduction in pain to a level of comfort that is acceptable to the patient *(continued next page)*	**Ambulation:** Ability to walk from place to place independently with or without assistive device **Ambulation: Wheelchair:** Ability to move from place to place in a wheelchair **Balance:** Ability to maintain body equilibrium **Body Mechanics Performance:** Personal actions to maintain proper body alignment and to prevent muscular skeletal strain **Body Positioning: Self-Initiated:** Ability to change own body position independently with or without assistive device **Coordinated Movement:** Ability of muscles to work together voluntarily for a purposeful movement **Client Satisfaction: Functional Assistance:** Extent of positive perception of nursing assistance to achieve mobility and self-care **Joint Movement: (Specify Joint):** Active range of motion of (specify joint) with self-initiated movement **Joint Movement Passive:** Joint movement with assistance *(continued next page)*

Nursing Diagnosis (NANDA): Mobility: Physical, Impaired; Mobility: Bed, Impaired; Mobility: Wheelchair Impaired *(continued)*		
Orthopaedic Conditions*	**Nursing Intervention Classifications (NIC)**	**Nursing Outcome Classifications (NOC)**
Chapter 13: Arthritis & Connective Tissue Disorders Juvenile Arthritis Rheumatoid Osteoarthritis Polymyalgia Rheumatica Gout **Chapter 15: Orthopaedic Trauma** Spine Fractures Pelvic Fractures Femur/Hip Fractures Amputations Soft Trauma Dislocations/Subluxations Strains Sprains **Chapter 18: The Shoulder** Impingement Syndrome Rotator Cuff Tears Arthritis Shoulder Instability Adhesive Capsulitis Sprains, Strains, Contusions, Separations Sprengel's Deformity Glenoid Hypoplasia Referred Visceral Somatic Pain **Chapter 21: The Hip, Femur & Pelvis** Hip Fractures Hip Arthroplasty Hip Resurfacing Arthroplasty Hemiarthroplasty/Bipolar Replacement Hip Arthroscopy Femoro-Acetabular Impingement Hip Dislocation Hip Girdlestone Psuedoarthrosis Proximal Femoral Osteotomy Femoral Shaft Fractures Pelvic Fracture **Chapter 22: The Knee** Osteoarthritis Overuse Syndrome Trauma and Soft Tissue Injuries Pediatric Knee Conditions **Chapter 23: The Foot & Ankle** Ankle Sprains Achilles Rupture Fractures Plantar Fasciitis Pes Planus Pes Cavus Foot Drop Amputations Osteoarthritis	**Positioning: Intraoperative:** Moving the patient or body part to promote surgical exposure while reducing the risk of discomfort and complications **Positioning: Wheelchair:** Placement of a patient in a properly selected wheelchair to enhance comfort, promote skin integrity, and foster independence **Self-Care Assistance:** Assisting another to perform activities of daily living **Self Care Assistance: Transfer:** Assisting a patient with limitation of independent movement to learn to change body location **Surveillance: Safety:** Purposeful and ongoing collection and analysis of information about the patient and the environment for the use in promoting and maintaining patient safety **Traction/Immobilization Care:** Management of a patient who has traction and/or a stabilizing device to immobilize and stabilizing device to immobilize and stabilize a body part **Teaching: Prescribed Activity/Exercise:** Preparing a patient to achieve and/or maintain a prescribed level of activity	**Mobility:** Ability to move purposefully in own environment independently with or without assistive device **Neurological Status: Central Motor Control:** Ability of the central nervous system to coordinate skeletal muscle activity for body movement **Skeletal Function:** Ability of the bones to support the body and facilitate movement **Transfer Performance:** Ability to change body location independently with or without assistive device

Nursing Diagnosis (NANDA): Nausea		
Orthopaedic Conditions*	**Nursing Intervention Classifications (NIC)**	**Nursing Outcome Classifications (NOC)**
Chapter 8: Orthopaedic Complications Postoperative Nausea and Vomiting	**Fluid/Electrolyte Management:** Regulation and prevention of complications from altered fluid and/or electrolyte levels **Medication Management:** Facilitation of safe and effective use of prescription and over-the-counter drugs **Nausea Management:** Prevention and alleviation of nausea **Nutritional Monitoring:** Collection and analysis of patient data to prevent or minimize malnourishment **Vomiting Management:** Prevention and alleviation of vomiting	**Appetite:** Desire to eat when ill or receiving treatment **Comfort Level:** Extent of positive perception of physical and psychological ease **Hydration:** Adequate water in the intracellular and extracellular compartments of the body **Nausea & Vomiting Control:** Personal actions to control nausea, retching, and vomiting symptoms **Nausea & Vomiting: Disruptive Effect:** Severity of observed or reported disruptive effects of nausea, retching, and vomiting on daily function

Nursing Diagnosis (NANDA): Noncompliance		
Orthopaedic Conditions*	**Nursing Intervention Classifications (NIC)**	**Nursing Outcome Classifications (NOC)**
Chapter 10: Therapeutic Modalities Braces/Orthotics/Orthoses Continuous Passive Motion (CPM) Machine **Chapter 17: The Spine** Scoliosis Kyphosis **Chapter 18 - The Shoulder** Impingement Syndrome Rotator Cuff Tears Arthritis Shoulder Instability Adhesive Capsulitis Fractures of the Shoulder Sprains, Strains, Contusions, Separations Glenoid Hypoplasia Referred Visceral Somatic Pain	**Caregiver Support:** Provision of the necessary information, advocacy, and support to facilitate primary patient care by someone other than a health care professional **Coping Enhancement:** Assisting a patient to adapt to perceived stressors, changes, or threats that interfere with meeting life demands and roles **Decision-Making Support**: Providing information and support for a patient who is making a decision regarding health care **Health Education:** Developing and providing instruction and learning experiences to facilitate voluntary adaptation of behavior conducive to health in individuals, families, groups, or communities **Health System Guidance:** Facilitating a patient's location and use of appropriate health services **Learning Facilitation:** Promoting the ability to process and comprehend information **Mutual Goal Setting:** Collaborating with patient to identify ad prioritize care goals, then developing a plan for achieving those goals **Nutritional Counseling:** Use of an interactive helping process focusing on the need for diet modification **Patient Contracting:** Negotiating an agreement with an individual that reinforces a specific behavior change **Self-Modification Assistance:** Reinforcement of self-directed change initiated by the patient to achieve personally important goals **Self-Responsibility Facilitation:** Encouraging a patient to assume more responsibility for own behavior **Support System Enhancement:** Facilitation of support to patient by family, friends, and community *(continued next page)*	**Adherence Behavior:** Self-initiated actions to promote wellness, recovery, and rehabilitation **Caregiver Performance: Direct Care:** Provision by family care provider of appropriate personal and health care for a family member **Caregiver Performance: Indirect Care:** Arrangement and oversight by family care provider of appropriate care for a family member **Compliance Behavior:** Persona actions to promote wellness, recovery, and rehabilitation based on professional advice **Compliance Behavior: Prescribed Diet:** Personal actions to follow food and fluid intake recommended by a health professional for a specific health condition **Compliance Behavior: Prescribed Medication:** Personal actions to administer medication safely to meet therapeutic goals as recommended by a health professional **Motivation:** Inner urge that moves or prompts an individual to positive action(s) **Treatment Behavior: Illness or Injury:** Personal actions to palliate or eliminate pathology

Nursing Diagnosis (NANDA): Noncompliance *(continued)*		
Orthopaedic Conditions*	**Nursing Intervention Classifications (NIC)**	**Nursing Outcome Classifications (NOC)**
(see page 652)	**Teaching: Disease Process:** Assisting the patient to understand information related to a specific disease process **Teaching: Individual:** Planning, implementation, and evaluation of teaching program designed to address a patient's particular needs **Teaching: Prescribed Diet:** Preparing a patient to correctly follow a prescribed diet **Teaching: Prescribed Medication:** Preparing a patient to safely take prescribed medications and monitor for their effects	*(see page 652)*

Nursing Diagnosis (NANDA): Nutrition, Imbalanced: Less than Body Requirements		
Orthopaedic Conditions*	**Nursing Intervention Classifications (NIC)**	**Nursing Outcome Classifications (NOC)**
Chapter 6: Orthopaedic Effects of Immobility Metabolic/Gastrointestinal Issues **Chapter 8: Orthopaedic Complications** Pressure Ulcer **Chapter 11: Pediatrics** Cerebral Palsy Physical Abuse **Chapter 13: Arthritis & Connective Tissue Disorders** Systemic Sclerosis **Chapter 14: Metabolic Bone Conditions** Osteoporosis Osteomalacia Rickets Primary Hyperparathyroidism Secondary and Tertiary Hyperparathyroidism Hypoparathyroidism **Chapter 15: Orthopaedic Trauma** Soft Trauma Dislocations/Subluxations Strains Sprains **Chapter 17: The Spine** Herniated Nucleus Pulposus Degenerative Disc Disease Spinal Stenosis Spondylosis Spondylolithesis Failed Back Surgery Syndrome Spinal Fractures **Chapter 21: The Hip, Femur & Pelvis** Hip Fractures Hip Resurfacing Arthroplasty Hemiarthroplasty/Bipolar Replacement	**Laboratory Data Interpretation:** Critical analysis of patient laboratory data in order to assist with clinical decision-making **Nutritional Counseling:** Use of an interactive helping process focusing on the need for diet modification **Nutritional Monitoring:** Collection and analysis of patient data to prevent or minimize malnourishment **Nutrition Therapy:** Administration of food and fluids to support metabolic processes of a patient who is malnourished or at high risk for becoming malnourished **Teaching: Prescribed Diet:** Preparing a patient to correctly follow a prescribed diet **Weight Gain Assistance:** Facilitating gain of body weight **Weight Management:** Facilitating maintenance of optimal body weight and percent of body fat	**Appetite:** Desire to eat when ill or receiving treatment **Compliance Behavior: Prescribed Diet:** Personal actions to follow food and fluid intake recommended by a health professional for a specific health condition **Gastrointestinal Function:** Extend to which foods (ingested or tube-fed) are moved from ingestion to excretion **Nutritional Status:** Extent to which nutrients are available to meet metabolic needs **Nutritional Status: Biochemical Measures:** Body fluid components and chemical indices of nutritional status **Nutritional Status: Nutrient Intake:** Nutrient intake to meet metabolic needs **Weight: Body Mass:** Extent to which body weight, muscle, and fat are congruent to height, frame, gender and age **Weight Gain Behavior:** Personal actions to gain weight following voluntary or involuntary significant weight loss

Nursing Diagnosis (NANDA): Nutrition, Imbalanced: More than Body Requirements; Nutrition, Imbalanced: Risk for More than Body Requirements		
Orthopaedic Conditions*	**Nursing Intervention Classifications (NIC)**	**Nursing Outcome Classifications (NOC)**
Chapter 6: Orthopedic Effects of Immobility Metabolic/Gastrointestinal Issues **Chapter 8: Orthopaedic Complications** Pressure Ulcer **Chapter 11: Pediatrics** Achondroplasia Myelomeningocele **Chapter 13: Arthritis & Connective Tissue Disorders** Osteoarthritis **Chapter 17: The Spine** Herniated Nucleus Pulposus Degenerative Disc Disease Spinal Stenosis Spondylosis Spondylolithesis Failed Back Surgery Syndrome Spinal Fractures	**Behavior Modification:** Promotion of a behavior change **Exercise Promotion:** Facilitation of regular physical activity to maintain or advance to a higher level of fitness and health **Mutual Goal Setting:** Collaborating with patient to identify and prioritize care goals, then developing a plan for achieving those goals **Nutritional Counseling:** Use of an interactive helping process focusing on the need for diet modification **Nutrition Management:** Assisting with or providing a balanced dietary intake of foods and fluids **Nutritional Monitoring:** Collection and analysis of patient data to prevent or minimize malnourishment **Self-Modification Assistance:** Reinforcement of self-directed change initiated by the patient to achieve personally important goals **Teaching: Prescribed Diet:** Preparing a patient to correctly follow a prescribed diet **Weight Reduction Assistance:** Facilitating loss of weight and/or body fat	**Adherence Behavior: Healthy Diet:** Personal actions to monitor and optimize a healthy and nutritional dietary regimen **Compliance Behavior: Prescribed Diet:** Personal actions to follow food and fluid intake recommended by a health professional for a specific health condition **Knowledge: Diet:** Extent of understanding conveyed about recommended diet **Nutritional Status: Food & Fluid Intake:** Amount of food and fluid taken into the body over a 24-hour period. **Weight Loss Behavior:** Personal action to loose weight through diet, exercise and behavior modification **Weight: Body Mass:** Extends to which body weight, muscle, and fats are congruent to height, frame, gender, and age **Weight Maintenance Behavior:** Personal actions to maintain optimal body weight

Nursing Diagnosis (NANDA): Pain, Acute		
Orthopaedic Conditions*	**Nursing Intervention Classifications (NIC)**	**Nursing Outcome Classifications (NOC)**
Chapter 8: Orthopaedic Complications Constipation Nosocomial Surgical Site Infections Compartment Syndrome Venous Thromboembolism Postoperative Urinary Retention **Chapter 9: Orthopaedic Infections** Osteomyelitis Septic Arthritis Prosthetic Joint Infection Skin and Soft Tissue Infections **Chapter 10: Therapeutic Modalities** Casts Continuous Passive Motion Machine External Fixator Traction *(continued next page)*	**Analgesic Administration:** Use of pharmacologic agents to reduce or eliminate pain **Coping Enhancement:** Assisting a patient to adapt to perceived stressors, changes, or threats that interfere with meeting life demands and roles **Environmental Management: Comfort:** Manipulation of the patient's surrounding for promotion of optimal comfort Heat/ Cold Application: Stimulation of the skin and underlying tissues with heat or cold for the purpose of decreasing pain, muscle spasm, or inflammation **Pain Management:** Alleviation of pain or a reduction in pain to a level of comfort that is acceptable to the patient Patient-Controlled Analgesia (PCA) Assistance: Facilitating patient control of analgesic administration and regulation **Positioning:** Deliberate placement of the patient or a body part to promote physiological and/or psychological well-being **Simple Guided Imagery:** Purposeful use of imagination to achieve relaxation and/or direct attention away from undesirable sensations *(continued next page)*	**Client Satisfaction: Pain Management:** Extent of positive perception of nursing care to relieve pain **Discomfort Level:** Extent of observed or reported mental or physical discomfort **Medication Response:** Therapeutic and adverse effects of prescribed medication **Pain Control:** Personal actions to control pain **Pain Level:** Severity of observed or reported pain

Nursing Diagnosis (NANDA): Pain, Acute *(continued)*		
Orthopaedic Conditions*	**Nursing Intervention Classifications (NIC)**	**Nursing Outcome Classifications (NOC)**
Chapter 11: Pediatrics Cerebral Palsy Neurofibromastosis Osteogenesis Imperfecta Legg-Calve-Perthes Disease Leg Length Discrepancies Osgood-Schlatter Disease Pediatric Fractures Slipped Capital Femoral Epiphysis **Chapter 13: Arthritis & Connective Tissue Disorders** Juvenile Arthritis Polymalgia Rhuematica Gout Lyme Disease Sytemic Lupus **Chapter 14: Metabolic Bone Conditions** Osteomalacia Paget's Disease **Chapter 15: Orthopaedic Trauma** Spine Fractures Pelvic Fractures Femur/Hip Fractures Amputations Soft Trauma Dislocations/Subluxations Strains Sprains **Chapter 16: Tumors of the Musculoskeletal System** Benign Lesions Primary Malignant Tumors Primary Sarcoma Bone Metastasis Multiple Myeloma **Chapter 17: The Spine** Herniated Nucleus Pulposus Degenerative Disc Disease Spinal Stenosis Spondylolysis and Spondylolisthesis Failed Back Surgery Syndrome Spinal Fractures **Chapter 18: The Shoulder** Tendinitis Rotator Cuff Tears Arthritis Fractures of the Shoulder Sprains, Strains, and Contusions Referred Visceral Somatic Pain *(continued next page)*	**Simple Massage:** Stimulation of the skin and underlying tissues with varying degrees of hand pressure to decrease pain, produce relaxation, and/or improve circulation **Simple Relaxation Therapy:** Use of techniques to encourage and elicit relaxation for the purpose of decreasing undesirable signs and symptoms such as pain, muscle tension, or anxiety **Splinting:** Stabilization, immobilization, and/or protection of an injured body part with a supportive appliance **Teaching: Prescribed Medication:** Preparing a patient to safely take prescribed medications and monitor for their effects	*(see page 654)*

Nursing Diagnosis (NANDA): Pain, Acute *(continued)*		
Orthopaedic Conditions*	**Nursing Intervention Classifications (NIC)**	**Nursing Outcome Classifications (NOC)**
Chapter 19: The Elbow Lateral and Medial Epicondylitis Pitcher's Elbow Olecranon Bursitis Distal Biceps Tendon Rupture Radial Head, Monteggia, Coronoid Process, and Olecranon Fractures Subluxation/Nursemaid's Elbow Supracondylar/Distal Humerus Fractures Elbow Dislocation Nerve Entrapments Osteochondritis of the Capitellum Elbow Arthroplasty **Chapter 20: The Hand & Wrist** Mallet Finger Boutonniere and Swan Neck Deformities Gamekeeper's Thumb Nail Bed Injuries DeQuervain's Replantation Arthroplasty Thumb Fractures—Bennett's and Rolando's Boxer's Fracture Scaphoid Fracture Distal Radius Fractures—Colles' and Smith's **Chapter 21: The Hip, Femur & Pelvis** Hip Fractures Hip Arthroplasty Hip Dislocation Hip Girdlestone Pseudoarthrosis Hip Arthrodesis Proximal Femoral Osteotomy Femoral Shaft Fractures Pelvic Fracture **Chapter 22: The Knee** Osteoarthritis Overuse Syndromes Trauma and Soft Tissue Injuries Pediatric Knee Conditions **Chapter 23: The Foot & Ankle** Ankle Sprains Achilles Tenosynovitis Achilles Tendon Rupture Plantar Fasciitis Corn, Verruca Plantaris, Onychocryptosis Hallux Valgus Amputations Interdigital Neuroma Toe Deformities Fractures Charcot Foot Diabetic Foot	*(see pages 654-55)*	*(see page 654)*

Nursing Diagnosis (NANDA): Pain, Chronic

Orthopaedic Conditions*	Nursing Intervention Classifications (NIC)	Nursing Outcome Classifications (NOC)
Chapter 8: Orthopaedic Complications Nosocomial Surgical Site Infections **Chapter 9: Orthopaedic Infections** Bone and Joint/Extrapulmonary Tuberculosis **Chapter 11: Pediatrics** Cerebral Palsy Legg-Calve-Perthes Disease Neurofibromatosis Osteogenesis Imperfecta Slipped Capital Femoral Epiphysis Torsional Issues **Chapter 13: Arthritis & Connective Tissue Disorders** Juvenile Arthritis Rheumatoid Arthritis Seronegative Spondyloarthropathies Ankylosing Spondylitis Psoriatic Arthritis Systemic Lupus Erythematosus Fibromyalgia Syndrome **Chapter 14: Metabolic Bone Conditions** Osteomalacia Paget's Disease **Chapter 15: Orthopaedic Trauma** Femur/Hip Fractures **Chapter 16: Tumors of the Musculoskeletal System** Benign Lesions Primary Malignant Tumors Primary Sarcoma Bone Metastasis Multiple Myeloma **Chapter 17: The Spine** Scoliosis Kyphosis Herniated Nucleus Pulposus Spinal Stenosis Degenerative Disc Disease Spondylolysis and Spondylolisthesis Failed Back Syndrome Spinal Fractures **Chapter 18: The Shoulder** Rotator Cuff Tears Impingement Syndrome Shoulder Instability Adhesive Capsulitis Arthritis Sprains, Strains, Contusions, Separations Sprengel's Deformity Glenoid Hyperplasia **Chapter 20: The Hand & Wrist** Trigger Thumb or Finger *(continued next page)*	**Behavior Modification:** Promotion of a behavior change **Cognitive Restructuring:** Challenging a patient to alter distorted thought patterns and view self and world more realistically **Coping Enhancement:** Assisting a patient to adapt to perceived stressors, changes, or threats that interfere with meeting life demands and roles **Medication Management:** Facilitation of safe and effective use of prescription and over-the-counter medications **Mood Management:** Providing for safety, stabilization, recovery, and maintenance of a patient experiencing dysfunctionally depressed or elevated mood **Pain Management:** Alleviation of pain or a reduction in pain to a level of comfort that is acceptable to the patient **Patient Contracting:** Negotiating an agreement with an individual that reinforces a specific behavior change **Self-Responsibility Facilitation:** Encouraging a patient to assume more responsibility for own behavior **Simple Guided Imagery:** Purposeful use of imagination to achieve relaxation and/or direct attention away from undesirable sensations **Simple Massage:** Stimulation of the skin and underlying tissues with varying degrees of hand pressure to decrease pain, produce relaxation, and/or improve circulation **Simple Relaxation Therapy:** Use of techniques to encourage and elicit relaxation for the purpose of decreasing undesirable signs and symptoms such as pain, muscle tension, or anxiety **Transcutaneous Electrical Nerve Stimulation (TENS):** Stimulation of skin and underlying tissues with controlled, low-voltage electrical vibration via electrodes	**Client Satisfaction: Pain Management:** Extent of positive perception of nursing care to relieve pain **Comfort Level:** Extent of positive perception of physical and psychological ease **Depression Level:** Severity of melancholic mood and loss of interest in life events **Depression Self-Control:** Personal actions to minimize melancholy and maintain interest in life events **Medication Response:** Therapeutic and adverse effects of prescribed medication **Pain: Adverse Psychological Response:** Severity of observed or reported adverse cognitive and emotional responses to physical pain **Pain Control:** Personal actions to control pain **Pain: Disruptive Effects:** Severity of observed or reported disruptive effects of chronic pain on daily functioning **Pain Level:** Severity of observed or reported pain

Nursing Diagnosis (NANDA): Pain, Chronic *(continued)*		
Orthopaedic Conditions*	**Nursing Intervention Classifications (NIC)**	**Nursing Outcome Classifications (NOC)**
Chapter 22: The Knee Osteoarthritis Overuse Syndromes Trauma and Soft Tissue Injuries Pediatric Knee Conditions **Chapter 23: The Foot & Ankle** Ankle Sprains Achilles Tendinitis Achilles Tendon Rupture Plantar Fasciitis Pes Planus Pes Cavus Toe Deformities Corns Verruca Plantaris Onychocryptosis Osteoarthritis	*(see page 657)*	*(see page 657)*

Nursing Diagnosis (NANDA): Parenting, Impaired; Parenting, Risk for Impaired		
Orthopaedic Conditions*	**Nursing Intervention Classifications (NIC)**	**Nursing Outcome Classifications (NOC)**
Chapter 8: Orthopaedic Complications Pressure Ulcer **Chapter 11: Pediatrics** Arthrogryposis Multiplex Congenita Physical Abuse **Chapter 13: Arthritis & Connective Tissue Disorders** Systemic Lupus Erythematosus **Chapter 18: The Shoulder** Fractures Sprengel's Deformity **Chapter 23: The Foot & Ankle** Pes Planus	**Anxiety Reduction:** Minimizing apprehension, dread, foreboding, or uneasiness related to an unidentified source of anticipated danger **Conflict Mediation:** Facilitation of constructive dialogue between opposing parties with a goal of resolving disputes in a mutually acceptable manner **Coping Enhancement:** Assisting the patient to adapt to perceived stressors, changes, or threats that interfere with meeting life demands and roles **Decision-Making Support:** Providing information and support for a patient who is making a decision regarding health care **Environmental Management: Safety:** Monitoring and manipulation of the physical environment to promote safety **Family Involvement Promotion:** Facilitating family participation in the emotional and physical care of the patient **Family Integrity Promotion:** Promotion of family cohesion and unity **Parenting Promotion:** Providing parenting information, support, and coordination of comprehensive services to high-risk families **Risk Identification:** Analysis of potential risk factors, determination of health risks, and prioritization of risk reduction strategies for an individual or group **Role Enhancement:** Assisting a patient, significant other, and/or family to improve relationships by clarifying and supplementing specific role behaviors *(continued next page)*	**Parenting Performance:** Parental actions to provide a child with a nurturing and constructive physical, emotional, and social environment **Parenting: Psychosocial Safety:** Parental actions to protect a child from social contacts that might cause harm or injury **Role Performance:** Congruence of an individual's role behavior with role expectations **Safe Home Environment:** Physical arrangements to minimize environmental factors that might cause physical harm or injury in the home **Social Support:** Reliable assistance from others

Nursing Diagnosis (NANDA): Parenting, Impaired; Parenting, Risk for Impaired *(continued)*		
Orthopaedic Conditions*	**Nursing Intervention Classifications (NIC)**	**Nursing Outcome Classifications (NOC)**
(see page 658)	**Support Group:** Use of a group environment to provide emotional support and health-related information for members **Support System Enhancement:** Facilitation of support to patient by family, friends, and community **Surveillance: Safety:** Purposeful and ongoing collection and analysis of information about the patient and the environment for use in promoting and maintaining patient safety	*(see page 658)*

Nursing Diagnosis (NANDA): Perioperative Positioning Injury, Risk For		
Orthopaedic Conditions*	**Nursing Intervention Classifications (NIC)**	**Nursing Outcome Classifications (NOC)**
Chapter 20: The Hand & Wrist Replantation Arthroplasty	**Circulatory Care: Arterial:** Promotion of arterial circulation **Circulatory Care: Mechanical Assist Device:** Temporary support of the circulation through the use of mechanical devices or pumps **Circulatory Care: Venous Insufficiency:** Promotion of venous circulation **Delirium Management:** Provision of a safe and therapeutic environment for the patient experiencing and acute confusional state **Embolus Precautions:** Reduction of the risk of embolus in a patient with thrombi by or risk for thrombus formation **Fluid Management:** Promotion of fluid balance and prevention of complications resulting from abnormal or undesired fluid levels **Positioning: Intraoperative:** Moving the patient or body part to promote surgical exposure while reducing the risk of discomfort and complications **Pressure Management:** Minimizing pressure to body parts	**Circulation Status:** Unobstructed, unidirectional blood flow at appropriate pressure through large vessels of the systemic and pulmonary circuits **Neurological Status: Spinal:** Ability of the spinal nerves to convey sensory and motor impulses **Physical Injury Severity:** Severity of injuries from accident and trauma **Sensory Function Status:** Extent to which an individual correctly perceives skin stimulation, sounds, proprioception, taste and smell, and visual images **Tissue Perfusion:** Peripheral: Adequacy of blood flow through the small vessels of the extremities to maintain tissue function

Nursing Diagnosis (NANDA): Peripheral Neurovascular Dysfunction, Risk for		
Orthopaedic Conditions*	**Nursing Intervention Classifications (NIC)**	**Nursing Outcome Classifications (NOC)**
Chapter 6: Orthopaedic Effects of Immobility Neurosensory Issues **Chapter 8: Orthopaedic Complications** Compartment Syndrome (Acute and Crush Syndrome) Venous Thromboembolism Compartment Syndrome **Chapter 10: Therapeutic Modalities** Braces/Orthotics/Orthoses Casts External Fixators Traction **Chapter 11: Pediatrics** Blount's Disease Developmental Dysplasia of the Hip GenuValgum/Genu Varum Leg Length Discrepencies Pediatric Fractures **Chapter 15: Orthopaedic Trauma** Spine Fractures Pelvic Fractures Soft Trauma Dislocations/Subluxations Strains Sprains **Chapter 17: The Spine** Herniated Nucleus Pulposus Spinal Stenosis Degenerative Disc Disease Spondylolysis and Spondylolisthesis Failed Back Syndrome **Chapter 19: The Elbow** Supracondylar/Distal Humerus Fractures Elbow Dislocation **Chapter 20: The Hand & Wrist** Replantation **Chapter 23: The Foot & Ankle** Charcot Foot Diabetic Foot	**Bed Rest Care:** Promotion of comfort and safety and prevention of complications for patients unable to get out of bed **Bleeding Reduction:** Limitation of the loss of blood volume during an episode of bleeding **Cast Care Maintenance:** Care of the cast after the drying **Cast Care: Wet:** Care of a new cast during the drying **Circulatory Care: Arterial Insufficiency:** Promotion of arterial circulation **Circulatory Care: Mechanical Assist Device:** Temporary support of the circulation through the use of mechanical devices or pumps **Embolus Precautions:** Reduction of the risk of an embolus in a patient with thrombi or at risk for thrombus formation **Neurologic Monitoring:** Collection and analysis of patient data to prevent or minimize neurologic complications **Pneumatic Tourniquet Precautions:** Applying a pneumatic tourniquet, while minimizing the potential for patient injury from use of the device **Pressure Management**: Minimizing pressure to body parts **Pressure Ulcer Prevention:** Prevention of pressure ulcers for a high-risk individual **Risk Identification:** Analysis of potential risk factors, determination of health risks, and prioritization of risk reduction strategies for an individual or group **Traction/Immobilization Care:** Management of the patient who has traction and/or a stabilizing device to immobilize and stabilize a body part	**Bone Healing:** Extent of regeneration of cells and tissues following bone injury **Burn Healing:** Extent of healing of a burn site **Circulation Status:** Unobstructed, unidirectional blood flow at an appropriate pressure through large vessels of the systemic and pulmonary circuits **Neurological Status: Peripheral:** Ability of the peripheral nervous system to transmit impulses to and from the central nervous system **Neurological Status: Spinal:** Ability of the spinal nerves to convey sensory and motor impulses **Sensory Function: Cutaneous:** Extent to which stimulation of the skin is correctly sensed **Sensory Function:** Extent to which an individual correctly perceives skin stimulation, sounds, proprioception, taste and smell, and visual images **Tissue Perfusion: Peripheral:** Adequacy of blood flow through the small vessels of the extremities to maintain tissue function

Nursing Diagnosis (NANDA): Post-Trauma Syndrome; Post-Trauma Syndrome, Risk for		
Orthopaedic Conditions*	**Nursing Intervention Classifications (NIC)**	**Nursing Outcome Classifications (NOC)**
Chapter 15: Orthopaedic Trauma Pelvic Fractures **Chapter 21: The Hip, Femur & Pelvis** Hip Fractures Hip Arthroplasty Hip Resurfacing Hemiarthroplasty/Bipolar	**Anger Control Assistance:** Facilitation of the expression of anger in an adaptive, nonviolent manner **Anxiety Reduction:** Minimizing apprehension, dread, foreboding, or uneasiness related to a an unidentified source of anticipated or perceived danger **Behavior Management: Self-Harm:** Assisting the patient to decrease or eliminate self-mutilating or self-abusive behaviors **Calming Technique:** Reducing anxiety in a patient experiencing acute distress **Coping Enhancement:** Assisting a patient to adapt to perceived stressors, changes, or threats that interfere with meeting life demands and roles **Counseling:** Use of interactive helping process focusing on the needs, problems, or feelings of the patient and significant others to enhance or support coping, problem solving, and interpersonal relationships **Emotional Support:** Provision of reassurance, acceptance, and encouragement during times of stress **Environmental Management: Safety:** Monitoring and manipulation of the physical environment to promote safety **Mood Management:** Providing for safety, stabilization, recovery, and maintenance of a patient experiencing dysfunctionally depressed or elevated mood **Grief Work Facilitation:** Assistance with the resolution of a significant loss **Guilt Work Facilitation:** Helping another to cope with painful feelings of actual or perceived responsibility **Music Therapy:** Using music to help achieve a specific change in behavior, feeling, or physiology **Progressive Muscle Relaxation:** Facilitating the tensing and releasing of successive muscle groups while attending to the resulting differences in sensation **Relaxation Therapy:** Use of techniques to encourage and elicit relaxation for the purpose of decreasing undesirable signs and symptoms such as pain, muscle tension, or anxiety **Suicide Prevention:** Reducing risk of self-inflicted harm with intent to end life **Support Group:** Use of a group environment to provide emotional support and health-related information for members **Support System Enhancement:** Facilitation of support to patients by family, friends, and community **Trauma Therapy: Child:** Use of an interactive helping process to resolve any trauma experienced by a child	**Anxiety Level:** Severity of manifested apprehension, tension, or uneasiness arising from an unidentifiable source **Comfort Status: Psychospiritual:** Psychospiritual ease related to self-concept, emotional well-being, source of inspiration, and meaning and purpose in one's life **Coping:** Personal actions to manage stressors that tax an individual's resources **Depression Level:** Severity of melancholic mood and loss of interest in life events **Fear Level:** Severity of manifested apprehension, tension, or uneasiness arising from an identifiable source **Fear Level: Child:** Severity of manifested apprehension, tension, or uneasiness arising from an identifiable source in children ages 1-17 **Health Beliefs: Perceived Threat:** Personal conviction that a threatening health problem is serious and has potential negative consequences for lifestyle **Impulse Self-Control:** Self-restraint of compulsive or impulsive behavior **Self-Mutilation Restraint:** Personal actions to refrain from intentional self-inflicted injury (non-lethal) **Stress Level:** Severity of manifested physical or mental tension resulting from factors that alter existing equilibrium

Nursing Diagnosis (NANDA): Powerlessness; Powerlessness, Risk for		
Orthopaedic Conditions*	**Nursing Intervention Classifications (NIC)**	**Nursing Outcome Classifications (NOC)**
Chapter 10: Therapeutic Modalities Ambulatory Devices and Techniques Braces/Orthotics/Orthoses Continuous Passive Motion Machine External Fixators Traction Wheelchairs **Chapter 13: Arthritis & Connective Tissue Disorders** Rheumatoid Arthritis Polymyalgia Rheumatica Fibromyalgia Syndrome **Chapter 16: Tumors of the Musculoskeletal System** Primary Sarcoma Bone Metastasis Multiple Myeloma **Chapter 17: The Spine** Scoliosis Kyphosis **Chapter 21: The Hip, Femur & Pelvis** Hip Fractures Hip Resurfacing Arthroplasty Hemiarthroplasty/Bipolar Replacement Hip Arthroscopy	**Cognitive Restructuring:** Challenging a patient to alter distorted thought patterns and view self and world more realistically **Decision Making Support:** Providing information and support for a patient who is making a decision regarding health care **Dying Care:** Promotion of physical comfort and psychological peace in the final phase of life **Emotional Support:** Provision of reassurance, acceptance, and encouragement during times of stress **Family Involvement Promotion:** Facilitating family participation in the emotional and physical care of the patient **Health Education:** Developing and providing instruction and learning experiences to facilitate voluntary adaptation of behavior conducive to health in individuals, families, groups, or communities **Health System Guidance:** Facilitating a patient's location of and use of appropriate health services **Hope Inspiration:** Enhancing the belief in one's capacity to initiate and sustain actions **Mood Management:** Providing for safety, stabilization, recovery, and maintenance of a patient experiencing dysfunctional depressed or elevated mood **Mutual Goal Setting:** Collaborating with patient to identify and prioritize care goals, then developing a plan for achieving those goals **Patient Rights Protection:** Protection of health care rights of a patient, especially a minor, incapacitated, or incompetent patient unable to make decisions **Self-Esteem Enhancement:** Assisting a patient to increase his/her personal judgment of self worth **Self-Responsibility Facilitation:** Encouraging a patient to assume more responsibility for own behavior **Values Clarification:** Assisting another to clarify her/his own values in order to facilitate effective decision-making	**Adaptation to Physical Disability:** Adaptive response to a significant functional challenge due to a physical disability **Depression: Self Control:** Personal actions to minimize melancholy and maintain interest in life events **Family Participation in Professional Care:** Family Involvement in decision-making, delivery, and evaluation of care provide by health care personnel **Health Beliefs:** Personal conviction that one can carry out a given health behavior **Health Beliefs: Perceived Ability to Perform:** Personal conviction that one can carry out a given health behavior **Health Beliefs: Perceived Control:** Personal conviction that one can influence a health outcome **Health Beliefs: Perceived Resources:** Personal conviction that one has adequate means to carry out a health behavior **Hope:** Optimism that is personally satisfying and life-supporting **Immobility Consequences: Psycho-Cognitive:** Severity of compromise in psycho-cognitive functioning due to impaired physical mobility **Participation in Health Care Decisions:** Personal involvement in selecting and evaluating health care options to achieve desired outcomes **Personal Autonomy:** Personal actions of a competent individual to exercise governance in life decisions

Nursing Diagnosis (NANDA): Resilience, Impaired Individual; Resilience, Readiness for Enhanced		
Orthopaedic Conditions*	**Nursing Intervention Classifications (NIC)**	**Nursing Outcome Classifications (NOC)**
Chapter 13: Arthritis & Connective Tissue Disorders Rheumatoid Arthritis Polymyalgia Rheumatica	**Anxiety Reduction:** Minimizing apprehension, dread, foreboding, or uneasiness related to an identified source of anticipated danger **Conflict Mediation:** Facilitation of constructive dialogue between opposing parties with the goal of resolving disputes in a mutually acceptable manner **Coping Enhancement:** Assisting a patient to adapt to perceived stressors, changes, or threats that interfere with meeting life demands and roles *(continued next page)*	**Coping:** Personal actions to manage stressors that tax an individual's resources **Depression Level:** Severity of melancholic mood and loss of interest in life events **Personal Resiliency:** Positive adaptation and function of an individual following significant adversity or crisis *(continued next page)*

Nursing Diagnosis (NANDA): Resilience, Impaired Individual; Resilience, Readiness for Enhanced *(continued)*		
Orthopaedic Conditions*	**Nursing Intervention Classifications (NIC)**	**Nursing Outcome Classifications (NOC)**
(see page 662)	**Decision-Making Support:** Providing information and support for patient making a decision regarding health care **Health System Guidance:** Facilitating a patient's location and use of appropriate health services **Mood Management:** Providing for safety, stabilization, recovery, and maintenance of a patient experiencing dysfunctionally depressed or elevated mood **Resiliency Promotion:** Assisting individuals, families, and communities in development, use, and strengthening of protective factors to be used in coping with environmental and societal stressors **Risk Identification:** Analysis of potential risk factors, determination of health risks, and prioritization of risk reduction strategies for any individual or group **Role Enhancement:** Assisting a patient, significant other, and/or family to improve relationships by clarifying and supplementing specific role behaviors **Support Group:** Use of a group environment to providing emotional support and health-related information for members **Support System Enhancement:** Facilitation of support to patient by family, friends, and community	*(see page 662)*

Nursing Diagnosis (NANDA): Role Performance, Ineffective		
Orthopaedic Conditions*	**Nursing Intervention Classifications (NIC)**	**Nursing Outcome Classifications (NOC)**
Chapter 10: Therapeutic Modalities Ambulatory Devices and Techniques **Chapter 13: Arthritis & Connective Tissue Disorders** Osteoarthritis **Chapter 18: The Shoulder** Impingement Syndrome Rotator Cuff Tears Arthritis Shoulder Instability Adhesive Capsulitis Fractures of the Shoulder Sprains, Strains, Contusions, Separations Sprengel's Deformity Glenoid Hypoplasia Referred Visceral Somatic Pain **Chapter 20: The Hand & Wrist** Replantation	**Anticipatory Guidance:** Preparation of patient for an anticipated developmental and/or situational crisis **Coping Enhancement:** Assisting the patient to adapt to perceived stressors, changes, or threats that interfere with meeting life demands and roles **Emotional Support:** Provision of reassurance, acceptance, and encouragement during times of stress **Hope Instillation:** Facilitation of the development of a positive outlook in a given situation **Mood Management:** Providing for safety, stabilization, recovery, and maintenance of a patient experiencing dysfunctionally depressed or elevated mood **Parenting Promotion:** Providing parenting information, support, and coordination of comprehensive services to high-risk families **Role Enhancement:** Assisting a patient, significant other, and/or family to improve relationships by clarifying and supplementing specific role behaviors **Self-Efficacy Enhancement:** Strengthening an individual's confidence in his/her ability to perform a health behavior	**Caregiver Lifestyle Disruption:** Severity of disturbances in the lifestyle of a family member due to caregiving **Caregiver Performance: Direct Care:** Provision by family care provider of appropriate personal and health care for a family member **Caregiver Performance: Indirect Care:** Arrangement and oversight by family care provider of appropriate care for a family member **Coping:** Personal actions to manage stressors that tax an individual's resources **Depression Level:** Severity of melancholic mood and loss of interest in life events **Parenting Performance:** Parental actions to provide a child with a nurturing and constructive physical, emotional, and social environment **Psychosocial Adjustment: Life Change:** Adaptive psychosocial response of an individual to a significant life change **Role Performance:** Congruence of an individual's role behavior with role expectations

Nursing Diagnosis (NANDA): Self-Care Deficit: Bathing/Hygiene, Dressing/Grooming, Feeding, Toileting		
Orthopaedic Conditions*	**Nursing Intervention Classifications (NIC)**	**Nursing Outcome Classifications (NOC)**
Chapter 10: Therapeutic Modalities Traction Ambulatory Devices/Techniques Braces/Orthotics/Orthoses External Fixators **Chapter 11: Pediatrics** Achondroplasia Arthrogryposis Multiplex Congenita **Chapter 13: Arthritis & Connective Tissue Disorders** Juvenile Arthritis Rheumatoid Arthritis Osteoarthritis Polymyalgia Rheumatica Psoriatic Arthritis Fibromyalgia Syndrome **Chapter 15: Orthopaedic Trauma** Pelvic Fractures Soft Trauma Dislocations/Subluxations Strains Sprains **Chapter 17: The Spine** Scoliosis Kyphosis Herniated Nucleus Pulposus Degenerative Disc Disease Spinal Stenosis Spondylosis Spondylolithesis Failed Back Surgery Syndrome Spinal Fractures **Chapter 18: The Shoulder** Impingement Syndrome Rotator Cuff Tears Arthritis Shoulder Instability Adhesive Capsulitis Fractures of the Shoulder Sprains, Strains, Contusions, Separations Sprengel's Deformity Glenoid Hypoplasia Referred Visceral Somatic Pain *(continued next page)*	**Environment Management:** Manipulation of the patient's surrounding for the therapeutic benefit, sensory appeal, and psychological well-being **Self-Care Assistance: Bathing/Hygiene:** Assisting another to perform personal hygiene **Self-Care Assistance: Dressing/Grooming:** Assisting patient with clothes and makeup **Self-Care Assistance: Feeding:** Assisting a person to eat **Self-Care Assistance: Toileting:** Assisting another with elimination	**Self-Care: Bathing/Hygiene:** Ability to cleanse own body independently with or without assistive devices and to maintain own personal cleanliness and kempt appearance independently with or without assistive device **Self-Care: Dressing:** Ability to dress self independently with or without assistive device **Self-Care: Eating:** Ability to prepare and ingest food and fluid independently with or without assistive device **Self-Care: Toileting:** Ability to toilet self independently with or without assistive device

Nursing Diagnosis (NANDA): Self-Care Deficit: Bathing/Hygiene, Dressing/Grooming, Feeding, Toileting *(continued)*		
Orthopaedic Conditions*	**Nursing Intervention Classifications (NIC)**	**Nursing Outcome Classifications (NOC)**
Chapter 19: The Elbow Lateral and Medial Epicondylitis Pitcher's Elbow Olecranon Bursitis Distal Biceps Tendon Rupture Radial Head, Monteggia, Coronoid Process, and Olecranon Fractures Subluxation/Nursemaid's Elbow Supracondylar/Distal Humerus Fractures Elbow Dislocation Nerve Entrapments Osteochondritis of the Capitellum Elbow Arthroplasty **Chapter 20: The Hand & Wrist** Boutonniere and Swan Neck Deformities Gamekeeper's Thumb Nail Bed Injuries Dupuytren's Contracture Distal Radius Fractures—Colles' and Smith's Mallet Finger Trigger Thumb/Finger DeQuervain's Ganglion Cyst Carpal Tunnel Syndrome Replantation Arthroplasty Thumb Fractures—Bennett's and Rolando's Boxer's Fracture Scaphoid Fracture **Chapter 21: The Hip, Femur & Pelvis** Hip Fractures Hip Arthroplasty Hip Resurfacing Arthroplasty Hemiarthroplasty/Bipolar Replacement Hip Arthroscopy Femoro-Acetabular Impingement Hip Dislocation Hip Girdlestone Psuedoarthrosis Proximal Femoral Osteotomy Femoral Shaft Fractures Pelvic Fracture **Chapter 22: The Knee** Osteoarthritis Overuse Injuries Traumas Pediatric Knee Conditions	*(see page 664)*	*(see page 664)*

Nursing Diagnosis (NANDA): Self-Concept, Readiness for Enhanced		
Orthopaedic Conditions*	**Nursing Intervention Classifications (NIC)**	**Nursing Outcome Classifications (NOC)**
Chapter 10: Therapeutic Modalities Ambulatory Devices and Techniques Braces/Orthotics/Orthoses External Fixators Traction Wheelchairs **Chapter 11: Pediatrics** Achondroplasia Blount's Disease GenuValgum/Genu Varum Leg Length Discrepencies Neurofibromatosis Torsional Issues **Chapter 15: Orthopaedic Trauma** Soft Trauma **Chapter 17: The Spine** Scoliosis Kyphosis Spondylosis Spondylolithesis Failed Back Surgery Syndrome Spinal Fractures **Chapter 18: The Shoulder** Arthritis Fractures of the Shoulder Sprengel's Deformity Referred Visceral Somatic Pain	**Amputation Care:** Promotion of physical and psychological healing before and after amputation of a body part **Body Image Enhancement:** Improving a patient's conscious and unconscious perceptions and attitudes toward own body **Developmental Enhancement: Adolescent:** Facilitating optimal physical, cognitive, social, and emotional growth of individuals during the transition from childhood to adulthood **Developmental Enhancement: Child:** Facilitating or teaching parents/caregivers to facilitate the optimal gross motor, fine motor, language, cognitive, social, and emotional growth of preschoolers and school-aged children **Role Enhancement:** Assisting a patient, significant other, and/or family to improve relationships by clarifying and supplementing specific role behaviors **Self-Awareness Enhancement:** Assisting a patient to explore and understand own thoughts, feelings, motivations, and behaviors **Self-Esteem Enhancement:** Assisting a patient to increase own personal judgment of self-worth	**Body Image:** Perception of own appearance and body functions **Personal Well-Being:** Extent of positive perception of one's health status **Self-Esteem:** Personal judgment of self-worth

Nursing Diagnosis (NANDA): Self-Esteem: Chronic Low; Self Esteem: Situational Low; Self-Esteem: Situational Low, Risk for		
Orthopaedic Conditions*	**Nursing Intervention Classifications (NIC)**	**Nursing Outcome Classifications (NOC)**
Chapter 10: Therapeutic Modalities Ambulatory Devices and Techniques **Chapter 17: The Spine** Scoliosis Kyphosis Spondylosis Spondylolithesis Failed Back Surgery Syndrome Spinal Fractures **Chapter 22: The Knee** Pediatric Knee Conditions **Chapter 23: The Foot & Ankle** Amputations	**Body Image Enhancement:** Improving a patient's conscious and unconscious perceptions and attitudes toward own body **Coping Enhancement:** Assisting the patient to adapt to perceived stressors, changes, or threats that interfere with meeting life demands and roles **Developmental Enhancement: Adolescent:** Facilitating optimal physical, cognitive, social, and emotional growth of individuals during the transition from childhood to adulthood **Developmental Enhancement: Child:** Facilitating or teaching parents/caregivers to facilitate the optimal gross motor, fine motor, language, cognitive, social, and emotional growth of preschoolers and school-aged children **Self-Esteem Enhancement:** Assisting a patient to increase personal judgment of self-worth	**Self-esteem:** Personal judgment of self worth

Nursing Diagnosis (NANDA): Self-Health Management, Ineffective		
Orthopaedic Conditions*	**Nursing Intervention Classifications (NIC)**	**Nursing Outcome Classifications (NOC)**
Chapter 13: Arthritis & Connective Tissue Disorders Juvenile Arthritis Osteoarthritis **Chapter 14: Metabolic Bone Conditions** Osteoporosis Osteomalacia Secondary and Tertiary Hyperparathyroidism Hypoparathyroidism Paget's Disease **Chapter 22: The Knee** Overuse Syndrome Trauma and Soft Tissue Injuries Pediatric Knee Conditions	**Behavior Modification:** Promotion of behavior change **Decision-Making Support:** Providing information and support for a patient who is making a decision regarding health care **Health System Guidance:** Facilitating a patient's location and use of appropriate health services **Mutual Goal Setting:** Collaborating with patient to identify and prioritize care goals, then developing a plan to achieve those goals **Patient Contracting:** Negotiating an agreement with an individual that reinforces a particular behavior change **Self-Modification Assistance:** Reinforcement of self-directed change initiated by the patient to achieve personally important goals **Teaching: Disease Process:** Assisting the patient to understand information related to a specific disease process **Teaching: Prescribed Diet:** Preparing a patient to correctly follow a prescribed diet **Teaching: Prescribed Medication:** Preparing a patient to safely take prescribed medications and monitor for their effects **Teaching: Procedure/Treatment:** Preparing a patient to achieve and/or maintain a prescribed level of activity	**Compliance Behavior:** Personal actions to promote wellness recovery and rehabilitation based on professional advice **Compliance Behavior: Prescribed Diet:** Personal actions to follow food and fluid intake recommendations from a health professional for a specific health condition **Compliance Behavior: Prescribed Medication:** Personal actions to administer medication safely to meet therapeutic goals as recommended by a health professional **Health Beliefs: Perceived Control:** Personal conviction that one can influence a health outcome **Medication Response:** Therapeutic and adverse effects of prescribed medication **Knowledge Treatment Regimen:** Extent of understanding conveyed about a specific treatment regimen **Participation in Health Care Decisions:** Personal involvement in selecting and evaluating health care options to achieve desired outcome **Symptom Control:** Personal actions to minimize perceived adverse changed in physical and emotional functioning **Symptom Control:** Personal actions to minimize perceived adverse changes in physical and emotional functioning

Nursing Diagnosis (NANDA): Sensory Perception: Tactile, Disturbed		
Orthopaedic Conditions*	**Nursing Intervention Classifications (NIC)**	**Nursing Outcome Classifications (NOC)**
Chapter 8: Orthopaedic Complications Delirium **Chapter 17: The Spine** Herniated Nucleus Pulposus Spinal Stenosis Degenerative Disc Disease Spondylolysis and Spondylolisthesis Failed Back Syndrome Spinal Fractures **Chapter 19: The Elbow** Lateral and Medial Epicondylitis Elbow Arthroplasty **Chapter 20: The Hand & Wrist** Nail Bed Injuries Thumb Fractures—Bennett's and Rolando's Replantation Arthroplasty **Chapter 23: The Foot & Ankle** Charcot Foot Diabetic Foot	**Amputation Care:** Promotion of physical and psychological healing before and after amputation of a body part **Environmental Management: Safety:** Monitoring and manipulation of the physical environment to promote safety **Lower Extremity Monitoring:** Collection, analysis, and use of patient data to categorize risk and prevent injury to the lower extremities **Neurological Monitoring:** Collection and analysis of patient data to prevent or minimize neurologic complications **Peripheral Sensation Management:** Prevention or minimization of injury or discomfort in the patient with altered sensation **Positioning:** Deliberative placement of the patient or a body part to promote physiological and/or psychological well-being **Pressure Management:** Minimizing pressure to body parts **Skin Surveillance:** Collection and analysis of patient data to maintain skin and mucous membrane integrity	**Neurological Status: Spinal Sensory/Motor Function:** Ability of the spinal nerves to convey sensory and motor impulses **Sensory Function: Cutaneous:** Extend to which stimulation of the skin is correctly sensed

Nursing Diagnosis (NANDA): Sexuality Patterns, Ineffective		
Orthopaedic Conditions*	**Nursing Intervention Classifications (NIC)**	**Nursing Outcome Classifications (NOC)**
Chapter 13: Arthritis & Connective Tissue Disorders Rheumatoid Arthritis	**Active Listening:** Attending closely to and attaching significance to a patient's verbal and nonverbal messages **Anxiety Reduction:** Minimizing apprehension, dread, foreboding, or uneasiness related to an identifiable source of anticipated or perceived danger **Behavior Management: Sexual:** Delineation and prevention of socially unacceptable sexual behavior **Body Image Enhancement:** Improving a patient's conscious and unconscious perceptions and attitudes toward own body **Role Enhancement:** Assisting a patient, significant other, and/or family to improve relationships by clarifying and supplementing specific role behaviors **Self-Awareness Enhancement:** Assisting a patient to explore and understand own thoughts, feelings, motivations, and behaviors **Sexual Counseling:** Use of an interactive helping process focusing on the need to make adjustments in sexual practice or to enhance coping with a sexual event/disorder **Teaching: Safe Sex:** Providing instruction concerning sexual protection during sexual activity **Teaching: Sexuality:** Assisting individuals to understand physical and psychosocial dimensions of sexual growth and development	**Physical Maturation: Female:** Normal physical changes in the female that occur with the transition from childhood to adulthood **Physical Maturation: Male:** Normal physical changes in the male that occur with the transition from childhood to adulthood **Sexual Identify:** Acknowledging and accepting own sexual identity

Nursing Diagnosis (NANDA): Shock, Risk for		
Orthopaedic Conditions*	**Nursing Intervention Classifications (NIC)**	**Nursing Outcome Classifications (NOC)**
Chapter 15: Orthopaedic Trauma Spine Fractures Pelvic Fractures Amputations	**Bleeding Precautions:** Reduction of stimuli that induce bleeding or hemorrhage in at-risk patients **Bleeding Reduction:** Limitation of the loss of blood volume during an episode **Bleeding Reduction: Wound:** Limitation of the blood loss from a wound that may be a result of trauma, incisions, or placement of a tube or catheter **Circulatory Care: Arterial:** Promotion of arterial circulation **Circulatory Care:** Venous Insufficiency: Promotion of venous circulation **Embolus Care: Pulmonary:** Limitation of complications for a patient experiencing, or at risk for, occlusion of pulmonary circulation **Hemorrhage Control:** Reduction or elimination of rapid and excessive blood loss **Hypovolemia Management:** Expansion of intravascular fluid volume in a patient who is volume-depleted **Infection Control:** Minimizing the acquisition and transmission of infectious agents **Oxygen Therapy:** Administration of oxygen and monitoring of its effectiveness **Respiratory Monitoring:** Collection and analysis of patient data to ensure airway patency and adequate gas exchange **Risk Identification:** Analysis of potential risk factors, determination of health risks, and prioritization of risk reduction strategies for an individual or group **Surveillance:** Purposeful and ongoing acquisition, interpretation, and synthesis of patient data for clinical decision-making **Vital Signs Monitoring:** Collection and analysis of cardiovascular, respiratory, and body temperature data to determine and prevent complications	**Blood Loss Severity:** Severity of internal or external bleeding/ hemorrhage **Blood Transfusion Reaction:** Severity of complications with blood transfusion reaction **Infection Severity:** Severity of infection and associated symptoms **Respiratory Status: Gas Exchange:** Alveolar exchange of carbon dioxide and oxygen to maintain arterial blood gas concentrations **Vital Signs:** Extent to which temperature, pulse, respiration, and blood pressure are within normal range **Tissue Perfusion: Cellular:** Adequacy of blood flow through the vasculature to maintain function at the cellular level

Nursing Diagnosis (NANDA): Skin Integrity, Impaired; Skin Integrity, Risk for Impairment		
Orthopaedic Conditions*	**Nursing Intervention Classifications (NIC)**	**Nursing Outcome Classifications (NOC)**
Chapter 6: Immobility Integumentary issues **Chapter 8: Orthopaedic Complications** Pressure Ulcer **Chapter 9: Orthopaedic Infections** Osteomyelitis Septic Arthritis Prosthetic Joint Infections **Chapter 10: Therapeutic Modalities** External Fixators Traction **Chapter 11: Pediatrics** Clubfoot Leg Length Discrepancies Metatarsus Adductus Myelomeningocele *(continued next page)*	**Bed Rest Care:** Promotion of comfort and safety and prevention of complications for a patient unable to get out of bed **Cast Care: Maintenance:** Care of a cast after the drying period **Cast Care: Wet:** Care of a new cast during the drying period **Diarrhea Management:** Management and alleviation of diarrhea **Incision Site Care:** Cleansing, monitoring, and promotion of healing in a wound that is closed with sutures, clips, or staples **Nutrition Management:** Assisting with or providing a balanced dietary intake of foods and fluids **Pressure Management:** Minimizing pressure to body parts *(continued next page)*	**Burn Healing:** Extent of healing of a burn site **Tissue Integrity: Skin and Mucous Membranes:** Structural intactness and normal physiological function of skin and mucous membranes **Wound Healing: Primary Intention:** Extent of regeneration of cells and tissue following intentional closure **Wound Healing: Secondary Intention:** Extent of regeneration of cells and tissue in an open wound

Nursing Diagnosis (NANDA): Skin Integrity, Impaired; Skin Integrity, Risk for Impairment *(continued)*		
Orthopaedic Conditions*	**Nursing Intervention Classifications (NIC)**	**Nursing Outcome Classifications (NOC)**
Chapter 13: Arthritis & Connective Tissue Disorders Gout Systemic Sclerosis **Chapter 15: Orthopaedic Trauma** Pelvic Fractures Femur/Hip Fractures Soft Trauma Dislocations/Subluxations Strains Sprains **Chapter 16: Tumors of the Musculoskeletal System** Benign Lesions Primary Malignant Tumors Primary Sarcoma Bone Metastasis Multiple Myeloma **Chapter 17: The Spine** Scoliosis Kyphosis Herniated Nucleus Pulposus Degenerative Disc Disease Spinal Stenosis **Chapter 18: The Shoulder** Fractures of the Shoulder Sprains, Strains, Contusions, Separations Sprengel's Deformity **Chapter 19: The Elbow** Elbow Arthroplasty **Chapter 20: The Hand &Wrist** Mallet Finger Trigger Thumb/Finger Nail Bed Injuries Dupuytren's Contracture Distal Radius Fractures—Colles' and Smith's Carpal Tunnel Syndrome Ganglion Cyst Carpal Tunnel Syndrome Replantation Arthroplasty Thumb Fractures—Bennett's and Rolando's Boxer's Fracture Scaphoid Fracture *(continued next page)*	**Pressure Ulcer Care:** Facilitation of healing pressure ulcers **Positioning: Intraoperative:** Moving the patient or body part to promote surgical exposure while reducing the risk of discomfort and complications **Self-Care Assistance** Bathing/Hygiene: Assisting another to perform personal hygiene **Skin Surveillance:** Collection and analysis of patient data to maintain skin and mucous membrane integrity **Wound Care:** Prevention of wound complications and promotion of wound healing **Wound Care: Burns:** Prevention of wound complications due to burns and facilitation of healing **Urinary Incontinence Care:** Assistance in promoting continence and maintaining perineal skin integrity	*(see page 669)*

Nursing Diagnosis (NANDA): Skin Integrity, Impaired; Skin Integrity, Risk for Impairment *(continued)*		
Orthopaedic Conditions*	**Nursing Intervention Classifications (NIC)**	**Nursing Outcome Classifications (NOC)**
Chapter 21: The Hip, Femur & Pelvis Hip Fractures Hip Arthroplasty Hip Resurfacing Arthroplasty Hip Arthroscopy Femoro-Acetabular Impingement Hip Dislocation Hip Girdlestone Psuedoarthrosis Proximal Femoral Osteotomy Femoral Shaft Fractures Pelvic Fracture **Chapter 22: The Knee** Osteoarthritis Trauma and Soft Tissue Injuries **Chapter 23: The Foot & Ankle** Fractures Charcot Foot Diabetic Foot	*(see pages 669-70)*	*(see page 669)*

Nursing Diagnosis (NANDA): Sleep Pattern, Disturbed		
Orthopaedic Conditions*	**Nursing Intervention Classifications (NIC)**	**Nursing Outcome Classifications (NOC)**
Chapter 8: Orthopaedic Complications Delirium **Chapter 10: Therapeutic Modalities** Casts Continuous Passive Motion Machine **Chapter 13: Arthritis & Connective Tissue Disorders** Psoriatic Arthritis Fibromyalgia **Chapter 23: The Foot & Ankle** Diabetic Foot	**Coping Enhancement:** Assisting the patient to adapt to perceived stressors, changes, or threats that interfere with meeting life demands and roles **Sleep Enhancement:** Facilitation of regular sleep/wake cycles **Environmental Management: Comfort:** Manipulation of the patient's surrounding for promotion of optimal comfort	**Personal Well-Being:** Extent of positive perception of one's health status and life circumstances **Sleep:** Natural periodic suspension of consciousness during which the body is restored

Nursing Diagnosis (NANDA): Social Interaction, Impaired		
Orthopaedic Conditions*	**Nursing Intervention Classifications (NIC)**	**Nursing Outcome Classifications (NOC)**
Chapter 6: Immobility Psychosocial/Mental Status **Chapter 10: Therapeutic Modalities** Ambulatory Devices and Techniques **Chapter 11: Pediatrics** Arthrogryposis Multiplex Congenita Physical Abuse **Chapter 17: The Spine** Herniated Nucleus Pulposus Spinal Stenosis Degenerative Disc Disease Spondylolysis and Spondylolisthesis Failed Back Syndrome	**Behavior Modification: Social Skills:** Assisting the patient to develop or improve interpersonal social skills **Complex Relationship Building:** Establishing a therapeutic relationship with a patient who has difficulty interacting with others **Family Integrity Promotion:** Promotion of family cohesion and unity **Family Process Maintenance:** Minimization of disruptive or adverse effects on the family process **Recreation Therapy:** Purposeful use of recreation to promote relaxation and enhancement of social skills **Socialization Enhancement:** Facilitation of a person's ability to interact with others **Therapeutic Play:** Purposeful and directive use of toys and other materials to assist children in communicating their perception and knowledge of their world and to help in gaining mastery of their environment	**Family Social Climate:** Supportive milieu as characterized by family member relationships and goals **Leisure Participation:** Use of relaxing, interesting, and enjoyable activities to promote well-being **Play Participation:** Use of activities by children ages 1-11 to promote enjoyment, entertainment, and development **Social Interaction Skills:** Personal behaviors that promote effective relationships **Social Involvement:** Social interactions with persons, groups, or organizations

Nursing Diagnosis (NANDA): Spiritual Distress; Spiritual Well-Being, Readiness for Enhanced		
Orthopaedic Conditions*	**Nursing Intervention Classifications (NIC)**	**Nursing Outcome Classifications (NOC)**
Chapter 16: Tumors of the Musculoskeletal System Primary Sarcoma Bone Metastasis Multiple Myeloma	**Coping Enhancement:** Assisting a patient to adapt to perceived stressors, changes, or threats which interfere with meeting life demands and roles **Decision-Making Support:** Providing information and support for a patient who is making a decision regarding health care **Hope Inspiration:** Enhancing the belief in one's capacity to initiate and sustain actions **Spiritual Support:** Assisting the patient to feel balance and connection with a greater power **Socialization Enhancement:** Facilitation of another person's ability to interact with others **Spiritual Growth Facilitation:** Facilitation of growth in patient's capacity to identify, connect with, and call upon the source of meaning, purpose, comfort, strength and hope in their lives **Values Clarification:** Assisting another to clarify own values in order to facilitate effective decision-making	**Dignified Life Closure:** Personal actions to maintain control during approaching end of life **Hope:** Optimism that is personally satisfying and life-supporting **Quality of Life:** Extent of positive perception of current life circumstances **Social Involvement:** Social interaction with person, groups, or organizations **Spiritual Health:** Connectedness with self, others, higher power, all life, nature, and the universe that transcends and empowers the self **Well-Being: Personal:** Extent of positive perception of one's health status

Nursing Diagnosis (NANDA): Surgery Recovery, Delayed		
Orthopaedic Conditions*	**Nursing Intervention Classifications (NIC)**	**Nursing Outcome Classifications (NOC)**
Chapter 8: Orthopaedic Complications Nosocomial Surgical Site Infection **Chapter 21: The Hip, Femur & Pelvis** Arthroplasty Hip Resurfacing Arthroplasty Hemi-Arthroplasty/Bipolar Hip Arthroscopy Femoro-Acetabular Impingement Hip Girdlestone Psuedoarthrosis Proximal Femoral Osteotomy Femoral Shaft Fractures Pelvic Fracture	**Bed Rest Care:** Promotion of comfort and safety and prevention of complications for a patient unable to get out of bed **Bleeding Reduction:** Limitation of the loss of blood volume during an episode of bleeding **Embolus Precautions:** Reduction of the risk of an embolus in a patient with thrombi or at risk for thrombus formation **Energy Management:** Regulating energy use to treat or prevent fatigue and optimize function **Exercise Therapy: Ambulation:** Promotion and assistance with walking to maintain or restore autonomic and voluntary body functions during treatment and recovery from illness or injury **Exercise Therapy: Joint Mobility:** Use of active or passive body movement to maintain or restore joint flexibility **Fluid Management:** Promotion of fluid balance and prevention of complications resulting from abnormal or undesired fluid levels **Hypovolemia Management:** Expansion of intravascular fluid volume in a patient who is volume-depleted **Hypervolemia Management:** Reduction in extracellular and/or intracellular fluid volume and prevention of complications in a patient who is fluid-overloaded **Incision Site Care:** Cleansing, monitoring, and promotion of healing in a wound that is closed with sutures, clips, or staples **Infection Control:** Minimizing the acquisition and transmission of infectious agents **Nausea Management:** Prevention and alleviation of nausea **Nutrition Management:** Assisting with or providing a balanced dietary intake of foods and fluids **Pain Management:** Alleviation of pain or a reduction in pain to a level of comfort that is acceptable to the patient **Self-Care Assistance:** Assisting another to perform activities of daily living **Vital Signs Monitoring:** Collection and analysis of cardiovascular, respiratory, and body temperature data to determine and prevent complications **Vomiting Management:** Prevention and alleviation of vomiting **Wound Care:** Prevention of wound complications and promotion of wound healing	**Ambulation:** Ability to walk from place to place independently with or without assistive device **Blood Loss Severity:** Severity of internal or external bleeding/hemorrhage **Endurance:** Capacity to sustain activity **Fluid Overload Severity:** Severity of excess fluids in the intracellular and extracellular compartments of the body **Immobility Consequences: Physiological:** Severity of compromise in physiological functioning due to impaired physical mobility **Immobility Consequences: Psycho-Cognitive:** Severity of compromise in psycho-cognitive functioning due to impaired mobility **Infection Severity:** Severity of infection and associated symptoms **Nausea and Vomiting Severity:** Severity of nausea, retching and vomiting symptoms **Pain Level:** Severity of observed or reported pain **Post-Procedure Recovery Status:** Extent to which an individual returns to baseline function following a procedure(s) requiring anesthesia or sedation **Self-Care: Activities of Daily Living (ADL):** Ability to perform the most basic physical tasks and personal care activities independently with or without assistive device **Wound Healing: Primary Intention:** Extent of regeneration of cells and tissue following intentional closure

Nursing Diagnosis (NANDA): Swallowing, Impaired		
Orthopaedic Conditions*	**Nursing Intervention Classifications (NIC)**	**Nursing Outcome Classifications (NOC)**
Chapter 13: Arthritis & Connective Tissue Disorders Systemic Sclerosis Polymyositis and Dermatomyositis	**Airway Suctioning:** Removal of airway secretions by inserting a suction catheter into the patient's oral airway and/or trachea **Aspiration Precautions:** Prevention or minimization of risk factors in the patient at risk for aspiration **Oral Health Maintenance:** Maintenance and promotion of oral hygiene and dental care for a patient at risk for developing oral or dental lesions **Positioning:** Deliberative placement of the patient or a body part to promote physiological and/or psychological well-being **Swallowing Therapy:** Facilitating swallowing and preventing complications of impaired swallowing	**Aspiration Prevention:** Personal actions to prevent the passage of fluid and solid particles into the lung **Swallowing Status: Esophageal Phase:** Safe passage of fluids and/or solids from the pharynx to the stomach **Swallowing Status: Oral Phase:** Preparation, containment, and posterior movement of fluids and/or solids in the mouth **Swallowing Status: Pharyngeal Phase:** Safe passage of fluids and/or solids from the mouth to the esophagus

Nursing Diagnosis (NANDA): Thermoregulation, Ineffective		
Orthopaedic Conditions*	**Nursing Intervention Classifications (NIC)**	**Nursing Outcome Classifications (NOC)**
Chapter 6: Orthopaedic Effects of Immobility Metabolic/Gastrointestinal Issues	**Emergency Care:** Providing life-saving measures in life-threatening situations **Fever Treatment:** Management of a patient with hyperpyrexia caused by nonenvironmental factors **Hypothermia Treatment:** Rewarming and surveillance of a patient whose core body temperature is below 35 degrees C **Malignant Hyperthermia Precautions:** Prevention or reduction of hypermetabolic response to pharmacological agents use during surgery **Temperature Regulation:** Attaining and/or maintaining body temperature within a normal range **Temperature Regulation: Intraoperative:** Attaining and/or maintaining desired intraoperative body temperature	**Thermoregulation:** Balance among heat production, heat gain, and heat loss

Nursing Diagnosis (NANDA): Tissue Integrity, Impaired		
Orthopaedic Conditions*	**Nursing Intervention Classifications (NIC)**	**Nursing Outcome Classifications (NOC)**
Chapter 8: Orthopaedic Complications Pressure Ulcer **Chapter 15: Orthopaedic Trauma** Spine Fractures Pelvic Fractures Amputations **Chapter 16: Tumors of the Musculoskeletal System** Benign Lesions Primary Malignant Tumors Primary Sarcoma Bone Metastasis Multiple Myeloma	**Infection Protection:** Prevention and early detection of infection in a patient at risk **Incision Site Care:** Cleansing, monitoring, and promotion of healing in a wound that is closed with sutures, clips, or staples **Oral Health Maintenance:** Maintenance and promotion of oral hygiene and dental health for the patient at risk for developing oral or dental lesions **Pressure Management:** Minimizing pressure to body parts **Pressure Ulcer Care:** Facilitation of healing and pressure ulcers **Pressure Ulcer Prevention:** Prevention of pressure ulcers in a high-risk individual **Wound Care:** Prevention of wound complications and promotion of wound healing	**Tissue Integrity: Skin and Mucous Membranes:** Structural intactness and normal physiological function of skin and mucous membranes **Wound Healing: Primary Intention:** Extent of regeneration of cells and tissue following intentional closure **Wound Healing: Secondary Intention:** Extent of regeneration of cells and tissue in an open wound

<table>
<tr><th colspan="3">Nursing Diagnosis (NANDA): Tissue Perfusion: Cardiac, Risk for Decrease; Tissue Perfusion: Cerebral, Risk for Ineffectiveness; Cardiac Perfusion, Risk for Decrease</th></tr>
<tr><th>Orthopaedic Conditions*</th><th>Nursing Intervention Classifications (NIC)</th><th>Nursing Outcome Classifications (NOC)</th></tr>
<tr><td>Chapter 8: Orthopaedic Complications
Fat Embolism Syndrome
Chapter 11: Pediatrics
Myelomeningocele
Chapter 13: Arthritis & Connective Tissue Disorders
Rheumatic Fever
Polymyositis/Dermatomyositis
Chapter 15: Orthopaedic Trauma
Pelvic Fractures
Amputations
Chapter 16: Tumors of the Musculoskeletal System
Primary Sarcoma
Bone Metastasis
Multiple Myeloma
Chapter 17: The Spine
Herniated Nucleus Pulposus
Degenerative Disc Disease
Spinal Stenosis
Spondylosis
Spondylolithesis
Failed Back Surgery Syndrome
Spinal Fractures
Chapter 21: The Hip, Femur & Pelvis Hip Fractures Hip
Arthroplasty
Hip Resurfacing Arthroplasty
Hemiarthroplasty/Bipolar Replacement</td><td>Acid-Base Monitoring: Collection and analysis of patient data to regulate acid-base balance
Embolus Care: Pulmonary: Limitation of complications for a patient experiencing, or at risk for, occlusion of pulmonary circulation
Hemodynamic Regulation: Optimization of heart rate, preload, afterload, and contractility
Oxygen Therapy: Administration of oxygen and monitoring of its effectiveness
Respiratory Monitoring: Collection and analysis of patient data to ensure airway patency and adequate gas exchange
Shock Management: Cardiac: Promotion of adequate tissue perfusion for a patient with severely compromised pumping function of the heart
Vital Signs Monitoring: Collection and analysis of cardiovascular, respiratory, and body temperature data to determine and prevent complications</td><td>Circulation Status: Unobstructed, unidirectional blood flow at an appropriate pressure through large vessels of the systemic and pulmonary circuits
Respiratory Status: Gas Exchange: Alveolar exchange of carbon dioxide and oxygen to maintain arterial blood gas concentrations
Tissue Perfusion: Cardiac: Adequacy of blood flow through the small vessels of the abdominal viscera to maintain organ function
Tissue Perfusion: Pulmonary: Adequacy of blood flow through pulmonary vasculature to perfuse alveoli/capillary unit
Vital Signs: Extent to which temperature, pulse, respiration, and blood pressure are within normal range</td></tr>
</table>

Nursing Diagnosis (NANDA): Tissue Perfusion: Peripheral, Ineffective		
Orthopaedic Conditions*	**Nursing Intervention Classifications (NIC)**	**Nursing Outcome Classifications (NOC)**
Chapter 8: Orthopaedic Complications Significant Blood Loss Venous Thromboembolism **Chapter 10: Therapeutic Modalities** Braces/Orthotics/Orthoses Casts External Fixators Traction **Chapter 11: Pediatrics** Blount's Disease Developmental Dysplasia of the Hip GenuValgum/Genu Varum Leg Length Discrepencies Pediatric Fractures **Chapter 15: Orthopaedic Trauma** Dislocations/Subluxations Strains Sprains **Chapter 17: The Spine** Kyphosis Herniated Nucleus Pulposus Spinal Stenosis Degenerative Disc Disease Spondylolysis and Spondylolisthesis Failed Back Syndrome **Chapter 19: The Elbow** Supracondylar/Distal Humerus Fractures Elbow Dislocation **Chapter 20: The Hand & Wrist** Replantation **Chapter 21: The Hip, Femur & Pelvis** Hip Fractures Hip Arthroplasty Hip Resurfacing Arthroplasty Hemiarthroplasty/Bipolar Replacement Hip Arthroscopy Femoro-Acetabular Impingement Hip Dislocation Girdlestone Psuedoarthrosis Proximal Femoral Osteotomy Femoral Shaft Fractures Pelvic Fracture **Chapter 23: The Foot & Ankle** Charcot Foot Diabetic Foot	**Circulatory Care: Arterial Insufficiency:** Promotion of arterial circulation **Circulatory Care: Mechanical Assist Device:** Temporary support of the circulation through the use of mechanical devices or pumps **Circulatory Care: Venous Insufficiency:** Promotion of venous circulation **Circulatory Precautions:** Protection of a localized area with limited perfusion **Fluid/Electrolyte Management:** Regulation and prevention of complications from altered fluid and/or electrolyte levels **Fluid Management:** Promotion of fluid balance and prevention of complications resulting from abnormal or undesired fluid levels **Hemodynamic Regulation:** Optimization of heart rate preload, afterload, and contractility **Hypervolemia Management:** Reduction in extracellular and/or intracellular fluid volume and prevention of complications in a patient who is fluid-overloaded **Neurologic Monitoring:** Collection and analysis of patient data to prevent or minimize neurologic complications **Peripheral Sensation Management:** Prevention or minimization of injury or discomfort in the patient with altered sensation **Shock Management:** Facilitation of the delivery of oxygen and nutrients to systemic tissue with removal of cellular waste products in patient with severely altered tissue perfusion **Skin Surveillance:** Collection and analysis of patient data to maintain skin and mucous membrane integrity	**Circulation Status:** Unobstructed, unidirectional blood flow at appropriate pressure through large vessels of the systemic and pulmonary circuits **Fluid Overload Severity:** Severity of excess fluids in the intracellular and extracellular compartments of the body **Sensory Function: Cutaneous:** Extent to which stimulation of the skin is correctly sensed **Tissue Integrity: Skin and Mucous Membranes:** Structural intactness and normal physiological function of skin and mucous membranes **Tissue Perfusion: Peripheral:** Adequacy of blood flow through the small vessels of the extremities to maintain tissue function

Nursing Diagnosis (NANDA): Transfer Ability, Impaired		
Orthopaedic Conditions*	**Nursing Intervention Classifications (NIC)**	**Nursing Outcome Classifications (NOC)**
Chapter 10: Therapeutic Modalities Ambulatory Devices and Techniques Braces/Orthotics/Orthoses External Fixators Traction Wheelchairs **Chapter 23: The Foot & Ankle** Amputations	**Exercise Promotion: Strength Training:** Facilitating regular resistive muscle training to maintain or increase muscle strength **Exercise Therapy: Ambulation:** Promotion and assistance with walking to maintain or restore autonomic and voluntary body functions during treatment and recovery from illness or injury **Exercise Therapy: Balance:** Use of specific activities, postures, and movements to maintain, enhance, or restore balance **Exercise Therapy: Joint Mobility:** Use of active or passive body movement to maintain or restore joint flexibility **Exercise Therapy: Muscle Control:** Use of specific activity or exercise protocols to enhance or restore controlled body movement **Fall Prevention:** Instituting special precautions with patient at risk for injury from falling **Self-Care Assistance: Transfer:** Assisting a patient with limitation of independent movement to learn to change body location	**Balance:** Ability to maintain body equilibrium **Body Positioning: Self-Initiated:** Ability to change own body position independently with or without assistive device **Coordinated Movement:** Ability of muscles to work together voluntarily for purposeful movement **Mobility:** Ability to move purposefully in own environment independently with or without assistive device **Transfer Performance:** Ability to change body location independently with or without assistive device

Nursing Diagnosis (NANDA): Urinary Retention; Urinary Elimination, Impaired		
Orthopaedic Conditions*	**Nursing Intervention Classifications (NIC)**	**Nursing Outcome Classifications (NOC)**
Chapter 6: Orthopaedic Effects of Immobility Genitourinary Issues **Chapter 8: Orthopaedic Complications** Postoperative Urinary Retention **Chapter 11: Pediatrics** Myelomeningocele **Chapter 15: Orthopaedic Trauma** Soft Trauma Dislocations/Subluxations Strains Sprains **Chapter 16: Tumors of the Musculoskeletal System** Multiple myeloma	**Urinary Catheterization:** Insertion of a catheter into the bladder for temporary or permanent drainage of urine **Urinary Elimination Management:** Maintenance of an **optimum urinary elimination pattern** **Urinary Retention Care:** Assistance in relieving bladder distention	**Urinary Continence:** Control of elimination of urine from the bladder **Urinary Elimination:** Collection and discharge of urine

Nursing Diagnosis (NANDA): Ventilation, Impaired Spontaneous		
Orthopaedic Conditions*	**Nursing Intervention Classifications (NIC)**	**Nursing Outcome Classifications (NOC)**
Chapter 9: Orthopaedic Infections Healthcare-Associated Infections	**Airway Management:** Facilitation of patency of air passages **Airway Suctioning:** Removal of airway secretions by inserting a suction catheter into the patient's oral airway and/or trachea **Aspiration Precautions:** Prevention or minimization of risk factors that put the patient at risk for aspiration **Bed Rest Care:** Promotion of comfort and safety and prevention of complications for a patient unable to get out of bed **Energy Management:** Regulating energy use to treat or prevent fatigue and optimize function **Environmental Management: Comfort:** Manipulation of the patient's surroundings for promotion of optimal comfort **Environmental Management: Safety:** Monitoring and manipulation of the physical environment to promote safety **Mechanical Ventilation Management: Invasive:** Assisting the patient receiving artificial breathing support through a device inserted into the trachea **Oxygen Therapy:** Administration of oxygen and monitoring of its effectiveness **Respiratory Monitoring:** Collection and analysis of patient data to ensure airway patency and adequate gas exchange	**Mechanical Ventilation Response: Adult:** Alveolar exchange and tissue perfusion are supported by mechanical ventilation **Respiratory Status: Gas Exchange:** Alveolar exchange of carbon dioxide and oxygen to maintain arterial blood gas concentrations **Respiratory Status: Ventilation:** Movement of air in and out of the lungs **Vital Signs:** Extent to which temperature, pulse, respiration, and blood pressure are within normal range

Nursing Diagnosis (NANDA): Walking, Impaired		
Orthopaedic Conditions*	**Nursing Intervention Classifications (NIC)**	**Nursing Outcome Classifications (NOC)**
Chapter 10: Therapeutic Modalities Ambulatory Devices and Techniques Braces/Orthotics/Orthoses External Fixators Traction **Chapter 13: Arthritis & Connective Tissue Disorders** Osteoarthritis Polymyalgia Rheumatica **Chapter 23: The Foot & Ankle** Charcot Foot Diabetic Foot	**Energy Management:** Regulating energy use to treat or prevent fatigue and optimize function **Exercise Therapy: Ambulation:** Promotion and assistance with walking to maintain or restore autonomic and voluntary body functions during treatment and recovery from illness or injury **Exercise Therapy: Balance:** Use of specific activities, postures, and movements to maintain, enhance, or restore balance **Exercise Therapy: Joint Mobility:** Use of active or passive body movement to maintain or restore joint flexibility **Exercise Therapy: Muscle Control:** Use of specific activity or exercise protocols to enhance or restore controlled body movement	**Ambulation:** Ability to walk from place to place independently with or without assistive device **Balance:** Ability to maintain body equilibrium **Coordinated Movement:** Ability of muscles to work together voluntarily for purposeful movement **Endurance:** Capacity to sustain activity **Joint Movement: Ankle, Hip, Knee:** Active range of motion of (specify joint) with self-initiated movement **Mobility:** Ability to move purposefully in own environment independently with or without assistive device

****Conditions listed with each nursing diagnosis represent those listed in this text and do not reflect all conditions for which the nursing diagnosis would be appropriate.***

References

Johnson, M., Moorehead, S., Bulecheck, G., Butcher, H., Maas, M., & Swanson, E. (2012). *NOC and NIC Linkages to NANDA-I and Clinical Conditions: Supporting Critical Reasoning and Quality Care* (3rd ed). Maryland Heights, MO: Elsevier Mosby.

NANDA International. (2012). *NANDA International Nursing Diagnoses: Definitions and Classifications 2012-2014.* Oxford, UK: Wiley-Blackwell.

Key Terms

Abduction: Lateral movement of a limb away from the median plane of the body.

Acute Phase Inflammatory Protein: Any of the plasma proteins whose concentration increases or decreases by at least 25% during inflammation. They help to mediate both positive and negative effects of acute and chronic inflammation. The erythrocyte sedimentation rate (ESR) or serum C-reactive protein (CRP) level is sometimes used as a marker of increased amounts of these proteins.

Adduction: Movement of a limb toward the median plane of the body.

Allogenic: Having a different genetic constitution but belonging to the same species.

American Academy of Nurse Practitioners (AANP): The first national organization created for nurse practitioners of all specialties. AANP formed in 1985 to provide NPs with a unified way to network and advocate for NP issues.

American Board of Nursing Specialties (ABNS): A nonprofit membership organization that focuses on improving patient outcomes and protection of consumers by advocating specialty nursing certification. ABNS member organizations represent more than 500,000 registered nurses throughout the world.

American Nurses Credentialing Center (ANCC): The largest nurse credentialing organization in the United States of America. ANCC has certified more than 250,000 nurses and 80,000 advanced practice nurses.

Ankylosing Spondylitis: A chronic progressive inflammatory disorder that involves primarily the joints between articular processes, costovertebral joints and sacroiliac joints, and occasionally the iris or the heart valves.

Ankylosis: Immobility of a joint. The condition may be congenital (sometimes hereditary), or it may be the result of disease, trauma, surgery, or contractures resulting from immobility.

Antagonist: Something that blocks, undoes, or produces the opposite effect of an action.

Antifibrinolysin: A substance that counteracts fibrinolysis.

Antinuclear Antibodies (ANA): An antibody, produced by B cells in response to altered "self" cells, that attacks and destroys these cells. Autoantibodies are the basis for autoimmune diseases such as rheumatoid arthritis and diabetes mellitus.

Atelectasis: A collapsed or airless condition of the lung.

Avulsion: A tearing away forcibly of a body part or structure. If surgical repair is necessary, a sterile dressing may be applied while surgery is awaited. If fingers, toes, feet, or even entire limbs are completely avulsed and separated, members are recovered.

Benign: Not recurrent or progressive; nonmalignant.

Biofilm: A thin coating of bacteria embedded in a moist, adhesive matrix that may cover mucous membranes and devices placed inside the body, including catheters and stents.

Biologic Response Modifier (BRM): An agent derived from or made of living tissues or cells and used in health care to arouse the body's response to an infection. Examples include monoclonal antibodies, interleukin-2, and interferon.

Bisphosphonate: Any of a class of medications that inhibit the resorption of bones by osteoclasts.

Borreliosis (Lyme Disease): A condition caused by a deer tick bite that transmits the spirochete bacteria Borrelia burgorferi, resulting in a rash and flu-like symptoms that progress to heart, nervous system, and arthritic problems if left untreated.

Breakthrough Pain: A brief increase in pain that occurs when background pain is controlled.

Burst Fracture: A fracture similar to a compression fracture but typically more severe and involving displacement of the bony fragments.

Calcitonin: A hormone produced by the human thyroid gland that is important for maintaining a dense, strong bone matrix and regulating the blood calcium level.

Cervical: Pertaining to or in the region of the neck.

Chance Fracture: A fracture that results in a horizontal splitting of the vertebra that begins with the spinous process or lamina and extends anteriorly through the pedicles and vertebral body, which tends to have a wedge compression fracture, while the posterior elements of the vertebra are distracted.

Chemotherapy: Drug therapy used to treat infections, cancers, and other diseases and conditions.

Chondroma: A slow-growing, painless cartilaginous tumor. It may occur wherever there is cartilage.

Clonus: A continuous rhythmic reflex tremor initiated by the spinal cord below an area of spinal cord injury, set in motion by reflex testing.

Comorbidity: A disease or pathological process occurring simultaneously with another.

Compression Fracture: A fracture of a vertebra by pressure along the long axis of the vertebral column. Such fractures, which may occur traumatically or as a result of osteoporosis, are marked by loss of bone height.

Condyle: A rounded protuberance at the end of a bone, forming an articulation.

Contamination: Exposure to environmental contaminants in doses sufficient to cause adverse health effects.

Contracture: Fibrosis of connective tissue in skin, fascia, muscle, or a joint capsule that prevents normal mobility of the related tissue or joint.

Controlled Release: Medication that is released slowly over a defined period of time

Cryotherapy: The removal of heat (e.g., use of ice compresses) from a body part to decrease cellular metabolism, improve cellular survival, decrease inflammation, decrease pain and muscle spasm, and promote vasoconstriction.

Debridement: The removal of foreign material and dead or damaged tissue, especially in a wound.

Decompression: The removal of pressure, as from gas in the intestinal tract.

Dementia: A progressive, irreversible decline in mental function, marked by memory impairment and, often, deficits in reasoning, judgment, abstract thought, registration, comprehension, learning, task execution, and use of language.

Disease-Modifying Anti-Rheumatic Drug (DMARD): A medication that acts on the immune system to slow the progression of rheumatoid arthritis.

Disuse Atrophy: A decrease in size of an organ or tissue from immobilization or the failure to exercise a body part.

Disuse Osteoporosis: A decrease in bone mass or bone funtionality due to the lack of normal functional stress on the bones such as during prolonged period of bedrest or as the result of being exposed to periods of weightlessness (e.g., astronauts in outer space).

Electrosurgery: An operative procedure with an instrument that converts electricity to heat used for cutting, cautery, coagulation, or coaptation of tissues.

Epidemiology: The study of the distribution and determinants of health-related states and events in populations, and the application of this study to the control of health problems.

Epiphysis: A secondary bone-forming (ossification) center separated from a parent bone in early life by cartilage, eventually becoming part of the larger parent bone.

KEY TERMS

Estrogen: Any natural or artificial substance that induces estrus and the development of female sex characteristics; more specifically, the estrogenic hormones produces by the ovary; the female sex hormones.

External Fixation: The use of external devices, such as pins, to keep fractured bone segments in place.

Exudate: Any fluid released from the body with a high concentration of protein, cells, or solid debris; classified as fibrinous, hemorrhagic, diphtheritic, purulent, and serous.

Facet: A small, smooth area on a bone or other hard surface.

Ferritin: An iron-phosphorus-protein complex containing about 23% iron. It is formed in the intestinal mucosa by the union of ferric iron with the protein apoferritin. Tissues store iron in this form, principally in the reticuloendothelial cells of the liver, spleen, and bone marrow.

Fibrinolysis: The breakdown of fibrin in blood clots and the prevention of the polymerization of fibrin into new clots.

Fibroma: A fibrous, encapsulated connective tissue tumor. It is irregular in shape, slow in growth, and has a firm consistency.

Fluid Challenge: A technique of giving a small amount of fluid in a short period of time to assess whether the patient has a preload reserve that can be used to increase the stroke volume with further fluids.

Giant Cell: An active, multinucleated phagocyte created by several individual macrophages that have merged around a large pathogen or a substance resistant to destruction (such as a splinter or surgical suture).

Gibbus: Hump; protuberance.

Hematogenous: Pertinaing to or originating in the blood.

Hemochromatosis: A genetic disease marked by excessive absorption and accumulation of iron in the body.

Hemodynamics: A branch of physiology that deals with the circulation of the blood.

Hemostatic Agent: A substance that arrests bleeding or circulation.

Hydroxyapatite: The calcium-phosphorus compound that constitutes the bulk of the mineral structure of bones and teeth.

Hypercalcemia: An excessive concentration of calcium in the blood.

Hypoplasia: Underdevelopment of a tissue organ or body.

Hypoplastic: Describes an incomplete or underdeveloped tissue or organ

Hypovolemia: An abnormal increase in the volume of circulating blood.

Idiopathic: Pertaining to illness whose cause is either uncertain or as yet undetermined.

Interleukin-6: A lymphokine produced by many cell types, including mononuclear phagocytes, T cells, and endothelial cells.

Intervertebral Discs: Any of the discs between the bodies of adjacent vertebrae. Also called intervertebral cartilage.

Isokinetic Exercise: An exercise with equipment that uses variable resistance to maintain a constant velocity of joint motion during muscle contraction, so that the force generated by the muscle is maximal through the full range of motion.

Kyphoscoliosis: Lateral curvature of the spine accompanying an anteroposterior hump.

Ligament: A band or sheet of strong fibrous connective tissue connecting the articular ends of bones, binding them together to limit motion.

Long Tract Signs: Neurologic signs such as clonus, muscle spasticity, or bladder involvement that usually indicate a lesion in the middle or upper parts of the spinal cord or in the brain.

Malar: Of or relating to the zygomatic bone or the cheek.

Malignant: Growing worse; resisting treatment, said of cancerous growths. Tending or threatening to produce death; harmful.

Malunion: The joining of the fragments of a fractured bone in a faulty position, forming an imperfect alignment, shortening, deformity, or rotation.

Metaphysis: The portion of a developing long bone between the diaphysis (or shaft) and the epiphysis; the growing portion of a bone.

National Association of Orthopaedic Nurses (NAON®): A nonprofit, volunteer organization that promotes the highest standards of orthopaedic nursing practice by educating its clinicians, promoting research, and encouraging communication between orthopaedic nurses and other groups with similar interests throughout the world. NAON® has nearly 6,000 members.

Neurosensory: Concerning a sensory nerve.

Nitrogen Balance: The difference between the amount of nitrogen ingested and excreted each day. If intake is greater, a positive balance exists; if less, there is a negative balance.

Olecranon: A large process of the ulna projecting behind the elbow joint and forming the bony prominence of the elbow.

Opioid/Opiate: A natural or synthetic medication that relieves pain by binding to the opioid receptor site in the nervous system.

Open Reduction and Internal Fixation (ORIF): Surgical treatment of bone fractures by placing the bones in their propoer position through surgery involving the use of internal wires, screws, or pins applied directly to fractured bone segments to keep them in place.

Orthopaedic Nurses Certification Board (ONCB®): An organization that advocates the highest standards of orthopaedic nursing practice through development, implementation, and coordination of all aspects of orthopaedic nursing certifications. The ONCB® first offered the Orthopaedic Nursing Certification (ONC®) exam in 1988.

Orthosis: Any device used externally to stabilize or immobilize a body part, prevent deformity, protect against injury, or assist with function.

Osteotomy: The operation of cutting through a bone.

Pannus: An inflammatory exudate overlying the synovial cells on the inside of a joint.

Pes Anserine: The combined tendinous expansions of the sartorius, gracilis, and semitendinosus muscles at the medial border of the tibial tuberosity.

Phagocytosis: A three-stage process by which phagocytes (neutrophils, monocytes, and marcophages) engulf and destroy microorganisms, other foreign antigens, and cell debris.

Phalanx: Any one of the bones of the fingers or toes; one of the set of plates of phalangeal cells (inner and outer) that forms the reticular membrane of the organ of Corti.

Plane: A flat surface formed by making a cut, imaginary or real, through the body or a part of it.

Play Therapy: The use of play, especially with dolls and toys, to allow children to express their feelings.

Positive Chvostek Sign: A spasm of the facial muscles following a tap on the facial nerve; seen in hypocalcemic tetany.

Preemptive Analgesia: The treatment of pain before an assumed painful event.

KEY TERMS

Pulley: Annular part of the fibrous sheathes of the fingers. These strong transverse bands of fibrous tissue, one in the vagina fibrosa of each finger, cross the flexor tendons at the level of the upper half of the proximal phalanges of the hand.

Radius: The outer and shorter bone of the forearm. It revolves partially about the ulna. Its head articulates with the capitulum of the humerus and with the radial notch on the ulna, and it is encircled by the annular ligament.

Range of Motion (ROM): An exercise that moves a joint through the extent of its limitations; it can be active, active assisted, or passive.

Renal Calculi: Kidney stones.

Rheumatoid Factor (RF): Antibodies raised by the body against immunoglobulins. They are present in roughly 80% of patients with rheumatoid arthritis and in many patients with other rheumatological and infectious illnesses. This factor is used, with other clinical indicators, in the diagnosis and management of rheumatoid arthritis.

Sequestra: A fragment of a necrosed bone that has become separated from the surrounding tissue.

Sequestration: Detachment of dead bone fragments from adjoining sound bone.

Subluxate: To partially dislocate.

Suppurative: Producing or associated with generation of pus.

Synovectomy: Excision of the synovial membrane.

Syringomyelia: A disease of the spinal cord characterized by the development of a cyst or cavities along the cord. It usually begins at the site of a congenital malformation of the cerebellum but sometimes results from spinal cord trauma, tumors, or spinal cord infection.

Tendon: Fibrous connective tissue serving as the attachment of muscles to bones and other parts.

Thermoregulation: Heat regulation.

Thrombus: A blood clot that adheres to the wall of a blood vessel or organ.

Time Out: A time of pause immediately before initiating an invasive procedure for all members of the procedure team to agree on correct patient identity, correct site, and correct procedure to be done.

Transverse: Lying at right angles to the long axis of the body; crosswise.

Triage: Sorting patients and setting priorities for their treatment in urgent care settings, emergency rooms, clinics, hospitals, health maintenance organizations, or in the field.

Tumor Staging: Also called Cancer Staging. The process of determining the severity of a person's cancer based on the extent of the original (primary) tumor and whether or not cancer has spread in the body.

Ulna: The larger bone of the forearm, between the wrist and the elbow, on the side opposite the thumb. It articulates with the head of the radius and humerus proximally, and with the radius and carpals distally.

Urinary Stasis: Stoppage of the normal flow of urine.

Valgus: Bent or turned outward from the midline of the body.

Varus: Angled or turned inward from the midline of the body.

Index

B

C

D

E

F

G

H

I

J

K

L

M

N

O

INDEX

P

Q

R

S

T

U

V

W

X

Y

Z